Estimated Safe and Adequate Daily Dietary Intakes of Additional Selected Vitamins and Minerals (United States)[a]

Age (years)	Vitamins	
	Biotin (μg)	Pantothenic Acid (mg)
Infants		
0–0.5	10	2
0.5–1	15	3
Children		
1–3	20	3
4–6	25	3–4
7–10	30	4–5
11 +	30–100	4–7
Adults	30–100	4–7

Age (years)	Trace Elements[b]				
	Chromium (μg)	Molybdenum (μg)	Copper (mg)	Manganese (mg)	Fluoride (mg)
Infants					
0–0.5	10–40	15–30	0.4–0.6	0.3–0.6	0.1–0.5
0.5–1	20–60	20–40	0.6–0.7	0.6–1.0	0.2–1.0
Children					
1–3	20–80	25–50	0.7–1.0	1.0–1.5	0.5–1.5
4–6	30–120	30–75	1.0–1.5	1.5–2.0	1.0–2.5
7–10	50–200	50–150	1.0–2.0	2.0–3.0	1.5–2.5
11 +	50–200	75–250	1.5–2.5	2.0–5.0	1.5–2.5
Adults	50–200	75–250	1.5–3.0	2.0–5.0	1.5–4.0

[a]Because there is less information on which to base allowances, these figures are not given in the main table of the RDA and are provided here in the form of ranges of recommended intakes.
[b]Because the toxic levels for many trace elements may be only several times usual intakes, the upper levels for the trace elements given in this table should not be habitually exceeded.

Source: *Recommended Dietary Allowances*, © 1989 by the National Academy of Sciences, National Academy Press, Washington, D.C.

Estimated Minimum Requirements of Sodium, Chloride, and Potassium

Age (years)	Sodium[a] (mg)	Chloride (mg)	Potassium[b] (mg)
Infants			
0.0–0.5	120	180	500
0.5–1.0	200	300	700
Children			
1	225	350	1000
2–5	300	500	1400
6–9	400	600	1600
Adolescents	500	750	
Adults	500	750	

[a]Sodium requirements are based on estimates of needs for growth and for replacement of obligatory losses. They cover a wide variation of physical activity patterns and climatic exposure but do not provide for large, prolonged losses from the skin through sweat.
[b]Dietary potassium may benefit the prevention and treatment of hypertension and recommendations to include many servings of fruits and vegetables would raise potassium intakes to about 3500 mg/day.

Source: *Recommended Dietary Allowances*, © 1989 by the National Academy of Sciences, National Academy Press, Washington, D.C.

B

Median Heights and Weights and Recommended Energy Intakes (United States)

Age	Weight		Height		Average Energy Allowance			
(years)	(kg)	(lb)	(cm)	(inches)	REE[a] (cal/day)	Multiples of REE[b]	cal per kg	cal per day[c]
Infants								
0.0–0.5	6	13	60	24	320		108	650
0.5–1.0	9	20	71	28	500		98	850
Children								
1–3	13	29	90	35	740		102	1300
4–6	20	44	112	44	950		90	1800
7–10	28	62	132	52	1130		70	2000
Males								
11–14	45	99	157	62	1440	1.70	55	2500
15–18	66	145	176	69	1760	1.67	45	3000
19–24	72	160	177	70	1780	1.67	40	2900
25–50	79	174	176	70	1800	1.60	37	2900
51 +	77	170	173	68	1530	1.50	30	2300
Females								
11–14	46	101	157	62	1310	1.67	47	2200
15–18	55	120	163	64	1370	1.60	40	2200
19–24	58	128	164	65	1350	1.60	38	2200
25–50	63	138	163	64	1380	1.55	36	2200
51 +	65	143	160	63	1280	1.50	30	1900
Pregnant (2nd and 3rd trimesters)								+300
Lactating								+500

[a]REE (resting energy expenditure) represents the energy expended by a person at rest under normal conditions.
[b]Recommended energy allowances assume light to moderate activity and were calculated by multiplying the REE by an activity factor.
[c]Average energy allowances have been rounded.
Source: *Recommended Dietary Allowances*, © 1989 by the National Academy of Sciences, National Academy Press, Washington, D.C.

U.S. RDA (used on food labels)

Nutrient	RDA for an Adult Man (1968)	RDA for an Adult Woman (1968)	U.S. RDA
Nutrients that *must* appear on the label[a]			
Protein (g), PER · casein[b]	45	—	45
Protein (g), PER < casein	65	55	65
Vitamin A (RE)	1,000	800	1,000
Vitamin C (ascorbic acid) (mg)	60	55	60
Thiamin (vitamin B_1) (mg)	1.4	1.0	1.5
Riboflavin (vitamin B_2) (mg)	1.7	1.5	1.7
Niacin (mg)	18	13	20
Calcium (g)	0.8	0.8	1.0
Iron (mg)	10	18	18
Nutrients that *may* appear on the label			
Vitamin D (IU)	—	—	400
Vitamin E (IU)	30	25	30
Vitamin B_6 (mg)	2.0	2.0	2.0
Folate (folic acid, folacin) (mg)	0.4	0.4	0.4
Vitamin B_{12} (μg)	6	6	6
Phosphorus (g)	0.8	0.8	1.0
Iodine (μg)	120	100	150
Magnesium (mg)	350	300	400
Zinc (mg)	—	—	15
Copper (mg)	—	—	2
Biotin (mg)	—	—	0.3
Pantothenic acid (mg)	—	—	10

[a]Whenever nutrition labeling is required. [b]PER is an index of protein quality. Source: Adapted from *Food Technology* 28, no. 7 (1974): 5.

■■■ F I F T H   E D I T I O N

Nutrition
CONCEPTS AND CONTROVERSIES

Eva May Nunnelley Hamilton   Eleanor Noss Whitney   Frances Sienkiewicz Sizer

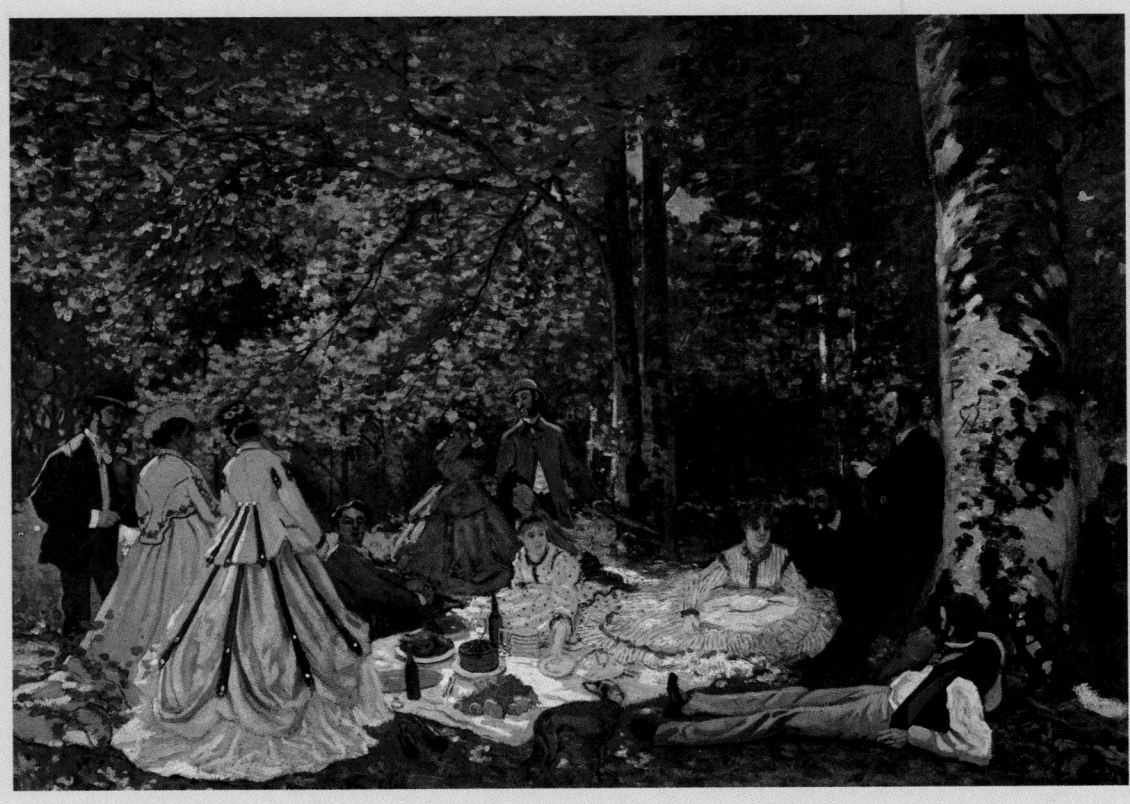

Fifth Edition Prepared by
Eleanor Noss Whitney
Frances Sienkiewicz Sizer

W E S T   P U B L I S H I N G   C O M P A N Y
St. Paul   New York   Los Angeles   San Francisco

▉▉▉ PRODUCTION CREDITS

Composition: Carlisle Communications
Copyediting: June Gomez
Dummy Artist: Kristen M. Weber
Index: Jo-Anne Naples, Naples Editing Services
Text and Cover Designer: Kristen M. Weber
Cover and Title Page Images: *Luncheon on the Grass* by Claude Monet The Pushkin Museum, Moscow, Scala/Art Resource, N.Y.

Library of Congress Cataloging-in-Publication Data

Hamilton, Eva May Nunnelley.
    Nutrition : concepts and controversies / Eva May Nunnelley Hamilton, Eleanor Noss Whitney, Frances Sienkiewicz Sizer. — 5th ed.
        p.   cm.
        Includes index.
        ISBN 0−314−81091−9 (soft)
        1. Nutrition.   2. Food.   I. Whitney, Eleanor Noss.   II. Sizer, Frances Sienkiewicz.   III. Title.
        QP141.H34   1990
        613.2 — dc20   90−47840
                                                                              CIP

▉▉▉ PHOTO CREDITS

2. © David Young–Wolff, PhotoEdit; 8 Roy Morsch, The Stock Market; 13 Ray Stanyard; 15 Ray Stanyard; 18 © Tony Freeman/PhotoEdit; 22 Marilyn Herbert; 27 © Williams and Edwards/The Image Bank; 36 (all) Courtesy of USDA; 41 (all) © Felicia Martinez/PhotoEdit; 42 (all) Ray Stanyard; 43 Ray Stanyard; 52 Felicia Martinez/PhotoEdit; 53 Felicia Martinez/PhotoEdit; 55 © Richard Kalvar, Magnum Photos, Inc.; 75 Courtesy of Dr. Susumu Ito; 77 Peter Menzel; 94 © Michael Skott/The Image Bank; 106 Ray Stanyard; 108 © Felicia Martinez/PhotoEdit; 114 Ray Stanyard; 120 © Tony Freeman, PhotoEdit; 123 Ray Stanyard; 137 (both) Ray Stanyard; 138 Felicia Martinez/PhotoEdit; 139 (all) Ray Stanyard; 145 Steve Niedorf/The Image Bank; 157 Human hemoglobin model constructed by Dr. Makio Murayama, NIH, Bethesda, Maryland (scaled to ½ inch to angstrom). Atomic coordinates were supplied for model by Dr. Max F. Perutz, Cambridge, England; 168 Ray Stanyard; 173 © Steve Maines/Stock, Boston; 177 (all) © Tony Freeman, PhotoEdit; 179 Ray Stanyard; 181 (all) © Felicia Martinez, PhotoEdit; 183 © Myrleen Ferguson/PhotoEdit; 196 David Farr; 198 © *Nutrition Today*, H. Stanstead, J. Carter, and W. Darby, Nutritional Deficiencies, Nutrition Today Aid #5 (Nutrition Today: Annapolis, MD) 1975; 199 Ray Stanyard; 201 Courtesy of Parke-Davis and Company 209 © *Nutrition To-*

day, C. Butterworth & G. Blackburn, Hospital Nutrition and How to Assess the Nutritional Status of a Patient. Nutrition Today Teaching Aid #18 (Nutrition Today: Annapolis, MD) 1975; 210 © *Nutrition Today*, C. Butterworth & G. Blackburn, Hospital Nutrition and How to Assess the Nutritional Status of a Patient. Nutrition Today Teaching Aid #18 (Nutrition Today: Annapolis, MD) 1975; 215 From C. Conn, The Specialties in General Practice, 2nd ed. (Philadelphia: Saunders, 1957); 217 (both) Ray Stanyard; 232 Anthony Vannelli; 241 Photo copyright © Camera M.D. Studios, Inc.; 250 © Felicia Martinez/PhotoEdit; 255 (both) Ray Stanyard; 258 © Felicia Martinez/PhotoEdit; 259 (both) Ray Stanyard; 261 Reproduced with permission of *Nutrition Today*, Magazine, P.O. Box 1829, Annapolis, MD 21404, March 1968; 262 Ray Stanyard; 263 Courtesy of H. Kaplan and V.P. Robbach; 269 Ray Stanyard; 272 Courtesy of Gjon Mili; 294 © Charles Gupton/ Stock, Boston; 301 Ray Stanyard; 314 Ray Stanyard; 318 © George S. Zimbel/ Monkmeyer Press; 334 © Daemmrich/Stock, Boston; 335 John Kelly/The Image Bank; 353 John Bahlik; 354 © Felicia Martinez/PhotoEdit; 359 Ray Stanyard; 374 Charles Feil/Stock, Boston; 378 © Derik Murray/The Image Bank; 388 © Michael Skott/The Image Bank; 390 Charles Feil/Stock, Boston; 393 Anthony Vannelli; 406 © Anthony Vannelli; 412 Streissguth, A.P., Clarren, S.K. & Jones K.L. (1985, July). National History of the Fatal Alcohol Syn-

drome: A ten-year follow up of eleven patients. *Lauret II*, 89-92; 415 Owen Franken, Sygma; 417 © Francis Wardle; 426 Courtesy of H. Kaplan and V.P. Rabbach; 429 Ray Ellis/Science Source Photo Researchers, Inc.; 438 (both) © Anthony Vannelli; 451 © Donald Dietz, Stock, Boston; 460 © Richard Hutchings/PhotoEdit; 466 © Owen Franken/ Stock, Boston; 469 George Ancona/International Stock Photography; 482 Peter Menzel/ Stock, Boston; 490 Ray Stanyard; 501 (both) Ray Stanyard; 503 © Alan Oddie/PhotoEdit; 506 Ray Stanyard; 518 Comstock; 520 © Tony Freeman/PhotoEdit; 521 ©Bill Thomas/PhotoEdit; 523 ©Tony Freeman/PhotoEdit; 531 © Rhonda Sidney/PhotoEdit; 533 © Ulrike Welsch/PhotoEdit; 535 (top) © Alan Oddie/PhotoEdit; (bottom) © Robert Brenner/PhotoEdit; 536 © Alan Oddie/PhotoEdit; 540 (top)Mark W. Richards/PhotoEdit; (bottom) Robert Rathe, Stock, Boston; 544 (top) © Tony Freeman/PhotoEdit; (bottom) © Alan Oddie, PhotoEdit; 546 Paul Conklin/PhotoEdit; 547 Comstock; 550 Courtesy of the U.S. Department of Agriculture

▉▉▉ ILLUSTRATION CREDITS

Sandra McMahon

64 Figure 3−1; 65 Figure 3−2; 66 Figure 3−3; 67 Figure 3−4; 68 Figure 3−5; 70 Fig-

Illustration credits continue following the index.

■■■ *To all families, and extended families, who stand by each other in both hard and joyful times— and especially to mine, including wonderful Tonya.*

Ellie

■■■ *To my sister Harriet Sienkiewicz, her achievements are inspirational; her caring gives me courage. Nothing stops her from loving.*

Fran

Eva May Nunnelley Hamilton received her B.S. in nutrition from the University of Kentucky in 1940 and then taught science to high school and college students for over 35 years. She received her M.S. in nutrition from The Florida State University in 1975. While she was there, West Publishing Company recruited her, with Eleanor Whitney, to create the first editions of *Understanding Nutrition* and *Nutrition: Concepts and Controversies,* which were published in 1977 and 1979. In addition, she authored *The Biochemistry of Human Nutrition: A Desk Reference.* Now retired, she remains vigorously active in community and church work and continues to share scientific interests with enthusiasm.

Eleanor Noss Whitney, Ph.D., R.D., received her B.A. in Biology from Radcliffe College in 1960 and her Ph.D. in Biology from Washington University, St. Louis, in 1970. Formerly on the faculty at the Florida State University, she now devotes full time to research, writing, and consulting in nutrition, health, and environmental issues. Her earlier publications include articles in *Science, Genetics,* and other journals. Her textbooks include *Understanding Nutrition, Understanding Normal and Clinical Nutrition, Nutrition and Diet Therapy,* and *Essential Life Choices,* among others.

Frances Sienkiewicz Sizer, M.S., R.D., attended Florida State University where, in 1980, she received her B.S., and in 1982, her M.S. in nutrition. She is a founding member and vice president of Nutrition and Health Associates, an organization of authors and educators in nutrition and health. Her current publications include *Nutrition Clinics,* a monograph series for health professionals. Her other textbooks include *Life Choices: Health Concepts and Strategies, Essential Life Choices,* and *The Fitness Triad: Motivation, Training, and Nutrition.* Among her professional memberships are the American Dietetic Association, the American Public Health Association, the American Alliance for Health, Physical Education, Recreation, and Dance, and others.

■■ CONTENTS IN BRIEF

▮▮▮ C O N T E N T S

ix

■■■ C H A P T E R   14

Food Technology and Food Safety   481

■■■ C H A P T E R   15

Hunger and Hope: Nutrition and the Environment, 1990s   517

■■■ A P P E N D I X E S

▌▌▌ PREFACE

For well over a decade, professors and students have been testing *Nutrition: Concepts and Controversies* in their classrooms. They have told us they appreciate our perspectives on established nutrition knowledge. They have liked taking glimpses with us into areas of rapid change, and they enjoy as we do the stories in nutrition that continue to intrigue us with their plot twists and surprise directions. In this fifth edition, we have updated our fundamentals with all available scientific advances in the field, including the (1989) *Recommended Dietary Allowances* and the latest dietary guidelines. To continue offering fast-breaking news, we have also written new Controversies on some beginnings of knowledge that are just now emerging from research scientists' reports. Some day, these may either develop fully into fundamentals of nutrition or retire to the pastures of the unproved.

We hope you will enjoy using this fifth edition. Along with its new topics come amenities such as airbrushed figures to lend clarity to nutrition concepts, cartoons that teach through humor, and photos of food that complement the book's accuracy, thoroughness, and personal style of writing.

Our new edition begins with a personal invitation to eat well, and to think in terms of how, when, and why people choose the foods they do. We also introduce the nutrients, and then move on to contrast sources of valid nutrition information with fraudulent claims. Chapter 2 brings together the concepts of diet planning through food grouping systems, the nutrient density concept, and exchange systems. Food labeling as a vehicle of nutrition and health information is a major topic of Chapter 2. Then Chapter 3 presents a brief but essential introduction to the workings of the body systems as they relate to nutrition. Chapters 4 through 6 are devoted to the energy-yielding nutrients—carbohydrates, lipids, and proteins. Chapters 7 and 8 present the vitamins, minerals, and water. Chapter 9 relates energy balance to the problems of overweight, obesity, and underweight, and presents life-long weight maintenance as a major new theme. For active people, and for those just starting exercise programs, Chapter 10 presents the relationships between fitness, physical activity, and nutrition. Chapter 11, new to this edition, describes how diet may be instrumental in the development of diseases. Chapters 12 and 13 point out the importance of nutrition throughout the lifespan, from gestation through old age. Chapter 14 considers the problems and advantages of food technology, and describes how to handle food safely at home. Chapter 15 touches on the vast problems of the global food supply—world hunger, contaminants and pesticides, environmental pollution, agribusiness, overpopulation, and the world's water supply—with an emphasis on solutions to these problems.

The Controversies of this book's title are optional readings printed on colored paper. Many are totally new to this edition, and the others have been updated. A few deserve special mention. Controversy 2 compares cuisines derived from many nations and religions and leaves it to the reader to answer its title question, "Who has the best way to eat?" Controversy 8, Osteoporosis and Calcium, debates whether adequate calcium intakes can help prevent development of osteoporosis in light of other contributing factors. Controversy 10 provides a glimpse into headline nutrition news that prompts researchers to ask the question, "Are fat calories more fattening?" Controversy 13 wonders aloud what effects nutrition might really have on the processes of aging. This book's final Controversy touches on a topic that may well turn out to be a key to survival in the next century.

The Food Feature sections that appear in Chapters 1, 2, and 4 through 14 act as bridges between theory and practice; they are personal applications of the concepts in the chapters. The Self-Study sections at the ends of the chapters offer the reader a means of comparing personal dietary habits to recommendations. Consumer Cautions in each chapter present information on supplements, other nutrition-related products, and marketplace choices to provide consumers with the information they need to make informed decisions.

New or major terms are defined in the margins of the pages where they are first used in the text. Each term is printed in boldface type at its first use, to call attention to its importance. The reader who wishes to locate any defined term may do so by consulting the index. The index lists in boldface type the page numbers of all terms defined in the text.

The appendixes have been updated to provide you with current references. Notice especially Appendix A, which presents the nutrient contents of well over 1000 foods; Appendix C, which presents aids to calculations in nutrition; and Appendix E which lists nutrition resources that provide materials for those interested in additional information.

As always, one of our tasks has been to present more updated information in fewer words and pages. To this end, we have removed older source notes to make room for the new, but anyone who wishes to check older sources can do so easily by consulting an older edition of this book, or by contacting our publisher, who will request them from us.

We hope that this edition of *Nutrition: Concepts and Controversies* proves useful to you in its classroom testing ground. We also hope that you enjoy using it.

Eleanor N. Whitney
Frances S. Sizer
October, 1990

▮▮▮ Acknowledgments

We are grateful to our associates, Linda DeBruyne, Sharon Rolfes, and Lori Turner for their continued assistance in our writing. Thanks to Linda De-Bruyne for Controversies 11 and 12 of this edition, and to Lori Turner for Chapter 9 of the text, much of the *Instructor's Manual,* and the special Instructor's Edition of the text. Linda Patton provided invaluable research and references throughout this edition. Our thanks, also, to Valerie West and Nancie Hopkins for their efficient word processing. We are grateful to Bob Celander, Bill Celander, and Gary Carroll who produced this edition's cartoons.

Our special thanks to our editors who supported us with their many efforts throughout this writing—Peter Marshall, Becky Tollerson, and Stacy Lenzen—and to their staff who supported them and who worked tirelessly to ensure the quality of this book. We thank also Jana Kicklighter for preparing the *Student*

Study Guide and the *Test Bank;* and also Margaret Hedley who prepared the Canadian portion of the Instructor's Manual. Thanks also to Bob Geltz and Betty Hands and their staff at ESHA research for creating the food composition table (Appendix A), and the computerized diet analysis program that accompanies this book. Thanks, too, to Kristen Weber for her creativity and style in design.

To May Hamilton, our continued thanks for infusing the first edition with her spirit and for her unending enthusiasm for our work. And to our reviewers, heartfelt thanks for your many good ideas.

▌▌▌ Reviewers and Affiliations

Sarah Ash
North Carolina State University

Dan Benardot
Georgia State University

Joanne Caid
California State University-Fresno

Carolyn Dunn
North Carolina State University

Chris Fideli
New York Institute of Technology

Art Gilbert
University of California-Santa Barbara

Margaret Harden
Texas Tech University

Margaret Hedley
University of Guelph

Mike Hudecki
SUNY University at Buffalo

Wendy Hunt
American River College

Janice Johnstone
University of Alberta

Younghee Kim
Bowling Green State University

Elena Kissick
California State University-Fresno

Bernard Marcus
Genesee Community College

William Morris
University of Tennessee-Knoxville

Peter Murano
Virginia Polytechnic and State University

Debra Pearce
Northern Kentucky University

Dennis Ponton
Buffalo State College

Emily Reid
McGill University

Nancy Sheard
University of Massachusetts-Amherst

Anne Smith
University of Utah

Sarah Strawn
Auburn University

Kathryn Sucher
San Jose State University

Simin Bolourchi Vaghefi
University of North Florida

Murray Weinstein
Erie Community College-City Campus

Elise West
Cornell University

Nutrients, Food Choices, and Human Health

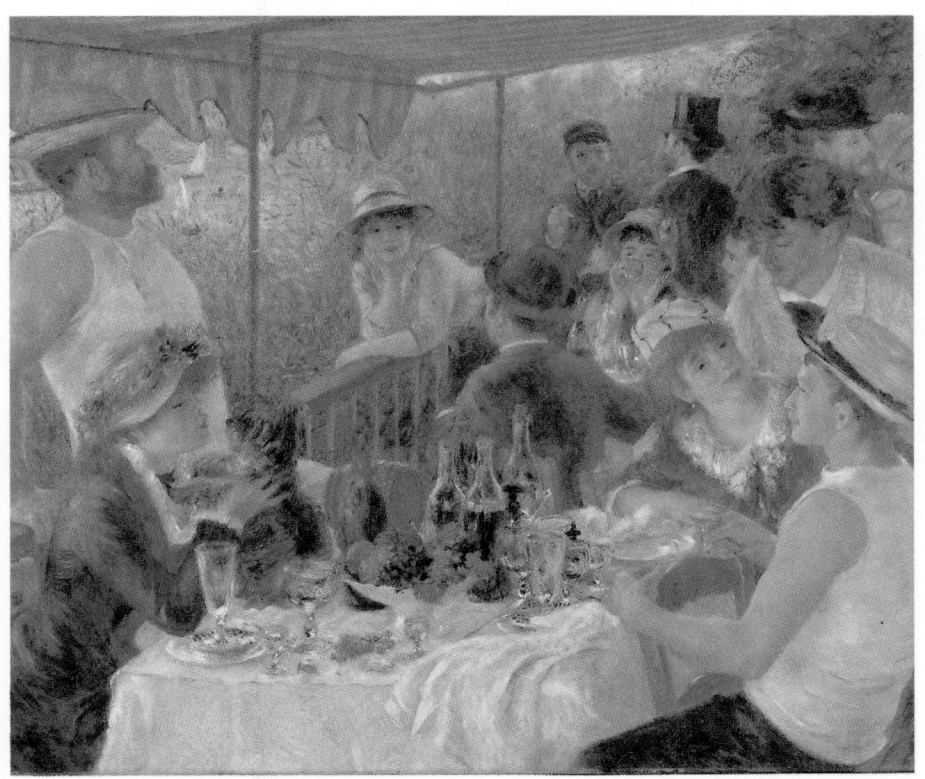

CONTENTS

The Luncheon of the Boating Party by Pierre Auguste Renoir. The Phillips Collection, Washington D.C.

energy: the capacity to do work. The energy in food is chemical energy. It can be converted to mechanical, electrical, heat, or other forms of energy in the body. Food energy can be measured in *calories*, described later.

nutrients: components of food that help to nourish the body, that is, to provide energy, to serve as building material, or to help maintain or repair body parts. The nutrients include carbohydrate, fat, protein, vitamins, minerals, and water.

If you live for 65 years or longer, you will have consumed more than 70,000 meals, and your remarkable body will have disposed of 50 tons of food. The effects on your body of the foods you choose accumulate. At 65 years of age you will see and feel those effects, if you know what to look for.

Your body renews its structures continuously, and each day it builds a little muscle, bone, skin, and blood, replacing old tissues with new. In this way some of the food you eat today becomes part of "you" tomorrow. The best food for you, then, is the kind that supports the growth and maintenance of strong muscles, sound bones, healthy skin, and sufficient blood to cleanse and to nourish all parts of your body.

Do you choose the foods that best meet your body's needs? If you are like most people, you may choose foods you like or that are most convenient whenever you feel hungry or thirsty or when the clock says it is mealtime. This strategy does at least one thing for you: it loosens the grip of hunger or thirst on your attention, freeing you to turn to higher purposes, such as studying for examinations.

Foods, however, must provide at least two other benefits besides relief from distraction. They must provide **energy** to fuel your activities, and they must offer at least some **nutrients** too. In fact, these two constituents of foods, their energy and their nutrients, occupy center stage in the study of nutrition. They are introduced formally later in this chapter, but before focusing on them, this chapter focuses on your food choices. After all, you choose foods, not nutrients—so how do you make your choices?

Do the foods you choose provide all the nutrients you need to maintain your body's structures? The answer is probably "sometimes." You must be doing something right because you have been eating for years and you are still here. You may be doing better than you think. For example, you may consider a meal at a pizza place an indulgence, a tasty but forbidden treat. Of course, experts do recommend that most people cut down on fat, and pizza can deliver a great deal of fat in sausages and cheese. But overall pizza provides a nourishing meal, contributing something from each food group: bread (the crust), vegetables (the tomato sauce and toppings), milk (the cheese), and meats. If you can order it with a whole-wheat crust, light on cheese and meat, and heavy on vegetables, so much the better. And if you balance the food energy it delivers by expending energy in physical activity, so much the better still. Your muscles, heart, and lungs thrive on activity as well as on energy and nutrients.

So that pizza you thought was just a treat turns out to be more than that. But that was just by chance, and leaving nutrition to chance may not work out optimally over 65 years or more. A diet of nothing but pizza would leave some of the body's needs unmet. A look at the health of the nation's older people makes clear that without sound nutrition, a person's chances for optimal health in later life are slim. The earlier you learn and begin to apply sound nutrition principles, the better your health will remain. In fact, in a 1988 report, the surgeon general remarked that only two lifestyle habits can influence your long-term health prospects more profoundly than your choice of diet. As you might expect, these two, both negative, are smoking and excessive drinking.[1] Many older people suffer from debilitating conditions that could have been largely prevented had they known and applied the nutrition and fitness principles that we know today throughout their lives.

We should hasten to say that not all of the so-called diseases of old age can be prevented by choice. The tendencies to develop heart disease, diabetes,

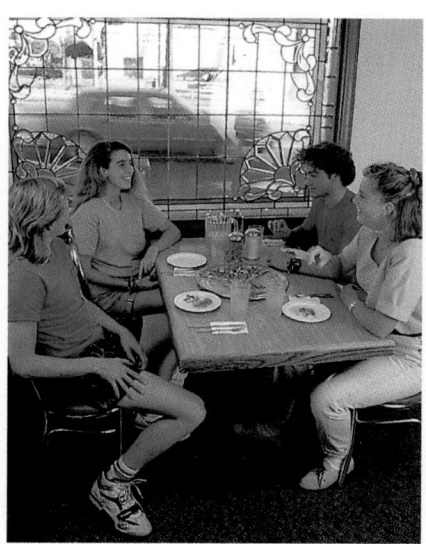

You may be doing better than you think.

some kinds of cancer, dental disease, and others do depend somewhat on people's genetic constitutions. However, within the range set by your inheritance, the likelihood that you will develop these diseases is strongly influenced by the lifestyle choices you make—whether to smoke; to consume alcohol; to eat a nutritious, balanced diet; and to engage in regular, physical activity. Figure 1–1 shows that many different diseases are responsive to nutrition to a greater or lesser extent, and Table 1–1 (next page) lists the nutrition measures you can take to help prevent these diseases.

The study of nutrition can help you to become more conscious of these issues. A place to begin the study is to take a look at how you choose foods. Why did you eat as you did today? Perhaps some life condition, such as a disease or special requirement, dictates your food choices each day. But more likely you can point to a variety of reasons for your choices. You ate the same food as yesterday, or you ate foods you are accustomed to, or perhaps you ate whatever the crowd was eating. Among factors people cite to explain food choices are:

■ Personal preference: You like them.
■ Habit: They are familiar; you always eat them.
■ Ethnic heritage or tradition: They are the foods of your ethnic group.
■ Social pressure: They are offered; you feel you can't refuse them.
■ Availability: There are no others to choose from.
■ Convenience: They are quick and easy to prepare.
■ Economy: They are within your means.
■ Positive associations: They are eaten by people you admire, or they indicate status, or they remind you of fun.
■ Emotional needs: Foods can make you feel better for awhile.
■ Values or beliefs: They fit your religious tradition, square with your political views, or honor the environmental ethic.
■ Nutritional value: You think they are good for you.

All but one of these reasons are behavioral and social reasons; only the last one reflects that you are conscious of nutrition's importance to your health.

Nutrition-unresponsive
(genetic) diseases

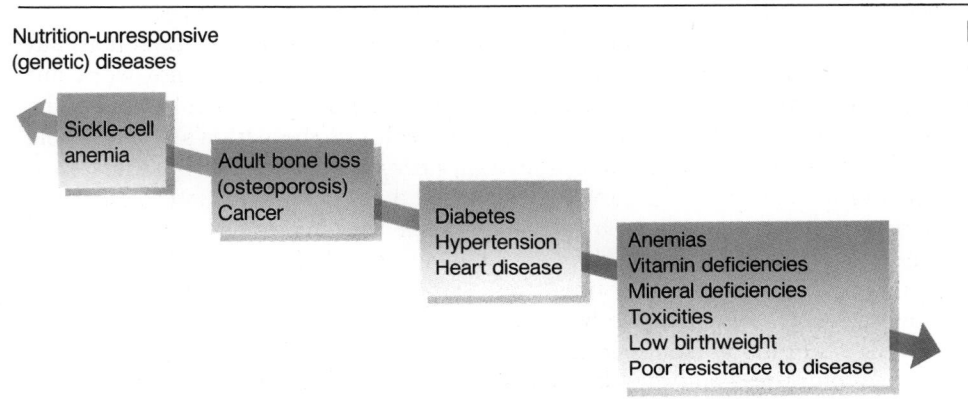

Nutrition-responsive diseases

■■■ Figure 1–1

Nutrition and Disease. Not all diseases are equally influenced by diet. Some are purely hereditary, like sickle-cell anemia. Some may be inherited (or the tendency to develop them may be inherited) but may be influenced by diet, like some forms of diabetes. Some are purely dietary, like the vitamin and mineral deficiency diseases.

■■■ **Table 1–1 Nutrition Measures to Prevent Diseases**

Adequate intake of essential nutrients, especially protein, and food energy helps
  prevent:
  In pregnancy:
    Low birthweight
    Poor resistance to disease
    Some forms of birth defects
    Some forms of mental/physical retardation
  In infancy and childhood:
    Growth deficits
    Poor resistance to disease
  In adulthood and old age:
    Poor resistance to infectious diseases
    Susceptibility to some forms of cancer

Moderation in food energy intake helps prevent:
  Obesity and related diseases, such as diabetes and hypertension

Moderation in fat intake helps prevent:
  Susceptibility to some cancers and atherosclerosis

Adequate fiber intake helps prevent:
  Digestive malfunctions such as constipation and diverticulosis and possibly colon
    or other cancers
  Possibly heart disease

Moderation in sugar intake helps prevent:
  Dental caries

Moderation in alcohol intake helps prevent:
  Liver disease
  Malnutrition

Adequate intake of any essential nutrient prevents:
  Deficiency diseases such as cretinism, scurvy, and folate-deficiency anemia

Moderation in intake of essential nutrients prevents:
  Toxicity states

Adequate calcium intake helps prevent:
  Adult bone loss

Adequate iron intake helps prevent:
  Anemia

Adequate fluoride intake helps prevent:
  Dental caries

Moderation in sodium intake helps prevent:
  Hypertension and related diseases of the heart and kidney

Adequate vitamin A intake helps prevent:
  Susceptibility to certain cancers

This is not to say that your behavioral and social reasons for choosing foods
are invalid or that the choices they lead you to make are bad for your health.
After all, food nourishes not only the body but the mind and spirit too. For
example, providing food can be a way of showing affection, such as parents
feeding children or friends inviting others to share a meal. Food can be fun or

traditional, such as hotdogs at ball games or turkey at Thanksgiving. Sharing food at times of bereavement serves both the giver's need to provide comfort and the receiver's need to be cared for and to interact with others. Buying vegetables from a local farmer's market costs less in fossil fuel and environmental pollution than buying food shipped in from far away. These and many other factors provide benefits to the eaters and are part of the health-promoting effects of food, just as the nutrients are. Still, the most basic role food plays is to nourish your body, and your awareness of how it does so can help you to promote and to prolong your good health.

It is important to realize that *single* foods are neither good nor bad for your nutritional health. What matters most is the way you use them within a total diet. No single food can reduce your likelihood of developing an illness, nor can any provide total nutrition, even if an advertisement seems to say that it does. The key to evaluating a food is to take lightly what people say about it but to weigh heavily its constituents and the nutrients and energy it contains and then to judge its appropriate role in the context of all your other food choices and your physical activity.

People who want to learn how best to choose foods to support their nutritional health have three objectives:

1. To learn the body's needs for energy and nutrients.
2. To learn what kinds and combinations of foods meet those needs.
3. To learn what kinds of claims are made by people who sell or write about nutrients and foods and how to tell whether the claims are valid.

This chapter introduces these themes, and the rest of the book develops them.

▌▌▌Energy and Nutrients

Foods are composed of hundreds of chemical substances, among which the nutrients usually predominate. Taken together, the nutrients of foods meet the following needs of cells. They provide:

■ Water (the environment in which cells live).
■ Fuel for energy (so that cells can do their work).
■ Building blocks (the nutrients cells use to build and to repair themselves).
■ Metabolic regulators (the nutrients cells use to coordinate life's processes).

The nutrients fall into six classes, and all six classes are found in most foods. Water usually predominates. Carbohydrate (including fiber), fat, and protein (to which the next section is devoted) are next in abundance; these provide the energy and building blocks on which the cells' lives depend. Last come the vitamins and minerals in smaller yet significant amounts; these are the metabolic regulators. (Some minerals also serve as building blocks for bones and teeth.)

The human body is made of these same materials in roughly the same order of predominance. If you weigh 150 pounds, your body contains about 90 pounds of water and (if 150 pounds is the proper weight for you) about 30 pounds of fat. The other 30 pounds are mostly protein, carbohydrate compounds, and the major minerals of your bones—calcium and phosphorus. Vitamins, other minerals, and incidental extras constitute a fraction of a pound.

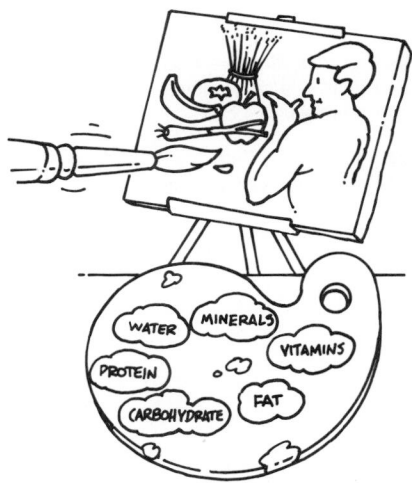

Foods and the human body are made of the same materials.

Basic nutrition needs:

■ Water.
■ Energy fuel.
■ Building blocks.
■ Metabolic regulators.

The six classes of nutrients:

■ Water.
■ Carbohydrate.
■ Fat.
■ Protein.
■ Vitamins.
■ Minerals.

organic: carbon containing. The four organic nutrients are carbohydrate, fat, protein, and vitamins.

oxidation: with respect to nutrients in the body, breakdown of a nutrient within a cell and combination of its parts with oxygen—a process that releases energy.

energy-yielding nutrients: the nutrients the body can use for energy (although they may also supply building blocks for body structures).

The energy-yielding nutrients:

- Carbohydrate.
- Fat.
- Protein.

- 1 g carbohydrate = 4 cal.
- 1 g fat = 9 cal or more.**
- 1 g protein = 4 cal.

- 1 g alcohol = 7 cal.
- More about alcohol in Controversy 11.

■■■ Figure 1–2

Elements in the Six Classes of Nutrients. The nutrients listed in the colored area are organic

	Carbon	Oxygen	Hydrogen	Nitrogen	Minerals*
Carbohydrate	x	x	x		
Fat	x	x	x		
Protein	x	x	x	x	
Vitamins	x	x	x		
Minerals					x
Water		x	x		

*Protein contains the mineral sulfur; vitamin B$_{12}$ contains the mineral cobalt.

Except for the minerals, which are pure atomic elements, all of the nutrients are composed of a framework of atoms of elements bonded together by energy, and all contain hydrogen and oxygen, the elements of which water is made (see Figure 1–2). Four nutrients also contain atoms of carbon and are therefore **organic** (carbon containing)—carbohydrate, fat, protein, and vitamins. This means that in a laboratory experiment or in a fire, they can undergo **oxidation**, or be burned (to carbon dioxide and water), and will release energy. But only three of these four—carbohydrate, fat, and protein—are **energy-yielding nutrients** from the body's point of view.

One of the most common misconceptions people have is that the vitamins in some way yield energy for human use. They may help in the energy-producing process, but they do not yield usable energy themselves. Taking vitamin pills for energy is a common mistake. The only significance to us of vitamins' being organic is that they are easily destroyed by chemical and physical agents such as heat and light. Therefore we have to be careful in cooking foods that contain vitamins. (Find out how to preserve vitamins in the Food Feature in Chapter 14.)

■▷ *Foods, as well as our own bodies, are made up primarily of six classes of nutrients—water, carbohydrate, fat, protein, vitamins, and minerals. All but water and minerals are organic, and three—carbohydrate, fat, and protein—yield energy that the body can use.*

The Energy-Yielding Nutrients

The energy in carbohydrate, fat, and protein can be measured in **calories**, familiar to everyone as something associated with foods that makes them fattening. This book uses the term *calories* as most people do. But properly speaking, the energy unit people are familiar with is really a **kilocalorie** or **kcal**,* a unit of 1000 calories. If you were to ask a chemist how many *calories* were in a large, double-patty, fast-food hamburger, the answer would be 570,000. How many in a cola? 144,000, But asked for kilocalories, the numbers provided would be 570 and 144, an amount more familiar to most people. Whenever you see the term calorie for the remainder of the book, keep in mind that the technical term is kilocalorie.

The energy values of the nutrients appear in the margin. Note that the energy-yielding nutrients are measured in **grams (g)**—units of weight—and that their energy values are expressed per gram.

The body may use energy from food in several ways: to produce heat, to build structures, to move muscles, or to store in body fat or other compounds for later use. Another compound also can contribute food energy—alcohol. Alcohol is not a nutrient because it cannot be used for any other purpose; it cannot promote growth, maintenance, or repair. It is a toxin that can be broken down for energy. When alcohol contributes a substantial portion of the energy in a person's diet, its effects are damaging.

Practically all foods contain mixtures of the three energy-yielding nutrients, although they are sometimes classified by the predominant nutrient. Thus it is incorrect to call meat a protein; it is a protein-rich food. A protein-rich food such as beef actually contains fat as well as protein. A carbohydrate-rich food

* Food energy can also be measured in *joules, kilojoules,* or *megajoules*. Conversions from calories to joules are in Appendix C.
** Chapter 5 reveals that a gram of fat may offer more than 9 calories to the body. For purposes of calculating calories from food, though, 9 remains the standard number of calories assigned to fat.

such as corn also contains fat (corn oil) and protein. Only a few refined foods are pure, single-nutrient foods, the common ones being sugar (which is almost pure carbohydrate) and oil (which is almost pure fat). It is also not correct to say that you are deriving "calories" from a food. You are deriving energy, and it is measured in calories. The energy and nutrients in over a thousand foods are shown in Appendix A, and the Self-Studies at the ends of the chapters direct you to look them up there.

▌▌▶ *Carbohydrate, fat, and protein contribute usable energy to the body, as does alcohol. But carbohydrate, fat, and protein are nutrients, whereas alcohol is a toxin. Most foods contain mixtures of carbohydrate, fat, and protein, as well as other nutrients.*

The Essential Nutrients

In nutrition the word *essential* is used to denote those nutrients that the body must obtain ready made from food. As examples, it cannot make any of the minerals, most vitamins, or certain lipids or amino acids. In contrast, there are some nutrients the body can make for itself if need be. As an example of the latter, the body can convert some of the amino acids (parts of protein) into carbohydrate. It can manufacture one of the vitamins—niacin—from a certain amino acid. It can make most of its fats and oils from any of several different raw materials. Thus the term *essential nutrients* means more than just "necessary nutrients." Many compounds the body makes for itself are necessary for good health, but *essential nutrient* means a necessary nutrient that can be obtained in sufficient quantities only from the diet. About 40 nutrients are now known to be essential for human beings, and more are still being discovered.

▌▌▶ *The essential nutrients are those that the body cannot make for itself from other raw materials.*

The task of cultivating your nutritional health can now be defined: obtain the necessary amounts of energy and essential nutrients from your diet. As mentioned earlier, people don't generally think in terms of nutrients; they buy, prepare, and eat *foods.* Their choices in doing so are influenced by the many factors also mentioned earlier—personal tastes, habits, traditions, and others. They say they are concerned about nutrition. In fact, most shoppers today, according to one source, name nutrition as their *primary* concern in making food choices.[2] However, when people's food choices are examined, they are found not to be entirely rational. Perhaps one reason for this is that consumers know too little about nutrition science to evaluate the claims that they encounter especially concerning supplements (see the Consumer Caution, next page).

---

calories: units of energy. A kilocalorie (**kcalorie, kcal**) or Calorie (with an upper-case "C") is the amount of heat necessary to raise the temperature of a kilogram (a liter) of water 1° C. This book uses the lower-case term *calorie* to mean the same thing.

grams: units of weight. A gram (g) is the weight of a cubic centimeter (cc) or milliliter (ml) of water under defined conditions of temperature and pressure.

Chapters 4, 5, and 6 discuss the energy-providing and other functions of carbohydrate, fat, and protein.

The essential nutrients:

- Some forms of carbohydrate.
- Certain constituents of fat (the essential fatty acids).
- Certain constituents of protein (the essential amino acids).
- 15 vitamins.
- About 25 minerals.
- Water.

Chapters 7 and 8 discuss the vitamins and minerals.

▌▌▌ Nutrition Information

The consumer who wants to judge correctly what is said about nutrition must learn to distinguish fact from fiction. Three major characteristics contribute to this distinction—the source of the information (how it is obtained), the recorder of it (where it is published), and the purveyor (who states it).

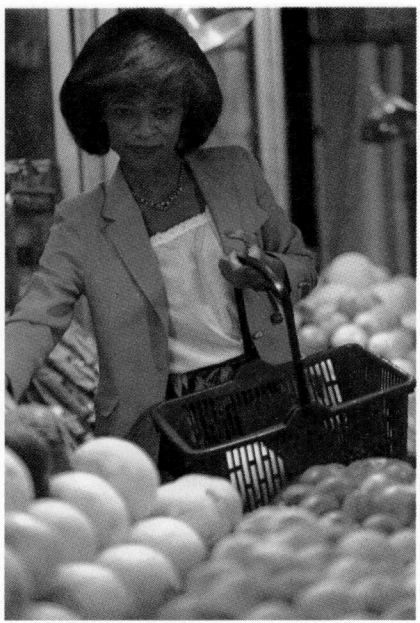

When you shop for food, you are really buying nutrients.

CONSUMER CAUTION ▐▐▐

Supplements

If what we are after from foods is simply nutrients, why shouldn't we just take supplements of nutrients and not bother with food? This represents an extreme argument that anyone could easily shoot down but gives us the opportunity to present some introductory remarks about supplements, which occupy a box like this in almost every chapter in this book. A question to start with: do we know all the nutrients people need?

We do know all the nutrients human beings need to *survive*, at least for a limited time. The 1970s and 1980s saw an explosion of interest and skill in the making of **elemental diets**—diets that are totally chemically defined, used for people in the hospital who cannot eat ordinary food. These formulas can be administered to severely ill people in amounts up to 3000 calories a day. They support not only continued life but recovery from malnutrition and infection and the healing of wounds.

However, these diets are not sufficient to enable people to *thrive*. Used experimentally in laboratory animals, they support life but not optimal growth and health.[3] Often people on all-synthetic diets develop nutrient deficiencies, as indicated by more than 100 separate reports.[4] Although each time this happens the nutrient deficiency can be detected and corrected, it makes clear that the definition of these diets is not yet perfectly worked out for all the settings in which they are used.

Even if all the basic nutrient needs were perfectly understood, there might be something else foods offer that nutrients do not. The story of a girl who could not eat illustrates this possibility. This girl had a severe intestinal disorder that had rendered her digestive tract almost completely nonfunctional. She had to be fed nutrient mixtures through a vein. Deficiencies did develop and were recognized and remedied. But still something was missing: she wanted to eat food. Her health care providers therefore occasionally allowed her to eat whatever she wanted, even though everything she ate had to be collected into a bag through an opening in her abdominal wall after only a few minutes in her intestines. Clearly she gained something important from real food:

continued on the next page

Valid Nutrition Information and Research Designs

The source of valid nutrition information is scientific research. Nutrition is a science, not an art, although it can be used artfully. It is a body of knowledge composed of facts that we believe to be true because they have proved true, time and again, in experiments designed to rule out all alternative possibilities. Each fact has been established by many different kinds of experiments. For example, we know that eyesight depends partly on vitamin A because animals deprived of that vitamin and only that vitamin begin to go blind; given it back soon enough, they regain their sight. The same fact (that eyesight depends on vitamin A) also is supported by several kinds of observations on human beings.

The type of study chosen for research depends upon what sort of information researchers require. Studies of individuals (**case studies**) yield observa-

Her psychological outlook was completely changed. She was happy. The tastes, sounds, sights, and smells of the food gave her great gratification. But, most especially, it was interesting to note the condition of her skin and hair improved and the pink on her cheeks and the look of 'wellness' returned.[5]

Whether the effect was physical or psychological remains unknown: "it was just something in food that gave this girl benefit, which we were not able to give through a needle."[6] The person reporting this was a physician with abundant knowledge and years of experience, not likely to ascribe mysterious powers to food without justification.

Some ingredient or characteristic of the food other than its nutrients may have been responsible for this health-promoting effect. This would not be surprising, since foods are composed of hundreds of chemicals, and we have much to learn about the effects of many of them on the body. Controversy 14 looks into the question of what else besides nutrients is present in foods that may affect our reactions to them.

Another explanation is possible. Human beings are complex, and their reactions to foods may be different than to supplements for reasons rooted in the nervous system. We have, after all, needs for pleasure that food gives in ways that supplements do not. We have needs for love, and the taking of nourishment is almost invariably associated with love from the first moment after birth when the baby is cradled and fed in loving arms. We have needs for stimulation and use of our nerves and muscles, and food stimulates the taste buds and requires chewing, as supplements do not. We have needs for social stimulation, and the taking of food is traditionally a social occasion among human beings.

For reasons like these, even if we don't understand them fully, it seems desirable to continue to rely as much as possible on real foods and as little as possible on supplements to meet our nutrient needs. Later chapters offer more information on supplements, but for the moment let us suggest the following strategy: for the most part, choose foods as whole and nutritious as possible.

elemental diets: diets composed of purified ingredients of known chemical composition such as amino acids, purified fats and sugars, vitamins, and minerals.

tions that may lead to the asking of useful questions and may suggest possible avenues of research. (A study of a man who ate gumdrops and became a famous dancer might suggest that gumdrops contained dance-enhancing power.)

Studies of whole populations in different areas of the world (**epidemiological studies**) provide another sort of information. Such a study can reveal a **correlation**. (For example, an epidemiological study might reveal no worldwide correlation of gumdrop-eating with fancy footwork but, unexpectedly, a correlation with tooth decay.)

Studies in which researchers actively intervene to alter people's eating habits (**intervention studies**) go a step further. In such a study, one set of subjects (the **experimental subjects**) receive a treatment and another set (the **control group**) go untreated or receive a sham treatment. If the two groups experience different effects, then the treatment's effect can be pinpointed. (For example,

fraud (quackery): conscious deceit, practiced for profit. (The word *quackery* comes from the old word "quacksalver," meaning a person who quacks loudly about a miracle product—a lotion or salve.)

an intervention study might show that withholding gumdrops, together with other candies and confections, reduced the incidence of tooth decay in an experimental population compared to that in a control population.)

Finally, **laboratory studies** can pinpoint the mechanism by which a nutrition effect acts. (What is it about the gumdrops: their size, shape, temperature, color, ingredients? Feeding variations on gumdrops to rats might yield the information that sugar, in a gummy carrier, promotes tooth decay.) In the laboratory, using animals or plants or cells, scientists can inoculate with diseases, induce deficiencies, and experiment with variations on treatments to obtain in-depth knowledge of the process under study. Intervention studies and laboratory experiments are among the most powerful research tools in nutrition research because they show the effects of treatments. Figure 1–3 sums up the research designs discussed here.

Our intent in discussing experimental design is not to make a research scientist out of you but to show you what a far cry real scientific validity is from the experience of someone who reports that they use "X vitamin" for "Y complaint" and it works every time. The terms shown in the accompanying Miniglossary of Research Terms (p. 12) will be used frequently throughout this text in explanations of how researchers gathered their information.

Other terms you will see in the Miniglossary refer to the design of intervention studies: **blind** and **double-blind**, **placebo**, and **randomization**. The purpose of the blind study is to ensure that experimental subjects' reactions will not be swayed by their knowledge that they are being treated. If they know they are being treated, they may react to the knowledge, not to the treatment. To keep them guessing about who in the study is receiving treatment and who is not, the researcher must devise placebos, fake treatments that fool the control group into thinking that they have an equal chance of receiving treatment. Furthermore, to best pull off the illusion, a researcher should also be in the dark as to who among the subjects is receiving genuine treatment and who is receiving the placebo—a double-blind study. One further check on the study's validity is the random selection of the experimental subjects. A researcher's nonrandom selections might bias the results.

Scientific facts are distinguished from fictions in a second way: they are published not just in newspapers and magazines but in professional journals. To be completely reliable, these journals must be **refereed journals** of the kind that employ **peer review** to screen the reports they publish. Even with safeguards like these, wrong facts are sometimes published; arguments appear in the scientific literature; and more experiments have to be conducted to resolve differences. Still, science proceeds haltingly but steadily in the direction of a more accurate picture of reality, and its body of knowledge grows greater. From it consumers can obtain useful guidelines as to how to manage their health and their lives.

A third way in which valid nutrition information can be recognized is that it is conveyed by reputable professional people whose education and credentials qualify them to speak knowledgeably on the subject. Nutrition experts have college and graduate degrees (MS, PhD) *in nutrition* from recognized universities, and they often have RD (registered dietitian)* or LD (licensed dietitian) credentials. Controversy 1, "Who Speaks on Nutrition?" gives details, and Appendix E provides a list of reliable nutrition resources.

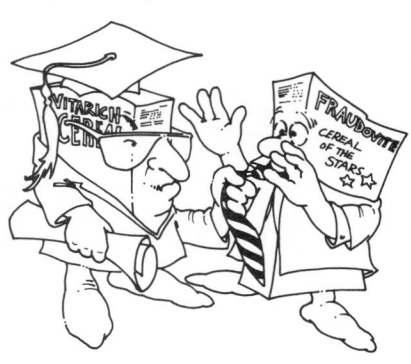

Fraudulant nutrition information is often packaged to resemble the real thing.

*The credentials to look for in Canada vary by province. Call the Canadian Dietetic Association (CDA) for local designations (CDA's phone number is in Appendix E).

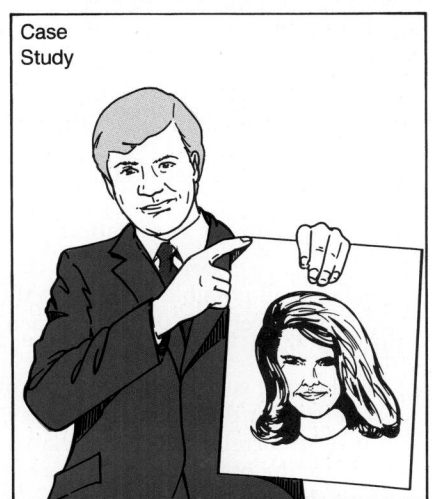

"This person eats too little of nutrient X and has illness Y."

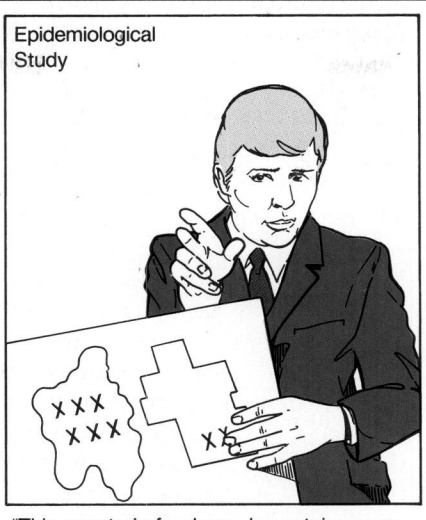

"This country's food supply contains more nutrient X, and these people suffer less illness Y."

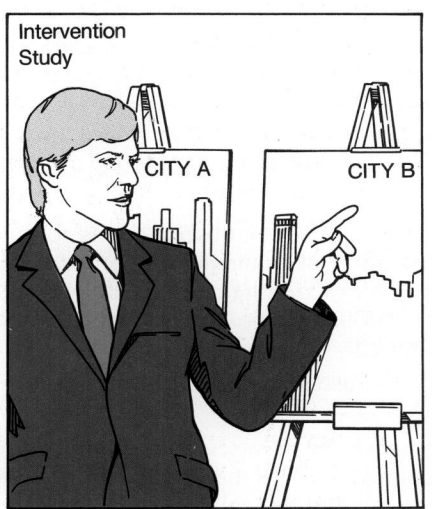

"Let's add foods containing nutrient X to city A's food supply and compare illness Y rates of city A with those of city B."

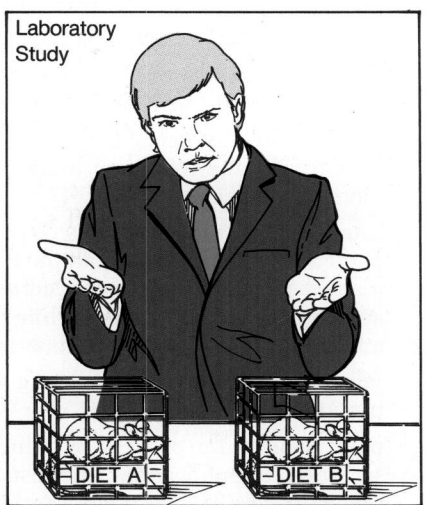

"Now let's prove that a nutrient X deficiency causes illness Y by inducing a deficiency in these rats."

■■■ Figure 1–3
Research Designs.

Fraudulent Nutrition Information—Nutrition Quackery

Nutrition **fraud** or **quackery** stands in contrast to reliable nutrition information. The field of nutrition is rife with fraud—multitudes of tricksters use skillful ploys to hoodwink consumers into handing over their money for worthless or even dangerous advice, products, and procedures.

Nutrition misinformation purveyed by quacks does not stick to facts derived from scientific research but makes claims that *sound* logical or true. It is not

▋▋▋Miniglossary of Research Terms

blind (experiment): an experiment in which the subjects do not know whether they are members of the experimental or the control group. See also *double-blind*.

case studies: studies of individuals, usually in clinical settings in which researchers can observe treatments and their apparent effects. To prove that a treatment has produced an effect requires simultaneous observation of an untreated similar subject (a *case control*).

control subjects: a group of individuals similar in all possible respects to the group being treated in an experiment but who receive a sham treatment instead of the real one. See also *intervention studies*.

correlation: the simultaneous change of two factors, such as the increase of weight with increasing height (a *direct* correlation) or the decrease of cancer incidence with increasing fiber intake (an *inverse* correlation). A correlation between two factors suggests that one may cause the other, but there may be no such relationship. Both may be caused by a third factor, or the correlation may be coincidental.

double-blind (experiment): an experiment in which neither the subjects nor the investigators know which subjects belong to which group until after the experiment is over.

epidemiological studies: studies of populations; often used in nutrition to search for correlations between dietary habits and disease incidence; a first step in seeking nutrition-related causes of diseases.

experimental subjects: the people or animals participating in an experiment who receive the treatment under investigation. See also *control subjects* and *intervention studies*.

intervention studies: studies of populations in which observation is accompanied by experimental manipulation of some of its members—for example, a study in which half of the subjects (the *experimental subjects*) follow diet advice to reduce fat intakes while the other half (the *control subjects*) do not, and both groups' heart health is monitored.

laboratory studies: studies using animals (usually) as subjects, designed to pinpoint causes and effects.

peer review: the process by which reports of new scientific findings are screened for publication. Scientists qualified to judge the validity of the work review it, and if it is poorly designed or appears invalid, they recommend against publication.

placebo (plah-SEE-bo): a sham treatment given to a control group; an inert, harmless medication that the group's members cannot recognize as different from the real thing. This will minimize the chance that an effect of the treatment will appear to have occurred due to the *placebo effect*: the healing effect that the act of treatment, rather than the treatment itself, often has.

randomization: a process of assigning members to experimental and control groups in a random fashion to reduce bias.

refereed journal: the journal of a reputable scientific society that does not publish reports of scientific findings until they have been reviewed and approved by two or more of the author's peers (*peer review*).

published in refereed journals (their reviewers would not accept it for publication) but solely in magazines, newspapers, and trade books. Some such sources have high standards for truthfulness, but even those may not be able to screen out all unreliable information. Writers making fraudulent claims are not credentialed professionals. If you look into their qualifications, you find they are only words on pretty pieces of paper. (There are exceptions, unfortunately. Occasionally a person with all the earmarks of the real thing turns out to be just plain dishonest. But for the most part these generalizations hold true.)

This book addresses fraudulent practices and products whenever it can, but it cannot deal with them all. To give you a head start and some tools of your own, Figure 1–4 offers a collection of "tags" to identify the tricks of quacks, and Table 1–2 lists some of the techniques of nutrition quackery. Wherever you recognize them, especially in a sales pitch, beware.

■■▶ *Valid nutrition information arises from scientific research that is published in refereed journals; credentialed professionals obtain and teach it. Fraudulent nutrition information is packaged to resemble the real thing.*

As you proceed with your study of nutrition principles, this background information will be useful. However, principles by themselves are no more nutritious than hot air. You have to take action before you will benefit from nutrition knowledge, and the action is no small thing.

Only if we arm ourselves with knowledge can we obtain from our food the nutrients we need. As an example of the difference that knowledge can make, two people might spend exactly the same amount of time and money planning, shopping, cooking, and cleaning up. Whereas one might spend most of those resources on a fancy, high-fat and high-sugar dessert that dominated the meal, the other might use the money and time to buy, peel, and slice vegetables for a stir-fry. The people who consumed the latter treat would be much better nourished.

■■■ Figure 1–4

Tags Identifying Questionable Nutrition Claims. The more of these tags you can tie on a package of nutrition information, the less likely it is to be valid.

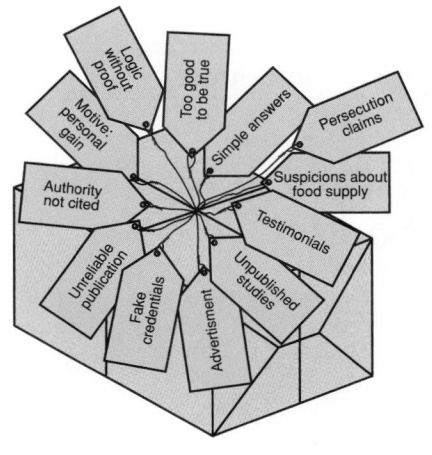

■■■ Table 1–2 Earmarks of Nutrition Quackery

To identify quackery, look for these signs:
1. Claims that sound too good to be true, with enticingly simple answers to complex problems often based on incomplete or bent truths or on logic. They say what most people want to hear, they sound magical but provide no real help.
2. Distrust of the current methods of medicine or suspicion of the regular food supply, with "alternatives" for sale (providing profit to the seller) under the guise that people should have freedom of choice. Beware of anyone claiming to be persecuted by the medical establishment—it means an amateur is making your diagnosis. They often try to convince you that physicians "want to keep you ill so that you will continue to pay for office visits."
3. Evidence in the forms of testimonials, case histories, and other nonscientific support for their claims.
4. Evidence from "unpublished studies." Valid scientific studies are published in reputable scientific journals.
5. In tiny print, somewhere on a page, the word "Advertisement."

SOURCE: Adapted from J. Ashley and R. Alfin-Slater, Position of the American Dietetic Association: Identifying food and nutrition misinformation, *Journal of the American Dietetic Association* 88 (1988): 1589–1591.

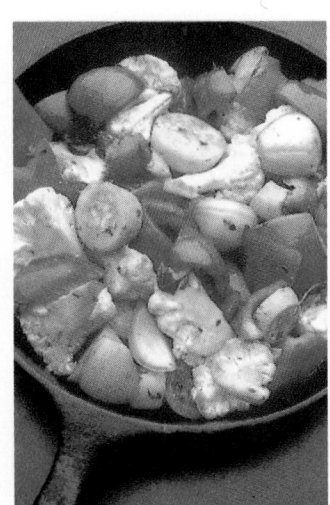

Would it take more time to prepare this dish than to prepare a batch of cookies? No, less time and less cleanup too.

To maximize the return on your investment of time, money, and energy, you must plan menus, shop, and cook and handle food with knowledge and a commitment to nutritional excellence. The Food Features to come can help you to do this. The first one, which follows, makes some basic distinctions about foods to help you with shopping.

 Food Feature

First Facts about Foods

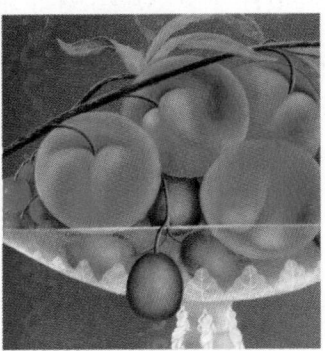

Shoppers encounter a bewildering variety of foods when they go to the grocery store—boxes, bottles, cans, jars, and bags, as well as arrays of fresh foods of all descriptions. What, exactly, should you be looking for at the store? The most nutritious foods, of course, but what does *that* mean? Natural foods? Fortified foods? Fresh foods? Which foods?

Before you even start to learn which foods are best, be sure to take note of this fact: to nourish you, the foods you choose must be *foods that you enjoy*. Food becomes nutrition, an old saying has it, only after it passes the lips. Buying nutritious foods will do you no good if they perish in your refrigerator. But within this constraint—that you must like them or be willing to learn to like them—what foods are best?

We wish we could use the term *natural* to describe the most nutritious foods because foods as taken originally from plants or animals have much to recommend them. Unfortunately, though, as used on *labels*, the term **natural food** is widely abused. The common meaning is often stretched by food companies who produce a myriad of highly processed foods that bear the word on their labels. Common examples are beer and wine claiming to be natural, even though no brand of beer or wine ever grew in the woods or on a farm. Another example is candy bars advertised as natural because they are made from sources like fruit sugar, honey, and carob beans rather than from cane sugar and chocolate. Candy bars are not made of whole fruits from plants; they are made of concentrated ingredients derived from those fruits. Only the sugar from the fruits has been used (leaving out the vitamins, minerals, and fiber), and only the fat from the beans (again, leaving out the nutrients and fiber). Hence they are high in calories, low in nutrients, and hardly natural at all.

Because of the widespread misuse of the word *natural* in food advertising and on labels, we are choosing to use a different term instead: **whole foods**. With one exception, in general, the less a food has been taken apart and the parts served separately, the more likely it is to have the characteristics experts agree are desirable: a high nutrient and fiber content relative to its calories and a low fat and sodium content. When this book speaks of whole foods, it means foods as similar as possible to the original, farm-grown products—and it often recommends them.

Foods from which the fat has been removed are the exceptions to the rule that foods should be whole. For adults who lead inactive lives and who cannot afford to eat much of foods that are high in fat, defatted products are desirable. They should seek lean meats and low-fat cheeses and other milk products.

In contrast to whole foods, many of the foods available today are *not* whole but are **partitioned foods**, that is, they are made of only parts of foods—sugar from beets or cane, refined flour from whole grains, butter from whole milk. Partitioning almost invariably yields products lower in nutrients than the original whole foods and sometimes virtually empty of nutrients, although usually high in calories. The food supply, which once consisted solely of whole foods, now offers *two-thirds of its calories* as partitioned foods almost completely stripped of nutrients: purified sugars, fats and oils, milled grains (primarily refined flour), and alcohol.[7] These items should probably not be allowed to contribute more than about 20 percent of the food energy for most healthy people eating a normal diet; they should occupy even less space in the diets of people whose energy intakes are low for reasons of dieting, illness, or aging.[8]

Notice that nothing has been said about **processed foods**. Processing is not the issue here; the nutritive value of foods is the issue. The term *processed* describes foods that have been subjected to any procedure during preparation— freezing, canning, dehydration, addition of additives, or even simply cooking. Processing may not affect the nutrient content of a food, may affect it only minimally, may destroy it, or may improve it. A totally unprocessed food like honey from a wild bee tree is *less* nutritious than a processed food like frozen spinach or canned salmon because the honey is almost pure sugar, while the other foods named come from a plant and a fish and their original nutrient content is little altered. On the other hand, processing may seriously diminish a food's quality, rendering it nearly nutrient-free and high in unwanted constituents such as salt and saturated fat. An example is chips made from originally nutritious potatoes. The question to ask is not whether a food has been processed or not but how it has been processed and how wholesome and nutritious it is now.

The addition of nutrients is described by two terms you often see on labels: **enriched** and **fortified**. The Consumer Caution of Chapter 4, "Refined, Enriched, and Whole-Grain Bread," explains the differences between these two terms. Examples of both are:

◼ Bread, whose grain has lost vitamins and minerals during refining, to which thiamin, riboflavin, niacin, and iron are added (this is enriched bread).
◼ Milk, to which vitamins A and D may be added (fortified).
◼ Soy milk, to which calcium and vitamin B_{12} are added (fortified).
◼ Salt, to which iodine is added (fortified).
◼ A sweetened drink, to which vitamin C is added (fortified).

Enriched and fortified foods may appear to be nutritious because their labels list many nutrients that have been added, but they may lack several dozen *other* nutrients that natural, whole foods contain. Whole foods have no labels that describe their abundant nutrient contents. To know whether a food is really nutritious, you have to know more than just what is on the label.

Among the most highly fortified of all foods on the market today are breakfast cereals, some of which boast additions of every vitamin and mineral you ever see named on a label. (The law requires that certain vitamins and minerals be listed on certain labels, those of the U.S. Recommended Dietary Allowances [U.S. RDA] table shown on the inside front cover, page C). When a food has nutrients added in amounts greater than 50 percent above the U.S. RDA standard, it has to be labeled a **supplement**, the same term that is used to identify a vitamin-mineral pill. Thus some breakfast cereals (those made from refined flour and described as supplements on their labels) are more like pills disguised as cereal than like whole grains. They are nutritious—with respect to the nutrients added—but they may not contain the full spectrum of nutrients that an unrefined whole food (or better, a mixture of such foods) might contain.

natural food: a term that has no legal definition. Turn to the definition of a *whole food*, which this book uses instead.

whole food: a food with all its naturally-occurring parts intact. Examples: a potato, an apple, a cut of meat, or a bowl of unpolished rice.

partitioned food: a food composed of part of a whole food, such as butter (from milk), sugar (from beets or cane), or corn oil (from corn).

processed food: a food subjected to any process, such as enrichment, milling, alteration of texture, addition of additives, cooking, or others.

enriched (fortified): terms referring to the addition of nutrients to a food.

supplement: a pill, liquid, or powder that contains nutrients. When used on food labels, this term means that nutrients have been added in amounts greater than 50% above the U.S. RDA.

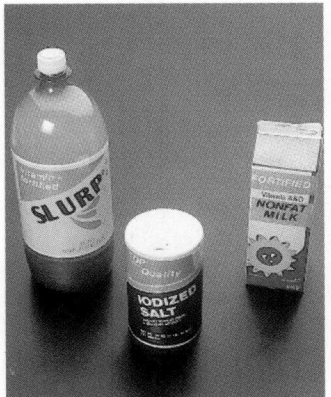

Fortified foods.

Some cereals are described as vitamin-mineral supplements on their labels.

staple food: a food used frequently or daily, for example, rice (in the East Indies) or potatoes (in Ireland).

In choosing processed foods, then, be sure that processing has improved them by adding nutrients you need, by rendering the foods safer to store and eat, or by removing unwanted constituents such as salt and fat. Avoid foods that have been processed by adding fat, sugar, and salt or by destroying or removing nutrients.

Wait, though: keep your favorite occasional treats *in* your food plan. In deciding whether to replace a favorite treat, ask yourself how much space it occupies in your food plan. There is no harm in indulging in any food now and then, but **staple food** items should be wholesome. For example, not every potato product you use must be recognizably a potato. But if potatoes are one of your staple foods, then whole potatoes with their skins are a better choice than potato chips.

Later chapters devote more space to foods but for now these guidelines will serve. Choose the most wholesome foods you like, especially for your staple foods, and most importantly—enjoy.

▌▌▌ SELF-STUDY

Record What You Eat

Our purpose in providing these exercises is to encourage you to study your own diet. Your reaction to them may be mixed. They will slow you down, and filling out all the forms can be tedious. Like your checkbook, they have to be done carefully, with frequent checking of arithmetic and tidy handwriting so that they will be accurate and meaningful.

The benefits, however, may well outweigh the drawbacks. Most students who do these activities with thoughtful attention report that unlike your checkbook, they are intriguing, informative, and often reassuring. They are also rewarding—in direct proportion to your accuracy.

In this first exercise you are to make a record of your typical food intake; in the subsequent exercises, you will analyze it for the nutrients it contains. You are undertaking this analysis before you have learned very much about the nutrients, but there is an advantage to that: having the results in front of you as you read will make the reading more meaningful. As you learn about each

nutrient and ask yourself how much of it you consume, you will already have the answer in front of you, ready for interpretation and action.

Use three copies of form 1 (Appendix F), and record on them all the foods you eat for a three-day period. If, like most people, you eat differently on weekdays than on weekends, then to get a true average you should probably record for two weekdays and one weekend day. Better still, make seven copies of form 1, and record your food intakes for a week. Fill in only columns 1 and 2 for the moment. The Self-Study at the end of Chapter 2 will instruct you to look up the nutrients in the foods.

As you record each food, make careful note of the amount. Estimate the amount to the nearest ounce, quarter cup, tablespoon, or other common measure. (Appendix C provides help with conversion factors.) In guessing at the sizes of meat portions, it helps to know that a piece of meat the size of the palm of your hand weighs about 3 or 4 ounces. If you are unable to estimate serving sizes, measure out servings the

size of a cup, tablespoon, and teaspoon onto a plate or into a bowl to see how they look. It also helps to know that a slice of cheese (such as sliced American cheese) or a 1 1/2-inch cube of cheese weighs about 1 ounce.

You may have to break down mixed dishes to their ingredients. However, many mixed dishes, including fast foods, are listed in Appendix A, where you will look up the foods. Other mixtures are simple to analyze. A ham-and-cheese sandwich, for example, can be listed as 2 slices of bread, 1 tablespoon of mayonnaise, 2 ounces of ham, 1 ounce of cheese, and so on. If you can't discover all the ingredients, estimate the amounts of only the major ones, like the beef, tomatoes, carrots, onions, and potatoes in a beef-vegetable soup.

You will, of course, make errors in estimating amounts. In calculations of this kind, errors of up to 20 percent are expected and tolerated. Still, you will have a rough approximation that will

continued on the next page

SELF STUDY *continued*

enable you to compare your nutrient intakes with the recommended ones.

Do not record any nutrient supplements you take. It will be interesting to discover whether your food choices alone deliver the nutrients you need. If they don't, you'll know better after analyzing your diet what supplement to choose.

You have now filled in columns 1 and 2 of form 1 in Appendix F. The next Self-Study will guide you in filling in the remainder of the form.

Notes

1. *The Surgeon General's Report on Nutrition and Health, Summary and Recommendations* (Washington, D.C.: DHHS [PHS] publication no. 88–50211, 1988).

2. D. T. Farr, Consumer attitudes and the supermarket, *Cereal Foods World* 32 (1987): 413–415.

3. R. L. Koretz and J. H. Meyer, Elemental diets—facts and fantasies, *Gastroenterology* 78 (1980): 393–410.

4. D. Rudman and P. J. Williams, Nutrient deficiencies during total parenertal nutrition, *Nutrition Reviews* 43 (1985): 1–13.

5. F. D. Moore, Current thoughts on malabsorption: Parenteral, enteral, and oral feeding (commentary), *Journal of the American Dietetic Association* 86 (1986): 1169–1170.

6. Moore, 1986.

7. D. R. Davis, Nutrition in the United States: Much room for improvement, *Journal of Applied Nutrition* 35 (1983): 17–29.

8. A. E. Harper, U.S. dietary goals: Against, *Journal of Nutrition Education* 9 (1977): 154–156.

Who Speaks on Nutrition?

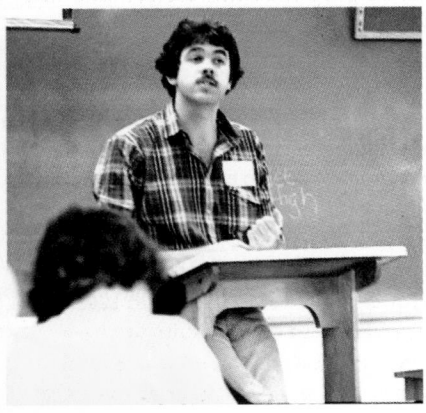

When you need nutrition advice, whom can you ask? Many people automatically ask the **doctor**, since "the doctor" is supposed to be an expert on everything related to health. But can you rely on your doctor (more correctly, your **physician**) to give you accurate information on nutrition? And if not, on whom can you rely? Do you have to go to a **nutritionist**? The answer, as you will see, is that the best-qualified expert on nutrition is a **registered dietitian**. However, because so many people rely on physicians to deliver nutrition information, this Controversy begins with "the doctor."

███ Physicians' Nutrition Know-how

Physicians have low credibility as nutrition experts. In 1974 Dr

Charles E. Butterworth published a shocking article in *Nutrition Today* titled "The Skeleton in the Hospital Closet."[1] In it he reported a high incidence of severe malnutrition in the hospital, which he called "physician-induced," or **iatrogenic**, malnutrition. He published pictures of emaciated people with signs of malnutrition, such as bleeding gums and sores on their skin, that could have been prevented by physicians' actions. He cited some of the causes: physicians often deprived their patients of food for days at a time so that they could give them medical tests; they seldom ordered vitamin and mineral supplements for them; and they often administered nutritionally inadequate clear fluids for long periods. The resulting malnutrition severely weakened patients, delayed their recovery, prolonged their hospital stays, and increased the cost of their treatment. Staff didn't notice their patients' weight losses because schedules for monitoring rotated frequently, no one was assigned ultimate responsibility, and physicians and dietitians didn't communicate.[2] The situation turned out to be typical of hospitals all across the country, with some hospitals reporting close to half of all patients having evidence of protein-energy malnutrition.[3]

Part of the blame for this deplorable situation was laid at the feet of the medical schools that educated the physicians. One physician remarked that "often doctors are trained in nutrition by doctors who heard it from another doctor who

made it up."[4] Another commented, "I would guess 90 percent of the graduates of our medical schools couldn't describe an adequate, nutritious diet."[5] Physicians were being taught how to give drugs and to perform surgery but not how to support people's health while they underwent these treatments.

Since then the medical schools have responded to these accusations by evaluating the situation, identifying deficits, and attempting to remedy them in a trend that resembled "a ground swell."[6] A medical journal reported that, "like sex, nutrition is increasingly discussed among physicians."[7]

Today the situation has improved somewhat but is still not fully remedied. Some physicians now specialize in nutrition.[8] A study of nutrition education in U.S. medical schools concluded that while schools teach nutrition as an academic subject, they still don't teach its application to cases in real practice. Many students graduate without being aware of how nutrition supports medical treatment, much less knowing how to apply nutrition's potential for prevention of diet-related diseases and maintenance of health.[9] Medical students are dissatisfied with the quality of nutrition instruction they are receiving.[10] Physicians in practice today still seldom use even simple tools, such as the RDA tables, to establish the needs of their patients, nor do they inquire about patients' food intakes.[11]

In response to these findings, the National Academy of Sciences has made several recommendations, among them the following:

That nutrition be a required science course in medical schools.

That 25 or more classroom hours be allocated to teaching its core concepts.

That nutrition be a distinct department with at least one full faculty position devoted entirely to it.

That the medical board examinations cover all nutrition areas in proportion to their importance.

In relation to the last item, a review of the board examinations showed that they asked no questions on such areas as osteoporosis, nutrition and cancer, and nutrient needs of the elderly.[12]

Not all physicians are untrained in nutrition. Some have received adequate training; some have sought it out on their own. Some are nationally recognized experts in nutrition. And many, recognizing that they cannot know everything about nutrition themselves, make use of properly credentialed nutrition experts as partners, consultants, or referrals.

■■■ Nutrition Support in the Hospitals

Currently, nutrition care in hospitals is uneven—excellent in some, poor to nonexistent in others. A 1986 study of 33 hospitals attempted to screen over 3000 clients' nutrition status but could not complete the job for 60 percent of them because the staff at admissions had not recorded critical nutrition data. The most important and simplest measures to record were height and weight, but they had not done even that. Of the 40 percent of clients whose data were available, more than half had below-normal values for one or more of the indicators studied.[13] This reflects extensive neglect of nutrition in the hospitals.

On the positive side, though, many hospitals have developed ways to deliver excellent nutrition care. A hospital entity called the **nutrition support team** has been defined—a team of selected physicians, nurses, dietitians, and pharmacists who work together to evaluate a client's nutrition status and to develop an individualized nutrition care plan.[14] Books have been published to guide nutrition support teams in the delivery of nutrition services,[15] and the computer is being recruited for the task of identifying the clients most in need of attention.[16] In short, it is now clear what hospitals should be doing to meet the need adequately, and some are doing it.

Outside the hospital, whom can people ask about nutrition for maintaining their health so that they will not have to *enter* the hospital? For people who are obese or too thin, who are living with heart disease or cancer or diabetes, who have food allergies or digestive disorders, or who simply want to ensure that their nutrition status is optimal, the dietitian is the person to see.

■■■ Dietitians' Credentials

The dietitian is educated specifically to understand nutrition needs and to deliver counsel and care. A dietitian who is the genuine article, that is, a registered dietitian, has an undergraduate degree requiring some 60 or so semester hours in nutrition and food science, has completed a year's clinical internship or the equivalent, has passed a national examination administered over six competency areas by the American Dietetic Association (ADA) or the Canadian Dietetic Association (CDA), and maintains up-to-date knowledge obtained through required continuing education activities (attending seminars, taking courses, or writing professional papers). Dietitians who have met these criteria may display the credential RD in the United States or **PDt** in Nova Scotia, Canada (other provinces vary), indicating **registration** with the ADA or CDA, should a consumer want to check on their credentials.

Dietitians work in a variety of settings and perform a multitude of duties. Dietitians can assume roles in clinical, administrative, consultant, public health, food service, research, and education settings. An example of the competencies of just one of these, the clinical dietitian, is provided in Table C1–1. Dietitians in other fields of practice have other competencies.

■■■ Table C1–1 Competencies of the Clinical Dietitian

Assesses nutrition status.
Develops individualized care plans.
Implements, monitors, and evaluates
   care plans.
Educates clients and families.
Communicates with physicians, nurses,
   and pharmacists regarding clients'
   nutrition status, needs, and
   treatment.
Directs food service personnel.
Supervises dietetic staff.
Participates in professional activities to
   enhance knowledge and skill.
Educates dietetics students and interns.

SOURCE: Adapted from P. M. Kris-Etherton and coauthors, A profile of clinical dietetics practice in Pennsylvania, *Journal of the American Dietetic Association* 83 (1983): 654–660. Material developed as part of the Continuing Professional Education Development Project, The Pennsylvania State University. Funding provided by the W. W. Kellogg Foundation.

Why, in talking about the dietitian, did we specify that the person had to be "the genuine article"? For reasons no one quite understands, nutrition is the field most riddled with quack practitioners.[17] Literally thousands of people possess fake nutrition degrees.

The documents many of these people display claim that they are dietitians (although they do not have the ADA-sanctioned RD credentials), or nutritionists, or dietists, to name a few. These titles are promoted as if they were equivalent in meaning to established credentials, but they are not.[18] That being the

■■■ Miniglossary

accreditation: approval; in the case of hospitals or university departments, approval by a professional organization of the educational program offered. There are phony accrediting agencies; the genuine ones are listed with the U.S. Department of Education.

correspondence school: a school from which courses can be taken and degrees granted by mail. Those that are accredited offer respectable courses and degrees. See also *diploma mills*.

dietitian: a person trained in nutrition, food science, and diet planning. See also *registered dietitian* and *professional dietitian*.

diploma mills: institutions that offer meaningless courses and degrees by mail.

doctor: see *physician, PhD*

iatrogenic (malnutrition): malnutrition caused by inadequate physician care (*iatro* means "doctor").

license to practice: permission under state or federal law, granted on passing an examination, to use a certain title (such as *medical doctor, osteopath, attorney*.

MS (master of science) degree: a degree beyond a bachelor's degree granted by an institution of higher learning that typically requires two to three years of course work, a research project or thesis, and passing a comprehensive set of examinations.

nutrition support team: a team of physicians, nurses, dietitians, and pharmacists who together evaluate a client's nutrition status and develop an appropriate nutrition care plan.

nutritionist: a person who specializes in the study of nutrition. Some nutritionists are registered dietitians, whereas others are self-described experts whose training is questionable. In states with responsible legislation in place, the term is legally reserved for people who have MS or PhD degrees from properly accredited institutions.

PhD (doctor of philosophy) degree: a degree beyond a master's degree that typically requires four to seven years of course work, a research thesis or dissertation, and passing a comprehensive set of examinations. A person with a PhD in any subject can be addressed as "doctor."

physician: a medical practitioner with an MD (medical doctor) or DO (doctor of osteopathy) degree from an accredited medical school.

professional dietitian (PDt): in Nova Scotia, an accredited member of the Canadian Dietetic Association who is entitled to practice dietetics under provincial law. Other designations vary by province.

public health nutritionist: a credentialed professional usually with a college degree in nutrition, employed by a government agency to serve the public need for nutrition services.

■■■ Miniglossary *continued*

registered dietitian (RD): a dietitian who has graduated from a program of dietetics approved by the American Dietetic Association (ADA), has passed the association's registration examination, has served in an internship program or the equivalent to practice the necessary skills, and maintains competencies through continuing education. Many states now require licensing for practicing dietitians.

registration: listing; with respect to health professionals, listing with a professional organization that requires specific course work, experience, and passing an examination.

case, if we are to turn to dietitians for our diet advice, we have two tasks on our hands: first, to tell the real ones from the fake ones, and second, to tell the good ones from the poor ones—since, as with other professionals, the possession of even a legitimate credential does not necessarily make a person a high-quality professional or even an honest human being.

A person who wants to visit a dietitian and obtain nutrition advice needs to know that in many states the title *dietitian* is no guarantee of professionalism. Many states allow use of the title by anyone who wants to use it, just as people can call themselves counselors. Some states have passed laws to allow only qualified individuals to call themselves dietitians and have specified that RDs or people with certain graduate degrees are the only ones who qualify. Many states now provide a further guarantee: the **license to practice**.[19] Licensing makes it still more difficult for unqualified people to advertise widely that they are experts.

Some states also regulate the use of the title *nutritionist*—a welcome development—since that title has enticed thousands of consumers into scams in which they have lost their health, their life savings, or both. If the term is to be meaningful, it should apply only to people who have an **MS (master of science) degree** or **PhD (doctor of philosophy) degree** in nutrition or related fields from accredited colleges or universities or the title **public health nutritionist**, not other forms of education. An MS or PhD in nutrition requires two to seven years of training in an accredited graduate school. A course of, for example, six to nine months at a **correspondence school** is simply not the same. Some schools are not even legitimate correspondence schools but **diploma mills**—places that essentially sell certificates of competency to anyone who pays their fees. Of course some untraditional universities teach adequate curriculum, and these are not the diploma mills referred to here, but diploma mills do exist, and you should beware.

Evidence of **accreditation** is important in the description of the institution from which the education comes. The most rampant abuse of credentials is in the display of master's and doctoral degrees. According to the *New York Times*, doctorates are available for around $2300; master's degrees for $1250; and bachelor's degrees for $800—with discounts for all three together. To obtain them a candidate need not read any books or pass any examinations. They are available from "accredited" schools, too, since there are 30 phony accrediting agencies.[20] To dramatize the situation, one writer enrolled for $82 in a nutrition diploma mill that billed itself as a correspondence school offering nutrition degrees. She made every attempt to fail the course, even purposely answering all of the examination questions incorrectly. Even so, she received a "nutritionist" certificate at the end of the course, together with a letter from the "school" explaining that they were sure she must have just misread the test.[21]

In a similar stunt, Ms Sassafras Herbert has been named a "professional member" of a professional association. For her efforts, Sassafras has received a wallet card and the privilege of being listed in a sort of fake *Who's Who* in nutrition that is distributed at health fairs and trade shows nationwide. Sassafras is a poodle; her master, Victor Herbert, MD, paid $50 to prove that she could win these honors merely by sending in her name. Mr Charlie

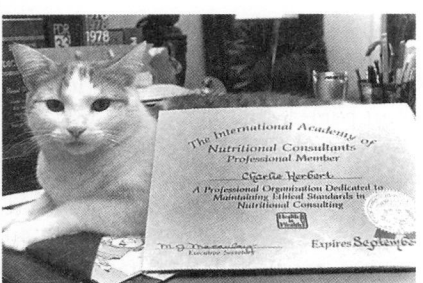

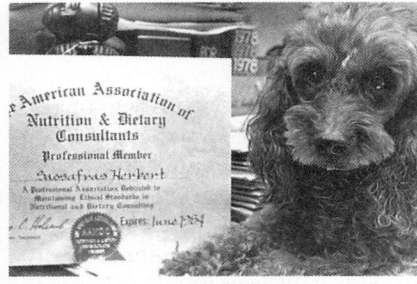

Charlie and Sassafras display their professional credentials.

Herbert also is a professional member of such an organization; Charlie is a cat.

To check a recommended provider's credentials, first look for the degrees listed by the person's titles. Then find out what you can about the reputations of the institutions from which the degrees were obtained. One of the best sources of information as to whether a school or other institution is legitimate or not is the National Council Against Health Fraud, whose address is in Appendix E. Also call and ask your state's health-licensing agency if dietitians are licensed in your state and (if so) if the person you are interested in has met licensure criteria.

Dietitians today are taking their rightful places among their peers—on nutrition support teams, on the staffs of wellness centers, in home health agencies, in long-term care institutions, in private practice, and in sports training centers, as well as in the hospital. The needs are there, and dietitians are the professionals who can meet them.

Notes

1. C. E. Butterworth, The skeleton in the hospital closet, *Nutrition Today*, March/April 1974, pp. 4–8.
2. Butterworth, 1974.
3. A. Fonaroff, Undernutrition (letter to the editor), *Journal of the American Medical Association* 237 (1977): 1825–1826.
4. J. B. Schorr, as quoted by L. Hofmann, ed., *The Great American Nutrition Hassle* (Palo Alto, Calif.: Mayfield, 1978), p. 399.
5. P. R. Lee, as quoted by Hofmann, 1978, p. 321.
6. W. J. Darby, The renaissance of nutrition education, *Nutrition Reviews* 35 (1977): 33–38.
7. Nutrition: No longer a stepchild in medicine (Medical News), *Journal of the American Medical Association* 238 (1977): 2245.
8. S. B. Heymsfield and coauthors, Biennial survey of physician clinical nutrition training programs, *American Journal of Clinical Nutrition* 42 (1985): 152–165.
9. Committee on Nutrition in Medical Education, Food and Nutrition Board, Commission on Life Sciences, National Research Council, *Nutrition Education in U.S. Medical Schools* (Washington, D.C.: National Academy Press, 1985), as reported in *American Journal of Clinical Nutrition* 43 (1986): 643–644.
10. R. L Weinsier and coauthors, Nutrition knowledge of senior medical students: A collaborative study of southeastern medical schools, *American Journal of Clinical Nutrition* 43 (1986): 959-968.
11. B. S. Levine and R. Tannenbaum, Frequency of nutritional considerations by practicing physicians (abstract), *American Journal of Clinical Nutrition* 43 (1986): 66.
12. Committee on Nutrition in Medical Education, 1985.
13. S. K. Kamath and coauthors, Hospital malnutrition: A 33-hospital screening study, *Journal of the American Dietetic Association* 86 (1986): 203–206.
14. C. J. Krazit and W. W. Turner, The nutrition support advisory committee: A council of hospital services for nutrition support, *Journal of the American Dietetic Association* 86 (1986): 1067–1068.
15. S. H. Krey and R. L. Murray, eds., *Dynamics of Nutrition Support: Assessment, Implementation, Evaluation* (Norwalk, Conn.: Appleton-Century-Crofts, 1986), reviewed in *Journal of the American Dietetic Association* 86 (1986): 1642; M. A. Bernard, D. O. Jacobs, and J. L. Rombeau, *Nutritional and Metabolic Support of Hospitalized Patients* (Philadelphia: Saunders, 1985), reviewed in *Journal of the American Dietetic Association* 86 (1986): 1318; D. B. A. Silk, *Nutritional Support in*

■■■ Other Health Care Professionals

These people's titles do not appear in this Controversy but are included here for those who might be curious about them. Their qualifications to practice their professions are not as clearly defined as those of the people discussed in this Controversy. Their knowledge of nutrition may be extensive or non-existent or anything in between. Some of these people may be out-and-out quacks.

acupuncturist: a practitioner who punctures the nerves of the body with needles to relieve pain and to achieve other effects. Acupuncture is an ancient art in China; in an expert's hands it can be useful in treatment of some kinds of pain.

chiropractor: a person who is trained to treat people with pain caused by misalignment of the skeleton. Chiropractic treatments involve manipulations of the joints that can, in the best of cases, relieve pressure on nerves. Provided that chiropractors stay within the bounds of their training and refer to other specialists clients whose problems are *not* caused by misalignment of the skeleton, they can offer a valuable service. Some chiropractors have only two years of college, two of training, and two of supervised practice, while others prepare more extensively for their profession.

clinical ecologist: a practitioner who claims to be able to cure people's illnesses by diagnosing and treating allergies they have developed to substances and materials in their environments.

homeopath: a practitioner who uses small doses of poisons to supposedly prevent or to relieve harm caused by those poisons (*homeo* means "same").

iridologist: a person who claims to be able to diagnose illnesses by studying the patterns of color in the iris of the eye. Training involves payment of $400 to purchase a chart of the iris and a list of diseases that various color patterns indicate.

naprapath: a person who treats connective tissue and ligament disorders by manipulation and massage (*napra* means "connective").

naturopath: a person who uses "natural" products such as foods and herbs to treat people's illnesses. Naturopaths distinguish themselves from traditional medical practitioners, whom they call *allopaths*—people who use medicine, surgery, x-ray examinations, and other "unnatural" tools to treat illnesses (*allo* means "other").

orthomolecular psychiatrist: a psychiatrist who uses "natural" treatments, especially vitamins and minerals, to rectify mental illnesses, assuming they are caused by wrong amounts of nutrient molecules in the system (*ortho* means "right amount").

Hospital Practice (Boston: Blackwell Scientific Publications, 1983), reviewed by M. J. Hall in *American Journal of Clinical Nutrition* 40 (1984): 1309–1310.

16. P. W. Bunton, Using the computer as a referral source to find the patient at nutritional risk, *Journal of the American Dietetic Association* 86 (1986): 1232–1233.

17. S. Barrett, Why licensing of "nutritionists" is needed, *Nutrition Forum*, May 1985, p. 40.

18. Barrett, 1985.

19. M. B. Haschke, Licensure for dietitians: The issue in context (President's Page), *Journal of the American Dietetic Association* 84 (1984): 454–457.

20. New York Times Service story in the *San Bernardino* (California) *Times*, 6 August 1985, as cited by *National Council Against Health Fraud Newsletter*, August 1985, p. 1.

21. V. Aronson, Bernardean University: A nutrition diploma mill, *ACSH News and Views*, March/April 1983, pp. 7, 11.

Nutrition Standards and Guidelines

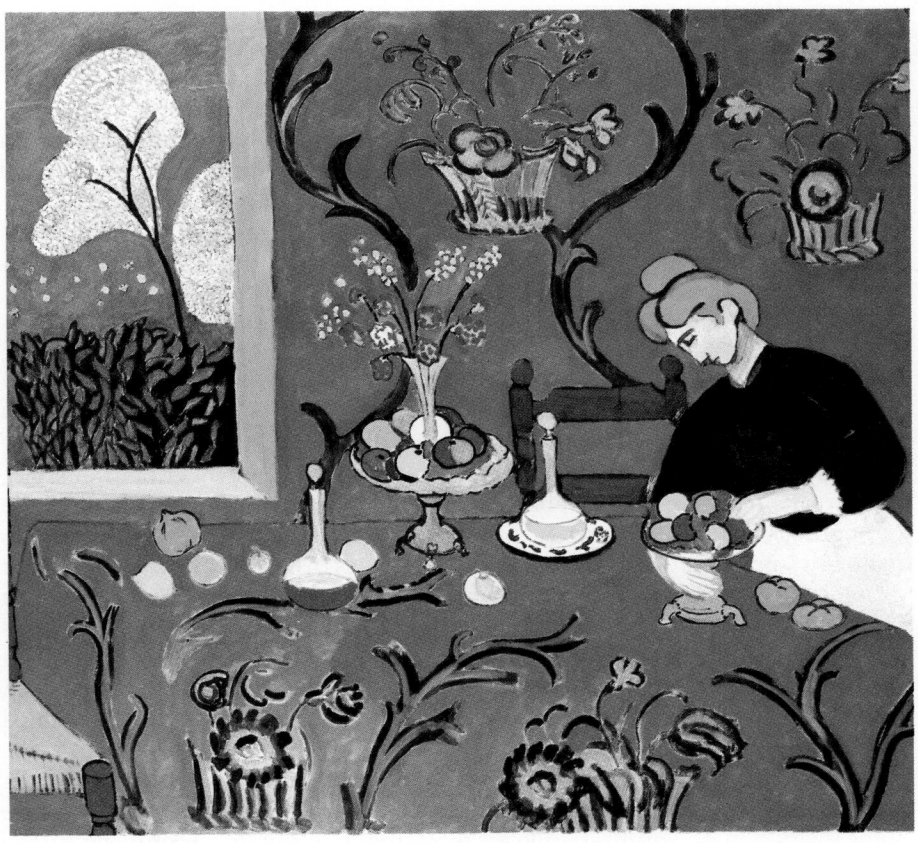

CONTENTS

The Red Room by Henri Matisse. George Roos/Art Resource, N.Y. Copyright 1990 Succession H. Matisse/ARS, N.Y.

malnutrition: any condition caused by excess or deficient food energy or nutrient intake or by an imbalance of nutrients. Nutrient or energy deficiencies are classified as forms of *undernutrition*; nutrient or energy excesses are forms of *overnutrition*.

adequacy: the description of a diet that provides all of the essential nutrients, fiber, and energy in amounts sufficient to maintain health.

balance: the description of a diet that provides foods of a number of types in proportion to each other, such that foods rich in some nutrients do not crowd out of the diet foods that are rich in other nutrients.

calorie control: control of energy intake, a feature of a sound diet plan.

moderation: the description of a diet that provides no constituent in excess.

variety: the description of a diet in which different foods are used for the same purposes on different occasions—the opposite of **monotony**.

Eating well is easy, in principle. All you need to do is to choose a selection of foods that supplies appropriate amounts of the essential nutrients, fiber, and energy. A few people do this automatically, but many do not. Many people are overweight, undernourished, and suffer from nutrient excesses or deficiencies that impair their health. In other words, they suffer from **malnutrition**. You may not think that this applies to you, but you may already be suffering ill effects from less-than-optimal nutrient intakes without knowing it. Accumulated over years, these can seriously impair the quality of your life. Putting it positively, you can enjoy the best of vim, vigor, and vitality if you learn now to nourish yourself optimally.

To master the task of meeting your nutrition needs, you may find it useful to learn the answers to several questions. How much energy and how much of each nutrient do you need? Which types of foods supply which nutrients? How much of each type of food do you have to eat to get enough? And how can you eat all these foods without gaining weight and without getting too much fat and salt? This chapter begins by identifying some dietary ideals and ends by showing how to achieve them. The last section shows how information on food labels can help you decide whether or not a packaged food supports dietary ideals.

▌▌▌ Dietary Ideals

The diet that meets your body's needs has all of the following characteristics: **adequacy** (it provides enough of each essential nutrient, fiber, and energy); **balance** (it does not overemphasize one food type or nutrient at the expense of another); **calorie control** (it provides the amount of energy you need to maintain appropriate weight—not more, not less); **moderation** (it does not provide excess intakes of fat, salt, sugar, or other constituents); and **variety** (it uses different foods to provide the needed nutrients rather than the same foods day after day). Importantly, too, it pleases you. That is, it consists of foods you enjoy eating and can easily obtain—foods that fit your tastes, personality, family and cultural traditions, lifestyle, and budget. At its best, a well-planned diet is a source of pleasure as well as of good health.

Any nutrient could be used to demonstrate the importance of dietary *adequacy*. Iron provides a familiar example. It is an essential nutrient; you lose some every day, so you have to keep replacing it; and you can only get it into your body by eating foods that contain it. If you eat too few of these foods, you can develop iron-deficiency anemia; you can feel weak, tired, and unenthusiastic, may have frequent headaches, and can do very little muscular work without disabling fatigue. If you make the needed correction and add iron-rich foods to your diet, you soon feel more energetic. Some foods are rich in iron; others are notoriously poor. Meat, fish, poultry, and legumes are in the iron-rich category, and an easy way to obtain the needed iron is to include these foods in your diet regularly.

To appreciate the importance of dietary *balance*, consider a second essential nutrient, calcium. Most foods that are rich in iron are poor in calcium. Calcium's best food sources are milk and milk products, which happen to be extraordinarily poor iron sources. A diet lacking calcium causes poor bone development during the growing years and increases a person's susceptibility to disabling bone loss in adult life. Children and adults are advised to consume enough milk, milk products, or other calcium-rich foods each day to meet their calcium needs—but not so much as to crowd iron-rich foods out of the diet.

Clearly, to obtain enough of both nutrients, which seldom appear together in the same foods, one has to balance one's food choices. Balancing the whole diet to provide enough but not too much of every one of the 40-odd nutrients the body needs for health is a juggling act that requires considerable skill. As you will see, food group plans can help you achieve dietary adequacy and balance because they recommend specific amounts of foods of each type.

To help with calorie control while attempting to balance the diet and to make it adequate, the planner is bound to find certain foods especially useful. These are foods that are rich in nutrients relative to their energy contents, that is, foods with high **nutrient density**. Consider calcium sources, for example. Ice cream supplies calcium, as does milk, but a cup of plain ice cream contributes about 300 calories and less calcium than a 90-calorie cup of milk. Or consider iron. A 3-ounce serving of high-fat beef pot roast offers about the same amount of iron as a 3-ounce serving of water-packed tuna, but the beef supplies over 300 calories, the tuna about 100.* Most people cannot, for their health's sake, afford to choose foods without regard to their energy contents. To help with diet planning, a person can use lists of foods that supply approximately equal amounts of nutrients and calories per portion. Such lists of interchangeable foods are presented later in this chapter.

Intakes of certain food constituents such as fat, cholesterol, sugar, and salt should be limited for health's sake (more on health effects in Chapter 11). Some people take this to mean that they must never indulge in a delicious beefsteak or hot-fudge sundae, but they are misinformed, since *moderation*, not elimination, is the key. A steady diet of ice cream and steak might be harmful; such a meal once a week as part of an otherwise moderate diet plan might have little impact; and a once-a-month treat of the food would have practically no effect at all. Moderation also means that limits for desirable food constituents are necessary. For example, while a certain level of fiber in foods contributes to the health of the digestive system, too much fiber causes nutrient losses, as described in Chapter 4.

As for *variety*, it is generally agreed that people should not eat the same foods day after day, for two reasons. One reason is that some less-known nutrients and some nonnutrient food components could be important to health; some foods may be better sources of these than others. Another reason is that a monotonous diet may deliver large amounts of undesirable food constituents, such as plant toxins or chemical contaminants. Each undesirable component of a food is diluted by all the other items eaten with it and is even further diluted if several days are skipped before it is eaten again. This is another reason why lists of interchangeable foods are useful—you can choose one today and a different one tomorrow to meet the same nutrient needs. Last, variety adds interest—trying new foods can be a source of pleasure.

nutrient density: a measure of nutrients provided per calorie of food.

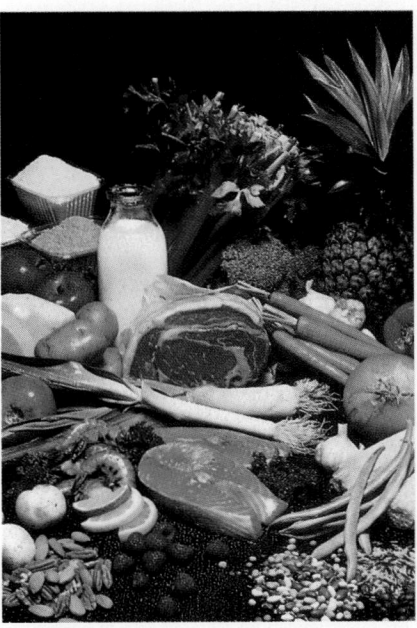

Variety helps to ensure an adequate and balanced diet.

❚❚▶ *A well-planned diet is adequate in nutrients, is balanced with regard to food types, is moderate in energy and unwanted constituents, and offers variety. Foods of high nutrient density form the foundation of such a diet.*

*These are approximate numbers; the actual values for these foods are listed in Appendix A.

The Canadian RNI are in Appendix B.

RDA are set for:

- Energy.
- Protein.
- Vitamins: A, C, D, E, K, thiamin, riboflavin, niacin, B_6, B_{12}, folate.
- Minerals: Calcium, phosphorus, magnesium, iron, zinc, iodine, selenium.

Estimated safe and adequate intakes are given in ranges for:

- Vitamins: biotin, pantothenic acid.
- Minerals (trace elements): copper, manganese, fluoride, chromium, molybdenum.

Estimated minimum requirements of healthy persons are given for:

- Sodium, potassium, chloride.

See inside front cover.

▐▐▐ Nutrient Recommendations

This section introduces the Recommended Dietary Allowances (RDA), used in the United States as a standard for healthy people's energy and nutrient intakes. The Canadian equivalent is the *Recommended Nutrient Intakes for Canadians* (RNI), and it is presented in Appendix B. (The U.S. RDA are standards used on food labels and are described later.)

The RDA

A committee of qualified nutrition experts appointed by the government publishes *recommendations* concerning appropriate nutrient intakes for the people in this country.* These are the **Recommended Dietary Allowances (RDA)**, and they are used and referred to so often that they are presented on the inside front cover of this book. As you can see, the main RDA table includes recommendations for protein, 11 vitamins, and 7 minerals, while the additional tables include 2 more vitamins and 8 more minerals as well as energy (calories). Periodically the committee on the RDA meets to reexamine and to revise these recommendations on the basis of new research regarding people's nutrient needs. It then publishes an updated set of RDA.[1]

The RDA have been much misunderstood. One young woman, on first learning of their existence, was outraged: "You mean Uncle Sam tells me that I must eat exactly 46 grams of protein every day?" This is not the committee's intention, and the RDA are recommendations, not commandments. The following facts will help put the RDA in perspective:

- The ongoing creation of the RDA is *funded* by the government, but the committee that determines the RDA is composed of scientists representing a variety of specialties.
- The RDA are based on reviews of available scientific research to the greatest extent possible and are revised periodically to keep them up to date.
- Except for sodium, potassium, and chloride, the RDA are not minimum requirements nor are they optimal intakes. They are safe and adequate intakes that include a generous margin of safety.
- They are average daily intakes set high enough to provide for full body nutrient stores to last through brief periods of inadequate intakes lasting a day or two for some nutrients and up to a month or two for others.
- They are most appropriately used to plan diets for populations such as school children or military personnel, but people like to use them to estimate the adequacy of their own individual intakes. They can be used this way if compared over a significant period of time.
- The RDA are for healthy persons only. Medical problems alter nutrient needs.

Separate recommendations are made for different sets of people: men, women, pregnant women, children, and other groups. They are also segregated by age. Children aged 4 to 6 years are distinguished from men and women aged 19 to 24 years, for example. Each individual can look up the recommendations for his or her own age and sex group.

*This is a committee of the Food and Nutrition Board (FNB) of the National Academy of Sciences/National Research Coucil (NAS/NRC).

No RDA is set for carbohydrate or fat. The assumption is that you will use a certain portion of your daily energy allowance meeting your protein RDA and then will distribute the remaining calories among carbohydrate and fat to meet your energy RDA. This chapter later shows how to balance energy sources to best support health (see "Food Groups and Exchange Lists"). The next two sections describe the process the committee goes through in selecting the RDA values, first for nutrients, then for energy.

II▶ *The RDA used in the United States and the RNI used in Canada represent suggested average daily intakes of energy and selected nutrients for healthy people in the population.*

The RDA for Nutrients

If you use the RDA to estimate the adequacy of your own diet, you need to be aware that individuals' nutrient needs vary and that the allowances are designed primarily for use with whole groups of people. A theoretical discussion will illustrate these points.

Suppose we were the committee members, and we had the task of setting an RDA for nutrient X (any essential nutrient). Ideally our first step would be to try to find out how much of that nutrient individuals need. We would review studies of deficiency states, of nutrient stores and their depletion, and of the factors influencing them. We would try to select the most valid data for use in our work. Among the experiments we might review or conduct would be measures of the body's intake and excretion (in the case of nutrients that aren't changed before they are excreted) to find out how much of an intake is required for balance (this is called a **balance study**). For each individual subject, we could determine a **requirement** for nutrient X. Below the requirement that person would slip into negative balance or experience declining stores that could, over time, lead to deficiency of the nutrient.

We would find that different individuals have different requirements. Mr A might need 40 units of the nutrient each day to maintain balance; Mr B might need 35; Mr C, 65. If we looked at enough individuals, we might find that their requirements were distributed as shown in Figure 2–1 —most near the midpoint, and only a few at the extremes.

balance study: a laboratory study in which a person is fed a controlled diet and the intake and excretion of a nutrient are measured. Balance studies are valid only for nutrients like calcium (chemical elements) that don't change while they are in the body.

requirement: that amount of a nutrient that will just prevent the development of specific deficiency signs; distinguished from the RDA, which is a recommended and generous allowance.

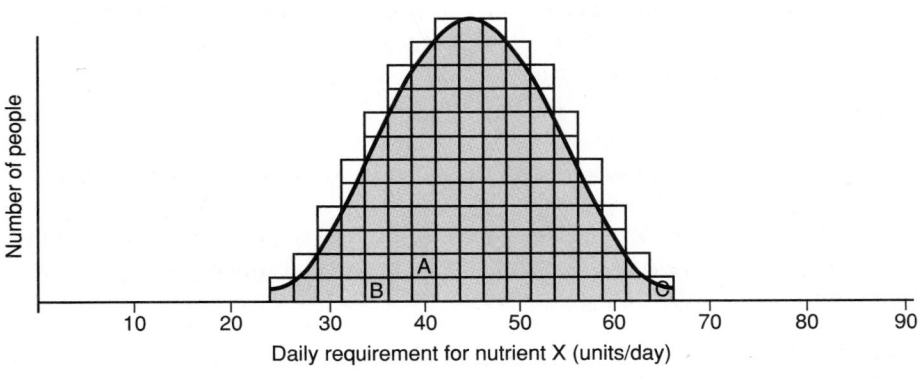

■■■ Figure 2–1

Individuality of Nutrient Requirements. Each square represents a person. A, B, and C are Mr A, Mr B, and Mr C.

Then, to set the RDA, we would have to decide what intake to recommend for everybody. Should we set it at the mean (shown in Figure 2–1 at 45 units)? This is the average requirement for nutrient X; it is probably the closest to everyone's need, assuming the distribution shown in Figure 2–1. (Actually the data for most nutrients other than protein indicate a distribution that is much less symmetrical.) But if people took us literally and consumed exactly this amount of nutrient X each day, half the population would begin to develop internal deficiencies and even possibly overt symptoms of them; Mr C would be one of those people.

Perhaps we should set the RDA for nutrient X at or above the extreme, say at 70 units a day, so that everyone would be covered. (Actually we didn't study everyone, so some individual we didn't happen to test might have a still higher requirement.) This might be a good idea in theory, but what about a person like Mr B, who needs only 35 units a day? He would be forced to consume twice his need, and to do so he might spend money needlessly on foods containing nutrient X to the exclusion of foods containing other nutrients he needs.

The choice we would finally make, with some reservations, would be to set the RDA at a reasonably high point so that the bulk of the population would be covered. In this example a reasonable choice might be to set it at 63 units a day. By moving the RDA further toward the extreme, we would pick up few additional people but inflate the recommendation for most people (including Mr A and Mr B).

The committee makes judgments of this kind when setting the RDA for nutrients. They set it well above the mean or average requirement as they can best determine it from the available information. In theory, relatively few healthy people's individual requirements, then, are not covered by the RDA.

For these reasons the RDA cannot be taken personally by any individual; that is, you can't know exactly what your own personal requirement may be. The committee makes several assumptions that may not apply to you at all. For example, they assume that you are eating a diet that includes protein, energy, and all the other nutrients. They assume, also, that you receive your nutrients in the form of foods, not supplements, because food components affect nutrient absorption. This may describe you exactly; then again, it may not. On the other hand, except as noted earlier, the RDA are not minimum requirements. R stands for "recommended," not for "required." The RDA are allowances, and they are generous. Even so, they do not necessarily cover every individual for every nutrient. One should probably try to get 100 percent or more of the RDA for every nutrient to ensure adequate intake.

Beyond a certain point, though, it is unwise to consume large amounts of any nutrient. It is naive to think of the RDA simply as a cutoff point. A more accurate view is to see your nutrient needs as falling within a range, with danger zones both below and above it. Figure 2–2 illustrates this point. The RDA reflect this consideration especially clearly in the tables for the trace minerals (inside front cover), which are stated in terms of "safe and adequate" ranges of intakes.

The RDA committee decided to estimate minimum requirements for sodium, potassium, and chloride. For sodium and its partner, chloride, there is danger in calling a high end of the intake scale "safe" because people differ in their sensitivities to salt. A level that may be harmless in one person could easily worsen high blood pressure in another. A range for potassium proved difficult to justify, so the committee also provided a minimum for potassium. For each

■■■ Figure 2–2

The Naive View versus the Accurate View of Optimal Nutrient Intakes. Consuming too much of a nutrient endangers health, just as consuming too little does; the RDA falls within a range of safe intake levels.

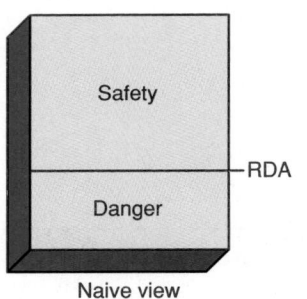

Naive view

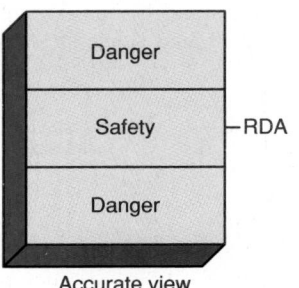

Accurate view

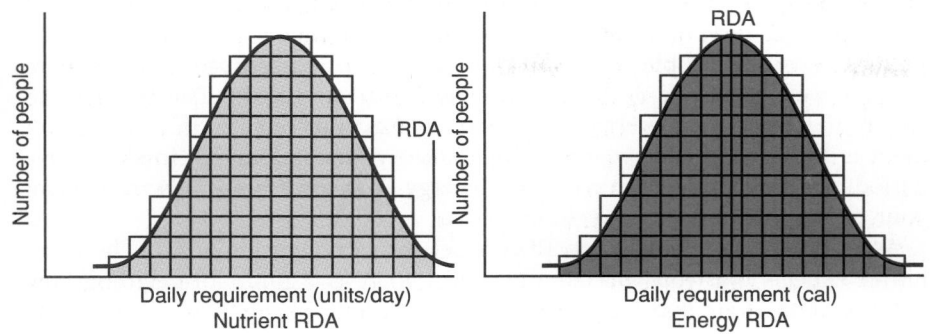

The Differences between the Nutrient RDA and the Energy RDA.
The nutrient RDA are set so that nearly all people's requirements will be met by them (boxes represent people). The energy RDA are set so that half the population's requirements will fall below and half above them.

of these three minerals, the committee estimated the amount needed for growth and to replace normal daily losses and set the minimum requirement at that level.

The RDA and other such recommendations are for the maintenance, not the restoration, of health. Under the stress of serious illness or malnutrition, a person may require a much higher intake of certain nutrients or may not be able to handle even the RDA amount. Therapeutic diets take into account medical conditions: they are for use after surgery, burns, fractures, or during recovery from illness or addictions.

With the understanding that they are approximate, flexible, and generous, we can use the RDA as a set of yardsticks to measure the adequacy of diets in whole populations, such as that of the United States. Such standards have been applied in a number of surveys to determine people's general nutrition status.

■■▶ *The RDA are a set of yardsticks for measuring the adequacy of nutrient intakes of groups of people and can also be used as a tool for evaluating people's individual intakes.*

The RDA for Energy

In setting allowances for food-energy intakes, the committee took a different approach than for the nutrients. The committee had set generous allowances for protein, vitamins, and minerals, believing that a little bit extra, for a nutrient, would keep body stores full to last through brief times of deficient intakes. However, extra energy, even a little bit extra, on a daily basis would be harmful because it would lead to obesity. The committee therefore centered the energy RDA around the median requirements for each age and sex group, with an acceptable variation of 20 percent above this amount to accommodate growth, large body size, or activity (these take more energy) or 20 percent below this amount for aging or small body size (these take less energy). Figure 2–3 above illustrates the difference between the nutrient and energy RDA set by the committee.

The energy RDA are thus recommendations for average persons within groups of a particular age, sex, height, weight, and activity level according to data from extensive surveys of the U.S. population. For example, the **reference**

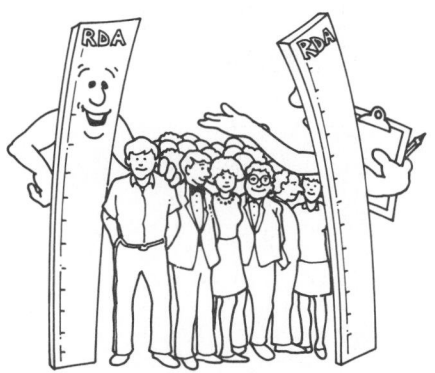

The RDA measure the adequacy of nutrient in takes of populations.

reference woman and man: actual median figures for heights and weights of people of each age-sex group in the U.S. population.

U.S. RDA: the RDA figures used on labels—the United States Recommended Dietary (or Daily) Allowances. In most cases the U.S. RDA for a nutrient is as high or higher than any individual person's RDA for that nutrient.

U.S. RDA—inside front cover, page C.

woman aged 19 to 24 years stands 5 feet 5 inches tall and weighs 128 pounds. The **reference man** of the same age stands 5 feet 10 inches tall and weighs 160 pounds. Very few people exactly fit the average for their groups, but as Figure 2–3 showed, most people's needs fall close to those shown. The best way to ensure that your food energy intake actually fits your own particular requirement is to monitor your weight compared to your food energy intake over a period of time. Chapter 9 revisits the energy RDA and shows how to control your energy intake to meet your needs.

As mentioned previously, no RDA is set for carbohydrate or fat. The committee expects that you will use the energy RDA as a guide for deciding how much carbohydrate and fat to include in your diet.

▯▮▷ *The energy RDA was set at the mean of people's needs so as to discourage overconsumption of food energy.*

The U.S. RDA

The **U.S. RDA** are a set of standard nutrient intakes designed especially for food labels, and, as the section on labels shows, much of the nutrient information provided on packages of food is expressed as percentages of the U.S. RDA. The U.S. RDA were developed by selecting from the 1968 RDA tables a single set of recommendations for an adult with high nutrient needs. For example, a woman's RDA for vitamin A is 800 retinol equivalents (RE). A man's is 1000 RE, so the single U.S. RDA value is set at 1000 RE, the higher of the two. The amount of vitamin A in a food is expressed as a percentage of that standard on the label. Thus instead of reading that a serving of the food contains "500 RE" of vitamin A, you read that it contains "50 percent of the U.S. RDA" for vitamin A. The advantage is that the consumer who wants information from a food label does not have to memorize all the different RDA, which are expressed in many different units (RE, milligrams, and others). If you read on a label that a serving of cereal provides 25 percent of the U.S. RDA for a nutrient, you can be sure that it will also provide at least 25 percent of *your* RDA. Your need, if it is different from the U.S. RDA, is almost surely lower. The U.S. RDA table is printed on page C, following the RDA on the inside front cover. A later section of this chapter explains how to read a food label.

▯▮▷ *The U.S. RDA are a single set of high nutrient values drawn from the RDA tables. Nutrient contents of packaged foods are stated on food labels as percentages of the U.S. RDA.*

Other Nutrient Standards

Different nations and international groups have published different sets of standards similar to the RDA. The RNI for Canadians are shown in Appendix B; they differ from the RDA in some respects, partly because of differences in interpretation of the data they were derived from and partly because people's food intakes and daily lives in Canada differ somewhat from those in the United States.

Besides the United States and Canada, many other countries have developed their own sets of recommendations. Many countries use recommendations developed by two international groups: the Food and Agriculture Organization (FAO) and the World Health Organization (WHO). The FAO/WHO recommendations are considered sufficient for the maintenance of health in nearly all people. They differ from the RDA because they are based on slightly different judgment factors and serve different purposes. The FAO/WHO recommendations, for example, assume that people will be eating protein of a quality lower than that commonly consumed in the United States, and so they recommend a higher intake than the RDA. They also take into consideration that worldwide, people are generally smaller and more physically active than the population of the United States. Nevertheless, the recommendations of different nations all fall within the same range.

Appendix E provides addresses for FAO, WHO, and other agencies.

▐▌▶ *Many nations and groups issue recommendations for nutrient intakes appropriate for specific groups of people.*

▌▌▌ Diet Recommendations

So far you know that the RDA is a standard for nutrient and energy intakes and that the U.S. RDA is a version of that standard used on food labels. Now why should it be necessary to have any other dietary standards? The reason is that while the RDA does much to ensure dietary *adequacy*, it does little for *moderation*. The RDA were developed to ensure adequate nutrient intakes, and so they make specific recommendations for protein, vitamin, and mineral intakes. They also make some general statements about energy intakes, but they do little to protect people from excess intakes of fat, salt, sugar, cholesterol, and alcohol.

To ensure dietary moderation where needed, the governments of many of the developed countries have published separate sets of recommendations. Among them are two from the United States and one from Canada: the so-called *NRCReport* of 1989, the *Surgeon General's Report* (1988), and the *Nutrition Recommendations for Canadians* (1988). The NRC and Canadian recommendations are shown in Tables 2–1 and 2–2 (next page); the Surgeon General's Report is presented in Chapter 11. Many other such recommendations have been published, but all present similar basic guidelines, as Table 2–3 demonstrates.

The agency that developed the *NRC Report* (Table 2–1) is the same one that originated the RDA, and the two documents are intended to be used together in planning diets that support health.[2] The RDA defines adequacy of nutrients in the diet, while the *NRC Report* describes the kinds of foods people should eat and also the kinds they should limit or avoid. The *NRC Report* also makes reference to weight maintenance and exercise.

Notice that the NRC recommendations do not require that you give up your favorite foods or eat strange, unappealing foods. Many studies show that almost anyone's diet, with minor adjustments, can fit the recommendations for health.[3] The secrets seem to be to cultivate the willingness to watch portion sizes (especially of fat-rich foods such as meat and dairy products), to omit or to limit just a few foods (especially pure fats, such as margarine), to make substitutions (such as nonfat for high-fat dairy products), and to make amplifications (more and larger servings of grains, fruits, and vegetables). These four tactics together can change almost anyone's diet into one that supports nutrition

■■■ Table 2–1 NRC Dietary Recommendations

Reduce total *fat* intake to 30% or less of calories. Reduce saturated fatty acid intake to less than 10% of calories and the intake of cholesterol to less than 300 milligrams daily.[a]

Increase intake of starches and other *complex corbohydrates*.[b]

Maintain *protein* intake at moderate levels.[c]

Balance food intake and physical activity to maintain appropriate *body weight*.

For those who drink *alcoholic beverages,* the committee recommends limiting consumption to the equivalent of less than 1 ounce of pure alcohol in a single day.[d] Pregnant women should avoid alcoholic beverages.

Limit total daily intake of *salt* (sodium chloride) to 6 grams or less.[e]

Maintain adequate *calcium* intake.

Avoid taking dietary *supplements* in excess of the RDA in any one day.

Maintain an optimal intake of *fluoride* particularly during the years of primary and secondary tooth formation and growth.

Note: Italics added to highlight the areas of concern.
[a]The intake of fat and cholesterol can be reduced by substituting fish, poultry without skin, lean meats, and low-fat or nonfat dairy products for fatty meats and whole-milk dairy products; by choosing more vegetables, fruits, cereals, and legumes; and by limiting oils, fats, egg yolks, and fried and other fatty foods.
[b]Every day eat five or more servings of a combination of vegetables and fruits, especially green and yellow vegetables and citrus fruits, and six or more daily servings of a combination of breads, cereals, and legumes.
[c]Meet at least the RDA for protein; do not exceed twice the RDA.
[d]The committee does not recommend alcohol consumption. One ounce of pure alcohol is the equivalent of two cans of beer, two small glasses of wine, or two average cocktails.
[e]Limit the use of salt in cooking, and avoid adding it to food at the table. Consume salty, highly processed, salt-preserved, and salt-pickled foods sparingly.
SOURCE: Adapted from the National Academy of Sciences report, *Diet and Health: Implications for Reducing Chronic Disease Risk* which was produced by the Committee on Diet and Health of the Food and Nutrition Board of the National Research Council and partially reprinted verbatim in *Nutrition Reviews* 47 (1989): 142–149.

■■■ Table 2–2 Nutrition Recommendations for Canadians

THE CANADIAN DIET SHOULD:
1. Provide energy consistent with the maintenance of body weight within the recommended range.
2. Include essential nutrients in amounts recommended in the RNI.
3. Include no more than 30 percent of energy as fat and no more than 10 percent as saturated fat.
4. Provide 55 percent of energy as carbohydrate from a variety of sources.
5. Reduce sodium contents.
6. Include no more than 5 percent of total energy as alcohol, or two drinks daily, whichever is less.
7. Contain no more caffeine than the equivalent of four regular cups of coffee per day.
8. Provide 1 milligram fluoride per litre of water.

SOURCE: Adapted from Scientific Review Committee and the Communications/Implementation Committee, *Nutrition Recommendations...A Call for Action* (Ottawa: Canadian Government Publishing Centre, 1989).

■■■ Table 2–3 Dietary Guidelines Compared

		AREAS OF RECOMMENDATIONS[a]							
YEAR	PUBLICATION NAME	VARY FOOD CHOICES	MAINTAIN IDEAL BODY WEIGHT	INCLUDE STARCH AND FIBER	LIMIT SUGAR	LIMIT FAT	LIMIT CHOLES-TEROL	LIMIT SALT	LIMIT ALCOHOL
1987	*National Cholesterol Education Program Guidelines*[b]	+	+	+		+	+		+
1988	*Dietary Guidelines for Cancer Prevention*[b]	+	+	+		+		+	+
1988	*The Surgeon General's Report on Nutrition and Health*[b]	+	+	+	+	+	+	+	+
1989	*Diet and Health: Implications for Reducing Chronic Disease Risk*[b]	+	+	+	+	+	+	+	+
1990	*Dietary Guidelines: for Americans, 3rd edition*[b]	+	+	+	+	+	+	+	+

[a]Other areas of recommendation include increase physical activity (1990); reduce intake of salt-cured or smoked foods (1988); use appropriate sources of fluoride, increase consumption of foods high in calcium and iron (1988); maintain adequate calcium intake, avoid supplements in excess of RDA, and maintain optimal fluoride intake (1989).

[b]The agencies putting forth these recommendations, in table order, are Department of Health and Human Services (DHHS) with National Heart, Lung, and Blood Institute; DHHS with National Cancer Institute; DHHS; National Research Council; United States Department of Agriculture and DHHS.

SOURCE: Adapted from *The Surgeon General's Report on Nutrition and Health: Summary and Recommendations,* DHHS (PHS) publication no. 88–50211 (Washington, D. C.: Government Printing Office, 1988), Appendix C.

and heart health superbly. You will see them again wherever diet changes are discussed.

If the experts who develop such documents were to ask us, we would add one more recommendation to their lists: choose foods that you enjoy. While it is of prime importance to choose foods that meet nutritional needs, it is equally important to seek out delicious foods that meet the needs for pleasure and fun. The joys of eating are physically beneficial to the body—they trigger health-promoting changes in the nervous, hormonal, and immune systems. They ensure that people will eat and thus obtain the nutrients to support those systems and also healthy skin, glossy hair, and the natural good looks that accompany health. People tend to repeat what brings them joy, and so they are much more likely to stick with foods they like. The remainder of this book refers often to the recommendations of Tables 2–1 and 2–2. When it does, remember this last recommendation: enjoy.

Dietary recommendations encourage health of individuals but are also best for the earth itself. Chapter 15 explores the relationships between people, their food, and the planet's well-being.

◧▷ *The* NRC Report, *the* Nutrition Recommendations for Canadians, *and other similar recommendations address the problems of overnutrition and under-nutrition, recommending weight control, reduced consumption of fat, and increased consumption of carbohydrate-rich foods. To implement the recommendations requires controlling portions, limiting intakes of fats, substituting nutrient-dense for fat-rich foods, and amplifying servings of low-fat grains, fruits, and vegetables.*

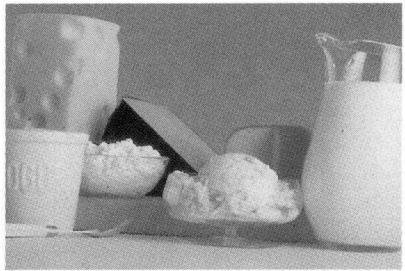

Milk and Milk Products
Calcium, riboflavin, protein, vitamin B_{12} (vitamin D and vitamin A, when fortified).
2 servings per day for adults.
3 servings per day for children.
4 servings per day for teenagers, pregnant/lactating women, women past menopause.
5 servings per day for pregnant/lactating teenagers.
Serving = 1 c milk or yogurt; ¼ c Parmesan cheese or process cheese spread; 2 c cottage cheese; 1 ½ c ice cream or ice milk; 2 oz process cheese food; 1 ⅓ oz cheese.
■ Nonfat milk, buttermilk, low-fat milk, plain yogurt.
☐ Whole milk, cheese, fruit-flavored yogurt, cottage cheese.
■ Custard, milk shakes, pudding, ice cream.

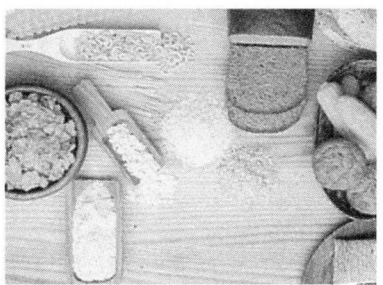

Breads and Cereals
Riboflavin, thiamin, niacin, iron, protein, magnesium, folate, fiber.
4 servings per day.
Serving = 1 slice bread; ½ to ¾ c cooked cereals, rice, or pastas; 1 oz ready-to-eat cereals.
■ Whole grains (wheat, oats, barley, millet, rye, bulgur) enriched breads, rolls, tortillas.
☐ Rice, cereals, pastas (macaroni, spaghetti), bagels.
■ Pancakes, muffins, cornbread, biscuits, presweetened cereals.

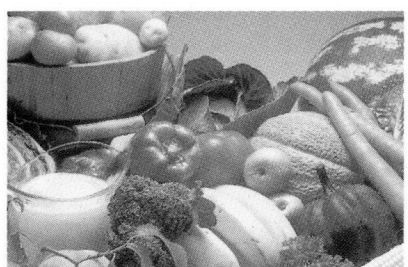

Vegetables and Fruits
Vitamin A, vitamin C, riboflavin, folate, iron, magnesium, low in fat, no cholesterol.
4 servings per day.
Serving = ½ c or typical portion (1 medium apple, ½ grapefruit, or 1 wedge lettuce).
■ Apricots, bean sprouts, broccoli, brussels sprouts, cabbage, cantaloupe, carrots, cauliflower, cucumbers, grapefruit, green beans, green peas, leafy greens (spinach, mustard, and collard greens), lettuce, mushrooms, oranges, orange juice, peaches, strawberries, tomatoes, winter squash.
☐ Apples, bananas, canned fruit, corn, pears, potatoes.
■ Avocados, dried fruit, sweet potatoes.

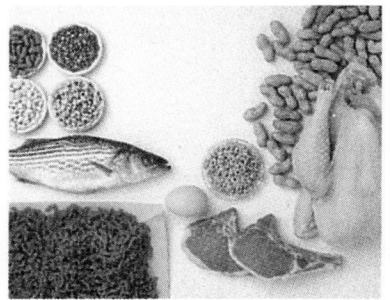

Meat and Meat Alternates
Protein, phosphorus, vitamin B_6, vitamin B_{12}, zinc, magnesium, iron, niacin, thiamin.
2 servings per day for adults, children, teenagers.
3 servings per day for pregnant/lactating women/teenagers.
Serving = 2 to 3 oz lean, cooked meat, poultry, or fish.
Note: 1 oz. meat, poultry, or fish = 1 egg, ½ to ¾ c legumes, 2 tbsp. peanut butter, ¼ to ½ c nuts or seeds.
■ Poultry, fish, lean meat (beef, lamb, pork), dried peas and beans, eggs.
☐ Beef, lamb, pork, refried beans.
■ Hotdogs, luncheon meats, peanut butter, nuts.

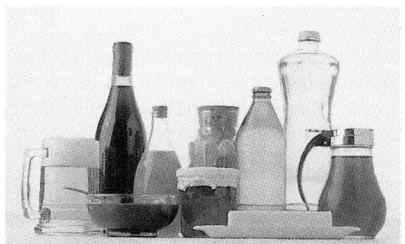

Miscellaneous Group
Sugar, fat (vitamin E), salt, alcohol, calories.
No serving sizes are provided because servings of these foods are not recommended. They provide few nutrients.
■ Miscellaneous foods, not high in calories, include spices, herbs, coffee, tea, and diet soft drinks.
■ Foods high in fat include margarine, salad dressing, oils, mayonnaise, cream, cream cheese, butter, gravy, and sauces.
■ Foods high in salt include potato chips, corn chips, pretzels, pickles, olives, bouillon, prepared mustard, soy sauce, steak sauce, salt, and seasoned salt.
■ Foods high in sugar include cake, pie, cookies, doughnuts, sweet rolls, candy, soft drinks, fruit drinks, jelly, syrup, gelatin desserts, sugar, and honey.
■ Alcoholic beverages include wine, beer, and liquor.

Key:
■ Foods generally highest in nutrient density.
☐ Food moderate in nutrient density.
■ Foods generally lowest in nutrient density.

▌▌▌ Diet Planning with Food Groups and Other Tools

Diet planning is the bridge between nutrition theory and the food on the table. To help people plan menus, two kinds of guides are available: **food group plans** to describe numbers of servings to choose and **exchange lists** of foods to identify specific foods to use.

Food Group Plans

The most famous and widely used of all food group plans is the Four Food Group Plan, shown in Figure 2–4. The foods in each group are notable contributors of certain key nutrients (see the figure), but of course they supply others as well. If you design your diet around this plan, it is assumed that you will have adequate amounts not only of the nutrients named on the figure but also of the other two dozen or so essential nutrients because they occur in the same groups of foods. This is true in theory, but in practice diet planners using this plan must be sure to choose mostly *nutrient-dense* foods in each group because some processes strip foods of some nutrients and add calories from fat (more about this in Chapter 14). With this caution, the Four Food Group Plan can provide a reasonable foundation for diet planning. Figure 2–4 provides a key to indicate a few foods within each group with high, moderate, and low nutrient densities to give you an idea of which are which. Chapters to come address nutrient density of foods directly and provide more help in making choices.

To use the plan most adults must choose at least four servings from the breads-and-cereals group, four from the vegetables-and-fruits group, two from the milk-and-milk-products group, and two from the meat-and-meat-alternates group. Many people use shorthand to remember the pattern: four, four, two, and two. These are the minimum numbers of servings. The plan's makers suggest that to meet additional energy needs, a person should choose more servings of foods from these four groups.

Some foods—such as butter, margarine, cream, sour cream, salad dressing, mayonnaise, potato chips, jelly, broth, coffee, tea, alcoholic beverages, and others—don't fit into any of the four food groups. Some of these contribute a few nutrients, but most primarily contribute energy; their nutrient contents have been greatly diluted by fat, sugar, alcohol, or water. They are grouped together into a miscellaneous category of extras that the plan's originators suggest should be used sparingly.

The beauty of the Four Food Group Plan lies in its simplicity. Also, although it may appear rigid, it can actually be very flexible once its intent is understood. For example, the user can substitute cheese for milk because both supply the key nutrients for the milk group. The user can choose legumes (beans) and nuts as alternatives to meats. One can adapt the plan to mixed dishes such as casseroles as well as to national and cultural cuisines.

The Four Food Group Plan does have drawbacks, however. For one thing, it does not specify calorie amounts. People who select the minimum number of servings from each food group and who strictly limit foods from the miscellaneous group can keep their energy intakes as low as 1000 calories a day, but people who use the higher calorie foods in each group and who eat large

food group plans: diet planning tools that sort foods of similar origin and nutrient content into groups and then specify that people eat certain minimum numbers of servings of foods from each group.

exchange lists: diet planning tools that organize foods with respect to their nutrient contents and calorie amounts. Foods on any single list can be used interchangeably.

■■■ **Table 2–4**

Canada's Food Guide

Milk and milk products—2 servings[a]
Meat, fish, poultry, and alternates—2 servings[b]
Fruits and vegetables—4 to 5 servings[b,c]
Breads and cereals—3 to 5 servings[b]

[a]A serving is 250 ml, or about 1 c. Milk group servings differ for children up to age 11—2 to 3 servings; adolescents—3 to 4 servings; pregnant and lactating women—3 to 4 servings.
[b]See Appendix D for foods and portion sizes.
[c]Include at least two vegetables.

SOURCE: *Canada's Food Guide Handbook,* revised (Health and Welfare Canada, 1985).

servings, even without miscellaneous foods added in, can easily obtain too many calories. In the cheese-for-milk substitution just mentioned, an amount of cheddar cheese sufficient to meet a day's calcium requirement would carry with it almost 700 calories, over 70 percent of them from saturated fat (compare this to the NRC Recommendation on fat in Table 2–1). A day's calcium from nonfat milk brings fewer than 350 calories, with hardly any fat. Less obvious but significant over time are energy differences between bread and biscuits, fish and hotdogs, or even green beans and sweet potatoes—all proper substitutions according to the Four Food Group Plan. High-calorie choices may be just what some people, such as athletes, need to meet their high energy requirements, but for others such choices can, over time, dramatically boost energy intakes and body weight.

Another criticism of the plan is that a person can follow all of the plan's rules, consistently make nutrient-poor choices, and fail to meet the day's needs for some nutrients—that of vitamin E, for example, because this vitamin is easily destroyed or refined out of foods. Other plans have been developed from time to time and may serve some people's needs more completely. Canada has developed such a plan, and it is shown in Table 2–4 in the margin.

Still another criticism is that the plan seems to be centered on meats and animal products such as milk, cheese, and eggs. It seems to ignore the needs of **vegetarians**. However, to think this is to misunderstand the plan. The food group that includes the meats also includes *meat alternates*—foods such as legumes and nuts. As for the food group that includes milk and milklike foods, people who choose not to use dairy foods can substitute soy "milk"—a product made from soybeans that fills the same nutrient needs, provided that it is fortified with calcium and vitamin B_{12}. In short, people who choose to eat no animal meats or products taken from animals can still use the Four Food Group Plan as a guide for making their diets adequate.

For these reasons, this book does not single out vegetarians as a separate class of eaters. Vegetarianism is merely an eating plan that selects plant foods to deliver its nutrients; it is not a religion like Buddhism or Hinduism. Some people make much of the distinctions between types of vegetarians—see the definitions of **lactovegetarians**, **ovovegetarians**, and **vegans** in the margin (facing page)—but these are not distinct classes of eaters. Many combinations and variations on these categories exist. Some people eat no red meat, but do eat chicken and fish. Some people eat fish only once a week, and use plant protein foods the rest of the time. Many people rely mostly on milk products to meet their protein needs, but eat fish occasionally, and so forth. To force people into the categories of "vegetarians" and "meat eaters" leaves out all these in-between styles of eating that represent large numbers of people and have a lot to recommend them. To the person just beginning to study nutrition, consider adopting the attitude that the choice to make is not whether to be a meat eater or a vegetarian, but where along the spectrum to locate yourself. Your preferences, whatever they are, should be honored and the only "should" that we would lay on you is to make your diet adequate.

■■▶ *Food group plans organize foods by their nutrients and origins to provide patterns of intake that cover nutrient needs.*

Exchange Lists

Exchange lists are lists of foods that can be used with food group plans. A plan may say, "Eat two portions of fruit"; an exchange system will list the foods that qualify as fruits and specify their portion sizes. Exchange systems are popular among careful diet planners, particularly people who wish to control calories as well as to obtain certain nutrients in desired quantities.

An exchange system can give you a "feel" for what is in the foods you choose to eat and a sense of which foods are similar to each other in energy and selected nutrient contents.* Several different systems are available for different purposes; people with hypertension use one that sorts foods according to their sodium contents, for example. The system used here was developed originally for use by people with diabetes but is now widely recognized as an excellent diet-planning tool for healthy people. It facilitates weight control; it also facilitates control of fat, saturated fat, fiber, and salt intakes for purposes of heart health and prevention of many diseases. It organizes foods into six lists according to their energy, carbohydrate, fat, and protein contents. Appendix D gives complete details of the U.S. and Canadian exchange systems.

A convenient way to remember the foods, portion sizes, and energy values of the six exchange lists is to keep in mind one typical member of each list. For example:

- Milk— 1 cup nonfat milk (90 calories).
- Vegetables— 1/2 cup cooked carrots (25 calories).
- Fruits— 1 small orange (60 calories).
- Starch/bread— 1 small potato/1 slice bread (80 calories).
- Meat— 1 ounce lean beef (55 calories).
- Fat— 1 teaspoon butter (45 calories).

Each food's associated number of calories is an average for the group. Individual foods on a list differ slightly in exact energy amounts but are close enough so that you can use the average values for them. Table 2–5 (next page) shows the carbohydrate, fat, protein, and calorie values that pertain to each list.

The exchange system pays strict attention to portions. Only if you measure a portion correctly do you obtain the number of calories and amounts of energy nutrients intended. All the food portions in a single list are treated as equal in calories and energy-nutrient contents. To use the system meaningfully, you must therefore become familiar with portion sizes, even if it means measuring your foods for awhile. Figure 2–5 (page 41) shows what some typical portions look like, and Figure 2–6 (pages 42–43) shows some of the foods that belong together in the exchange lists.

Foods are not always listed in an exchange system where you might expect them to be because the system is based on their contents of carbohydrate, fat, and protein, and not on other characteristics such as their vitamin and mineral contents. For example, notice that cheese is classed as a meat in the exchange system because its protein and fat contents are similar to those of meat. (In the Four Food Group Plan cheese is classed with milk because of its calcium

vegetarians: people who eat no meat.

lactovegetarians: vegetarians who use milk and milk products.

ovovegetarians: vegetarians who use eggs.

vegans: vegetarians who include no animal-derived products in their diets, also called *strict vegetarians*.

---

*The exchange system being described here is the one developed originally by the American Dietetic Association and the American Diabetes Association.

content; in Canada's Food Group System it is permitted to serve either role but not both at any one time.) Also, most people say corn is a vegetable, but the exchange system lists it with starch/breads as a "starchy vegetable." Similarly, olives are not classed as a "fruit," as a botanist would claim; they are a "fat" because they are more like butter than berries in fat content. Bacon is also a member of the fat list because it is more like fat than like meat.

To help control fat and food energy intake, the user of the exchange system is taught to think of nonfat milk as milk and of whole milk as milk with fat added. The vegetable list includes only low-calorie vegetables prepared without added fat, so a half cup of any of them will provide about 25 calories. The fruit list specifies "no added sugar or sugar syrup"; if you eat sugar, you have to keep track of its extra calories. Portion sizes are adjusted so that fruit portions are equal in calories. One-half cup canned peaches or one-half a small banana counts as one fruit. A piece of cherry pie is not a fruit. It includes a fruit if it contains ten large cherries, but it also includes bread and fat exchanges and added sugar. (Thus it might be counted as one fruit, two bread, and three fat, with two tablespoons added sugar.) Lima beans, potatoes, and other starchy vegetables are listed with the breads, not the vegetables, because they are similar to breads in calorie and carbohydrate content. The starch/bread list also makes clear which grain products contain added fat, such as muffins and cookies.

Perhaps most important of all, milks, meats, and cheeses are separated into three categories by their fat contents. Milks are classed as nonfat, low-fat, and whole products; meats and cheeses as lean, medium-fat, and high-fat items. A warning: the items listed under Meats and Meat Alternates in the exchange system are single ounces, much smaller than the typical serving on a dinner plate. The exchange system does not necessarily recommend that you eat only

■■■ Table 2–5 The Six Exchange Lists

LIST	PORTION SIZE	CARBOHYDRATE (g)	PROTEIN (g)	FAT (g)	ENERGY (cal)
Starch/bread[a]	1 slice	15	3	Trace	80
Meat[b]	1 oz				
Lean		—	7	3	55
Medium-fat		—	7	5	75
High-fat		—	7	8	100
Vegetable[c]	½ c	5	2	—	25
Fruit	1 portion	15	—	—	60
Milk	1 c				
Nonfat		12	8	Trace	90
Low fat		12	8	5	120
Whole		12	8	8	150
Fat	1 tsp	—	—	5	45

Note: This is the U. S. exchange system. The complete details, and those of the Canadian system, are shown in Appendix D.
[a]This list includes starchy vegetables such as lima beans and corn, as well as cereal, bread, pasta, and other grain products. For portion sizes see Appendix D.
[b]This list includes cheese and peanut butter as well as meat.
[c]This list includes low-calorie vegetables only.

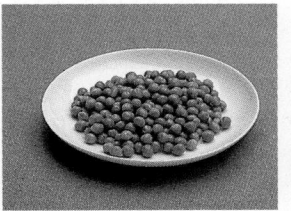

100 grams peas (about ½ cup).

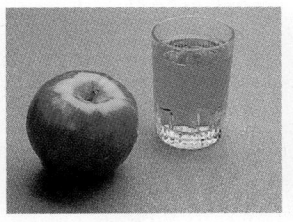

100 ml juice (about ½ cup).

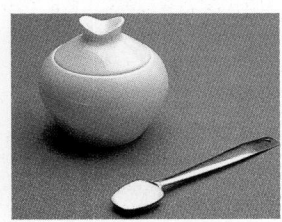

5 grams sugar (about 1 teaspoon).

■■■ **Figure 2–5**

Portion Sizes. Portions in the exchange system are specific. Shown here are three typical portions: 100 grams of a food (which is about the same as ½ cup), 100 milliliters of a juice (which is also about the same as ½ cup), and 5 grams of a powder, sugar (which is about the same as a teaspoon). Cooks who like to switch back and forth between the British and metric systems have learned to use these values interchangeably.

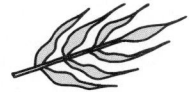

Fiber symbol.   Sodium symbol.

one ounce of meat at a given meal but that you note the number of ounces that you eat in a serving. To further help you keep track of your fat intakes, the fat list includes items such as cream, cream cheese, nuts, coconut, and avocados, high-fat foods that you might not recognize as such.

The exchange lists point out fiber and sodium, too, wherever they exist in significant quantities. In Appendix D, foods high in fiber can be picked out by the wheat symbol they bear (use them often). The saltshaker symbol identifies foods high in sodium, so that people who must avoid them can do so.

■■▶ *Unlike the Four Food Group Plan, the exchange system facilitates calorie control because the foods on each list provide approximately equal amounts of carbohydrate, fat, and protein, and therefore energy. It is an excellent tool to use whenever these nutrient intakes need to be balanced in diet planning.*

The exchange system booklets identify foods high in fiber and sodium with these symbols, so that users can choose foods wisely. In Appendix D these foods are identified using miniature versions of the same symbols. To obtain the original booklet, which is handy to carry around, write to the American Dietetic Association (ADA) at the address given in Appendix E.

Using Food Group Plans with Exchange Lists

The Four Food Group Plan helps you to be sure to include all classes of nutritious foods. The exchange lists enable you to make your food selections with an eye to their energy nutrient contents. By using the two together, you can easily achieve the goals of a good diet mentioned at the start of the chapter: adequacy, balance, calorie control, moderation, and variety.

Table 2–6 (page 44) shows that when you use the Four Food Group Plan as a pattern and the exchange lists as guides for choosing the items to eat, you can meet the plan's requirements and still eat as few as 1000 calories. Even if you are only moderately active, you would still be entitled to eat some 500 to 1000 more calories in the day's allowance, and the more active you are, the higher the energy allowance you "earn." A wise choice would be to invest many of those additional calories in additional vegetables, legumes, fruits, and whole-grain foods and only a few in luxury items such as sweet desserts, butter, margarine, oil, or alcohol. If you make these additions, make them by choice rather than through the unintentional use of high-calorie foods.

With judicious selections the diet can meet the need for all the nutrients and provide some luxury items as well. The final plan might be like one of those outlined in Table 2–7 on page 45 (many variations are possible). Diet planners use different patterns of exchanges for different energy levels. The table shows

▓▓▓ Figure 2–6

The Exchange System.

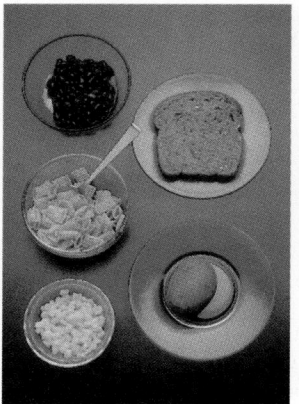

1. Starch/breads
1 slice bread is like:
¾ c ready-to-eat cereal.
⅓ c cooked beans.
½ c corn.
1 small (3-oz) potato.
(1 bread = 15 g carbohydrate, 3 g protein, trace of fat, and 80 cal).

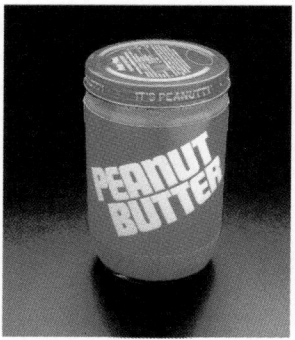

2e. Peanut butter
Peanut butter is like a meat in terms of its protein content. It is estimated as:
1 tbsp peanut butter = 1 high-fat meat
(1 tbsp peanut butter = 7 g protein, 8 g fat, and 100 cal.)
(Don't stop reading now, and don't swear off peanut butter, necessarily. You'll need to read about the polyunsaturated character of its fat in Chapter 5, and the B vitamin contributions it makes in Chapter 7 before deciding how much of a place it should have in your diet.)

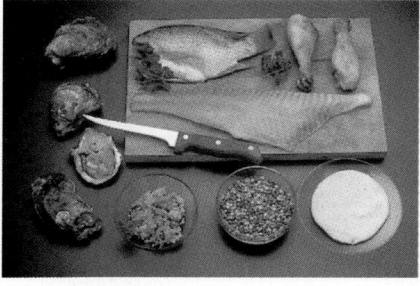

2a. Meats (lean)
1 oz lean meat is like:
1 oz chicken meat without the skin.
1 oz any fish.
¼ c canned tuna.
1 oz low-fat cheese.[a]
(1 lean meat = 7 g protein, 3 g fat, and 55 cal.)
(One 3-oz portion of meat such as a hamburger patty = 3 meat exchanges.)
(One meat exchange = ⅓ of a 3-oz hamburger patty.)

[a]Cheeses are grouped with milk in food group plans because of their calcium content but with meats in this system because, like meat, they contribute calories from protein and fat and have negligible carbohydrate content.

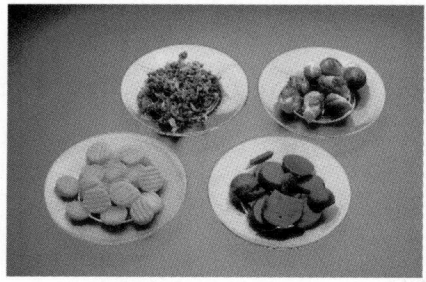

3. Vegetables
½ c carrots is like:
½ c greens.
½ c brussels sprouts.
½ c beets.
(1 vegetable = 5 g carbohydrate, 2 g protein, and 25 cal.)

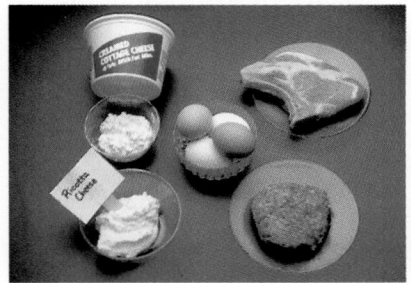

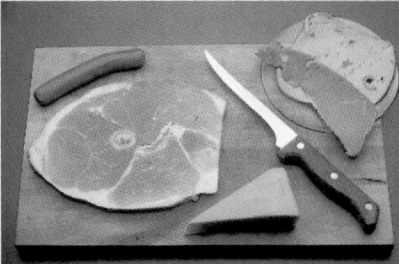

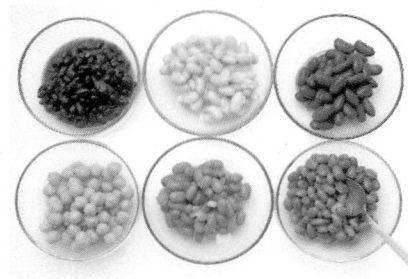

2b. Meats (medium-fat)

1 oz medium-fat meat is like 1 oz lean meat in protein content, but has 5 g fat (2 g more fat than lean meat). Examples:
1 oz pork loin.
1 egg.
¼ c creamed cottage cheese.[a]
(1 medium-fat meat = 7 g protein, 5 g fat, and about 75 cal.)

2c. Meats (high-fat)

1 oz high-fat meat is like 1 oz lean meat in protein content but is estimated to have an **extra "1 fat"**—that is, to have the 3 g fat of a lean meat and 5 g additional fat. Examples:
1 oz country-style ham.
1 oz cheddar cheese.[a]
1 small hotdog (frankfurter).[b]
(1 high-fat meat = 7 g protein, 8 g fat, and 100 cal.)

[b]The frankfurter counts as 1 high-fat meat exchange plus 1 fat exchange.

2d. Legumes

Legumes are an odd kind of plant food. They are like meats because they are rich in protein and iron, but many are lower in fat than meat. Besides, they contain a lot of starch. For this reason the exchange system lists them with the starch/breads, although they are often used as meat substitutes. Examples:
¼ c baked beans.
⅓ c other beans.

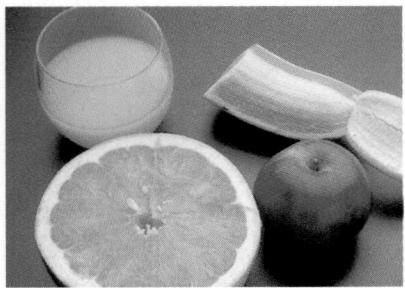

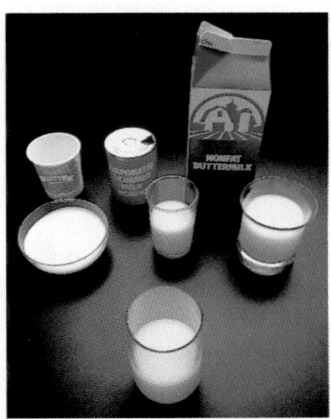

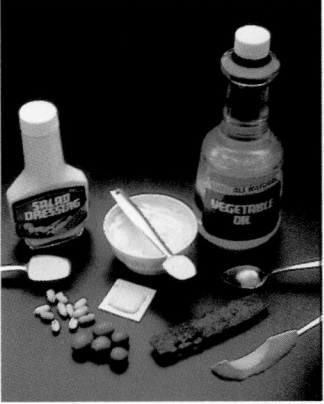

4. Fruits

½ small banana is like:
1 small apple.
½ grapefruit.
½ c orange juice.
(1 fruit = 15 g carbohydrate and 60 cal.)

5. Milks

1 c nonfat milk is like:
1 c nonfat yogurt, plain.
1 c nonfat buttermilk.
½ c evaporated nonfat milk.
(1 milk = 12 g carbohydrate, 8 g protein, trace of fat, and 90 cal.)

6. Fats

1 tsp butter is like:
1 tsp margarine.
1 tsp any oil.
1 tbsp salad dressing.
1 strip crisp bacon.
5 large olives.
10 whole Virginia peanuts.
(1 fat = 5 g fat and 45 cal.)

■■■ Table 2–6 ■ Diet Planning with the Exchange System Using the Four Food Group Pattern

PATTERN FROM FOUR FOOD GROUP PLAN	SELECTIONS MADE FROM THE EXCHANGE LISTS	EXAMPLE	ENERGY COST (cal)
Grains—4 servings	Starches/grains— select 4 items[b]	2 breads; 2 starchy vegetables	320
Meat—2 servings (2 to 3 oz each)	Meat list—select 6 items[a]	6 oz lean meat	330
Fruits and vegetables—4 servings	Fruit and vegetable lists—select 4 items from the lists	2 vegetables; 2 fruits	50 120
Milk—2 c	Milk list—select 2 items	2 c nonfat milk	180
			Total: 1000

[a]In the Four Food Group Plan, 1 serving is 2 to 3 oz. On the exchange lists, the unit of measure is 1 oz.
[b]Because the starchy vegetables are on the same list with the grains, some of them can be substituted for grains.

that a person eating 3000 calories per day could use considerably more bread portions, for example, than a person eating 1500 calories per day.

■■▷ *Food group plans and exchange lists, used together, ease diet planning. Food group plans provide the framework that ensures adequacy and balance; exchange lists supply the items to go in the frame, permitting calorie control, moderation, and variety.*

■■■ Food Labels

A potato is a potato and doesn't bear a label to tell you so, but a package of potato chips is potato, fat, and salt, and you may have to read its label to find that out. You can use packaged foods artfully in diet planning only if you can interpret their labels. It is worth some effort to do so, since food labels have much to tell consumers. Labels have been regulated by many agencies over the years, and the result is that they are complex, some say unnecessarily so.[4] Still, they carry valuable information. According to law, every food label must state:

■ The common or usual name of the product.
■ The name and address of the manufacturer, packer, or distributor.
■ The net contents in terms of weight, measure, or count.

Then, unless the food has a standard of identity (explained later), the label must list in ordinary language:

■ The ingredients, in descending order of predominance by weight.

■■■ Table 2–7 Diet Plans for Different Energy Intakes

| | ENERGY LEVEL (cal) | | | | | | | |
EXCHANGES	1000	1200	1500	1800	2000	2200	2600	3000
Starches/grains	3	4	6	8	10	11	13	15
Vegetables	2	3	4	4	4	6	6	6
Fruits	3	3	4	5	5	5	5	6
Milks	2	2	2	2	2	2	3	3
Meats	4	5	5	5	6	6	7	8
Fats	3	4	5	7	7	8	10	12

[a]These patterns of exchanges supply about 30% of the calories as fat, in accordance with the view that a moderate fat intake is desirable. For higher-energy patterns, such as athletes might need, see Chapter 10.

Nutrition Information on Labels

Many labels provide much more than just the basics, and if you know how to read the front and side of a package, you are many steps ahead of the naive buyer. Consider the mandatory ingredient list. Whatever is listed first is the ingredient that predominates, by weight. Compare the ingredient list on an orange powder that reads, "sugar, citric acid, orange flavor. . . ." You can tell that sugar is the chief ingredient. Now look at a canned juice whose ingredient list reads, "water, orange juice concentrate, pineapple juice concentrate. . . ." This product is clearly made mostly of juice. Now look at a cereal whose entire list contains just one item: "100 percent rolled oats." No question, this is a natural, whole-grain food. Finally, compare a cereal that contains "puffed milled corn, sugar, corn syrup, honey, dextrose, salt. . . ." If you can recognize that sugar, corn syrup, honey, and dextrose are all different versions of sugar (and you will, after Controversy 4), you'll know that this product is similar to the orange powder, mostly sugar. Skill in reading ingredient lists is indispensable to consumers who want to know what they are getting in packaged food.

Generally, food labels must provide an additional information panel if a nutrient is added to a food (for example, vitamin C to improve the nutritional quality of a breakfast drink), or if a nutrition-related claim is made (for example, that a food is high in protein). In those cases the law requires more information in the following format under the heading "Nutrition Information":

■ Serving or portion size.
■ Servings or portions per container.
■ Food energy (in calories) per serving.
■ Protein (grams) per serving.
■ Carbohydrate (grams) per serving.
■ Fat (grams) per serving.
■ Sodium (milligrams) per serving.
■ Protein, vitamins, and minerals as percentages of the U.S. RDA. (No claim may be made that a food is a significant source of a nutrient unless it provides at least 10 percent of the U.S. RDA of that nutrient in a serving.)

The side panel of the box of cooked cereal provides all this information; Figure 2–7 demonstrates the reading of such a label.*

*On November 8, 1990, the President signed a new labeling law that is expected to take effect in May 1992. This discussion describes the labeling requirements at the time of this book writing—current until the new law takes effect. Figure 2-7 presents nutrient information characteristic of both the old and the new requirements.

With an understanding of the U. S. RDA (introduced earlier), you can extract a lot of information from a nutrition label. Recall that the U.S. RDA states the highest probable requirement for a healthy adult and that nutrient contents are stated on labels as percentages of the U.S. RDA. The table of U.S. RDA amounts appears on page C of the inside front pages of this book. If you want

■■■ Figure 2–7

How to Read a Food Label.

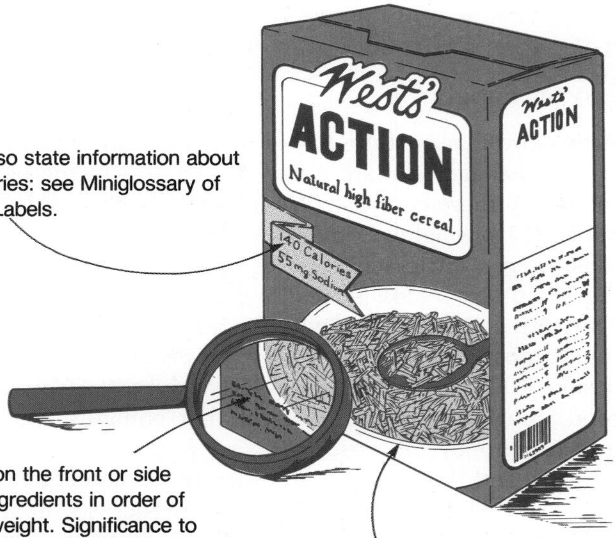

The label may also state information about sodium and calories: see Miniglossary of Terms on Food Labels.

The ingredient list on the front or side panel names the ingredients in order of predominance by weight. Significance to you, the consumer: what appears first is present in the largest quantity. Only products with standards of identity (recipes defined by law) have no ingredient list.

The package must always tell you the product name, the name and address of the company, and the weight or measure; and it may list the ingredients

Nutrition Information (per serving)[a]
Serving Size = ½ c
Servings per Container = 10

	Cereal	With ½ c nonfat milk (Vitamins A- and D-fortified)[b]
Calories	140	180
Calories from fat	9	9
Protein (g)[c]	4	8
Total carbohydrates (g)[d]	32	38
Simple sugars (g)	11	17
Complex carbohydrates (g)	17	17
Fiber (g)	4	4
Fat (g)[e]	1	1
Saturated fat	0	0
Cholesterol	0	0
Sodium (mg)[f]	55	120
Percentage of U.S. Recommended Daily Allowances (U.S. RDA)[g]		
Protein	6	15
Vitamin A	4	10
Vitamin C	*	2
Thiamin	25	30
Riboflavin	25	35
Niacin	25	25
Calcium	2	15
Iron	25	25

*Contains less than 2% of the U.S. RDA of this nutrient.

Some currently required information will become optional; for example, the U.S. RDA for protein and most vitamins and minerals. Vitamins A and C, and the minerals iron and calcium will remain.

[a]The nutrition information panel tells you the nutrients in a serving. The serving size may or may not be the same as the amount you eat. Check the servings per container to get an idea if it is.
[b]The nutrient contents in the food are listed and can be listed also as served (after adding milk, in this example).
[c]The energy-yielding nutrients are given in grams (units of weight). This is especially meaningful with respect to protein, because you need 40 to 80 g/day, depending on your size and other factors. Protein is also given in percentage of U.S. RDA in the list below.
[d]The carbohydrate breakdown tells you how much simple sugar, starch, and dietary fiber is in the product.
[e]A fat breakdown may also be listed, including saturated fat, unsaturated fat, and cholesterol.
[f]Sodium is listed in milligrams. A safe minimum intake is 500 mg sodium/day; recommendations limit salt intake to 6,000 mg salt/day (2,400 mg sodium/day). A teaspoon of salt contains just over 2,000 mg sodium.
[g]Protein, vitamins, and minerals are given in percentages of U.S. RDA (see inside front cover, page c). Significance to you, the consumer: if it meets 10% of the U.S. RDA, it almost undoubtedly meets at least 10% of your daily needs.

███ **Terms on Food Labels**

Cholesterol terms:

- ■ **cholesterol-free**: containing fewer than 2 mg of cholesterol per serving.
- ■ **low-cholesterol**: containing fewer than 20 mg of cholesterol per serving.
- ■ **reduced cholesterol**: processed to reduce the cholesterol by at least 75% compared with the original.

Energy terms:

- ■ **diet, dietetic**: terms used to indicate that a food is either a *low-calorie* or a *reduced-calorie* food.
- ■ **light, lite**: for alcoholic beverages, containing 20 percent fewer calories than regular products; for meat products, 33 percent fewer. For other foods the terms have no definition but can mean light in color, texture, taste, or weight, or it can mean reduced in some component.[a]
- ■ **low-calorie**: containing no more than 40 calories per serving or 0.4 cal/g.
- ■ **reduced-calorie**: containing at least a third fewer calories than the most similar food of the same type.

Fat terms (these apply only to meat and poultry products):

- ■ **extra lean**: containing not more than 5% fat by weight.
- ■ **lean or low-fat**[b]: containing not more than 10% fat by weight.
- ■ **leaner, lower-fat**: reduced in fat by 25% when compared to the company's regular product.

Sodium terms:

- ■ **low-sodium**: containing 140 mg or less sodium per serving.
- ■ **reduced-sodium**: processed to reduce the usual level of sodium by 75%.
- ■ **sodium-free**: containing less than 5 mg sodium per serving.
- ■ **unsalted, no added salt, salt-free**: having no salt added during processing, but not necessarily low in sodium.
- ■ **very-low-sodium**: containing 35 mg or less sodium per serving.

Sugar terms:

- ■ **sugar-free, sugarless, no added sugar**: free of sucrose (table sugar), but possibly containing other energy-providing sweeteners.

[a]For example, a "Light French" frozen cheesecake may be light in texture but may have more calories than an original frozen cream cheesecake; a fast food "light" taco is "light" only because it is made with a fried flour tortilla instead of a tougher, but lower-calorie, corn tortilla.

[b]The word *lean* as part of the brand name (as in "Lean Supreme") indicates that the product is 25 percent lower in fat than the regular variety. Lean ground beef can be up to 22.5 percent fat by weight.

to know exactly how much of a nutrient is in a serving, you can do a simple calculation. Suppose a label says that a serving provides 25 percent of the U.S. RDA for vitamin A. The U.S. RDA table lists 1000 RE as the U.S. RDA for that vitamin. Twenty-five percent of the U.S. RDA thus equals 250 RE Vitamin A.

What if, in addition to the net contents and company address, the label says nothing more than a name, such as *mayonnaise*? For these and other products

standards of identity: standards for the recipes manufacturers must use if they are to be permitted to use certain common names (for example, *mayonnaise*) on labels.

imitation (food): a food that imitates another food and is nutritionally inferior to it with respect to vitamin, mineral, or protein content. Nutritional inferiority is defined by law as having "a reduction in the content of an essential vitamin or mineral or of protein that amounts to 10 percent or more of the U.S. RDA."

substitute (food): a food that is designed to replace another and is its nutritional equal.

natural food: a food that has been altered as little as possible from the original farm-grown state. As used on labels, this term may misleadingly imply unusual power to promote health. It has not been legally defined.

health food: a misleading term used to imply unusual power of a food to promote health. This term has no legal meaning.

organic food: the chemist's definition of *organic* is given on page 6. The popular definition is a food or nutrient produced without the use of chemical fertilizers, pesticides, or additives. Some states are beginning to define this term to limit its misuse.

the law provides **standards of identity** and excuses manufacturers from the requirement of listing ingredients. Standards of identity exist for some familiar foods to ensure that commercial products have approximately the same composition as recipes that once were followed in the home. Certain ingredients must be present in specific percentages before the food may be called by the standard name.

Some foods are imitations of familiar foods. If you read **imitation** on a label, you can conclude that the food is a poor imitation nutritionally. This may be of no consequence when the food is an incidental item in your diet, such as vanilla, because you do not depend on vanilla for any nutrients. But if it is a drink that you drink daily, for example, imitation chocolate milk, then the label may alert you to note the nutrient differences to determine if you need a change.

Although imitation foods are inferior in some ways, many may also be superior in some ways to traditional foods. For example, some imitation cheeses are lower in saturated fat and cholesterol than regular cheeses, and dietary recommendations urge people to reduce their intakes of these constituents. Imitation foods are, however, also inferior in one or more nutrients, and the law requires that the word imitation be used on the label in those cases. A food that is designed to replace another and is its nutritional equal can be called a **substitute** (for example, fat-free egg substitutes). The larger the space a food occupies in your diet the more important distinctions like this are.

Some terms on labels only have meaning because people generally agree on their meanings, not because they are legally defined. One such term is **natural food**, already discussed in Chapter 1, sometimes used to describe such "unnatural" products as chewing gum, flavored drink mixes, pan spray coating, and even purified sugars. Other such terms are **health food** and **organic food**. The term *health food* is always misleading on labels—no food has special powers to promote health. The term *organic* was defined earlier; it describes any substance that contains atoms of carbon, but it also has a popular definition that refers to the way a food is grown. An organically grown food by the popular definition is one grown without the use of pesticides and with only such fertilizers as compost, not the concentrated fertilizers of isolated compounds made in factories. Such foods may not be more nutritious for the eater than are regular, farm-raised products; but if produced honestly, organic foods contain no pesticide residues above those that occur naturally in plants. Ethical practices are not a certainty, though, and a label that says *organic* is no guarantee that a food is pesticide-free, since monitoring of organic foods does not surpass that of regular foods. Foods labeled *organic* are often more expensive than their ordinary grocery-store counterparts, and they are sometimes (as in the case of herbal preparations) even dangerous to use.

One strong plus attends the production of organic foods: their cultivation is much more conservative of the earth's resources than is regular farming. Under a new name, *sustainable agriculture*, organic farming is gaining a new respectability today, and Chapter 15 delves into the reasons why.

Health Messages on Labels

The law permits scientifically based health statements on labels, subject to FDA's approval.[5] The statements must emphasize the importance of the total diet without claiming that a single food can confer health benefits. A label can state, for example, that "a high-fiber diet may reduce your risk of some kinds of cancer." The statement is true—a high-fiber *diet* can reduce your risks; a high-fiber *cereal*, though, cannot make this claim. In fact, a cereal, even a high fiber cereal, may pull in the opposite direction. If the cereal in the box should contain large amounts of fat, as some high-fiber cereals do, then the cancer-promoting effects of the fat may outweigh the benefits from the fiber in this regard. Therefore the claim must be stated in terms of total diet. In this way labels are held to claims that are truthful, and they are not supposed to be misleading; but you can see from this example that consumers have to be well-informed to keep from being misled.[6]

FDA has two concerns about health messages on food labels.[7] The first is that they may lead people to act inappropriately after reading labels. For example, some people might forgo needed medical treatment for, say, hypertension, based on information provided on a food label. FDA's second concern is how to encourage food manufacturers to print truthful, responsible health messages. Most people would like to find such nutrition information on labels, but presently, FDA has no reliable way to sort truthful from misleading statements.

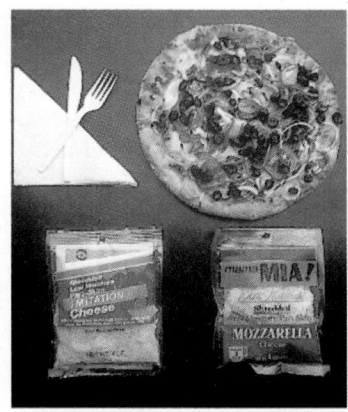
An imitation food is nutritionally inferior to the real thing.

Based on these concerns, and taking into account suggestions from individuals, consumer groups, health and medical professional groups, and food industry representatives, FDA has proposed the following health-message criteria:

■ The label statement must be truthful and not misleading, must not imply that the food should be used as a treatment, and must not overemphasize or distort the role of food in promoting good health. (In determining whether food label statements are misleading, the proposal instructs FDA to look not only at what *is* said, but also at what is *not* said.)

■ The label must make the statement in terms of total diet.

■ The label statement must agree with recognized medical and nutrition principles.

■ The label must refer consumers to FDA-approved summaries, available separately, of complete and balanced information about the nutrition and health interaction referred to on the label.

■ A label with a health message must also meet full nutrition labeling requirements.

In addition, the current proposal limits health messages to the six areas addressed by the *NRC Report* and the *Surgeon General's Report* of 1988.*

Finally, FDA would like to establish a special committee who would develop label statements that manufacturers could use on appropriate products. Under the current proposal, manufacturers would not be permitted to create their own health-related statements, but would be required to use the committee's statements. The proposed committee would also develop detailed research summaries to support each of the health messages, to be distributed to consumers upon their request. If implemented, these proposals will go a long way toward providing valid nutrition information to consumers in a form they can easily use.

*The six topic areas are: calcium and osteoporosis; dietary fiber and cancer; lipids and cardiovascular disease; lipids and cancer; sodium and hypertension; and dietary fiber and cardiovascular disease.

▌▐▌ Food Feature

Choosing Foods with High Nutrient Density

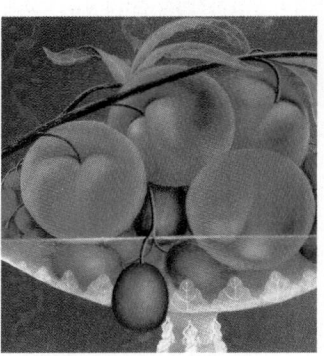

To demonstrate how meals differ from day to day, Figure 2–8 (pages 52–53) illustrates a playful contrast between two days' meals. One, labeled "Monday's Meals," shows the result of following some of the recommendations cited in this chapter; it contains abundant plant foods, nonfat milk, and modest amounts of meats, seafood, and legumes. The second, "Tuesday's Meals," emphasize meats, eggs, and fats at every meal.

The two sets of meals were made similar in energy, so that the other differences would stand out. Both add up to 1750 calories. Monday's choices provided more carbohydrate and more-than-adequate protein, with only 24 percent of the calories from fat. Tuesday's choices supplied less carbohydrate, more protein, and 44 percent of the calories from fat. The contrast is dramatic, and some of the reasons for it are obvious, but for the moment, just notice the food choices made on these two days. Suspend judgment on their implications until later chapters have filled in needed information on the nutrients.

The Controversy that follows adds a new twist to diet planning. It asks the question whether we can eat according to ethnic hertiage and still meet dietary recommendations.

▌▐▌ SELF-STUDY

Calculate Your Nutrient Intakes

This Self-Study takes up where the last one left off and directs you to calculate your nutrient intakes for the period in which you wrote down what foods you ate. Refer to Appendix C if you need help with the calculations.

1. Pick up Form 1 again (you copied it from Appendix F and filled out the first two columns in Self-Study 1). Using Appendix A, enter in the remaining columns of the form the amounts of nutrients each food contributed. If the foods you have eaten are not included in Appendix A, read the label on the package, or use your ingenuity to guess their composition, using the most sim-

ilar food you can find as a guide. (You may need to convert these values to the units used on the form; this is explained below).

Be careful in recording the nutrient amounts in odd-sized portions. For example, if you used a quarter cup of milk, then you will have to record a fourth of the amount of every nutrient listed for a cup of milk. (Again, refer to Appendix C if you need help). And note the units in which the nutrients are measured:

☐ Energy is measured in calories (cal), as explained on p. 6. Keep in mind that the terms *kilocalorie* and *calorie* are

used to mean the same thing in this text.

☐ Protein, carbohydrate, fiber, fat, and fatty acid breakdown are measured in grams (g).

☐ Cholesterol, calcium, iron, zinc, thiamin, riboflavin, niacin, vitamin B_6, and vitamin C (ascorbic acid) are measured in milligrams (mg)—thousandths of a gram (0.001 gram). Folate is measured in micrograms (mcg or μg)—thousandths of a milligram or millionths of a gram (0.001 milligram or 0.000001 gram). Thus 800 milligrams calcium is the same as 0.8 grams calcium, and 400 micrograms folate is the same as 0.4 milligrams

continued on the next page

▌▌▌ SELF STUDY *continued*

folate. Be sure to convert all calcium amounts to milligrams and all folate amounts to micrograms before calculating.

☐ Vitamin A is sometimes measured in international units (IU) and sometimes in retinol equivalents (RE); 1 RE equals 3 IU of vitamin A from animal foods, 10 IU of vitamin A from plant foods,* or, on the average, 5 IU (for mixed dishes). Appendix A lists vitamin A in RE to ease comparison with the RDA, which is also in RE. If you find vitamin A listed in IU on a label, be sure to convert to RE before calculating.

If you eat a packaged food whose label lists nutrient amounts as "percent of U.S. RDA," use the table on the inside front cover, page C, to convert to grams, milligrams, micrograms, or RE. Suppose a food portion contains 25 percent

---

*One IU of vitamin A is equal to 0.344 microgram of crystalline vitamin A acetate or 0.6 microgram of all-*trans* beta-carotene.

of the U.S. RDA of iron, for example. The table shows that the U.S. RDA for iron is 18 milligrams. The food portion therefore contributes a fourth of 18 milligrams, or 4.5 milligrams of iron.

Now, still using Form 1, total the amount of each nutrient you've consumed for each day.

2. Transfer your totals from Form 1 to Form 2 in Appendix F. Form 2 provides a convenient means of deriving a three-day average intake for each nutrient.

3. As a final step, transfer your average intakes to Form 3 in Appendix F for future reference. For comparison, enter the intakes recommended for a person of your age and sex using either the RDA (on the inside front cover) or the Canadian Recommended Nutrient Intakes (RNI; see Appendix B), whichever you prefer. Note that no recommendations are made for intakes of fat or carbohydrate. Guidelines for these nutrients will be presented and discussed later, and tentative standards for fiber and cholesterol are provided on the

form. Succeeding Self-Studies will guide you in focusing on each of the nutrients provided by your diet.

Suspend judgment about the adequacy of your diet for the moment. You have much to learn about your individuality, the nutrients, and the recommendations before you can reach any reasonable conclusions.

4. What percentage of the calories you consumed come from protein, fat, and carbohydrate? (Use Form 4 in Appendix F to calculate; use Appendix C if you need help doing the calculation.) Is your diet in line with current recommendations in this respect? The suggested balance is about 10 to 15 percent of the calories from protein, about 30 percent (not more) from fat, and the remainder from carbohydrate.

5. You can get an indication of whether your diet is balanced on any particular day by using the Food Selection Scorecard (Form 5 in Appendix F—one copy for each day). How does your diet score by these criteria?

■■■ **Figure 2–8a**

Monday's Meal Selections

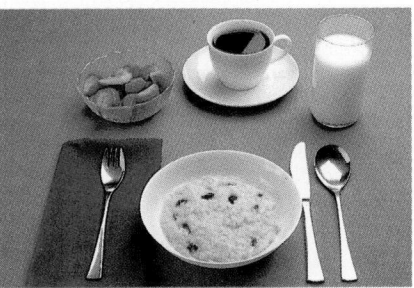

A student prepares breakfast:
  1 c coffee
  1 c oatmeal with ¼ c raisins
  1 c nonfat milk
  1¼ c strawberries

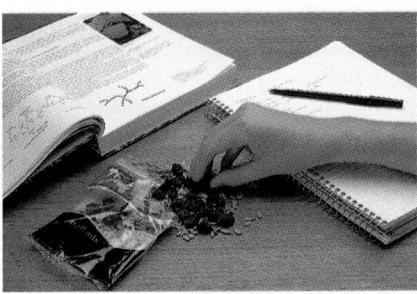

and grabs a snack:
  2 tbsp raisins
  2 tbsp sunflower seeds

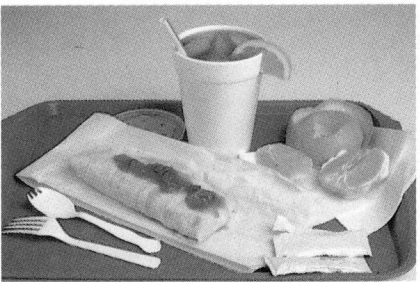

and takes along an orange to eat with lunch.
Lunch is fast-food fare:
  1 beef and bean burrito
  Iced tea with sugar and lemon
  1 orange

After classes, the student plays a quick game of racquetball and heads home. Later that evening, the student visits a friend for dinner. The friend serves:
A salad made with:
  1 c raw spinach leaves
  1 tbsp sesame seeds
  ¼ c fresh mushroom slices
  ¼ c water chestnuts
  ⅓ c garbanzo beans
  1 tbsp vinaigrette dressing
A dinner of:
  4 oz broiled salmon garnished with
  ⅛ lemon
  1 c broccoli
  ½ c noodles tossed with 2 tsp
  butter and ¼ c parsley
  ¼ tomato
  1 c nonfat milk
And, for dessert:
  ½ c sherbet

Total cal: 1750
57% cal from carbohydrate
24% cal from fat
19% cal from protein

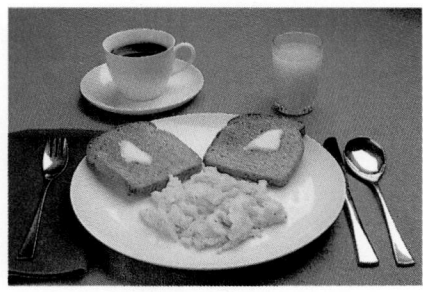

Today, the student starts the day with
    1 c coffee
    ½ c orange juice
    2 scrambled eggs
    2 pieces whole-wheat toast with 2
    tsp butter

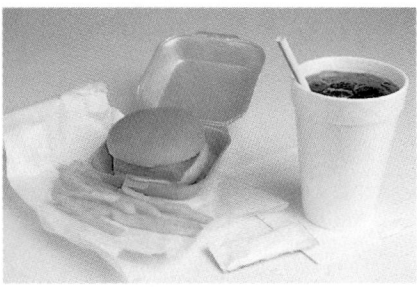

Between classes, the students buys a
fast-food meal:
    1 hamburger
    15 french fries
    12 oz diet cola

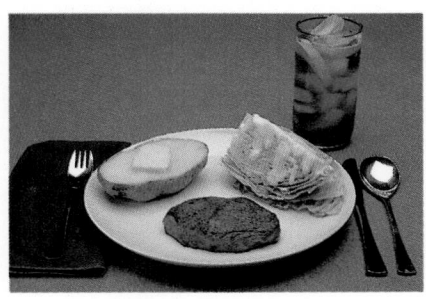

The student joins a friend to prepare
an evening meal:
A salad made with:
    1 c iceberg lettuce
    1 tbsp ranch salad dressing
A main course of:
    6 oz. steak
    ½ baked potato with 2 tsp butter
    A glass of iced tea with 1 tsp sugar
    and ⅛ lemon

Total cal: 1750
33% cal from carbohydrate
44% cal from fat
23% cal from protein

Notes

1. Food and Nutrition Board, *Recommended Dietary Allowances*, 10th ed. (Washington, D.C.: National Academy of Sciences, 1989).

2. Food and Nutrition Board, 1989, p. 9.

3. J. Hallfrisch and coauthors, Acceptability of a 7-day higher-carbohydrate, lower-fat menu: The Beltsville Diet Study, *Journal of the American Dietetic Association* 88 (1988): 163–168.

4. ADA Timely Statement: Nutrition information on food labels, *Journal of the American Dietetic Association* 89 (1989): 266–268.

5. T. P. Labuza, A perspective on health claims in food labeling, *Cereal Foods World*, 32 (1987): 256–267.

6. ADA timely statement, 1989.

7. Food and Drug Administration, Food labeling; health messages and label statement; reproposed rule, *Federal Register* 55 (1990): 5176–5192.

Cultural and Religious Cuisines: Which Ethnic Group Has the Best Way to Eat?

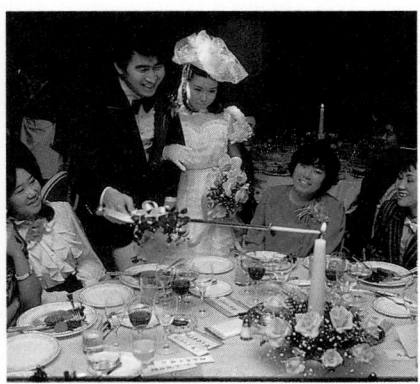

The last chapter presented nutrient guidelines and dietary recommendations and then showed how some meal patterns can meet them. It stopped short, though, of suggesting *foods* to meet those plans. What foods? Whose foods? People eat differently, depending on many influences, including ethnic background, the local food supply, local **cuisine**, religious restrictions, and the other factors affecting food choices named in Chapter 1. Do some **foodways** better meet human dietary needs

than others? Which are best? Here we can present only a few possible ethnic foodways but these suffice to show that basic diet planning principles can be successfully applied to all sorts of cuisines and foodways.

How does a culture decide what to eat among the many plants and animals that surround it? This depends, at least partly, on the answers of its people to a series of questions:

☐ Would eating this plant or animal injure us? If a plant or animal is poisonous when eaten then it is not edible. Even if it is only *believed* to be harmful it may become **taboo**.
☐ Is this plant or animal considered food for animals or for people? A U.S. citizen would probably consider insects appropriate food for fish or chickens but not for people, while other cultures consider certain insects a delicacy. In France, corn is used to feed cattle, not people.
☐ Does the group to which I belong eat this food? Some cultures may eat horse meat, but others do not. Some people eat variety meats, such as tripe, chitterlings, or brains, but others do not.
☐ Is this a food that I eat? If I like it, if I can afford to buy it, if it is allowed by my religion and is consistent with other values, and if it is not restricted for health reasons, this is food I eat.[1]

Foods that meet these criteria comprise a person's diet within a culture. However, as individual tastes and circumstances change, a culture may try new foods, too, and adopt them as standard fare.

Every country, and in fact every region of a country, has its own typical foods and ways of combining them into meals. Immigrants to North America have brought those ways with them, and they have evolved here into patterns that we call—for lack of a better term—**ethnic diets** or cuisines. As generations have passed and people have migrated from one region of North America to another, these cuisines have melded together into combinations of the characteristics of many different diets.

Some cultures or ethnic groups are relatively pure, and so are their foodways. However, in the United States, many ethnic groups have mingled, so U.S. foodways are influenced by many subcultures. A menu in an "American-style" restaurant might list everyday foods with many different ethnic origins—spaghetti (Italian), nachos (Mexican), hot dogs with sauerkraut (German), french fried potatoes (French), peanuts (African), popcorn (Native American), and egg rolls (Chinese). These and other ethnic foods have become integral in the "American diet;" further some ingenious cross-cultural recipes have yielded fanciful creations, such as tofu lasagne and Tex-Mex wonton.

Ethnic influences have extended the lists of foods that people recognize as food that they eat. This helps people to achieve variety in their meals, one of the five basic characteristics of a healthy diet, presented in Chapter 2. However, when you include ethnic foods in your diet, be sure to choose them not only for variety but also with an eye to their nutrient density to achieve adequacy, calorie control, and moderation. For balance, attend first to fat, as we do in this Controversy. Whether a food enhances or detracts from your nutritional health often depends on the amount and kind of fat it delivers. With these principles in mind, we turn to the cuisines of just a few groups whose foodways have helped to shape eating habits in the United States.

▪▪▪ Northern Europe

Immigrants from northern Europe vastly influenced traditional American home cooking. For example, an evening meal of a hearty portion of fine roast meat; side dishes of mashed potatoes or boiled cabbage, and bread; and fruit pie for dessert characterizes the cuisine of Germany, England, and Ireland. But such a meal is also typical of suppers across the United States because immigrants from those countries brought this meal plan with them to the New World. Many variations of this meal are based on the same foods, prepared differently. For example, a New England boiled dinner may include a corned (spiced and cured) cut of beef boiled together with potatoes, carrots, and cabbage. Plates are typically filled with large portions of the meat with the vegetables on the side; however, diners who wish to eat this meal and meet dietary recommendations would be wise to fill their plates with the tasty vegetables, and limit

the meat to a 3-ounce portion. This way, the meal would provide plenty of carbohydrate, adequate protein, and not too much fat.

Many other familiar foodways are also of northern European derivation. The traditional breakfast of eggs with bacon and biscuits was also originally derived from England, as was tea as a beverage. (An aside: the English serve baked beans with breakfast, not potatoes or grits.) The familiar three-meal-a-day plan, with breakfast as the lightest meal, lunch somewhat more substantial, and supper contributing the bulk of the day's food is also a northern European import.

Every eating style has advantages and drawbacks, and northern European is no exception. This style of eating provides abundant protein, and ensures adequacy of all the nutrients associated with meat. However, it also delivers a lot of fat and is short on fiber and the vitamins and minerals associated with fruits and vegetables. People who adhere to foodways that resemble those of the northern European countries can improve their nutrition by reducing meat portion sizes (see Chapter 6 if you worry about consuming enough protein), by cutting down on added fats, and by choosing more whole grains, fruits, and vegetables.

The famed cuisines of France influenced the foodways of both the British Isles and Ireland, but French immigrants to the United States were relatively few in number, and most were assimilated fully into the

new culture. One group, the French Acadians from Canada who settled in southern Louisiana preserved their French country-cooking heritage and easily adapted it to the local Louisiana food supply. Today their descendants, the Cajuns, have made their foodways popular with people across the nation.

A gradual blending of Acadian and African American cultures produced the unique Cajun cuisine with both French with African influences. Cajun dishes include spicy, thick soups (gumbo, jambalaya), sausages, *Tabasco* pepper sauce, red beans and rice, dirty rice (rice made brown with chopped chicken livers and seasonings), and seafood. Cajun coffee is flavored with chicory root, and many people enjoy this distinctive brew. More French in nature are the puffed, sugared doughnuts known as beignets and the familiar French toast.

Many Cajun foods are perfectly suited to meeting the *NRC Recommendations* introduced in Chapter 2. Nutritionists agree with enthusiastic diners that red beans and rice is a classic dish—delicious because it is full of flavor from expert use of spice and nutritious because it is high in carbohydrate, protein, and fiber, while low in fat. Stews of seafood, tomatoes, vegetables, and rice seasoned with a little strong-flavored sausage are packed with vitamins and minerals, adequate in protein, rich in carbohydrate, while usually low in fat. Overall, many Cajun foods can support efforts to meet dietary guidelines deliciously.

▓▓▓ Southern Europe

Almost everybody enjoys one or another of the Italian foods brought to the United States by the millions of Italian immigrants. What teenager would turn down a slice of pizza, a food native to Naples? Who wouldn't like spumone—ice cream with fruits, nuts, and flavorings?

The foods of Italy bear regional characteristics. Generally people living in the northern regions of that country consume abundant animal-derived food—meat, butter, cheese, eggs, and cream. In the southern regions, wheat pastas accompany vegetables such as artichokes, eggplants, peppers, and tomatoes; these foods are served more with beans than meat and are seasoned with olive oil, not butter. Even pasta, a favorite in both the north and south, varies by region—northern pastas are egg-based and usually ribbon shaped, while southern varieties are made without eggs and are shaped more like macaroni.

Nutritionally Italian favorites receive high marks in balance and adequacy. Chapter 1 depicted some students who chose pizza for supper and thus enjoyed a food that offered something from each of the four food groups. Other Italian dishes can do equally well: eggplant parmesan served with a side dish of pasta supplies vegetables, cheese, grain, and perhaps a bit of meat in the sauce. Pastas with meaty tomato sauces and a sprinkling of cheese also meet the four food-group recommendations. However, for the sake of moderation, the eater of Ital-ian foods must introduce modifications to reduce the fat in many original recipes. It helps especially to reduce the amounts of oil and high-fat cheeses added to the foods of southern Italian origin and to substitute low-fat ingredients for the high-fat cream and butter used in foods of the northern regions. The Food Feature of Chapter 5 gives general principles for reducing fat in foods of all origins. Some Italian dishes such as pasta prima vera, a mixture of colorful vegetables and pasta, and minestrone, a bean and pasta soup are high in nutrient density and appealing in both taste and appearance without modifications.

▓▓▓ West Africa

When you spread peanut butter on your bread, do you think you are eating an African food? Actually peanut *butter* is considered an American food, invented by George Washington Carver, an agricultural scientist. However, peanuts and peanut paste were and still are staple foods of Africa and were brought to U.S. soil by African slaves. If you have ever eaten boiled peanuts, today a southern specialty, you have partaken of a dish that emerged with the origins of humankind in Africa. Similarly, okra and blackeye (cow) peas are of African origin.

Most black Americans are the descendants of ancestors who came to the United States from western Africa by force, not by choice. Although generations of blacks suffered slavery, segregation, and persecution, their unique culture strongly influenced today's general U.S. culture, especially in music, art, and in its foodways.

Within the possibilities allowed them, enslaved Africans held tenaciously to their familiar, ancient foodways and adapted them to the foods they encountered in their new world. They offered their agricultural expertise to the landowners, too, so that a blending of cultures took place. African crops tended on Southern agricultural plantations were eaten by slaves and owners alike, often in combination with native American greens, sweet potatoes, and wild fish and game.

Today's rural southern cuisine varies little between blacks and whites, and it offers both nutritional advantages and disadvantages. It provides ample vitamins and minerals found in green leafy vegetables, meats, and corn. Sweet potatoes are a rich source of vitamin A and are naturally low in fat and high in carbohydrate. Cajun seafood gumbo (similar to an African dish of the same name) was already described as a nutritious mixture of low-fat foods. However, many foods of the rural South are perilously fat-rich: some dishes are traditionally flavored with lard or are fried in other fats. Biscuits, a favored bread, are made with almost as much shortening as flour and are often served with butter or fat-rich gravy. Preferred meals also include large servings of high-fat meats, such as fried chicken, pork cuts or sausages, and spareribs, greatly overemphasizing protein and fat in the diet while diminishing the role of the carbohydrates whole grains, fruits, and vegetables. The trick to choosing health-promoting rural southern food is to choose the vegetables, beans, and cornbread; go easy on fatty meats, biscuits, and gravies.

▓▓▓ Mexico

In a Mexican restaurant you can order beautiful plates of complex food mixtures—tortillas filled with meats and cheeses, some fried and crisp and others baked and soft, along with flavored rice, refried beans, sour cream, guacamole (avocado sauce), and salsa (tomato sauce). These foods are of Mexican origin, but they are not the day-to-day fare of Mexican families, although they are typical of festive foods prepared for special occasions. A typical Mexican meal is simple, consisting of a stew of beans, meat, and potatoes served with tortillas or bread and tomato salsa. A Mexican breakfast might include tortillas and eggs with a beverage while lunch and supper might consist of beans and rice or a stew served with a lettuce and tomato salad or a cooked vegetable.[2]

As American as the hamburger place, taco stands sell fast food to millions of U.S. diners each day. If carefully chosen, these foods can make valuable contributions to the diet. Many Mexican dishes (even the fast-food type) provide beans in abundance. Beans are high in nutrient density and fiber while low in fat (more about beans in Chapter

6), although the refried variety may be cooked with lard. Without care in choosing, though, you can obtain an extraordinarily high-fat meal, such as a fried tortilla shell filled with commercial-grade, high-fat ground beef and topped with cheese and sour cream. Just as tasty, but higher in nutrient density, are soft corn tortillas filled with beans, lettuce, and salsa with a side order of rice.

For the special occasion described earlier, the wise diner avoids adding sour cream, and skips the fried varieties of stuffed tortillas. A dish called fajita—lean meats, marinated and sizzled on a grill, wrapped in soft tortillas with chili salsa toppings deserves consideration. As for guacamole, you will see in Chapter 5 that even though they are high in fat you needn't avoid avocados altogether. The type of fat avocados contain is not implicated in disease causation, although they are fattening and should be limited by people who tend to gain weight. Salsa is rich in vitamins and zest but adds no fat burden to the meal.

You may be beginning to see that the diner's choices within an ethnic frame, and not the frame itself, determine whether a meal benefits the diner's health. One cuisine, though, reliably presents many interesting dishes that meet nutrient needs extraordinarily well. It is the Chinese cuisine.

▓▓▓ China

Tried and true, the diet of China has supported the health of people

there for thousands of years. The foodways of China reflect that economy is essential in a land crowded with more than 1000 people per acre and where only 10 percent of the land can be used to grow food. China's population numbers well over a billion people, of whom about 75 percent are involved in agriculture. Contrast this to the United States: population density— 113 per acre; land in farms—about 50 percent; population—250 million; farmers—1 to 2 percent.

There seems to be little malnutrition or obesity among Chinese people, even though they consume 20 percent more calories of food each day than do people in the United States. One source reported that, on the whole, Chinese people eating traditional foods consume three times the fiber of people eating the American way, take in about half the fat, and have blood cholesterol values about half of what they are in the United States.[3] It seems worthwhile to study the fine points of a diet so conservative of resources yet so superbly supportive of health— not to convince you to eat all Chinese meals but perhaps to encourage you to adopt some of its governing principles and to apply them to foods of all origins.

Chinese meals do not follow the separate meat-vegetable-starch pattern of northern European origin. The vegetables and meats are cooked together. The total amount of meat (or fish or egg) in a Chinese dish is very small by Western standards; instead, there is abundant rice at almost every meal. The Chi-

■■■ Table C2-1 Characteristics of Selected Ethnic Diets

GROUP AND PLACE OF ORIGIN	STAPLE FOODS	FOODS EXCLUDED	STRENGTHS AND WEAKNESSES OF THE DIET
Hispanic Americans from Cuba, Haiti, Puerto Rico	Steamed white rice; many varieties of beans; wheat breads; starchy vegetables such as cassavas, yuccas, yams, breadfruit, plantains, and green bananas; green peppers; tomatoes; garlic; dried, salted fish; chicken; pork; lard; olive oil; sugar; jams and jellies; sweet pastries; sugared fruit juices; coffee	Green leafy vegetables; milk as a beverage for adults; fish other than dried and salted	Provides adequate protein, many other nutrients, and fiber; may provide too much fat, especially animal fat; may lack calcium
Hispanic Americans from Mexico, Central America	Many varieties of beans; steamed rice; corn products such as tortillas made from lime-soaked cornmeal; chili peppers; tomatoes; mangoes; prickly pear fruit; potatoes; meat and sausages; fish; poultry; eggs; milk cheeses; milk custards and bread puddings; lard; sweet chocolate and coffee drinks; cakes; pastries	Green leafy vegetables; yellow vegetables; milk as a beverage for adults	Is high in calories and fat, especially saturated fat, and high in sugar; most nutrients can be obtained, but with many calories
Black Americans from West Indies, Central or South America and recent African immigrants	Dumplings or gruel made from millet, corn, wheat, rice, or barley; starchy roots such as cassavas, yams, plantains, and bananas; coconuts; peanuts; fresh fruits; hot peppers; tomatoes; onions; okra; palm oil; fruit wine; tea; coffee; honey; molasses	Milk and milk products (meat and fish limited use)	Is low in calcium, iron, and vitamin B_{12}; is potentially low in protein, depending on availability of foods; is low in fat and salt; is high in fiber
Southern black Americans from West Africa (many generations in United States)	Hominy grits; biscuits; cornmeal and corn bread; rice; legumes; potatoes; onions; tomatoes; hot peppers; green leafy vegetables; okra; sweet potatoes; squashes; corn; cabbage; melons; peaches; pecans; smoked pork; fresh meats and poultry; fish; thick stews; butter, shortening, and lard; sugar; bread puddings; pies and sweets	Milk and milk products; yeast breads	Provides ample nutrients of meat; provides excess protein; is high in calories; provides excess fat, especially saturated fat; is high in salt; is low in calcium
Chinese Americans from China (diets vary sometimes with region)	Rice and rice gruel; wheat noodles; corn; green vegetables, especially from the cabbage family; squashes; cucumbers; eggplant; leafy vegetables; various shoots, including bamboo, mung, and soy; sweet potatoes; radishes; onions; peas and pods; mushrooms; roots; many local, seasonal vegetables; pickled vegetables; sea vegetables; plums; peaches; tangerines; kumquats and other citrus fruits; litchis; longans; mangoes; papayas; pomegranates; soybean products such as tofu (soybean curd), soy sauces, bean noodles, and soy milk; tiny portions of meat, fish with bones, or poultry; seafood; soup or tea as beverage; sugar as seasoning	Milk and most milk products	Depending on availability of protein-rich foods, protein and iron may be low; is low in fat; is high in fiber and many nutrients; see text for further discussion of the Chinese diet
Japanese Americans from Japan	Rice; vegetables; pickled vegetables; soy as miso (soup), tofu, bean paste, and soy sauce; fruits; salads; fish with bones; sugar as seasoning; sea vegetables; seafood; ginseng	Milk and milk products	Provides abundant nutrients with little fat; is high in salt

■■■ Table C2-1 Characteristics of Selected Ethnic Diets *continued*

GROUP AND PLACE OF ORIGIN	STAPLE FOODS	FOODS EXCLUDED	STRENGTHS AND WEAKNESSES OF THE DIET
Korean Americans from South Korea	Rice; noodle; many leafy vegetables; kimchi (extremely hot pickled cabbage); sea vegetables; hot peppers; seasonal fruits; mushrooms; small fish with bones; large servings of grilled beef; chicken; fresh or dried squid, octopus, and lobster; fish with bones; mussels; eggs; lard and vegetable fat for frying; sesame oil; nuts and seeds; ginger; sugar as seasoning	Milk and milk products	Is high in fat and adequate in protein; is monotonous in winter (kimchi is served at each meal, to the exclusion of other vegetables); without the traditional small fish with bones, calcium can be lacking
Vietnamese Americans from Vietnam	Rice, rice noodles; french bread and croissants with butter; hot peppers; curries of asparagus and potatoes; salads; tropical fruits and vegetables; lemons and limes; small portions of poultry; eggs; fish pâtés; nuoc nam (a strong, fermented fish sauce); sweets, candies, sweetened drinks; coffee; tea	Milk and milk products	Can be low in iron or calcium
Native Americans (Indians)	*Southeast:* corn; cornmeal; coontie (flour from a palmlike plant); fried breads; swamp cabbage (now illegal to harvest); pumpkins; squashes; papayas; alligator, snake, wild hog, duck, fish, and shell fish. *Northeast:* blueberries; cranberries; beans; corn; pumpkins; fish; lobster; wild game; maple syrup. *Midwest:* bison; beans; corn; melons; squashes; tomatoes. *Southwest:* corn (many colors and varieties); beans; squash; pumpkins; chili peppers; melons; pinenuts; cactus. *Northwest:* salmon; caviar; other fish; otter; seal; whale; bear; elk; other game; wild fruits; acorns (and other wild nuts); wild greens.	Milk and milk products	Varies with region; may be low in calcium.

nese also usually partake of soup or tea throughout each meal. Meals center on a staple starch food (every diner has a personal rice dish) with other foods chosen according to each person's appetite (from serving dishes).

Vegetables and fruits provide tremendous variety in the Chinese diet. The nutrients in the foods are undiluted by fat and sugar. Nor do alcohol calories have a significant place, although the Chinese do make and drink a wine on special occasions.

The subtle flavors that make Chinese dishes appealing come largely from the seasonings and sauces used in their preparation. Among the seasonings are ginger root, almonds, scallions, sesame seed oil, rice wine, and garlic. Among the sauces are soy, hoisin, oyster, bean, and plum sauce. Most Chinese seasonings are fat-free, and cooks use just a tablespoon or two in an entire dish. Most sauces add tasty flavors but no fat, unlike our gravies, butter, or sour cream. The Chinese mode of cooking employs very little oil. Chinese dishes do have a nutrition drawback, though: they are likely to be high in sodium. (Details about sodium are presented in Chapter 8.)

Cooking foods the Chinese way tends to preserve nutrients. The water in which the rice is cooked may absorb nutrients, but then it soaks back into the rice rather than being drained away, so the nutrients are retained. All food is cut into bite-sized pieces before cooking so that it will be easy to eat with chopsticks; cooking finely cut-up food requires only short times and so destroys few nutrients. No extra water is used, and none is thrown away, so nutrients are not lost that way either.

The Chinese diet and cooking techniques are also land efficient, as they must be in view of the scarcity of agricultural land and fuels. Nearly all of the calories come from plants rather than animals. A million calories in wheat or rice can be produced on less than an acre of land; a million calories in beef require 17 acres. In a world in which fuel and land are becoming increasingly scarce, the Chinese way of eating offers a model to nations. You should be aware, though, if you choose rice as a staple food in your diet, that polished rice is highly refined in this country and loses nutrients such as iron, B vitamins, and other nutrients in the refining process. Therefore you should choose unpolished brown rice, or, to regain at least some of the depleted nutrients, choose rice that has been enriched. (Chapter 4 describes the processes of refining and enriching grains. Chapter 15 and Controversy 15 explore further the links between world resources and people's foodways.)

Many other cuisines and foodways are of interest. Table C2-1 lists some of them, with a brief description of some foods that characterize each.

■■■ Religious Dietary Traditions

A discussion of ethnic foodways would not be complete without mention of foodways practiced by the world's major religious groups. Religions help people to answer the questions, "Why am I here?" "What purpose do I serve?" "What is the reason for my existence?" To ask such universal questions seems to be essential to human mental and emotional health.[4] According to many religions, ritual and ceremony surrounding food can provide nourishment for the spirit as well as for the body. Special foodways also help give religious groups, like national groups, their distinct identity.

The Jewish laws set forth an extensive set of dietary rules. These laws are obeyed by Orthodox Jews worldwide: they eat only foods that are **kosher**. Many people, on hearing the word *kosher*, think of foods such as pickles, bagels and lox, corned beef, or matzoh crackers. However, kosher is not a cuisine but is instead a set of restrictions placed on the selection and preparation of animal-derived foods. Jewish cuisines vary among Jews whose families emigrated from different countries. Jews from Eastern Europe, Germany, the Soviet Union, the Middle East, or India eat differently, but all may apply the kosher rules to their foods.[5]

The laws of kosher permit some foods and exclude others, such as allowing beef but not pork or permitting fin fish but not shellfish, and they dictate handling methods for permitted foods. Blood is forbidden as food, and thus meats must be specially prepared to remove the blood. Rules govern the method of animal slaughter, cuts that may be eaten, and preparation rituals. Processed foods that have been made according to kosher laws are identified by an insignia; a "U" or a "K" on the label means that the food has been deemed kosher by a rabbi. Kosher law prohibits Jews from consuming milk and meat in the same meal. This leads some kosher cooks to replace milk with nondairy creamer in meals that include meat. Nutritionally, however, creamers do not replace milk, and they carry more of the type of fat implicated in heart disease. A better choice is to use soy "milk" products that are formulated to resemble the nutrient and cooking qualities of milk products.

In addition to kosher laws for daily meals, holidays call for traditional feasting on foods rich with religious symbolism. For example, a traditional Passover dinner includes a special salad of apples, nuts, cinnamon, and wine that symbolizes the mortar that Jewish slaves used to build Egyptian pyramids and palaces.

Just as with other cuisines, Jewish cuisines and kosher foods can be

■■■ Miniglossary

cuisine: style of cooking or preparing food.

foodways: the sum of the food habits, customs, beliefs, and preferences of a culture.

taboo: forbidden or banned; for food, usually a food believed to be sacred or cursed.

ethnic diets: foodways and cuisines typical of national origins, cultural heritages, or geographic locations.

kosher: foods fit to eat according to the Jewish bible, the *Torah*, which sets the laws.

evaluated according to dietary standards. A Jewish meal of European cuisine might be improved by reducing schmaltz (chicken fat) used in cooking, or by frying latke (potato pancakes) in nonstick pans, not in oil. Bagels with lox (but without cream cheese) are an excellent breakfast choice—bagels are naturally low in fat, and lox are a form of salmon. (Chapter 5 presents details of the special oils found in salmon and other fish.) A person dining on European Jewish cuisine would do well to keep servings of meat (usually beef) to the 3- to 4-ounce serving sizes recommended in Figure 2–4 of Chapter 2, and to fill in the meal with grains such as noodle pudding (without butter), and with fruit and vegetables. For Indian Kosher cuisines, emphasize grains and legumes over fats.

Occasionally someone suggests that the laws of kosher originated for reasons of health, that kosher food was "clean" and therefore kept people safe from foodborne illnesses. However, religious commitment is the sole intent of those who keep kosher, and few of the rules of kosher offer special benefits to health.

Food symbolism abounds in most other religions as well. Among Christians, a revered expression of faith is the sacrament of eating a bite of bread or bread wafer and taking a sip of grape juice or wine, symbolizing the last supper of Jesus Christ. During certain days of Lent, the period prior to Easter, many Christians eat only vegetarian dishes, giving up meat until Easter dinner. Eastern Orthodox Christians observe many fast days on which they consume no animal products at all. Some Christian faiths prohibit or promote certain dietary habits. The Mormon faith does not allow alcohol, coffee, or tea. Many Seventh-day Adventists consume no meat but include eggs and milk products and also shun alcohol, coffee, and tea. In addition, Seventh-day Adventist doctrine advises fol-

lowers to avoid strong spices such as mustard or pepper and discourages between-meal snacks.

Other faiths, such as Islam, Hinduism, and Buddhism, prohibit some dietary practices while promoting others. Dietitians know that to honor a person's cultural or religious foodways honors the person. Sometimes, respecting a person's foodways can provide nourishment of self-esteem, and this can be as important to health as nourishment for the body.

Notes

1. Adapted from P. G. Kittler and K. Sucher, *Food and Culture in America* (New York, 1989: Van Nostrand Reinhold), p. 13.
2. S. J. Algert and T. H. Ellison, Mexican American Food practices, customs, and holidays, *Ethnic and Regional Food Practices* (series) (Chicago and Alexandria, VA: American Dietetic Association and American Diabetes Association, 1989).
3. L. Roberts, Diet and health in China, *Science* 240 (1988): 27.
4. L. S. Chapman, Developing a useful perspective on spiritual health: Love, joy, peace and fulfillment, *American Journal of Health Promotion*, Fall 1987, pp. 12–17.
5. C. Higgins and H. S. Warshaw, Jewish food practices, customs, and holidays, *Ethnic and Regional Food Practices* (series) (Chicago and Alexandria, VA: American Dietetic Association and American Diabetes Association, 1989).

■■■ CHAPTER 3

The Remarkable Body

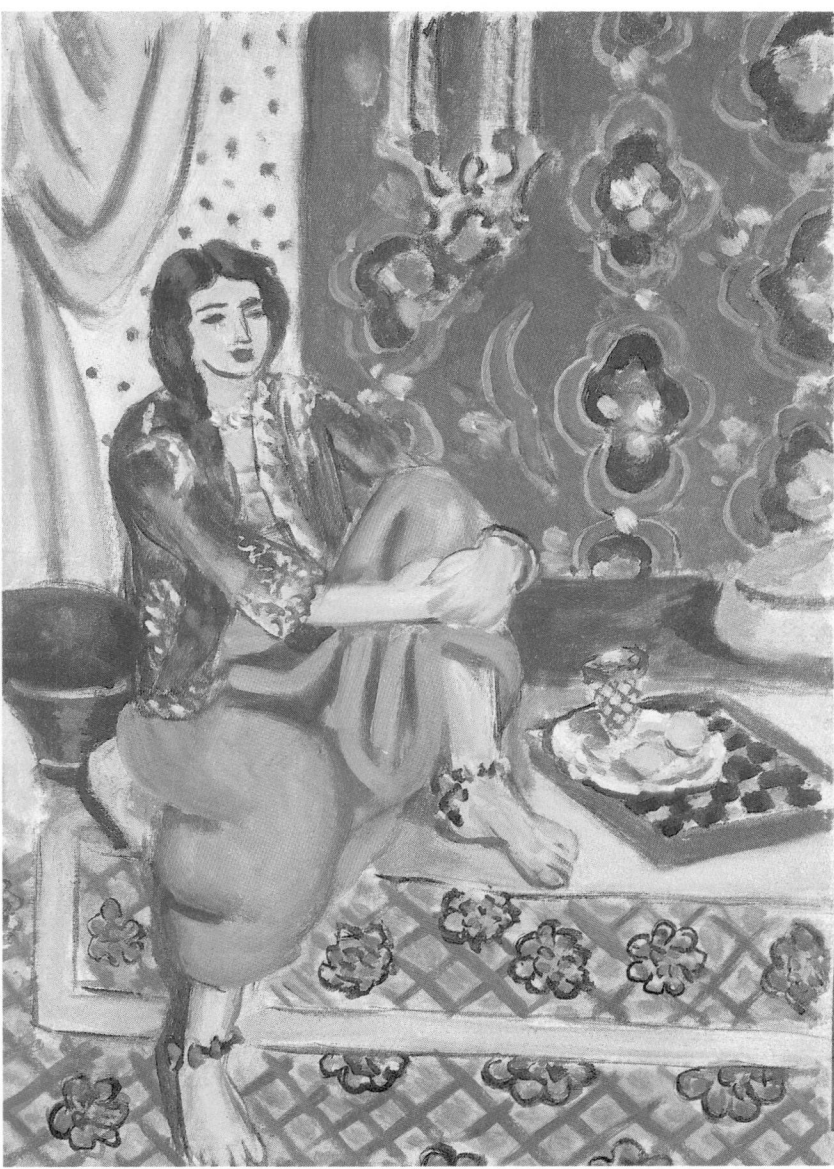

Seated Odalisque, Left Knee Bent, Ornamental Background and Checkerboard by Henri Matisse. The Baltimore Museum of Art: The Cone Collection, formed by Dr. Claribel Cone and Miss Etta Cone of Baltimore, Maryland (Photograph by Tennant). BMA 1950. 255.

CONTENTS

cells: the smallest units in which independent life can exist. All living things are single cells or organisms made of cells.

Your body is composed of billions of cells, and none of them knows anything about food. *You* may get hungry for fruit, milk, or bread, but each cell of your body needs nutrients—the vital components of foods. How they cooperate to obtain the nutrients and to help each other use them are the subjects of this chapter. The brief anatomy lessons that follow review the body systems and terminology that underlie this book's treatment of nutrition.

The Body's Cells

Each of the body's **cells** is a self-contained, living entity (Figure 3–1), although each depends on the rest of the body to supply its needs. Each cell keeps itself alive just as its single-celled ancestors did, living alone in the ocean 3 billion years ago, by taking up the substances it needs from the surrounding fluid and releasing the wastes it produces into that fluid.

Among the cells' most basic needs are energy fuel and the oxygen with which to burn it. Cells also need water to maintain the environment in which they live. They need building blocks and control systems to maintain themselves. They especially need the ones they cannot make for themselves, the essential nutrients, which must be supplied preformed from food. The first principle of diet planning is that whatever foods we choose, they must provide energy, water, and the essential nutrients.

Figure 3–1

A Typical Cell (simplified diagram).

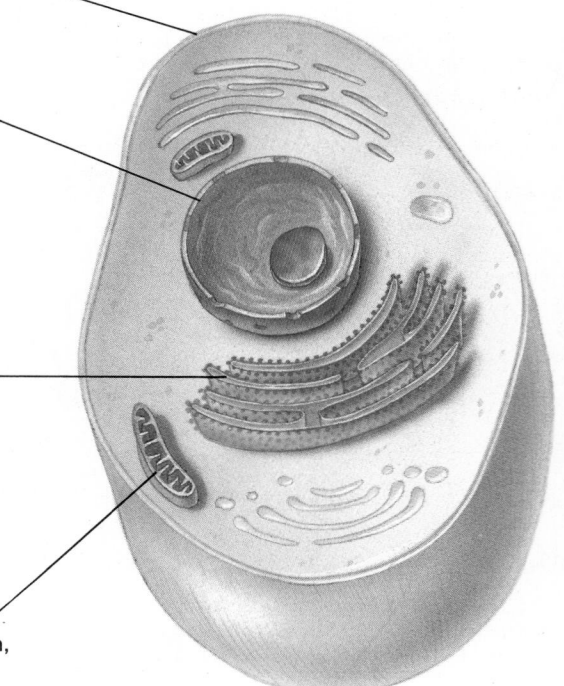

A membrane encloses each cell's contents.

A separate inner membrane encloses the cell's nucleus. Inside the nucleus is the hereditary material, which contains the genes. The genes control the inheritance of the cell's characteristics and its day-to-day workings. They are faithfully copied each time the cell duplicates itself.

Many other structures lie within the cell. In these systems of membranes, for example, instructions from the genes are translated into proteins that perform functions in the body.

Many other cell structures are present. This is a mitochondrion, a structure that takes in nutrients and releases energy from them.

In the human body every cell works in cooperation with every other to support the whole. The cell's **genes** determine the nature of that work. Each gene is a blueprint that directs the making of a piece of protein machinery—most often an **enzyme**—that helps to do the cell's work. Each cell contains a complete set of genes, but different ones are active in different types of cells. For example, in some intestinal cells, the genes for making digestive enzymes are active; in some of the body's fat cells, the genes for making enzymes that make and break down fat are active.

Cells are organized into **tissues** that perform specialized tasks governed by the genes that are active in them. For example, some cells are joined together to form muscle tissue, which can contract. Tissues also are organized in sets to form whole **organs**. In the heart organ, for example, muscle tissues, nerve tissues, connective tissues, and other types all work together to pump blood. Some jobs around the body require that several related organs cooperate to perform them. The organs that join together to work on a function are parts of a **body system**. For example, the heart, lungs, and blood vessels all work to deliver oxygen and nutrients to the body tissues as parts of the cardiovascular system. The next few sections present some body systems with special significance to nutrition.

gene: a unit of a cell's inheritance, made of a chemical, DNA, that directs the making of a protein do the body's work. (Proteins are described fully in Chapter 6.)

enzyme: a protein catalyst. A catalyst is an agent that facilitates a chemical reaction without itself being altered in the process.

tissues: systems of cells working together to perform specialized tasks.

organs: discrete structural units made of tissues that perform specific jobs.

body system: a group of related organs that work together to perform a function composed of several organs' jobs.

❚❚▶ *The body's cells need energy fuel, oxygen, water, and essential nutrients to remain healthy and to do their work. Genes direct the making of each cell's machinery, including enzymes. Specialized cells are grouped together to form tissues and organs; organs work together in body systems.*

❚❚❚ The Body Fluids and the Cardiovascular System

Every cell of the body needs a continuous supply of oxygen, energy, water, and building materials. The body fluids supply these necessities, bathing the outsides of all the cells much as the water of the ancient ocean bathed their one-celled ancestors (Figure 3–2). Every cell continuously uses up oxygen and

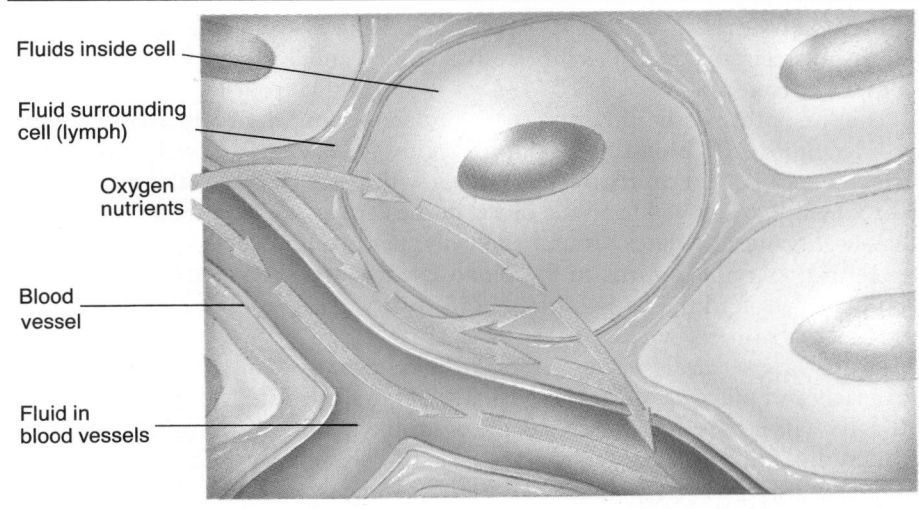

Fluids inside cell

Fluid surrounding cell (lymph)

Oxygen nutrients

Blood vessel

Fluid in blood vessels

Carbon dioxide wastes

❚❚❚ Figure 3–2

One Cell and the Associated Fluids

■■■ Figure 3–3

How the Body Fluids Circulate Around Cells.

A. Portion of body tissue.
  1. Blood enters tissues by way of an artery.
  2. Blood circulates among cells by way of capillaries.
  3. Blood collects into veins for return to heart.
B. Detail of A.
  1. Lymph filters out of capillary.
  2. Exchange of materials takes place between cell fluid and lymph.
  3. Lymph circulates away, later reentering bloodstream in a vein.

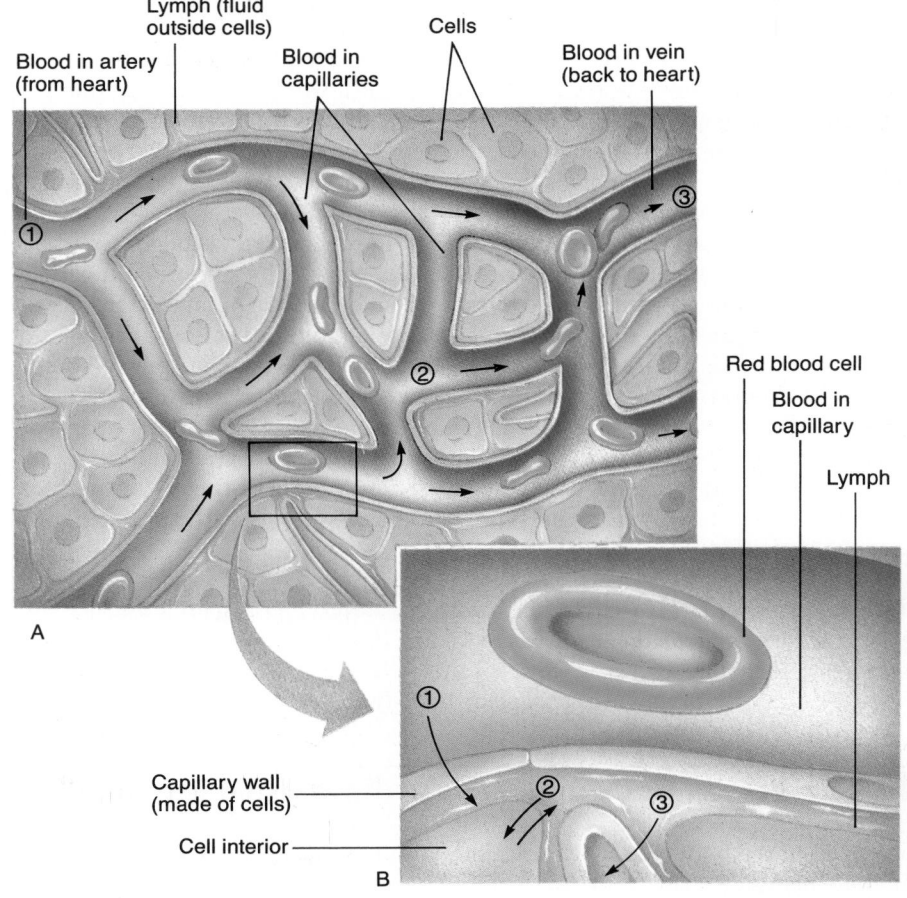

nutrients (producing carbon dioxide and other waste products). The body fluids must circulate to pick up fresh supplies and to deliver the wastes to points of disposal.

The fluids that bathe the cells and circulate around the body are the extra-cellular fluids, the **blood** and **lymph** (Figure 3–3). Blood travels within the **arteries**, **veins**, and **capillaries**, as well as within the heart's chambers (Figure 3–4). Lymph is derived from the blood in the capillaries; it squeezes out across their walls and circulates around the cells, permitting exchange of materials. Some of the lymph returns to the blood farther along the capillaries, and the rest travels around the body by way of its own vessels, eventually returning to the bloodstream elsewhere.

As the blood travels through the cardiovascular system, it delivers needed materials and picks up wastes. Figure 3–4 shows its route, which ensures that all cells will be served. The blood picks up oxygen in the **lungs** and releases carbon dioxide there, as Figure 3–5 (page 68) shows. All the blood circulates to the lungs, then returns to the heart, where it receives powerful impetus from the pumping heartbeats that push it out to all the other body tissues. Thus all tissues receive oxygenated blood fresh from the lungs.

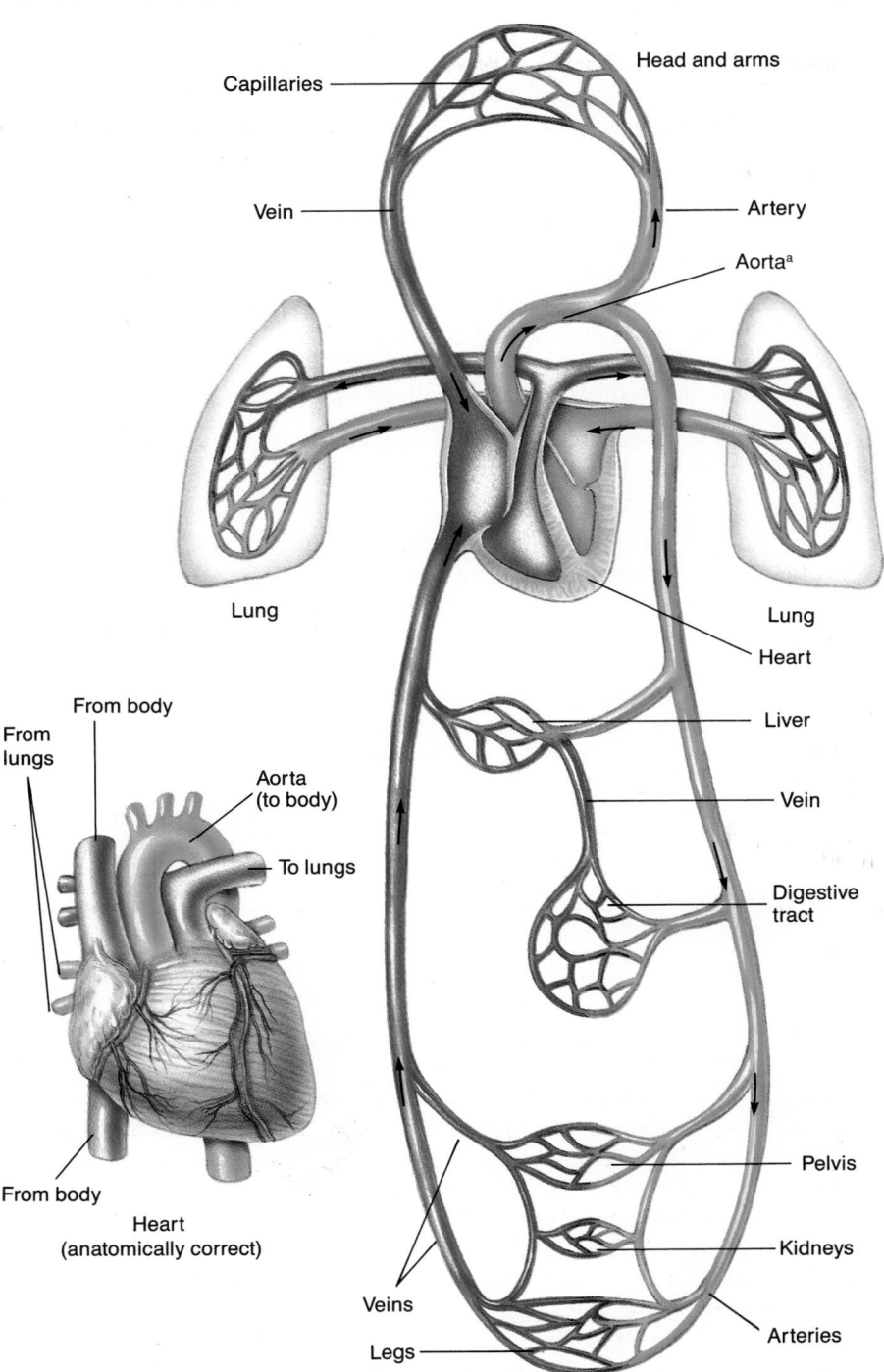

Capillaries

Head and arms

Vein

Artery

Aorta[a]

Lung

Lung

Heart

Liver

Vein

Digestive tract

Pelvis

Kidneys

Arteries

Veins

Legs

From body

From lungs

Aorta (to body)

To lungs

From body

Heart (anatomically correct)

[a]The aorta is the main artery that launches blood on its course through the body. The picture is not anatomically correct but is drawn this way for clarity. The aorta actually arises behind the left side of the heart and arcs upwards, then divides. See detail of heart.

■■■ **Figure 3–4**

Cardiovascular System. Blood leaves right side of heart, picks up oxygen in lungs, and returns to left side of heart. Blood leaves left side of heart, goes to head or digestive tract and then to liver or lower body, and then returns to right side of heart.

blood: the fluid of the cardiovascular system—composed of water, red and white blood cells, other formed particles, nutrients, oxygen, and other constituents.

lymph (LIMF): the fluid that bathes the cells, derived from the blood by being pressed through the capillary walls. Lymph moves through tissue spaces and travels in its own vessels, which eventually drain back into the bloodstream.

arteries: blood vessels that carry blood containing fresh oxygen supplies from the heart to the tissues. See Figure 3–4.

veins: blood vessels that carry used blood from the tissues back to the heart. See Figure 3–4.

capillaries: minute, weblike blood vessels that connect arteries to veins and permit transfer of materials between blood and tissues. See Figures 3–3 and 3–4.

lungs: the organs of gas exchange. Blood circulating through the lungs releases its carbon dioxide and picks up fresh oxygen to carry to the tissues.

intestine: a long, tubular organ of digestion and the site of nutrient absorption.

liver: a large, many-lobed organ that lies under the ribs. It filters the blood, removing and processing nutrients, manufacturing materials for export to other parts of the body, and destroying toxins or storing them out of circulation.

kidneys: the organs that filter the blood to remove waste material and forward it to the bladder for excretion out of the body.

Details on the intestines, liver, and kidneys are presented later.

Chapter 10 describes the nutrition implications of sweating.

As it passes the digestive system, the blood delivers oxygen to the cells there and picks up nutrients from the **intestine** for distribution elsewhere. All blood leaving the digestive system must go directly to the **liver**, which has the special task of chemically altering the absorbed materials to make them better suited for use by other tissues. Later, in passing through the **kidneys**, the blood is cleansed of wastes.

As it flows through the skin, the blood also helps regulate the body temperature in two ways. First, heat generated by the internal organs is carried by blood to the skin, where it radiates into the surroundings. Second, fluid from lymph is used to make sweat, which carries off large amounts of heat when it evaporates. After being cooled, the blood returns to the deep body core, where it siphons off additional excess heat. (There's more on temperature regulation in a later section.)

In summary, the blood is routed as follows (look again at Figure 3–4):

■ Heart to body to heart to lungs to heart (repeat). The portion of the blood that flows by the intestine travels from:
■ Heart to intestine to liver to heart.

To ensure efficient circulation of fluid to all your cells, you need an ample fluid intake. This means drinking sufficient water to replace the water you necessarily lose every day. You also need to maintain your cardiovascular fitness, a project that requires combined attention to nutrition and physical activity. Moreover, you need healthy red blood cells because these carry oxygen to all the other cells, enabling them to burn their fuels for energy. Since red blood cells are born, live, and die within about four months, you need to replace them constantly, a manufacturing process that requires many essential nutrients from food. Many kinds of blood disorders are caused by dietary deficiencies of vitamins or minerals; the blood is very sensitive to malnutrition.

■■■ **Figure 3–5**

Oxygen-Carbon Dioxide Exchange in the Lungs.

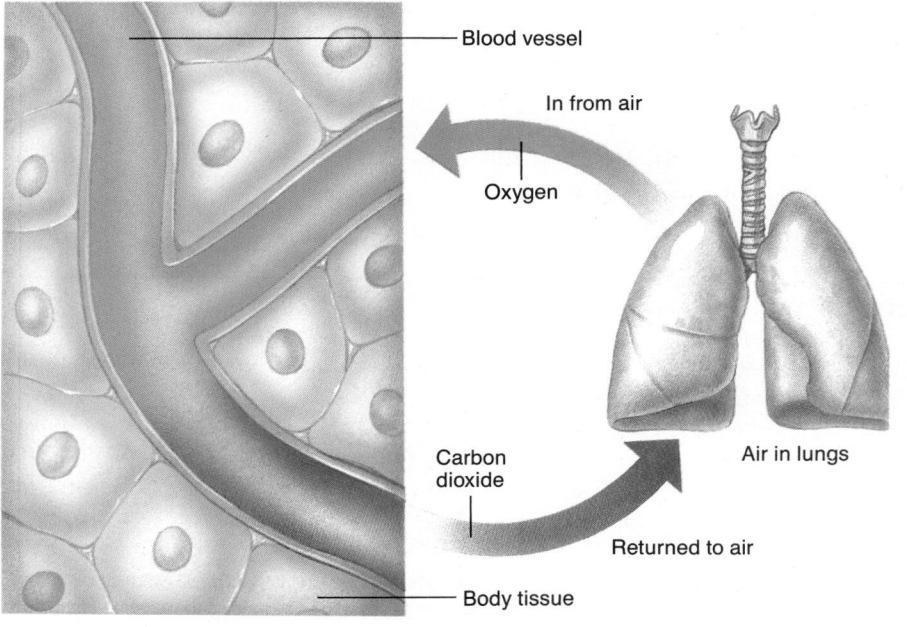

◼◼▶ *Blood and lymph deliver oxygen and nutrients to all the body's cells and carry waste materials away from them. The cardiovascular system ensures that these fluids circulate among all the organs, enabling each organ to contribute and to remove materials.*

◼◼◼ The Immune System

Many of the body's cells cooperate to maintain its defenses against infection. The skin presents a physical barrier, and the body's cavities (lungs, digestive tract, and others) are lined with membranes that resist penetration by invading **microbes** or unwanted substances. The body's linings are easily damaged by nutrient deficiencies, and clinicians inspect both the skin and the inside of the mouth to detect signs of malnutrition. (The chapters on protein, vitamins, minerals, and energy present details of the signs of deficiencies.)

When a wound or infection penetrates these first lines of defense (the skin and linings), the lymph and blood present internal defenses: cells and proteins that can inactivate, remove, or destroy microbes and foreign substances. Special cells are able to recognize the chemical structures of some foreign materials and to remember them for a time so that they can quickly mobilize their defenses when they see them again. This ability confers **immunity** against many diseases that you have previously fought and conquered. Some immune cells produce proteins that act as ammunition (**antibodies**) designed to destroy specific targets (**antigens**), and still other cells can gobble up and digest the injured invaders—to clean up the battlefield, so to speak.

Immune system components reside in tissues all over the body—in the linings of the bones, in the digestive tract, in the blood vessels, in the lymph glands, and in glands of their own. They are in constant flux, being made and dismantled rapidly, and their maintenance requires a continuous supply of nutrients. A deficiency or an overdose of any nutrient is likely to affect the immune system adversely, and a deficiency of nutrients early in an infant's development can weaken that individual's immune defenses against infection for years.

◼◼▶ *The immune system confers ability to resist disease. Its successful functioning depends on an adequate nutrient supply.*

◼◼◼ The Hormonal and Nervous Systems

In addition to nutrients, oxygen, wastes, immune cells, and proteins, the blood also carries chemical messages from one system of cells to another. These communicate changing conditions that demand responses. The chemical messages, or **hormones**, are secreted and released into the blood by organs known as glands. For example, when the **pancreas** (a gland) experiences a high concentration of the blood's sugar, glucose, it releases **insulin** (a hormone). Insulin stimulates the liver, muscles, and fat cells to remove glucose from the blood and to store it. When the blood glucose level falls, the pancreas secretes another hormone to which the liver responds by releasing glucose into the blood once again.

---

microbes: bacteria, viruses, or other organisms invisible to the naked eye; some cause disease.

immunity: the ability to successfully resist a disease, conferred on the body by way of the immune system's memory of previous exposure to that disease and its ability to mount a specific defense promptly and swiftly.

antibodies: proteins made by the immune system, expressly designed to combine with and to inactivate specific antigens. (For more on proteins, see Chapter 6.)

antigens: microbes or substances that are foreign to the body.

hormones: chemicals that are secreted by glands in response to conditions in the body that require a response. These chemicals serve as messengers, acting on other organs to change those conditions.

pancreas: an organ with two main functions. One is an *endocrine* function—the making of hormones such as insulin, which it releases directly into the blood (*endo* means "into" the blood). The other is an *exocrine* function—the manufacture of digestive enzymes, which it releases through a duct into the small intestine to assist in digestion (*exo* means "out" into a body cavity or onto the skin surface).

insulin: a hormone from the pancreas that helps glucose get into cells (more in Chapter 4).

Chapter 11 offers more on nutrition's contributions to the body's defense systems.

Chapter 4, whose subject is carbohydrates, describes the regulation of blood glucose in greater detail.

hunger: the physiological need to eat, experienced as an unpleasant sensation that demands relief.

appetite: the psychological desire to eat, experienced as a pleasant sensation that accompanies the sight, smell, or thought of certain foods.

cortex: the outermost layer of something. The brain's cortex is that part of the brain in which conscious thought takes place.

hypothalamus (high-poh-THAL-uh-mus): a part of the brain that senses a variety of conditions in the blood, such as temperature, glucose content, salt content, and others. It signals other parts of the brain or body to change those conditions when necessary.

Hunger and appetite usually occur together, but either may occur without the other (more in Chapter 9). More about women's hormones and appetite in Chapters 12 and 13.

▮▮▮ Figure 3–6

The Brain's Hypothalamus and Cortex. The hypothalamus monitors the body's conditions and sends signals to the brain's thinking portion, the cortex, which decides on actions.

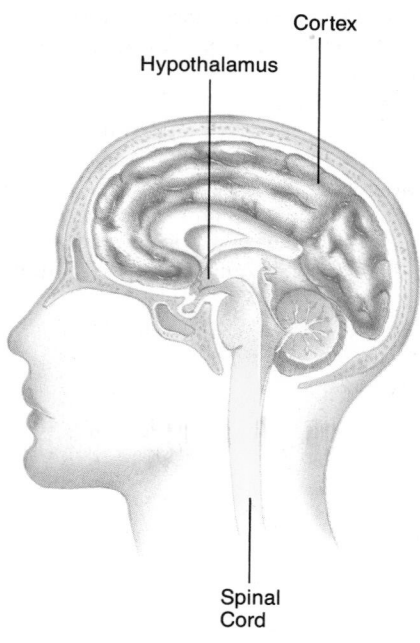

Glands and hormones abound in the body. Each gland monitors a condition and produces one or more hormones to regulate it. Each hormone acts as a message that stimulates certain organs to take appropriate action. Examples of the working of these hormones appear throughout this book.

Nutrition affects the hormonal system. Fasting, feeding, and exercise alter hormonal balances. People who become very thin have an altered hormonal balance that makes them unable to maintain their bones. People who eat high-fat diets have hormone levels that make them susceptible to certain cancers.

Hormones also affect nutrition. Along with the nervous system, they regulate **hunger** and affect **appetite**. Hormones also regulate the menstrual cycle in women, and they affect women's appetites differently at different times in the cycle and in pregnancy. An abnormal hormonal state is probably at least partly responsible, too, for the loss of appetite that sick people experience. Hormones also regulate the body's reaction to stress, suppressing hunger and the digestion and absorption of nutrients. Whenever questions about a person's nutrition are asked, the state of that person's hormonal system is always part of the answer.

The body's other major communication system is, of course, the nervous system. With the brain and spinal cord as central controllers, the system receives and integrates messages from sensory receptors all over the body— sight, hearing, touch, smell, taste, and others—which all communicate to the brain the state of both the outer and inner worlds, including the availability of food and the need to eat. The system then returns instructions to the muscles and glands, telling them what to do.

The nervous system's part in hunger regulation is coordinated by the brain. The sensations of hunger and appetite are experienced in the **cortex** of the brain, the thinking, outer layer. However, much of the brain's regulatory work goes on without the person's (or the cortex's) awareness in the deep brain centers. An organ there, the **hypothalamus** (Figure 3–6), monitors many body conditions, including the availability of nutrients and water. The digestive tract sends messages to the hypothalamus via hormones and nerves that signal the physiological need for food. The signals also stimulate the stomach to intensify its contractions and secretions, creating hunger pangs (and gurgling sounds). Becoming conscious of hunger, then, you eat. The conscious mind of the cortex can override such signals, and a person can delay eating, despite hunger, or eat when hunger is absent.

▮▮▶ *The hormonal and nervous systems facilitate regulation of body processes through communication among all the organs. They respond to the need for food, govern the act of eating, and regulate digestion.*

▮▮▮ The Digestive System

When your body needs food, your brain and hormones alert your conscious mind to the sensation of hunger. Once you have eaten, your brain and hormones then direct the many organs of the digestive system to digest and to absorb the complex mixture of chewed and swallowed food that you have delivered to them. This section presents only an introduction to the digestive system, but later chapters come back to its roles in digesting and absorbing individual nutrients.

A diagram of the digestive tract and associated organs appears in Figure 3-7. The tract itself is a flexible, muscular tube measuring about 26 feet in length from the mouth, through the throat, esophagus, stomach, small intestine, large

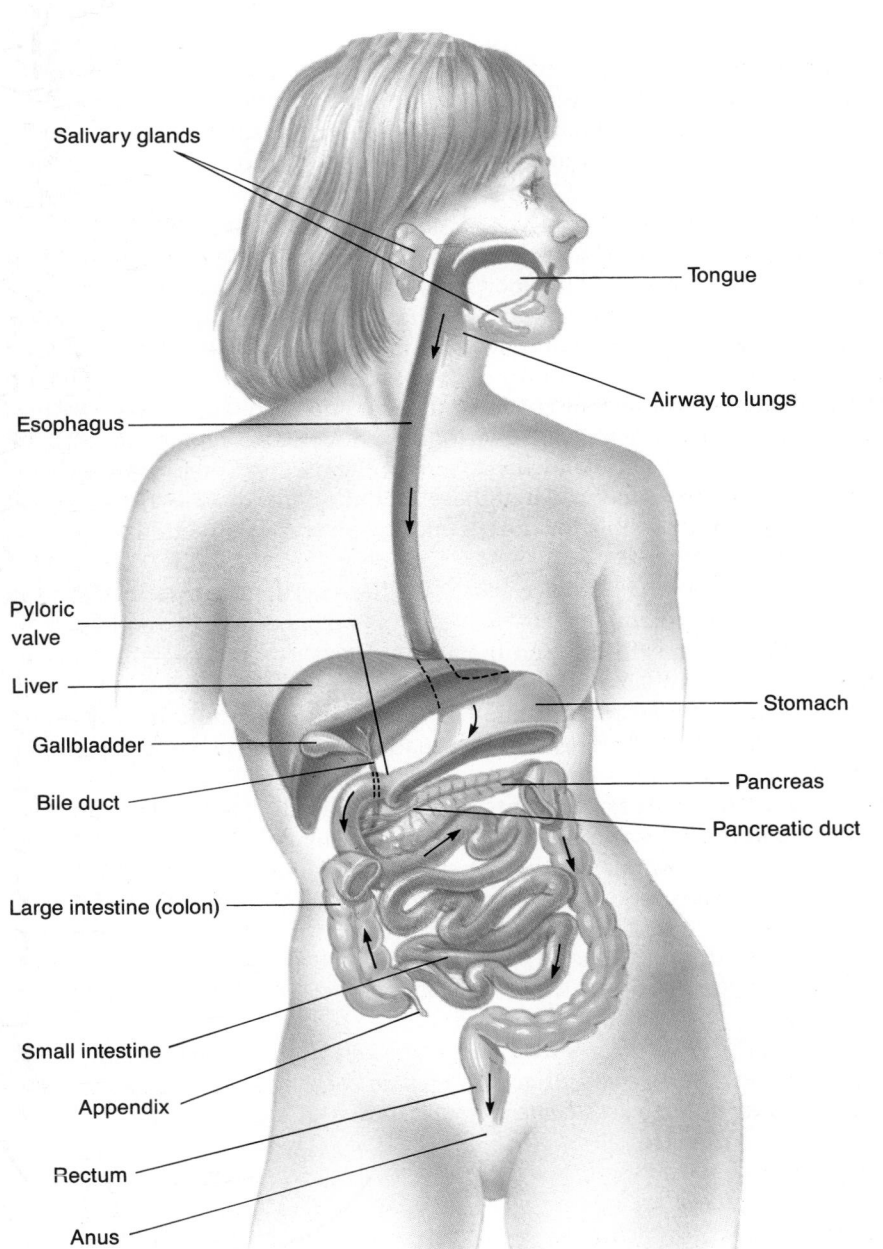

■■■

The Digestive System.

Mouth:
    Chews and mixes food with saliva
    Donates mainly starch-digesting enzymes
Esophagus:
    Passes food to stomach
Stomach:
    Adds acid, enzymes, and fluid
    Churns, mixes, and grinds food to a liquid mass
Small intestine:
    Secretes enzymes that digest all food to small nutrient particles
    Cells of wall absorb nutrients into blood and lymph
Liver:
    Manufactures bile, a detergentlike substance, to help digest fats
Gall bladder[a]
    Stores bile until needed
Bile duct:
    Conducts bile into small intestine
Pancreas:
    Manufactures enzymes to digest food and bicarbonate to neutralize stomach acid
Pancreatic duct:[b]
    Conducts pancreatic juice into small intestine
Large intestine (colon):
    Reabsorbs water and minerals
    Passes undigested waste (fiber, bacteria, and some water) to rectum
Rectum:
    Stores waste prior to elimination
Anus:
    Holds rectum closed
    Opens to allow elimination

[a]The gallbladder is a sac embedded in the liver that stores bile. The gallbladder releases bile through a duct into the small intestine whenever fat is present there.
[b]In some people, the pancreatic duct merges with the bile duct before they open into the small intestine. The common portion is called the *common bile duct*.

peristalsis (perri-STALL-sis): the wavelike squeezing motions of the esophogus, stomach, and intestines that push their contents along.

stomach: a muscular, elastic, sacklike portion of the digestive tract that grinds and churns swallowed food.

small intestine: a 20-foot length of small-diameter intestine that is the major site of digestion of food and absorption of nutrients.

pyloric valve (pye-LORE-ick): the circular muscle of the lower stomach that regulates the flow of partly digested food into the small intestine.

large intestine (colon): the portion of the intestine that completes the absorption process.

intestine, and rectum to the anus. In a sense the human body is itself a tube that surrounds this series of digestive organs. When you have swallowed something, it still is not inside your body; it is only inside the inner bore of this tube. Only when a nutrient or other substance penetrates the digestive tract wall does it actually enter the body's tissues; many things pass into the body and out again, unabsorbed.

The digestive system's job is to render food into its component nutrients and then to absorb those nutrients, leaving behind the substances that are appropriate to excrete. To do this the system works at two levels—one, mechanical; the other, chemical.

The Mechanical Aspect of Digestion

The mechanical job of digestion is to chew and to crush foods and to add sufficient water to them so that the digestive enzymes can gain access to all of the component molecules. This job is accomplished first by chewing and the addition of saliva and then by various grinding and squeezing actions of the stomach and intestines. The best known of these actions is **peristalsis**, a series of squeezing waves that pass all the way down the digestive tract from the top of the esophagus to the rectum, pushing the contents through the tract. Besides these actions, the **stomach** grinds the swallowed food into a fine paste, and the stomach and intestines also add water, so that the paste becomes progressively more dilute as it moves along. All of these actions divide and mix the intestinal contents, making it possible for the chemical processes of digestion to proceed efficiently.

Chemical digestion takes place mostly in the **small intestine**, beyond the stomach, and is so complicated that only small amounts of foods can be processed at one time. To this end the stomach acts as a holding tank, and its **pyloric valve**, a circular muscle constricting the stomach at its lower end, controls the exit of the contents, allowing only a little at a time to be squirted forcefully into the small intestine. Gradually the stomach empties itself by means of these powerful squirts.

By the time the intestinal contents have arrived in the **large intestine** (also called the **colon**), digestion is nearly complete. The colon's task is mostly to absorb water and minerals, leaving a paste of fiber and other undigested materials suitable for excretion. The fiber provides bulk against which the muscles of the colon can work. The rectum then stores this material to be excreted at intervals.

⫿▷ *The digestive tract renders food into absorbable nutrients by mechanical and chemical means. The mechanical actions include chewing, grinding by the stomach, and moving of the tract's contents by peristalsis. After digestion and absorption, wastes are excreted.*

The Chemical Aspect of Digestion

Several organs of the digestive system secrete special juices that contain enzymes to disintegrate food into its component parts: the salivary glands, the stomach, the pancreas, the liver, and the small intestine. Table 3–1 summarizes their secretions.

The digestive juices and enzymes within the digestive tract might digest the tract's own cellular lining were it not for cells of that lining that specialize in protecting it. These cells secrete a thick, viscous substance known as **mucus**, which coats the digestive tract lining and ensures that it will not itself be digested.

Digestion begins in the mouth, where a salivary enzyme starts breaking down starch. It proceeds further in the stomach, where protein digestion begins. But the process gets under way in earnest in the small intestine; it is "the" organ of digestion and absorption; and it finishes the job the mouth and stomach have started.

The small intestine works with the precision of a laboratory chemist. As the thoroughly liquefied and partially digested nutrient mixture arrives there, hormonal messages tell the gallbladder to send its **emulsifier**, **bile**, in amounts matched to the amount of fat present. Other hormones notify the pancreas to release **bicarbonate** in amounts precisely adjusted to neutralize the stomach acid, as well as enzymes of the appropriate kinds and quantities to continue dismantling whatever large molecules remain.

Meanwhile the pancreatic and intestinal enzymes act on the bonds that hold the large nutrients together so that smaller and smaller pieces appear in the intestinal fluids. Finally, nutrients that can be absorbed and that the cells can use are released. Nutrients released early in the digestive process or those requiring no special handling, such as sugars or some vitamins, are absorbed

mucus (MYOO-cus): a slippery coating of the intestinal tract lining (and other body linings) that protects the cells from exposure to digestive juices (and other destructive agents). The adjective form is *mucous* (same pronunciation). The *mucous membrane* is the digestive tract lining.

emulsifier (ee-MULL-sih-fire): a compound with both water-soluble and fat-soluble portions that can attract fats and oils into water solution.

bile: a compound made by the liver, stored in the gallbladder, and secreted into the small intestine when needed. It emulsifies fats and oils to ready them for enzymatic digestion.

bicarbonate: a commonly occurring chemical that neutralizes acid; a secretion of the pancreas.

■■■ **Table 3–1 Summary of Digestive Secretions**

This is a summary of the main functions of the secretions of the digestive organs. Chapters 4, 5, and 6 discuss the digestion of the energy nutrients; Chapters 7 and 8 discuss the effects of digestive processes on vitamins and minerals.

Salivary glands:
  Saliva (fluid).
  Enzyme (breaks down starch).

Stomach glands:
  Gastric juice (fluid).
  Hydrochloric acid (uncoils protein).
  Enzyme (breaks down protein).
  Mucus (thick coating that protects the stomach wall from these secretions).

Pancreas:
  Bicarbonate (neutralizes acid fluid from stomach so that intestinal and pancreatic enzymes can work).
  Pancreatic enzymes (break down carbohydrate, fat, and protein).

Liver:
  Bile (emulsifier that separates fat into small particles that enzymes can attack).

Gallbladder:
  (Stores bile from liver until needed in small intestine.)

Small intestine:
  Enzymes (break down carbohydrate and protein).
  Mucus (thin coating that protects the intestinal wall).

villi (VILL-ee, VILL-eye): fingerlike projections of the sheet of cells that line the intestinal tract; the villi make the surface area much greater than it would otherwise be (singular: *villus*).

microvilli (MY-croh-VILL-ee, MY-croh-VILL-eye): tiny, hairlike projections on each cell of every villus that can trap nutrient particles and transport them into the cells (singular: *microvillus*).

bladder: the sac that holds urine until time for elimination.

high in the small intestine; nutrients that are released slowly or that do require special handling are absorbed further down. Chemical digestion is essentially complete by the time the intestinal contents enter the colon. However, water, fiber, and some minerals remain.

The digestive system can adjust to whatever mixture of foods is presented to it. People sometimes wonder if the digestive tract has trouble digesting certain foods in combination, for example, fruit and meat. The fad of "food combining" claims that the digestive tract cannot handle more than one task at a time, but this is a gross underestimation of the body's capabilities. The truth is that all foods, regardless of identity, are broken down by enzymes into the basic units that make them up. Whether the nutrients occurred originally in a banana or in a chili dog makes little difference to the digestive tract, which can polish off either or both with dispatch.

▌▌▶ *Chemical digestion begins in the mouth, where food is mixed with saliva that acts on carbohydrate. It proceeds in the stomach, where stomach juices break down protein. It continues in the small intestine, where the liver and gallbladder donate bile that emulsifies fat and where the pancreas and small intestine both donate enzymes that continue chemical digestion.*

Absorption and Transport of Nutrients

Once the digestive system has broken food down to its nutrient components, it must deliver them to the rest of the body. The cells of the intestinal lining absorb nutrients from the mixture within the intestine and deposit them in the blood and lymph. Every molecule of nutrient must traverse one of these cells if it is to enter the body fluids. The cells are selective: they can recognize the nutrients needed by the body. The cells are also extraordinarily efficient: they absorb enough nutrients to nourish all the body's other cells.

The intestinal tract lining is composed of a single sheet of cells, and the sheet pokes out into millions of finger-shaped projections (**villi**). Each villus has its own capillary network and a lymph vessel so that as nutrients move across the cells, they can immediately mingle into the body fluids. On every villus every cell has a brushlike covering of tiny hairs (**microvilli**) that can trap the nutrient particles. Figure 3–8 and Figure 3–9 provide a close look at these details.

The small intestine's lining, villi and all, is wrinkled into thousands of folds, so that its absorbing surface is enormous. If the folds, and the villi that cover them, were spread out flat, the total area would equal a third of a football field in size. The billions of cells of that surface, although they weigh only 4 to 5 pounds, absorb enough nutrients in a few hours a day to nourish the other 150 or so pounds of body tissues.

The blood and lymph then take over the job of transporting nutrients to their ultimate consumers, the body's cells. The lymph at first carries most of the products of fat digestion and a few vitamins, later delivering them to the blood. The blood carries the products of carbohydrate and protein digestion, most vitamins, and the minerals. Thanks to these two transportation systems, every nutrient arrives at the place where it is needed.

The process of rendering foods into nutrients and absorbing them into the body fluids is remarkably efficient. In a healthy body about 90 percent of the carbohydrate, fat, and protein that pass through the intestinal tract are digested to their component parts in time to be absorbed.

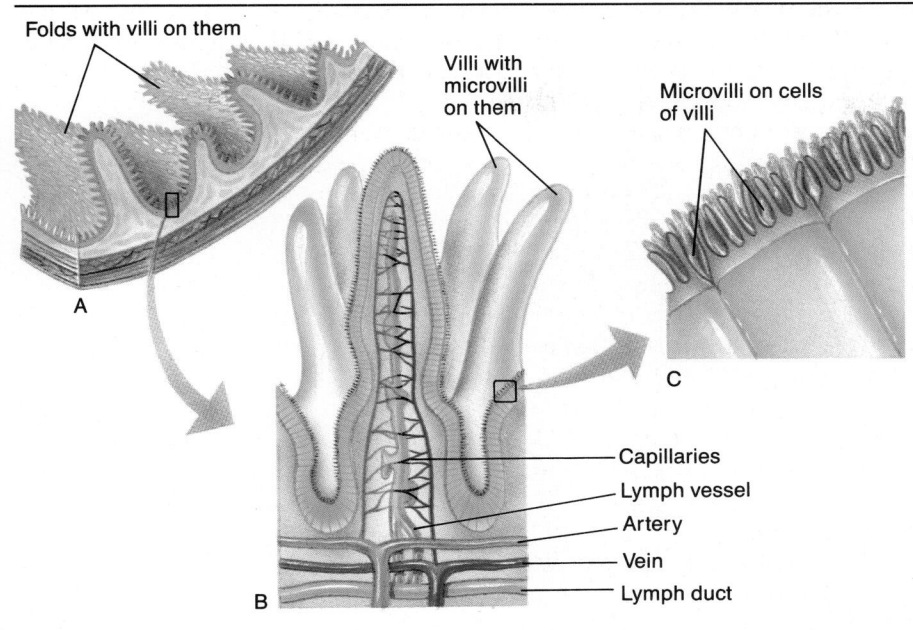

Folds with villi on them

Villi with microvilli on them

Microvilli on cells of villi

A

B

C

Capillaries
Lymph vessel
Artery
Vein
Lymph duct

■■■ **Figure 3–8**

Details of the Lining of the Small Intestine. The wall of the small intestine is wrinkled into thousands of folds and is carpeted with villi (part A). Each villus, in turn (part B), is covered with even smaller projections, the microvilli (part C).

The digestive system's millions of specialized cells are themselves sensitive to an undersupply of energy, nutrients, or dietary fiber. In cases of severe undernutrition, the absorptive surface of the small intestine shrinks and may be reduced to a tenth of its normal area, making it impossible to obtain what few nutrients a limited food supply may provide. Without sufficient fiber, the digestive tract muscles have too little bulk to push against and so get too little exercise, becoming weak. Malnutrition that impairs digestion is self-perpetuating because impaired digestion makes malnutrition worse.

❚❚▶ *The digestive system feeds the rest of the body and is itself sensitive to malnutrition. The folds and villi of the small intestine enlarge its surface area to facilitate nutrient absorption through uncountable microvilli on individual cell surfaces. Blood and lymph deliver nutrients to body cells.*

■■■ The Excretory System

To dispose of waste, the kidneys straddle the cardiovascular system and filter the passing blood, as Figure 3–10 shows. Waste materials removed with water are collected as urine in tubes that deliver them to the urinary **bladder**, which is periodically emptied. Thus the blood is purified continuously throughout the day, and dissolved materials are excreted as necessary (including sodium, to help keep blood pressure from rising too high). As you might expect, the kidneys' work is regulated by hormones secreted by glands that respond to conditions in the blood (such as the sodium concentration).

Whatever supports the health of the kidneys supports the health of the whole body because the kidneys cleanse the blood. A strong cardiovascular

■■■ **Figure 3–9**

Microvilli of the Small Intestine. The two dark objects are individual cells of two neighboring villi; the fingerlike projections that border them are microvilli. This photograph was taken through an electron microscope at a magnification of 51,000 times.

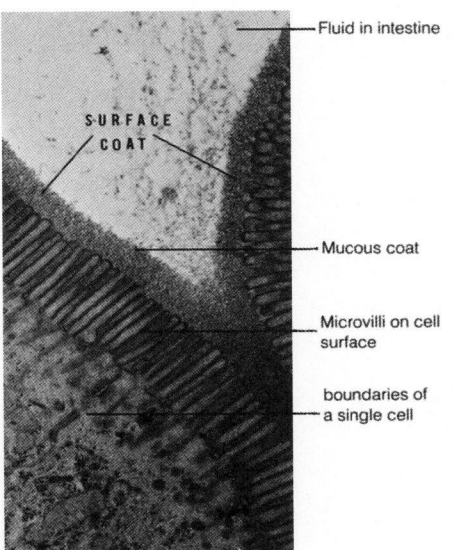

Fluid in intestine

SURFACE COAT

Mucous coat

Microvilli on cell surface

boundaries of a single cell

■■■ **Figure 3–10**

The Excretory System.
1. Blood enters kidney by way of arteries, and disperses into capillaries.
2. Kidney filters waste from blood and sends it as urine to the bladder.
3. Bladder periodically eliminates urine.

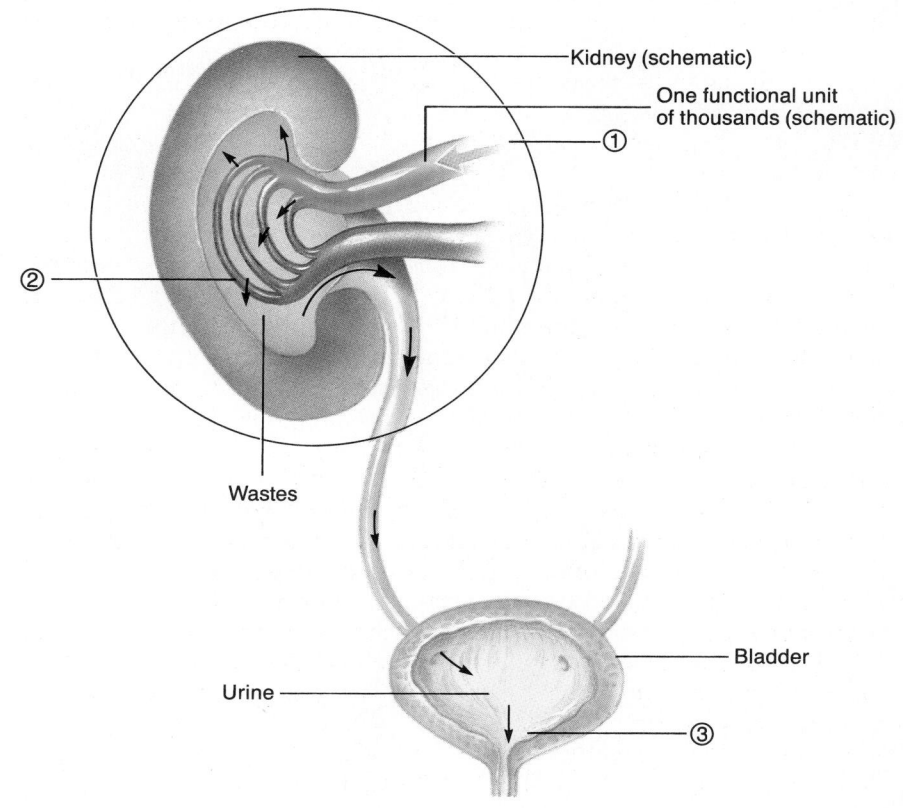

Kidney (schematic)

One functional unit of thousands (schematic) ①

②

Wastes

Urine

Bladder

③

system is important to keep blood flushing swiftly through the kidneys. Abundant water is also needed. In addition, the kidneys need sufficient energy to do their complex sifting and sorting job, and many vitamins and minerals serve as the cogs in their machinery. Exercise and nutrition are vital to healthy kidney function.

◧▶ *The kidneys adjust the blood's composition in response to the body's needs. Nutrients, including water, and exercise help keep them healthy.*

■■■ Storage Systems

A meal eaten in half an hour will provide nutrients that will reach the body fluids over a span of about four hours. However, as already mentioned, the cells of the body need their nutrients around the clock. Providing a constant flow of the needed nutrients to them requires the cooperation of many body systems. These systems store and release nutrients to meet the cells' needs between meals.

Nutrients collected from the digestive system sooner or later all move through a vast network of capillaries that weave among the liver cells, an arrangement that ensures that the cells may have access to the newly arriving nutrients. The liver cells process these nutrients. Later chapters provide the details, but it is important to know now that the liver converts excess energy-containing nutrients into two forms. It makes some into **glycogen** and some into **fat**. It stores the glycogen to use for the body's ongoing glucose needs, and it ships out the fat in packages (see Chapter 5) to be picked up by all cells that need it. All body cells may withdraw fat from these packages, and the excess fat winds up being stored in the **fat cells**, which hold it to meet long-term energy needs.

The liver's glycogen provides a reserve supply of glucose and thus can sustain cell activities if the intervals between meals become so long that glucose absorbed from ingested food is exhausted. But without food to replenish it, the liver's glycogen supply dwindles within one day and can be effectively depleted within as little as three to six hours. Similarly, fat tissue stores a reserve supply of fat, the body's other principal energy nutrient; but unlike the liver, the fat tissue has virtually infinite storage capacity. It can continue to supply fat for days, weeks, or possibly even months when no food is eaten.

These storage systems for glucose and fat ensure that the cells will not go without energy even if the body is hungry for food, except under extreme conditions. Body stores also exist for many other nutrients, each with a characteristic capacity. For example, the liver and fat cells store many vitamins, and the bones provide reserves of calcium, sodium, and other minerals that can be drawn on to keep the blood levels constant and to meet cellular demands.

Some nutrients are stored in the body in much larger quantities than are others. For example, stored amounts of certain vitamins can reach toxic levels if too-large quantities are eaten. Other nutrients, the ones that are stored in only small amounts, can readily be depleted. As this book discusses the body's handling of various nutrients, it pays particular attention to how they are stored so that you can know your tolerance limits. For example, you needn't eat fat at every meal, since fat is stored in virtually unlimited quantities in your body. On the other hand, you normally do need to have a source of carbohydrate at intervals throughout the day because the liver stores less than one day's worth of glycogen before becoming depleted.

❚❚▶ *The body stores large quantities of some nutrients, small quantities of others. Its energy stores are of two principal kinds: fat in the fat cells (in potentially large quantities) and glycogen in the liver cells (in smaller quantities).*

❚❚❚ Other Systems

In addition to the systems described above, the body has many more: the bones, the muscles, the reproductive organs, and others. All of these cooperate, enabling each cell to carry on its own life. Each system ensures, through hormonal or nerve-mediated messages, that its needs will be met by the others, and each contributes to the welfare of the whole by doing its own specialized work. Each needs a continuous supply of many specific nutrients to maintain itself and to carry out its work: calcium is particularly important for the bones, for example; iron for the muscles; glucose for the brain. But all systems need all nutrients, and every system is impaired by an undersupply or oversupply of them. And each responds to exercise—the bones and muscles by becoming stronger, the brain and reproductive organs by remaining healthy.

glycogen: a storage form of carbohydrate energy (gluclose), described more fully in Chapter 4.

fat: a storage form of lipid energy (triglycerides), described more fully in Chapter 5.

fat cells: cells that specialize in the storage of fat.

Chapter 9 describes what happens during fasting. Chapter 10 describes how the muscles also store glycogen for their own use.

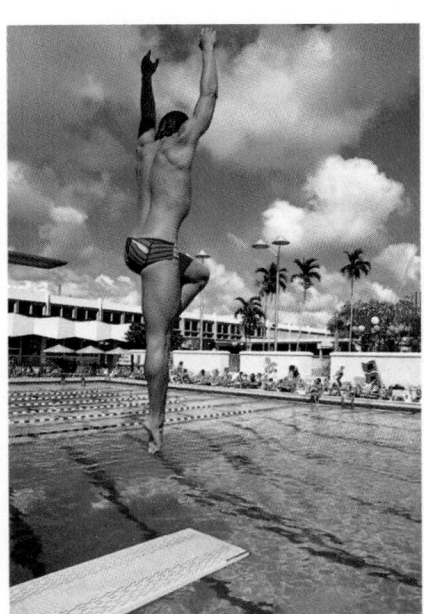

For the health of all body systems, people need exercise.

While external events clamor and vie for attention, the body remains quiet in its life-sustaining work. Of the billions of cells in the body, only a small percentage make up the cortex of the brain, in which the conscious mind resides. These cells receive messages from other cells when they require you to "become conscious" of a need for decision and action. In modern life the need may be as complex as, for example, noticing that you feel anxious and deciding to consult an advisor; or it may be a "simple" need, such as "I'm hungry, I guess I'd better eat."

Most of the body's work is done automatically by the other, unconscious portions of the brain and nervous system, and this work is finely regulated to achieve a state of well-being. But you need to involve your cortex—your consciousness—so as to cultivate an understanding and appreciation of your body's needs. Try to be mindful of its needs, and attend to nutrition first. The rewards are liberating—ample energy to tackle life's tasks, a robust attitude, and the glowing appearance that comes from the best of health. Indulge yourself in the foods available to you. But before you decide what is healthiest for you, read on, and learn to let nutrition principles guide your choices.

❚❚▶ *To achieve optimal function, the body's systems require nutrients from outside, and these have to be supplied through a human being's conscious food choices.*

This chapter has no Food Feature and no Self-Study.

▰▰▰ C O N T R O V E R S Y   3 ▰▰▰

Our Ancestors' Diet: Is It Best for Us?

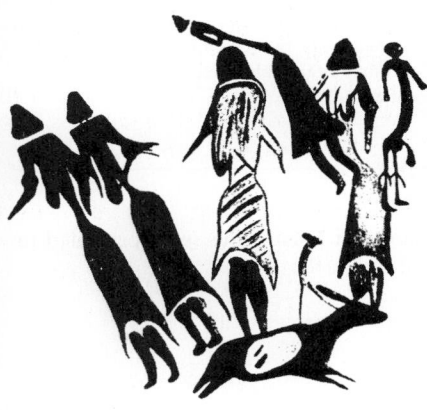

You may be clothed in the latest fashions, and your car may be the maker's latest model, but the body you live in is of prehistoric design. You have come a long way from the Stone Age in many ways: in language skills, in the arts, in medicine, and especially in the use of machinery. But in the ways your body handles food, bacteria, environmental pollutants, and other stresses, there have been hardly any changes. You have virtually the same body and brain today as your ancestors had 20,000 years ago.

Although the body has remained the same, the world has changed vastly, especially in the last hundred years. The earth is far more crowded than it used to be. In 1900 the world's population was 1 billion; now it is over 5 billion. Today hunger and starvation are a greater threat than ever before in the developing countries and even for some in the devloped countries. Some 15 million infants and children die each year from malnutrition and related causes.[1]

At the same time, abundance is also extreme, especially in the developed countries, since the technological era has brought great advantages. In much of the United States and Canada, for example, the food supply is abundant and relatively low in cost. The luxuries of convenience foods and high-speed cooking equipment, massive transportation and communication networks, and widespread economic security have made food so easily available that they have created problems of a different kind for people's health. People's diets are often much higher in fat, salt, and sugar and lower in fiber, vitamins, and minerals than those of the best-nourished people of the past. Most people's lifestyles offer much less physical activity than did the lives of their ancestors. Many people face new technological byproducts in their environments: smog, water pollution, and other forms of contamination. Your Stone Age body is stressed by contending with these new problems.

Thanks to modern technology, you have far greater freedom to choose foods from a far greater variety in local stores than ever before. But with freedom comes both risk and responsibility; you have to make choices. One of the questions you might be inclined to ask is, "Should I eat as my ancestors did?"

Some people think you should. They say that the diet of the typical, prosperous, middle-class North American consumer today is not suited to the body's needs. It is too high in fat, sugar, and salt; and it is too low in fiber, vitamins, and minerals. It is unnatural because most foods today are domesticated, refined, and processed to the point where they resemble very little the wild, natural, whole foods of earlier times. Some modern foods, they say, are even fabricated entirely from synthetic ingredients.

Others favor the way we eat today. They say that our foods can be combined into one of the most healthful, nutritious diets people have ever consumed. Our ancestors died young of a host of diseases, including food poisoning and malnutrition, without knowing how to prevent them. We know how to keep foods safe, and we know our nutrient needs, so we can meet them—if not with foods alone, then with foods and appropriate supplementation. There is no reason why we should go back to the primitive foods of the past when we can enjoy all the benefits of modern technology and eat delicious foods besides.

Who is right? Before arriving at any conclusions, it is necessary to know what our ancestors ate and how healthy they were. We have to begin by deciding which ancestors to study—our farmer forebears of

200 years ago, the early agricultural people who preceded them, or the hunter-gatherer people who lived still longer ago.

The people we should study are probably the earliest ones, the hunter-gatherers. They were the people of the Stone Age, the **paleolithic period**.[2] Their way of life and diet persisted for close to half a million years, vastly longer than the mere 10,000 years since the dawn of agriculture. Compared with the time since the beginning of the industrial era (about 1800), human beings have practiced agriculture for 10,000 years or more, 50 times longer. Ten thousand years may seem long, but try a second comparison. Imagine all of human existence on earth to have occurred within the last 24 hours. Then the agricultural era would have begun only 3 1/2 minutes ago, and the industrial era would have begun 4 *seconds* ago. People who grow their own food have thus occupied the earth for "only" a few *hundred* generations, while people who hunted for their food roamed the earth for *thousands* of generations. Figure C2–1 depicts the magnitude of the differences between the earlier people's times on earth and our time.

Enough time elapsed during hunter-gatherer times to permit natural selection of genes for traits that favored survival in the life and with the diet of the time, generation after generation. Many of the genes for these traits persist in our inheritance today. They are thousands of years old, and they still support

physical characteristics in us that would favor our survival in the conditions of those early times. In the few generations that have passed since then, not much evolutionary change has taken place.[3]

The more we know about the Stone Age people, then, the better we can understand our bodies' needs today. The publication of several popular novels in the *Earth's Children* series by Jean Auel*[1] has made it possible for people to learn informally not only about food and activities of those times but also about what the culture, traditions,

The Clan of the Cave Bear, The Valley of Horses, The Mammoth Hunters, and *The Plains of Passage* had been published at the time of this writing.

■■■ Figure C3–1

A Perspective on Modern Human Beings' Time on Earth. The *space* occupied in the pyramid is proportional to the *time* spent on earth

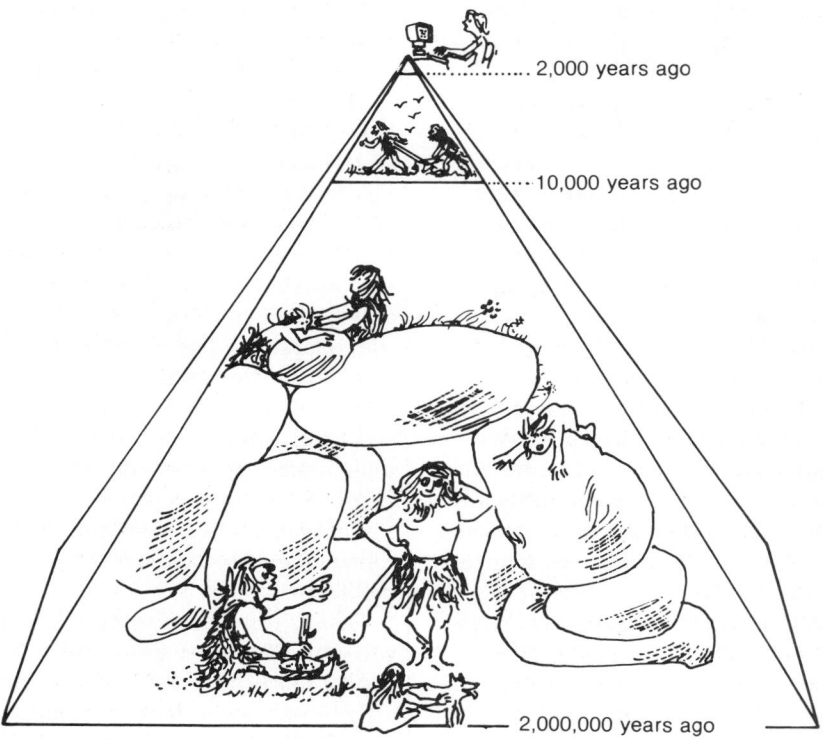

- - - - 2,000 years ago

- - - - 10,000 years ago

- - - - 2,000,000 years ago

SOURCE: Inspired by A. Leaf and P. C. Weber, A new era for science in nutrition, *American Journal of Clinical Nutrition* 45 (1987): 1048–1053.

and daily experiences of those people may have been like. The stories in the novels are fictional, but the descriptions are based on anthropological facts.

■■■ The Ancient Body in the Modern World

Food was not available all the time for the Stone Age people. Times of plenty alternated with times of famine. The human body was well adapted to this state of affairs. It was the body of an **omnivore**—a creature able to digest and to use the nutrients from both plants and animals. This made wide food choices possible and presented the least likelihood of starvation in the face of a food supply that depended on the geographical location and season. The body could also store excess energy-yielding nutrients when food was plentiful and then draw on these nutrients when threatened by starvation from famine or debilitating illness.

Our bodies still have those capabilities today. We can eat and derive nourishment from any of many different kinds of food. We also efficiently store surplus energy in body fat. Today, however, this ability confers less of an advantage because in food-abundant societies, the times of famine never come. The storage of surplus energy in body fat that served the Stone Age person so well now produces conditions that may shorten life. Obesity is responsible for many of today's ills. It precipitates diabetes

in susceptible people, it aggravates high blood pressure, it increases the likelihood of certain kinds of cancers, it worsens arthritis, and it harms health in many other ways.

The body feels hungry at approximately four- to six-hour intervals, even though it may have sufficient fat stores to last for many days. This adaptation also served the Stone Age people well, since it drove them to continue stocking fuel within their bodies as often as their digestive systems could perform the task, even when they had sufficient reserves for temporary needs. Thus they never had to dip deeply into those stores until the food supply ran out. Furthermore, their appetites were stimulated whenever they encountered foods that were likely to be especially important for them to consume when available. Among these foods were those that were rich in food energy—those with the taste of energy-rich fat or the sweetness of concentrated sugar. Other foods that appealed to their taste buds were those that tasted of salt, since pure salt was rarely available in the very early times and since the essential nutrient sodium was harder to come by then than now. Novel foods also appealed to them. For long periods their diets might have been monotonous; their curiosity and willingness to try new foods probably helped to ensure that they would obtain the nutrients their regular diet might have lacked.

We have the same traits today. We keenly feel hunger every four to six hours during the day, whether we

need to eat or not. We experience appetite on seeing, smelling, or tasting certain foods, even when we are not hungry—especially if the foods presented to us are rich in fat, sugar, or salt, or are foods that we don't often get the chance to eat. These traits still benefit people in many parts of the world where starvation and malnutrition are ever-present threats; but in food-abundant societies they contribute to overeating on the part of people who are already overfat.

Another adaptation of early human beings was the ability to respond to emergencies by instantly calling forth stored fuel and preparing to use it for maximum physical exertion. The surge of energy this gave our ancestors frequently helped them in overcoming or outrunning enemies. The ability to react this way to physical danger, known as the **fight-or-flight reaction** or as the **stress reaction**, is present with only minor variations in all animals, showing how universally important it is to survival. In human beings it is a magnificently well-coordinated response. The moment danger is detected, nerves and glands pour forth the stress hormones, and every organ of the body responds. The pupils of the eyes widen so that you can see better; the muscles tense up so that you can jump, run, or struggle with maximum strength; breathing quickens to bring more oxygen to the lungs. The heart races to rush oxygen to the muscles, and the blood pressure rises to deliver efficiently the fuel the muscles need for

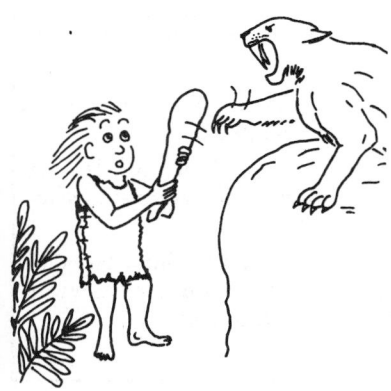

The fight-or-flight reaction

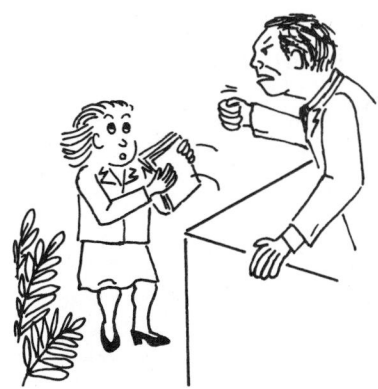

The stress reaction.

energy. The liver pours forth glucose from its stored supply, while the fat cells release fat, another fuel. The digestive system shuts down to permit all the body's systems to serve the muscles and nerves. With all of its action systems at peak efficiency, the body can respond with amazing speed and strength to whatever threatens it.

This adaptation serves people well in modern times, too, but only in war or in sport, when the stresses they face are physical. However, the stress reaction is called forth whenever any danger is perceived, even if it is an intangible, psychological, or economic threat. What stresses you today may be a boss who threatens to fire you or a teacher who gives you an undeserved low grade. You can't eliminate these threats by fighting or running, as your early ancestors did; in fact, you may have to smile at the enemy and suppress your fear or anger. But your heart still races, you feel it pounding, and

hormones still flood your bloodstream with glucose and fat fragments to support muscular action. At such a time, if you don't engage in vigorous exercise, eventually your body gets the message that these fuels are not needed, and it packs away both the glucose and fat fragments to be stored as fat. Your blood pressure stays high for a long time after the event, and your digestion is upset. People today have to learn to manage stress by learning to perceive events as not so alarming and by learning to work off their accumulated tension physically.

In other ways, too, the body is adapted to the conditions of earlier times. Heredity has given each human being a body that can *develop* to run after prey, to fight enemies, or to carry heavy burdens long distances; it responds to physical exertion by becoming stronger and swifter. Among the muscles that become stronger in response to exercise are the heart muscles, and they

also (like all muscles) become weaker without exercise. In ancient times, there was little likelihood that anyone would sit around for months at a time, but today people have to make special efforts to plan exercise into their daily routines if their muscles, including their heart muscles, are not to become weak.

Still another difference between the world our bodies are adapted for and the one they actually live in is the new chemicals present in our environments. The body has always had to defend itself against harmful substances ingested by mistake. The sense of taste is part of this defense; you refuse foods that do not taste right. A second part is the stomach's rejection response; you vomit up or wash out via diarrhea whatever "disagrees" with the digestive system. A third defense is the liver's filtering and detoxifying systems; toxins that get into the bloodstream are removed from it by the liver cells, which put some away in permanent storage and render others harmless and then release them for excretion.

For example, protection against the harmful effects of one ancient and familiar substance, alcohol, is built into your genes. Alcohol has been around ever since the first fruit ripened and fermented, so there have been thousands of generations for natural selection to mold a detoxifying system for it. Two of your genes code for two enzymes that in your liver convert alcohol into substances the body can use or excrete (Controversy 11 provides details). As long as the alcohol doses are small enough, the body can handle them because it is adapted to detoxify alcohol.

Today, however, many pollutants and toxins that are new to the body occur in our environment and get into food. If the body cannot efficiently excrete them, it may accumulate them in harmful quantities or convert them to odd, unfamiliar substances that can interfere with metabolism or cause cancer or birth defects. It may not even recognize them: for example, it possesses no sense to detect radioactivity.

All of these differences add up to a set of circumstances that challenge your body and mind to maintain health against many odds. You are living with the food, the labor-saving devices, the medical miracles, the contaminants, and all the other pleasures and problems of the twentieth century. However, you are housed in a body adapted to another world in which the weak died before they could reproduce and in which strong men and women survived on simple foods obtained through hard physical labor. You now have the freedom to choose many different kinds of foods, to eat often or seldom, to exercise a lot or a little. There is no guarantee that your diet and exercise routine, haphazardly chosen, will meet the needs of your Stone Age body.

Only with your brain can you compensate for these disadvantages of modern life. The Stone Age people used their brains to discover ways to obtain food; you must use

---

■■■ Miniglossary

fight-or-flight reaction: the body's instinctive, hormone- and nerve-mediated reaction to danger, also known as the *stress reaction.*

omnivore: an animal that eats both plant foods and the flesh of animals—for example, a human being. (Plant eaters are *herbivores*; flesh eaters are *carnivores*.)

paleolithic period: the Stone Age, the period from 10,000 to about 500,000 years ago, before agriculture, when human beings were hunter-gatherers and used stone tools (*paleo* means "ancient"; *lith* means "stone").

stress reaction: see *fight-or-flight reaction.*

---

yours, sometimes, to refuse delicious food and to battle the ancient instincts that cry out for you to eat. Stone Age people used their ingenuity to spare their energy when they could; you may have to use yours to find ways to increase your energy expenditure so that you can maintain appropriate weight and keep your heart and muscles fit. You have an advantage, though: you have access to more knowledge. Unlike your ancestors, you have the opportunity to learn how your body works and what it needs from food.

Researchers have turned to asking what the Stone Age people actually ate. We can learn from differences between the diet they ate long ago and the diets we eat today and can try to discern the significance those differences might have for us.

■■■ The Stone Age Diet

The probable diet of the Stone Age people has been analyzed to dis-

cover what foods they ate and how much of each nutrient they received. Although the figures are undoubtedly not exact, it is interesting to compare them with those of today. They probably consumed 3000 calories per day and were never obese. (Today we consume fewer than 2000 calories a day and still many of us are obese because we get so little exercise.)

Within their large energy allowances, the Stone Age people were able to meet all of their nutrient needs well. For example, although they drank no milk and made no cheese, their intakes of calcium were probably close to 1500 milligrams a day, thanks to the fruits and vegetables they consumed. Today we fall short of 800 milligrams, although recommendations state that many people (and especially young people) need more than 1000 milligrams to preserve the integrity of their bones. Stone Age people probably consumed close to 400 milligrams a day of vitamin C, whereas we take in less than 100 milligrams.

They ingested much more fiber than we do today, 45 grams or so, as compared with our 20 grams or less. They did this using only two of the four groups of foods we think of as important: meat and fruits/vegetables. Their intakes of meat, and therefore of protein, were two to five times higher than ours are today, but most of their meats were lean, whereas many of ours are high in fat. They apparently consumed cereal grains rarely, if at all, and they had no dairy foods whatsoever.[4] (Remember, this was before the development of agriculture.)

Although their total energy intakes were higher than ours, the people of the Stone Age had lower intakes of two no-no's that plague modern eaters: fat and sodium. Their cholesterol intakes were similar to ours, however, because even lean meat contains cholesterol. Also, their diet seldom contained concentrated sweets such as honey, and there was no such thing as purified, refined sugar.

Was this diet healthier for them than ours is for us? Stone Age people died younger than we do, but from causes we no longer face today. Our longer lives, however, are not the only reason that degenerative diseases have become more common.[5] Judging from the evidence available on primitive people living today (tribes in Africa and other places whose diets and ways of life resemble those of the Stone Age people), their way of life and diet can enable them to attain the age of 60 years relatively free of de-generative diseases.[6] The differences between their diets and ours are those that most concern medical experts today. The heart associations, cancer societies, diabetes associations, and even political governing bodies of many developed nations agree on these recommendations. To remain healthy into old age, they say, people should eat less fat, cholesterol, sugar, and salt and eat more foods rich in fiber, vitamins, and minerals than they do (see Chapter 2).

What does all of this mean in practice? Does it mean we should abandon the use of grains and dairy products and eat only meat and fruits/vegetables? The answer lies in the differences between foods of the Stone Age and those of today. Our meats are different in character and especially in the amount and type of fat they contain. Our fruits and vegetables are totally different. In fact, the question of whether we should eat as the Stone Age people did is purely academic, since the foods they ate are no longer available today. The environment they experienced no longer exists for us.

Still, even if we cannot eat the same foods they did, we can attempt to duplicate their activity and nutrient intake levels using the foods available to us. Clearly we should emulate them in incorporating more physical activity into our days. If we exercise more, we can eat more without getting fat; if we eat more, we can obtain more nutrients; and if we obtain nutrients, we are better protected against deficiencies.

In conclusion, no one can go back to the days of the Stone Age people and really live as they did. We can learn from them, though, the importance of getting more exercise and of eating wholesome foods that will support our health as well as, or even better than, theirs did.

Notes

1. D. R. Gwatkin, How many die? A set of demographic estimates of the annual number of infant and child deaths in the world, *American Journal of Public Health* 70 (1980): 1286–1289.

2. S. B. Eaton and M. Konner, Paleolithic nutrition, a consideration of its nature and current implications, *New England Journal of Medicine* 312 (1985): 283–289.

3. Eaton and Konner, 1985.

4. Eaton and Konner, 1985.

5. A. Leaf and P. C. Weber, A new era for science in nutrition, *American Journal of Clinical Nutrition* 45 (1987): 1048–1053.

6. Eaton and Konner, 1985.

The Carbohydrates: Sugar, Starch, Glycogen, and Fiber

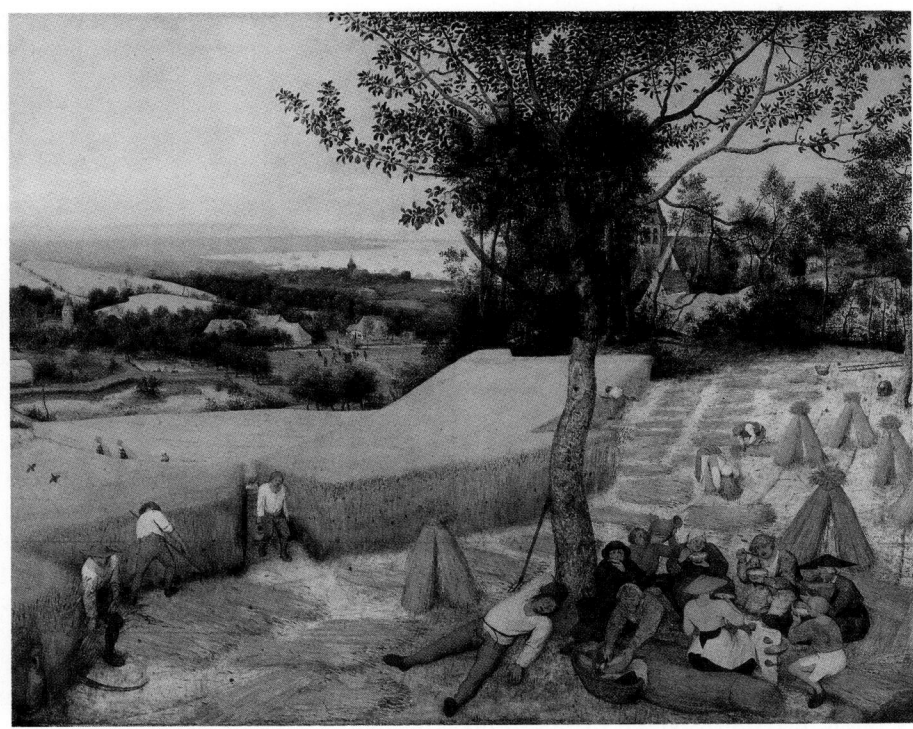

CONTENTS

The Harvesters by Pieter Bruegel, the Elder, © The Metropolitan Museum of Art, Rogers Fund, 1919 (19. 164). Photo by Eric Pollitzer.

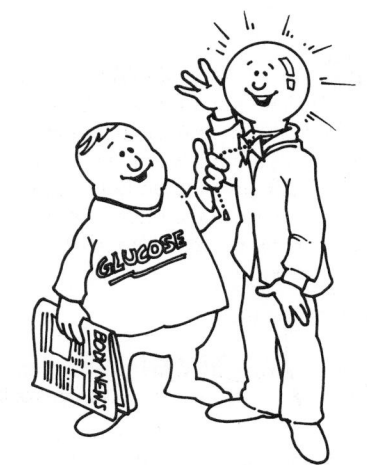

Glucose provides energy to the brain.

████ This chapter is the first of a series of three on the energy-yielding nutrients: it deals with the **carbohydrates**, including fiber. These nutrients, together with fat and protein, give bulk to foods and provide energy to the body. It is impossible to single out the most important nutrient: nutrients work together, in harmony, each affecting the functions of many others. However, carbohydrate is ideal to meet your body's energy needs, to keep your digestive system fit, to feed your brain and nervous system, and (and this may come as a surprise) to keep your body lean. Years of false propaganda about the evils of carbohydrate's supposed "fattening powers" have misled millions of weight-concious people to avoid carbohydrate-rich foods—a counterproductive tactic. People who wish to lose fat and maintain lean tissue can do no better than to design their diets around foods that supply carbohydrates in abundance. Consider the Chinese population who consume many more calories of food a day than do westerners, but who remain lithe and lean. Researchers believe that their high-carbohydrate, low-fat diet promotes their leaness. But all carbohydrates are not equal as far as nutrition is concerned.

This chapter invites you to learn to distinguish between the **complex carbohydrates** (starch and fiber), which are put to good use in the body, and the **simple carbohydrates** (sugars), whose value is questioned. The Controversy then asks whether the sugar added to foods harms health.

███ A Close Look at Carbohydrates

Carbohydrates contain the sun's radiant energy, captured in a form that living things can use to drive the processes of life. Thus they form the first link in the food chain that supports all life on earth. Carbohydrate-rich foods are obtained almost exclusively from plants; milk is the only animal-derived food that contains significant amounts of carbohydrate.

Green plants make carbohydrate through **photosynthesis**. In this process water from the plant's roots and carbon dioxide absorbed into its leaves combine in the presence of **chlorophyll** to yield the sugar **glucose**. Scientists know the reaction in the minutest detail, and yet it has never been reproduced from scratch; it requires green plants to make it happen (Figure 4–1).

Energy from the sun drives the photosynthesis reaction, and is trapped in the chemical bonds that hold six atoms of carbon in the special configuration that is glucose. The capture of energy in glucose is the part that is important to our survival. The sun's energy so caught and held will remain there until some agent (perhaps an animal's enzyme or one of yours) breaks the bonds, freeing the energy. The next few sections describe the forms that carbohydrates take, with their treasures of stored energy awaiting use in the human body.

██▷ *Through photosynthesis, plants combine carbon dioxide, water, and the sun's energy to form glucose. Carbohydrate is made of carbon, hydrogen, and oxygen held together by energy-containing bonds: carbo means "carbon"; hydrate means "water."*

Sugars and Starch

Glucose is a member of the chemical family known as **sugars**, or simple carbohydrates. These sugars, made in the leaves of green plants, provide energy for the work of all plant cells—those of the stem, roots, flowers, and fruits. For example, in the roots, far from the energy-giving rays of the sun, each cell takes some of the glucose made in the leaves, breaks it down (to carbon dioxide and water), and uses the energy thus released to fuel its own growth and water-gathering activities.

The last chapter of this book delves into humankind's relationship with the earth's food chain.

Plants make other sugar molecules—for example, **fructose**, the sweet sugar of fruit—by rearranging the atoms in glucose molecules. Fructose occurs mostly in fruits; in honey; and as part of another sugar, table sugar, to be described in a moment. Glucose and fructose are the most common single sugars, or **monosaccharides**, in nature. Another, monosaccharide, **galactose**, has the same numbers and kinds of atoms, but they are arranged still differently. Galactose is one of the two single sugars bound together to form the pair that make up the sugar of milk. It does not occur free in nature; it is instead tied up in milk sugar until it is freed during digestion.

Some sugars are pairs of sugars, **disaccharides**, made by linking two monosaccharides together. One is the sugar of milk, just mentioned—**lactose**, which consists of glucose linked to galactose. Another disaccharide, **maltose**, consists of two glucose units. Maltose appears wherever starch is being broken down. It occurs in germinating seeds and arises during the digestion of starch in the human body. When fructose and glucose are bonded together, they form **sucrose**, or table sugar, the product most people think of when they use the term *sugar*. This sugar is usually obtained by refining the juice from sugar beets or sugar cane, but it occurs naturally in many vegetables and fruits. It is of such major importance in human nutrition that Controversy 4 is devoted to it. Table 4–1 (next page) summarizes the sugars, the three monosaccharides, and the three disaccharides just named.

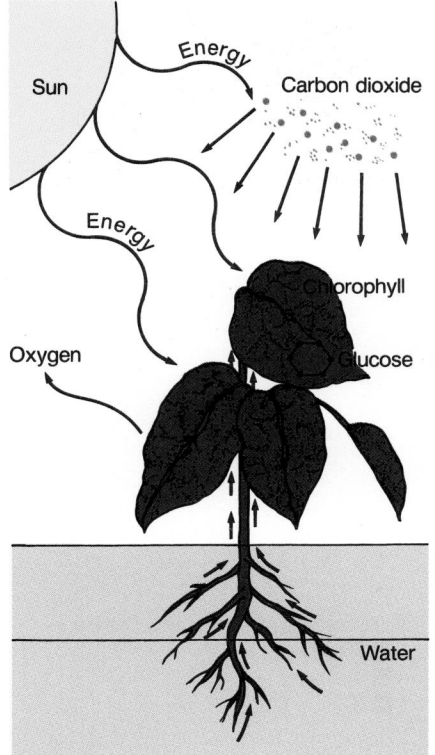

■■■ **Figure 4–1**

Carbohydrate—Mainly Glucose—Is Made by Photosynthesis. The sun's energy becomes part of the glucose molecule—its calories, in a sense. In the molecule of glucose here, dots represent the carbon atoms; bars represent the chemical bonds that contain energy.

Carbohydrates:
- ■ Sugars.
- ■ Starch.
- ■ Fiber.

Simple carbohydrates (sugars):
- ■ Single sugars (monosaccharides).
- ■ Paired sugars (disaccharides).

■■■ **Miniglossary of Carbohydrate Terms**

carbohydrates: compounds composed of single sugars or multiples of them.

complex carbohydrates: long chains of sugars arranged as starch or fiber. (The basic *sugar* unit is a molecule containing six carbon atoms, together with oxygen and hydrogen atoms.) Also called *polysaccharides*.

simple carbohydrates: sugars, both single sugar units and pairs of sugars linked together.

photosynthesis: the synthesis of carbohydrates by green plants from carbon dioxide and water using the green pigment chlorophyll to trap the sun's energy (*photo* means "light"; *synthesis* means "making").

chlorophyll: the green pigment of plants, which traps energy from sunlight and uses this energy in photosynthesis.

glucose (GLOO-koce): a single sugar used in both plant and animal tissues for quick energy; sometimes known as blood sugar; also called *dextrose*.

sugars: *simple carbohydrates*, that is, molecules of either single sugar units or pairs of those sugar units bonded together.

fructose (FROOK-toce): a monosaccharide, sometimes known as fruit sugar (*fruct* means "fruit"; *ose* means "sugar").

monosaccharides: single sugar units (*mono* means "one").

galactose (ga-LACK-toce): a monosaccharide; part of the disaccharide lactose, milk sugar.

disaccharides: two-sugar units (*di* means "two").

lactose: a disaccharide composed of glucose and galactose—milk sugar (*lact* means "milk"; *ose* means "sugar").

maltose: a disaccharide composed of two glucose units—malt sugar.

sucrose (SOO-crose): a disaccharide composed of glucose and fructose—table, beet, or cane sugar.

▪▪▪ Table 4–1 The Sugars (Simple Carbohydrates)

Monosaccharides:	
Glucose	⬡
Galactose[a]	GAL
Fructose	FRU
Disaccharides:	
Sucrose (glucose + fructose)	⬡–FRU
Maltose (glucose + glucose)	⬡–⬡
Lactose (glucose + galactose)	⬡–GAL

[a]Galactose does not occur in foods singly but as part of lactose.

When you eat a food containing sugars, enzymes in your intestine must split the disaccharides into separate monosaccharides so that they can enter your bloodstream, which delivers them to your liver. Your liver then quickly converts fructose or galactose to glucose or to smaller pieces that can serve as building blocks of either glucose or fat. Glucose is the most important monosaccharide inside the body.

When people learn that fruit's energy comes from sugars, they may think that eating fruit is the same as eating concentrated sweets such as candy or cola beverages. However, fruits differ from concentrated sweets in nutrient density. The sugars of fruits arrive in the body diluted in large volumes of water, packaged in fiber, and mixed with many vitamins and needed minerals. In contrast, all types of refined sugars, even honey, arrive in the body as concentrated sugar, practically devoid of nutrients. This chapter's Controversy distinguishes between sugar and honey with regards to nutrient density, see the cartoon and accompanying text.

Glucose occurs not only in pairs in sugars but may also be strung together in long strands of thousands of glucose units to form the **polysaccharides**. Starch is one of these; glycogen is another; some of the fibers are others.

Starch is a plant's storage form of glucose. As a plant matures it provides not only energy for its own needs but also food for the next generation. For example, after a corn plant reaches its full growth and has many leaves manufacturing glucose, it begins to store in its seeds surplus energy for the growth of new plants next season. It can't store the glucose in its sugar form because glucose is soluble in water and would be washed away by the winter rains. Instead it must form an insoluble substance that will stay with the seed and nourish it until it puts out shoots with leaves that can catch the sun's rays. This storage form of glucose is **starch**, and a kernel of corn is really a seed embedded in this nutritive material. It is nutritive for human beings also because they can digest the starch back to glucose and extract the sun's energy from its chemical bonds. Figure 4–2 depicts starch, and a later section describes starch digestion in full.

The human body stores glucose, too, as **glycogen** (shown in Figure 4–3). Glycogen is like starch in that it consists of glucose molecules linked together, but its chains are longer and are highly branched. Figures 4–2 and 4–3 compare starch with glycogen, and a later section describes the body's handling of these packages of stored glucose.

Complex carbohydratees (polysaccharides):
- ◼ Starch.
- ◼ Glycogen.
- ◼ Fiber.

▪▪▪ Figure 4–2

Starch. Glucose units are linked in long, occasionally branched chains to make starch. Human digestive enzymes can digest these bonds, retrieving glucose. Real glucose units are so tiny that you can't see them, even with the highest-power light microscope.

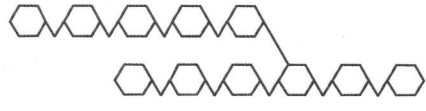

The story of carbohydrate turns out to be a cycle. Carbon dioxide, water, and energy are combined in plants to form glucose; the plants may store the glucose in the polysaccharide starch. Then a person eats the plant. In the body the starch becomes glucose again, and the liver and muscles may store it as the polysaccharide glycogen. Ultimately the glucose delivers the sun's energy to fuel the body's activities; the waste products, carbon dioxide and water, are excreted to be used again by a plant.

▌▌▷ *Glucose is the most important monosaccharide in the human body. Most other monosaccharides and disaccharides become glucose in the body. Starch is a storage form of glucose in plants. Glycogen is the storage form of glucose in human beings and animals.*

Fiber

The **fibers** of a plant contribute the supporting structures of its leaves, stems, and seeds. Most fibers are polysaccharides made of glucose, just as starch is, but with the glucose units held together by bonds that cannot be broken by human digestive enzymes. Thus fibers are "the nonstarch polysaccharides in foods."[1] The best known of these polysaccharides are **cellulose** (shown in Figure 4–4, next page), **hemicellulose**, and **pectin**.* The first two are found in the familiar strings of celery, the skins of corn kernels, and the membranes separating the segments in citrus fruits. In the body they provide **roughage**, which aids in digestion and elimination. The last one, pectin, when isolated from plants, may be used to thicken jelly, to keep salad dressing from separating, and to otherwise alter texture and consistency.

The term *dietary fiber* describes substances that cannot be broken down by human digestive enzymes. Some dietary fiber, however, can be digested by the living inhabitants of the human digestive tract—the resident bacteria. Digestion of fiber by these bacteria yields products related to fats that the body can absorb and use to provide a little energy.[2] (The other main product, gas, may make people want to avoid fiber-containing foods altogether. Don't give up on fiber foods, but gradually increase the amounts you eat, chew foods thoroughly to break up hard-to-digest lumps that can ferment in the intestine, and try many fiber-rich foods until you find some that do not cause the problem.)

Some animals, such as cattle, depend heavily on their intestinal bacteria to make available the energy of glucose derived from fiber. When we eat beef, we receive indirectly some of the sun's energy that was originally stored in the fiber of the plants the cattle ate. Beef, of course, contains no fiber itself; no meats or dairy products contain fiber.

Fibers are classified by how readily they dissolve in water. Some are called soluble fibers; some, insoluble fibers. Each type of fiber exerts important effects on people's health, and these are described in a later section.

▌▌▷ *Fiber is not much digested by people for energy. Some fiber is changed by the intestinal bacteria into products that are absorbed; most fiber passes through the digestive tract unchanged.*

*Other fibers are gums, mucilages, and lignins.

polysaccharides: another term for complex carbohydrates, compounds of long strands of glucose units linked together (*poly* means "many," and *saccharide* means "sugar unit").

starch: a plant polysaccharide composed of glucose, digestible by human beings.

glycogen (GLY-co-gen): a polysaccharide composed of glucose, made and stored by liver and muscle tissues of human beings and animals as a storage form of glucose. Glycogen is not a significant food source of carbohydrate and is not counted as one of the complex carbohydrates in foods.

fibers: the indigestible residue of food, composed mostly of the polysaccharides **cellulose**, **hemicellulose**, and **pectin**.

roughage (RUFF-idge): the rough parts of food, an imprecise term that has been largely replaced by the term *fiber*.

■■■ **Figure 4–3**

Glycogen. The bonds between glucose units are the same as in starch, but the chains are longer and more highly branched.

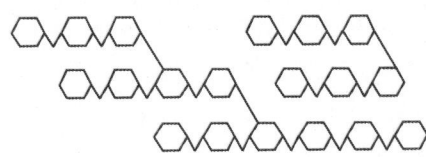

■■■ **Figure 4–4**

Cellulose. The bonds that link glucose units together are different from the bonds in starch and glycogen. Human enzymes cannot digest them.

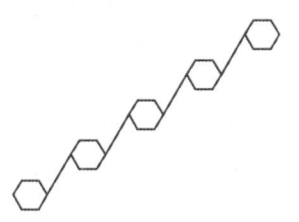

The Need for Starch and Fiber

Carbohydrate is the preferred fuel for most body functions. There are only three other energy sources available to the body—protein, fat, and alcohol. Protein-rich foods are usually expensive and provide no advantage over carbohydrates when used to make fuel for the body. In fact, their overuse has disadvantages, as explained in Chapter 6. Fat is not normally used as fuel by the brain and central nervous system, and diets high in fat are associated with many disease states. Alcohol has the same disadvantage as fat, to say nothing of its well-known undesirable side effects. Thus of all the possible alternatives, carbohydrate is the preferred energy source. It is especially important as the chief fuel of nerve cells, including those of the brain.

The human brain never ceases its activity. Day and night it depends exclusively on carbohydrate for its energy whenever that fuel is available. And because the mind resides in the brain, to some extent your attitude toward life, the world, and other people is affected by your brain's glucose supply.

For years carbohydrate was wrongly accused of being "the" fattening ingredient of foods. Some people are still startled to hear that we need to consume more starchy food rather than less. Yet much evidence supports this assertion. The Senate committee that produced the *Dietary Goals for the United States* made the observation that a young man's weight-reducing diet could include as many as 12 slices of bread in a day and still allow him to lose more than a pound a week.[3] The report urged consumption of all kinds of foods rich in starch, such as potatoes, pasta, and rice. On the other hand, the Senate committee recommended that we reduce our intakes of refined sugar. The National Research Council (NRC) recommendations (Chapter 2) echoed these suggestions. The Canadian government made similar recommendations to its people, as have the governments of several other countries.

Foods containing starch offer additional benefits by way of fiber, which comes with the starch. Fiber, as mentioned, benefits health in many ways. To sum them all up, fiber:

■ Promotes feelings of fullness and reduces energy consumption because high-fiber foods absorb and swell with water while donating little energy. Some fibers also delay the emptying of the stomach so that you feel fuller longer. By displacing calorie-dense concentrated fats and sweets from the diet, fiber can help in weight control.

■ Prevents **constipation**, **hemorrhoids**, and other intestinal problems by keeping the contents of the intestine moving along easily.

■ Helps prevent bacterial infection of the appendix (**appendicitis**) by the same mechanism.

■ Is associated with reduced incidence of colon cancer (see Chapter 11) possibly because it speeds transit of cancer-causing materials through the colon.

■ Stimulates the muscles of the digestive tract so that they retain their health and tone; this prevents **diverticulosis** (in which the intestinal walls become weak and bulge out in places).

■ May reduce the risks of heart and artery disease by lowering blood cholesterol in several ways. Some insoluble fibers bind cholesterol compounds and carry them out of the body with the feces so that the whole body content of cholesterol is lowered. The digestion of soluble fiber by bacteria in the colon yields products that may inhibit the body's production of cholesterol, and enhance its clearance from the blood.[4] High-fiber foods may also lower cholesterol by displacing fatty, cholesterol-raising foods from the diet.[5]

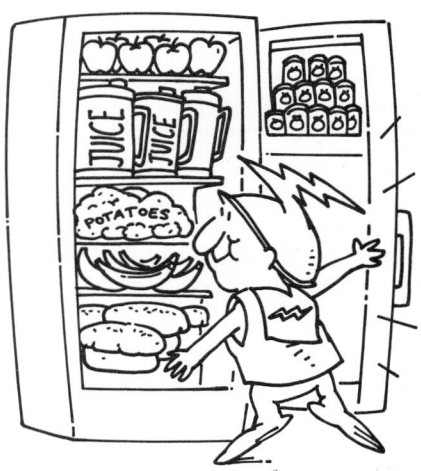

For energy, the body prefers carbohydrates.

■■■ **Table 4–2 Characteristics, Health Effects, and Sources of Fiber**

FIBER TYPE	MAJOR FOOD SOURCES	POSSIBLE HEALTH EFFECTS
Water Soluble:[a]	Fruits	Lowered blood cholesterol
	Vegetables	
	Oats	
Hemicellulose[b]	Barley	Slowed glucose absorption
	Legumes	
Pectins	Seeds	
	Rye	
Water Insoluble:	Fruits	Softened stools
	Vegetables	
Cellulose	Whole grains, such as wheat	Regulation of bowel movements
Hemicellulose	Seeds	
	Legumes	
	Brown rice	

[a]Gums and mucilages are also water soluble. Psyllium, a fiber laxative and a cereal additive under study for safety by the FDA, has both soluble and insoluble properties.
[b]Some hemicelluloses are water soluble, and others are water insoluble.

constipation: hardness and dryness of bowel movements, associated with discomfort in passing them.

hemorrhoids (HEM-or-oids): swollen, hardened (varicose) veins in the rectum, usually caused by the pressure resulting from constipation.

appendicitis: inflammation and/or infection of the appendix, a sac protruding from the large intestine.

diverticulosis (dye-ver-tic-you-LOH-sis): outpocketing of weakened areas of the intestinal wall, like blowouts in a tire.

diabetes (dye-uh-BEET-eez): a hereditary disease (technically termed *diabetes mellitus*) characterized by inadequate or ineffective insulin, which renders a person unable to regulate the blood-glucose level normally. A later section gives details.

■ Also improves the body's handling of glucose, even in people with **diabetes**, perhaps by slowing the digestion or absorption rate of carbohydrate.[6] A high-fiber meal eaten for breakfast still exerts regulatory effects on people's blood glucose after lunch.[7]

When people choose high-fiber foods in hopes of receiving some of these benefits, they must choose with care. Wheat bran, which is composed mostly of cellulose, has no cholesterol-lowering effect, whereas oat bran and the fibers of legumes, apples, and carrots may lower blood cholesterol. On the other hand, the cellulose of wheat bran in muffins or whole wheat bread is one of the most effective stool-softening fibers. Table 4–2 shows the diversity of effects of different fibers; it also shows that most unrefined plant foods contain a mix of fiber types. To consumers this means that although a food may play a star role in providing one type of fiber, that food is never the only source of that fiber. For example, while oatmeal is much advertised as a source of soluble fiber, less-celebrated grains and also legumes are equally rich sources, and both these classes of foods are rich in insoluble fiber as well. Thus to receive the whole range of fiber benefits while best meeting *other* nutrient needs, choose a variety of whole foods each day, and do not rely on purified forms of fiber. This chapter's Consumer Caution provides more information about choosing among grain foods for fiber and other nutrients.

❚❚▶ *Carbohydrate is the preferred energy source for the body; the brain and nerves prefer glucose as fuel. Fiber helps to maintain the health of the digestive tract, and helps to prevent or to control certain diseases.*

Fiber Recommendations

Undoubtedly, including fiber-rich foods in a daily meal plan offers benefits—but how much is enough? Like any other substance, if taken in excess, fiber has the potential to cause harm. Fiber carries water out of the body and can cause

chelating (KEE-late-ing) agents: molecules that surround other molecules and are therefore useful in either preventing or promoting movement of substances from place to place. Chelating agents are often sold by quacks to "remove poisons" from the body, although there are some valid medical uses.

dehydration. Iron is absorbed mostly high in the intestinal tract, and excess fiber, by speeding up the transit of foods through the digestive system, may limit iron's absorption. Binders in some fibers act as **chelating agents** and link chemically with the minerals calcium, zinc, and others and carry them out of the body. Some fibers interfere with the body's use of carotene to make vitamin A (the conversion is described in Chapter 7).[8] Too much bulk in the diet could limit the total amount of food consumed and cause deficiencies of both nutrients and energy. The malnourished, the elderly, and vegan children are especially vulnerable to this chain of events.

The average fiber intake in the United States is lower than has previously been thought. On any given day about half the population reports an intake of less than 10 grams per day. Women eat more fiber than do men, and most adults eat more as they grow older; but most do not consume as much as they need for their health.[9] There is no Recommended Dietary Allowance (RDA) for fiber, but the Committee on RDA acknowledges the need for fiber and states that it should be met by adding a variety of unprocessed, fiber-containing foods to the diet and *not* by adding refined fiber such as bran.[10] Although uncertainties remain, one reliable source recommends from 20 to 35 grams of dietary fiber daily as a desirable intake.[11] The diet can supply that amount, given ample choices of whole foods, as Table 4–3 demonstrates. To do this, though,

■■■ Table 4–3 Foods to Provide 25 Grams Dietary Fiber per Day

Choose enough of these foods to provide 25 g of fiber each day:		
Fruits (with skins): about 2 g of fiber per portion.		
apple, 1 small	cherries, 16 large	pear, ½ small
banana, 1 small	cantaloupe, ½ mellon (flesh only)	prunes, 2
strawberries, ¾ c	peach, 1	
Grains and cereals: about 2 g of fiber per portion.[a]		
whole-wheat bread, 1 slice	Grape-Nuts, ⅓ c	oatmeal, cooked, 1 c
Rye Crisp, 2 crackers	barley, ½ c	Puffed Wheat, 1½ c
cracked-wheat bread, 2 slices	Cornbran (cereal), ¼ c	popcorn, popped, 2 c
Shredded Wheat, ½ biscuit		
Vegetables (cooked): about 2 g of fiber per portion.		
broccoli, ½ c	celery, 1 c	green beans, ⅔ c
brussels sprouts, ½ c	corn, ⅓ c	potato, 1 small
carrots ½ c	lettuce, raw, 2 c	tomato, 1 large
Legumes (cooked): about 8 g of fiber per portion.		
garbanzo beans, ½ c	dried peas, 1 c	lentils, 1 c
kidney beans, ½ c	baked beans, canned, ½ c	lima beans, 1 c
Miscellaneous: about 1 g of fiber per portion.		
peanut butter, 2 ½ tsp	walnuts, ¼ c	strawberry jam, t tbsp
peanuts, 7 nuts	pickle, 1 large	

[a]Small amounts of purified cereal fibers and high-fiber cereals also contribute about 2 g of fiber per portion: All-Bran (1 tbsp), Wheat bran (1 tsp), or oat bran (2 tsp), for example. However whole-food sources of fiber are preferred, as explained in the text.

SOURCE: Values for barley, Puffed Wheat, celery, lettuce, garbanzo beans, walnuts, pickles, and jam from Recommendations for a high-fiber diet, *Nutrition and the MD,* July 1981, in turn adapted from D. A. T. Southgate and coauthors, A guide to calculating intakes of dietary fiber, *Journal of Human Nutrition* 30 (1976): 303–313; value for popcorn from Appendix A; all others from: E. Lanza and R. R. Butrum, A critical review of food fiber analysis and data, *Journal of the American Dietetic Association* 86 (1986): 732–743.

| CONSUMER CAUTION ||| | Refined, Enriched, and Whole-Grain Bread |

For many people bread supplies much of the carbohydrate, or at least most of the starch, in a day's meals. Any food used in such abundance in the diet should be scrutinized closely, and if it doesn't measure up to high nutrition standards, it should be replaced with a food that does. For people who eat bread, the meanings of the words associated with the wheat flour that makes up the bread—**refined**, **enriched**, and **whole grain**—hold the key to understanding this product in which they invest many calories per day. See the special section on page 95 entitled "Terms that Describe Grain Foods."

The part of the wheat plant that is made into flour and then into bread and other baked goods is the seed or kernel. About 50 kernels cluster in the grain head, where they stick tightly until fully ripe. These kernels are first separated from the stem and then further broken apart by the milling process.

The wheat kernel (a whole grain) has four main parts: the **germ**, the **endosperm**, the **bran**, and the **husk**, as shown in Figure 4–5. The germ is the part that grows into a wheat plant, and so it carries with it concentrated food to support the new life. It is especially rich in vitamins and minerals. The endosperm is the soft, white, inside portion of the kernel, containing starch and proteins. The bran, a protective coating around the kernel, similar in function to the shell of a nut, is also rich in nutrients and fiber. (The husk, commonly called chaff, is unusable for most purposes except for animal feed.)

In earlier times people milled wheat by grinding it between two stones, then blowing or sifting out the inedible chaff but retaining the nutrient-rich bran and germ as well as the endosperm. Improved milling machinery made it possible to remove the dark, heavy germ and bran as well, leaving a whiter, smoother-textured flour. People came to look on this flour as more desirable than the crunchy, dark brown, "old-fashioned" flour but were unaware of the nutrition implications at first.

Bread eaters suffered a tragic loss of needed nutrients in turning to white bread. Many people suffered from deficiencies of iron, thiamin, riboflavin, and niacin, nutrients that they had formerly received from bread. Finally the problem was recognized, and a law was passed to correct it. The Enrichment Act of 1942 provided standards regarding levels of iron, niacin, thiamin, and riboflavin that must be added to refined grain products before they are sold. This doesn't make a single slice of refined bread "rich" in these nutrients, but people who eat several or many slices of bread a day obtain significantly more of them than they would from unenriched white bread, as Figure 4-6 shows. Today you can almost take for granted that all breads; grain products such as rice, macaroni, and spaghetti; and cereals of all types have been enriched with these four nutrients.

To a great extent the enrichment of grain products eliminated these four known deficiency problems, but many other deficiencies went undetected for years more. The trouble with *enriched* flour is that it is comparable to whole grain only with respect to these four nutrients and not with respect to others.

continued on the next page

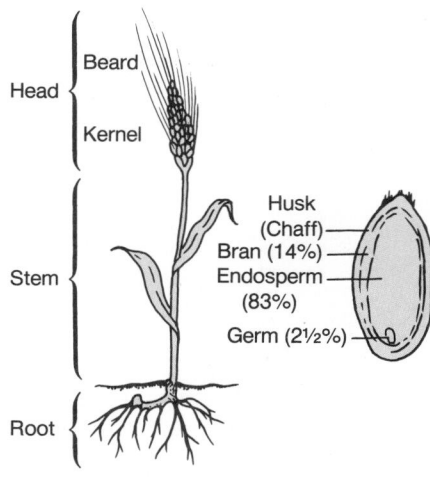

■■■ Figure 4–5

A Whole Wheat Plant and a Single Kernel

Head — Beard, Kernel
Stem
Root

Husk (Chaff)
Bran (14%)
Endosperm (83%)
Germ (2½%)

A wheat plant.   A kernel of wheat.

■■■ **Figure 4–6**

Nutrients in Whole-grain, Enriched White, and Unenriched White Breads

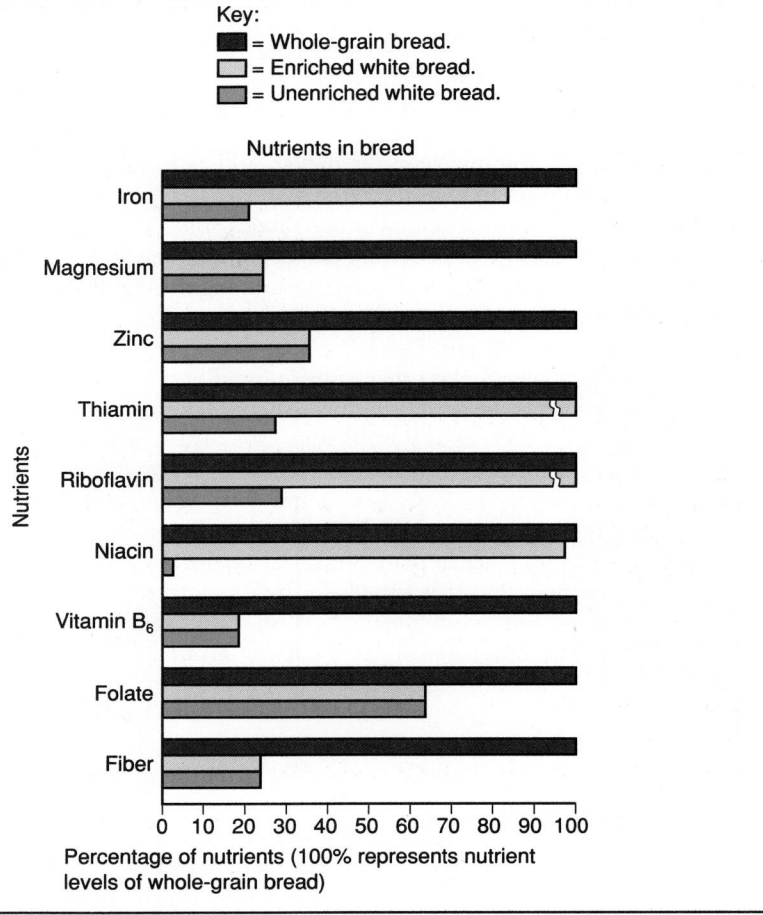

Key:
■ = Whole-grain bread.
▢ = Enriched white bread.
▨ = Unenriched white bread.

Nutrients in bread

Percentage of nutrients (100% represents nutrient levels of whole-grain bread)

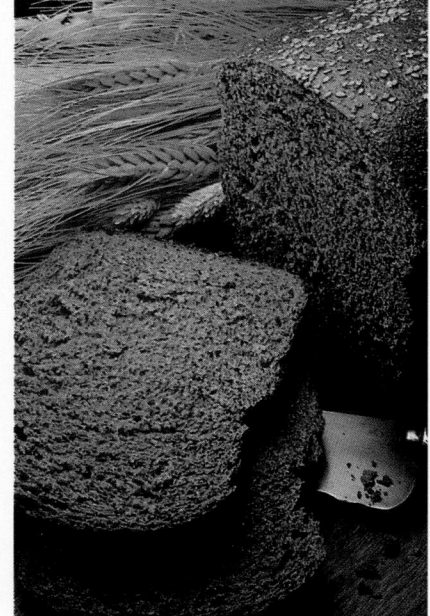

Learn to like the hearty flavor of whole grains.

Only *whole-grain* flour contains all nutritive portions of the grain. Notice, too, the distinctions between **wheat flour** and **whole wheat flour**; **white flour** and **unbleached flour** among the terms that follow.

When a grain is refined, many nutrients, not just four, are lost. Similar losses occur in other foods subjected to refinement. For example, fiber needs go unmet as fiber is refined out of many foods. Some experts have attributed a few cases of diabetes to deficiency of a mineral that is refined out of processed foods—chromium, essential for insulin to act. Therefore, although the enrichment of refined grain products does improve them, it may not improve them enough. Whole-grain items are still preferable even to the enriched products because they are likely to contain more magnesium, zinc, folate, vitamin B₆, fiber, vitamin E, chromium, and many other nutrients. If bread is a staple food in your diet—that is, if you eat it every day— you would be well advised to learn to like the hearty flavor of whole-grain bread.

☐☐☐ Terms that Describe Grain Foods

bran: the chief fiber donator of a grain.

endosperm: the bulk of the edible part of a grain, the starchy part.

enriched: refers to addition of nutrients to a refined food product. As originally defined by law, this term means that thiamin, riboflavin, niacin, and iron have been added to refined grains and grain products at specified levels. After enrichment, a grain product has approximately the same amount of thiamin, niacin, and iron and about twice as much riboflavin as the original whole-grain product. (The term *enriched* can refer to addition of more nutrients than just these four; read the label.)

germ: the nutrient-rich inner part of a grain.

husk: the outer, inedible part of a grain.

refined: refers to the process by which the coarse parts of food products are removed. For example, the refining of wheat into flour involves removing three of the four parts of the kernel—the chaff, the bran, and the germ—leaving only the endosperm (starch, with only a little protein).

unbleached flour: a tan-colored endosperm flour with texture and nutritive qualities approximately the same as regular white flour.

wheat flour: any flour made from wheat, including white flour.

white flour: an endosperm flour that has been refined and bleached for maximum softness and whiteness.

whole grain: refers to a grain milled in its entirety (all but the husk), not refined.

whole wheat flour: flour made from whole wheat kernels; a whole-grain flour.

---

the diet must be high in fruits, vegetables, and grains, and relatively low in meats, fats, and concentrated sugar—the same recommendations put forth by the NRC Recommendations.

The addition of purified fiber (such as oat or wheat bran) to foods is ill advised because it is so easily taken to extreme. A recent report tells of a man who required sudden intestinal surgery for the removal of a blockage formed by too many oat bran muffins; the excessive bran had overwhelmed his digestive system's ability to work.[12] A less extreme concern lies in what else purified fiber might displace from the diet. Whole foods deliver many fiber types and nutrients, with all of their associated benefits. Refined fiber could be compared in one way to refined sugar: the nutrients that normally accompany it have been lost. Furthermore, a purified fiber, such as cellulose, may not have the same effect in the body as the cellulose in whole grains.[13] This chapter's Food Feature shows where the fiber is found in an ordinary day's meals.

▌▶ *People probably need 20 to 35 grams of fiber each day. Fiber needs are best met with whole foods, which also deliver needed nutrients; purified fiber can be harmful in large doses and should be avoided.*

∎∎∎ Figure 4–7

How Carbohydrate in Food Becomes Glucose in the Body. Not shown here, salivary enzymes in the mouth partially break down some of the starch before it reaches the intestine.
a. Starch and disaccharides enter the intestine.
b. Enzymes digest the starch to disaccharides.
c. Enzymes on surface of intestinal wall cells split disaccharides to monosaccharides.
d. Monosaccharides enter capillary.
e. Capillary delivers monosaccharides to liver.
f. Liver converts galactose and fructose to glucose.
g. Fiber travels unchanged to the colon.
More about digestion in Chapter 3.

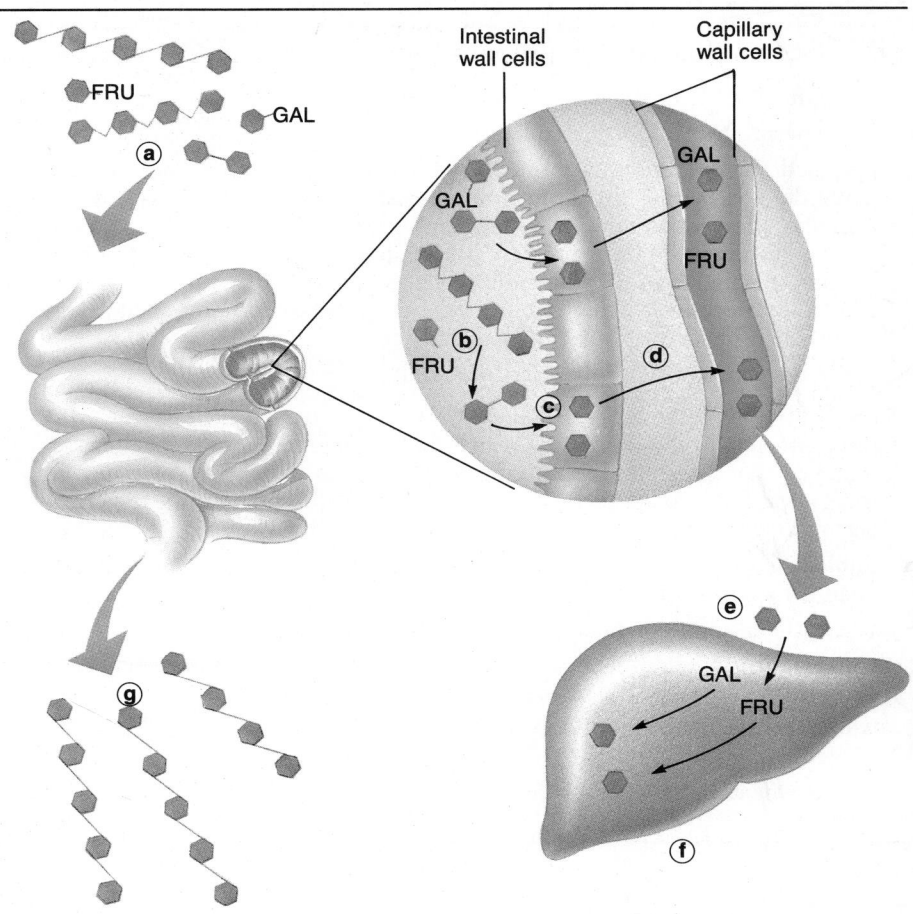

∎∎∎ The Body's Use of Glucose

Just as glucose is the original unit from which the wide variety of carbohydrate foods are made, so also is glucose the basic carbohydrate unit that each cell of the body uses. Cells cannot use foods such as bread or even whole molecules of lactose, sucrose, or starch; they require glucose. The task of the various body systems, then, is to make glucose available to the cells.

Digestion and Absorption of Carbohydrate

To provide glucose, the digestive system must first render food carbohydrate into monosaccharides that can be absorbed through the lining of the small intestine. The largest of the carbohydrate molecules, starch, requires the most extensive breakdown. Disaccharides, on the other hand, must be split only once before they can be absorbed.

Digestion of starch begins in the mouth, where salivary enzymes mix with food and begin to split starch into maltose. You may have noticed while chewing a bite of bread the slightly sweet taste as maltose is liberated from starch by salivary enzymes. The mouth is the only digestive organ that communicates information about its contents to the conscious brain through one of the senses—taste.

The salivary enzymes continue to act on the starch in your swallowed bite of bread until all the chewed lumps have been churned and mixed thoroughly with the secretions of the stomach. As proteins, the salivary enzymes eventually succumb to the protein-digesting stomach secretions; starch digestion ceases when the salivary enzymes are themselves digested. Starch digestion resumes in the small intestine, where many more starch-splitting enzymes from the pancreas break starch down entirely into disaccharides.

Sucrose and lactose from food and maltose freed from starch undergo one split to yield free monosaccharides before they can be absorbed. The conversion of a bite of bread to nutrients for cells is completed when monosaccharides traverse the cells of the lining of the small intestine and are washed away in a rush of circulating blood that carries them to the waiting liver. Figure 4–7 presents a quick review of the events of carbohydrate digestion.

Once in the body, the absorbed carbohydrates follow one of many paths to the cells and may be used in any of several ways. The liver converts fructose and galactose to glucose or derivatives of glucose (such as fat), and the circulatory system transports the glucose and fat to the cells. Cells may store circulating glucose as glycogen or split it for energy. Similarly they may store circulating fat or use it for energy.

Molecules of fiber are not changed by human digestive enzymes. Fiber travels to the colon, where it provides bulk and holds water. There fiber encounters billions of resident bacteria whose digestive processes release from fiber small amounts of nutrients the colon can absorb, along with some gas, usually unnoticeable and odorless.

❚❚▶ *With respect to starch and sugars, the task of the various body systems is to convert them into glucose to fuel the cells' work.*

Storing Glucose as Glycogen

If the blood delivers more glucose than the cells need, the hormone insulin signals the liver, and muscles take up the surplus. From some of it they build the polysaccharide glycogen. The muscles hoard two-thirds of the body's total store of this carbohydrate and use it just for themselves during intensive exercise. (Chapter 10 gives many details about how glycogen supports exercise, and it gives tips on how athletes can make the most of glycogen stores.) The liver stores the other one-third and is more generous with it: it makes it available as glucose when the brain or other organs need to draw on the supply.

Glycogen is wondrously designed for its task of releasing glucose on demand. Instead of having long chains with occasional branches, such as starch, which is cleaved one unit after the other during digestion, glycogen is highly branched so that hundreds of ends stick out at its surface. On the tip of each chain is a glucose, whose attachment to the next glucose is easily accessible to the glycogen-splitting enzymes. When glucose energy is needed by the cells, a hormone, **glucagon**, floods the bloodstream. Thousands of enzymes within the liver cells respond by attacking a multitude of ends simultaneously, and they release an abundance of glucose into the blood for use by all the other body cells. Another hormone, epinephrine, does the same thing as part of the body's defense mechanism in times of danger.

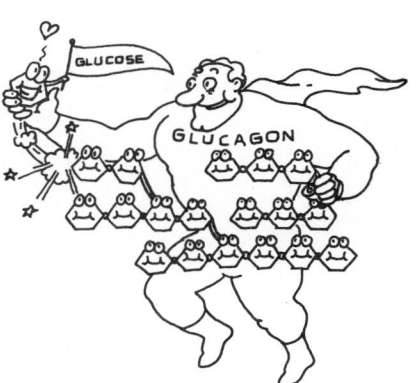

Glucagon liberates glucose from storage.

glucagon: a hormone of the pancreas that acts on the liver when blood-glucose concentration dips, stimulating the release of glucose into the blood.

This section refers to many body organs and hormones. If you want to review them, turn to Chapter 3.

■■■ **Figure 4–8**

The Breakdown of Glucose Yields Energy and Carbon Dioxide. The bonds between the carbon atoms in glucose are split apart by human-cell enzymes, liberating the energy stored there for the cell's use. The carbon atoms are combined with oxygen and released into the air, via the lungs, as carbon dioxide. Although not shown here, water is also produced at each step.

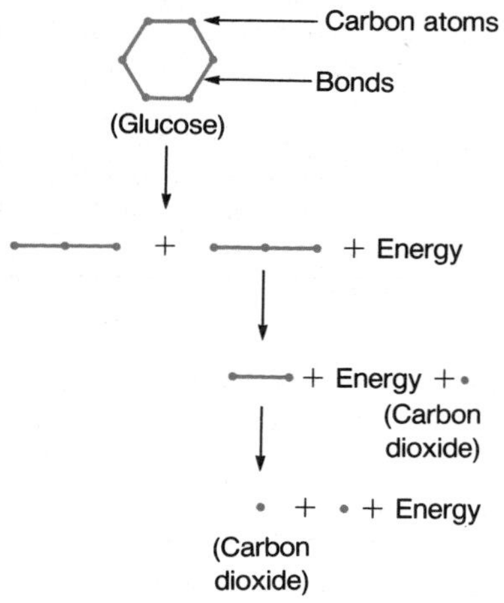

To a person living in the Stone Age, an internal source of quick energy was obviously an advantage. Life was fraught with physical peril. The person who stopped and ate before running from a man-eating tiger did not survive to produce our ancestors. The quick-energy response in a stress situation works to our advantage today as well. (One example: It accounts for the energy you suddenly have to clean up your room when you learn that a special person is coming to visit.) To meet such emergencies, we are well advised to eat and to store carbohydrate every four to six hours when we are awake.

You might rightly ask, "What kind of carbohydrate?" Knowing only that you need energy, you might become convinced that the best source of energy is a concentrated sugar food, such as a candy bar or a sugary beverage. These do supply sugar energy quickly, but they are not the best choices. Starchy food will provide glucose, along with an assortment of other nutrients needed by the cells to use their glucose.

▶ *Glycogen is the body's form of stored glucose; the liver stores it for use by the whole body. Muscles have their own private glycogen stock for muscle use only. The hormone glucagon acts to liberate stored glucose from the liver.*

Splitting Glucose for Energy

Glucose fuels the work of most of the body's cells. When a cell splits glucose for energy, it performs an intricate sequence of maneuvers that are of great interest to the biochemist—and of no interest whatever to most people who eat bread and potatoes. There is only one fact that everybody needs to understand about the process, and it may help to give the punch line before telling the story: there is no good substitute for carbohydrate. There is a point at which glucose is forever lost to the body, and this can have serious consequences. The following details are given only for the purpose of making this point clear.

Inside the cell, glucose breaks in half, releasing some energy. These halves have two pathways open to them. They can be put back together to make glucose, or they can be further broken apart into smaller fragments. If they are broken into smaller fragments, they can never again be reassembled to form glucose. They can yield still more energy and in the process break down completely to carbon dioxide and water; or they can be hitched together into units of body fat. Figure 4–8 shows how glucose is broken down to yield energy and carbon dioxide.

Although glucose can be converted into body fat, body fat can never be converted into glucose to feed the brain adequately. This is one reason why fasting and low-carbohydrate diets are dangerous. When there is a severe carbohydrate deficit, the body has two problems. Having no glucose, it has to turn to protein to make some (it has this ability), thus diverting protein from vitally important functions of its own. Protein's importance to the body is so great that carbohydrate should be kept available precisely to prevent this use of protein for energy. This is called the **protein-sparing action** of carbohydrate. For another thing, without sufficient carbohydrate, the body can't use its fat in the normal way. (Carbohydrate is needed to combine with the fat fragments so that they can be used for energy.) So the body has to go into **ketosis** (using fat without the help of carbohydrate), a condition in which unusual products of fat breakdown (**ketone bodies**) accumulate in the blood. Ketosis during pregnancy can cause brain damage and irreversible mental retardation in infants; but even in nonpregnant adults it is a condition to avoid because it disturbs the body's normal acid-base balance.

The minimum amount of carbohydrate needed to ensure complete sparing of body protein and avoidance of ketosis is around 100 grams a day in an average-sized person. This has to be digestible carbohydrate, and considerably more (two or three times more) than this minimum is recommended.[14] This chapter's Food Feature shows how to estimate grams of carbohydrate in foods.

◼◼▷ *Without glucose the body is forced to use protein and fat differently. The body breaks down its own muscles and other protein tissues to make glucose and converts its fat into ketone bodies, incurring ketosis.*

Maintaining the Blood Glucose Level

The maintenance of a normal blood-glucose level depends on two safeguards. When the level gets too low, it can be replenished by drawing on liver glycogen stores. When it gets too high, it can be corrected by siphoning off the excess into the liver, to be converted to glycogen or fat, and into muscle, to be converted to glycogen.

The elevation of blood-glucose concentration has already been mentioned. The hormone glucagon, also mentioned earlier, triggers the release of glucose from liver glycogen. Other hormones also act in this manner, including epinephrine (the stress hormone) and some that promote the conversion of protein into glucose. However, the liver's glycogen can be depleted within half a day, and as for protein, none can be spared without cost. When body protein is used, it has to be taken from muscle, organ, or blood proteins—no surplus of protein is stored for emergencies. As for fat, you have already seen that it can't regenerate enough glucose to make a difference.

Obviously, when the blood-glucose level falls and stores are depleted, a meal or a snack can replenish the supply. The meal or snack you choose may, however, flood the blood with glucose, requiring the body to protect itself against too *high* a blood-glucose concentration.

When the blood-glucose level rises, the body adjusts by storing the excess. The first organ to detect the excess glucose is the pancreas, which releases the hormone **insulin** in response. Most of the body's cells respond to insulin by taking up glucose from the blood. As already shown, they dispose of it by making glycogen or fat. Thus the blood-glucose concentration is quickly brought back down to normal as the body stores the excess. The whole process of glucose regulation is summed up in Figure 4–9.

If you eat a meal or snack that is unusually high in concentrated sugar and low in fiber, fat, or protein, your blood-glucose concentration may rise so high that the pancreas oversecretes insulin and drives glucose into the cells too fast. Then the blood-glucose level may fall low enough to cause symptoms such as fatigue. The effect of food on a person's blood glucose and insulin response is called the **glycemic effect**—how fast and how high the blood glucose rises and how quickly the body responds by bringing it back to normal. Most people can quickly readjust, but people with abnormal carbohydrate metabolism should avoid foods with a strong glycemic effect.

protein-sparing action: the action of carbohydrate and fat in providing energy that allows protein to be used for other purposes.

ketosis (kee-TOE-sis): an undesirably high concentration of ketone bodies, such as acetone, in the blood and urine.

ketone (KEE-tone) **bodies**: the product of the incomplete breakdown of fat when carbohydrate is not available.

insulin: a hormone secreted by the pancreas in response to a high blood-glucose concentration; it assists cells in drawing glucose from the blood.

glycemic (gligh-SEEM-ic) **effect**: a measure of the extent to which a food raises the blood-glucose level as compared with pure glucose.

Chapter 5 offers details of fat storage.

■■■ **Figure 4−9**

Glucose Regulation. The close regulation of the blood glucose level shows how important a constant supply of glucose is to the body.

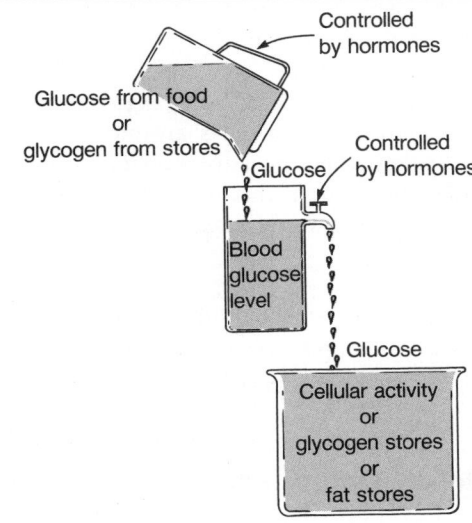

It has long been thought that starch elicits a weaker glycemic effect than does simple sugar, but the old axiom "avoid sugar and eat starch" oversimplifies the case. The effects of different foods on blood glucose apparently depend on many factors:

■ The digestibility of the starch in the food.
■ The form of the food (dry, paste, or liquid; coarsely or finely ground; cooked or raw).
■ How quickly the food empties from the stomach into the intestine. (The longer it takes to empty, the lesser the food's glycemic effect.[15])
■ Interactions of the starch with the protein, fat, sugar, and fiber in the food.
■ The presence of other constituents, such as molecules that bind starch.

These factors work together to determine a food's glycemic effect, and the result is not always what a person might expect.[16] Ice cream, for example, produces less of a response than potatoes; legumes are notable for keeping blood glucose remarkably steady.[17] Most importantly, a food's glycemic effect differs when it is eaten alone or as part of a mixed meal. To the above list of factors that influence a food's glycemic effect, add:

■ The *combination* of foods consumed at a given time.

This factor is significant, considering that most people eat a variety of foods in a meal.

The glycemic effect of foods is of interest to people with abnormalities of blood-glucose regulation, notably diabetes or hypoglycemia (see later section). These people might benefit from avoiding foods that produce too great a rise and too sudden a fall in blood glucose. For their use, researchers have produced a "glycemic index" that ranks foods according to their effects on blood glucose. For most people, however, the glycemic index is of little value in meal planning. To control blood glucose, dietitians employ other methods of meal planning, such as controlling energy intake.

▌▐ ▶ *Blood-glucose regulation depends mainly on the hormones insulin and glucogen. Certain carbohydrate foods are absorbed more quickly than others, producing a sudden rise and fall in blood glucose. Eating well-spaced, carefully chosen meals can prevent rapid falls in blood-glucose levels.*

> **lactase:** the intestinal enzyme that splits the disaccharide lactose to monosaccharides during digestion.

Converting Glucose to Fat

When food is tempting, people may continue to eat beyond the amount they need. After filling glycogen stores to capacity and meeting the body cells' immediate energy needs, the body takes a third path for disposing of incoming carbohydrate. Say you have eaten. Now you are sitting, watching a ball game on television, eating pretzels, and drinking beer. Your digestive tract is delivering molecules of glucose from the pretzels and of alcohol from the beer to your bloodstream, and your blood is carrying these molecules to your liver. The liver breaks the extra energy compounds into small fragments and puts them together into the more permanent energy-storage compound—fat. (This would happen if you were eating excess protein or fat, too.) The fat is then released into the blood, carried to the fatty tissues of the body, and deposited there. Unlike the liver cells, which can store only about half a day's worth of glycogen, the fat cells can store unlimited quantities of fat. Moral: you had better play the game if you are going to eat the food.

The beginning of this chapter told of carbohydrate's role in the maintenance of body weight and lean tissue. Researchers are just beginning to understand the issues involved, but the results of the work are fascinating, and presented in full in Controversy 10. The punchline seems to be that, calorie for calorie, carbohydrate-rich foods contribute much less to body fatness than do fat-rich foods. Another way of saying this is that a person who wishes to eat until full, never skip a meal, and yet remain lean should make every effort to eat foods that combine to provide a diet with 55 percent or more of its calories from carbohydrate, 30 percent or less from fat. The Food Feature of this chapter provides the first set of tools required for the job of designing such a diet. Once you have learned to identify the carbohydrates in foods, you must then learn where the fats come in (Chapter 5's Food Feature), and how to ensure adequate protein without overdoing it (Chapter 6).

▌▐ ▶ *The liver converts extra energy compounds into fat, a more permanent and less limited energy-storage compound than glycogen.*

▌▌▌ Abnormal Use of Carbohydrate

Some people have physical conditions that cause abnormal handling of carbohydrates in their bodies. Two are common: lactose intolerance and diabetes. A third, hypoglycemia, is rare as a true disease condition, but many people believe they experience the symptoms at times.

Lactose Intolerance

Many people, as they age, lose the ability to produce enough of the enzyme **lactase** to digest lactose, the sugar of milk. Thereafter, on drinking milk or

lactose intolerance: inability to digest lactose due to a lack of the necessary enzyme; often sets in at age four in children of nonwhite races and makes them unable to drink milk.

eating lactose-containing products, these people will experience nausea, pain, diarrhea, and excessive gas because the intestinal bacteria will use the undigested lactose for their own energy, a process that produces gas and intestinal irritants. This condition, **lactose intolerance**, appears in many cases to be a racial trait, inherited by about 80 percent of the world's people, including most Africans, Greeks, and Asians. It also can develop temporarily in anyone who is malnourished or sick, making avoidance of milk and milk products temporarily necessary. Lactose intolerance affects people to differing degrees, and some can tolerate small quantities of milk.

Because milk is an almost indispensable source of calcium for growth, a milk substitute must be found for a child who becomes lactose intolerant. Sometimes yogurt or cheese makes an acceptable substitute: these products contain less lactose because the sugar is already fermented by the bacteria that make them.

Sometimes sensitivity to milk is due not to lactose intolerance but to an allergic reaction to the protein in the milk. Children and adults with this problem often cannot tolerate cheese or yogurt either, and they have to find nondairy calcium sources, such as calcium-fortified soy milk, oysters, sardines, and legumes to compensate. Controversy 8 examines the topic of milk in adult diets in relation to the bone disease of old age, osteoporosis.

❚❚▷ *A common condition in which the body uses carbohydrate abnormally is lactose intolerance. People with lactose intolerance lack the enzyme lactase and so are unable to properly digest the sugar in milk, leaving it available for bacterial use.*

Diabetes

Diabetes can lead to or contribute to any of a number of other diseases (see Chapter 11). Several diseases have been called diabetes, but by far the most common ones, and the only ones most people hear of, are the two forms of **diabetes mellitus** described here. They are disorders of blood-glucose regulation.

Diabetes takes two main forms. In the first, less common type (about 20 percent of all cases), the person's own immune system attacks the cells of the pancreas that normally synthesize the hormone insulin. Soon, the pancreas can no longer produce insulin, and, after each meal, blood glucose remains elevated, even though body tissues are simultaneously starving for glucose. The person must inject insulin periodically to assist the cells in taking up the needed glucose from the blood; therefore this type of diabetes is called **insulin-dependent diabetes mellitus (IDDM), or Type I diabetes**. (Insulin must be injected, either by daily shots or by an insulin pump that delivers insulin through an implanted needle. Insulin is made of protein, and if it were taken orally, the digestive system would digest it.)

The second, predominant, type of diabetes mellitus (80 percent of all cases) is characterized by insulin resistance of the body's cells, including fat cells. Insulin is present, often in abnormally large amounts, and it does move glucose into cells, but slowly. Blood glucose rises too high, as in IDDM, but insulin is also high, not absent. This type of diabetes is therefore called **non-insulin-dependent diabetes mellitus (NIDDM), or Type II diabetes**. (People may be given insulin or insulin-inducing agents to supplement their own supply of

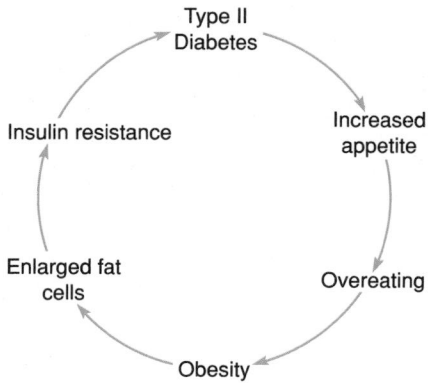

■■■ **Figure 4–10**

The Obesity-Diabetes Cycle.

■■■ **Table 4–4 The Warning Signs of Diabetes**

Excessive urination and thirst.
Weight loss with nausea, easy tiring, weakness, or irritability.
Craving for food, especially sweets.
Frequent infections of the skin, gums, or urinary tract.
Vision disturbances; blurred vision.
Pain in the legs, feet, or fingers.
Slow healing of cuts and bruises.
Itching.
Drowsiness.

SOURCE: Adapted from J. M. Couric, Diabetes is a controllable disease with a growth factor, *FDA Consumer,* November 1982, pp. 21–23.

diabetes (DYE-uh-BEET-eez) **mellitus** (MELL-ih-tus): a disorder of blood-glucose regulation usually caused by insufficiency or relative ineffectiveness of insulin.

Type I diabetes, or **insulin-dependent diabetes mellitus (IDDM):** the type of diabetes in which the person produces no insulin at all, also known as **juvenile-onset diabetes,** although some cases arise in adulthood.

Type II diabetes, or **non-insulin-dependent diabetes mellitus (NIDDM):** the type of diabetes in which the fat cells resist insulin, also called **adult-onset diabetes.**

glucose tolerance: the ability of the body to respond to dietary carbohydrate by regulating its blood-glucose concentration promptly to a normal level.

hyperglycemia (HIGH-per-gligh-SEEM-ee-uh): an abnormally high blood-glucose concentration—above about 170 mg/100 ml (*hyper* means "too much"; *glyce* means "glucose"; *emia* means "in the blood").

insulin, but they do not absolutely require these, as do people with IDDM.) NIDDM tends to set in later in life, and people with the disease often become obese because they overeat due to their cells' resistance to insulin—while they are waiting for their cells to be fed, so to speak. Figure 4–10 shows that this becomes a cycle: the larger the fat cells become, the more insulin resistant they become, and the obesity worsens insulin resistance just as insulin resistance worsens obesity.[18] The incidence of this type of diabetes also increases with increasing age, for in all people, pancreatic cells (which produce insulin) progressively lose their function with time.[19] In some people this age-related decline in cell function is more rapid or more severe than in others, and these are the people who need especially to beware of weight gain.

Diabetes can be diagnosed by means of a **glucose tolerance** test, in which the body is challenged to handle a sudden, large amount of glucose. After fasting overnight, the subject is fed a large, sugary drink. Four or six hours later, when blood glucose should be normal, the person with diabetes will show a blood-glucose level that is still elevated (**hyperglycemia**). Table 4–4 lists warning signs of diabetes.

Although its symptoms are controllable for the most part, diabetes should not be taken lightly. Its effects can be severe: impaired circulation leading to disease of the feet and legs, sometimes necessitating amputation; kidney disease sometimes requiring hospital care or kidney transplant; impaired vision or blindness due to cataracts; nerve damage; and strokes and heart attacks. The root cause of all these conditions is the same. Diabetes causes blockage or destruction of the small arteries that feed the tissues, and tissues die from lack of nourishment. The person is also advised to control all possible risk factors that might contribute to heart and blood vessel disease (atherosclerosis and hypertension, as discussed in Chapter 11).

The exchange system used throughout this book was originally developed for people with diabetes but has often been praised as the best possible system for people in perfect health to manage their diets. A diet constructed of a balanced pattern of foods from the exchange lists is best for weight control. (Weight Watchers and other reputable weight control systems use it.) Such a diet also has all the characteristics most important in disease prevention and well meets the recommendations of most guidelines. It is adequate (deficiencies in trace minerals, especially chromium, may hasten diabetes onset), it has ample fiber; it is low in concentrated sugar; and it is high in complex carbo-

hypoglycemia: an abnormally low blood-glucose concentration, a symptom that may indicate any of several diseases, including impending diabetes (NIDDM).

epinephrine: the major hormone that elicits the stress reaction.

norepinephrine: a hormone related to epinephrine that helps to elicit the stress reaction.

reactive hypoglycemia: hypoglycemia experienced simultaneously with epinephrine-induced symptoms four to six hours after a meal.

fasting hypoglycemia: hypoglycemia that occurs after 8 to 14 hours of fasting.

nonhypoglycemia: a term used to describe people who think they have hypoglycemia but don't.

hydrates (thought to assist in blood-glucose regulation). Furthermore, it is low in fat and not too high in protein (helping to protect against cardiovascular disease). A person threatened with diabetes can do no better than to adopt such a diet long before any symptoms appear.

Exercise is important too. It not only helps to maintain a desirable body weight, but it also heightens tissue sensitivity to insulin (more on this effect in Chapter 10).

◖◖▶ *Diabetes is an example of the body's abnormal handling of glucose. Inadequate or ineffective insulin leaves blood-glucose levels high and cells undersupplied with glucose energy and causes blood vessel and tissue damage. Weight control is the most effective prevention for the predominant form of diabetes and the ills that accompany it.*

Hypoglycemia

Strictly speaking, the term **hypoglycemia** simply means "low blood glucose." Minor hypoglycemia can arise in any healthy person who goes without food for a longer time than usual, or it can be a symptom of a number of disease conditions.[20] When blood sugar drops extremely low, symptoms occur, some of which may be uncomfortable. True hypoglycemia brings on symptoms similar to those of an anxiety attack: weakness, rapid heartbeat, sweating, anxiety, hunger, and trembling. This is not surprising, since these symptoms are caused by the emergency hormones, **epinephrine** and **norepinephrine**. Normally, these symptoms do not occur. Most people, after eating, experience a rise in their blood-glucose level, followed by a gradual decline, during which time fuel storage is taking place—the physiological condition characteristic of the "fed state." Once no more glucose enters the body from the small intestine, metabolism shifts gently into the reverse condition, the "fasting state," in which rather than storing glucose the liver starts to release it from stored glycogen for the body's use. Throughout, blood glucose remains in the normal range, and the transition is not noticeable. However, in some people, the transition is rough, the emergency hormones are secreted to push glucose into the blood, and the person feels the symptoms of alarm that go with actual emergencies, the symptoms of **reactive hypoglycemia.**

Reactive hypoglycemia can be experimentally produced in just about everyone. Its symptoms include impaired thought processes, memory, and psychomotor activity.[21] To produce even mild reactive hypoglycemia and its symptoms, though, requires administering drugs that overwhelm the body's sensitive glucose control team—insulin and glucagon. Without such intervention, those hormones rarely fail to keep blood glucose within normal limits, and symptoms people ascribe to reactive hypoglycemia hardly ever correlate to low blood glucose in blood tests.[22]

A different kind of hypoglycemia exists in a person who has symptoms while well advanced into the fasting state (for example, overnight). The symptoms of **fasting hypoglycemia** are different from those of reactive hypoglycemia: headache, mental dullness, fatigue, confusion, amnesia, and even seizures and unconsciousness.

True hypoglycemia can have a multitude of causes, and no one treatment is appropriate for everyone. Still, many dishonest or ill-informed practitioners "diagnose" hypoglycemia on the basis of their clients' verbal reports alone and "prescribe" all sorts of "remedies" for it with transparently thin rationale. People also diagnose themselves so commonly that physicians have identified a special category for their condition: **nonhypoglycemia**. Hypoglycemia can be identified by directly testing the blood-glucose concentration at intervals.

There is no doubt that some people may be more sensitive than others to slight changes in glucose levels and may experience symptoms even when their blood glucose reaches a low level within the range considered normal. Two findings are relevant to these people:

1. People with *normal* glucose regulation can develop the symptoms of reactive hypoglycemia if they take a large dose of simple sugar after three days of following a low-carbohydrate diet.
2. Some people who appear to have reactive hypoglycemia by traditional testing do not have it after mixed meals—only after a simple-sugar load.

This means that if you experience symptoms that you attribute to hypoglycemia, you can try to eliminate them by eating regular mixed meals rather than sugar snacks. If you are *not* prone to such symptoms, you may bring them on if you deprive your system of carbohydrate for days and then dump in a large dose all at once. Eat regularly, eat balanced meals, and some problems may clear right up.

 Everyone can experience symptoms from low blood sugar. Spontaneous hypoglycemia is a rare medical condition in which the blood-glucose level is constantly too low.

This Food Feature illustrates something the exchange system can do for you. It can show you where the carbohydrates are in your meals and how much you are getting. You can use it the same way to find fat and protein in meals, as the next two chapters will show.

Breads, cereals, vegetables, fruits, and milk—these are the foods noted for their contributions of valuable energy-yielding carbohydrates: starches and dilute sugars. To learn how much starch and sugars these foods offer, consult the exchange lists, and remember that all of the foods on any one list are treated as interchangeable with respect to carbohydrate, fat, and protein. Within a list you can trade one food for another without altering your carbohydrate intake. Carbohydrate-containing foods appear in four of the six lists; Figure 4–11 (next page) provides details.

THE STARCH/GRAIN LIST. A slice of whole-wheat bread contains 15 grams of carbohydrate as starch. Equivalent foods are other breads, cereals, potatoes, rice, pasta, corn, peas, limas and other beans (legumes), and many other foods that are predominantly complex carbohydrate. Be aware that starchy vegetables such as corn and green peas actually resemble breads more closely than vegetables in their starch content. People who like breads and starchy vegetables are happy to learn that it is considered desirable to use them freely. They know that if calories are a problem, they should cut out fat, not complex carbohydrate foods. However, some foods in this group, especially baked goods, such as biscuits, muffins, and snack crackers, do contain fat. Chapter 5 gives more information about the fats in foods.

Food Feature

Meeting Carbohydrate Needs

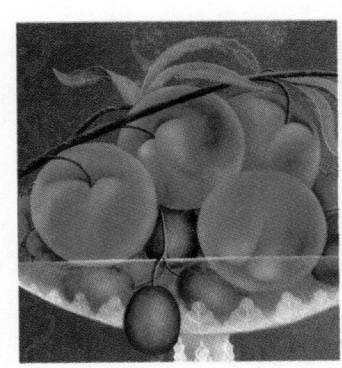

■■■ Figure 4–11

Carbohydrate in Foods. Four of the six exchange lists contain carbohydrate, so you need only know four values and learn a value for concentrated sugar (which is not on the exchange lists). The lists identify a few items that are especially high in fiber with a logo, but all whole plant foods are valuable fiber contributors if you eat enough of them.

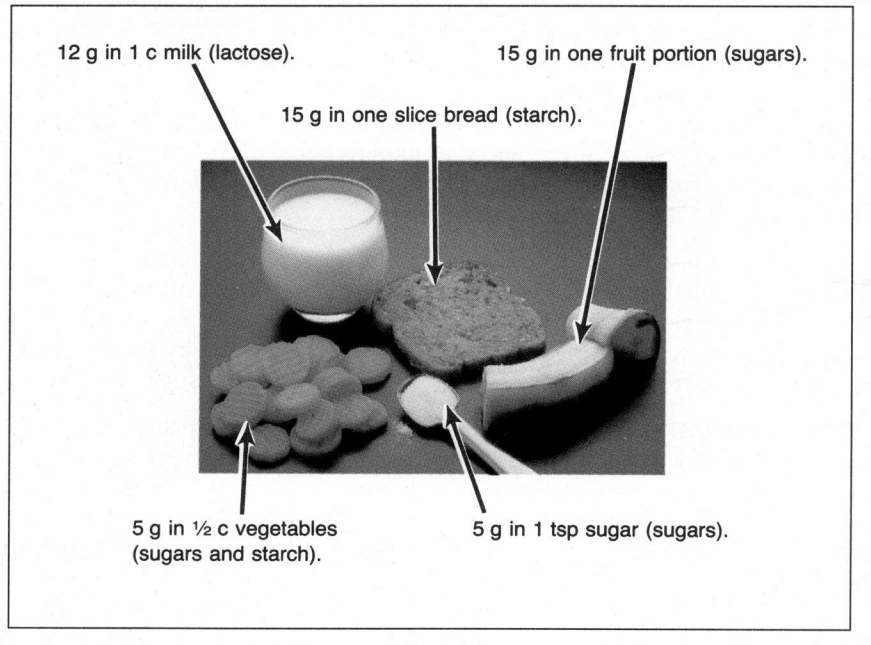

12 g in 1 c milk (lactose).

15 g in one slice bread (starch).

15 g in one fruit portion (sugars).

5 g in ½ c vegetables (sugars and starch).

5 g in 1 tsp sugar (sugars).

ONE EXCHANGE	CARBOHY-DRATE (g)
Starches/grains	15
Vegetables	5
Fruits	15
Milks	12
Sugar	5
Meats	0
Fats	0

More about the exchange lists and "free foods" in Chapter 2 and Appendix D.

THE VEGETABLE LIST. The exchange list portions of vegetables are small, only a half cup, a vestige from the days when people thought that meat should be the center of a meal and that vegetables should only decorate the plate. The opposite now seems to be a healthier strategy, so you are encouraged to double your servings to 1-cup portions of vegetables.

A half-cup portion of carrots or any other vegetable on this list contains 5 grams of carbohydrate as a mixture of starch and sugars. Such a portion is called a vegetable exchange. The vegetable exchanges include tomatoes, greens, okra, onions, summer squash, beets, and others. Each of these foods also contributes a little protein and no fat. Some vegetables are so low in carbohydrate and calories that the exchange system calls them "free foods." Among these are lettuce, parsley, and radishes.

THE FRUIT LIST. A typical fruit portion, such as a half cup of orange juice, contains 15 grams of carbohydrate, mostly as sugars, including the fruit sugar fructose. Fruits vary greatly in their water and fiber content, and therefore their sugar concentrations vary also. The portion sizes of different fruits are adjusted so that each contains 15 grams of carbohydrate. Thus in a diet plan they are interchangeable; you can "exchange" any fruit portion for any other without altering the amount of carbohydrate you eat. Among the fruit exchanges are one-third cup pineapple juice, one-half cup applesauce, and half of a small banana. The fruits contain insignificant amounts of fat and protein.

THE MILK LIST. A portion (1 cup) of milk or the equivalent is a generous contributor of carbohydrate, donating 12 grams. It also contributes high-quality protein (a point in its favor), as well as several important vitamins and minerals. (Milk products vary in fat content, an important consideration in choosing among them; Chapter 5 provides the details.) Similar to milk in these respects are the other items on the milk list:

- 1 cup buttermilk.
- 1 cup yogurt (plain).
- 1/3 cup dry milk powder.
- 1/2 cup canned, evaporated milk, undiluted.

Cream and butter, although dairy products, are *not* on the milk list because they contain little or no carbohydrate and insignificant amounts of the other nutrients important in milk. They are found on the fat list instead.

SUGAR. The exchange lists do not include concentrated sugar (not surprisingly, since the exchange system was originally designed for use by people with diabetes). But since we know that sweets supply carbohydrate, we need a portion size and calorie amount for them:

- 1 teaspoon brown sugar.
- 1 teaspoon molasses.
- 1 teaspoon corn syrup.
- 1 teaspoon honey.
- 1 teaspoon jam.
- 1 teaspoon jelly.
- 1 teaspoon any candy.
- 1 teaspoon maple syrup.

Each of these teaspoons is equivalent in sugar content to a teaspoon of white sugar and can be assumed to supply about 20 calories. Actually most contribute less, but in the case of concentrated sweets, it is better to overestimate than to underestimate their energy contributions so as to encourage moderation in their use. (We repeated the 1 *teaspoon* with each item to reemphasize that each is like white sugar, in spite of many people's belief that some are different or "better.")

For a person who uses ketchup liberally, it may help to remember that a tablespoon of it contains a teaspoon of sugar. And for the soft-drink user, a 12-ounce can of a sugar-sweetened cola contains about 8 teaspoons of sugar. Controversy 4 offers more information on the sugar contents of foods.

CARBOHYDRATES IN A DAY'S MEALS. Chapter 2 introduced the basic tools to ensure that your diet provided at least the RDA for nutrients. There is, however, no RDA for carbohydrate, nor is there one for fiber. It is left to you to plan to get enough.

According to dietary guidelines, people would do well to obtain 55 to 60 percent of their daily energy from complex carbohydrate. The sample diet plans of Table 2–7 (p. 45) provided amounts close to that, so they take care of the caloric carbohydrate—starch. But what about the *other*, noncaloric, complex carbohydrate—fiber? Happily fiber follows other carbohydrates into the diet. As long as the choices are made of whole foods, such as whole grains, potatoes with skins, or apples with peels, no special effort need be spent on obtaining fiber.

The choice of whole foods, including whole grains, is especially important for staple foods, as already emphasized. Does this mean that you should never eat white rolls, potato chips, or apple jelly? No. An occasional white roll, like

■■■ Figure 4–12

Estimating Carbohydrate Intake using the Exchange System. This day's meals provide an ideal percentage of total energy from carbohydrate. A total of 264 grams of carbohydrate times 4 calories per gram is 1056 calories from carbohydrate, about 57% of the day's total 1750 calories. These meals also provide well over the recommended 20 to 35 grams of fiber, yet the eater made no special effort to do so and did not include refined fiber.

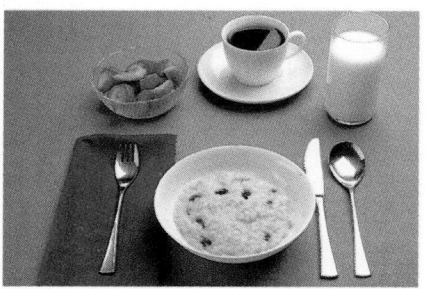

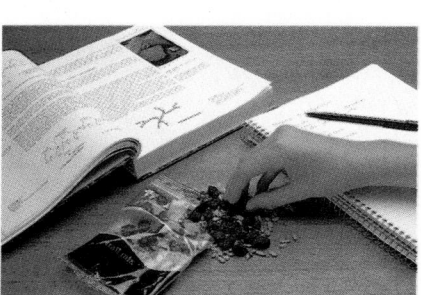

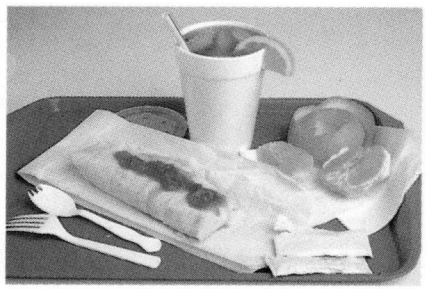

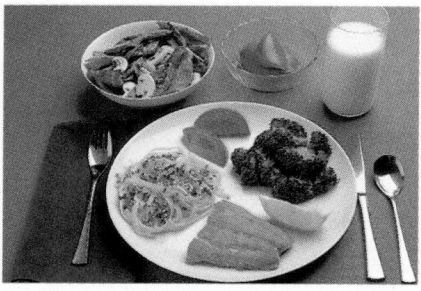

	TOTAL CARBOHYDRATE (GRAMS)	FIBER (GRAMS)
BREAKFAST		
1 c oatmeal = 2 starch/grains	30	4
¼ c raisins = 2 fruits	30	2
1 c nonfat milk = 1 milk	12	0
1 ¼ c strawberries = 1 fruit	15	5
MORNING SNACK		
2 tbsp raisins = 1 fruit	15	1
2 tbsp sunflower seeds = 2 fats		1
LUNCH		
1 beef and bean burrito		
(1 lg tortilla = 2 starch/grains	30	2
⅓ c beans = 1 starch/grains	15	6
+ ½ high-fat meat)		0
1 orange = 1 fruit	15	3
1 packet sugar	10	0
DINNER		
4 oz broiled salmon = 4 lean meats		0
1 c broccoli = 2 vegetables	10	6
½ c noodles = 1 starch	15	2
2 tsp butter = 2 fats		0
¼ c parsley = ¼ vegetable		
¼ tomato = ¼ vegetable	5	1
¼ c mushrooms = ¼ vegetable		
¼ c water chestnuts = ¼ vegetable		2
1 c fresh spinach = 1 vegetable	5	2
1 tbsp sesame seeds = 1 fat		0
1 tbsp vinaigrette and oil dressing = 1 fat		0
1 c nonfat milk = 1 milk	12	0
⅓ c garbanzo beans = 1 starch/grain	15	3
½ c sherbet = 2 starch/grains	30	0
Day's totals	264 g	40 g

an occasional candy bar, will not ruin a diet's adequacy; but for the bulk of the diet, the best choices are whole foods, and their fiber contributions are one of the reasons why. Constructed of whole foods, the diet can easily supply 15 to 30 grams of dietary fiber daily. One slice of whole-grain bread, a cup of vegetables (raw or cooked), and two portions of fruit (fresh or dried) will provide 15 to 30 grams of fiber. Using such foods as those recommended in Table 4–3 (p. 92), you can plan to receive about 25 grams a day of dietary fiber. Appendix A lists the amounts of fiber in each of over 1000 foods.

If high-fiber foods are new to you, your digestive system may need some time to adjust. Start slowly. Eat small amounts of salad and fresh cooked vegetables at first. Choose breads made with a mixture of white and whole-grain flours (these appear as light tan breads with flecks of brown). Try whole-wheat crackers, bread sticks, or puffed grain cakes, which are especially easy to like. Experiment with several whole-grain breakfast cereals (the kind to which *you* add the sugar) to find one that appeals to you. One trick to add fiber and the nutrients of whole grain to your day's foods, especially if you are having trouble adjusting to whole-grain products, is to use **wheat germ** liberally in toppings, coatings, and mixed dishes as well as on cereal. Wheat germ, unlike purified fiber, is rich in fiber and nutrients, but it also contains oil and so is high in calories; you might use it as a stepping stone to whole grains rather than as a permanent substitute.

Figure 4–12 redisplays the set of meals, first shown in Chapter 2, that a hypothetical student ate on a Monday. They were excellent choices nutritionally, partly because they contained abundant carbohydrate and fiber. The figure uses exchange system estimates for the amounts of carbohydrate and fiber in each food; if you were to look them up in Appendix A you would obtain different, but similar, numbers. You have to become familiar with the exchange system before this technique saves time, but a few practice sessions are enough to make estimating carbohydrate grams easy. To estimate the fiber, use the symbols and notes in Appendix D and remember that all vegetable list items donate between 2 and 3 grams per serving.

Carbohydrate is important, but it is only a part of the story. The next two Food Features will provide information on limiting fat and on obtaining enough, but not too much, protein.

wheat germ: the germ (see p. 93) of the wheat grain.

continued on the next page

SELF-STUDY

Examine Your Carbohydrate Intake

Having read Chapter 4, you are in a position to study your carbohydrate intake. From Forms 1 through 4 in Appendix F that you filled out earlier, answer the following questions. If you need help with calculations, turn to Appendix C.

1. How many grams of carbohydrate do you consume in an average day? (You calculated this on Form 2.)
2. How many calories does this represent (Form 4)? Remember, 1 gram of carbohydrate contributes 4 calories.
3. It is estimated that you should have at least 100 grams, and ideally much more, of carbohydrate in a day. How does your intake compare with this minimum?
4. What percentage of your total calories is contributed by carbohydrate (Form 4)?

▌▌▌ SELF STUDY *continued*

5. How does this figure compare with the recommendation that 60 percent of the calories in your diet should come from carbohydrate? (Note: If you are on a diet to lose weight, then this goal does not apply to you. See the exercises in Self-Study 9, "Practice Diet Planning.")

6. Another dietary goal is that no more than 10 percent of total calories should come from refined and other processed sugars and foods high in such sugars. To assess your intake against this standard, sort the carbohydrate-containing food items you listed on the copies of Form 1 into three groups:

☐ Foods containing complex carbohy-drate (foods found on the bread/starchy vegetable exchange lists).

☐ Nutritious foods containing simple carbohydrate (foods on the milk and fruit lists).

☐ Foods containing mostly concentrated simple carbohydrate (sugar, honey, molasses, syrup, jam, jelly, candy, cakes, doughnuts, sweet rolls, soft drinks, etc). Estimate and include such sources as the syrup of canned fruit, the sugars of flavored yogurts, and other sugars added during processing.

How many grams of carbohydrate did you consume in each of these three categories? How many calories (grams times 4)? What percentage of your total calories comes from concentrated sugars? From other simple carbohydrates? Does your concentrated sugar intake fall within the recommended maximum of 10 percent of total calories?

7. Estimate how many pounds of sugar (concentrated simple carbohydrate) you eat in a year (1 pound = 454 grams). How does your yearly sugar intake compare with the estimated U.S. average of about 125 pounds per person per year?

8. You may be interested in evaluating your fiber intake as well. Compare your fiber intake with the recommendation of 25 grams dietary fiber per day.

Notes

1. D. A. T. Southgate, The relation between composition and properties of dietary fiber and physiological effects, in *Dietary Fiber: Basic and Clinical Aspects*, eds. G. V. Vahouny and D. Kritchevsky (New York: Plenum Press, 1986), pp. 35–48.

2. M. I. McBurney and L. U. Thompson, Dietary fiber and energy balance: Integration of the human ileostomy and in vitro fermentation models, *Animal Feed Science and Technology* 23 (1989): 261–275.

3. U.S. Senate, Select Committee on Nutrition and Human Needs, *Dietary Goals for the United States*, 2d ed. (Washington, D.C.: Government Printing Office, 1977).

4. W. J. L. Chen and W. J. Anderson, Hypocholesterolemic effects of soluble fiber, in *Dietary Fiber*, 1986, pp. 275–286.

5. J. F. Swain and coauthors, Comparison of the effects of oat bran and low-fiber wheat on serum lipoprotein levels and blood pressure, *New England Journal of Medicine* 322 (1990): 147–152.

6. J. W. Anderson, Dietary fiber in nutrition management of diabetes, in *Dietary Fiber*, 1986, pp. 343–360.

7. S. M. Saheen and S. E. Fleming, High-fiber foods at breakfast: Influence on plasma glucose and insulin responses to lunch, *American Journal of Clinical Nutrition* 46 (1987): 804–811.

8. Dietary fiber reduces B-carotene utilization, *Nutrition Reviews* 45 (1987): 350–352.

9. E. Lanza and coauthors, Dietary fiber intake in the U.S. population, *American Journal of Clinical Nutrition* 46 (1987): 790–797.

10. Food and Nutrition Board, *Recommended Dietary Allowances*, 10th ed. (Washington, D.C.: National Academy of Sciences, 1989), p. 42.

11. Position of the American Dietetic Association: Health Implications of dietary fiber, *Journal of the American Dietetic Association* 88 (1988): 216.

12. S. G. Cooper and E. J. Tracey, Small-bowel obstruction caused by oat-bran bezoar, *New England Journal of Medicine* 320 (1989): 1148–1149.

13. J. L. Slavin, Dietary fiber: Classification, chemical analyses, and food sources, *Journal of the American Dietetic Association* 87 (1987): 1164–1171; D. M. Klurfeld, The role of dietary fiber in gastrointestinal disease, *Journal of the American Dietetic Association* 87 (1987): 1172–1177.

14. Food and Nutrition Board, Food and Nutrition Board, 1989, p. 41

15. J. Mourot and coauthors, Relationship between the rate of gastric emptying and glucose and insulin responses to starchy foods in young healthy adults, *American Journal of Clinical Nutrition* 48 (1988): 1035–1040.

16. G. M. Reaven, Parma symposium: Current controversies in nutrition, *American Journal of Clinical Nutrition* 47 (1988): 1078–1082.

17. D. J. A. Jenkins and coauthors, Simple and complex carbohydrates, *Nutrition Reviews* 44 (1986): 44–49.

18. S. Lillioja and coauthors, Impaired glucose tolerance as a disorder of insulin action, *New England Journal of Medicine* 318 (1988): 1217–1225.

19. G. F. Cahill, Beta-cell deficiency, insulin resistance, or both? *New England Journal of Medicine* 318 (1988): 1268–1270.

20. Much of this section was adapted from E. N. Whitney and S. R. Rolfes, Hypoglycemia and nonhypoglycemia, *Nutrition Clinics*, (Philadelphia: Lippincott, 1986).

21. A. B. Stevens and coauthors, Psychomotor performance and counterregulatory responses in healthy volunteers, *Diabetes Care* 12 (1989): 12–17.

22. V. Marks, Functional Hypoglycemia: Fact or fancy, *Hypoglycemia* (New York: Raven Press, 1987), pp. 1–17.

CONTROVERSY 4

Sugar: Is It "Bad" for You?

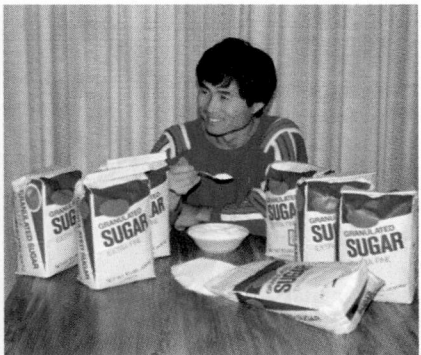

People today are said to be eating 125 pounds of sugar a year—amounting to about 25 percent of the energy they consume. Over half of this sugar is added by people directly from the sugar bowl or during food preparation at home. The other half is added by food manufacturers, mostly as fructose in **corn syrup**.[1] A century ago people's sugar intakes amounted to only 20 pounds per year, all from whole-food sources, and purified sugar was almost unknown. Since that time the amount of sugar in the diet has crept upward, as Figure C4–1 shows.

Figure C4–1 does *not* show that consumption of artificial sweeteners also rose dramatically within this time frame. The original purpose for artificial sweeteners, which are discussed in Controversy 5, was to replace some of the sugar in the diet, but this did not happen. People seem to be choosing both.

Does the large place of sugars in the diet harm people's health? Some

people think so. In fact, sugars stand accused of causing several diseases. When they are scientifically investigated, how valid do these accusations prove to be? And if any are valid, are sugar substitutes a better choice? This Controversy addresses these questions.

The Evidence

Sugar is thought, among other things, to (1) promote and maintain obesity, (2) cause and aggravate diabetes, (3) increase the risk of heart disease, (4) disrupt behavior in children and adults, (5) cause dental decay and gum disease, and (6) cause malnutrition. Is it guilty or innocent of these charges?

1. Does sugar cause obesity? Evidence from population studies shows that in many countries obesity rises as sugar consumption increases. But this evidence does not all point to sugar as the sole cause. Wherever sugar intake has increased, usually fat and total calorie intakes have also risen. Simultaneously, physical activity has decreased. Obesity also occurs where sugar intake is low, and fat people in many instances eat less sugar than thin people. Studies of populations do not, by themselves, make it possible to separate the effects of eating sugar from those of eating excess calories or of exercising too little.

Concentrated sweets do make it easy for people to consume large amounts of calories fast, however, and that is why most diet plans recom-

mend avoiding them. Some people believe that eating small amounts of sugar triggers binges; for them, conscientious sugar avoidance is an important part of weight-loss dieting.[2] For others the inclusion of small amounts of sugar in a weight-loss plan makes the plan easier to follow.[3] In short, the effects of sugar on a person's eating style and weight depend on the user.

2. Does sugar cause or contribute to diabetes? Recall from the chapter that in diabetes, insulin secretion or tissue responsivity to it becomes abnormal, and this, of course, affects the body's ability to manage sugar. At one time it was thought that eating sugar caused diabetes by "overstraining the pancreas," but this is now known not to be the case. More related than diet to diabetes is

Figure C4–1

U.S. Sugar Intakes

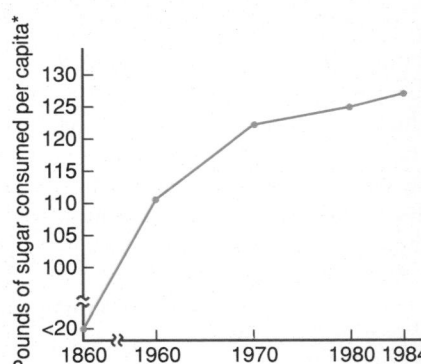

* Note: These amounts reflect both table sugar added at home and sugar sweeteners added in processing

source: C. Lecos, Our Insatiable sweet tooth, *FDA Consumer,* October 1985, p. 25.

body fatness. High rates of diabetes have not been reported in any society in which obesity is rare.[4] Still, it can be asked whether people with the genetic tendency to develop this type of diabetes should avoid eating sugar. The evidence on this point is conflicting and interesting.

In populations around the world, a profound increase—by as much as tenfold—in the incidence of diabetes has occurred simultaneously with an increase in sugar consumption. This has been true for the Japanese, Israelis, Africans, native Americans, Eskimos, Polynesians, and Micronesians. Yet in other populations, no relation has been found between sugar intake and diabetes. Wherever starch, rather than sugar, is the major carbohydrate in the diet, diabetes is rare; but this does not prove that sugar causes diabetes or that starch prevents it. The apparent protective effect of starch might be due to the chromium or fiber that comes with it, for example. Sugar is thought not to raise blood glucose levels any more than do starches.[5] The fairest conclusion that can be drawn is that obesity is a major causal factor but that sugar may share in the guilt as a contributor to diabetes.

Once a person has diabetes, is it all right to use moderate amounts of sugar? As recently as 1983 it was thought so because sucrose-containing foods seemed to elicit no more of a glycemic response (see p. 99) in many instances than did starchy foods. The American Diabetes Association published a state-

ment that "consumption of a modest amount of sucrose is acceptable, contingent on maintenance of metabolic control."[6] However, *other* body responses had not been looked at. Since then researchers have shown that people with diabetes eating a diet that contains a moderate amount of sucrose experience many undesirable metabolic effects, among them raised blood lipid levels suggesting an increased risk of heart disease. The amount of sucrose was similar to that eaten by most U.S. citizens today, and the researchers concluded that for people with diabetes, this was too much.[7] Not all researchers agree; perhaps if the diet is low enough in fat and high enough in fiber, some sugar will do no harm.[8] The jury is still out on this question.

3. Does eating sugar raise the risk of heart disease? Logic says that sugar turned to fat and transported through the bloodstream might cause the sort of fat deposits in the arteries that are known to lead to heart disease. (More about heart disease appears in Chapter 11.) Fat is clearly the major dietary culprit in the heart disease susceptibility of most people, but there is a hereditary condition in 10 to 20 percent of the population that is characterized by carbohydrate sensitivity. People with this condition tend to develop raised blood lipid levels in response to carbohydrate and alcohol in their diets, and their blood lipid patterns are associated with heart disease. If their heart disease risk seems high, they are told to

restrict their intakes of carbohydrate and alcohol.[9] Some research has appeared to indicate that the blood lipid response is especially marked after these people eat the sugar fructose—or sucrose, which contains it.[10] However, this sensitivity may apply to complex as well as to simple carbohydrate. The foods to avoid are those that elicit the greatest glycemic response, and they are sometimes sugary, sometimes starchy foods.[11]

Sugar may also have a relationship to high blood pressure, which contributes to heart disease. From studies of rats and monkeys, it appears that animals retain sodium when they are fed sucrose and that this raises their blood pressure (Chapter 8 explains how sodium raises blood pressure). From studies of people it is known that human beings excrete large amounts of sodium and water at first if they fast or restrict their carbohydrate intakes. When they resume eating carbohydrate (glucose, sucrose, or especially fructose), it causes them to regain both sodium and water.[12] However, the hormonal regulation of fluid balances quickly adjusts to different carbohydrate intakes, and within a few days the effect on blood pressure is gone. Such transient fluctuations are different from the dangerous, sustained hypertension associated with heart disease. A high-sugar diet does not cause a significant sustained increase in blood pressure in healthy subjects.[13]

Animal experiments implicating sugar in heart and artery disease have used diets so high in sugar that the results may not reflect effects of people's real sugar intakes. No one has shown conclusively, throughout many years of research, that moderate amounts of sugar (10 to 20 percent of total calories) affect the disease process in human beings.

4. What about sugar and behavior? In the 1970s and early 1980s, many claims appeared that eating sugary foods caused children to become unruly and adolescents and adults to exhibit antisocial and even criminal behavior.[14] Sugar has been called a toxin and an addictive drug, and people have been warned that their lives would be destroyed if they allowed themselves or their children to consume it. A criminal defense was even won on the argument that the defendant was in the habit of eating high-sugar "junk food," notably Twinkies, therefore had become hypoglycemic, and therefore was not responsible for his actions. Is there any truth to these claims?

The idea that nutrition influences behavior is a popular one. There are many ways in which it might do so—by altering the levels of chemicals in the brain that affect mood, by delivering substances to which people are allergic, by way of nutrient deficiencies, and others. The relationships of nutrition in general to behavior and mood are reviewed in Controversy 6, but the specific relationship of sugar to behavior is dealt with here. It has been proposed, specifically, that sugar adversely affects behavior by altering brain function. The brain is dependent on blood glucose for its energy, and according to the logic used by proponents of the sugar-behavior idea, eating sucrose causes wide fluctuations in blood glucose level, with frequent hypoglycemia and resultant irrational and violent behavior.

These ideas have generated a proliferation of research, all of which has yielded negative, or at most inconclusive, results. Some reports have simply not been based on valid research techniques (using hair analysis, for example, to diagnose hypoglycemia). One study claimed to show that abnormal glucose tolerance occurred at a higher-than-normal frequency among violent offenders, but it failed to take into account the probability that many of them were long-term alcohol abusers, a factor known to produce abnormal glucose tolerance test results, to say nothing of causing brain damage.[15]

In a study of 13 children hospitalized for psychiatric disorders, researchers gave the children either plain orange juice or orange juice sweetened with pure sucrose or fructose. The children given the sugar-added drinks became more active and exhibited more inappropriate behavior, but the researchers critiqued their own study, saying that it showed only that added calories permit children to exert more energy, not that sugar, specifically, has a negative effect on behavior.[16] They made a follow-up attempt to demonstrate that a high sucrose intake tended to make children distractable, but they again critiqued their own study, showing other possible reasons for the weak but apparently real relationship they found.[17]

Clearly, though, sugary food, like any energy-containing food, will enable children to do more of whatever they do, including misbehave. The "Halloween effect" is an example: tired children, overstimulated by the excitement of costumery and late-night gallivanting, may act up afterward. Sugar has been accused of making them do so, but this has not been proven. It is more likely and more reasonable to suppose that Halloween makes them excited and sugar simply gives them the energy to act that way.

In contrast to these inconclusive studies, one well-controlled study has shown that sugar calms children down, a finding consistent with convincing biochemical evidence. The subjects used were 21 boys whose parents described them as behaving badly after eating sugar. The study was designed to keep the parents' and the boys' expectations from influencing the results; none of them was told whether the boys were receiving glucose, sucrose, or a substitute (saccharin). The behavioral and physiological tests performed during the five hours following showed clearly that the boys were significantly *less* active after receiving the sugar than the substitute.[18] A follow-up study, using glucose, sucrose, saccharin, and aspartame in preschool children, showed no differences in activity, school performance, or emotional state in response to the four substances.[19]

Other studies have similarly failed to demonstrate any effects of sucrose on behavior either in normal or hyperactive children.[20] One analysis showed a difference between sugar and substitute in only one of 37 different measures, with children performing *better* on the sugar day.[21]

In the midst of all these inconclusive reports, one case stands out in which a hyperactive boy was found to become irritable, hyperactive, and headachy when he received a sugary drink but not when he received the same drink artificially sweetened. The physician tested in the same way the next 50 hyperactive children he saw but found no other cases in which this sensitivity to sucrose showed up.[22] In conclusion, very occasional behavioral reactions to sugar are not unheard of, but that sugar directly affects behavior adversely in most children or adults has been ruled out.

5. Does sugar cause **dental caries**? Caries are a serious public health problem. They afflict nearly everyone in the country, half by the time they are two years old. One of the most successful measures taken to reduce the incidence of dental decay is fluoridation of community water (see Chapter 8), but sugar has something to do with dental caries too.

Caries develop as acid produced by bacterial growth in the mouth eats into tooth enamel. Bacteria establish colonies known as **plaque** whenever they can get a foothold on tooth surfaces, and they multiply and affix themselves more and more firmly unless they are brushed, flossed, or scraped away. Eventually the acid of plaque creates pits that deepen into cavities. Below the gum line, plaque works its way down until it erodes the roots of teeth and the jawbone they are embedded in, loosening the teeth and infecting the gums. Gum disease severe enough to threaten tooth loss afflicts 95 percent of our population by their later years.[23]

Bacteria thrive on food particles, especially carbohydrate. Logic based on this point says that sugar might cause cavities. However, starch also supports bacterial growth if the bacteria are allowed sufficient time to work on it. Of prime importance is the length of time the food stays in your mouth, and this depends on the food's composition, how sticky it is, how often you eat it, and on whether you brush your teeth afterwards.[24] Bacteria produce acid for 20 to 30 minutes after exposure to sugar. Thus if you were to eat three pieces of candy, one right after the other, your teeth would be exposed to approximately 30 minutes of acid demineralization. Should you eat the candy pieces at half-hour intervals though, the acid exposure time would be 90 minutes. Likewise, slowly sipping a sugary soft drink may be more harmful than drinking quickly and emptying the mouth of sugar. A better choice is milk or water drunk with a meal to help wash the carbohydrate off the teeth. One large and well-controlled two-year study (979 children) showed that presweetened cereals eaten for breakfast did not increase cavities, probably because they were eaten at mealtimes and with milk.[25]

Mechanically disturbing bacteria by flossing every 24 hours may effectively prevent formation of cavities, regardless of the carbohydrate content of the diet. And some people may *never* get cavities because they have inherited resistance to them. Thus in this matter, as in the others, sugar may not be the extreme villain that some have made it out to be. Still, it is clear that sugar is the best energy source for the bacteria that cause tooth decay and that when exposure is sufficient, it is guilty as charged.[26]

■■■ Personal Strategy

Concentrated sugar is new in the human environment, and we are not biologically adapted to cope with it. It has been estimated that over a third of the calories in our diet now comes from sugars and visible fats, and sugar is our number one additive today. Our consumption of it is not entirely voluntary; two-thirds of the sugar we eat comes already added to foods during processing.[27] To reduce such a high intake to half or less of the present level would surely do no harm and might well do some good. However, sugar offers some benefits.

Sugar is valuable to some people precisely because it is a delicious, concentrated source of calories. After all, although many people in our society need to lose weight, some need to gain, and sugary treats can be useful in a weight-gain effort. A growing teenage boy, for example, may need up to 4000 calories a day, and as long as he eats enough nutritious foods first, the addition of the calories of sweets to his intake can help meet his vast energy needs. Sugar is also useful to an athlete in an endurance event, as Chapter 10 shows, although before the event starch seems to enable the athlete to store more glycogen in muscle than does sugar.[28]

The question of whether sugar harms health is less in the news these days, partly because evidence against sugar has been inconclusive.[29] Still, scientists continue their research to determine whether sugar directly affects health.

Sugar does, however, displace nutrient-dense foods from the diet.

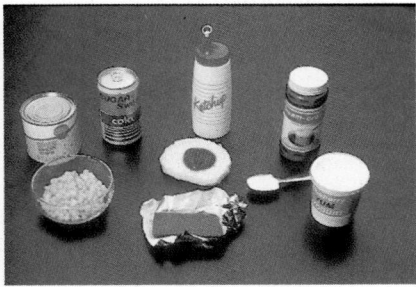

5 oz canned corn = 3 tsp sugar.
12 oz cola = 8 tsp sugar
1 tbsp ketchup = 1 tsp sugar.
1 tbsp creamer = 2 tsp sugar.
8 oz yogurt = 7 tsp sugar.
2 oz chocolate = 8 tsp sugar.

Processed foods contain surprisingly large amounts of sugar.

■■■ Miniglossary of Dental Terms

dental caries: decay of the teeth (*caries* means "rottenness").

plaque (PLACK): a mass of microorganisms and their resultant deposits on the crowns and roots of the teeth, a forerunner of dental caries and gum disease. (The term *plaque* is used in another connection—arterial plaque in atherosclerosis. See Chapter 11.)

Purified, refined white sugar, sucrose, contains no other nutrients—protein, vitamins, or minerals—and so can be termed an empty-calorie food. If you choose 400 calories of sugar in place of 400 calories of starchy food like whole-grain bread, you lose not only the starch but also the vitamins, minerals, and fiber of the bread. You can afford to do this only if you have already met your nutrient needs for the day and still have calories to spend. For teenage girls and others who have limited calorie budgets and who obtain too few nutrients, high-sugar, empty-calorie foods can be said to be contributing to their malnutrition.

Aside from malnutrition, a high-sugar diet may affect those with a tendency to develop kidney stones. Large amounts of sugar promote the excretion of calcium and magnesium, and these two minerals build up in the kidney to form stones.[30] For them, sugar is best used only moderately.

What about using a product such as **molasses** in place of white sugar? Molasses contains over 3 milligrams of iron per tablespoon and so if used frequently can make a major contribution of this important and, for women, hard-to-get nutrient. However, it is less sweet than the other sweeteners and so does not satisfy the "sweet tooth" of people who like sugar. Also, its iron comes from the iron machinery in which the molasses is made: it is a salt not easily absorbed by the body.

What about substituting **raw sugar** or **brown sugar**, **fructose**, or **honey** for white sugar? These sugars are virtually empty of other nutrients, just as white sugar is. The monosaccharide fructose is sold in purified, crystalline form, billed as a **"natural" sweetener** that, unlike the nasty, unnatural sugar sucrose, "won't cause ugly weight gain." This is just a sales pitch. What's natural about *any* purified, concentrated sugar? The calories in fructose are used for energy just as those in ordinary table sugar are—and too much of either can make you fat.

Some people believe that honey is better for health than white sugar because it is "natural." As a matter of fact, chemically they are almost indistinguishable. Honey contains the two monosaccharides glucose and fructose in approximately equal amounts. Sugar contains the same monosaccharides but joined together in the disaccharide sucrose. In the body, after digestion, sugar and honey are identical. Spoon for spoon, however, sugar contains

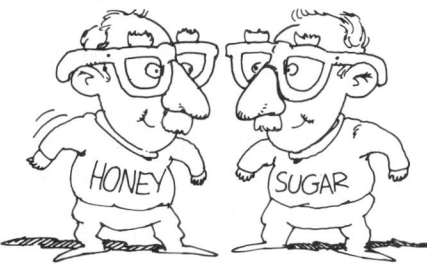

Honey has twice as much energy as the same amount of sugar, but in terms of nutrients there is no significant difference between them.

fewer calories than honey because the dry crystals of sugar take up more space than the sugars of honey dissolved in its water. Many other sugars try to lay claim to being "more healthy" than white sugar, but they too are white sugar's nutritional equivalents.

It would be absurd to rely on any sugar for nutrient contributions because one would have to eat so much to obtain significant nutrients. Thus if you choose molasses, brown sugar, or honey, choose them not for their nutrient contributions but for the pleasure they give. Tricks to get the most sweetness for the calories:

■ Serve sweet food warm (heat augments the perception of sweet taste).
■ Add sweet spices such as cinnamon, nutmeg, allspice, or cloves.
■ Add a tiny pinch of salt; it will enhance a food's sweetness.
■ Try reducing the sugar added to recipes by one third; this amount usually has little or no effect on the finished product except to diminish calorie content.

▪▪▪ Sugar Terms

Note: The term *sugars* here refers to all of the monosaccharides and disaccharides. On a food label the term *sugar* means sucrose. See Controversy 5 for *artificial sweeteners* and *sugar alcohols*.

brown sugar: white sugar with molasses added, about 95% pure sucrose.

confectioner's sugar: finely powdered sucrose, 99.9% pure.

corn sweeteners: corn syrup and sugar solutions derived from corn.

corn syrup: a syrup, mostly glucose, partly maltose, produced by the action of enzymes on cornstarch. **High-fructose corn syrup (HFCS)** is mostly fructose; glucose (dextrose) and maltose make up the balance.

dextrose: an older name for glucose.

fructose, galactose, glucose: the monosaccharides (see Chapter 4).

granulated sugar: common table sugar, crystalline sucrose, 99.9% pure.

honey: a concentrated solution primarily composed of glucose and fructose produced by enzymatic digestion, by bees, of the sucrose in nectar.

invert sugar: a mixture of glucose and fructose formed by the splitting of sucrose in an industrial process. Sold only in liquid form, sweeter than sucrose, invert sugar forms during certain cooking procedures and works to prevent crystallization of sucrose in soft candies and sweets.

lactose, maltose, sucrose: the disaccharides (see Chapter 4).

levulose: an older name for fructose.

maple sugar: a concentrated solution of sucrose derived from the sap of the sugar maple tree—mostly sucrose. This sugar was once common but is now usually replaced by sucrose and artificial maple flavoring.

molasses: a syrup left over from the refining of sucrose from sugar cane; a thick, brown syrup. The major nutrient in molasses is iron, a contaminant from the machinery used in processing it.

natural sweeteners: a term used freely, without legal definition, to refer to any sugar or sweetener except refined sucrose.

raw sugar: the first crop of crystals harvested during sugar processing. Raw sugar cannot be sold in the United States because it contains too much filth (dirt, insect fragments, and the like). Sugar sold as "raw sugar" domestically is not actually raw, but has gone through over half of the refining steps.

turbinado (ter-bih-NOD-oh) **sugar**: raw sugar from which the filth has been washed; legal to sell in the United States.

white sugar: pure sucrose, produced by dissolving, concentrating, and re-crystallizing raw sugar.

Also:

■ Learn to enjoy the natural sweetness of whole nutrient-dense foods—fruits, melons, and berries. You'll be eating sugars but in smaller quantities, and you'll get more nutrients with them.

■ Use all concentrated sugars in small quantities, including white sugar, brown sugar, **raw sugar**, honey, and syrups.

■ Eat limited amounts of foods containing added sugars— foods such as candy, soft drinks, ice cream, cakes, and cookies.

■ Select fresh fruits, fruit juice, or fruits canned without sugar or in light syrup rather than heavy syrup.

■ Use sugar substitutes that don't cause dental caries in place of sucrose and glucose in some foods, especially in snacks.

■ Read food labels for clues on sugar content—if the names for sugar—*sucrose, glucose, maltose, dextrose, fructose, or syrups*—appear first or if several appear anywhere on the ingredient list, then the food contains a large amount of sugar.

■ For snacks between meals, use sugar-free foods and beverages, or brush your teeth after sweet snacks. Remember, how frequently you eat sugar is as important as, and perhaps more important than, how much sugar you eat.

Finally, enjoy whatever sugar you do eat. Sweetness is one of life's great sensations, and you need not forego it completely. The person who cares about nutrition and loves sweets can artfully combine the two by using moderate amounts of sugar with creative imagination to enhance the flavors of nutritious foods.

Notes

1. C. Lecos, Our insatiable sweet tooth, *FDA Consumer*, October 1985, p. 25.

2. M. A. Gannon and J. E. Mitchell, Subjective evaluation of treatment methods by patients treated for bulimia, *Journal of the American Dietetic Association* 86 (1986): 520–521.

3. D. K. Cowley and F. S. Sizer, *Fad diets: Fact and Fiction? Nutrition Clinics,* (Philadelphia: Lippincott, 1987).

4. K. M. West, Prevention and therapy of diabetes mellitus, in *Nutrition Reviews' Present Knowledge in Nutrition*, 4th ed. (Washington, D.C.: Nutrition Foundation, 1976), pp. 356–364.

5. W. H. Glinsmann, H. Irausquin, and Y. K. Park, Evaluation of health aspects of sugars contained in carbohydrate sweeteners; Report of Sugars Task Force, *Journal of Nutrition* 116 (1986): S1-S216.

6. A. M. Coulston, How safe is sucrose for patients with NIDDM? *Nutrition and the MD*, January 1987, p. 1.

7. Coulston, 1987.

8. D. B. Peterson and coauthors, Sucrose in the diet of diabetic patients— just another carbohydrate? *Diabetologia* 29 (1986): 216–220, as cited by *Modern Medicine*, October 1986, pp. 117, 120.

9. Nutritionists say revaluation of sucrose "appears to be warranted," *Food Chemical News*, 21 February 1983, pp. 3–4.

10. J. Hallfrisch, S. Reiser, and E. S. Prather, Blood lipid distribution of hyperinsulinemic men consuming three levels of fructose, *American Journal of Clinical Nutrition* 37 (1983): 740-748.

11. D. J. A. Jenkins and coauthors, Low glycemic index carbohydrate foods in the management of hyperlipidemia, *American Journal of Clinical Nutrition* 42 (1985): 604–617.

12. T. Rebello R. E. Hodges and J. L. Smith, Short-term effects of various sugars on antinatriuresis and blood pressure changes in normotensive young men, *American Journal of Clinical Nutrition* 38 (1983): 84–94.

13. H. B Affarah and coauthors, High-carbohydrate diet: Antinatriuretic and blood pressure response in normal men, *American Journal of Clinical Nutrition* 44 (1986): 341–348.

14. J. F. Wallace and M. J. Wallace, *The Effects of Excessive Consumption of Refined Sugar on Learning Skills, Behavior Attitudes and/or Physical Condition in School-Aged Children* (a booklet available from Parents for Better Nutrition, 33 North Central, Room 200, Medford, OR 97501); S. Buchanan, The most ubiquitous toxin, *American Psychologist*, November 1984, pp. 1327–1328, as cited by R. Milich, S. Lindgren, and M. Wolraich, The behavioral effects of sugar: A comment on Buchanan, *American Psychologist*, February 1986, pp. 218–220.

15. D. H. Morris, Diet and behavior: Sugar (sucrose) and criminal behavior, *Food and Nutrition News* 58, no.1 (1986): 5–6.

16. C. K. Conners and A. G. Blouin, *Journal of Psychiatric Research* 17 (1982/83): 193, as cited in Nutrition update: Sugar, *Dairy Council Digest*, July/August 1984.

17. R. J. Prinz and D. B. Riddle, Associations between nutrition and behavior in 5-year-old children, *Nutrition Reviews* (supplement), May 1986, pp. 151–158.

18. D. Behar and coauthors, *Nutrition and Behavior* 1 (1984): 277, as cited in Nutrition update: Sugar, 1984.

19. J. L. Rapoport, Diet and hyperactivity, *Nutrition Reviews* (supplement), May 1986, pp. 158–162.

20. H. B. Ferguson, C. Stoddart, and J. G. Simeon, Double-blind challenge studies of behavioral and cognitive effects of sucrose-aspartame ingestion in normal children, *Nutri-*

tion Reviews (supplement), May 1986, pp. 144–150; M. L. Wolraich and coauthors, Dietary characteristics of hyperactive and control boys, *Journal of the American Dietetic Association* 86 (1986): 500–504.

21. Milich, Lindgren, and Wolraich, 1986.

22. M. G. Gross, Effect of sucrose on hyperkinetic children, *Pediatrics* 74 (1984): 876–878.

23. Gum disease largest threat to dental health, *Tallahassee Democrat*, 12 March 1987.

24. B. G. Bibby and coauthors, Oral food clearance and the pH of plaque and saliva, *Journal of the American Dental Association* 112 (1986): 333–337.

25. R. L. Glass and S. Fleisch, Diet and dental caries, *Journal of the American Dental Association* 88 (1974): 807–813.

26. S. M. Garn, M. A. Solomon, and A. Schaefer, Internal validation of sugar-food intakes in obese adoles-

cents (letter to the editor), *American Journal of Clinical Nutrition* 33 (1980): 1890.

27. Institute of Food Technologists' Expert Panel on Food Safety and Nutrition, Sugars and nutritive sweeteners in processed foods, *Food Technology* 33 (May 1979): 101–105.

28. D. L. Costill and coauthors, The role of dietary carbohydrates in muscle glycogen resynthesis after strenuous running, *American Journal of Clinical Nutrition* 34 (1981): 1831–1836; Dietary contributions to endurance athletics, *Nutrition and the MD*, September 1986; Sugar: Don't eat it to win, *Health*, June 1985, p. 12.

29. B. Szepesi, Carbohydrates, *Present Knowledge In Nutrition*, 6th ed. (Washington, D.C.: Nutrition Foundation, 1990), pp. 47–55.

30. Glinsmann, Irausquin, and Park, 1986.

▌▌▌C H A P T E R 5

The Lipids: Fats and Oils

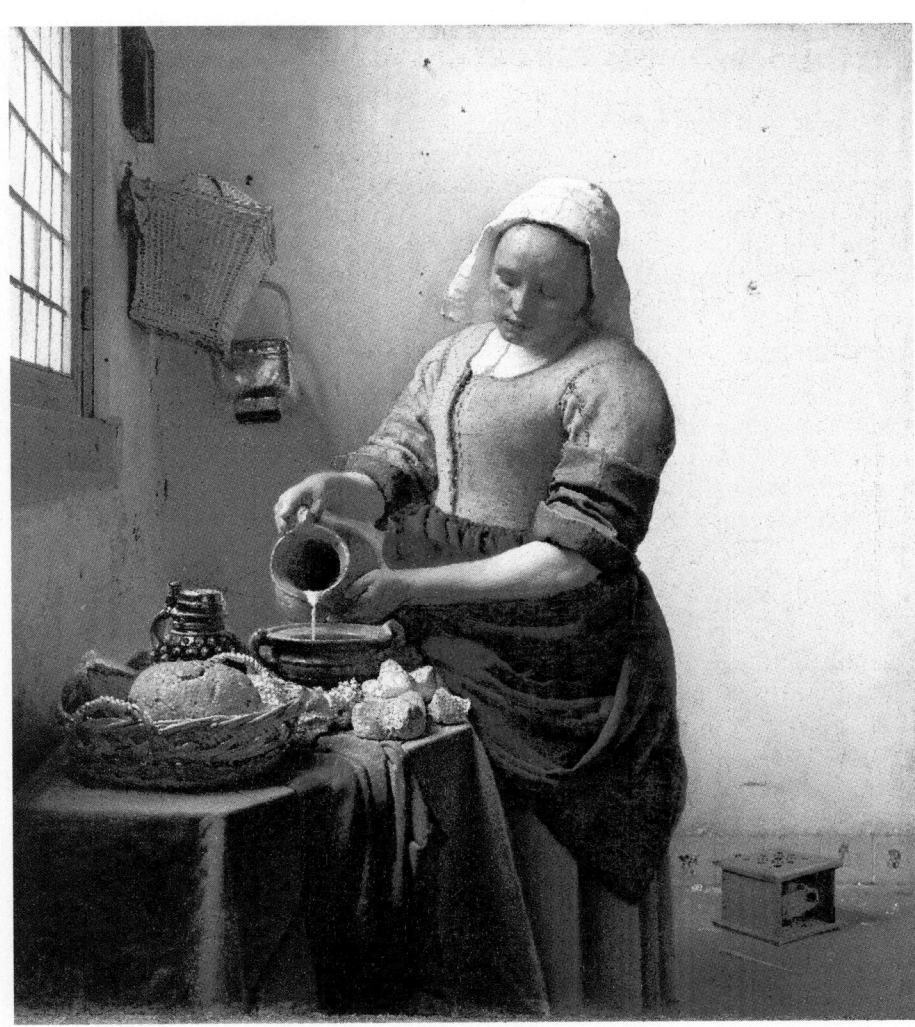

CONTENTS

Jan Vermeer, *The Kitchenmaid*, Rijkmuseum, Amsterdam (A2344).

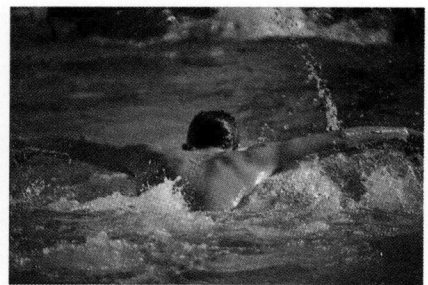

Body fat supplies much of the fuel these muscles need to do their work.

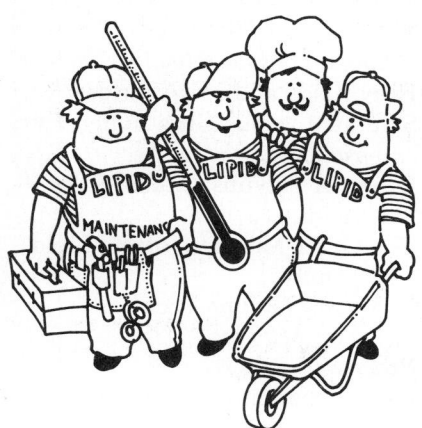

Lipids perform tasks that are absolutely necessary to the body.

▌▌▌ Your bill from a medical laboratory reads, "Blood **lipid** profile—$125." A health care provider reports, "Your blood **cholesterol** is high." Your physician advises, "You must cut down on the **fats** in your diet." A health-food store advertisement recommends, "Use fish **oils** to lower your blood cholesterol." Blood lipid profile, cholesterol, fats, fish oils—it is the mission of this chapter to provide an understanding of these and other terms related to fats, oils, and lipids and to make clear that they both contribute to health and detract from it.

▌▌▌ Introduction to Fats

No doubt you have been expecting to hear that the fat in the diet has the potential to harm your health. It may come as a surprise to hear that lipids are also valuable—more than valuable. In fact, they are absolutely necessary, and some lipids must be present in the foods you eat for you to maintain good health. Luckily at least a trace of fat is present in almost all foods; so you needn't make it a point to eat any extra.

Usefulness of Fats

Fat is the body's chief storage form for the energy from food eaten in excess of need. The storage of fat is a valuable evolutionary mechanism for people who must live a feast-or-famine existence: stored during times of plenty, it enables them to remain alive during times of famine. In addition, fats provide most of the energy needed to perform much of the body's work, especially muscular work.

▌▌▌ **Figure 5–1**

A Fat Cell. Within the fat cell, lipid is stored in a droplet. This droplet can greatly enlarge, and the fat cell membrane will grow to accommodate its swollen contents. More about fat cells and obesity—Chapter 9.

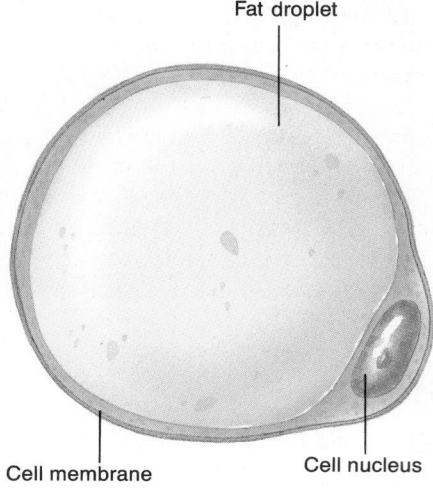

Fat droplet

Cell membrane   Cell nucleus

Most body cells can store only limited fat, but the fat cells seem able to expand almost indefinitely. The more fat they store the larger they grow, and an obese person's fat cells may be many times the size of a thin person's. A fat cell is shown in Figure 5–1.

You may be wondering why glucose is not the body's major form of stored energy. You will remember from Chapter 4 that the stored form of carbohydrate is glycogen. One characteristic of glycogen is that it holds a great deal of water, and as a result, it is quite bulky. The body cannot store enough glycogen to provide energy for very long. Fats, however, pack tightly together without water and can store much more energy in a small space. The body fat found on a normal-weight, healthy person contains sufficient energy to fuel a marathon runner or a long-distance swimmer to the finish or to give a sick person who cannot eat the energy to battle disease with minimum assistance from food.

By the same token, foods rich in fat are valuable in many situations. A gram of fat or oil delivers over twice as many calories as a gram of carbohydrate. A hunter or hiker needs to consume a large amount of food energy to travel long distances or to survive in intensely cold weather. As Figure 5–2 shows, such a person can carry more energy in fat-rich foods than in carbohydrate-rich foods.

On the other hand, high-fat foods may deliver many *unneeded* calories in only a few bites to the person who is not expending much energy in physical work. Overeating high-fat foods is especially likely because fat also carries with it many of the dissolved compounds that give foods enticing aromas and flavors, such as the aroma of frying bacon or french fries. In fact, when a person's appetite is poor, foods flavored with some fat may tempt that person to eat again. Some fat in food also slows digestion, lending **satiety** to a meal. People feel fuller longer after eating a meal with a little fat in it.

Fat pads in the body surround and cushion the vital organs. They serve as shock absorbers, so that you can ride a horse or a motorcycle for many hours with no serious damage to internal organs. The fat blanket under the skin also insulates the body from extremes of temperature, thus assisting with internal climate control. Some essential nutrients are soluble in fat and therefore are found mainly in foods that contain fat. These nutrients are the **essential fatty acids** and the fat-soluble vitamins—A, D, E, and K. A later section explains that essential fatty acids serve as raw materials from which the body makes molecules it needs. Vitamins are examined in Chapter 7.

Fat is important to all the body's cells as part of their surrounding envelopes—the cell membranes. Many dangerous household chemicals do their deadly work on the fat in cell membranes. Kerosene, gasoline, and paint thinners are a few of the substances that dissolve fat in human tissue when they come in contact with it. Such chemicals can injure the skin of the hands or (if swallowed) the digestive tract membranes. This is why people must keep these substances out of the reach of small children. Harsh soaps have an excess of alkali, which combines chemically with the fat of the skin cells and washes it away, leaving the hands dry and cracked. One must then apply an oily salve in an effort to replace the lost fat and to prevent further damage to the skin.

▌▌▶ *Lipids not only provide energy reserves but also lend satiety to meals, enhance food's aroma and flavor, cushion vital body organs, protect the body from temperature extremes, carry the fat-soluble nutrients, serve as raw materials, and provide the major material of which cell membranes are made.*

---

lipid (LIP-id): a family of compounds soluble in organic solvents but not in water. Lipids include triglycerides (fats and oils), phospholipids, and sterols.

cholesterol (koh-LESS-ter-all): one of the sterols; see page 122.

fats: lipids that are solid at room temperature (70°F or 25°C).

oils: lipids that are liquid at room temperature (70°F or 25°C).

satiety (sat-EYE-uh-tee): the feeling of fullness or satisfaction after a meal. Fat provides more satiety than carbohydrate or protein because it slows the stomach's motility.

essential fatty acids: fatty acids needed by the body but not synthesized in the body in amounts sufficient to meet physiological need.

■ 1 g carbohydrate = 4 cal
■ 1 g fat = 9 cal (but see page 136 and Controversy 10)
■ 1 g protein = 4 cal

■■■ Figure 5–2

Two Lunches. Both lunches contain the same number of calories, but the fat-rich lunch takes up less space and weighs less.

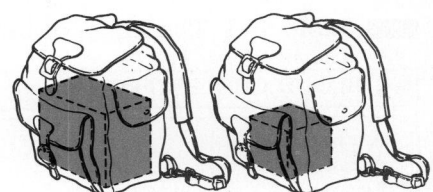

Carbohydrate-rich foods   High-fat foods

triglycerides (try-GLISS-er-ides): one of the three main classes of dietary lipids and the chief form of fat in foods. A triglyceride is made up of three units known as fatty acids and one unit called glycerol. More on fatty acids and glycerol later.

phospholipids (FOSS-foh-LIP-ids): one of the three main classes of lipids; lipids similar to a triglyceride but having a phosphorus-containing acid in place of one of the fatty acids.

lecithin (LESS-ih-thin): a phospholipid, a major constituent of cell membranes, manufactured by the liver and also found in many foods.

sterols (STEER-alls): one of the three main classes of lipids; lipids with a structure similar to that of cholesterol.

cholesterol: one of the sterols, a soft waxy substance manufactured in the body for a variety of purposes and also found in animal-derived foods.

cardiovascular disease (CVD): disease of the heart and blood vessels. The two most common such diseases are *atherosclerosis* and *hypertension* (Chapter 11).

Terminology

The lipids in foods and in the human body fall into three classes. About 95 percent are **triglycerides**. Other members of the lipid family are the **phospholipids** (of which lecithin is one) and the **sterols** (**cholesterol** is the best known of these).

Other terms of interest in connection with lipids relate mostly to health. A medical test, the blood lipid profile, reveals the amounts of various lipids (especially triglycerides and cholesterol) found in the blood and identifies the carriers in which these lipids are traveling. The results of this test tell much about a person's risk of heart and artery disease, or **cardiovascular disease** (**CVD**). The blood cholesterol level is especially telling, and it bears on the question of whether people should avoid foods containing fat, those containing cholesterol, or both. Chapter 11 addresses issues of diet and CVD in depth, but some distinctions are important now.

Most important in regard to CVD is *blood* cholesterol.* A person's blood level of cholesterol is considered to be a predictor of that person's likelihood of suffering a fatal heart attack or stroke.[1] Table 5–1 shows that blood cholesterol is one of the three major risk factors for CVD (the other two are smoking and high blood pressure, or hypertension) The higher the blood cholesterol, the earlier in life a person may suffer from heart or vascular disease. Reducing it by a third may cut a person's risk by half.[2]

The importance of blood cholesterol cannot be overstressed, but oddly enough, cholesterol in *foods* is of far less importance in relation to CVD. Food *fats* (triglycerides) raise blood cholesterol more than food *cholesterol* does. People often fail to understand this point, and the question arises again and again: "Should I eat cholesterol?" When told, "It doesn't matter as much as total dietary fat," the questioner often jumps to the wrong conclusion—the conclusion that cholesterol in general doesn't matter. It does matter. High *blood* cholesterol is an indicator of risk for CVD. The main food factor associated with elevated blood cholesterol is a high *fat intake*; dietary cholesterol makes only a minor contribution in comparison.†

One more distinction must be made clear about food fats as they relate to CVD. Fats come in two varieties, saturated and unsaturated, and the saturated type is most implicated in raising blood cholesterol. A later section describes the differences between saturated and unsaturated fats.

Food fats include visible fats and oils, such as butter, the oil in salad dressing, and the fat you trim from a steak. It also refers to some fats you can't see, such as the fat that marbles meat or the fat that is hidden in foods such as nuts, cheese, biscuits, avocados, olives, and fried foods. The photos of Figure 5–3

■■■ Table 5–1 The Effect of Blood Cholesterol and Other Risk Factors on Age of Onset of CVD

BLOOD CHOLESTEROL	200 mg/100 ml[a]	250 mg/100 ml	300 mg/100 ml
Age of nonsmoker	70	60	50
Age of smoker	60	50	40
Age of smoker with hypertension	50	40	30

The age listed is the hypothetical age of onset of the critical phase of CVD risk (60% coverage of artery surfaces by atherosclerosis).

The table shows that a nonsmoker with normal blood pressure and cholesterol of 200 would reach the critical phase at age 70. A smoker with high blood pressure and cholesterol of 300 would reach that phase at age 30.

[a]Milligrams cholesterol per 100 ml of blood.

SOURCE: Data from S. M. Grundy, Cholesterol and coronary heart disease, *Journal of the American Medical Association* 256 (1986): 2849–2858.

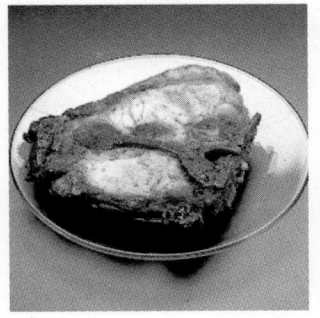

Small pork chop with ½ inch of fat (25 grams fat, 352 calories).

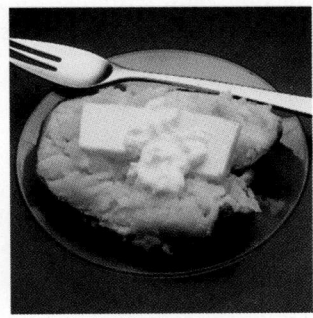

Large potato with 1 tablespoon butter and 1 tablespoon sour cream (14 grams fat, 350 calories).

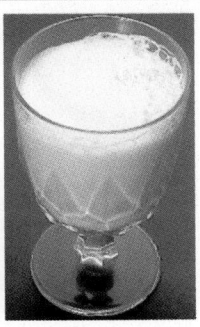

Whole milk, 1 cup (8 grams fat, 150 calories).

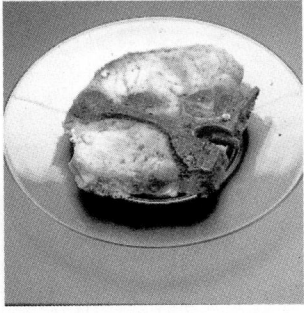

Small pork chop with fat trimmed off (13 grams fat, 265 calories).

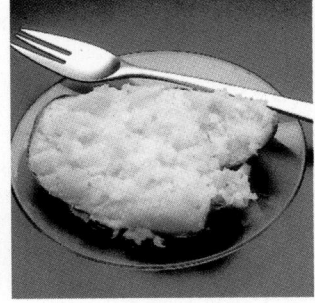

Plain large potato (less than 1 gram fat, 220 calories).

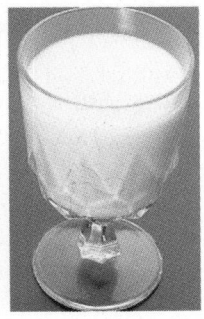

Nonfat milk, 1 cup (less than 1 gram fat, 90 calories).

■■■ **Figure 5–3**

Fat and Calories. Fat hides calories in food. When you trim fat, you trim calories.

show that when you remove the fat from foods, you also remove much of the energy. A small pork chop with a one-half-inch border of fat provides 352 calories; the same chop with the fat border trimmed off provides 265 calories. A baked potato with 1 tablespoon each of butter and sour cream has double the calories of a plain potato. Choosing nonfat milk over whole milk provides a large saving of fat and calories, and so it goes. The single most effective step you can take to reduce the energy value of a food is to eat it without the fat. This step is also an effective dietary weapon against high blood cholesterol.

*Blood, plasma, and serum cholesterol all refer to about the same thing; this book uses the term blood cholesterol. Plasma is blood with the cells removed; in serum the clotting factors are also removed. The concentration of cholesterol is not much altered by these treatments.

†Heredity modifies everyone's ability to handle food cholesterol somewhat, but a few individuals have inherited a total inability to clear from their blood the cholesterol they have eaten and absorbed. This condition is rare but well known because the study of it led to the discovery of how cholesterol is transported in the body. People with hereditary high blood cholesterol must refrain from eating cholesterol in foods; perhaps this is where the general public's fear of food cholesterol has come from. The majority of people can eat eggs, shellfish, and other cholesterol-containing foods without fear of incurring high blood cholesterol.

fatty acids: organic acids composed of carbon chains of various lengths. Each fatty acid has an acid end and hydrogens attached all along its length.

glycerol (GLISS-er-all): an organic compound, three carbons long, of interest here because it serves as the backbone for triglycerides.

▌▌▶ *An important distinction: total fat intake, and especially saturated fat intake, is the major dietary factor that raises blood cholesterol. Elevated blood cholesterol is a risk factor for cardiovascular disease.*

▌▌▌ A Close Look at Fats

Much of the fat in most people's diets comes from animals. Animal fat, in turn, may have come from the fats and oils in plants or from the carbohydrates or protein in plants. When an animal eats food and does not put all of its energy nutrients to work right away, it stores the excess energy as fat. Your body does the same thing. To convert carbohydrate or protein to fat, you first digest food and absorb the digested nutrients. Then your tissues may either use the protein or carbohydrate immediately or store some as is. The rest is broken down by the tissues into fragments—small molecules made of carbon, hydrogen, and oxygen. These fragments are then linked together into chains of carbon atoms known as **fatty acids**.

Fatty Acids and Triglycerides

Very few fatty acids are found free in the body or in foods. Usually the fatty acids have been incorporated into large, complex compounds: triglycerides, the chief form of fat. The name almost explains itself: three fatty acids (*tri*) are attached to a molecule of **glycerol**. Figure 5–4 shows how glycerol and three fatty acids combine to make a triglyceride molecule. Finally, triglycerides are transported to the fat depots—muscles, breasts, the insulating fat layer under the skin, and others—and are stored there.

Fatty acids may differ from one another in two ways: in chain length and in degree of saturation (explained next). Depending on which fatty acids are incorporated into a triglyceride, the resulting fat will be soft or hard. Those that contain the shorter chain fatty acids or the more unsaturated ones are softer and melt more readily. Each species of animal (including people) has its own characteristic kinds of triglycerides; but within limits, fats in the diet can affect the types of triglycerides made. For example, animals raised for food can be fed diets with different fats in them to give them softer or harder fat, whichever consumers demand.

▌▌▶ *The body combines three fatty acids with one glycerol to make its storage form of fat, triglycerides.*

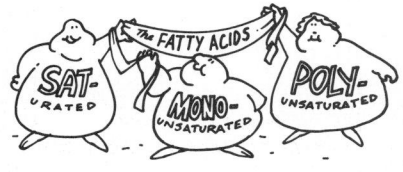

This trio of fatty acids is introduced chemically in Figure 5–5.

▌▌▌ Figure 5–4

Triglyceride Formation. Glycerol, a small, water-soluble carbohydrate, plus three fatty acids equals a triglyceride.

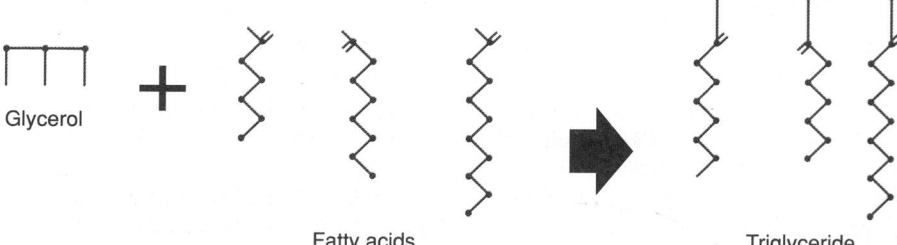

Saturated versus Unsaturated Fatty Acids

Saturation, a term that was mentioned earlier in relation to CVD, refers to the chemical structure—specifically to the number of hydrogens the fatty-acid chain is holding. If every available bond from the carbons is holding a hydrogen, the chain is a **saturated fatty acid**—filled to capacity with hydrogen. The first zigzag structure in Figure 5–5 represents a saturated fatty acid.

Sometimes, especially in the fatty acids in plants and fish, there is a place in the chain where hydrogens are missing, an "empty spot," or **point of unsaturation**. A chain that possesses one or more points of unsaturation is an **unsaturated fatty acid**. If there is one point of unsaturation (as in **oleic acid**), then it is a **monounsaturated fatty acid**; the second structure in Figure 5–5 is an example. If there are two or more points of unsaturation, then it is a **polyunsaturated fatty acid** (see the third structure in Figure 5-5). You sometimes see polyunsaturated fatty acids abbreviated on food labels as **PUFA**.

◗▶ *Fatty acids are energy-rich carbon chains that can be saturated (filled with hydrogens) or monounsaturated (with one point of unsaturation) or polyunsaturated (with more than one point of unsaturation).*

Essential Polyunsaturated Fatty Acids

The human body can synthesize all the fatty acids it needs from carbohydrate, fat, or protein, except two—**linoleic acid** and **linolenic acid**. These two, which are both polyunsaturated fatty acids that the body needs for its basic functions, cannot be made from other substances in the body or from each other. They must be supplied by the diet, and they are therefore essential fatty acids. Linoleic and linolenic acids are widely distributed in plant and fish oils and are readily stored in the adult body, so deficiencies are unlikely. Both serve as raw materials from which the body makes hormonelike substances that regulate a wide range of body functions, including blood pressure. Research is currently exploring the possibility that adequate amounts in the diet protect against hypertension.[3]

Of the two essential fatty acids, linoleic acid is an **omega-6 fatty acid,** and it is related to a whole series of other omega-6 acids—its family, so to speak. Linolenic acid is an **omega-3 fatty acid,** with a similar family of its own, including DHA and EPA seen on supplement labels. Linoleic acid has long been known to be essential; the essentiality of linolenic acid has only recently been appreciated.

---

saturated fatty acid: a fatty acid carrying the maximum possible number of hydrogen atoms (having no points of unsaturation). A saturated fat is a triglyceride that contains three saturated fatty acids.

point of unsaturation: a site in a molecule where the bonding is such that additional hydrogen atoms can easily be added.

unsaturated fatty acid: a fatty acid in which one or more points of unsaturation occur. An unsaturated fat is a triglyceride that contains one or more unsaturated fatty acids.

oleic (oh-LAY-ic) acid: a monounsaturated fatty acid found in animal and vegetable oils.

monounsaturated fatty acid: a fatty acid containing one point of unsaturation.

polyunsaturated fatty acid (PUFA): a fatty acid in which two or more points of unsaturation occur.

For a possible relationship between polyunsaturated fatty acids and cancer, see Chapter 11.

■■■ **Figure 5–5**

Three Fatty Acids.

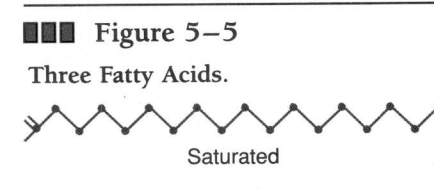

Saturated

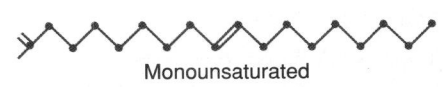

Monounsaturated

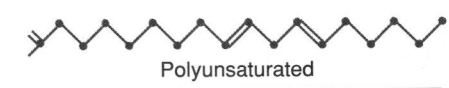

Polyunsaturated

■■■ Miniglossary of Polyunsaturated Fatty Acid Terms

DHA, EPA: omega-3 fatty acids made from linolenic acid in the body tissues of fish.

linoleic (lin-oh-LAY-ic) acid and **linolenic (lin-oh-LEN-ic) acid:** polyunsaturated fatty acids, essential for human beings.

omega: the last letter of the Greek alphabet (ω) used by chemists to refer to the position of the endmost double bond in a fatty acid.

omega-6 fatty acid: long recognized as important in nutrition, a polyunsaturated fatty acid with its endmost double bond six carbons from the end of the carbon chain.

omega-3 fatty acid: relatively newly recognized as important in nutrition, a polyunsaturated fatty acid with its endmost double bond three carbons from the end of its carbon chain.

■■■ Table 5–2 Dietary Sources of Omega Fatty Acids

FATTY ACID	FOOD SOURCES
Omega-6 family Linoleic acid	Safflower oil, sunflower oil, corn oil, soybean oil, peanut oil, meats
Omega-3 family Linolenic acid	Leafy vegetables, canola (rapeseed) oil, soybean oil, walnuts or walnut oil, fish and seafoods (including canned tuna)[a]

[a] Particularly good sources are herring, sardines, mackerel, water-packed white albacore tuna, trout, and salmon. These "fat fish" store their fat in their muscles; in contrast, lean fish (such as cod) store their fat in the their livers, which people generally do not eat. Chapter 11 lists other fish that are rich in omega-3 acids.

Each of the omega-3 and omega-6 fatty acid families plays a distinct role in the structure and function of body cells and systems. Together they or their hormonelike derivatives help regulate the formation of blood clots, blood pressure, blood lipid levels, the immune response, the inflammation response to injury and infection, and many other body functions.‡ They also become part of the structure of cell membranes.

The deficiency of any of these fatty acids in the diet leads to observable changes in the cells, some more subtle than others. When the diet is deficient in *all* of the polyunsaturated fatty acids, symptoms of growth retardation, reproductive failure, skin abnormalities, and kidney and liver disorders appear. Luckily these deficiency disorders are seldom seen except when intentionally induced in research. They sometimes do arise, however, when inadequate diets are provided by mistake—for example, in hospital clients who have been fed through a vein a formula that provides no polyunsaturated fatty acids for long periods or in infants fed exclusively on a formula that lacks polyunsaturated fatty acids.

Restoring omega-6 fatty acids corrects all of the symptoms of deficiency, and omega-3 fatty acids appear to be at least partially effective. Normal food, and especially a balanced diet that includes leafy vegetables and fish, supplies all the needed forms of fatty acids in abundance and prevents deficiencies. Table 5–2 lists some sources of both omega-6 and omega-3 fatty acids.

Given linoleic acid, the first member of the omega-6 family, in the diet, the body can convert it to the other members of its omega-6 family. One of these plays a critical role as part of cell membranes that define and protect each body cell. Any diet that contains vegetable oils and meats supplies enough linoleic acid to meet the body's needs. Linoleic acid need only contribute about 3 percent of daily calories to meet the need, and almost everyone eats enough.

Linolenic acid, a member of the omega-3 family, has been thought until recently to only duplicate some of the tasks performed by linoleic acid. It seemed dispensable as long as plenty of linoleic acid was available. However, someone thought to ask the question why the native people of Greenland, who eat a diet very high in fat, have such a low death rate from heart disease. The trail led to the abundance of fish they eat, then to the oils in those fish, and finally to the omega-3 fatty acids in the oils. Now researchers recognize distinct roles for compounds that the body makes from linolenic acid. Their presence

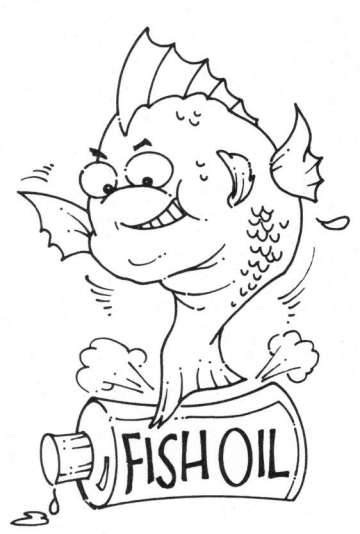

Eat fish; don't rely on fish oil. See Chapter 11.

‡The hormonelike derivatives referred to here are *eicosanoid* (eye-COSS-a-noid) compounds, such as prostaglandins and thromboxanes.

is evident in many tissues, and they are thought to be superbly adept at protecting membranes from destruction by oxygen, especially in the retina of the eye. In rats the concentration of linolenic products diminishes with age, leading researchers to wonder if age-related vision changes might be partly due to insufficient linolenic acid.[4] It also plays roles in the cerebral cortex of the brain and in male reproductive tissue.

The body converts linolenic acid into its derivatives inefficiently.[5] The rate of conversion suffices only to meet the body's minimum needs, not to store any extra. To build up body stores, we must consume omega-3 fatty acids directly, and many people eating regular diets in North America do not obtain enough to store any extra. They do, however, receive plenty of the omega-6 fatty acids—perhaps undesirably high amounts. A comparison with the fish-eating people of Greenland is illuminating. They eat more calories, and more of those calories come from omega-3 acids. We eat fewer calories, and more of ours come from omega-6 acids. Indeed, we eat about twice as many omega-6 and half as many omega-3 acids as the Greenlanders. Researchers have speculated that this may be why we have so many more heart attacks than they do.

Our high intakes of seed oils (rich in omega-6 acids) and our limited intakes of wild fish, wild plants, and wild game (rich in omega-3 acids) create a deficit of omega-3 acids in our diets.[6] Unfortunately human habitation and activity has devoured the wilderness and polluted oceans and lakes to the point where there is little remaining wild food to go around, and when we domesticate wild species, we often change the character of their fat from the omega-3 type to omega-6. Pond catfish are an example: in the wild, catfish eat lake-bottom weeds and animals from which they make omega-3 acids, but on a fish farm they are fed corn meal, from which they make omega-6 fatty acids. Some omega-3 fatty acid sources other than wild species exist, and these may become increasingly important as more discoveries about requirements are made. There is no Recommended Dietary Allowance (RDA) for omega-6 and omega-3 fatty acids, but scientists may agree on one to include in the next edition of the RDA. Meanwhile it is thought that we should try to include some fish in our diets, as well as vegetable oils, in order to balance omega-3 and omega-6 intakes.§[7]

▐▌▶ *Two polyunsaturated fatty acids, linoleic acid (an omega-6 acid) and lino-lenic acid (an omega-3 acid), are essential nutrients, used to make hormonelike substances that play regulatory roles in the body. The omega-6 family includes linoleic acid; seed oils are rich sources. The omega-3 family includes linolenic acid; fish oils are rich sources.*

The Other Members of the Lipid Family

The foregoing sections have dealt with one of the three classes of lipids—the triglycerides and their component fatty acids. The emphasis is appropriate because they represent 95 percent of all the lipids in the diet and in the body. The word *fat*, used properly, refers to the triglycerides.

§The recommendation is to try to obtain about 1 gram of omega-3 fatty acids for each 4 to 10 grams of omega-6 fatty acids.

emulsifier: a substance that mixes with both fat and water and that permanently disperses the fat in the water, forming an *emulsion*.

bile: an emulsifier made by the liver from cholesterol and stored in the gallbladder. Bile does not digest fat as enzymes do but emulsifies it so that enzymes in the watery fluids may contact it and split the fatty acids from their glycerols for absorption.

| CONSUMER CAUTION ▐▐▐ | **Lecithin Supplements** |

Lecithin periodically receives noisy attention in the popular press, being credited with great good deeds. You may hear that it is a major constituent of cell membranes (true) and that you must therefore purchase bottles of lecithin and give yourself daily doses (false). You might as well believe that to have healthy hair you must take supplements made from hair! One of the digestive enzymes takes most of the lecithin apart before it passes into the body fluids anyway, so not much of the lecithin you eat reaches the body tissues intact. All the lecithin you need for building cell membranes is made by your liver from scratch; in other words, lecithins are not essential nutrients. Furthermore, although once thought to be harmless, excess lecithin is now known to be potentially harmful. Even slightly higher-than-normal doses of lecithin fed to pregnant rats produce offspring with nervous system defects and retarded development. And large doses of lecithin taken by people have caused gastrointestinal upsets, sweating, salivation, and loss of appetite. These symptoms should serve to warn people to stop self-dosing with lecithin.

Some pill manufacturers claim that taking lecithin can unplug clogged arteries and lower blood cholesterol in people with CVD. Unfortunately, well-designed studies on lecithin show no such effect; supplements of lecithin do nothing to reverse CVD or to reduce people's blood cholesterol.

▐▐▐ **Figure 5–6**

A Molecule of Lecithin. A molecule of lecithin is like a triglyceride but contains only two (polyunsaturated) fatty acids. The third position is occupied by choline (a compound related to the B vitamins). The identity of the two fatty acids can vary, and all of the possible combinations are lecithins.

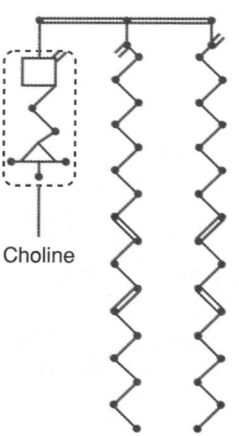

Choline

The other two classes—phospholipids and sterols—merit a moment's attention, though, because they play important roles in the body. A phospholipid, like a triglyceride, consists of a molecule of glycerol with fatty acids attached, but it contains two rather than three fatty acids. In place of the third is a molecule containing phosphorus, which makes the phospholipid soluble in water while its fatty acids make it soluble in fat. This versatility permits any phospholipid to play a role in mixing fats with water; it can serve as an **emulsifier**.

Lecithins and other phospholipids also play key roles in the structure of cell membranes. Because they are emulsifiers, they have both water-loving and fat-loving characteristics, which enable them to help fats back and forth across the lipid-containing membranes of cells into the watery fluids on both sides. Almost magical health-promoting properties are sometimes attributed to the group of lipids called lecithin, but the people making such claims are those selling supplements, as the above Consumer Caution makes clear. A molecule of lecithin is shown in Figure 5–6.

As for the sterols, they are large, complicated molecules consisting of interconnected *rings* of carbon atoms with side chains of carbon, hydrogen, and oxygen attached. The most familiar one, already named many times, is cholesterol, which serves as the raw material for making another important emulsifier, **bile**. Other sterols are vitamin D (made from cholesterol, and described in Chapter 7) and several important hormones—the so-called *steroid* hormones, including the sex hormones. These appear in later sections of this chapter and in other chapters.

Another claim made for lecithin is that it helps to improve people's memories. If only this were true, we could all benefit by eating lecithin; but if it is true at all, it seems to be so only for people with a specific kind of memory disorder. Even in those people, high doses are needed along with other drugs, suggesting that lecithin's effect is like that of a drug, not a nutrient. Lecithin probably works by contributing choline, but when researchers try to test its effects on neurological disorders results are disappointing. Memory weakness is not a sign of lecithin deficiency. When you hear someone making claims for lecithin, especially someone recommending that you take it to escape deficiency, ask yourself, "Do I really need this? What is the evidence that my body is likely to be deficient?" In the case of lecithin, as with the overwhelming majority of other products that are hawked this way, such evidence is lacking.

SOURCES: Anon, Dietary lecithin may pose hazard to unborn, abstract, *California Council Against Health Fraud Newsletter*, Jan/Feb 1984, p. 7; Can lecithin unplug arteries? *Tufts University Diet and Nutrition Letter*, October 1989; J. L. Wood and R. G. Allison, Effects of consumption of choline and lecithin on neurological and cardiovascular systems, *Federation Proceedings* 41 (1982): 3015–3021; S. Vida, L. Gauthier, and S. Gauthier, Canadian collaborative study of tetrahydroaminoacridine (THA) and lecithin treatment of Alzheimer's disease, *Canadian Journal of Psychiatry* 34 (1989): 165–170; J. Fitten and coauthors, Treatment of Alzheimer's disease with short- and long-term oral THA and lecithin, *American Journal of Psychiatry* 147 (1990): 239–242.

Cholesterol is an important sterol in the structure of brain and nerve cells. In fact, cholesterol is a part of every cell. Like lecithin, cholesterol can be made by the body, so it is not an essential nutrient. But while it is widespread in the body and necessary to its function, it is also the major part of the plaques that narrow the arteries in atherosclerosis, the underlying cause of heart attacks and strokes (see Chapter 11).

▌▌▶ *Phospholipids, including lecithin, play key roles in cell membranes; sterols play roles as part of bile, vitamin D, the sex hormones, and other important compounds.*

▌▌▌ Processed Fats

When manufacturers process foods, they often alter the fats in them. One of the major processes they subject them to is hydrogenation; another is emulsification.

Hydrogenation of Fats

Points of unsaturation in fatty acids are like weak spots in that they are vulnerable to attack by oxygen. When the unsaturated points are oxidized, the oils become rancid. This is why oils should be stored in tightly covered containers. If stored for long periods, they need refrigeration to retard the oxidation reaction.

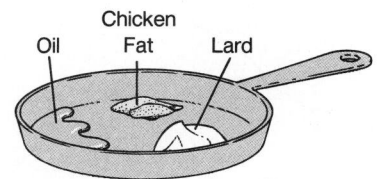

The more unsaturated a fat, the more liquid it is at room temperature.

hydrogenation (high-droh-gen-AY-shun): the process of adding hydrogen to unsaturated fat to make it solid and resistant to chemical change of oxidation.

antioxidant (anti-OX-ih-dant): a compound that protects other compounds from oxygen by itself reacting with oxygen (*anti* means "against"; *oxy* means "oxygen").

monounsaturated fats: triglycerides in which one or more of the fatty acids is monounsaturated.

polyunsaturated fats: triglycerides in which one or more of the fatty acids is polyunsaturated.

smoking point: the temperature at which fat gives off an acrid blue gas.

■■■ **Figure 5–7**

Nondairy Creamer. Some vegetable oils are saturated.

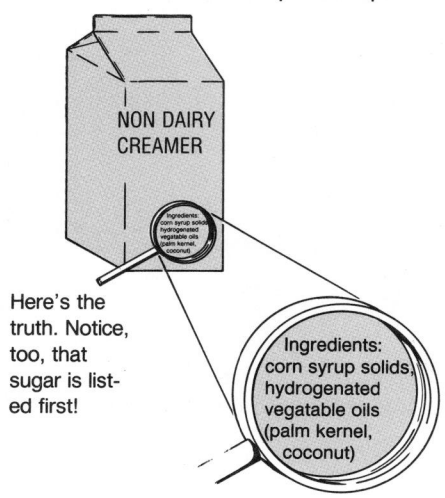

Sales pitch:
Nondairy creamer contains vegetable fat—and 20 calories per tablespoon.

NON DAIRY CREAMER

Ingredients: corn syrup solids, hydrogenated vegatable oils (palm kernel, coconut)

Here's the truth. Notice, too, that sugar is listed first!

One way to prevent spoilage of unsaturated fatty acids and also to make them harder is to change them chemically by **hydrogenation**. When food producers want to use a polyunsaturated oil such as corn oil to make a spreadable margarine, for example, they hydrogenate it. They force hydrogen into the oil, some of the unsaturated fatty acids accept the hydrogen, and the oil becomes harder. The product that results is more saturated and more spreadable than the original oil.

Once hydrogenated, oils lose their unsaturated character and the health benefits that go with it. An alternative to hydrogenation is to add a chemical preservative that will compete for the oxygen and thus protect the oil. Such an additive is called an **antioxidant**. Examples are the well-known additives BHA and BHT listed on snack food labels and the natural antioxidant vitamin E. A third alternative, already mentioned, is to keep the product refrigerated.

The presence of unsaturated fatty acids in a fat affects the temperature at which the fat melts. Generally the more unsaturated a fat the more liquid it is at room temperature. In contrast, the more saturated a fat the firmer it is. Thus of three fats—lard (which comes from pork), chicken fat, and safflower oil—lard is the most saturated and the hardest; chicken fat is less saturated and somewhat soft; and safflower oil, which is the most unsaturated, is an oil at room temperature. Chicken is recommended over pork for people avoiding saturated fats. Thus if your health care provider tells you to use **monounsaturated** or **polyunsaturated** fats, you can judge by the hardness of the fats which ones to choose. If you wish to see whether the oil you use contains saturated fats, place the oil in a clear container in the refrigerator and watch for cloudiness—the least saturated oils remain clear.

Generally speaking, vegetable and fish oils are rich in polyunsaturates, whereas olive oil is rich in monounsaturates, and the harder fats, generally animal fats, are more saturated. But you have to know your oils; it is not enough to prefer plant oils over animal fats. Not all vegetable oils are polyunsaturated. If you were looking for a substitute for cream, you might choose a nondairy creamer made from vegetable oil; but many nondairy creamers substitute coconut oil (one of the so-called tropical oils) for cream (butterfat). Coconut oil does come from a plant, but it disobeys the rule that plant oils are more liquid than animal fats; coconut oil is actually more saturated than cream and seems to add to heart disease risk.

Some manufacturers of processed food have taken steps to reduce or to eliminate tropical oils from their products in response to public demand (see Figure 5–7). Whether or not this is beneficial to heart health depends on the effects of the oils. Palm oil, used frequently in food processing, is highly saturated but seems not to add to heart disease risk.

Other oils have other effects. Olive oil may be beneficial to heart health, if the people of the Mediterranean are any indication; they consume large quantities of it and their cardiovascular health is good.[8] Lately canola oil (also called rapeseed oil), a rich source of monounsaturated fatty acids, has appeared on grocers' shelves. It, too, seems to benefit health when used in place of saturated fat.[9] Figure 5–8 compares fats and oils with regard to their percentages of saturated, monounsaturated, polyunsaturated, and omega-3 and omega-6 series fatty acids.

If you, the consumer, are looking for polyunsaturated oils to include in your diet, hydrogenated oils will not meet your need. A hydrogenated oil is easy to handle, stores well, has a high **smoking point**, and is suitable for purposes

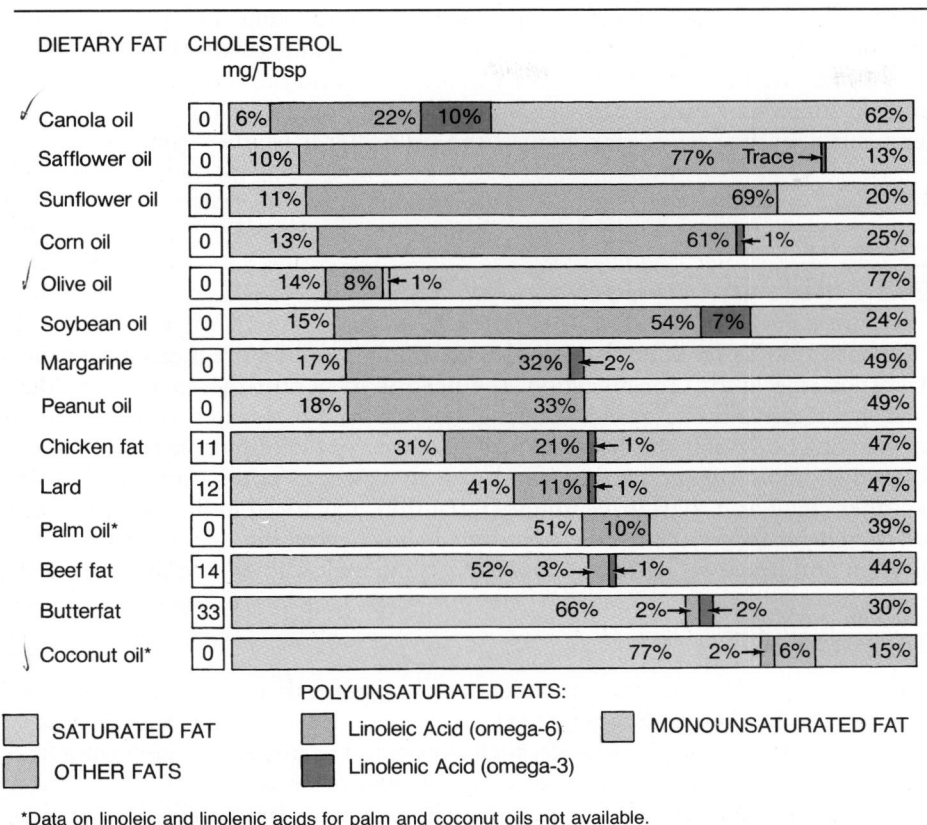

DIETARY FAT	CHOLESTEROL mg/Tbsp				
✓ Canola oil	0	6%	22%	10%	62%
Safflower oil	0	10%	77%	Trace→	13%
Sunflower oil	0	11%	69%		20%
Corn oil	0	13%	61% ←1%		25%
✓ Olive oil	0	14%	8% ←1%		77%
Soybean oil	0	15%	54%	7%	24%
Margarine	0	17%	32% ←2%		49%
Peanut oil	0	18%	33%		49%
Chicken fat	11	31%	21% ←1%		47%
Lard	12	41%	11% ←1%		47%
Palm oil*	0	51%	10%		39%
Beef fat	14	52%	3%→ ←1%		44%
Butterfat	33	66%	2%→ ←2%		30%
╲ Coconut oil*	0	77%	2%→ 6%		15%

POLYUNSATURATED FATS:

☐ SATURATED FAT   ☐ Linoleic Acid (omega-6)   ☐ MONOUNSATURATED FAT

☐ OTHER FATS   ☐ Linolenic Acid (omega-3)

*Data on linoleic and linolenic acids for palm and coconut oils not available.
Sources: Canola oil: data on file, Procter & Gamble. All others: J. B. Reeves and J. L. Weihrauch, *Composition of Foods, Agriculture Handbook No. 8–4.* Washington, D.C.: United States Department of Agriculture, 1979. Reprinted with permission from Procter & Gamble Copyright © 1987.

such as frying, but it is more saturated than the oil it was made from. In contrast, margarines that list liquid oil as the first ingredient are usually the most polyunsaturated. Margarines that are sold in tubs and labeled "soft" are sometimes less saturated than the stick varieties.[10]

Newest among the fats are the artificial fats, which hold promise for solving some of the problems just described. Food technologists have been working for years to develop substances that duplicate the taste and cooking functions of fats but that contribute none of the calories or risks of fats. This chapter's Controversy presents the current status of artificial fats.

■■▶ *The degree of saturation of the fatty acids in a fat and the crystal size in a solid fat affect how the fat behaves. Vegetable margarines are partially hydrogenated oils that are more saturated than the oils they are made from.*

Emulsification of Fats

No doubt you have encountered salad dressings that separate to form two layers—vinegar on the bottom, oil on top. You have to shake them to blend them before pouring them on your salad. No doubt you are acquainted, too,

monoglycerides (mon-oh-GLISS-er-ides): a product of the digestion of lipids; glycerol molecules with one fatty acid attached to it (*mono* means "one"; *glyceride* means "a compound of glycerol").

Chapter 3 presented details of the digestive system.

with other dressings made from vinegar and oil that never separate—mayonnaise, for example. Food chemists accomplish the mixing of ingredients in mayonnaise the same way the body does: they blend the vinegar and oil with a third ingredient that mixes well with both fatty oil and watery vinegar—an emulsifier. In the case of mayonnaise, the emulsifier is lecithin from egg yolks.

▮▮▶ *Emulsified fats have their fats mixed permanently with water.*

▮▮▮ Lipids in the Body

The body needs to mix lipids with its own watery fluids before it can digest and transport the lipids. For digestion, the need is to permit the enzymes in the watery digestive fluids to mix thoroughly with lipid molecules to break them down. The body uses the emulsifier bile to disperse food lipids into the watery digestive fluids. After digesting and absorbing these lipids, the body faces another challenge: to package lipids so that they may travel in the watery fluids of the circulatory system. The next two sections give the details of lipid digestion and transport, with an emphasis on the major lipids, the triglycerides.

Digestion of Fats

When you partake of animal products, such as meat, fish, poultry, milk, cheese, or eggs, the energy-yielding nutrients you are eating are fat and protein. When you eat oil-containing plant foods, such as coconut or olives, you are eating fat, protein, and carbohydrate. Of the fats and oils in foods, 95 percent are triglycerides that have been made in living tissues, mostly from carbohydrate, the same way you make them.

Food fat can end up in fat stores in your own body, but first it has to be digested, absorbed, and transported to its cell destinations. Once the food has been chewed and swallowed, it travels to the stomach, where the fat separates from other components and floats as a layer on the top. Since fat does not mix with the stomach fluids, little fat digestion takes place.

▮▮▮ **Figure 5–9**
The Action of Bile in Fat Digestion.

A. In the stomach, fat floats in a layer.

B. In the small intestine, bile attracts both water and fat, emulsifying them.

C. Enzymes from the pancreas can attack fat after emulsification by bile.

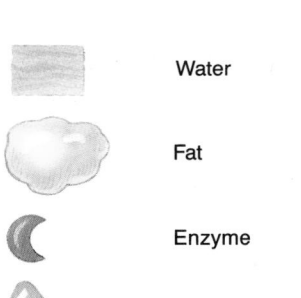

Water

Fat

Enzyme

Bile

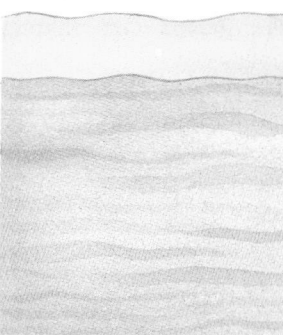 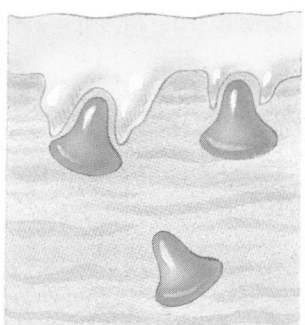 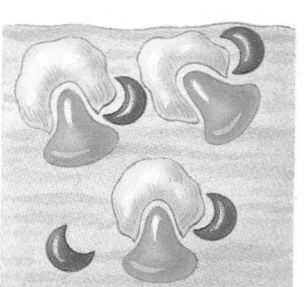

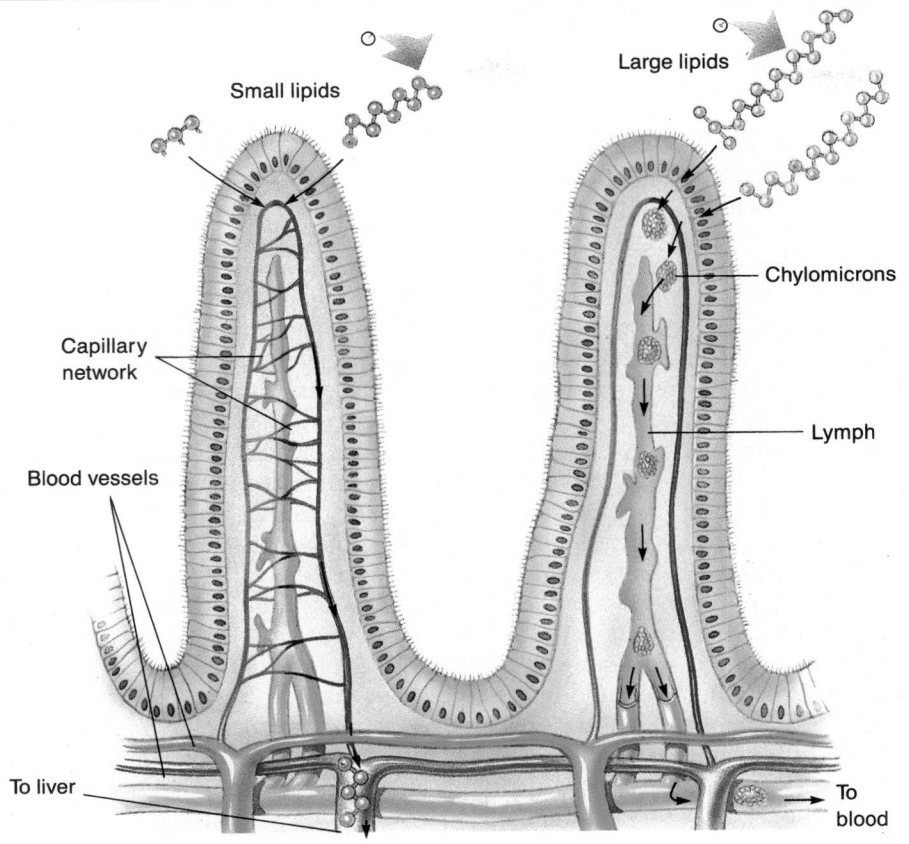

Small lipids

Large lipids

Capillary
network

Chylomicrons

Blood vessels

Lymph

To liver

To
blood

■■■ Figure 5–10

Absorption and Transport of Lipids.
The villus on the right shows that
large lipids such as monoglycerides
and long-chain fatty acids must be
incorporated into chylomicrons that
can travel through the lymph. The
villus on the left shows that glycerol
and short-chain fatty acids can move
directly into the bloodstream. In this
the diagram, molecules of fatty acids
are shown as large objects, but in
reality, molecules of fatty acids are too
small to see, even with a powerful
microscope, while villi are visible to
the naked eye.

Once the fat enters the small intestine, the gallbladder, which stores up the
liver's output of bile, contracts to squirt bile into the intestinal contents. Bile
emulsifies the fat and holds it suspended as tiny particles until the enzymes
contributed by the pancreas and other glands can split them for absorption.
Figure 5–9 shows that one end of the bile molecule attracts and holds fat,
while the other end is attracted to and held by water. People sometimes wonder
how a person who has had the gallbladder removed can eat. Even without the
gallbladder, the liver still produces bile and delivers it directly into the small
intestine, where it works on fat.

Once the intestine's contents are emulsified, fat-splitting enzymes are free to
act on triglycerides and to split the fatty acids from their glycerol backbones.
Free fatty acids, glycerol, and **monoglycerides** are small enough to pass
through the cells of the digestive tract lining and to enter the vessels therein.
From here the body must transport the fat particles through the blood and
lymph to the tissues that need them. Glycerol and shorter chain fatty acids can
travel in the bloodstream without help; other fats require special handling for
transport. Absorption and transport of lipids are depicted in Figure 5–10.

❙❙▶ *In the stomach, fats separate from other food components. In the small intestine, bile emulsifies them, enzymes digest them, and the intestinal cells absorb
them.*

Lipid Transport in the Body Fluids

Within the body many fats always travel from place to place mixed with protein particles—that is, as **lipoproteins**. For example, the monoglycerides and long-chain fatty acids liberated from digested food fat are too large to be released directly into the bloodstream—they would separate out and float in globules, disrupting the blood's normal functions. Instead the intestinal cells allow them to cluster together, and before release, they combine them with protein, forming a type of lipoprotein. The protein in the cluster acts somewhat like an emulsifier in that it is attracted to both water and fat. Its association with both substances enables the fats to travel in the watery body fluids. That way, when the tissues of the body need energy from fat, they can extract what they need from these clusters. What is left, the remnants, are picked up by the liver, which dismantles them and reuses their parts. Figure 5–11 depicts a lipoprotein.

Lipoproteins are very much on the minds of health care providers who measure people's blood lipid profiles. They are interested not only in the types of fats in the blood (triglycerides and cholesterol) but also in the lipoproteins that carry them. One distinction among types of lipoproteins is of great importance because it has implications for the health of the heart and blood vessels; that is the distinction between **low-density lipoproteins** (**LDL**) and **high-density lipoproteins** (HDL).[||] The more protein in the lipoprotein molecule, the higher the density; the more lipids, the lower the density. Both LDL and HDL carry lipids around in the blood, but the LDL are larger, lighter, and more lipid filled; the HDL are smaller, denser, and carry less lipid. Raised LDL concentrations in the blood are a sign of high heart-attack risk, whereas raised HDL concentrations are associated with a low risk. The next section clarifies this relationship.

■■■ Figure 5–11

A Lipoprotein. An LDL has a higher ratio of lipid to protein; an HDL has more protein relative to its lipid content.
Source: Adapted from D. Kritchevsky, An update on lipids, lipoproteins and fat metabolism, in *The Medicine Called Nutrition,* Medical Education (Meded) Programs, Ltd. (Englewood Cliffs, N.J.: Best Foods, 1979), p. 61.

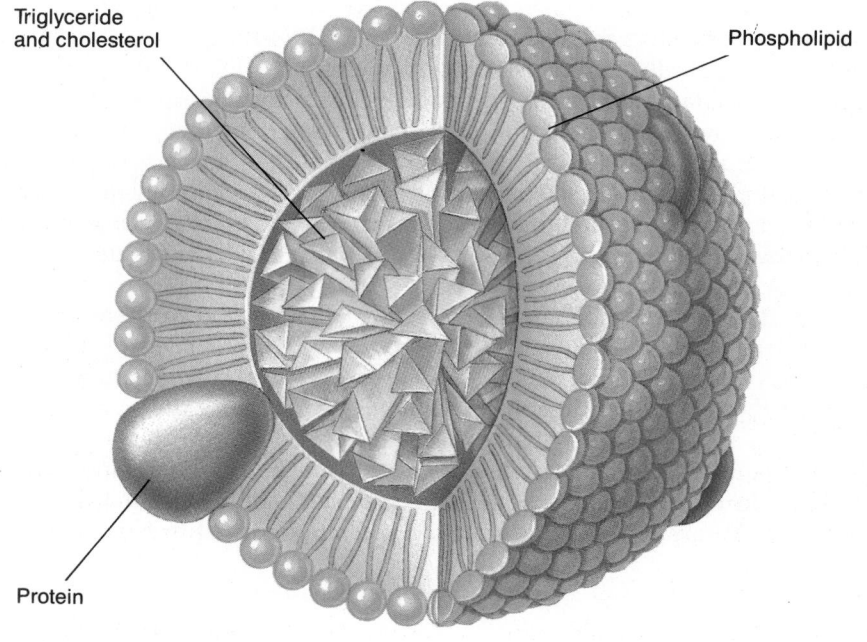

❚❚▶ *Blood and other body fluids are watery, so non-water-soluble fats need a special transport system to carry them around the body—the lipoproteins. Among lipoproteins, the HDL are unique in that a high blood concentration indicates a reduced heart-disease risk.*

Significance of LDL and HDL

The beginning of this chapter made clear that although the cholesterol in foods does contribute somewhat to cholesterol in the blood and it is prudent to avoid excesses, dietary cholesterol is not as influential as total dietary fat, and especially saturated fat, in raising blood cholesterol—actually, LDL. It is LDL that forecasts heart and artery disease. Fortunately, the changes in diet that reduce blood cholesterol concentrations mostly do so by reducing LDL. HDL remain unaffected.

Among the most influential dietary factors that *raise* LDL are total fat, saturated fat, and high calories.[11] Among those that lower LDL are monounsaturated fats, including those of olive oil and rapeseed oil, and polyunsaturated fats, including those of other vegetable oils and fish oils. As for dietary cholesterol itself, it raises LDL slightly, depending on the amount eaten and on the body's ability to compensate by making less. Generally guidelines recommend that we eat no more than 30 percent of calories as fat, with no more than a third of this fat as saturated fat; that we partially substitute polyunsaturated and monounsaturated fats for saturated fats; and that we limit our cholesterol intakes to less than 300 milligrams per day.

Some say all adults should take steps to reduce their blood cholesterol; others say only those medically identified as at risk for heart disease should do so. The question remains open, but it seems likely that most people need not make efforts to reduce their intakes of food cholesterol very stringently. Eggs, shellfish, liver, and other cholesterol-containing foods are nutritious and, used in moderation, have little blood cholesterol-raising effect. Cholesterol is unlike salt and sugar in this respect: you cannot omit it from the diet without omitting nutritious foods. On the other hand, it may be advisable for most people to control their *fat* intakes; this will help some people's health and probably harm no one.

❚❚▶ *Dietary measures most effective in reducing the risk of heart disease are reducing total fat and saturated fats and partially substituting polyunsaturated fats. A third measure, perhaps effective to a lesser degree, is to reduce cholesterol intake. Don't omit cholesterol-containing foods altogether; they are nutritious. To lower LDL and to raise HDL further, stop smoking and exercise regularly.*

Use of Stored Fat for Energy

When a person's body starts to run out of fuel from food, it begins to use its stored fat for energy and also its glycogen, as the last chapter showed. Fat cells respond to the call for energy by starting to dismantle stored fat molecules and

---

‖ These are just two of the known lipoproteins. Others include chylomicrons (the clusters of protein and lipid made in the intestines, referred to earlier), and very-low-density lipoproteins (VLDL).

■■■ **Figure 5-12**

Glucose to Fat. Glucose can be used for energy or can be changed into fat. Glucose is broken down into fragments (A), and the fragments can provide immediate energy for the tissues. If the tissues need no more energy, the fragments can be reassembled (B), not back to glucose but into fatty acid chains.

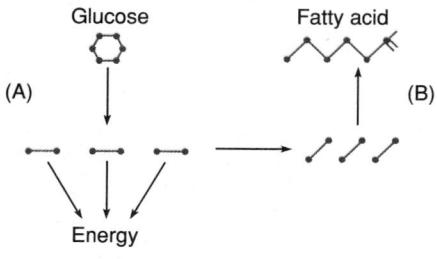

releasing their components into the blood. When energy-hungry cells receive these components, they break them down further into small fragments. Finally, each fat fragment combines with a fragment derived from glucose, and oxidation proceeds to yield energy, carbon dioxide, and water.

Thus whenever you break down your body fat, you need carbohydrate to do so. Without carbohydrate, ketosis will occur, as described in the last chapter, and products of incomplete fat breakdown (ketones) will appear in the blood and urine. Because this process and its consequences are so important in weight control, Chapter 9 describes them in greater detail.

It may be that fat is a more efficient fuel than glucose.[12] Tests performed in the laboratory to measure how many calories a substance contains use the same method for all fuels—the fuels are completely burned, and the heat energy they release is measured in calories. But the body is different from a laboratory in that it treats energy substances in different ways, depending on the substance and on body conditions. To be stored as fat, glucose must undergo many chemical conversions in the body, each requiring energy to perform (see Figure 5-12). Fat, on the other hand, requires fewer conversions. The body may spend less energy assimilating fat than assimilating carbohydrate. Thus it can store more calories when fat is eaten than it can store from the same number of calories (according to laboratory measurement) of carbohydrate. In short, you may get fatter on fat calories than on the same number of carbohydrate calories. Controversy 10 revisits this emerging theory and tells what, if any, significance it holds to planners of meals who wish to control energy from fat in the diet.

■■■ Fat in the Diet

The remainder of this chapter will help you to apply what you have learned about fats—that is, how to choose foods that supply enough, but not too much, of the right kinds of fat to support optimal health and to provide pleasure in eating. To start, you must know where the fats are in the food groups.

Three food groups—fats and oils; meat, poultry, and fish; and dairy products—have traditionally accounted for about nine-tenths of the fat in the North American diet. However, recently there has been some shift from animal fats to fats of vegetable origin. The increasing consumption of vegetable fats and oils has come about because of three factors: (1) their increased use by fast-food chains serving fried foods such as french fries and chicken, (2) a shift away from the use of lard, and (3) a shift from butter to margarine. A healthy trend is appearing: people are increasing the proportion of unsaturated to saturated fat in their diets.[13] This is countered, though, by a high overall fat intake. Remember, though, that the total amount of fat in the diet, even more than the degree of saturation of that fat, most profoundly affects health.

The exchange lists show exactly where the fats are in foods. Two groups always contain fat (the fats and the meats), and two sometimes contain fat (the milks and the breads). The unprocessed vegetables and fruits are, for the most part, fat free. Figure 5-13 illustrates the fat values of foods.

The Fats

One portion of fat contains about 5 grams of fat, donating 45 calories and negligible protein and carbohydrate. Examples are:

1 oz = 28.4 g (dietitians often use "about 30 g" for an ounce).
1 oz meat = about 30 g meat, containing about 7 g protein and from 3 to 15 g of fat.

■■■ **Table 5–3 Some Examples of Lean, Medium-, and High-Fat Meats**

LEAN MEAT	MEDIUM-FAT MEAT	HIGH-FAT MEAT
Beef tenderloin, round steak	Corned beef, chuck	Hamburger; club or rib steaks
Chicken or turkey without skin	Ground round steak	Fried chicken or fish patties as in fast food
Leg of Lamb	Pork roast, liver, heart, kidney	Breast of lamb
Fish	Eggs, creamed cottage cheese	Duck, goose
Dry cottage cheese		Cold cuts
		Hot dogs
		Cheddar cheese

- A teaspoon of butter or margarine.
- One-eighth of an avocado or five small olives.
- Two large whole pecans or 1 tablespoon of french dressing.
- Two tablespoons of sour cream or 1 tablespoon of heavy cream.
- Ten large peanuts.
- A strip of crisp bacon.

Many are surprised to find crisp bacon listed as a fat. They expect to find bacon fat included but think of bacon as meat. It is classified as a fat, however, because its protein content is negligible, even if it is fried crisp and the melted fat is drained away.

■■▶ *Fats occur naturally in milk products and meats. In their natural states, grains are like fruits and vegetables in that they contain little or no fat. However, fat is often added to grains to produce products such as cakes, breakfast cereals, and muffins.*

The Meats

Meats conceal much of the fat that people unwittingly consume. Many people, when choosing a serving of meat, don't realize that they are electing to eat a large amount of fat. To help people "see" the fat in meats, the exchange lists present the meats in three categories according to their fat contents: low-fat, medium-fat, and high-fat meats. Meats in all three categories contain about equal amounts of protein; but because they differ in amounts of fat, their calorie amounts vary significantly. Table 5–3 lists some examples of lean, medium-fat, and high-fat meats. The complete meat lists are in Appendix D.

A unit of meat on the exchange lists is only 1 ounce of meat. This is a very small amount of meat and is not a serving size. A small fast-food hamburger, for example, weighs about 3 ounces (three exchanges), and 3 or 4 ounces of meat is thought of as a normal serving size for meal planning. Of course, your judgment of what is normal differs from other people's, and you might have to weigh a serving or two of meat to see how much you are eating.

People think of meat as protein food, but calculation of its nutrient content shows a surprising fact. A quarter-pound (4-ounce) hamburger contains 28 grams of protein and 23 grams of fat. Because protein offers 4 calories per gram

■■■ **Figure 5–13**

Fat in Foods.
3 g in 1 oz lean meat.

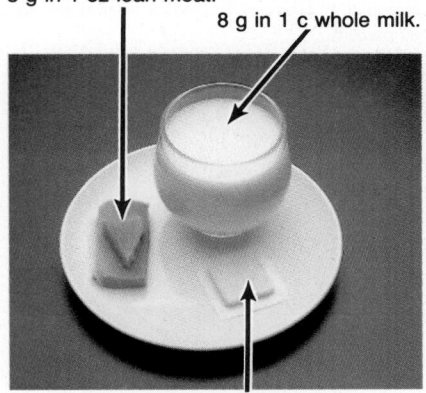

5 g in 1 pat butter or margarine.

EXCHANGE ONE	FAT (G)
Milk (1 c)	
Nonfat	Trace
2%	5
Whole	8
Meat (1 oz)	
Lean	3
Medium fat	5 ½[a]
High fat	8
Peanut butter (1 tbsp)	8 (unsaturated)
Fat (1 tsp)	
Butter, margarine, or oil	5
Vegetables	0
Fruits	0
Breads and starchy vegetables	0
Sugar	0

[a]This is often rounded off to 5 g for purposes of diet planning.

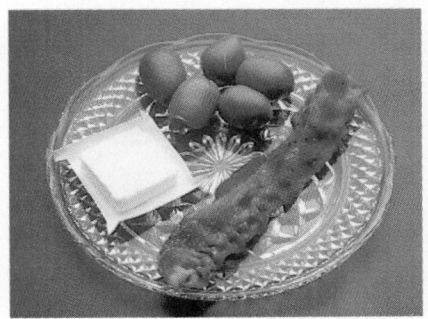

Fat exchanges. Each contributes 5 g fat.

■■■ Figure 5–14

Estimating Fat Intake using Exchange System.

A total of 46 grams of fat times 9 calories per gram is 414 calories from fat, about 24 percent of the day's total 1,750 calories. This is well below the recommended 30 percent.

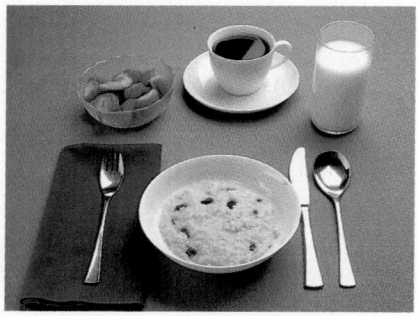

BREAKFAST	**FAT (GRAMS)**
1 c oatmeal = 2 starch/grains	Trace
¼ c raisins = 2 fruits	—
1 c nonfat milk = 1 milk	Trace
1¼ c strawberries = 1 fruit	—

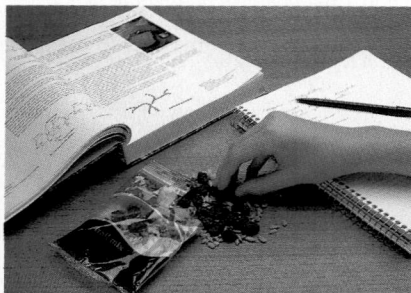

MORNING SNACK	
2 tbsp raisins = 1 fruit	—
2 tbsp sunflower seeds = 2 fats	10

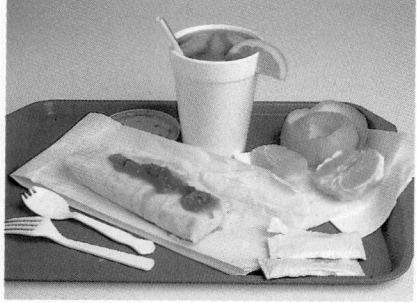

LUNCH	
1 beef and bean burrito	
(1 lg tortilla = 2 starch/grains	Trace
⅓ c beans = 1 starch/grain +	Trace
½ high-fat meat)	4
1 orange = 1 fruit	—
1 packet sugar	—

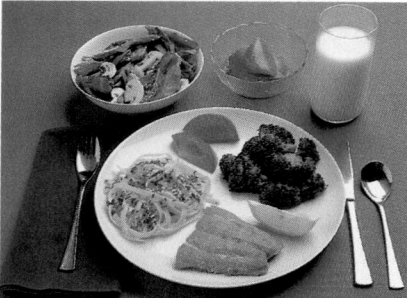

DINNER	
4 oz broiled salmon = 4 lean meats	12
1 c broccoli = 2 vegetables	—
½ c noodles = 1 starch/grain	Trace
2 tsp butter = 2 fats	10
¼ c parsley = ¼ vegetable	—
¼ tomato = ¼ vegetable	—
¼ c mushrooms = ¼ vegetable	—
¼ c water chestnuts = ¼ vegetable	—
1 c fresh spinach = 1 vegetable	—
1 tbsp sesame seeds = 1 fat	5
1 tbsp vinaigrette dressing = 1 fat	5
⅓ c garbanzo beans = 1 starch/grain	Trace
½ c sherbet = 2 starch/grains	Trace
1 c nonfat milk = 1 milk	Trace
Day's total	46 g

and fat offers 9, the hamburger provides 112 calories from protein and 207 calories from fat. The total is over 300 calories, 65 percent of them from fat. A hotdog is even higher in fat, which contributes 84 percent of its calories. People who overeat on meat find weight control difficult because so much of the energy in a meat eater's diet is hidden from view—unrecognized.

Recently some animal breeders have begun producing beef and pork that is lower in fat. This is a help to those people who choose lean cuts—they get less fat in the same quantity of meat. For the person choosing a hamburger, hotdog, or sausages, though, the change would not be significant—fat is ground together with the lean, negating any changes in the fat content of the lean. When choosing beef or pork, look for lean cuts named *loin* or *round* from which the fat can be trimmed. Eat small portions, too.

Chickens have also been bred to be leaner, but the nature of chicken meat remains mostly unchanged—chicken fat lies mainly under the skin, not within the meat tissue. If you skin an ordinary chicken, you end up with a product that is much lower in fat than a lean-bred chicken with the skin left on. In the same way, watch out for commercial ground turkey or chicken products. Many of these have the skin ground in, and they can be much higher in fat than many other meats, even lean beef! Their labels may state "lower in fat," but ask yourself "lower than what?" The box of terms that appeared on Chapter 2's page 47 provided some definitions concerning the fat levels of meats.

◗◗▶ *Many meats harbor high levels of fat, especially those that are marbled or have the fat ground in. Ground meats, and even ground turkey, are usually higher in fat than lean meat cuts from which the fat can be trimmed.*

Other Foods

Figure 5–13 showed that some milk products contain fat. The exchange system views nonfat milk as milk and whole milk as milk with "added" fat. This is because in homogenizing whole milk, milk processors blend in the cream, which otherwise would float and could be removed by skimming. The portion size is 1 cup. A cup of whole milk, then, contains the protein and carbohydrate of skim milk but in addition contains 8 grams (about 70 calories) of fat. A cup of low-fat (2 percent) milk is halfway between whole and nonfat, with 5 grams of fat. The fat occupies only a teaspoon of the volume but more than doubles the calories in the milk.

Milk and yogurt appear on the milk list, but cream and butter do not. Milk and yogurt are rich in calcium and protein, but cream and butter are not. Cream and butter are on the fat list, which also includes whipped cream, sour cream, and cream cheese.

Bread products also sometimes contain fat. Notable are granola cereal, croissants, biscuits, corn bread, dinner rolls, quick breads, french-fried potatoes, potato chips, snack and party crackers, muffins, pancakes, and waffles. Breakfast bars are most like candy bars in their fat and sugar contents. People are often surprised to learn of the high fat content of these foods.

Figure 5–14 redisplays the set of meals, first shown in Chapter 2, that a hypothetical student ate on a Monday. Chapter 4 analyzed these meals for carbohydrate and fiber, and praised them for providing both in abundance. Now you can see that these meals are also low in fat and fit the National Research Council (NRC) recommendations. The figure uses exchange system

Meat exchanges. Fat in these varies:

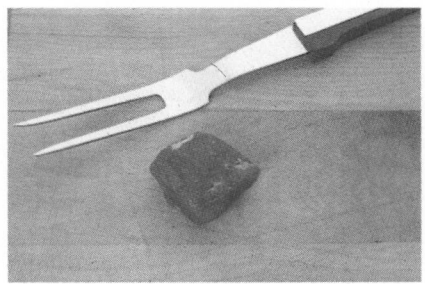

1 oz lean meat = 3 g fat.

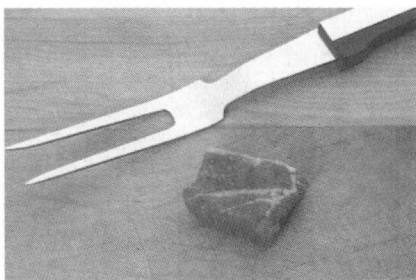

1 oz medium-fat meat = 5½ g fat.

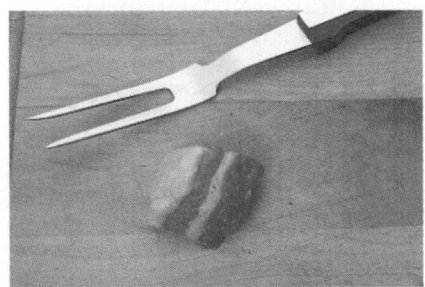

1 oz high-fat meat = 8 g fat.

estimates for the amounts of fat in each food. Vegetables, fruit, grains, and starchy vegetables can be assumed to contain no fat, so the only foods to inspect are the meats, milk, and fats.

Another useful feature of the exchange lists is that they separate the polyunsaturated fat items from the saturated fat items. Of course, which of these you eat makes no difference in the total calories coming from fat, but it may make a difference in the unseen condition of your arteries.

▌▌▶ *People are eating more fat than they did 100 years ago. Fats, oils, meats, and dairy products contribute large amounts of fat to the diet.*

▌▌▌ Food Feature

Defensive Dining

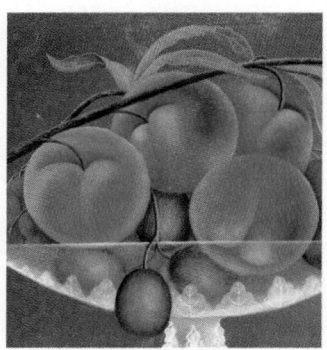

You can find fat listed on a label as: Vegetable fat, lard, animal fat, shortening, oil, butter, margarine, cream. Watch out also for mayonnaise, dressings, coconut, olives, cheese, nuts, and meats—they carry fat into foods, too.

To meet the single most important recommendation of almost every nutrition authority—to reduce dietary fat—requires of most people that they make changes according to five principles:

▪ Eliminate fat as a seasoning and in cooking.
▪ Cut down on intake of red meat.
▪ Remove the fat from high-fat foods.
▪ Substitute high-fat foods with specially manufactured lower fat versions of those foods.
▪ Replace high-fat foods with natural low-fat alternatives.[14]

With these principles in mind, you can begin to make choices about foods in your diet.

The first arena of choice consumers face is the grocery store. The right choices here can save many grams of fat at the dinner table. Food labels can tell you much about a processed food's fat content. The margin lists some words that can alert you to the presence of fat. Conveniently, the ingredients are listed in order of predominance in the product; if fat is one of the first ingredients listed, you know you are holding in your hands a high-fat product. Remember, though, that even if fat is third or fourth on the label, its high energy density may make it a significant calorie contributor. Whether or not to choose a high-fat product depends on how you intend to use it in your diet: as a staple item or as an occasional treat.

Some labels are especially useful in that they list grams of fat and number of calories per serving. Given these numbers, you can easily compare a food to the NRC's limit of "not more than 30 percent of calories from fat." Here's how to get a rough estimate of the percentage of fat in a given food: compare the grams fat per serving listed on the label to the calories per serving, and look for a 3:100 ratio. Three grams fat per 100 calories of food equals about 30 percent of calories from fat. If the food you are considering has more fat than this, you shouldn't necessarily bypass the food, particularly if it is a nutritious choice such as peanut butter.** Include the food in moderation, but keep in mind that it must be balanced with foods having fewer than 3 grams per 100 calories to achieve a day's worth of food whose cumulative average compares well with the recommen-

---

**About 80% of the calories of peanuts are from fat, but the fat is polyunsaturated, a better choice than many meat fats. Peanut butter, if hydrogenated, loses this advantage, but peanut butter is also rich in vitamins and still a good choice on that basis. Use it sparingly, but use it.

dation. In the case of peanut butter, two teaspoons spread on a big slice of bread produces a sandwich that comes to *less* than 30 percent of *total* calories from fat.

Once at home, limit the fats that you add in cooking and serving foods. Use an air popper for popcorn, and sprinkle the popcorn with butter flavoring, if you like it. Keep that flavoring on hand together with other low-fat cooking substitutes such as diet margarine, low-fat salad dressings, and nonstick spray for frying in nonstick pans. To replace high-fat ingredients in recipes, check Table 5–4 for hints. These replacements will not change the finished product too much, except for dramatically lowering its content of fat.

If you must add fats, be sure that they are detectable in the food and that you enjoy them. For example, if you use strongly flavored fat, a little goes a long way. Sesame oil, peanut butter, and the fats of strong cheeses are equal in calories to others, but they are so strongly flavored that you can use much less. Try small amounts of grated sapsago, romano, or other hard cheeses to replace larger amounts of less flavorful cheeses. Butter and regular margarine contain the same number of calories (45 per teaspoon); diet margarine contains fewer calories because water and fillers have been added. Substitute imitation butter flavoring that contains no fat and few calories.

If you do use oils, trade off to obtain the benefits different oils offer. Peanut and safflower oils are especially rich in vitamin E. Olive and canola oil present the heart-health benefits associated with monounsaturates mentioned earlier, and canola also contains omega-3 fatty acids. High temperatures, such as those of frying, destroy omega-3 acids.

Here are some other tips to help you apply the five principles listed earlier while updating old high-fat recipes:

1. *Eliminate fat as a seasoning and in cooking.*

■ Grill, roast, broil, boil, bake, stir fry, microwave, or poach foods. Don't fry.
■ Add a little water to thick, bottled salad dressings—you'll use less each time, and they'll go farther this way.

On a food label, look for 3 or fewer grams of fat per serving for each 100-calorie serving.

■■■ **Table 5–4 Substitutes for High-Fat Ingredients**

USE	INSTEAD OF
Nonfat milk products	Whole milk products
Evaporated nonfat ("skim") milk (canned)	Cream
Yogurt[a]	Sour cream
Reduced-calorie margarine; butter replacers	Butter
Wine, lemon juice, or broth	Butter
Fruit butters	Butter
Part-skim ricotta; low-fat cottage cheese	Whole-milk ricotta
Part-skim or low-fat cheeses	Regular cheeses
1 tbsp cornstarch (for thickening sauces)	1 egg yolk
Reduced-calorie mayonnaise	Regular mayonnaise
Low- or reduced-calorie salad dressing (for salads and marinades)	Regular salad dressing
Water-packed canned fish and meats	Oil-packed fish and meats
Lean ground meat and grain mixture	Ground beef

[a]If the recipe is to be boiled, the yogurt or cottage cheese must be stabalized with a small amount of cornstarch or flour.

■ Use nonstick pans without fat for frying.

■ Use eye appeal to enhance enjoyment of the meal—vary colors, textures, temperatures on the plate, and use garnishes to complement food.

2. *Cut down on intake of red meat.*

■ Choose lean cuts, such as round or loin; have the butcher grind it without the fat. Then cut recipe amounts of the meat in half; the meat price per recipe will be as economical as that of high-fat hamburger. Fill in the lost bulk with shredded vegetables, legumes, pasta, grains, or other low-fat items.

3. *Remove the fat from high-fat foods.*

■ If you use oil-packed tuna or chicken, place in a wire strainer, and rinse with hot water to remove much of the fat.

■ Trim all visible fat and skin from meat and poultry.

■ Refrigerate meat pan drippings and broth, and lift off the fat when it solidifies. Then add the defatted broth to a recipe.

4. *Substitute high-fat foods with specially manufactured lower fat versions.*

■ When you add butter, margarine, or cream cheese at the table, use the whipped types—they contain half the calories of the regular types.

■ Choose oil-free dressings and reduced calorie mayonnaise.

■ Use spray-on pan coating to grease pans or to fry instead of oil or shortening. (Use a pump spray, though, to avoid releasing environmentally harmful gases. See Chapter 15.)

■ Use low-fat yogurt instead of sour cream.

■ Use evaporated nonfat milk to replace sweet cream.

■ Use commercial butter-flavored granules to replace butter.

5. *Replace high-fat foods with natural low-fat alternatives.*

■ Use oil-free flavorings instead of fats: herbs, lemons, spices, fruits, oil-free dressings.

■ Use wine, lemon juice, or broth to replace butter.

All of these suggestions work well when a person carefully plans, selects, purchases, and prepares each meal with the loving attention it deserves. But in the real world, people sometimes fall behind schedule and don't have time to cook—they eat fast food. Fast foods can be extraordinarily high in fat because so many items are high in meat, are fried, or are made with whole milk. But they need not do you in.

The first question to ask about fast foods is, How often do I use them? If you visit a fast-food type restaurant only once a week, then the food consumed there accounts for only 1 meal out of 21 and can easily fit into an otherwise low-fat diet. The more often you visit fast-food places, the more important are the choices you make.

Fast foods are regrettably high in sodium—so high, in fact, that people on sodium-restricted diets have to stay away from them altogether. For those who can eat them, the old hamburger, french fries, and soft-drink–fast-food meal provides *more* than adequate protein, several of the B vitamins, and iron. Many fast-food places offer abundant vegetables and salads. Here are some considerations for choosing:

■ Except for pizza, fast-food meals are likely to be low in calcium. Choose low-fat milk for your beverage, or make sure to include milk or milk products in your other meals for the day.

■ Hamburger/fries meals are low in vitamin A and folate. The amount of lettuce and tomato provided in a typical hamburger, for example, doesn't make a dent on your need for these nutrients. Your next meal should be a large salad or should include a generous serving of dark green vegetables.

■ To save calories, the salads are a good choice (use only about a quarter of the dressing provided). If you are really hungry, choose a salad with meat, cheese, or egg. (Fast food salads are a boon to people who need to lose weight and who are short on time.) Figure 5–15 compares two fast-food meals.

■ Fried fish or chicken sandwiches are at least as high in fat as hamburgers. Broiled sandwiches are far less fatty if you eat them without spreads or dressings.

Because fast foods are short on variety, let them be part of a lifestyle in which they complement the other parts. Eat differently, often, elsewhere.

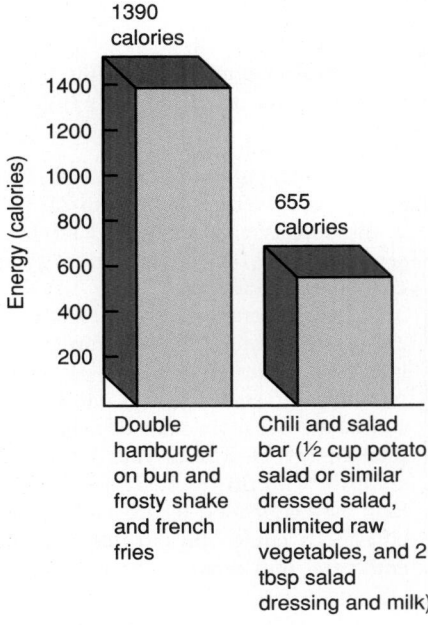

■■■ Figure 5–15

Calories in Fast-Food Choices.

■■■ Indulgence

By this time you may be wondering if you can realistically make all the changes listed above and give up all high-fat foods permanently. Be assured that most of the changes easily can become habits after a few repetitions. As for giving up all high-fat foods, the famous French chef Julia Childs makes this point about moderation:

An imaginary shelf labeled INDULGENCES is a good idea. It contains the best butter . . . heavy cream, marbled steaks, sausages and pates, hollandaise and butter sauces, French butter-cream fillings, gooey chocolate cakes, and all those lovely items that demand disciplined rationing. Thus, with these items high up and almost out of reach, we are ever conscious that they are not everyday foods. They are for special occasions, and when that occasion comes we can enjoy every mouthful.

—Julia Childs, *The Way to Cook*, 1989.

You decide what the treats should be and then choose them judiciously, just for pure pleasure. Meanwhile, make sure that your everyday, ordinary choices are those whole, nutrient-dense foods suggested throughout this book. Use the five fat-reducing principles presented here to achieve a *diet* with an ideal percentage of fat, with room left over for favorite foods. That way you'll meet all your body's needs for nutrients and never feel deprived.

▌▌▌ SELF-STUDY

Examine Your Fat Intake

These exercises make use of the information you recorded on Forms 1 to 4 in Appendix F.

1. How many grams of fat do you consume on an average day (Form 2)?
2. How many calories does this represent (Form 4)? Remember, 1 gram of fat contributes 9 calories.
3. What percentage of your total energy is contributed by fat? You calculated this earlier on Form 4.
4. A recommendation says fat should contribute not more than 30 percent of total energy. How does your fat intake compare with this level? If it is higher, look over your food records: what specific foods could you cut down on or eliminate, and what foods could you add to your diet to bring your total fat intake into line?
5. How much linoleic acid do you consume? (Refer to Form 1, polyunsaturated fatty acid column, and assume that most of this fatty acid is linoleic acid.) Remembering that linoleic acid is a lipid (energy value, 9 calories per gram), calculate the number of calories it gives you. What percentage of your total energy comes from linoleic acid? A guideline recommends 1 to 3 percent of *total* calories.
6. Appendix A does not show omega-3 fatty acids in foods, nor has the committee on RDA yet published a standard for intake. However, you can take a guess at the adequacy of your intake by answering the following questions. Do you eat leafy vegetables, fish and seafoods, or walnuts? Do you use canola oil for home cooking and for salads? If you include just one of these categories of foods each day, you may receive enough omega-3 fatty acids. If you never eat these foods, you might want to find ways to include them.
7. How much cholesterol do you consume daily? How does your cholesterol intake compare with the suggested limit of 300 milligrams a day? If your intake is high, you might want to read Chapter 11 before arriving at any conclusions regarding the importance of this limit.

Notes

1. S. W. Corbett, J. S. Stern, and R. E. Keesey, Energy expenditure in rats with diet-induced obesity, *American Journal of Clinical Nutrition* 44 (1986): 173–180.
2. Lipid Research Clinics Program, The Lipid Research Clinics coronary primary prevention trial results: I. Reduction in incidence of coronary heart disease, *Journal of American Medical Association* 251 (1984): 351–364.
3. Lipid Research Clinics Program, The Lipid Research Clinics coronary primary prevention trial results: II. The relationship of reduction in incidence of coronary heart disease to cholesterol lowering, *Journal of American Medical Association* 251 (1984): 365–374.
4. E. M. Berry and J. Hirsch, Does dietary linolenic acid influence blood pressure? *American Journal of Clinical Nutrition* 44 (1986): 336–340.
5. Anon, Age decreases the omega-3 polyunsaturated fatty acids of the retina, *Nutrition Reviews* 47 (1989): 87–89.
6. A. Leaf and P. C. Weber, Cardiovascular effects of n-3 fatty acids, *New England Journal of Medicine* 318(1988): 549–555.
7. L. D. McBean, Nutritional and health effects of unsaturated fatty acids, *Dairy Council Digest* 59 (1988): 1–6.
8. P. J. Nestel, Polyunsaturated fatty acids (n-3, n-6), *American Journal of Clinical Nutrition* 45 (1987): 1161–1167; M. Neu-ringer, G. J. Anderson, and W. E. Connor, The essentiality of n-3 fatty acids for the development and function of the retina and brain, *Annual Review of Nutrition* 8 (1988): 517–541.
9. Consensus conference: Lowering blood cholesterol to prevent heart disease, *Journal of the American Medical Association* 253 (1985): 2080–2086.
10. R. Goor and coauthors, Nutrient intakes among selected North American populations in the Lipid Research Clinics Prevalence Study: Composition of fat intake, *American Journal of Clinical Nutrition* 41 (1985): 299–311.
11. Is it the olive oil? Cardiovascular benefits of the 'Mediterranean diet,' *Nutrition and the MD*, September 1987, p. 4.
12. F. H. Mattson, A changing role for dietary monounsaturated fatty acids, *Journal of the American Dietetic Association* 89 (1989): 387–391.
13. M. Burros, Margarine choices: A guide for consumers, *New York Times*, 21 November 1984.
14. The five principles listed here and a validated food questionnaire that correlates well with fat intakes are found in A. R. Kristal, A. L. Shattuck, and H. J. Henry, Patterns of dietary behavior associated with selecting diets low in fat: Reliability and validity of a behavioral approach to dietary assessment, *Journal of the American Dietetic Association* 90 (1990): 214–220.

▓▓▓ C O N T R O V E R S Y   5 ▓▓▓

Sugar Substitutes and Artificial Fats

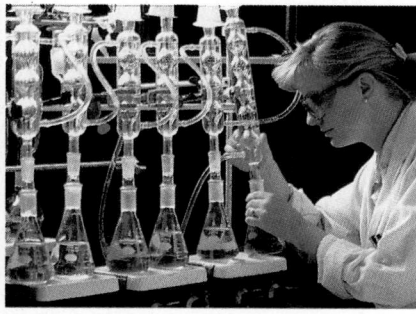

People dream of calorie-less doughnuts, ice cream with the calories of skim milk, and french fries as fat-free as a baked potato. At the same time, consumers insist that no risks to health accompany calorie savings. The desire of most people to control body weight while eating as they like provides the push for research to discover or to invent artificial sweeteners and fats. This Controversy explores issues surrounding the currently available artificial sweeteners and then explores the possibility that calorie-free artificial fats may partially replace energy-rich fats.

▓▓▓ Sugar Substitutes

People who want to avoid sugar may choose from two sets of alternative sweeteners. One set is the sugar alcohols, which are energy-yielding sweeteners sometimes referred to as nutritive sweeteners; the other is the artificial sweeteners, which provide virtually no energy, also referred to as nonnutritive sweeteners.

▓▓▓ Sugar Alcohols

The sugar alcohols are familiar to people who use special dietary products. Among them are **maltitol, mannitol**, **sorbitol**, and **xylitol**. The body either absorbs these carbohydrates more slowly or metabolizes them to glucose more slowly than most of the other sugars. For this reason they were once used by people with diabetes who could not handle large amounts of glucose efficiently and so had to restrict their intakes of ordinary sweets. However, their associated side effects and their energy contributions make them unsuitable for managing diabetes. A proven benefit of sugar alcohols is that ordinary mouth bacteria cannot metabolize them as rapidly as they metabolize sugar, so sugar alcohols do not contribute as much to dental caries. All the sugar alcohols provide as much energy as sucrose (4 calories per gram).

Mannitol is the least satisfactory of the sugar alcohols just named. Because it is less sweet than sucrose, large amounts have to be used to obtain the same sweetness (see Table C14–1). It lingers unabsorbed in the intestine for a long time, available to intestinal bacteria for their energy. As the bacteria consume the mannitol, they multiply, they attract water, and they produce irritating waste, which causes diarrhea.

More practical than mannitol, sorbitol sweetens sugar-free gums and candies; but it, too, has drawbacks. It is only half as sweet as sucrose, so twice as much sorbitol (with twice the calories) must be used to deliver an equivalent amount of sweetness. Also, like mannitol, it can cause diarrhea when consumed in large quantities.

Xylitol is popular, especially in chewing gums, thanks to reports that it helps to prevent dental caries. (It not only doesn't support caries-producing bacteria; it actually inhibits their growth.) Xylitol occurs in foods, and the body produces some xylitol during normal metabolic processes; it is not a foreign substance. Xylitol is widely used in many Western European countries and in Canada; however, reports that it may cause tumors in animals have led to the voluntary curtailing of its use by U.S. food producers.

Maltitol has a sweetness equal to about 75 percent that of sucrose. It is used in some carbonated beverages and canned fruits, as well as in Japanese bakery products and other sweets that are promoted as not causing tooth decay. At first thought not to be absorbed from the gastrointestinal tract, maltitol was recommended for use in food products for dieters and for people with diabetes.

The validity of the claim that maltitol is not absorbed is doubtful, however; maltitol probably donates as much energy to the body as does sugar. Maltitol is expensive, and cost limits its use.

The person who wishes to reduce energy intake should be aware that the sugar alcohols *do* provide as much energy per gram as sucrose. In spite of this, products that contain them are labeled "sugar-free." The reason they are suitable for people who must limit their intakes of ordinary sugars is that the body handles them differently, not that they are calorie-free. The person who is limiting energy intake must limit sugar alcohols just as carefully as sugars. For this person, artificial sweeteners may offer a preferable alternative.

■■■ Artificial Sweeteners

Like the sugar alcohols, artificial sweeteners make foods taste sweet without promoting dental decay. Unlike sugar alcohols, they have the added attraction of being calorie-free. But are they safe? All substances are toxic if a high enough dose is consumed, so it is of little surprise that large doses of artificial sweeteners (or their components or metabolic by-products) have toxic effects. The question to ask is whether they are harmful to human beings at normal use and potential overuse levels.[1]

The big three synthetic sweeteners are **saccharin**, **cyclamate**, and **aspartame**. Table C5–1 showed

that their sweetness per unit of weight far exceeds that of the sugar alcohols. Saccharin has been around since before 1900, and it dominated the market for the first half of this century. In the 1950s and 1960s, cyclamate came into wide use. Aspartame was approved by the Food and Drug Administration (FDA) in 1981 and swept the market.[2]

The cases of saccharin and cyclamate illustrate some general points about additives and food safety that are worth a moment's attention here. Saccharin is now consumed by some 50 million Americans— primarily in soft drinks, secondarily as a tabletop sweetener. Questions about its safety surfaced in 1977, when experiments suggested it caused bladder tumors in rats, and the FDA proposed banning it as a result. The public outcry in favor of retaining it was so loud, however, that Congress placed a moratorium on any action, and the moratorium

has since been repeatedly renewed. Products containing saccharin are required to carry the warning label, now familiar to all consumers of diet beverages, that "use of this product may be hazardous to your health. This product contains saccharin, which has been determined to cause cancer in laboratory animals."

Does saccharin cause cancer? The evidence that it does so in animals is as follows. When male and female rats are fed diets containing saccharin from the time of weaning to adulthood and are then mated and their offspring are also fed saccharin throughout life, the offspring have a higher incidence of bladder tumors than comparable animals not fed saccharin.[3] It wasn't clear whether the tumors were cancerous. In Canada, on the basis of these findings and in the face of public outcry as loud as that in the United States, all uses of saccharin were banned ex-

■■■ Table C5–1 Sweetness of Sugar Alternates

SUGAR ALTERNATE	RELATIVE SWEETNESS[a]
Sucrose	100
Sorbitol	50
Mannitol	70
Maltitol	75
Xylitol	100
Cyclamate	1,500–5,000
Aspartame	15,000–25,000
Saccharin	24,000–50,000

[a]The relative sweetness depends on the temperature and acidity of the foods in which the substance occurs. Sucrose is the standard by which the approximate sweetness of sugar substitutes is compared.

SOURCE: Adapted from D. B. Drucker, Sweetening agents in food, drinks and medicine: Cariogenic potential and adverse effects, *Journal of Human Nutrition* 33 (1979): 114–124.

cept use as a tabletop sweetener to be sold in pharmacies, and Canada permits those sales only with a warning label.

One large-scale population study involving 9,000 people showed a distinctly greater risk of cancers in some groups such as women who drank two or more diet sodas a day and in people who both smoked heavily and used artificial sweeteners heavily. Another study involving over 1,000 people showed little or no excess risk of bladder cancers but of course could not conclude that there was no risk at all. As of now, two alternative conclusions are possible:

1. Saccharin causes tumors, possibly cancerous, in rats but not in people.
2. Saccharin is a weak carcinogen in people, and its effects will take more years of exposure to become apparent.

Cyclamate has had a shorter life than saccharin, dominating the artificial sweetener market for only 20 years. The 1970 ban on its use in the United States, although repeatedly appealed, has been continued even though, like saccharin, cyclamate has never been conclusively proven guilty of causing cancer in human beings. In Canada, saccharin use is restricted, and cyclamate is restricted to use as a tabletop sweetener on the advice of a physician and as a sweetening additive in medicines.

As for aspartame, within only a few years of receiving the FDA's approval it appeared in dozens of

■■■ PKU Miniglossary

phenylketonuria (PKU): an inborn error of metabolism in which the amino acid phenylalanine cannot follow its normal pathways in the body. Unusual products made from phenylalanine build up in the tissues and damage them. PKU is devastating to the infant brain, causing irreversible, progressive brain damage if untreated early. All newborns in the United States are tested for PKU, and the treatment is to limit dietary intake of phenylalanine.

inborn errors of metabolism: hereditary diseases caused by inheritance of faulty genes, which make people unable to conduct body processes normally. Inborn errors usually have implications for nutrition.

food products. Worldwide, people gratefully accepted aspartame as NutraSweet in diet drinks, chewing gum, presweetened cereal, gelatins, and pudding and as Equal, a powder to use at home in place of sugar. Aspartame sales have well surpassed the sales of saccharin and are also encroaching on sugar sales in some markets.

This amazing popularity is mostly due to aspartame's flavor, which is almost identical to that of sugar. Another lure drawing people to aspartame is the hope that it may be completely harmless, unlike the other sweeteners, whose laboratory records are tarnished. Furthermore, aspartame is touted as safe for children, so families wishing to limit sugar are turning to it. Finally, as a sweet-toothed, overweight population, many people perceive sugar substitutes as the only way to cheat the scales.

Aspartame is a simple chemical compound: two protein fragments (the amino acids phenylalanine and aspartic acid) joined together. In the digestive tract the two protein frag-

ments are split apart, absorbed, and used to build protein or are burned for energy, just as they would be if they had come from protein in food. The flavors of the components give no clue to the combined effect; one of them tastes bitter, and the other is tasteless. But aspartame is incredibly sweet—200 times sweeter than sucrose.

The disease **phenylketonuria (PKU)** poses some interesting problems with regard to aspartame. People with PKU have the hereditary inability to dispose of phenylalanine when it is eaten in excess of the need for building proteins. Therefore they cannot use unlimited amounts of the sweetener. They can use some, but there is a compelling reason why PKU children should not get their phenylalanine from this source. Phenylalanine occurs in such protein-rich and nutrient-rich foods as milk and meat, and the PKU child is allowed only a limited amount of these foods. Such a child can obtain only with difficulty the many essential nutrients—such as calcium, iron, and the B vitamins—

found along with phenylalanine in these foods. To suggest that such a child squander any of the limited phenylalanine allowance on the purified phenylalanine of aspartame, with none of the associated vitamins or minerals essential for normal growth, would be to invite nutritional disaster. People with PKU need to know which products now contain aspartame and how to avoid them. Product labels offer a special warning for people with PKU.

In people with normal metabolism, large doses of phenylalanine can stimulate production of prolactin, a hormone associated with lactation in women. A recent study dispelled fears that aspartame, made partly from phenylalanine, may affect hormone production. Aspartame had no influence on prolactin or other hormone production when taken in amounts commonly used.[4]

A concern about aspartame's safety has to do with its chemical structure. During aspartame's metabolism, a toxic chemical, methyl alcohol, is momentarily formed. Methyl alcohol is quickly converted to formaldehyde, another toxic compound, and finally to carbon dioxide. The quantities generated from normal use of aspartame are below the threshold at which these compounds cause harm. But in the testing of aspartame, that threshold had to be determined and its acceptability evaluated.

Still another concern is about the product that aspartame breaks down to a chemical called **DKP***.

*The chemical is **diketopiperazine**.

Long-term studies using animals have directly tested DKP and have eliminated it as a source of concern. Still another concern was over the effect aspartame use might have on the brain. Experiments with rats, monkeys, and human beings were performed, and none showed any cause for concern. The monkey study involved infant monkeys given up to 3,000 milligrams of aspartame per kilogram of body weight for nine months and showed no ill effects on growth, development, health, or behavior either during the test or on the withdrawal of aspartame.[5] The conclusion reached was that aspartame is safe except for people with PKU. Some 500 individual complaints received after its approval were reviewed by the Centers for Disease Control, which concluded that some individuals may exhibit vague but not dangerous symptoms due to unusual sensitivity to aspartame but that the product is considered generally safe.[6]

Every day, millions of people use artificial sweeteners. Every day millions of people have headaches. Anyone who claimed, on this basis, that artificial sweeteners caused headaches is using logic to jump to conclusions rather than using science to probe for answers. In the case of sweeteners and headaches, only a correlation, not a cause, has been shown.

An analogy may help to make clear the distinction between correlations and causal relationships. Suppose that there is an outbreak of arson and the police are searching for the suspect. Police observe that a

certain person, Mr. Tagalong, is always in the neighborhoods when the fires start, and they accuse him of arson. However, another sneaky individual, Ms. Match, is the real arsonist; Mr. Tagalong is only following her around. Mr. Tagalong is associated with, but is not a causal agent in, the setting of fires. The evidence against him is only circumstantial (correlational). If the police can show that whenever Mr. Tagalong is in jail there are no fires and that whenever he is let out the fires start again, the evidence against him will strengthen. Better yet, if they catch him pouring gasoline and lighting the match, they will know for sure.

To return to the case at hand—suppose there is an outbreak of headaches, and researchers are searching for the suspect. They observe that some of the people with headaches use artificial sweeteners. It would be premature to accuse the artificial sweeteners of causing the headaches. Some of the headache sufferers might indeed be reacting to the artificial sweeteners, but they might also be reacting to another substance in the same or other foods or to factors in their lives unrelated to foods. The evidence against artificial sweeteners is, at most, only correlational.

As it happens, even the correlation does not hold up. It turns out that some people with headaches do not use artificial sweeteners and that some people use artificial sweeteners without getting headaches. The sweeteners still might be causing some headaches in a few sensitive people, of course, but until researchers can show that these head-

■■■ Miniglossary of Sugar Substitutes

acesulfame (AY-see-sul-fame) **potassium** (**acesulfame K**): a zero-calorie sweetener recently approved by the FDA.

aspartame: a compound of phenylalanine and aspartic acid that tastes like the sugar sucrose but is much sweeter. It provides 4 cal/g, as does protein, but because so little is used, it is virtually calorie-free. In powdered form it is mixed with lactose, however, so a 1-g packet contains 4 cal. It is used in both the United States and Canada.

cyclamate: a zero-calorie sweetener banned in the United States and used restrictively in Canada.

diketopiperazine (dye-KEY-toe-pie-PER-a-zeen), or **DKP**: a product to which aspartame breaks down during metabolism.

maltitol, **mannitol**, **sorbitol**, **xylitol**: sugar alcohols, which can be derived from fruits or commercially produced from dextrose; absorbed more slowly and metabolized differently than other sugars in the human body and not readily used by ordinary mouth bacteria.

saccharin: a zero-calorie sweetener used freely in the United States but restricted in Canada.

aches come and go with sweetener use, they have no consistent correlation: the evidence remains weak.

The FDA has approved aspartame based on the assumption that no one will consume more than 50 milligrams per kilogram of their body weight in a day. This maximum daily intake is not impossible to obtain: for a 132-pound person, it adds up to 80 packets of Equal. About 15 soft drinks sweetened only with aspartame provide this maximum amount. The company that produces aspartame estimates that if all the sugar and saccharin in the U.S. diet were replaced with aspartame, 1 percent of the population would be consuming the FDA maximum.[7] Some people actually do consume this amount, however. A child who drinks a quart of Kool-Aid on a hot day and who also has pudding, chewing gum, cereal, and other products with aspartame that day packs in more than the FDA maximum level.

In an attempt to give a guideline for a safe level of aspartame, an advisory group to the World Health Organization has recommended a maximum of 40 milligrams per kilogram of body weight for adults.[8] A much more conservative limit of three to four packets of Equal per day is suggested by the Canadian Diabetes Association as a safe and useful level.[9] The newsletter for physicians called *Nutrition and the M.D.* states that it is not known if aspartame is safe for children under two years old, and it points out that there are "very few if any reasons to use a sugar substitute in infants and young children."[10] It is unfortunate but not uncommon to see infants' bottles filled with soft drinks instead of juices. Until aspartame has been around for a longer time, it would be best not to cast infants as unwitting "testers" of aspartame's safety.

The FDA has recently approved the artificial sweetener **acesulfame potassium** (or acesulfame K), which has been used without reported health problems in several other countries.[11] Marketed under the trade name Sunette, this sweetener is about as sweet as aspartame and has been approved for use in chewing gum, beverages, instant coffee and tea, gelatins, and puddings. Unlike aspartame, acesulfame K holds up under cooking, and since it continues no phenylalanine, it need bear no warnings to people with PKU. Like its predecessors, acesulfame potassium is being challenged by consumer groups concerned about its safety. Further research and consumer acceptance will determine its place on the grocery shelves.

Current evidence seems to suggest that artificial sweeteners ingested at normal-use concentrations pose no health risks. For persons choosing to use them, the American Dietetic Association advises that their use be moderate as a part of a well-balanced nutritious diet.[12]

■■■ Artificial Fats

Given that heart disease and obesity are two major health problems linked to dietary fat, artificial fats

■■■ Miniglossary of Artificial Fats

olestra: a noncaloric artificial fat made from sucrose and fatty acids; formerly called *sucrose polyester*.

Simplesse: the trade name for a protein-based, low-calorie artificial fat, approved by the FDA for use in foods. (If Simplesse had a chemical name, it would simply be "protein.")

offer hope for the prevention and treatment of both. Food chemists have been working on artificial fats since the 1960s, and recently two have come into the spotlight. These artificial fats are not the same as granules that mimic the flavors of butter, cheese, or sour cream. Although such flavors have been available for years and they replicate the *taste* of fats, they lack the feeling of richness provided by the fatty foods themselves. Artificial fats are designed to provide the entire experience of eating fat—the creaminess as well as the taste—but without the calories.

One product the FDA has had under consideration for approval is a calorie-free fat replacement formerly known as **sucrose polyester** (SPE), now known by its generic name **olestra** (with a lower case "o"). Olestra is a synthetic combination of sucrose and fatty acids, but unlike either, it is indigestible. Because the body cannot digest it, olestra passes through the digestive tract unabsorbed. Its presence in the digestive tract reduces blood cholesterol concentrations by interfering with cholesterol's absorption.

Olestra looks, feels, and tastes like dietary fat and can substitute for fats and oils without diminishing the flavor of food, adding calories to the food, or raising blood lipid concentrations. It has the same cooking properties as fats and oils and can be used in products such as shortenings, oils, margarines, snacks, ice creams, and other desserts.

Scientific research on animals and human beings seems to support the safety of olestra as a partial replacement for dietary fats and oils.[13] An undesirable side effect of olestra is its interference with vitamin E absorption. One proposed solution to this problem is to supplement olestra products with vitamin E. Studies suggest that, for people routinely using olestra, an intake of two times the RDA of vitamin E might be appropriate. Early studies of olestra found it to cause diarrhea in some people, but this fault seems to have been corrected.

The other fat substitute is made from protein and its trade name is **Simplesse.** It has been approved by the FDA for use in certain products, such as frozen desserts, mayonnaise, and salad dressings. Simplesse is fabricated in a process called microparticulation, which heats and blends proteins from egg whites or milk into tiny round particles. This method counters the normal changes that occur when a protein is subjected to heat. The naturally occurring proteins are altered in Simplesse so that they create the *perception* of fat; the tongue perceives creaminess because of the extremely small size of the protein particles.

Olestra and Simplesse differ in that olestra is a sucrose polyester, while Simplesse is made of protein. Both the body and the chef use the products differently, too. In the body, Simplesse is digested and absorbed, contributing to energy intake, while olestra passes through essentially unchanged. Simplesse provides 1 1/3 calories per gram—a substantial reduction from fat's 9 calories per gram but more than olestra's zero calories. In the kitchen, Simplesse is unsuitable for frying or baking because it gels when heated, while olestra is a partial replacement for cooking fats.

The ideal fat replacement would look, taste, and cook like fat but would not add fat's calories. This is a tall order, but it looks as if food chemists are close to filling it with these two and other related products.[14] Artificial fats are taking their place on grocer's shelves and may become as commonplace as artificial sweeteners. Some health professionals still wonder whether fat substitutes will really better people's nutrition. They may help to increase the nutrient density of the diet, but on the other hand, their availability may encourage the consumption of more nutrient-poor foods.[15] In any case, consumers are eagerly awaiting them.

Notes

1. L. D. Stegink, The aspartame story: A model for the clinical testing of a food additive, *American Journal of Clinical Nutrition* 46 (1987): 204–215.

2. C. Lecos, The sweet and sour history of saccharin, cyclamate, aspartame, *FDA Consumer,* September 1981, pp. 8–11.

3. Council on Scientific Affairs, American Medical Association, Saccharin: Review of safety issues, *Journal of the American Medical Association* 254 (1985): 2622–2624.

4. H. Carlson and J. Shah, Aspartame and its constituent amino acids: Effects on prolactin, cortisol, growth hormone, insulin, and glucose in normal humans, *American Journal of Clinical Nutrition* 49 (1989): 427–432.

5. Council on Scientific Affairs, American Medical Association, Aspartame, review of safety, *Journal of the American Medical Association* 254 (1985): 400–402.

6. Council on Scientific Affairs, Aspartame, 1985.

7. *A Health Care Practitioner's Guide,* a pamphlet (1987): available from The NutraSweet Company, P.O. Box 1111, Skokie, IL 60076.

8. Joint FAO/WHO Expert Committee on Food Additives, International Programme on Chemical Safety, Toxicological evaluation of certain food additives, WHO technical report series no. 669 (Geneva: World Health Organization, 1981), pp. 25–32.

9. G. S. Wong, Aspartame and its safe use, *Diabetes Dialog* 29 (1982): 3.

10. Questions readers ask, *Nutrition and the MD*, January 1984.

11. FDA OKs new sweetener, *Nutrition and the MD*, March 1989, p. 4.

12. Position of the American Dietetic Association: Appropriate use of nutritive and non-nutritive sweeteners, *Journal of the American Dietetic Association* 87 (1987): 1689–1690.

13. M. Kroger, Can we have our cake and eat it too? *Priorities*, Winter 1989, pp. 37–39.

14. No regulatory clearance needed for NutriFat (abstract), *Journal of the American Dietetic Association* 89 (1989): 426.

15. L. McBean, Fat/cholesterol: An update, *Dairy Council Digest* 60 (1989): 7–12.

The Proteins and Amino Acids

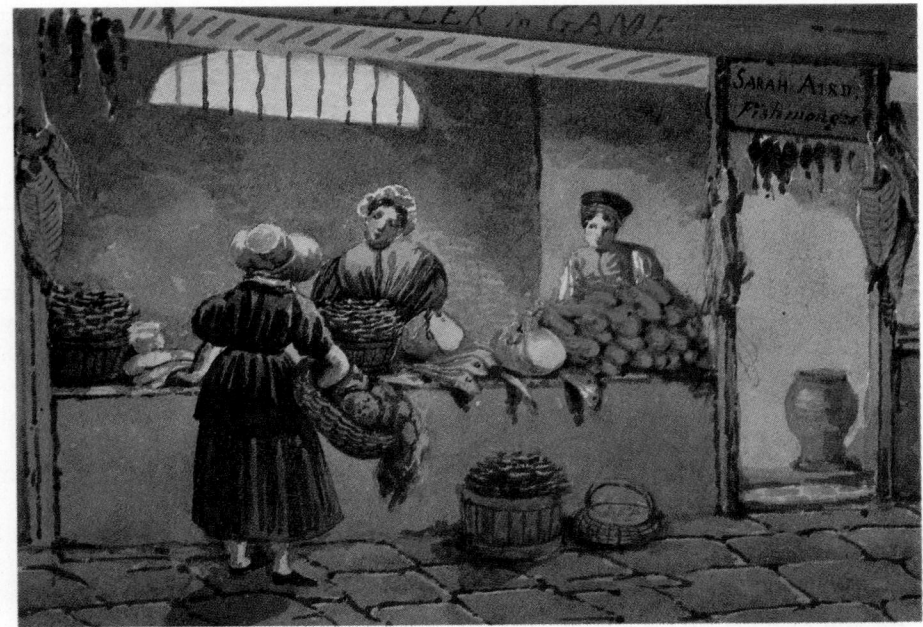

CONTENTS

Fish Stall in St. John's Market, Liverpool, 1832 by Mary Ellen Best. Reproduced from THE WORLD
OF MARY ELLEN BEST, published by Chatto & Windus, London.

proteins: compounds—composed of carbon, hydrogen, oxygen, *and* nitrogen—arranged as a strand of amino acids. Some amino acids also contain the element sulfur.

amino (a-MEEN-o) acids: building blocks of protein: each has an amine group at one end, an acid group at the other, and a distinctive side chain.

amine (a-MEEN) group: the nitrogen-containing portion of an amino acid.

essential amino acids: amino acids that cannot be synthesized at all by the body or that cannot be synthesized in amounts sufficient to meet physiological need.

The **proteins** are amazing, versatile, and vital cellular machines. Without them, life would not exist. First named 150 years ago after the Greek word *proteios* ("of prime importance"), proteins have revealed countless secrets of the ways living processes take place, and they account for many nutrition concerns. Why do we need to eat certain chemical substances (nutrients) and not others? How do we grow? How do our bodies replace the materials they lose? How does blood clot? What gives us immunity to diseases we have encountered? Understanding the nature of the proteins gives us many of the answers to these questions.

Protein machinery comes in many forms: enzymes, antibodies, transport vehicles, cellular "pumps," oxygen carriers, tendons and ligaments, scars, the cores of bones and teeth, the filaments of hair, the materials of nails, and more. But before describing the individual roles of protein, it is necessary to describe what all protein molecules have in common.

The Structure of Proteins

To appreciate the many vital functions of proteins, we must understand their structure. One key difference from carbohydrate and fat, which contain only carbon, hydrogen, and oxygen atoms, is that protein contains nitrogen atoms. These nitrogen atoms give the name *amino* (nitrogen-containing) to the **amino acids** of which protein is made. Another key difference is that in contrast to the carbohydrates, whose repeating units—glucose molecules—are identical, the amino acids in a strand of protein are different from one another. A protein is a strand of individual amino acids of 20 *different* kinds.

Amino Acids and Their Side Chains

All amino acids have a simple chemical backbone with an **amine group** (the nitrogen-containing part) at one end and an acid group at the other end. This backbone is the same for all amino acids. The differences between them depend on a distinctive structure, the chemical side chain, that is attached to the backbone (Figure 6–1). It is the nature of the side chain that gives identity and chemical nature to each amino acid. Twenty amino acids with 20 different side chains make up most of the proteins of living tissue. Other rare amino acids appear in a few proteins.

The side chains vary in complexity. This makes the amino acids differ in size, shape, and electrical charge. Some are negative, some are positive, and some have no charge (they are neutral). The first part of Figure 6–2 is a diagram of three different side chains attached to amino acid backbones. The rest of the figure shows how amino acids link up to form protein strands. The side chains ultimately help to determine the shapes and behaviors of the large protein molecules they link together.

The body can make about half of the amino acids for itself, given the needed parts: nitrogen to form the amine group and backbone fragments derived from carbohydrate or fat. But there are others that the healthy adult body cannot make. These are the **essential amino acids**. If the diet does not supply them, the body cannot make the proteins it needs to do its work. The indispensability of the essential amino acids makes it necessary to eat often the foods that provide them.

▪▪▪ Figure 6–1

An Amino Acid. The "backbone" of the amino acid is similar to that of carbohydrates (p. 98) and fats (p. 136)—two carbon atoms joined together. The side chain differs from one amino acid to the next. The nitrogen is in the amine group.

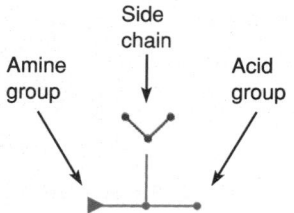

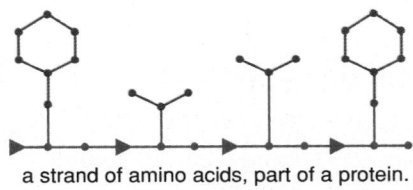

Valine   Leucine   Tyrosine

Single amino acids with different side chains...

can bond together to form...

a strand of amino acids, part of a protein.

■■■ **Figure 6–2**

Different Amino Acids Join to Make Proteins.

The distinction between essential and nonessential amino acids is not quite as clear-cut as the list in the margin makes it appear. Histidine often appears not to be essential, perhaps because the diet supplies it in abundance; now, however, it has been added to the list of essential amino acids.[1] Arginine may, under some conditions, be synthesized too slowly to fully meet the human need.[2] Cysteine and tyrosine normally are not essential because the body makes them from methionine and phenylalanine; but if there is not enough of these precursors to make them from, then they have to be supplied in the diet. Another amino acid, taurine, is not listed with the standard 20 acids because it is not used in protein strands. However, it is used to make materials important in brain and eye function and in the digestion of fat. Its concentration in human milk is high, and under special circumstances, human infants may require an external dietary source. States of illness can interfere with amino acid transformations in the body and so may make other amino acids essential for individual human beings who suffer from such conditions.

The body also breaks protein molecules apart and reuses the amino acids from which they were made. When protein molecules have finished their cellular work and are no longer needed, they are dismantled to liberate their component amino acids. Pools of such amino acids provide the cells with raw materials from which they can build protein molecules they need, or they can break the amino acids down further for energy and discard their nitrogen atoms as wastes. By reusing amino acids, the body recycles and conserves a valuable commodity while easing its waste disposal burden.[3]

The body's protein recycling system also provides a sort of emergency fund of amino acids that tissues can draw on in times of fuel or protein deprivation.

The essential amino acids:

■ Histidine.
■ Isoleucine.
■ Leucine.
■ Lysine.
■ Methionine.
■ Phenylalanine.
■ Threonine.
■ Tryptophan.
■ Valine.

Other amino acids important in nutrition:

■ Alanine.
■ Arginine.
■ Aspartic acid.
■ Cysteine.
■ Cystine.
■ Glumatic acid.
■ Glutamine.
■ Glycine.
■ Proline.
■ Serine.
■ Tyrosine.

enzymes (EN-zimes): protein catalysts (as mentioned in Chapter 3). A catalyst is a compound that facilitates a chemical reaction without itself being altered in the process. (Additional details about digestive enzymes were listed in Table 3–1 of Chapter 3.)

For more about the neurotransmitters, read Controversy 6.

When the diet fails to provide sufficient energy or protein, tissues break down many more proteins, sacrificing working molecules before their time to supply building materials and energy to body tissues.

Not only do amino acids supply raw material from which tissues build proteins and energy to support work, they also perform their own important tasks. For example, the amino acid tyrosine forms part of the neurotransmitters epinephrine and norepinephrine that relay nervous system messages throughout the body. Tyrosine also forms the brown pigment melanin responsible for skin, hair, and eye color, and it forms the hormone thyroxin that helps regulate the body's metabolic rate. The amino acid tryptophan serves as starting material for the neurotransmitter serotonin and the vitamin niacin. All of these and other functions rely on the availability of the amino acids from which the active molecules are made.

❚❚ ▷ *Proteins, unique among the energy nutrients because they possess nitrogen-containing amine groups, are composed of 20 different amino acid units. Some amino acids are essential, and some are essential only in special circumstances.*

Proteins: Strands of Amino Acids

In the first step of making a protein, each amino acid is hooked to the next (this was shown in Figure 6–2). A bond, called a peptide bond, is formed between the amino end of one and the acid end of the next. The side chains bristle out from the backbone of the structure, and these give the protein molecule its unique character.

A strand of protein is not a straight chain. Figure 6–2 showed only the first step in making proteins—the linking of from several dozen to as many as 300 amino acid units with peptide bonds. The amino acids at different places along the strand are attracted to each other, and in the second step of making a protein, this attraction causes the strand to coil into a shape reminiscent of a metal spring. To complete the protein the coiled chains are attracted to, or repelled from, one another, causing the entire coil to fold back on itself this way and that, the last step to forming a globular structure. The amino acids whose side chains are electrically charged are attracted to water, and in the body fluids, they orient themselves on the outside of the protein structure. The amino acids whose side chains are neutral are repelled by water and are attracted to one another; these tuck themselves into the center, away from the body fluids. All these interactions among the amino acids and the surrounding fluid result in the unique architecture of each type of protein. One final step may be needed for the protein to become functional. Several strands may gather together and depend on one another to function, or a metal ion (mineral) or a vitamin may be needed to complete the unit and to activate it.

The dramatically different shapes of proteins enable them to perform different tasks in the body. Those of globular shape, such as some proteins of the blood, are water soluble. Some are hollow balls, which can carry and store materials in their interiors. In proteins that give strength and elasticity to body parts, several springs of amino acids coil together and form rope-like fibers. Some, such as those that form tendons, are more than ten times as long as they are wide, forming stiff, rodlike structures that are somewhat insoluble in water and very strong. Still others act like glue. Among the most fascinating are the

enzymes, which act on other substances to change them chemically. The variety of proteins is endless. A photo of a model of a single, large, globular protein molecule, the one that carries oxygen in the red blood cells, is shown in Figure 6–3 below.

The great variety of proteins in the world is due to the infinite number of sequences of amino acids that is possible. If you consider the size of the dictionary, in which all of the words are constructed from just 26 letters, you can visualize the variety of proteins that are designed from 20 or so amino acids. The letters in a word must alternate between consonant and vowel sounds, but the amino acids in a protein need follow no such rules. Also, there is no restriction on the length of the chain of amino acids. Thus there are many more possible proteins than possible English words. There may be as many as 10,000 different proteins in a single human cell, each one present in thousands of copies.

The sequences of amino acids that make up a protein molecule are specified by heredity with exquisite order and precision. For each protein there is only one proper sequence. If the wrong amino acid is inserted or if one is out of place, the result may be disastrous.

Sickle-cell disease—in which hemoglobin, the oxygen-carrier protein of the red blood cells, is abnormal—is an example of an inherited mistake in the amino acid sequence. Normal hemoglobin contains two kinds of chains. One of the chains in sickle-cell hemoglobin is an exact copy of that in normal hemoglobin. But in the other chain, the sixth amino acid, which should be glutamine, is replaced by valine. The character and shape of the protein are so much affected by this difference that the protein is unable to carry and to release oxygen. The red blood cells collapse into crescent shapes instead of remaining disk shaped as they normally do. If too many abnormal hemoglobins appear in the blood, the result is illness and death. One of the methods of

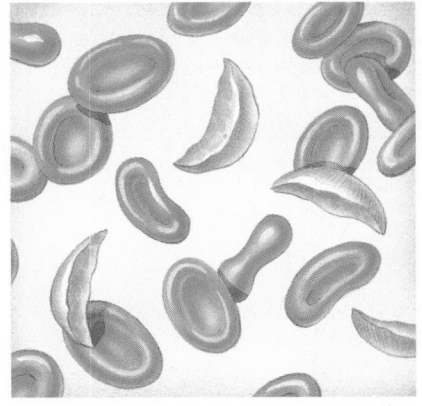

Normal cells (disk shaped) and sickle cells (crescent shaped).

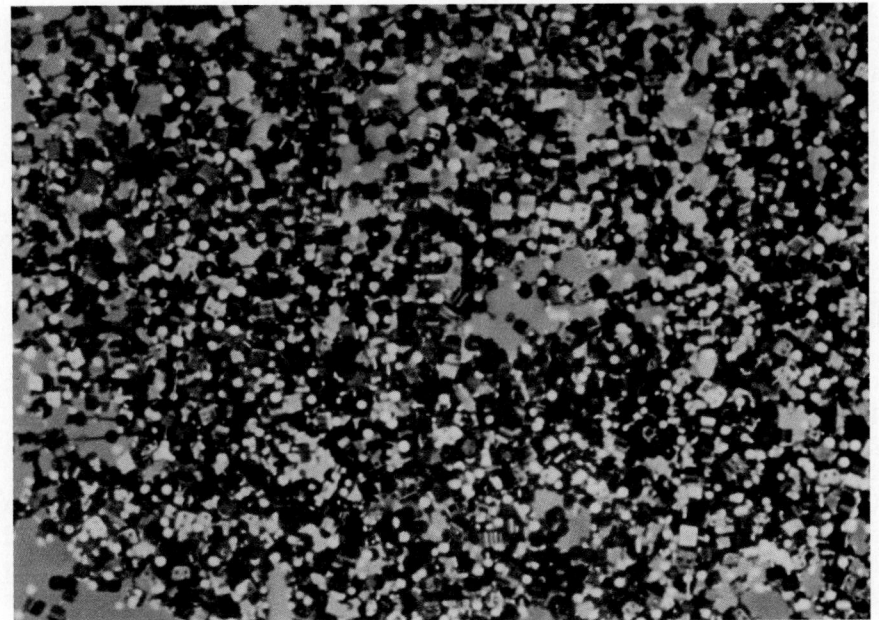

■■■ **Figure 6–3**

The Protein Hemoglobin. Each ball is an atom; the red cubes are iron atoms. This model represents one molecule of hemoglobin magnified 27 million times.

denaturation: the change in shape of a protein brought about by heat, acid, base, alcohol, heavy metals, or other agents.

detecting the disease is to observe under the microscope the altered shape of the red blood cells.

You are different from any other human being. What makes you unique are minute differences in your body proteins. These differences are determined by the amino acid sequences of your proteins, which are written into the genetic code you inherited from your parents and they from their ancestors. Each person receives at conception a unique combination of genes. The genes, passed down to a cell from its parent cell, direct the making of all the body's proteins, as shown in Figure 6–4. Notice that genes determine the sequences of the amino acids in the finished protein. Figure 6–5 on page 160 takes a broader view to show the whole picture of how a cell makes protein.

▐▐▶ *Amino acids link into long strands that fold or coil to make a wide variety of different proteins. Each type of protein has a distinctive sequence of amino acids and so has great specificity.*

Denaturation of Proteins

Proteins can undergo **denaturation** (that is, distortion of shape) by heat, alcohol, acids, or the salts of heavy metals. Chemical reactions can be harmful or useful because of their effects on protein. The denaturation of a protein is the first step in its destruction; thus excess acidity or alkalinity in the body is dangerous because it damages the body's proteins. However, denaturation is useful to the body in digestion. During the digestion of a food protein, an early step is denaturation by the stomach acid, which opens up the protein's structure, permitting digestive enzymes to get at it. Cooking an egg denatures the proteins of the egg and makes it more appetizing. Perhaps more importantly, cooking denatures two raw-egg proteins: one that binds the B vitamin biotin and the mineral iron and another that slows protein digestion. Thus cooking eggs liberates biotin and iron and aids digestion.

Many well-known poisons are salts of heavy metals like mercury and silver; these alter the structure of proteins wherever they touch them. The common first-aid remedy for swallowing ·a heavy-metal poison is to drink milk. The poison then acts on the protein of the milk rather than on the protein tissues of the mouth, esophagus, and stomach. Later, vomiting is induced to expel the poison.

▐▐▶ *Proteins can be denatured by heat, acid, alcohol, or the salts of heavy metals.*

▐▐▐ Digestion and Absorption of Protein

Each protein is designed for a special purpose in a particular tissue of a specific kind of animal or plant. When a person eats food proteins, whether from cereals, vegetables, beef, fish, or cheese, the body must alter them by breaking them down into amino acids before rearranging them into its own unique sequences.

Other than being crushed and moistened with saliva, nothing happens to protein until it reaches the very strong acid of the stomach. There the acid helps to uncoil (denature) the protein's tangled strands so that the stomach enzymes can attack the bonds. You might expect that the stomach enzymes themselves, being proteins, would be denatured by the stomach's acid; but

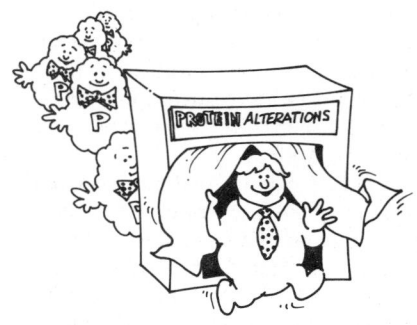

By recycling amino acids the body conserves valuable protein and eases its waste burden.

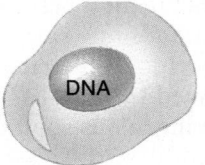

1. DNA is in the
nucleus of each cell.

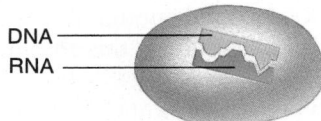

DNA
RNA

2. DNA makes a copy
of that portion of itself
that has the instructions
for the protein the
cell needs.

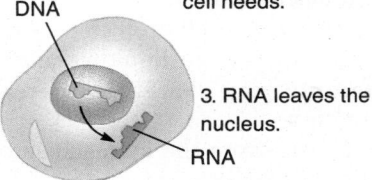

DNA

3. RNA leaves the
nucleus.

RNA

Protein-
making
machinery

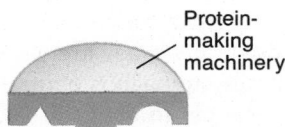

4. RNA attaches itself to the protein-
making machinery of the cell.

Messenger   Transfer
RNA   RNAs

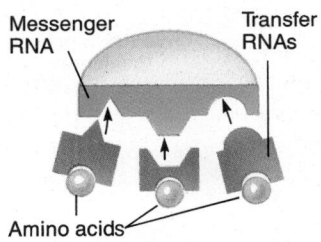

Amino acids

5. Transfer RNAs carry their
amino acids to the
messenger RNA, where they
are snapped into place.

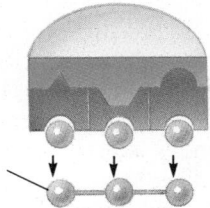

6. The completed protein
strand is released, and
the messenger RNA is
degraded.

■■■ **Figure 6–4**

Protein Synthesis. The instructions for making every protein in a person's body are transmitted in the genetic information he or she receives at conception. This body of knowledge is filed away in a master file in the nucleus of every cell. The master file is the DNA (deoxyribonucleic acid), which never leaves the nucleus. Every cell within an individual contains identical DNA. Each specialized cell has access to the total inherited information but calls on only the instructions needed for its own functions.

To inform the cell of the proper sequence of amino acids for a needed protein, a "photocopy" of the appropriate portion of DNA is made. This copy is messenger RNA (ribonucleic acid), which, unlike DNA, is able to escape through the nuclear membrane. In the cell fluid it seeks out and attaches itself to one of the ribosomes (a protein-making machine, itself composed of RNA and protein). Thus situated, the messenger presents the specifications for the amino acids to be linked into a protein strand.

Meanwhile, other forms of RNA, called transfer RNAs, collect amino acids from the cell fluid and bring them to the messenger. For each amino acid there is a specific transfer RNA. Thousands of these transfer RNAs, each carrying its amino acid, cluster around the ribosomes, like donors bearing gifts to a host. When an amino acid is called for by the messenger, the transfer RNA carrying it snaps into position. Then the next and the next and the next loaded transfer RNAs move into place. Thus the amino acids are lined up in the right sequence. Then an enzyme bonds them together.

Finally, the completed protein strand is released, the messenger is degraded, and the transfer RNAs are freed to return for another load. It takes many words to describe these events, but in the cell, 40 to 100 amino acids can be added to a growing protein strand in only a second.

pH: a measure of acidity on a point scale. A solution with a pH of 1 is a strong acid; a solution with a pH of 7 is neutral; and a solution with a pH of 14 is a strong base.

dipeptides (dye-PEP-tides): protein fragments two amino acids long. A *peptide* is a strand of amino acids (*di* means "two").

tripeptides (try-PEP-tides): protein fragments three amino acids long (*tri* means "three").

polypeptides: protein fragments of many (more than ten) amino acids bonded together. (A chain of between three and ten is called an *oligopeptide*.)

unlike most enzymes, stomach enzymes function best in an acid environment. Their job is to break apart the protein strands into smaller pieces. The stomach lining, which is also made partly of protein, is protected against attack by acid and enzymes by a coat of mucus, secreted by its cells.

The whole process of digestion is an ingenious solution to a complex problem. Proteins (enzymes), when activated by acid, digest proteins (food) denatured by acid. The mucous coating of the stomach wall protects *its* proteins from being affected by either acid or enzymes. The acid in the stomach is so strong (**pH** 2) that no food is acid enough to make it stronger (the pH of pure vinegar is about 3). It is obvious from this that the stomach is supposed to be acid to do its job.

Television commercials promote antacids for relief of "acid indigestion," but antacids only put the burden on the stomach to produce even more acid to restore its normal balance. Antacids are useful to protect ulcers from stomach acid but are not needed by normal, healthy people. It is normal to have an acid stomach. Sometimes the stomach acid backs up and burns the lining of the esophagus or throat, which are not as well protected by mucus as the stomach. When this happens repeatedly, the person shouldn't take an antacid but should consult a physician. The cause may simply be overeating, but it may be serious—a hernia or obstruction.

By the time most proteins slip from the stomach into the small intestine, they are already broken into different-sized pieces. Some are single amino acids; many are strands of two, three, or more amino acids (**dipeptides, tripeptides, polypeptides**); and a few are whole proteins. In the small intestine the acid delivered by the stomach is neutralized by alkaline juice from the pancreas. The raising of the pH to about 7 enables the next enzyme team to accomplish the final breakdown of the strands. Digestion continues until al-

■■■ Figure 6–5

Cells Absorb Amino Acids and Build Their Own Proteins.

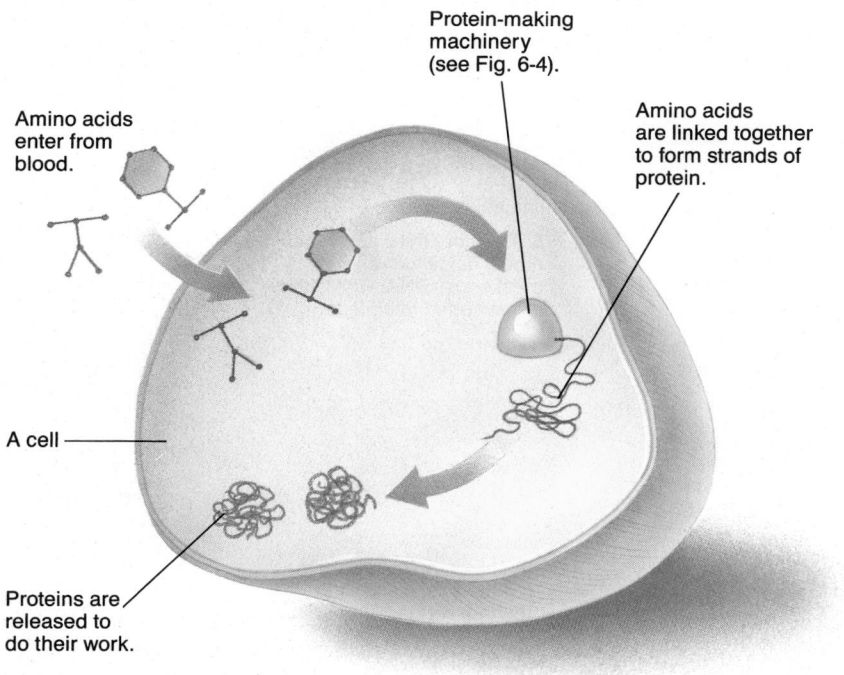

Amino acids enter from blood.

Protein-making machinery (see Fig. 6-4).

Amino acids are linked together to form strands of protein.

A cell

Proteins are released to do their work.

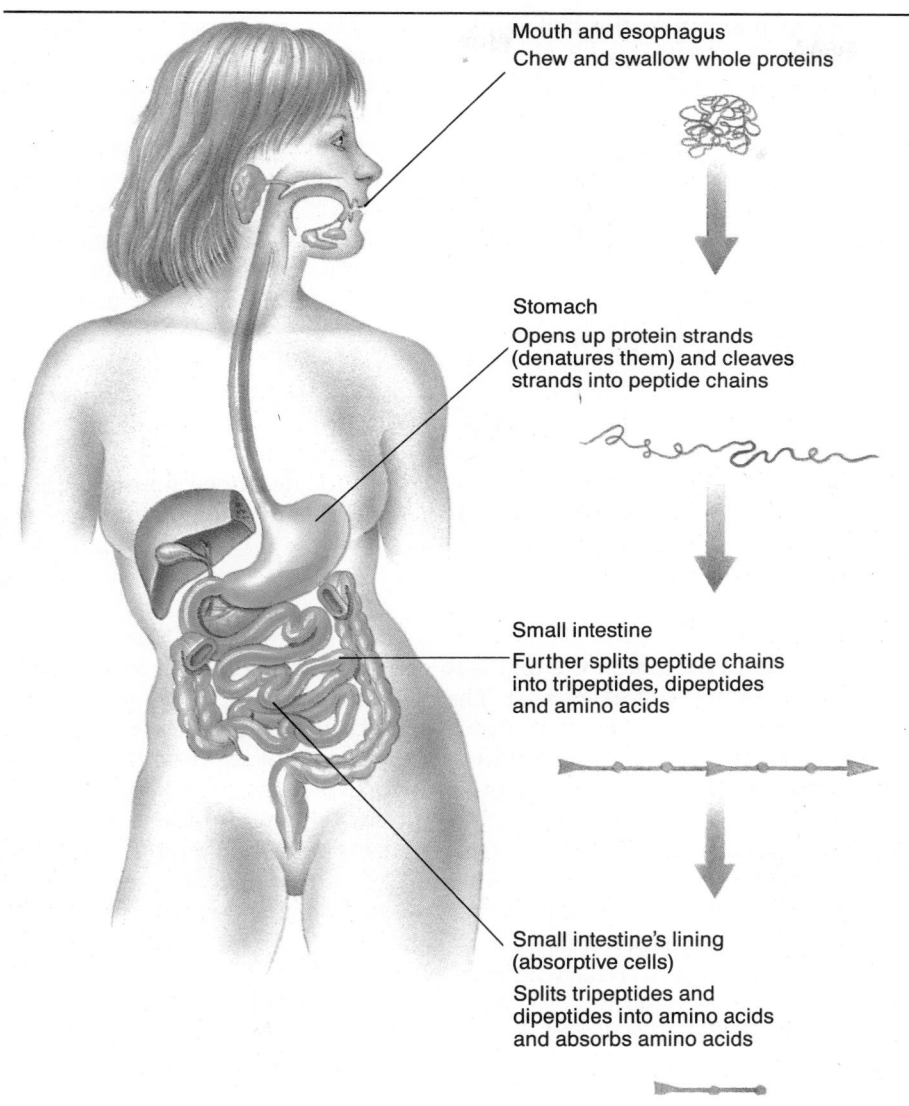

Mouth and esophagus
Chew and swallow whole proteins

Stomach
Opens up protein strands
(denatures them) and cleaves
strands into peptide chains

Small intestine
Further splits peptide chains
into tripeptides, dipeptides
and amino acids

Small intestine's lining
(absorptive cells)
Splits tripeptides and
dipeptides into amino acids
and absorbs amino acids

■■■ **Figure 6–6**

Protein Digestion and Absorption.

most all pieces of protein are broken into small fragments and more free amino acids. The whole process is summarized in Figure 6–6.

The cells all along the small intestine absorb single amino acids. As for dipeptides and tripeptides, the cells that line the small intestine capture them on their surfaces, split them into single amino acids, and absorb them, too. Then the cells release all the single amino acids into the bloodstream. A few whole proteins, or large portions of them, escape the digestion process altogether, and these slip across the digestive tract wall to enter the bloodstream. It is thought that these large particles may provide the body with information about the environment and may play a role in food allergy via the immune response.[4]

The cells of the small intestine possess different sites for the absorption of different classes of amino acids. Amino acids of the same class compete for the same carriers. This means that when a person ingests a large dose of any single

More about food allergy in Chapter 13.

hormone: as defined in Chapter 3, a chemical messenger that is secreted by one of a number of body organs in response to a condition that requires regulation. Each hormone affects a specific organ or tissue and elicits a specific response.

antibodies (AN-tee-bod-ees; introduced in Chapter 3): large proteins of the blood, produced by the immune system in response to invasion of the body by foreign substances (antigens); they combine with and inactivate them.

immunity (introduced in Chapter 3): specific disease resistance, derived from the immune system's memory of prior exposure to specific disease agents and its ability to mount a swift defense against them.

amino acid, absorption of others in its class may be limited (see the Consumer Caution entitled "Protein and Amino Acid Supplements" later in this chapter). Once they are circulating in the bloodstream, amino acids are available to be taken up by any cell of the body. The body cells then make proteins, either for their own use or for secretion into lymph or blood for other uses. Alternatively the body cells can use amino acids for energy.

▮▮▶ *Digestion of protein involves denaturation by stomach acid, followed by enzymatic digestion by the stomach and small intestine to amino acids, dipeptides, and tripeptides. The cells of the small intestine complete digestion, absorb the amino acids, and release them into the blood.*

▮▮▮ The Roles of the Body's Proteins

Only a few of the many roles proteins play will be described here to give an appreciation of their versatility and importance. Primary among their functions is the support of growth.

Growth and Maintenance

One function of protein in the diet is to ensure that amino acids are available to build the proteins of new tissue. The new tissue may be in an embryo; in a growing child; in new blood needed to replace that which has been lost in burns, hemorrhage, or surgery; in the scar tissue that heals wounds; or in new hair and nails. Not so obvious is the protein that helps to replace worn-out cells. Each of the millions of red cells of the blood is useful for three or four months, and then each must be replaced by a new cell, produced in and released by the bone marrow. The millions of cells that line the intestinal tract live for only three days and are constantly being shed and replaced. You have probably observed that the cells of your skin die and rub off and that new ones grow from underneath. Nearly all cells arise, live, and die this way, and while they are living, as described earlier, proteins within each cell are constantly being made and broken down. Amino acids from food must be supplied to support new growth and maintenance of cells and of the working parts within them.

Enzymes and Hormones

Enzymes are among the most important of the proteins formed in living cells. Enzymes are catalysts—they help chemical reactions take place. There are thousands of enzymes inside a single cell, each one facilitating a specific chemical reaction.

Figure 6–7 shows how an enzyme might work. Chemicals A and B are attracted to the enzyme's active site and park there for a moment. The two chemicals are "made for each other" and so bond together and leave the enzyme a new compound AB (a substance that is needed in some way). It could be that A and B, because they were both swimming around in the cell fluid, would have eventually discovered each other and combined without help. However, the enzyme attracted them and snapped them into the exact position for bonding. In this way the enzyme speeded up the reaction time. A single en-

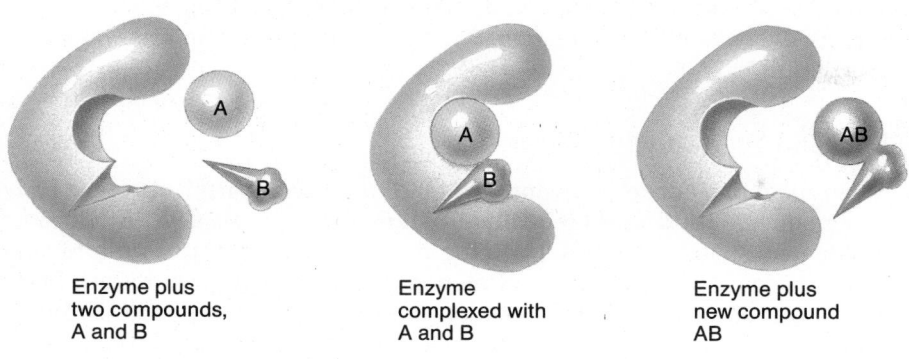

Enzyme plus
two compounds,
A and B

Enzyme
complexed with
A and B

Enzyme plus
new compound
AB

Figure 6–7

Enzyme Action. Each enzyme facilitates a specific chemical reaction.

zyme can facilitate several hundred such syntheses in a second. Other enzymes break apart compounds into two or more products or rearrange the atoms in one compound to make another one.

The body's many **hormones** are messenger molecules, and some are made from amino acids. Various glands in the body release hormones in response to changes in the internal environment, and the hormones elicit the appropriate responses to restore normal conditions. Among the hormones is the thyroid hormone that regulates the metabolic rate of the body. An opposing pair of hormones, insulin and glucagon, maintain blood glucose levels, as was described in Chapter 4. Many other hormones are at work in the body regulating equally critical body functions. Figure 6–8 shows the amino acid sequence of human insulin.

The thyroid hormone contains iodine, and insulin associates with zinc; these minerals are helper nutrients (see Chapter 8).

Figure 6–8

Amino Acid Sequence of Human Insulin. This picture shows a refinement of protein structure not mentioned in the text. The amino acid cysteine (cys) has a sulfur-containing side group in it, and these groups on two cysteine molecules can bond together, creating a bridge between two protein strands or two parts of the same strand. Insulin contains three such bridges.

Antibodies

Of all the great variety of proteins in living organisms, the **antibodies** demonstrate that proteins are specific for one organism. Antibodies, as first described in Chapter 3, are formed in response to the presence of foreign particles (usually proteins) that invade the body. The foreign protein may be part of a bacterium, a virus, or a toxin, or it may be present in a food that causes allergy. The body, after recognizing that it has been invaded, manufactures antibodies, and they inactivate the foreign protein.

One of the most fascinating aspects of this response is that each antibody is designed specifically to destroy one invader. An antibody that has been manufactured to combat one strain of influenza would be of no help in protecting a person against another strain. Once the body has learned to make a particular antibody, it remembers; and the next time it encounters that same invader, it will be equipped to destroy it even more rapidly. In other words, it develops an **immunity**. This molecular memory is the principle underlying immunizations— injections of drugs made from destroyed and inactivated microbes or their products, which activate the body immune defenses more or less permanently. Some immunities are lifelong; others, such as that to tetanus, must be renewed.

In some cases the immune response can cause harm. If a transfusion should accidentally deliver the wrong blood type, the body would make antibodies to inactivate the foreign blood proteins. The first time this happened, the body might be able to tolerate or to get rid of the gradual accumulation of inactivated

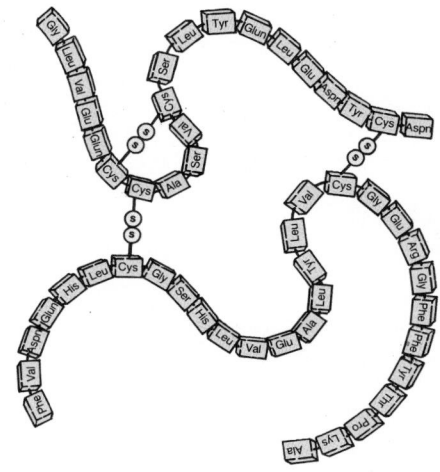

foreign blood cells. But with a second transfusion of the wrong type, the body would be overwhelmed by an immediate, massive immune response, and death would result.

Fluid and Electrolyte Balance

Proteins help to regulate the quantity of fluids in the compartments of the body to maintain the **fluid and electrolyte balance**. To remain alive, a cell must contain a constant amount of fluid. Too much might cause it to rupture, and too little would make it unable to function. Although water can diffuse freely into and out of the cell, proteins cannot—and proteins attract water. By maintaining a store of internal proteins, the cell retains the fluid it needs (it also uses minerals this way). Similarly, the cells secrete proteins (and minerals) into the spaces between them to keep the fluid volume constant in those spaces. The proteins secreted into the blood can't cross the vessel walls, and thus they maintain the blood volume in the same way. (The control of water's location by particles is called *osmosis* and is discussed further in Chapter 8.)

Not only the quantity but also the composition of the body fluids is vital to life. Transport proteins in the membranes of all the cells respond sensitively to small changes in the circulating fluids and work to maintain equilibrium by transferring substances into and out of cells. Thus, for example, sodium is concentrated outside the cells, and potassium is concentrated inside—a condition that is especially critical to the functioning of nerve and muscle cells (Figure 6–9). A disturbance of the fluid and electrolyte balance can impair the action of the indispensable heart, lungs, and brain, triggering a major medical emergency. Cell proteins work daily to avert such a disaster by holding fluids and electrolytes in their proper chambers.

Acid-Base Balance

Normal processes of the body continually produce **acids** and their opposite, **bases**, which must be carried by the blood to the organs of excretion. The blood must do this without allowing its own **acid-base balance** to be affected. This magical feat is another trick of the proteins in the blood, which act as **buffers**. They pick up hydrogens (acid) when there are too many and release them again when there are too few. The secret is that the negatively charged side chains of the amino acids can accommodate additional hydrogens (which are positively charged) when necessary.

The acid-base balance of the blood is one of the most rigidly controlled conditions in the body. If it changes too much, the dangerous condition **acidosis** or the opposite, basic condition **alkalosis** can cause coma or death. The hazard of these conditions is due to their effect on proteins. When the proteins' buffering capacity is exceeded—when they have taken on board all the acid hydrogens they can accommodate—additional acid deranges their structure by pulling them out of shape: that is, it denatures them. Knowing how indispensable the structures of proteins are to their functions and how vital their functions are to life, you can imagine how many body processes would be halted by such a disturbance.

These are but a sampling of the major roles proteins play in the body but should serve to illustrate their versatility, uniqueness, and importance. No wonder their discoverers called them the primary material of life.

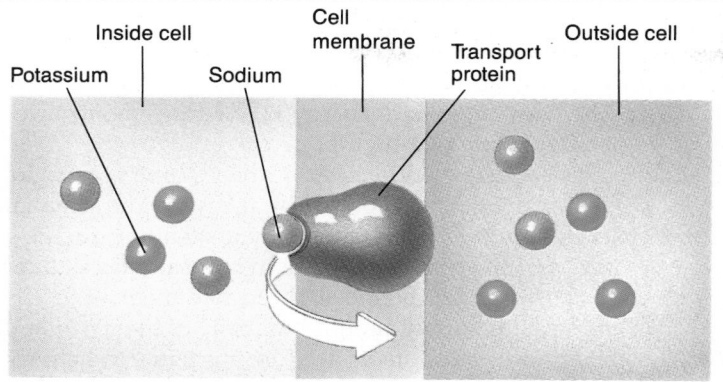

Potassium · Inside cell · Sodium · Cell membrane · Transport protein · Outside cell

(Protein flips)

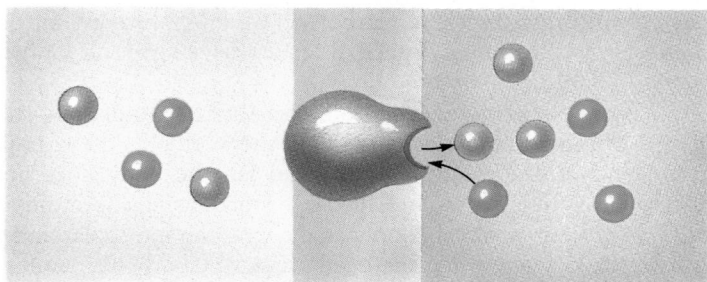

(Molecules trade places)

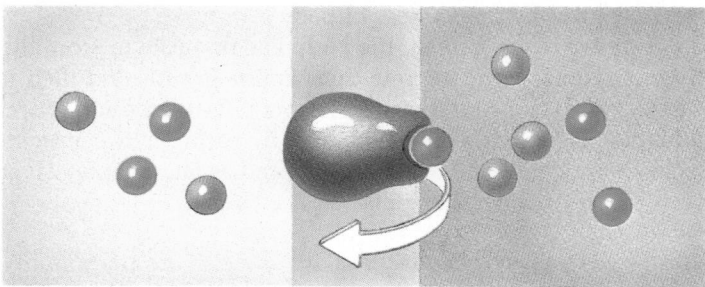

(Protein flips)

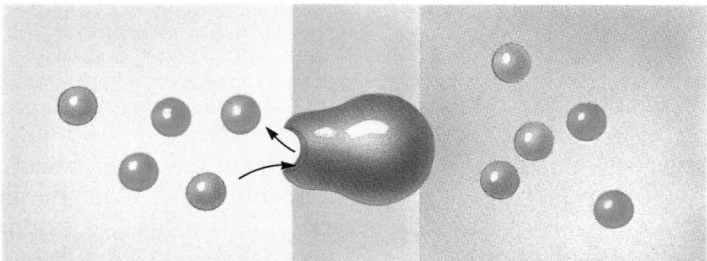

■■■ **Figure 6—9**

Proteins Transport Substances into and out of Cells. A transport protein within a cell membrane acts as a sort of revolving door—it picks up substances on one side of the membrane and flips them to the other side without leaving the membrane itself. The substances being transported here are sodium and potassium. The significance of their movement in and out of cells is discussed in Chapter 8.

urea (yoo-REE-uh): the principal nitrogen-excretion product of metabolism, generated mostly by removal of amine groups from unneeded amino acids or from amino acids being sacrificed to a need for energy.

Energy

Only protein can perform all the functions described earlier, but it will be sacrificed to provide needed energy if insufficient fat- and carbohydrate-rich foods are eaten. The body must have energy to live from moment to moment, and so it gives obtaining energy a high priority.

When amino acids are degraded for energy, their amine groups are stripped off and used elsewhere or are incorporated by the liver into **urea** and sent to the kidney for excretion in the urine. The fragments that remain are composed of carbon, hydrogen, and oxygen, as are carbohydrate and fat, and can be used to build those substances or can be metabolized like them.

Not only can amino acids supply energy, but many of them can be converted to glucose, as fat can never be. Thus if need be, protein can help to maintain a steady blood-glucose level and so serve the energy needs of the brain.

A perspective on the three energy-yielding nutrients—their similarities and differences—should now be clear. Carbohydrate offers energy; fat offers concentrated energy; and protein, if needed, can offer energy plus nitrogen (see Figure 6–10).

Only if the protein-sparing energy from carbohydrate and fat is sufficient to power the cells will the amino acids be used for the work only they can perform—making proteins. Unlike for carbohydrate and fat, the body does not make a specialized storage form for protein. Glucose is stored as glycogen, fats as triglycerides, but body protein is available only as the working molecular and structural components of the tissues. When the need arises, the body dismantles its tissue proteins, each in its own time, first those of the liver, and then those of the muscles and other organs and burns them for energy. Thus energy deficiency (starvation) is always accompanied by the wasting of body lean tissue.

If amino acids are oversupplied, the body has no place to store them. It has no choice but to remove and excrete their amine groups and then to convert the residues to glycogen or fat for energy storage. Athletes and exercisers take note: you cannot build extra muscle tissue by eating extra protein, because protein excesses are converted to fuel and stored as fat. Chapter 10 gives more details about protein needs of exercisers.

❚❚▷ *Proteins serve many diverse functions, all of which are essential to life. When sufficient carbohydrate and fat are consumed to meet the body's energy need, food protein and body protein are sacrificed to supply energy. The nitrogen part is removed from each amino acid, and the resulting fragment is oxidized for energy.*

❚❚❚ Use of Amino Acids Inside Cells

To review the body's handling of amino acids, let us follow the fate of an amino acid that was originally part of a protein-containing food. When the amino acid arrives in a cell, it may be used in several different ways, depending on the needs of the cell at the time.

The amino acid may be used as is and become part of a growing protein. Alternatively, the cell may dismantle it and use its amine group to build a different amino acid. The remainder may be used for fuel or, if not needed, converted to and stored as fat.

Nearly the same fate awaits the amino acid present in a cell that is screaming for energy but has no fuel in the form of glucose or fatty acids. Even though

❚❚❚ **Figure 6–10**

Three Different Energy Sources. Carbohydrate offers energy; fat offers concentrated energy; and protein, if necessary, can offer energy plus nitrogen.

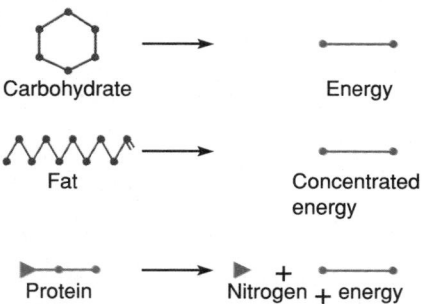

Carbohydrate → Energy

Fat → Concentrated energy

Protein → Nitrogen + energy

this amino acid may be needed to build a vital protein, the energy need will be given top priority. Without energy, the cell dies. Therefore this valuable amino acid will be stripped of its amine group, and the remainder of its structure will be used for energy. The amine group will be excreted from the cell and, finally, from the body in the urine.

Another circumstance in which amino acids are used for energy is when there is a surplus of amino acids and energy-yielding nutrients. In this case the body does not waste this resource. It takes the amino acid apart, excretes the amine group, converts the rest to fat, and then stores the fat in the fat cells. In this way valuable, expensive, protein-rich foods can contribute to obesity.

In summary, amino acids in the cell can be used to:

- Synthesize protein.
- Provide glucose (many of them can be converted to glucose).
- Provide nitrogen in the form of amine groups to build nonessential amino acids.
- Provide energy if there is a scarcity of energy nutrients.
- Increase the stores of fat.

Amino acids are wasted (not used to build protein) whenever there is:

- Not enough energy from carbohydrate and fat.
- An imbalance, with not enough essential amino acids (low-quality protein, see following section).
- Too much protein so that not all is needed.
- Too much of any amino acid from a supplement.

Factors that must be supplied in the diet for the body to be able to synthesize protein include:

- All essential amino acids in the proper amounts.
- An adequate total amount of protein (to supply amine groups to synthesize ₍ne nonessential amino acids).
- Adequate energy-yielding carbohydrate and fat (to spare the protein).

▐▌▶ *Amino acids can be metabolized to protein, glucose, nitrogen + energy, or fat. They will be metabolized to protein only if sufficient energy is present from other sources. The diet should supply all essential amino acids. If an essential amino acid is consistently lacking, protein synthesis stops, and other amino acids are degraded.*

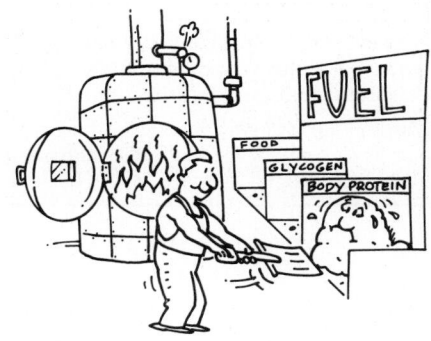

In times of energy deficiency, the body dismantles its own protein tissues for fuel.

▮▮▮ Food Proteins: Quality, Use, and Need

The body responds to different proteins in different ways, depending on many factors: the body's state of health, the food source of the protein, its digestibility, the other nutrients taken with it, and its amino acid assortment. Protein will be used most efficiently if accompanied by carbohydrate, fat, and the full array of vitamins and minerals. To know whether, say, 30 grams of a protein is enough to meet a person's daily needs, it is necessary to know how all these other factors affect the body's use of the protein.

Regarding a person's state of health, malnutrition or infection may greatly increase the need for protein while making it harder to meet. In malnutrition,

complete proteins: proteins containing
all the essential amino acids in the
right balance.

incomplete proteins: proteins lacking,
or low in, one or more of the essential
amino acids.

protein digestion and absorption are impaired because digestive enzyme secretion is reduced, and the absorptive surfaces of the digestive tract degenerate.
Diarrhea may result, causing further protein losses. In infection, protein is
needed to make antibodies as well as to support normal functioning, and this
increases the need.

In making a protein, the cells need a full array of amino acids from food,
from their own amino acid pools, or from both. If a *nonessential* amino acid
(that is, one the cell *can* make) is unavailable from food, the cell will synthesize
it and continue attaching amino acids to the strand. If an *essential* amino acid
(one the cell *cannot* make) is missing, the cells dismantle their own proteins to
obtain the needed amino acids, and protein synthesis proceeds. Should a shortage of essential amino acids become chronic, though, the building of protein
would be halted. Partially completed proteins are not held for completion at a
later time when the diet may improve. Rather, the partial structures are dismantled, and the component amino acids are returned to the circulation to be
made available to other cells. If they are not soon inserted into protein, their
amine groups are removed and excreted, and the residues are used for other
purposes. The need that prompted the calling for that particular protein will
not be met, and since the amino groups are excreted, the body cannot resyn-
thesize the amino acids later.

It follows that all the essential amino acids must be consumed in a balanced
diet before the body pools of the essential amino acids dwindle to the point at
which body organs are compromised. This presents no problem to people who
regularly eat **complete proteins**, such as those of meat, fish, poultry, cheese,
eggs, or milk. The proteins of these foods contain ample amounts of all the
essential amino acids. An equally sound choice is to eat two **incomplete
protein** foods from plants, each of which supplies the amino acids missing in
the other. This strategy is described in the section entitled "Vegetarian Protein
Choices."

Concern about the quality of individual food proteins is of only theoretical
interest in settings where food is abundant. Most people in the United States
and Canada would find it next to impossible *not* to meet their protein requirements, even if they ate no meat, fish, poultry, eggs, or cheese—provided only
that they ate a variety of other nutritious foods to meet their energy needs—
not, say, just cookies, potato chips, and alcoholic beverages. (While *protein* is
usually sufficient in North American diets, Chapters 7 and 8 point out the *other*
nutrients to which people must attend.)

However, protein quality can make the difference between health and disease when food energy intake is limited (where malnutrition is widespread) or
when the selection of foods available is severely limited (where a single food
such as potato or rice provides 90 percent of the calories). Even then, protein
intake may be adequate, but it may not be. In these cases the primary food
source of protein must be checked, since its quality is of great importance.

Measuring Protein Quality

Researchers have developed many different methods of evaluating the quality
of food protein. The generalizations that follow come from such research.

Amino acids from animal proteins are best absorbed (over 90 percent).
Those from legumes follow (about 80 percent). Those from grains and other

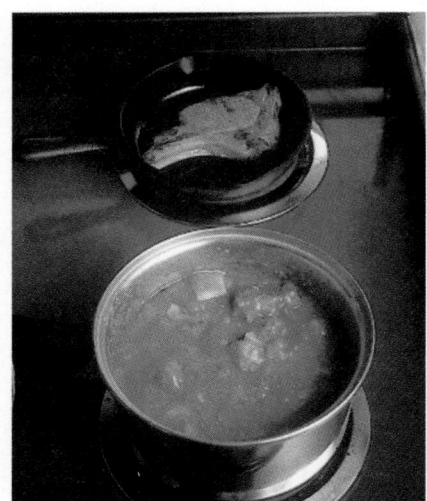
Cooking with moist heat improves
protein digestibility.

plant foods vary (from 60 to 90 percent). Cooking with moist heat generally improves protein digestibility, whereas dry heat methods may impair it.

All other things being equal, a protein that supplies all the essential amino acids in exactly the right ratio will be most completely used. If an essential amino acid is in short supply in the diet, it limits the use of all the others for building protein. A protein that almost entirely lacks an essential amino acid does not, by itself, support protein synthesis.

When amino acids are wasted, their amine groups (which contain their nitrogen) can't be stored. Therefore the efficiency of a protein in supporting maintenance of body tissue can be assessed experimentally by measuring the net loss of nitrogen from the body when that protein is fed by itself. The higher the amount of nitrogen retained, the higher the quality of the protein. This is the basis for determinations of the **biological value (BV)** of proteins.

A high-quality protein by this standard is egg protein. It has been designated the **reference protein** and given a score of 100; other proteins are scored against this standard. Three other ways of scoring protein quality are in common use. One is **chemical scoring**—a pencil-and-paper method of calculating which amino acid is in shortest supply relative to human physiological need. The second is **net protein utilization (NPU)**—a measure of the amount of protein retained from that ingested. The third is **protein efficiency ratio (PER)**—a method that involves feeding the protein to young, growing rats and measuring their weight gains per unit of protein. These different methods of evaluating proteins give different results. The chemical scores and NPUs of several proteins are listed in Table 6–1 to illustrate this point.

The PER is used as a standard for food labeling. The U.S. RDA recommends two different daily intakes of protein, depending on the quality. If the protein is of a quality as high as milk protein (casein) or higher, then 45 grams a day is considered sufficient for an adult; if the protein's quality is lower than that, then 65 grams a day is recommended. (See inside front cover, page C for the U.S. RDA table.)

Protein scores are of great importance in dealing with widespread malnutrition. For the average well-fed North American, however, perhaps the most relevant lesson to be learned from them is that although animal proteins tend to have slightly higher scores than plant proteins, the two overlap considerably. The best guarantee of amino acid adequacy is to eat mixtures of foods containing protein in the presence of adequate amounts of vitamins, minerals, and energy from carbohydrate and fat.

▐▌▷ *Protein use depends on the user's health, the protein's digestibility, the nutrients eaten with it, and its amino acid assortment. The quality of a protein is measured by how much of its nitrogen is retained by the body or by how well the protein supports growth.*

The Protein RDA

Protein is at the heart of a good diet. Menu planners build their meals around the RDA for protein. The RDA is designed to cover the need to replace protein-containing tissue people lose and wear out every day. Therefore it depends on body size: larger people have a higher protein RDA. The protein RDA also is adjusted to cover additional needs for building new tissue and so is higher for

biological value (BV): a measure of protein quality, assessed by determining how well a given food or food mixture supports nitrogen retention.

reference protein: egg protein, the standard with which other proteins are compared to determine biological value.

chemical scoring: a method of evaluating protein quality by comparing its chemically determined amino acid composition, on paper, with human amino acid requirements.

net protein utilization (NPU): a method of evaluating protein quality by comparing the amount animals retain to the amount they ingest.

protein efficiency ratio (PER): a measure of protein quality assessed by determining how well a given protein supports weight gain in laboratory animals.

▐▐▐ Table 6–1 Chemical Scores and NPUs of Various Proteins

PROTEIN	CHEMICAL	NPU
Eggs	100	100
Milk	93	75
Rice	86	67
Beef	75	80
Fish	75	83
Corn	72	56

SOURCE: Adapted from the Assessment of proteins, *Nutrition and the MD*, June 1985, pp. 3–4.

■■■ **Table 6–2 The Protein RDA (1989)**

AGE (yr)	RDA (g/kg)[a]
0–½	2.2
½–1	1.6
1–3	1.2
4–6	1.1
7–14	1.0
15–18 (males)	0.9
15–18 (females)	0.8
19 and up	0.8

[a]The RDA is 10 g/day higher during pregnancy, 15 g/day higher during the first six months of lactation, and 12 g/day higher during the remainder of lactation.

The RDA tables are on the inside front cover.

Protein RDA (adult) = 0.8 g/kg.

To figure your protein RDA:

1. Find your body weight.
2. Convert pounds to kilograms (pounds divided by 2.2 lb/kg equals kilograms).
3. Multiply by 0.8 g/kg to get your RDA in grams per day.

For example:

1. Weight = 110 lb.
2. 110 lb ÷ 2.2 lb/kg = 50 kg.
3. 50 kg × 0.8 g/kg = 40 g.

growing children and pregnant and lactating women. The Canadian recommendation for protein is similar and is based on similar assumptions.

Underlying the protein RDA are **nitrogen balance** studies, which measure nitrogen lost by excretion compared with nitrogen eaten in food. In healthy adults nitrogen-in must equal nitrogen-out. The laboratory scientist measures the body's daily nitrogen losses in urine, feces, sweat, and skin under controlled conditions and can then estimate the amount of protein needed to replace these losses. The average amino acid is 6.25 times as heavy as the nitrogen it contains, so as a rule of thumb, the scientist multiplies the nitrogen weight by 6.25 to estimate the protein's weight.

Under normal circumstances healthy adults are in nitrogen equilibrium, or zero balance—that is, they have at all times the same amount of total protein in their bodies. When nitrogen-in exceeds nitrogen-out, they are said to be in positive nitrogen balance; this means that somewhere in their bodies more proteins are being built than are being broken down and lost. When nitrogen-in is less than nitrogen-out, they are said to be in negative nitrogen balance; they are losing protein.

Growing children add to their bodies new blood, bone, and muscle cells every day. These cells contain protein, so children must have in their bodies more protein (and therefore more nitrogen) at the end of each day than they had at the beginning. A growing child is therefore in positive nitrogen balance. Similarly, when a woman is pregnant she is, in essence, growing a new person; she too must be in positive nitrogen balance. When she is lactating, she may be in equilibrium again, but it is a sort of enhanced equilibrium. She is eating more protein than before to make her milk and is secreting it whenever the baby nurses.

Negative nitrogen balance occurs when muscle or other protein tissue is broken down and lost. Consider the situation when people have to rest in bed for a long time. Their muscles degenerate, and they suffer a net loss of protein. One of several problems faced by the nutritionists responsible for the welfare of astronauts involves the negative nitrogen balance that occurs if astronauts spend many days in the space capsule. Without the exercise of supporting their bodies' weight, their muscles may waste and weaken. To maintain the muscles, special exercises are assigned. (The same is true for the bones and calcium as discussed in Controversy 8.)

For healthy adults the Recommended Dietary Allowance (RDA) for protein has been set at 0.8 grams for each kilogram (or 2.2 pounds) of body weight. Athletes need slightly more, but the increased need is well covered by a regular diet (see Chapter 10). For children who are growing, the RDA is higher per unit of body weight; for infants it is highest of all (see Table 6–2).

The protein RDA listed in the RDA tables are intended for the mythical creatures of Chapter 2—the man and woman who are "average" figures for our population. Real, live people may have a hard time discovering how the RDA apply to them. This is not surprising: recall that all the RDA are values for *populations*, not individuals. Still, they can yield a rough, ballpark estimate of protein needs for people of appropriate weight for height.

Very little attention has been paid to the protein needs of obese people. This is because once excess fat tissue is established it does not require extra protein, and the obese person's protein need is usually assumed to be about the same as that of a normal-weight person of the same height. (*Building* fat tissue does require protein, probably for constructing new blood vessels and cellular proteins.) Similarly, the underweight person who lacks fat but not lean tissue probably also needs the same amount of protein as the normal-weight person of the same height.

It would be easier to state people's protein needs if there were an easy way to measure lean tissue. Weight does not reveal much about lean tissue. The very inactive fat person may have a severely underdeveloped lean body and so need less protein than the person's weight seems to imply; the heavy-weight football player may have a greatly overdeveloped lean body and so need much more than the inactive person of the same weight. In the absence of other guidelines, the best way to estimate protein needs seems to be to use the RDA and the person's *appropriate* weight—another frustratingly rough approximation (see Chapter 9).

In making its recommendations for protein intakes, the members of the Committee on RDA took into consideration that the protein in a normal diet would be mixed—that is, a combination of animal and plant protein. They also recognized that not all proteins are used with 100 percent efficiency and that individuals use protein with different efficiencies. Accordingly, the committee made the RDA quite generous. Many normal people can consume less than the RDA for protein and still meet their bodies' needs. What this means in terms of food selections is presented in this chapter's Food Feature.

The RDA must be interpreted with caution. For the present, perhaps the most important point is that the RDA are generous recommendations and that the healthy person need not exceed them. A look at food sources of protein will show that the foods people normally eat supply it in abundance.

▌▌▶ *The amount of protein needed daily depends on size and stage of growth. The RDA for adults is 0.8 grams of protein per kilogram of body weight.*

nitrogen balance: the amount of nitrogen consumed compared with the amount excreted in a given time period.

protein-energy malnutrition (PEM), also called **protein- calorie malnutrition (PCM)**: the world's most widespread malnutrition problem, including both kwashiorkor and marasmus and states in which they overlap.

kwashiorkor (kwash-ee-OR-core, kwash-ee-or-CORE): the deficiency disease caused by inadequate protein in the presence of adequate energy.

marasmus (ma-RAZ-mus): the calorie-deficiency disease; starvation.

▌▌▌ Protein and Health

With all the attention that has been paid in recent years to the health effects of starch, sugars, fibers, fats, oils, and cholesterol, protein has been slighted. Protein deficiency effects are well known because, together with energy deficiency, they are the world's main form of malnutrition. But the health effects of too much protein, and particularly the effects of proteins of different kinds, are far less well known. Let us consider each in turn: deficiency, excess, and type of protein.

Protein-Energy Malnutrition

Protein deficiency and energy deficiency go hand in hand so often that public health officials have given a name to the pair: **protein-energy malnutrition (PEM)**. The two diseases and their symptoms overlap all along the spectrum, but the extremes have names of their own. Protein deficiency is **kwashiorkor**, and energy deficiency is **marasmus**.

Kwashiorkor is the Ghanaian name for "the evil spirit that infects the first child when the second child is born early." In countries where kwashiorkor is prevalent, parents customarily give their newly weaned children watery cereal rather than the food eaten by the rest of the family. The child has been receiving its mother's breast milk containing high-quality protein designed beautifully to support growth. Suddenly the child receives only a weak drink with

edema (eh-DEEM-uh): the swelling of body tissue caused by leakage of fluid from the blood vessels, seen in (among other conditions) protein deficiency.

dysentery (DISS-en-terry): an infection of the digestive tract that causes diarrhea.

scant protein of very low quality. Small wonder the just-weaned child sickens when the new baby arrives.

The child who has been banished from its mother's breast faces this threat to life by engaging in as little activity as possible. Apathy is one of the earliest signs of protein deprivation; the body is collecting all its forces to meet the crisis and so cuts down on any expenditure of protein not needed for the heart, lungs, and brain. As the apathy increases, the child doesn't even cry for food. Growth ceases; the child is no larger at four than at two. New hair grows without the protein pigment that gave it its color. The skin also loses its color, and when sores open, they fail to heal. Digestive enzymes are in short supply, the digestive tract lining deteriorates, and absorption fails. The child can't assimilate what little food is eaten. Proteins and hormones that previously kept the fluid correctly distributed among the compartments of the body now are diminished, so that fluid leaks out of the blood (**edema**) and accumulates in the belly and legs. Blood proteins, including hemoglobin, diminish, so the child becomes anemic; this increases the weakness and apathy. The kwashiorkor victim often develops a fatty liver, caused by lack of the protein carriers that transport fat out of the liver. The liver damage diminishes the organ's ability to clear poisons from the body, prolonging their toxic effects.[5] Antibodies to fight off invading bacteria are degraded to provide amino acids for other uses; the child becomes an easy target for any infection. Then **dysentery**, an infection of the digestive tract that causes diarrhea, further depletes the body of nutrients, especially minerals. Measles, which might make a healthy child sick for a week or two, kills the kwashiorkor child within two or three days.

If the child is taken into the hospital, this starved condition may not be obvious. Water in the tissues may cause the body to look almost fat. Only when the fluid balance is restored will it be seen that the child is just a skeleton thinly covered with skin.

If caught in time, a kwashiorkor child's life may be saved by careful nutrition therapy. The fluid balances are most critical. Diarrhea will have depleted the body's potassium stores and upset other salt balances. Careful remediation of these critical balances will prevent sudden death from heart failure about half the time. Only later can nonfat milk, containing protein and carbohydrate, be safely given; then comes fat, when body protein is sufficient to provide carriers. If kwashiorkor is prolonged, some damage may not be reversible.

Children with marasmus suffer symptoms similar to those of children with kwashiorkor, since both cause loss of body protein tissue, but there are also differences between the two. Kwashiorkor children retain some of their stores of body fat; marasmic children consume too few calories and burn off body fat stores. Kwashiorkor children accumulate fat in their livers because they have insufficient protein to carry it away; marasmic children receive enough protein to handle what little fat they take in. Kwashiorkor children develop edema because protein is needed for fluid balance; marasmic children may develop edema, or they may not if their meager food contains a little protein. The livers of marasmus children retain the ability to clear toxins from the blood; the livers of kwashiorkor children may lose this ability. Marasmus children experience ketosis to conserve body protein, while kwashiorkor children do not because they are receiving some carbohydrate; so kwashiorkor is actually a less-balanced state and a more fatal disease than marasmus for children at any given age.

A marasmic child looks like a wizened little old person—just skin and bones. The child is often sick because resistance to disease is low. All the muscles are wasted, including the heart muscle, and the heart is weak. Me-

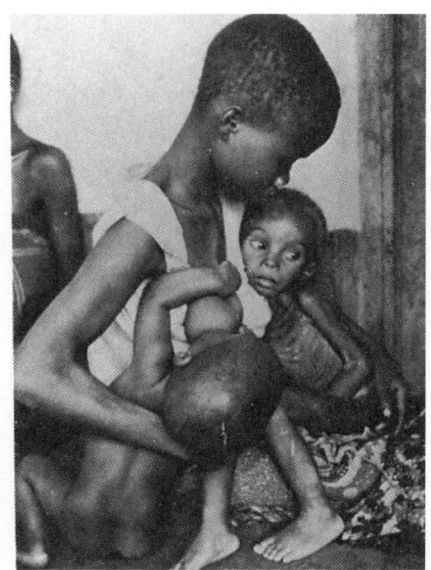

Kwashiorkor.

tabolism is so slow that body temperature is subnormal. There is little or no fat under the skin to insulate against cold. The experience of hospital workers with victims of this disease is that their primary need is to be wrapped up and kept warm. They also need love because they have often been deprived of parental attention as well as food.

Unlike the kwashiorkor child, who is fed milk until weaning, the marasmic child may have been neglected from early infancy. The disease occurs most commonly in children from 6 to 18 months of age in all the overpopulated city slums of the world. Since the brain normally grows to almost its full adult size within the first two years of life, marasmus, if chronically untreated, impairs brain development and may have a permanent effect on learning ability.

Kwashiorkor occurs not only in Ghana but in other African countries, Central America, South America, the Near East, and the Far East. Cases have also been reported on the Indian reservations and in the poor inner cities of the United States. Both marasmus and kwashiorkor also occur in adults in countries where PEM is prevalent. In recent years PEM has also been recognized in many undernourished hospital patients and is the major threat to the person with anorexia nervosa (Controversy 9). Malnutrition worldwide is a political and economic problem, discussed further in Chapter 15.

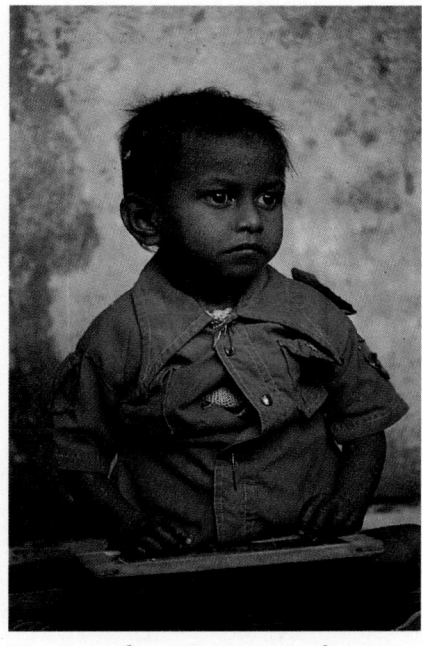

Protein malnutrition impairs learning.

❚❚▶ *Protein deficiency symptoms are always observed when either protein or energy is deficient. Extreme protein deficiency with ample energy is kwashiorkor; extreme energy deficiency is marasmus. The two diseases overlap most of the time and together are called PEM.*

Protein Excess

Many of the world's people struggle to obtain enough food and enough protein to keep themselves alive, but in the developed countries protein is so abundant that problems of protein excess are seen. There are no benefits, and there are risks associated with the overconsumption of protein. For one thing, as we have said before, protein-rich foods are often high-fat foods that contribute to obesity, with its accompanying health risks. In addition to the effects of fat, high levels of animal protein itself may raise cholesterol levels, thus contributing to heart disease.[6] In addition, infants and children do not adjust well to diets containing large amounts of protein; their body composition is altered. Animals fed high-protein diets experience a "protein overload effect," seen in the enlargement of their livers and kidneys. In human beings, high-protein diets eaten over a lifetime may cause problems in kidney function.

Animals experimentally fed high-protein diets of the same nature as those that Americans typically eat also experience losses of the essential mineral zinc from their tissues as they age.[7] Such zinc excretion is also seen in pregnant women and in infants on protein supplements. The use of such supplements during pregnancy may do more harm than good, even to undernourished women.[8] In infants their use has been linked to deficits in cognitive development.[9]

Protein also creates a demand for certain vitamins for its metabolism; vitamin B_6 is an example. An overabundance of protein without accompanying vitamin B_6 can cause a deficiency of the vitamin, and such deficiencies are suspected of contributing to our population's high incidence of atherosclerosis.[10] High dietary protein also increases the tendency to obesity, a finding in direct contrast to the popular belief that such diets cause people to "burn off fat." Fed *low-protein* diets, even with ample calories from carbohydrate, obese subjects can lose weight.[11]

Diets high in protein may also increase the body's excretion of calcium, depleting the bones of their chief mineral.[12] Some argue that *food* sources of excess protein do not promote calcium excretion but that protein or amino acid supplements do so.[13] In keeping with the first possibility, the Committee on RDA has suggested an upper limit for protein intake of no more than twice the RDA amount. In a world in which protein deficiency is such a threat to so many, it is ironic that some people in developed countries should be overconsuming protein.

While eating excess protein is clearly ill advised, taking protein or amino acid supplements (except for abnormal conditions, on competent medical advice) is even more so. The accompanying Consumer Caution, "Protein and Amino Acid Supplements," tells why.

▍▍▶ *Health risks follow the overconsumption of protein foods.*

Chapter 10 describes how the body *really* builds muscle.

| CONSUMER CAUTION ▍▍▍ | **Protein and Amino Acid Supplements** |

Why do people take protein supplements? Athletes take them to build muscle. Dieters take them to spare their bodies' protein while losing weight. Women take them to improve the strength of their fingernails. People take individual amino acids, too—to cure herpes, to make themselves sleep better, to relieve pain and depression. Do protein and amino acid supplements really do any of these things? Almost never. Are they safe? No.

Muscle work builds muscle; protein supplements do not, and athletes do not need them. Food energy spares body protein; fat and carbohydrate serve this purpose equally well, and carbohydrate is safer (see Chapter 10 for details). Fingernails remain unaffected by protein supplements, provided the diet is otherwise adequate in protein. This chapter demonstrates that no decent diet fails to supply enough protein, so protein supplements never are needed by the normal, healthy person.

Furthermore, protein supplements are expensive and less well digested than protein-rich food; and when used as a replacement for such food, they are often downright dangerous. The "liquid protein" diet, advocated some years ago for weight loss, caused death in many users, and even the physician-supervised protein-sparing modified fast (also based on liquid protein) can cause abnormal heart rhythms.

As for amino acid supplements, they, too, are unnecessary, and the body is not adapted to handle them. The body is designed to handle whole proteins best. It breaks them into manageable pieces (dipeptides and tripeptides), then splits these a few at a time, simultaneously absorbing them into the blood. When proteins are predigested in a laboratory and served up as mixtures of single amino acids, they are less well digested and absorbed because

continued on the next page

they overwhelm the absorptive mechanism and not all can be accommo-
dated. When amino acids are presented singly, severe imbalances and toxicities can occur. Groups of chemically similar amino acids compete for the
carriers that absorb them into the blood, and an excess of one can create such
demand for a carrier that it prevents the absorption of another. The result is
a deficiency. Many amino acids are toxic when taken in excess. In some cases
"excess" means not very much above normal daily intake levels.

In two cases recommendations for amino acids have led to widespread
public use—lysine to prevent or to relieve the infections that cause herpes
sores on the mouth or genital organs and tryptophan to relieve pain, depression, and insomnia. In both cases enthusiastic, popular reports and careful
scientific experiments are at odds. Lysine does not relieve or cure herpes
infections, and if long-term use helps prevent them, it does so only in some
individuals and with unknown associated risks. Tryptophan does have some
interesting effects with respect to pain and sleep in responsive individuals, as
Controversy 6 explains further, but people taking large doses may be damaging their livers. In fact, a blood disorder characterized by severe muscle
and joint pain, limb swelling, extremely high fever, and, in at least one case,
death has been linked to tryptophan supplements.* The Food and Drug
Administration (FDA) has requested a recall of tryptophan supplements, and
if you own a bottle of tryptophan pills, throw it out. It is safer to take amino
acids in protein foods with a little carbohydrate to facilitate their use—a
turkey sandwich, for example.

Many of the chapters of this book present evidence on purified nutrients
added to foods or taken singly. The Consumer Caution of Chapter 4 showed
that the enrichment of a nutritionally inferior food (refined bread) with four
added nutrients left it still deficient in many others. The Chapter 5 Consumer
Caution showed that an excess of lecithin provides no benefits and causes
side effects. With amino acids, the same thing is true. Even with all that we
know about science, it is hard to improve on nature.

Sources: R. A. Lantigua and coauthors, Cardiac arrhythmias associated with a liquid protein
diet for the treatment of obesity, *New England Journal of Medicine* 303 (1980): 735–738;
N. J. Benevenga and R. D. Steele, Adverse effects of excessive consumption of amino acids,
Annual Review of Nutrition 4 (1984): 157–181; Myth of the month: Lysine for herpes,
Nutrition and the MD, December 1984, p. 4; L. J. Fitten, J. Profita, and T. G. Bidder,
L-tryptophan as a hypnotic in special patients, *Journal of the American Geriatrics Society* 33
(1985): 294–297; M. E. Trulson and H. W. Sampson, Ultrastructural changes of the liver
following L-tryptophan ingestion, *Journal of Nutrition* 116 (1986): 1109–1115;
Eosinophilia-myalgia syndrome and L-tryptophan-containing products—New Mexico,
Minnesota, Oregon, and New York, 1989, *MMWR—Morbidity and Mortality Weekly Report*
38 (1989): 785–788.

Animal versus Vegetable Protein

Protein from animals is invariably accompanied by fat; that from land animals
by saturated fat mostly. Protein from plants is likely to have little lipid with it,
and that lipid is mostly oil. Scientists studying heart disease and cancer have
observed that people who ate large amounts of meat had higher disease rates
than people who ate large amounts of vegetables, and the difference has usually

*About 20,000 cases of tryptophan-induced eosinophilia-myalgia syndrome have been reported.

legumes (leg-GYOOMS, LEG-yooms): plants of the bean and pea family having roots with nodules that contain special bacteria. These bacteria can trap nitrogen from the air in the soil and make it into compounds that become part of the seed. The seeds are rich in high-quality protein compared with those of most other plant foods.

mutual supplementation: the strategy of combining two protein foods in a meal so that each food provides the essential amino acid(s) lacking in the other.

complementary proteins: two or more proteins whose amino acid assortments complement each other in such a way that the essential amino acids missing from each are supplied by the other.

▌▌▌ Figure 6–11

A Legume. The legumes are the seeds of such plants as the kidney bean, soybean, garden pea, lentil, black-eyed pea, and lima bean. Bacteria in the root nodules can "fix" nitrogen, contributing it to the beans. Ultimately, thanks to these bacteria, the plant leaves in the soil more nitrogen than it takes out. So efficient at trapping nitrogen are the legumes that farmers often grow them in rotation with other crops to fertilize fields. For a variety of legumes used in cooking, see photographs in Figure 2–6 of Chapter 2.

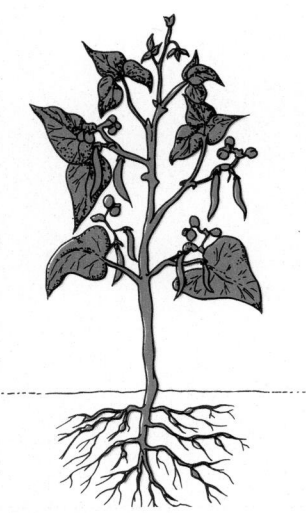

been attributed to the lipids in those diets. When the lipids are factored out, though, it becomes clear that independently of the accompanying lipids, animal and plant proteins may act on risk factors and associated diseases.

One difference observed experimentally is that diets containing purified proteins from animal sources raise blood cholesterol higher than do similar diets containing purified vegetable proteins. When fed diets based on purified animal protein for a long time, experimental animals are more prone to develop atherosclerosis than their vegetable-protein–fed counterparts.[14] It is suggested that people with high blood cholesterol can bring it down by altering the ratio of the animal-to-vegetable protein in their diets. The typical ratio is 2 to 1; the suggested altered ratio 1 to 1. In animals, the 1-to-1 ratio maintains blood cholesterol as low as a diet containing vegetable protein alone. For people with blood cholesterol in the lower ranges, though, no effect is seen, and some investigators believe that the type of dietary protein is of little significance in this regard.[15]

The question of whether animal or vegetable proteins, by themselves, raise or lower blood cholesterol may not be directly applicable to people's food choices, since people eat foods, not purified proteins. The purified proteins most often used in experiments that involve dietary protein and raised blood cholesterol are milk protein (casein) and soy protein. If the whole foods are used instead of the isolated proteins, the contrast is not seen. Milk *lowers* blood cholesterol just as soy does.

▌▌▶ *The use of diets high in animal protein may be associated with increased risks of heart disease.*

▌▌▌ Vegetarian Protein Choices

A person who eats animal products such as meat, milk, or eggs is more likely to consume too much protein than too little because these foods deliver abundant protein of high quality. Those who eat an all-plant diet might give some thought to their protein intakes because plant proteins—at least individually—are of lower quality, and they offer protein in less abundance. Notice in Table 6–3 that although meats provide protein in a concentrated form, other foods, including vegetables, can donate a surprising amount of their own protein to the diet. Especially protein-rich are the **legumes**. Figure 6–11 shows that their specially adapted root system enables them to produce abundant protein.

Vegans (see p. 39) have long known how to combine plant proteins to obtain a balanced assortment of essential amino acids. In this strategy, called **mutual supplementation**, the two protein-rich foods are combined to yield **complementary proteins**, that is, proteins containing all the essential amino acids in amounts sufficient to support health. Such combinations of foods are shown in Figure 6–12.

When researchers first studied human protein needs, they concluded that vegans could easily become protein deficient unless they balanced their amino acids gram for gram at every meal. Later research showed this investment of effort to be unnecessary, but the original dictate carried over for years. Researchers still agree that obtaining adequate amounts of all the essential amino acids is essential to life, but they now think that the timing is less critical. Evidence shows that the liver monitors the amino acid composition of protein

■■■ Table 6–3 Protein Sources and the Energy They Provide

Each of the following provides about 7 grams of protein:
  1 ounce lean meat, poultry, fish—about 55 calories

And so do these:
  ½ cup legumes— 80 calories
  1 cup egg noodles— 160 calories
  1 cup broccoli or Brussels sprouts— 50 calories
  7 ounces milk or yogurt— 80 calories
  1 ounce cheese[a]— 100 calories
  ¼ cup cottage cheese— 55 calories
  2 tablespoons peanut butter[a]— 200 calories
  1–2 ounces nuts or seeds[a]— 175 to 250 calories
  ¼ cup tofu— 75 calories

Each of these provides about 3 grams protein:
  1 slice bread— 80 calories
  ½ cup most cooked cereals and grains— 80 calories
  ⅓ cup cooked rice— 80 calories

And these provide about 2 grams protein each:
  ½ cup cooked vegetables— 25 calories
  1 cup raw vegetables— 25 calories

[a]These are high-fat choices.

Choose from two or more of these columns to obtain complete protein.[a]

GRAINS	LEGUMES	SEEDS AND NUTS	VEGETABLES
Barley	Dried beans	Sesame seeds	Leafy greens
Bulgur	Dried lentils	Sunflower seeds	Broccoli
Cornmeal	Dried peas	Walnuts	Others (see exchange lists)
Oats	Peanuts	Cashews	
Rice	Soy products	Other nuts	
Whole-grain		Nut butters	
breads			
Pasta			

■■■ Figure 6–12

Complimentary Protein Combinations

Create delicious meals such as these:

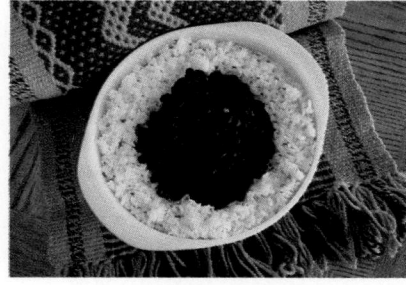

⅓ c black beans + ⅔ c rice
= 9 g complete protein

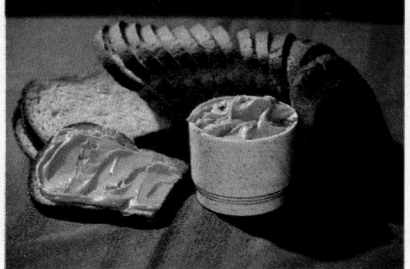

2 slices bread + 1 tbsp peanut butter
= 13 g complete protein

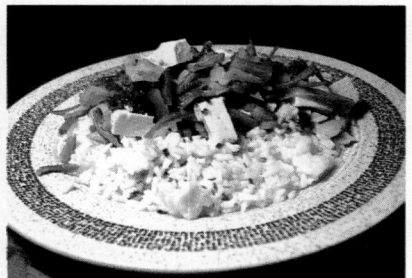

4 oz tofu + ½ c vegetables + ⅔ c rice
= 15 g complete protein

[a]Protein estimates from the Exchange System of Appendix D.

eaten at a meal, and if the meal is low in an essential amino acid, the liver breaks down its own proteins to supply it and then replenishes its protein to be ready for the next occasion. Thus if a protein source such as corn (low in tryptophan, but not in other amino acids) is eaten alone on occasion, the liver will donate extra amino acids, including tryptophan, thus allowing protein synthesis to continue temporarily. In a well-nourished person, protein functions continue normally, even if incomplete proteins are eaten alone on occasion.

In practice, the possibility of a protein deficiency from unbalanced amino acid consumption is remote. Only when fruits and certain vegetables define the core of the diet, severely limiting the *quantity and quality* of its protein, might protein deficiency result. Fruits provide adequate energy, but most are low in protein. Even advocates of a fruitarian diet include nuts and seeds regularly. The root vegetable cassava that people of many developing countries use daily contains adequate energy but inadequate protein. A steady diet of fruit or cassava would soon deplete the body's essential amino acid pool, and protein deficiency would ensue.

▌▌▶ *Almost any diet that provides a variety of nutrient-dense foods can provide enough protein. The body compensates for day-to-day variations in amino acid intakes.*

▐▐▐ **Food Feature**

Enough, But Not Too Much, Protein

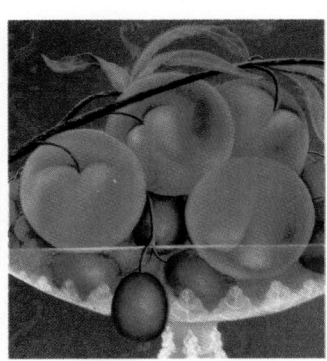

People who learn of the dire consequences of protein deficiency may, understandably, become concerned about their own intakes. For people in developed nations, however, that concern may be misdirected, for such people usually eat ample protein. The protein RDA is generous: it more than adequately covers the estimated needs of most people, even those with unusually high requirements.

The meat list is one of two lists of foods in the exchange system that contributes an abundance of high-quality protein; the milk list is the other. Two others—the vegetable and grain lists—contribute smaller amounts of proteins, but they can add up to significant quantities. The protein values assigned to each of the exchange lists permit you to estimate the protein content of foods (Figure 6–13).

To illustrate how easy it is to overconsume protein, assume that *your* protein RDA is 50 grams per day. This would divide easily into three meals: 10 grams at breakfast, 20 grams at lunch, and 20 grams at dinner. An egg, a slice of toast, and a glass of milk at breakfast would add up to 18 grams, almost double the allowance for that meal. At lunch a chef's salad with an egg, an ounce of ham, and an ounce of cheese accompanied by a roll would deliver 24 grams—and the greens would be additional. For supper, a 4-ounce piece of chicken, a potato, and vegetable would contribute 33 more. By the time you added more vegetables, the second milk serving, and two more bread/cereal servings as suggested by the Four Food Group Plan, you would have added about 20 grams more, exceeding your protein needs for the day by far. Finally, if you also included a cup of legumes, you would add over 10 grams more protein to your day's meals, for a total of more than 100 grams. No wonder most people get more than twice the protein they need.

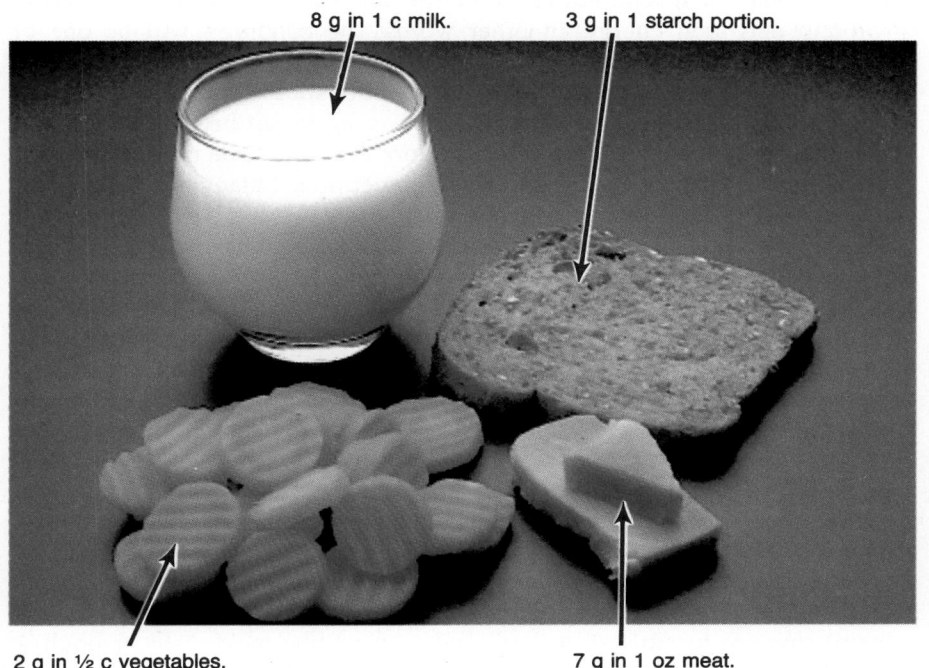

8 g in 1 c milk.

3 g in 1 starch portion.

2 g in ½ c vegetables.

7 g in 1 oz meat.

■■■ Figure 6–13

Protein in Foods.

ONE EXCHANGE	PROTEINS (g)
Milk (1 c)	8
Vegetable (½ c)	2
Fruit (1 portion)	0
Bread and starchy vegetable (1 slice or ½ c)	3
Sugar	0
Meat (1 oz)	7
Fat	0

Protein is critical in nutrition, but overemphasis on protein-rich foods in the diet can easily lead to nutrient imbalances. Protein-rich foods carry with them a characteristic array of vitamins and minerals, including vitamin B_{12} and iron. By the same token, they are notoriously lacking in others—vitamin C and folate, for example (more about these nutrients in the next two chapters). To overemphasize protein-rich foods, then, would be to ensure an overabundance of vitamin B_{12} and iron while shortchanging vitamin C and folate. In addition, many protein-rich foods such as meat are high in calories, and to overconsume them is to invite obesity.

In Figure 2–7 of Chapter 2, two days' meals were compared. They both contained the same amount of protein, but the meat-and-potatoes meals delivered far less carbohydrate, more fat, and a more limited variety of other nutrients than the other meals which included many more vegetables. The person eating such meals, which are typical of Western developed nations, cannot improve that diet by simply adding nutritious foods on top of it. If the person added milk, whole grains, or vegetables; the protein would far exceed the need. To keep from vastly overconsuming protein (and calories), the person must delete something, and the obvious "something" to delete is some of the meat.

Is it at all possible, then, that a person may have trouble meeting protein needs? Yes, if the person fails to consume adequate *food*, or if the person overemphasizes nonnutritious energy foods such as pure fats or sugars, or if the person drinks much alcohol. Also, someone who overemphasizes one group of foods, especially the fruits or even certain vegetables (cassava root, for example), at the expense of others could conceivably create a protein deficiency. More often, though, people who eat too few protein-rich foods will

textured vegetable protein: processed soybean protein used in product formulated to look and to taste like meat, fish, or poultry.

tofu (TOE-foo): a curd made from soybeans, rich in protein and often rich in calcium, used in many Asian and vegetarian dishes in place of meat.

suffer from *many* deficiencies—calcium, iron, and many of the vitamins as well as protein and food energy. In other words, the condition will be one of starvation.

Once you have the confidence that you will not short yourself with respect to protein, planning meatless or reduced-meat meals can become a pleasure. Many interesting, novel sources of protein are available. One class of protein-rich foods other than meats has already been mentioned many times: the plant family known as the legumes.

The protein of legumes is of a quality almost comparable to that of meat. Legumes are also excellent sources of fiber, many B vitamins, iron, calcium, and other minerals. A cup of cooked legumes contains 31 percent of the protein and 42 percent of the iron recommended daily for an adult male. Like meats, though, legumes do not offer every nutrient, and they do not make a complete meal by themselves. They contain no vitamin A, vitamin C, or vitamin B_{12}, and their balance of amino acids can be improved by using grains and other vegetables with them.

Soybeans are versatile legumes, and people make many products from them. However, the heavy use of soy products in place of meat severely inhibits iron absorption. The effect can be alleviated by using small amounts of meat and/or foods rich in vitamin C in the same meal with the soy products.[16] Vegetarians sometimes use convenience foods made from **textured vegetable protein** (soy protein) that are formulated to look and to taste like meat, fish, or poultry. Many of these are designed to match the known nutrient contents of animal-protein foods, but often they fall short. Instead of relying solely on these products, a wise vegetarian would learn to use combinations of whole foods as suggested earlier.

Another form in which the nutrients of soybeans are available is as bean curd, or **tofu**, a staple used in many Asian dishes. Thanks to the way some tofu is made, it can be high in calcium.

The key to getting enough but not too much protein seems to be to use a variety of foods in ample quantities, to de-emphasize meats, and to emphasize vegetables, grains, legumes, and nonfat milk and milk products. If you have followed the Food Features so far, you may now see that the recommendations for the three energy-yielding nutrients go hand in hand—if you reduce fat and increase carbohydrate, protein totals automatically come into line with the requirements. To estimate the amounts of protein in meals such as those shown here, assign each food to the appropriate exchange list, and note its protein value. (This is done in Figure 6–14 for the meals that were used as examples in Chapters 2, 4, and 5.) The fruits and fats can be assumed to contain no protein, so the only foods to inspect are the meats, milks, grains, starchy vegetables and breads, and vegetables. This method underestimates the protein in foods such as sunflower seeds (listed with fats and assigned no protein value) and peas and beans (listed with the breads for their high carbohydrate contents). Still, if you looked up every food in Appendix A, divided the amount you ate by the amount listed there, and then computed the actual protein grams in these meals, the total would come to 86 grams—a number very close to the 82.5 grams obtained much more conveniently with the exchange system. For macronutrients such as protein, a difference of just a few grams in the day's total is not significant, and the exchange system allows for a quick tally.

■■■ **Figure 6–14**

Estimating Protein Intake Using the Exchange System

	PROTEIN (GRAMS)

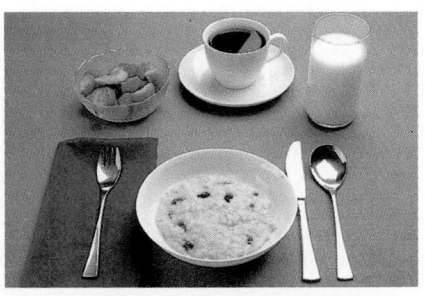

BREAKFAST

1 c oatmeal = 2 starch/grains	6
¼ c raisins = 2 fruits	—
1 c nonfat milk = 1 milk	8
1¼ c strawberries = 1 fruit	0

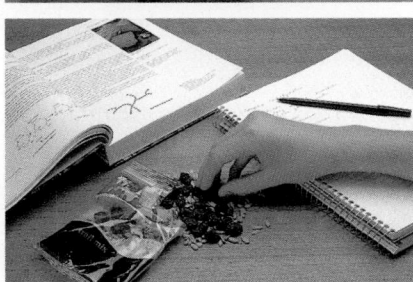

MORNING SNACK

2 tbsp raisins = 1 fruit	—
2 tbsp sunflower seeds = 2 fats	

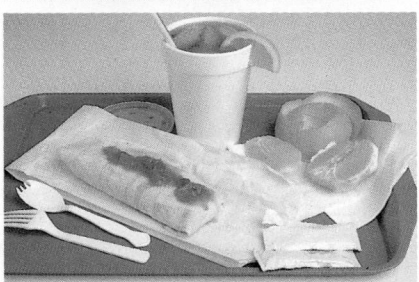

LUNCH

1 beef and bean burrito	6
(1 lg tortilla = 2 starch/grains	
⅓ c beans = 1 starch/grain	3
½ high-fat meat)	3½
1 packet sugar	—
1 orange = 1 fruit	—

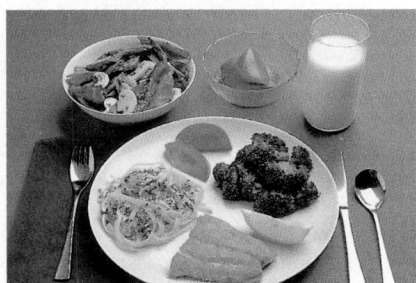

DINNER

4 oz broiled salmon = 4 lean meat	28
1 c broccoli = 2 vegetable	4
½ c noodles = 1 starch/grain	3
2 tsp butter = 2 fats	—
¼ c parsley = ¼ vegetable	
¼ tomato = ¼ vegetable	2
¼ c mushrooms = ¼ vegetable	
¼ c water chestnuts = ¼ vegetable	
1 c fresh spinach = 1 vegetable	2
1 tbsp sesame seeds = 1 fat	—
⅓ c garbanzo beans = 1 starch/grain	3
1 tbsp vinaigrette dressing = 1 fat	—
1 c nonfat milk = 1 milk	8
½ c sherbet = 2 starch/grains	6
Day's totals	82.5g

A total of 82.5 grams of protein times 4 calories per gram is 330 calories from protein, about 19 percent of the day's total 1750 calories. This 82.5 grams is well above most people's RDA for protein but is not more than double that amount, and so meets the National Research Council (NRC) recommendation to hold protein to less than twice the RDA.

▌▌▌ SELF-STUDY

Evaluate Your Protein Intake.

For this exercise, refer to the information you previously recorded on Forms 1 to 4 in Appendix F.

1. How many grams of protein do you consume on an average day (Form 2)?
2. How many calories does this represent (Form 4)? Remember, 1 gram of protein contributes 4 calories.
3. What percentage of your total energy is contributed by protein? You calculated this earlier, using Form 4.
4. One source suggests that protein should contribute about 10 to 15 percent of total energy.† How does your protein intake compare with this recommendation? (Note: If you are on a calorie-restricted diet, then a higher percentage of your calories should come from protein. See the Self-Study

for Chapter 9.) If your protein intake is out of line, what foods could you consume more of—or less of—to bring it into line?
5. Calculate your protein RDA (see p. 170). Is it similar to the RDA for the "average" person of your age and sex, as shown in the RDA tables (inside front cover)?
6. Compare your average daily protein intake with your RDA. On the average, about what percentage of your RDA for protein are you consuming each day? If you are healthy, the RDA is probably a generous recommendation for you, and yet you may be eating more than that amount. The NRC recommendations of Chapter 2 suggest that you eat no more than twice your RDA of protein. If you are eating more than this, you are—

spending protein prices for an energy-yielding nutrient and are displacing other important foods with too many protein-rich foods. What substitutions could you make in your day's food choices so that you would derive from carbohydrate, rather than from protein, the energy you need?
7. How many of your protein grams are from animal, and how many from plant foods? Assuming that the animal protein is all of high quality, no more than 20 percent of your total protein need come from this source. Should you alter the ratio of plant to animal protein in your diet? If you did, what effect would this have on the total *fat* content of your diet?

†The source is the U.S. *Dietary Goals*.

Notes

1. S. A. Laidlaw, Indispensable amino acids, *Nutrition and the MD*, August 1986, pp. 1–3; K. C. Hayes, Taurine requirements in primates, *Nutrition Reviews* 43 (1985): 65–70.
2. W. J. Visek, Arginine needs, physiological state and usual diets: A reevaluation, *Journal of Nutrition* 116 (1986): 36–46.
3. G. E. Mortimore and A. R. Pösö, Intracellular protein catabolism and its control during nutrient deprivation and supply, *Annual Reviews of Nutrition* 7 (1987): 539–564.
4. M. L. G. Gardner, Gastrointestinal absorption of intact proteins, *Annual Reviews of Nutrition* 8 (1988): 329–350.
5. J. B. Coulter and coauthors, Aflatoxins in liver biopsies from Sudanese children, *American Journal of Tropical Medicine and Hygiene* 35 (1986): 360–365.
6. K. K. Carroll, Dietary protein and heart disease, *Nutrition and the MD*, June 1986, p. 1.
7. A. R. Sherman, L. Helyar, and I. Wolinsky, Effects of dietary protein concentration on trace minerals in rat tissues at different ages, *Journal of Nutrition* 115 (1985): 607–614.
8. H. H. Sandstead, Zinc: Essentiality for brain development and function, *Nutrition Today*, November/December 1984, pp. 26–30; B. Worthington-Roberts, Nutrition and maternal health, *Nutrition Today*, November/December 1984, pp. 6–19.
9. E. Pollitt and N. Lewis, Nutritional and educational achievement, *Food and Nutrition Bulletin* 2 (1980): 33–37, as cited by C. G. Neumann and E. F. P. Jelliffe, Effects of infant feeding,

Chapter 44, pp. 529–574 in E. F. P. Jelliffe and D. B. Jelliffe, eds., *Adverse Effects of Foods* (New York: Plenum Press, 1982), p. 549.
10. R. B. Alfin-Slater, Vitamin B₆ and coronary heart disease, *Nutrition and the MD*, March 1983, p. 4.
11. Dietary protein and body fat distribution, *Nutrition Reviews* 40 (1982): 89–90.
12. M. G. Holl and L. H. Allen, Comparative effects of meals high in protein, sucrose, or starch on human mineral metabolism and insulin secretion, *American Journal of Clinical Nutrition* 48 (1988): 1219–1225; M. B. Zemel, Calcium utilization: Effect of varying level and source of dietary protein, *American Journal of Clinical Nutrition* 48 (1988): 880–883.
13. H. Spencer, L. Kramer, and D. Osis, Do protein and phosphorous cause calcium loss? *Journal of Nutrition* 118 (1988): 657–660.
14. Carroll, 1986.
15. S. M. Grundy and J. J. Abrams, Comparison of actions of soy protein and casein on metabolism of plasma lipoproteins and cholesterol in humans, *American Journal of Clinical Nutrition* 38 (1983): 245–252; A. C. Beynen and coauthors, Dietary soybean protein and serum cholesterol, *American Journal of Clinical Nutrition* 39 (1984): 840–841.
16. Soyfoods and iron bioavailability, *Nutrition and the MD*, March 1983, pp. 4–5.

Food, Mood, and Time of Day

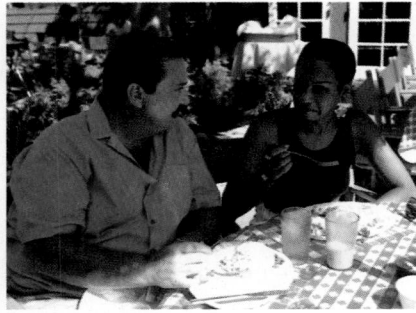

Why do you feel like eating a steak at one meal and a donut at another? Why do you feel sleepy after lunch and not after dinner? Why does depression cause some people to eat more and others less than they usually do? Or, putting these questions in general terms, does what you eat affect your mood? Does your mood affect what you eat? Researchers no longer doubt that food affects mood and the reverse, and they are beginning to understand how and why. Investigations into the effects have been more and more intense recently, and their focus is, of course, the brain.

The brain has its own survival at stake in directing the body when and what to eat. It is encased in the skull, a hard, inelastic helmet, for its own protection and so cannot expand and contract as can, say, the liver or adipose tissue. It cannot store its own reserve energy supply in glycogen, fat, or other molecules because those molecules take up space, and it cannot store oxygen with which to oxidize those fuels. Therefore the brain must depend on the passing blood supply for its oxygen and fuels. Furthermore, its needs for those substances are extraordinary. It comprises only 2 percent of the adult's body weight, but at any given time the brain contains 15 percent of the body's blood, and it devours 20 to 30 percent of the fuels that support the basal metabolism. Its rapid metabolism makes its temperature a degree higher than that of the rest of the body. Should the blood deliver too little oxygen or glucose, coma would occur within minutes; should the blood supply be interrupted altogether, coma would ensue within 10 seconds.[1] The brain also depends on the blood supply for amino acids from which it makes its messenger molecules; for electrically charged minerals that it uses to transmit its electrical impulses; for vitamins and other minerals to facilitate these processes; for lipids to repair its cell membranes; and for water. Figure C6–1 shows how one cell within the brain communicates with another.

The brain is also extremely sensitive to fluctuations in its internal chemical composition. To protect itself from them, it has its own molecular sieve through which the blood must pass. The blood vessels that feed the brain differ from those that feed other organs in that they are lined with highly selective cells. These cells form a barrier known as the **blood-brain barrier**, which allows desired constituents to enter the brain tissue while restricting others. Whereas the environment outside the body may fluctuate widely in temperature, humidity, and chemical composition, the blood changes only a little, and the brain's internal milieu hardly fluctuates at all.

Because of its dependence on the blood supply, the brain continuously monitors it and sends messages to other organs when it needs their help in regulating it. At one time the brain may need glucose; at another, protein. Should body stores be inadequate to supply the amounts needed, indications are that the brain may be able to direct eating to obtain carbohydrate at one time and protein at another, depending on its needs. It is known that animals regulate the proportions of protein and carbohydrate that they consume. A possible explanation of how people may do so comes largely from research using animals and is presented here as an example of research into the connections between brain chemistry and food choices.

One of the ways the brain may be able to tell whether it needs carbohydrate or protein is by the amounts of **monoamines**—a type of **neurotransmitter**—available for its use. The monoamines are made in the nerve cells from single amino acids by modifying them slightly.

The monoamines are an exception to the rule that the brain's internal chemistry hardly fluctuates at all. The amino acid building blocks

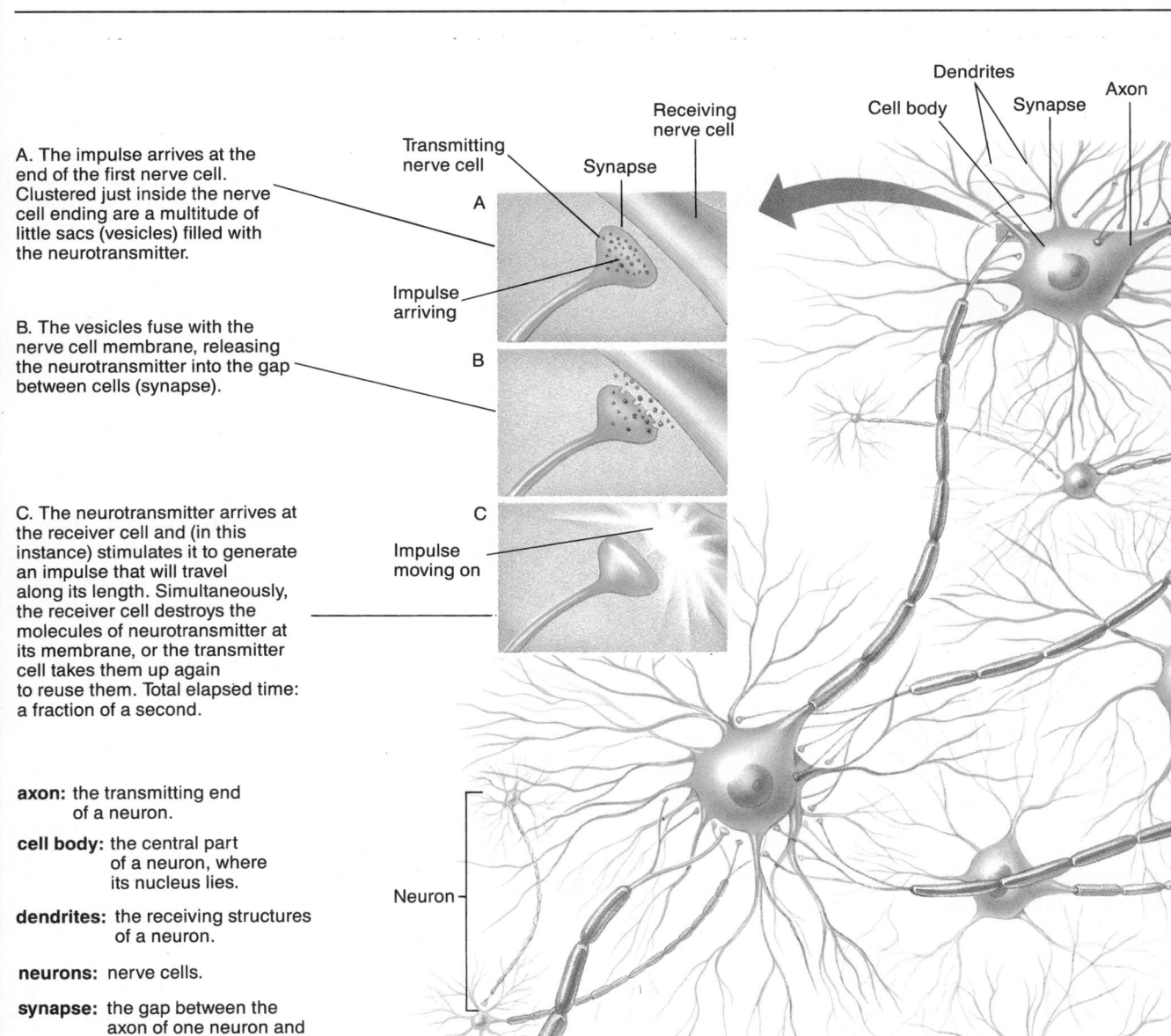

A. The impulse arrives at the end of the first nerve cell. Clustered just inside the nerve cell ending are a multitude of little sacs (vesicles) filled with the neurotransmitter.

B. The vesicles fuse with the nerve cell membrane, releasing the neurotransmitter into the gap between cells (synapse).

C. The neurotransmitter arrives at the receiver cell and (in this instance) stimulates it to generate an impulse that will travel along its length. Simultaneously, the receiver cell destroys the molecules of neurotransmitter at its membrane, or the transmitter cell takes them up again to reuse them. Total elapsed time: a fraction of a second.

Transmitting nerve cell

Receiving nerve cell

Synapse

Impulse arriving

Impulse moving on

Dendrites

Cell body

Synapse

Axon

Neuron

axon: the transmitting end of a neuron.

cell body: the central part of a neuron, where its nucleus lies.

dendrites: the receiving structures of a neuron.

neurons: nerve cells.

synapse: the gap between the axon of one neuron and the dendrites of the next.

■■■ Figure C6–1

Communication within the Brain. The mature human brain is composed of about 10 billion nerve cells, or **neurons**, which communicate with one another using a combination of electrical and chemical signals.[a] Each neuron is a long, slim cell with receiving structures (**dendrites**) at one end; a transmitting structure (the **axon**) at the other; and a bulge, the **cell body**, between. Electrical impulses arise in the dendrites, pass through the cell body, and continue down the axon to its terminal. At the point where the terminal makes contact with the next nerve, it bulges slightly; many such bulges are shown in this figure, and one is enlarged.

The electrical impulses that travel along nerve cells can, in some cases, jump unaided across the gap (called a **synapse**) from one cell to the next, but in most cases the gap between cells prevents electrical transmission. Communication across synapses usually requires the release of a chemical substance, or neurotransmitter, which flows across the gap. The first nerve cell (the one sending the impulse) releases a quantity of these molecules, and they diffuse across the synapse to reach the second (receiving) nerve cell. On arrival, they may make the receiving nerve cell either *more* or *less* likely to fire. Thus a neurotransmitter can either *stimulate* or *inhibit* the postsynaptic nerve. If it stimulates it and the nerve fires, then an electrical impulse starts up and travels along the nerve to the other end, the next synapse. Thus messages are carried along nerves by electrical impulses and from one nerve to the next by chemical compounds until they result in action (storage or integration of information, or contraction of a muscle) or die away.

A nerve cell "decides" to fire based on inputs from all the other cells in contact with it. If the amount of stimulation relative to the amount of inhibition is great enough to initiate an impulse, then the nerve cell will fire.

[a]The brain's billions of neurons are surrounded by many more billions of supporting cells, known as *glial cells,* whose purpose is to provide for the needs of the neurons.

(precursors) from which they are made, unlike most molecules, are able to penetrate the blood-brain barrier and do so in quantities that depend on their concentrations in the bloodstream. Thus the food a person eats can influence the brain chemistry by producing high or low concentrations of the precursor nutrients in an available form. Furthermore, once in the brain, these precursor nutrients exert **precursor control**, that is, the nerve cells respond to a larger or smaller supply of building blocks by making larger or smaller amounts of monoamines from them. These facts link eating directly to brain chemistry and, as you will see in a moment, to mood and other sensations.

One monoamine whose brain concentration is especially sensitive to changes in precursor supply has been studied in depth: **serotonin**, made from its precursor, the amino acid tryptophan (see Figure C6–2).

Ordinary meals of the kind people eat every day raise or lower the concentration of serotonin in the brain, depending on the meal's protein and carbohydrate content. Serotonin concentration in turn affects sensations and mood, so the ingredients of meals have real effects on how people feel afterwards. A lack of tryptophan flowing into the brain can manifest itself in wakefulness and enhanced sensitivity to pain. Animals that have been made tryptophan deficient have a lowered threshold for pain; when they are given a single injection of tryptophan, their pain threshold becomes normal as their brain serotonin level is restored.[2]

The amount of tryptophan that enters the brain does not depend only on the amount the person eats but also on the total amounts of protein *and carbohydrate* the person eats. If tryptophan is eaten by itself, as a single amino acid, then its concentration in the blood rises, it flows into the brain, and brain serotonin increases proportionately. But normally, whole proteins containing tryptophan are eaten. In this case some of the other large amino acids in the proteins compete with tryptophan for entry into the brain because they use the same transport mechanism to get across the blood-brain barrier.* In this situation tryptophan fails to enter the brain in increased quantities and so does not effectively enhance brain serotonin

*The amino acids that share this transport system are tyrosine, phenylalanine, leucine, isoleucine, and valine. These amino acids also compete for absorption in the digestive tract.

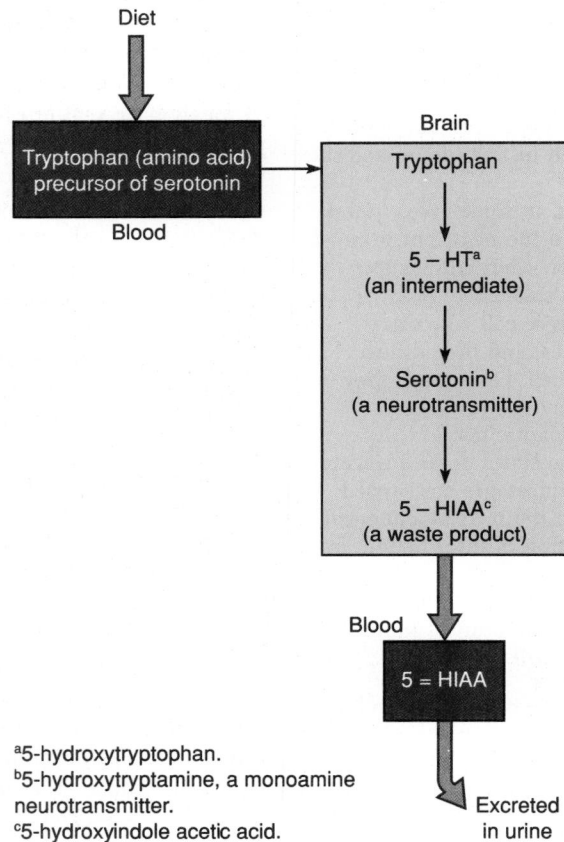

■■■ Figure C6–2

Serotonin Synthesis in the Brain.

[a]5-hydroxytryptophan.
[b]5-hydroxytryptamine, a monoamine neurotransmitter.
[c]5-hydroxyindole acetic acid.

synthesis. If carbohydrate is fed along with protein, however, it can "help" the protein to deliver tryptophan to the brain because it elicits the secretion of the hormone insulin. Insulin drives the other amino acids, but not tryptophan, into body cells, leaving the tryptophan free to enter the brain without competition. Thus, paradoxically, a meal high in carbohydrate, but not one high in protein, eases tryptophan's transport into the brain and so promotes serotonin synthesis. It is not the total amount of tryptophan, then, but the amount relative to the competing amino acids that affects the brain's serotonin level.

These facts may help explain how animals and human beings may know which kind of diet they have eaten last and what to eat next time. According to one theory, a high-carbohydrate meal raises their brain serotonin, makes them feel good, and so reduces their need for carbohydrate. They therefore eat more protein at the next meal. A high-protein meal creates a serotonin deficit, a loss of the good feeling, and therefore a craving for carbohydrate.[3]

One of the chief appeals of this theory is that it seems to account for what is observed to happen often with weight-control diets. The harder dieters try to restrict carbohydrate the more they seem to crave it. The effect is accentuated if they are insulin resistant, as is likely if they are obese. When an insulin-resistant person eats carbohydrate, insulin's normal actions do not follow. The person's cells continue to be hungry for glucose; furthermore, brain serotonin does not rise, and so the carbohydrate craving is intensified.

The theory also helps explain why some people describe themselves as anxious, tense, and depressed before eating carbohydrate and peaceful or relaxed afterward. The amino acid tryptophan given by itself has similar effects, consistent with the notion that it is the agent of carbohydrate's effect. This doesn't mean people should dose themselves with tryptophan, of course. The last chapter warned that to do so is to imperil your health. Besides, tryptophan occurs in virtually all proteins, so all you need is a balanced assortment of amino acids from protein. An excess of any one could cause deficiencies of others, with consequent upsets of mood and much worse. The Consumer Caution on pages 174–175 gave many reasons why amino acid supplements are a poor choice.

Not all the evidence supports the theory that links serotonin to the appetite for carbohydrate. For example, under some circumstances when animals eat tryptophan, they then eat *less* protein. This cannot be explained by changes in blood tryptophan, brain tryptophan, or brain serotonin levels.[4] Ongoing research should ultimately help to untangle this problem, but chances are that it will become more knotty before it becomes less so. Other hormones are probably involved. For example, carbohydrate and protein intakes affect not only insulin secretion but also the secretion of insulin's opposing hormone, glucagon, and glucagon influences the synthesis of neurotransmitters too.[5] Other hormones that affect the brain—or that are synthesized inside the brain—after eating include cholecystokinin (the messenger that, outside the brain, communicates the arrival of fat to the gallbladder and pancreas) and calcitonin (a hormone that responds to the blood calcium level).

Carbohydrate or tryptophan can also induce fatigue or sleepiness. The effect of tryptophan in inducing sleep is particularly well known; 43 studies have now demonstrated it in people and animals.[6] Carbohydrate or tryptophan can also reduce sensitivity to mild pain and (in people over 40 years) increase the error rate in performance tests.[7] Brain serotonin may reduce aggression too.[8]

Other avenues of investigation into such effects are also interesting, although many are just opening up and offer no more than tantalizing bits of information. For example, men and women may react differently to carbohydrates. A high-carbohydrate meal makes women sleepier and men calmer. Sugar, especially, makes women sleepy.[9] Perhaps this is because women secrete more estrogen hormones than men. Estrogens can reduce serotonin synthesis in the brain, may favor a higher ratio of blood tryptophan to its competing amino acids, and may increase the number of serotonin receptors in the brain.[10] The monthly fluctuation of estrogen secretion may make women react differently to carbohydrate at different times of the month—women's appetites for carbohydrate are keener during the ten days prior to menstruation than during the ten days after. Chapter 13 gives more details about the effects of menstruation on appetite.

The time of day also modulates these reactions: a high-starch meal eaten for breakfast has less effect than the same meal eaten at lunch.[11] Time-of-day effects like this influence both mood and eating behavior in many ways, as the next section shows.

■■■ Time of Day, Mood, and Eating Behavior

Whenever researchers have tried to study the effects of meals on how people feel, they have had to contend with a multitude of complications. How a meal affects a person seems to depend not only on the time of day, the composition of the meal, and the sex of the person, but on the time of the *year*, the composition of the *last* meal, and on other aspects of the nature of the person.[12] What all this means, practically speaking, is that when a person claims that particular kinds of meals typically affect him or her in ways quite unlike the listener's experience, the claims may well be valid.

Time-of-day effects seem to have a lot to do with our evolutionary history. The postlunch dip that many people experience, for example, seems to be a consequence of the need our ancestors had to rest during the hot tropical noontime. It happens when the temperature is high and rising, and it happens regardless of exactly what time a person eats lunch, though the effect is greater the more carbohydrate the person eats.[13] Many other things vary with a daily rhythm:

- ■ Sleep and wakefulness.
- ■ Cognitive and motor performance.
- ■ Body temperature.
- ■ Blood hormone (including sex hormone) levels.
- ■ Volume and composition of urine excreted.
- ■ Susceptibility to medicines, other drugs, and toxic agents.
- ■ Many nerve activities—photoreception, excitability, receptor sensitivities.[14]

The question of how these daily rhythms work has fascinated researchers for years, and their investigations have led to the conclusions reported here.

Naturally, because we live in a world in which day and night alternate on a regular 24-hour cycle, human beings do many things at intervals timed accordingly—a person typically sleeps at night, wakes in the morning, eats, performs tasks efficiently until after lunch, becomes sleepy and perhaps naps, performs efficiently again late in the day, eats again, and later sleeps. It used to be thought that sunlight and darkness were responsible for our cyclic behaviors, but it has now been found that the brain operates on such a cycle anyway. Kept in isolation, away from the light-dark cycle for weeks, both human beings and animals continue to perform these activities with a periodicity of about 25 (not 24) hours. The cycle, called **circadian rhythm** (*circa die* means "about a day"), is thus built in, and its basis in the brain is a sort of timer device that has been named the **biological clock**. The location of the clock has even been pinpointed. It is in a part of the hypothalamus connected to the retina of the eye. This location permits the eye to synchronize the internal clock with the day-night cycle. Since the earth's clock is faster, it normally overrides the person's clock, but if for any reason the person does not perceive the external day, the approximate rhythm will still be maintained. Influences other than light can also change the internal clock's setting, particularly temperature and, in human beings, social cues.[15]

The nerves of the clock manufacture a monoamine, **norepinephrine**, in small quantities during the day and in large quantities at night. One of the centers with which they communicate is the **pineal gland**, a small gland in the brain that resembles the retina of the eye. (The Greeks named it the "third eye" when they first discovered it, and they thought it to be the seat of the soul.) When the pineal gland experiences the surge in norepinephrine level that occurs at night, it responds by intensifying its secretion of a hormone of its own, **melatonin**, which it makes from serotonin—almost all of it at night.[16] Melatonin, in turn, affects (among many things) the synthesis of a neurotransmitter, **dopamine**, that regulates (among many things) the ability to pay attention.

The chemistry and behavior of the brain at night are therefore different from its chemistry and behavior by day. Normally people sleep at night. If they are awake, they are sleepy and subdued. If deprived of sleep for long (**insomnia**), they may become emotionally disturbed. Should the clock itself be abnormal, as it is in some people, they manifest sleep disorders, many abnormalities of hormone synthesis, and mental disorders.[17]

The body's chemistry is also different at different times of day, as is evident from its responses to drugs. Tumors are much more sensitive to anticancer drugs at certain times of day than at others, so the schedules on which the drugs are administered are adjusted accordingly.[18]

A phenomenon familiar to everyone connected to daily rhythms is **jet lag**. It occurs when rapid travel across time zones suddenly forces people to reset their biological clocks by more than an hour or two. In reaction, people may feel dazed, become unable to concentrate, have trouble sleeping, and feel physically and emotionally depressed.

People who must travel frequently can learn some tricks to help reset their bodies' clocks and to prevent the worst of the jet lag effect. For example, a man who must fly from New York to California can start to adjust a few days before the trip by forcing himself to stay up late, wake up late, and eat late according to New York standards. On arrival in California, he'll function easily on the new schedule. Of course, he goes through the same amount of disruption, but by making the adjustment before his trip, his first few days in California are more pleasant, and he can think and work much more efficiently than he would otherwise. Alternatively, such a traveler can plan to arrive a day early and use that day to adjust without work pressure.

Depressed mood is linked in many other ways to eating behavior and time of day. In general, mood is depressed when people are hungry, as it is when they lack sleep or have to work too hard for too long. People's performance under such conditions deteriorates.[19] Many more specific connections also exist between depression, nutrition, and time. For example, some people have an abnormal way of sleeping, awaken several times a night, and invariably go and eat.[20] In other people, when severe depression occurs it disturbs both their diets and their sleep patterns.[21]

Psychiatrists studying such connections describe the relationship between depression and eating behavior as "robust."[22] It is particularly strongly manifested in connection with the eating disorders, anorexia nervosa, bulimia, and obesity. Again, there are connections to the mood-regulating neurotransmitter serotonin. Even after recovery, people with bulimia have lower than normal levels of the serotonin product 5-HIAA† (see Figure C6–2 on page 186) in their brains. Certain subgroups of depressed people also have low 5-HIAA. It is believed that in people with bulimia, this may impair their ability to experience satiety after eating a reasonable amount of food. Depression, in fact, is an invariable accompaniment to bulimia, and altered serotonin synthesis "may be of major significance in mediating the prominent clinical symptoms in bulimia."[23] This possibility is revisited in Controversy 9.

Another type of depression, known as major depression, affects the appetite in the opposite way and causes weight loss. Still another connection of eating behavior with depression is seasonal; it is sometimes called winter depression, or

†5-hydroxyindole acetic acid

■■■ Table C6–1 The Mental Symptoms of Anemia[a]

Lack of appetite
Apathy, listlessness
Clumsiness
Behavior disturbances
Shortened attention span
Hyperactivity
Irritability
Learning disorders (vocabulary, perception)
Lowered IQ
Low scores on latency and associative reactions
Reduced physical work capacity
Repetitive hand and foot movements

[a]These symptoms are not caused by anemia itself but by iron deficiency in the brain. Children with much more severe anemias from other causes, such as sickle-cell anemia and thalassemia, show no reduction in IQ when compared with children without anemia.

SOURCE: E. N. Whitney and L. K. DeBruyne, *Nutrition and Behavior,* a monograph (1987) available from Stickley Publishing Company, 210 W. Washington Sq., Philadelphia, PA 19106, with permission.

more clinically, seasonal affective disorder (SAD). Most people who have it have increased appetites, mostly for carbohydrate.[24]

■■■ Vitamins, Trace Minerals, and the Brain

The discussion thus far has suggested that only the energy-yielding nutrients, particularly carbohydrate and protein, affect neurotransmitter synthesis and mood. However, in the synthesis of neurotransmitters—whether norepinephrine, dopamine, or serotonin—other nutrients are involved. Iron is needed in one of the first steps. Vitamin B_6 and riboflavin are needed in later steps. These nutrients are but three among many; deficiencies of them are reflected in depressed or otherwise

disturbed mood.[25] Many of them cause anemia, which produces mental symptoms of its own (see Table C6–1):

■ Protein-energy deficiency causes apathy, fretfulness, lack of energy, and lack of interest in food.

■ Thiamin deficiency causes confusion, uncoordinated movements, depressed appetite, irritability, insomnia, fatigue, personality changes, and depression.[26]

■ Riboflavin deficiency causes depression, hysteria, psychopathic behavior, lethargy, and hypochondria evident before clinical deficiency is detected.[27]

■ Niacin deficiency causes irritability, agitated depression, headaches, sleeplessness, memory loss, emotional instability (early signs of pellagra onset), and mental confusion

▰▰▰ Miniglossary

biological clock: the structure within the brain that governs an organism's circadian rhythm, known to reside within the hypothalamus.

blood-brain barrier: a barrier composed of the cells lining the blood vessels in the brain, which are so tightly glued to each other that substances can only get through the lining by crossing the cell bodies themselves. Thus the cells can use all their sophisticated equipment and be highly selective in permitting entry.

circadian rhythm: the cyclic rhythm of about 24 to 25 hours in duration that many body functions (such as temperature and blood pressure) follow.

dopamine: a neurotransmitter derived from melatonin that (among other things) regulates ability to pay attention.

insomnia: inability to sleep, sleep disruption.

jet lag: disruption of a person's normal circadian rhythm, caused by rapid (jet) travel from one time zone to another.

melatonin: a hormone derived from serotonin that acts on the ovaries, produced by the pineal gland mostly at night.

monoamines: derivatives of single amino acids that, in the brain, serve as neurotransmitters.

neurotransmitter: a substance that is released at the end of one nerve cell when a nerve impulse arrives there, diffuses across the gap to the next nerve cell, and alters the membrane of that cell in such a way that it becomes either less or more likely to fire (or does fire).

norepinephrine: a compound related in structure to (and made from) the amino acid tyrosine. When secreted by the adrenal gland, it acts as a hormone; when secreted at the ends of nerve cells, it acts as a neurotransmitter.

pineal (pine-EE-ul) gland: a small gland within the brain that produces melatonin.

precursor control: control of a compound's synthesis by the availability of that compound's precursor. (The more precursor there is, the more of the compound is made.)

serotonin: A compound related in structure to (and made from) the amino acid tryptophan; it serves as one of the brain's principal neurotransmitters.

progressing to psychosis or delirium.

■ Vitamin B_6 deficiency causes irritability, insomnia, weakness, depression, abnormal brainwave patterns, convulsions, the mental symptoms of anemia (Table C6-1), fatigue, and headaches.[28]

■ Folacin deficiency causes the mental symptoms of anemia (Table C6-1), tiredness, apathy, weakness, forgetfulness, mild depression, abnormal nerve function, irritability, headache, disorientation, confusion, and inability to perform simple calculations.[29]

■ Vitamin B_{12} deficiency causes degeneration of the peripheral nervous system and anemia.

■ Vitamin C deficiency causes hysteria, depression, listlessness, lassitude, weakness, an aversion to work, hypochondria, social introversion, possible anemia, and fatigue.

■ Vitamin A deficiency causes anemia.

■ Iron deficiency causes fatigue, weakness, headaches, pallor, listlessness, irritability, and the mental symptoms of anemia (Table C6-1).

■ Magnesium deficiency causes apathy, personality changes, and hyper-irritability.

■ Copper deficiency causes iron-deficiency anemia.

■ Zinc deficiency causes poor appetite, failure to grow, iron-deficiency anemia, irritability, emotional disorders, and mental lethargy.[30]

Nutrients affect brain function in many other ways, but this list should suffice to show how dramatically the way people eat can affect how they feel. Apparently the saying "You are what you eat" is true not only physically but also emotionally.

▰▰▰ Food and Learning

One of the most important things the brain does is learn. Until recently it has not been known that food had anything to do with learning other than the obvious things—that nutrient deficiencies or low blood glucose impair the brain's function in general, including its ability to learn. Now, however, some specific connections are appearing between eating and remembering. For example, hungry mice, fed immediately after learning a task, later remember how to perform that task better than do mice fed before the learning session or after a lag time. In terms of evolution, this makes sense: if an animal learns a new trick and it leads to food, the trick is worth remembering; it has survival value.[31]

How does food facilitate remembering? The details are not yet known, but it is known that the digestive hormone cholecystokinin is involved. The hormone apparently activates memory by stimulating nerve fibers that lead from the stomach to the brain.[32] It is also known that polyunsaturated fat enables animals to learn better than does saturated fat.[33] On the other hand, neither the now-familiar neurotransmitter precursor tryptophan nor sugar seems to affect factors associated with learning, such as vigilance or memory.[34] Chapter 5 mentioned that in specific brain disorders, choline compounds may be beneficial.

Snacking habits may also play a role in the mind's ability to pay attention. A recent study of college-age men found that subjects given energy-rich afternoon snacks were able to learn better and work faster than those given just noncaloric soft drinks.[35] Sweet confections and fla-vored yogurt were equally effective in improving both the ability to remember newly learned information and in performing mathematical computations. Many people experience a slump in attention in the hours after noon, and if you are one of them, you may want to try eating an afternoon snack. Just be sure to plan your snack so that it contributes nutrients and not too much fat, and that you adjust the energy in the day's other meals to avoid gaining weight.

Another factor that affects vigilance, of course, is caffeine. Students often use coffee or cola beverages, or wake-up pills to prolong their attention spans. The wake-up effect probably works through prolonging the action of the neurotransmitter epinephrine.[36] No harm results from moderate use of caffeine-containing beverages, but excessive use or use of wake-up pills, like excess stress, is harmful physiologically.

Research into the roles of nutrients in the brain is relatively new but has branched out into many lines of investigation. The more investigators learn, the more they want to find out because so much territory remains to be explored. It is hoped that research into these areas will continue to be supported, not only because they are of interest but also because they have great potential for enhancing human life.

Notes

1. M. B. Krassner, Diet and brain function, *Nutrition Reviews/Supplement*, May 1986, pp. 12–15.
2. J. D. Fernstrom, Effects of the diet on brain neurotransmitters, *Metabolism* 26 (1977): 207–223; S. H. Zeisel and J. H. Growdon, Diet and brain neurotransmitters, *Nutrition and the MD*, April 1980.
3. J. D. Fernstrom, Acute and chronic effects of protein and carbohydrate ingestion on brain tryptophan levels and serotonin synthesis, *Nutrition Reviews/Supplement*, May 1986, pp. 25–36.
4. Fernstrom, 1986.
5. W. M. Lovenberg, Biochemical regulation of brain function, *Nutrition Reviews/Supplement*, May 1986, pp. 6–11.
6. E. L. Hartmann, Effect of L-tryptophan and other amino acids on sleep, *Nutrition Reviews/Supplement*, May 1986, pp. 70–73.
7. R. J. Wurtman, Ways that foods can affect the brain, *Nutrition Reviews/Supplement*, May 1986, pp. 2–6.
8. S. N. Young, The effect on aggression and mood of altering tryptophan levels, *Nutrition Reviews/Supplement*, May 1986, pp. 112–122.
9. E. E. A. Pivonka and K. K. Grunewald, Aspartame- or sugar-sweetened beverages: Effects on mood in young women, *Journal of the American Dietetic Association* 90 (1990): 250–254.
10. B. J. Spring and coauthors, Effects of carbohydrates on mood and behavior, *Nutrition Reviews/Supplement*, May 1986, pp. 51–60.
11. Spring, 1986.
12. A. Craig, Acute effects of meals on perceptual and cognitive efficiency, *Nutrition Reviews/Supplement*, May 1986, pp. 163–171.

13. M. J. Thompson and D. W. Harsha, Our rhythms still follow the African sun, *Psychology Today*, January 1984, pp. 50–54.

14. J. S. Takahashi and M. Zatz, Regulation of circadian rhythmicity, *Science* 217 (1982): 1104–1110.

15. Takahashi and Zatz, 1982.

16. Takahashi and Zatz, 1982.

17. M. C. Moore-Ede, C. A. Czeisler, and G. S. Richardson, Circadian timekeeping in health and disease, *New England Journal of Medicine* 309 (1983): 469–476; 530–536.

18. W. Hrushesky, physician, University of Minnesota, as cited in Chemotherapy goes circadian, *American Health*, June 1986, pp. 10, 12.

19. Spring, 1986.

20. I. Oswald and K. Adam, Rhythmic raiding of refrigerator related to rapid eye movement sleep, *British Medical Journal* 292 (1986): 589.

21. P. E. Mullen, C. R. Linsell, and D. Parker, Influence of sleep disruption and calorie restriction on biological markers for depression, *Lancet*, 8 November 1986, pp. 1051–1055.

22. T. D. Brewerton, M. M. Heffernan, and N. E. Rosenthal, Psychiatric aspects of the relationship between eating and mood, *Nutrition Reviews/Supplement*, May 1986, pp. 78–88.

23. Brewerton, Heffernan, and Rosenthal, 1986.

24. Brewerton, Heffernan, and Rosenthal, 1986.

25. Unless otherwise cited, all of the listed symptoms can be found in R. S. Goodhart and M. E. Shils, eds., *Modern Nutrition in Health and Disease,* 6th ed. (Philadelphia: Lea and Febiger, 1980).

26. Marginal vitamin deficiency, *Nutrition and the MD*, July 1983, p. 3; D. Lonsdale and R. J. Shamberger, Red cell transketolase as an indicator of nutritional deficiency, *American Journal of Clinical Nutrition* 33 (1980): 205–211.

27. R. Sterner and W. Price, Restricted riboflavin: With subject behavioral effects in humans, *American Journal of Clinical Nutrition* 26 (1973): 150–160.

28. Marginal vitamin deficiency, 1983.

29. J. H. Pincus, E. H. Reynolds, and G. H. Glaser, Subacute combined system degeneration with folacin deficiency, *Journal of the American Medical Association* 221 (1972): 496–497; Neurological disease in folic acid deficiency, *Nutrition Reviews* 39 (1981): 337–338.

30. A. S. Prasad, Clinical, biochemical and nutritional spectrum of zinc deficiency in human subjects: An update, *Nutrition Reviews* 7 (1983): 197–206.

31. S. Weisburd, Eat to remember, *Science News*, 23 May 1987, p. 327.

32. Weisburd, 1987.

33. Brainfood, *Science News*, 11 January 1986, p. 24.

34. Spring and coauthors, 1986.

35. R. B. Kanarek and D. Swinney, Effects of food snacks on cognitive performance in male college students, *Appetite* 14 (1990): 15–27.

36. H. R. Lieberman, B. J. Spring, and G. S. Garfield, The behavioral effects of food constituents: Strategies used in studies of amino acids, protein, carbohydrate and caffeine, *Nutrition Reviews/Supplement*, May 1986, pp. 61–70.

■■■ CHAPTER 7

The Vitamins

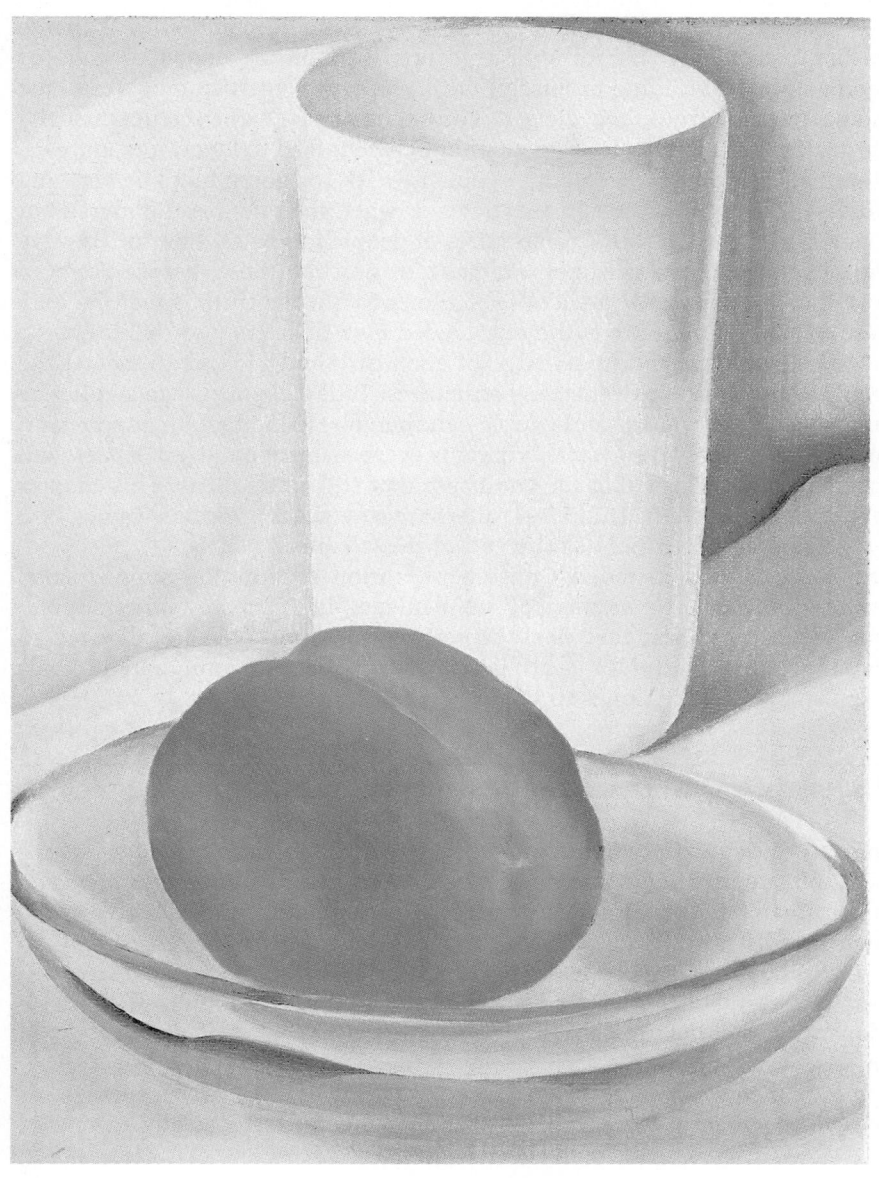

Peach and Glass, 1927, Georgia O'Keeffe. Philadelphia Museum of Art: Gift of Dr. Herman Lorber.

CONTENTS

vitamins: organic compounds, vital to life, indispensable to body function, needed in minute amounts; noncaloric essential nutrients.

precursors: compounds that can be converted into active vitamins; also known as provitamins.

The only disease a vitamin will cure is the one caused by a deficiency of that vitamin.

■■■ Table 7–1 Vitamin Names

Fat-soluble vitamins
    Vitamin A
    Vitamin D
    Vitamin E
    Vitamin K
Water-soluble vitamins
    B vitamins
        Thiamin
        Riboflavin
        Niacin
        Vitamin B_6
        Folate
        Vitamin B_{12}
        Pantothenic acid
        Biotin
    Vitamin C

■■■ At the turn of this century, the romance and thrill of discovery of the first **vitamins** captured the world's heart. People loved the vitamins. Catapulted from the shrouded mystery of folk cures to the technological era that brings us vitamin pills, they seemed a perfect answer to people who were looking for an easy way to good health. Today, scientists are stepping back from their microscopes to appreciate the complexity of the interactions of vitamins in the body. The media bombard us with a never-ending stream of advertisements for "miracle vitamins," and the supplement business is a multi*billion* dollar industry.

From a review of the history of vitamin discoveries, it is easy to see why people are so impressed. The story line has been repeated over and over with the discovery of each new vitamin. Whole groups of people are unable to walk (or are going blind or bleeding profusely) until an alert scientist stumbles onto the substance missing from their diets. According to the plot, the scientist usually confirms the discovery by feeding vitamin-deficient feed to laboratory animals. The animals respond by becoming unable to walk (or going blind or bleeding profusely). Then, miraculously, they recover when the one missing ingredient is restored to their diet. Miraculous cures of people follow as they, too, receive the missing vitamin. On reading dramatic stories like these, people come to believe that vitamins will cure a host of ailments. But the truth is that the only disease a vitamin will cure is the one caused by a deficiency of that vitamin.

It took a sophisticated knowledge of chemistry and biology to isolate the vitamins and to learn their chemical structures. Today, chemists can synthesize vitamins in the laboratory, and people can therefore take them in supplement form. As they were discovered, vitamins were named or given letters and numbers or both. This led to the confusion that still exists today. This chapter uses the names shown in Table 7–1; alternative names are given in Tables 7–2 and 7–3 on pages 218–223 at the end of this chapter.*

Previous chapters included Consumer Caution sections on supplements. This one does, too—on vitamin B_6 supplements, but so many other supplements of vitamins exist that this chapter's entire Controversy is devoted to explaining them all. Read it to learn when you may need vitamin (and mineral) supplements and which ones to take.

■■■ Definition and Classification of Vitamins

A child once defined a vitamin as "what, if you don't eat, you get sick." Although the grammar left something to be desired, the definition was accurate. Less imaginatively, a vitamin is defined as an essential, noncaloric, organic nutrient needed in tiny amounts in the diet. The role of many vitamins is to help make possible the processes by which other nutrients are digested, absorbed, and metabolized, or built into body structures. Although small in size and quantity, the vitamins accomplish mighty tasks, some of which are still being discovered.

Some of the vitamins occur in foods in a form known as **precursors**, or **provitamins**. Once inside the body, these are changed chemically to one or

*The vitamin names used here are those agreed to by the Committee on Nomenclature of the American Institute of Nutrition and published in Nomenclature policy: Generic descriptors and trivial names for vitamins and related compounds, *Journal of Nutrition* 112 (1982): 7–14.

more active forms. Thus in measuring the amount of a vitamin found in food, it is often most accurate to count not only the amount of the true vitamin but also the vitamin activity potentially available from its precursors. Tables 7–2 and 7–3 show which vitamins have precursors.

The vitamins fall naturally into two classes—fat soluble and water soluble. Solubility imparts on vitamins many of their characteristic behaviors and determines how they are absorbed into and transported around the bloodstream, whether they can be stored, and how easily they are lost from the body. In general, fat-soluble vitamins are absorbed like other fats, into the lymph, and travel in the blood associated with protein carriers. Fat-soluble vitamins can be stored with other fats in fatty tissues, and because they are stored, they can build up to toxic concentrations. The water-soluble vitamins, on the other hand, are generally absorbed directly into the bloodstream, where they travel freely. They are not stored in tissues to any great extent; rather, excesses are excreted in the urine. Thus immediate toxicities are not as likely as for fat-soluble vitamins, except in cases of extremely high doses. This chapter addresses first the fat-soluble vitamins and later the water-soluble ones. Some of the most important facts will be discussed separately for each vitamin, and the tables at the end of the chapter sum up the basic facts about all of them.

▌▌▶ *Vitamins are essential, noncaloric nutrients, needed in tiny amounts in the diet, that serve as helpers in cell functions. The fat-soluble vitamins are vitamins A, D, E, and K; the water-soluble vitamins are the B vitamins and vitamin C.*

▐▐▐ The Fat-Soluble Vitamins

The fat-soluble vitamins—A, D, E, and K—generally occur together in the fats and oils of foods. Like the lipids, these vitamins require bile for digestion, and once absorbed, they are not as readily excreted as water-soluble substances are. They remain stored in the liver and fatty tissues until the body needs them. For this reason the body can easily survive weeks of consuming foods that lack them, as long as the diet as a whole provides *average* amounts that approximate the Recommended Dietary Allowances (RDA).[1] The capacity to be stored also sets the stage for toxic buildup, should an excess be taken in, especially in the form of supplements; excesses of vitamins A, D, and K can especially easily reach toxic levels. As you read about each, you may want to refer to the table in Controversy 7 that lists safe doses for these vitamins.

Deficiencies of the fat-soluble vitamins are likely when the diet is consistently low in them or when they are inadvertently lost from the digestive tract mixed with undigested fat; any disease that produces fat malabsorption (such as liver disease that prevents bile production) can bring about deficiencies of them. A person who uses mineral oil (which the body can't absorb) as a laxative risks losing the fat-soluble vitamins by excretion.

The fat-soluble vitamins are diverse, as you will see. Vitamin A is, among many other things, a visual pigment. Vitamin A and also D can act somewhat like hormones, directing cells to convert one substance to another, to store this, or to release that. Vitamin E swarms all over the body, preventing oxidative destruction of tissues. Vitamin K helps in blood clotting. Each is worth a book in itself, but each receives only a section here.

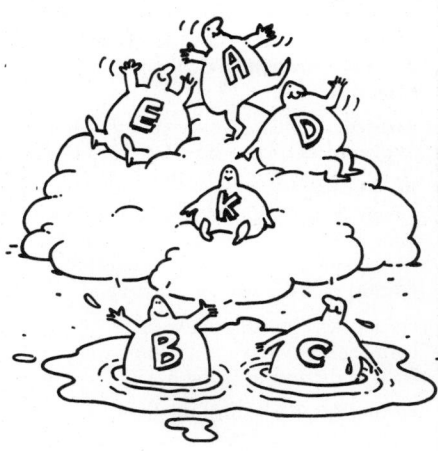

Vitamins fall into two classes—fat soluble and water soluble

Fat-soluble vitamins:

- ▪ Vitamin A.
- ▪ Vitamin D.
- ▪ Vitamin E.
- ▪ Vitamin K.

Water-soluble vitamins:

- ▪ B vitamins.
- ▪ Vitamin C.

retinol: one of the active forms of vitamin A made in animal and human bodies.

carotene: a vitamin A precursor found in plants; an orange pigment.

RE (retinol equivalent): a measure of vitamin A activity; the amount of retinol that the body will derive from a food containing vitamin A (preformed retinol) or its precursor carotene.

retina (RET-in-uh): the layer of light-sensitive nerve cells lining the back of the inside of the eye.

cornea (KOR-nee-uh): the hard, transparent membrane covering the outside of the eye.

rhodopsin: the light-sensitive pigment of the cells in the retina; it contains vitamin A (*rhod* refers to the rod-shaped cells; *opsin* means "visual protein").

Vitamin A

Vitamin A has the distinction of being the first fat-soluble vitamin to be recognized. It is certainly one of the most versatile, with roles in such diverse functions as vision, immune defenses, the stress response, metabolism, the nervous system, maintenance of body linings and skin, the making of blood, bone growth, body growth, and reproduction. In short, it is everywhere. It is the most flashy too; the active form **retinol** is yellow, and the precursor form **carotene** is bright orange, calling attention to its presence in fruits and vegetables. When carotene is converted to retinol in the body, losses occur, so rather than expressing the amounts of carotene in foods, nutrition scientists use the **retinol equivalent (RE)**—the amount of retinol the body actually derives from a plant food after conversion. The body can make one unit of retinol from about three of carotene. The liver stores vitamin A and makes it available to the bloodstream and thereby to the cells of the body.

Perhaps the most familiar function of vitamin A is in eyesight. Vitamin A plays two indispensable roles in the eye—in the events of light perception at the **retina** and in the maintenance of a healthy, crystal-clear outer window, the **cornea**.

When light falls on the eye, it passes through the clear cornea and strikes the retina, bleaching many molecules of the pigment **rhodopsin** that lie within them. Vitamin A is a part of the rhodopsin molecule. The vitamin is broken off when bleaching occurs, initiating the signal that conveys the sensation of sight

▪▪▪ Figure 7–1

Night Blindness. This is one of the earliest signs of vitamin A deficiency.

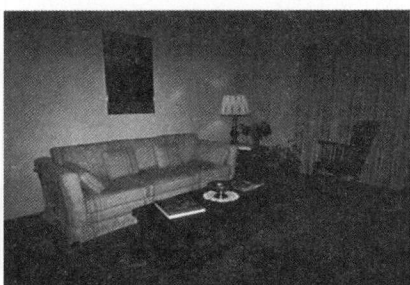

In dim light, you can make out the details in this room.

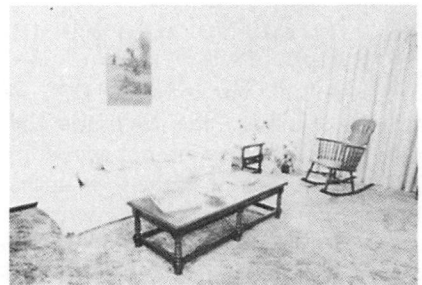

A flash of bright light momentarily blinds you as the pigment in the retina is bleached.

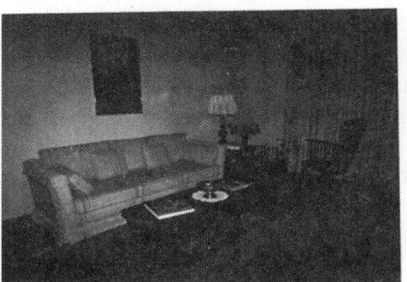

You quickly recover and can see the details again in a few seconds.

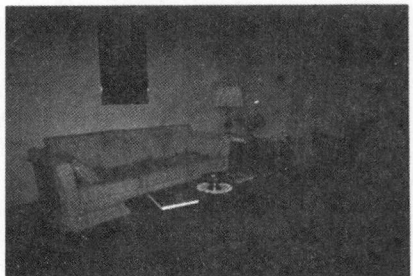

With inadequate vitamin A, you do not recover but remain blind for many seconds; this is night blindness.

to the optic center in the brain. The vitamin then reunites with the pigment, but a little vitamin A is destroyed each time this reaction takes place, and fresh vitamin A arriving in the blood regenerates the supply. If the supply is low, a lag occurs before the eye can see again after a flash of bright light at night (Figure 7–1). This lag in the recovery of night vision, termed **night blindness**, may indicate a vitamin A deficiency. A bright flash of light can temporarily blind even normal, well-nourished eyes, but if you experience a long recovery period before vision returns, you may want to check your diet for vitamin A adequacy.

A deficiency of vitamin A that has progressed well beyond the night blindness stage may be reflected in an accumulation of a protein, **keratin**, which clouds the eye's outer vitamin A-dependent part, the cornea. The condition is known as **keratinization**, and it can progress to **xerosis** (drying) and then to thickening and permanent blindness—**xerophthalmia**. Tragically, vitamin A-deprived children often become blind from this preventable condition. If the deficiency is discovered early, it can be reversed by two or three capsules of vitamin A a year.

The body's defenses against infections also depend on vitamin A; the cells of immunity require vitamin A to function.[2] When the body's defenses are weakened, especially in vitamin A-deficient children, an illness such as measles can become severe. A downward cycle of malnutrition and infection can set in— the child's body must devote its scanty store of vitamin A to fight measles viruses. But without adequate vitamin A, the infection worsens, more vitamin A is needed for the fight, but it is unavailable and the infection gains ground. Even if the child lives through the measles infection, blindness is likely. The corneas, already damaged by the chronic vitamin A shortage, degenerate rapidly as even their meager supply is diverted to the immune system. Vitamin A deficiency-induced blindness often occurs following bouts of infection.[3]

Vitamin A is needed by all **epithelial tissue** (external skin and internal linings), not just the cornea. The skin and all of the protective linings of the lungs, intestines, vagina, urinary tract, and bladder serve as barriers to infection from bacteria or to damage from other sources. If vitamin A is deficient, some of the cells in these areas are displaced by cells that secrete keratin, which is normally produced only in the hair and fingernails. Keratin makes the surfaces dry, hard, and vulnerable to infection (Figure 7–2). The cells then cannot perform their jobs; they die, accumulate on the surface, and become hosts to bacterial infection. In the cornea, as described, keratinization leads to xerophthalmia; in the lungs, the displacement of mucus-producing cells makes respiratory infections likely; in the vagina, the same process leads to vaginal infections.

Adequate vitamin A has been shown to be important in the prevention of certain cancers. Healthy skin and internal linings are able to interrupt the process by which cancers get started, but vitamin A deficiency handicaps this defense. Skin, lung, bladder, and larynx cancers become more likely when vitamin A or carotene is lacking.

Vitamin A also assists in bone growth, as Figure 7–3 shows. Normal children's bones grow longer, and the children grow taller by remodeling of each old bone into a new, bigger version. To do this requires dismantling the old bone structures and replacing them with new, larger bone parts. Growth cannot take place just by adding on to the small bone; vitamin A is needed in the critical dismantling steps. By helping reshape the jawbone as it grows, vitamin A permits normal tooth spacing. Crooked teeth and poor dental health can

night blindness: slow recovery of vision after flashes of bright light at night; an early symptom of vitamin A deficiency.

keratin (KERR-uh-tin): a water-insoluble protein; the normal protein of hair and nails.

keratinization: accumulation of keratin in a tissue, a sign of vitamin A deficiency.

xerosis: a second stage of vitamin A deficiency in the cornea—drying.

xerophthalmia (ZEER-ahf-THALL-me-uh): hardening of the cornea of the eye in advanced vitamin A deficiency that can lead to blindness (*xero* means "dry"; *ophthalm* means "eye").

epithelial (ep-ih-THEE-lee-ull) **tissue:** the layers of the body that serve as selective barriers to the environment. Examples are the cornea, the skin, the respiratory lining, and the lining of the digestive tract.

A vitamin A drug is also used to fight acne; see Chapter 13.

Chapter 11 offers more on vitamin A and cancer.

■■■ **Figure 7–2**

The Skin in Vitamin A Deficiency.
The hard lumps reflect accumulations
of keratin in the epithelial cells.

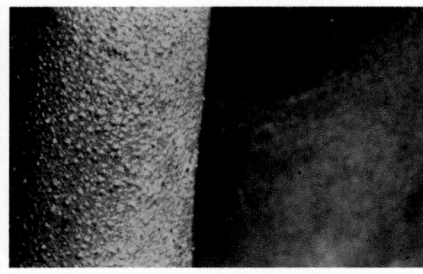

■■■ **Figure 7–3**

Vitamin A in Bone Growth. As bone
lengthens, vitamin A helps remove old
bone (arrows).

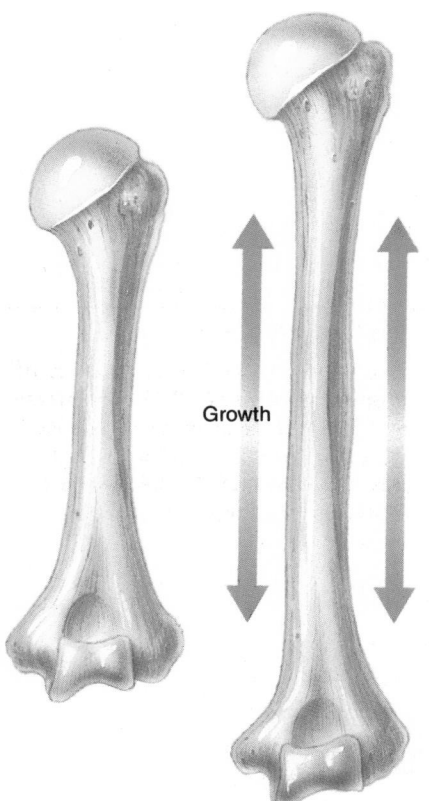

Growth

result from a deficiency in prenatal or early postnatal life. In children, failure to grow is one of the first signs of poor vitamin A status; when such children receive vitamin A supplements, they gain weight and grow taller.[4]

Although relatively rare in developed countries, vitamin A deficiency is a vast problem worldwide, causing a quarter of a million new cases of blindness a year in Asia alone and placing a heavy burden on society. More than 5 million of the world's children suffer from less obvious signs of vitamin A deficiency— stunted growth, poor appetite, and impaired immunity with resulting infections. In one small country (Indonesia), vitamin A deficiency is charged with the deaths of 150,000 preschool children each year, and in other countries the toll is many times greater.[5] To prevent all this sickness and death would cost only a few pennies per child per year, since vitamin A capsules are inexpensive.

Toxicity presents a danger equal to that of deficiency for people who take excess vitamin A in supplements. Its many symptoms include hair loss, joint pain, stunted growth, bone and muscle soreness, cessation of menstruation, nausea, diarrhea, rashes, and enlargement of the liver and spleen. Taken during pregnancy, vitamin A megadoses can cause major birth defects; much smaller doses given to animals during pregnancy cause permanent learning disabilities in their offspring, implying that they may do so in human children too.[6] Early symptoms of overdoses in children are loss of appetite, growth failure, and itching of the skin. Healthy people can eat vitamin A-rich foods in large amounts without causing toxicity symptoms, with the possible exception of liver. One report has described children falling ill after eating too much liver daily for years, but this is a medical rarity.[7] Inuit people and arctic explorers know that polar bear livers, because the bears eat fish whole (and thus fish livers), contain large amounts of the vitamin and are therefore a dangerous food source. Carotene from plant foods is not converted to the active form of vitamin A completely enough to be hazardous but has been known to turn people bright yellow if they eat too much. Carotene builds up in the fat just beneath the skin and imparts a yellow cast.

Experts argue about how much preformed vitamin A is too much. Some authorities think people in general take too much vitamin A in supplements and that "we may be on the verge of an epidemic of vitamin A toxicity."[8] Other authorities point to a relatively low supplemental dose (five to ten times the RDA) given over many years as a cause of toxicity in the long run. Still others cite evidence that it takes 40 to 120 times the RDA to achieve an acute toxic dose. A table in Controversy 7 lists a safe dose of vitamin A that will not be toxic even over a long period of time, but the best way to ensure a safe vitamin A intake is to steer clear of supplements and instead, to eat foods to obtain it.

Some foods with animal fat in them contain the active vitamin retinol. Among the richest sources are liver, cod-liver oil, butter, egg yolks, whole or fortified milk, cream, and cheeses made from whole milk or cream.

Many foods from plants contain carotene, the orange pigment that is a precursor to vitamin A. They are so brightly colored that they decorate the plate. Carrots, sweet potatoes, pumpkins, cantaloupe, and apricots are all rich sources. Another colorful group, *dark* green vegetables such as spinach, other greens, or broccoli, owe their color to chlorophyll and carotene: the two pigments together give a deep, murky, dark green color to the vegetables. Other colorful vegetables can fool you into thinking they contain carotene—iceberg lettuce, beets, and sweet corn—but these derive their color from other pigments and are poor sources of carotene, along with the "white" plant foods such as grains and potatoes, which have none. Recommendations state that a person should eat *dark* green or *deep* orange vegetables and fruits at least every other day. Figure 7–4 shows a sampling of the richest food sources of vitamin A, and this chapter's Food Feature discusses the best ways to obtain sufficient amounts of all of the vitamins.

Studies of typical fast-food meals indicate that these foods are particularly lacking in vitamin A. Recently, however, even fast-food restaurants have been offering salads with cheese, carrots, and other carotene-rich foods as alternatives to the plain burgers, fries, and cola meals of yesterday. These selections greatly improve the nutritional quality of fast-food meals, for historically, fast foods have lacked vitamin A.

The amount of vitamin A a person needs is proportional to the person's body weight. Although the RDA for vitamin A is given as a daily amount, the vitamin need not be consumed every day. For example, a person who eats the one whole carrot listed in Appendix A (page A–66) easily meets two days' needs of vitamin A. An average intake that meets the daily RDA over several months is sufficient. According to the RDA, a man needs a daily average of about 1000 RE and a woman about 800 RE. Needs increase during lactation; children need less.

Vitamin A recommendations are expressed in RE, but some food tables still express vitamin A contents using a different unit, the **IU** (**international unit**). Note that this book's Appendix A uses RE for your convenience, but be careful to notice whether other food tables or supplement labels do, and see Appendix C for help in converting the units. Not everything in nutrition is arranged for the consumer's convenience; people working with the amounts of vitamin A in foods have to remember to make sure that they are all expressed in the same units before making comparisons.

▌▶ *Vitamin A is essential to vision, integrity of epithelial tissue, growth of bone, reproduction, and more. Vitamin A deficiency causes blindness, sickness, and death and is a major problem worldwide. Overdoses are possible and cause many serious symptoms. Brightly colored plant foods are richest in carotene, a vitamin A precursor. Liver and milk are rich animal sources.*

> **IU (international unit):** a measure of fat-soluble vitamin activity.

The RDA tables are on the inside front cover.

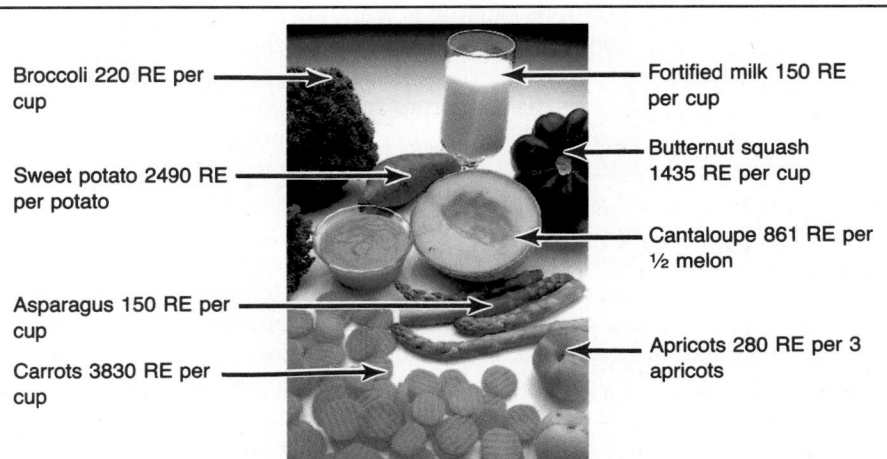

Broccoli 220 RE per cup

Sweet potato 2490 RE per potato

Asparagus 150 RE per cup

Carrots 3830 RE per cup

Fortified milk 150 RE per cup

Butternut squash 1435 RE per cup

Cantaloupe 861 RE per ½ melon

Apricots 280 RE per 3 apricots

■■■ **Figure 7–4**

A Sampling of Rich Food Sources of Vitamin A. A man's RDA for vitamin A is 1000 RE; a woman's is 800 RE. A 3-ounce portion of beef liver (not shown) contains 9120 RE. See also this chapter's Food Feature and Appendix A.

rickets: the vitamin D deficiency disease in children, characterized by abnormal growth of bone, manifested in bowed legs or knock-knees, outward-bowed chest, and knobs on the ribs.

osteomalacia (OS-tee-o-mal-AY-shuh): the vitamin D deficiency disease in adults (*osteo* means "bone"; *mal* means "bad"). Symptoms include bending of the spine and bowing of the legs.

Chapter and Controversy 8 present more about bone minerals and their regulation.

Osteoporosis, another bone-weakening disease, is discussed in Controversy 8.

Vitamin D

In a sense, vitamin D is not an essential nutrient because food sources are scarce and because the body can make all it needs with the help of sunlight. Given enough sun, you need consume no vitamin D at all in the foods you eat. Vitamin D is also more like a hormone than a vitamin in that it stimulates maturation of cells, including cells of the immune system.[9] Folk wisdom has it that sunshine promotes health and recovery from diseases. People of past generations observed the recovery from diseases effected by the immune system's response to vitamin D long before scientists worked out the details.[10] However, keep in mind that too much sun is dangerous—it can increase a person's risk of skin cancer.

The best-known role of vitamin D is as a member of a large and interacting team of nutrients and hormones that continuously maintain blood calcium levels and thereby bone integrity, especially during growth. Vitamin D ensures that sufficient calcium and phosphorus are available in the blood to feed the growing bone structure. Calcium is also indispensable to the proper functioning of all the tissues of the body; cells of muscles, nerves, glands and others all draw it from the blood as they need it. The skeleton serves as a vast warehouse of stored calcium, and it is tapped when the blood supply begins to run low. Calcium to raise the blood level can be drawn from only two other places: from the digestive tract, where food brings it in, and from the kidney, which recycles it into the body from the blood filtrate destined to become urine. Vitamin D acts, when needed, at all three locations to raise the blood calcium level.

The most obvious sign of vitamin D deficiency is abnormality of the bones. The disease **rickets**, caused in children by vitamin D deficiency, has been recognized for several centuries, and even in the 1700s it was known to be curable by cod-liver oil. More than a hundred years later, a Polish physician linked sunlight exposure to prevention and cure of rickets, and at the turn of this century, enough was finally known about rickets to reproduce it in laboratory animals. Today the bowed legs, knock-knees, and pigeon breasts of children with rickets are no longer common sights.

Adult rickets, or **osteomalacia**, occurs most often in women with low calcium intakes and little exposure to the sun (therefore little opportunity to make vitamin D) and who have repeated pregnancies and then breast-feed their babies. Under these conditions calcium is withdrawn from the bones but is not picked up efficiently from the intestine or saved by the kidney. The bones lose their minerals and protein understructure, becoming porous, soft, and easy to break. The bones of the legs may soften to such an extent that a young woman who is tall and straight at age 20 may, after several pregnancies, be bowlegged and bent by age 30. Deafness, too, can result from vitamin D deficiency because sounds are transmitted to the brain along tiny ear bones, and these bones also degenerate when vitamin D is lacking.[11]

Vitamin D is the most toxic of all vitamins. Ingestion of as little as four to five times the recommended daily intake can cause toxicity symptoms including diarrhea, headache, and nausea. If overdoses continue, the vitamin raises the blood mineral level to dangerous extremes, forcing calcium to be deposited in soft tissues such as the heart and kidneys. If calcium deposits form in the arteries of the heart, the consequence of overdosing is death.

The likeliest victims of vitamin D poisoning are infants whose mothers have been so misguided as to think that if some is good, more is better. People who

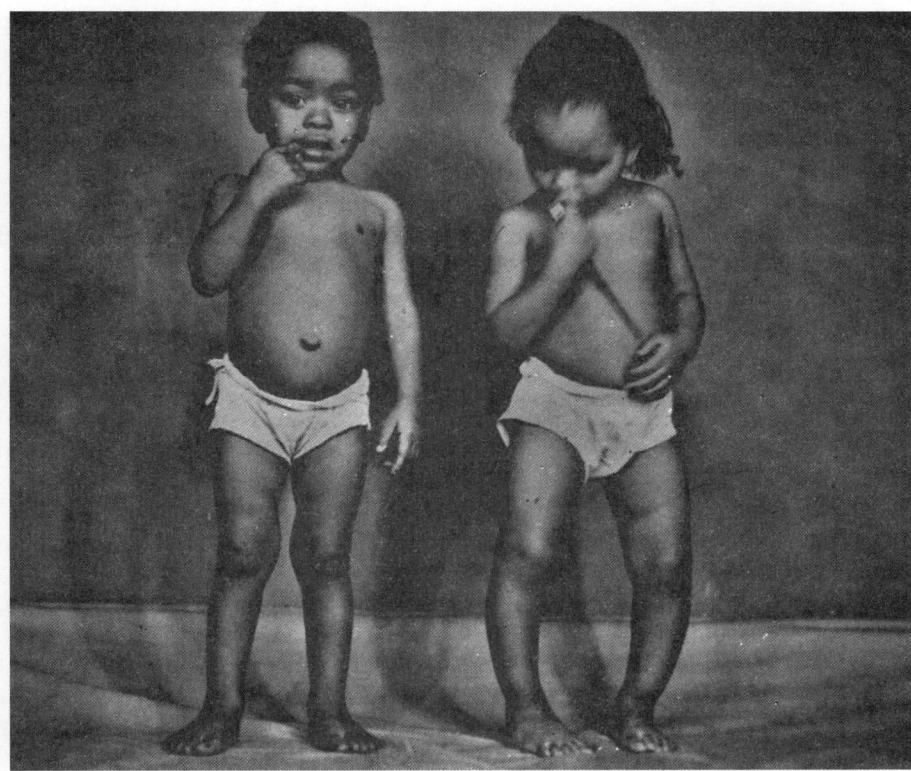

The child on the right has the vitamin D deficiency disease rickets.

take supplements containing vitamin D may also easily overdose, not realizing that their tissues are building up stockpiles of the vitamin. The amounts found in foods are safe, but concentrated supplements should be treated with respect and used only on the advice of a physician.

The best way to obtain vitamin D may not be to eat it but rather to make it yourself. When the sun shines on a cholesterol compound in human skin, the compound is transformed into a vitamin D precursor and is absorbed directly into the blood. (The liver and kidneys finish converting the precursor to the active vitamin.) Worldwide most people meet their need for vitamin D this way; the sun presents no risk of toxicity. Even lifeguards on southern beaches are safe from vitamin D toxicity from the sun because the skin breaks down any excess vitamin made there. The body shows wisdom in handling of the vitamin D it makes; supplements bypass the body's safeguards and easily induce toxicity.

Of course, long sun exposure has *other* undesirable consequences such as premature wrinkling of the skin and the increased risk of skin cancer mentioned earlier, but these dangers may be somewhat reduced by using sunscreens. Unfortunately, sunscreens with sun protection factors (SPF) of 8 and above also prevent vitamin D synthesis. A strategy to solve this dilemma is to apply sunscreen after enough time has elapsed to provide sufficient vitamin D. Production of vitamin D doesn't demand idle hours of sunbathing, though. Just being outdoors, even in lightweight clothing, is sufficient.

The ultraviolet rays of the sun that promote vitamin D synthesis may be filtered—by clouds, smoke, smog, heavy clothing, window glass, and even window screens. Dark-skinned people require long exposure to direct sun (up to 3 hours, depending on the climate) for a full day's supply of vitamin D, while light-skinned people need much less time (10 or 15 minutes).[12] Some types of tanning booths also stimulate vitamin D synthesis, but the Food and Drug Administration (FDA) warns that these may be hazardous if they are not properly filtered, and users risk burns, damage to blood vessels, and damage to the eyes.[13] Daily doses of vitamin D or even of sunshine are not necessary because synthesis of vitamin D continues for days *after* exposure to sun and because the body stores enough vitamin D to last through dark winter months.

There was a time when rickets seemed almost absent from developed countries, but since the 1970s it has been creeping back, with cases being reported in inner-city children, especially blacks; in children breastfed for an exceptionally long time; and in vegetarian children.[14] The slower vitamin D production in dark-skinned people may account for most of today's cases of rickets. In the United States and Canada, almost all cases show up in dark-skinned people who live in smoggy northern cities or who lack exposure to sunlight. Worldwide, rickets is still a major health problem, especially in people of societies that traditionally clothe themselves in concealing garments.

The few significant food sources of vitamin D are butter, cream, egg yolks, and liver and medicinal cod-liver oil. In the United States and Canada, milk, whether fluid, dried, or evaporated, is usually fortified with vitamin D, so that a daily quart or liter will supply the amount recommended for a younger adult. That way the young adult who drinks the recommended 2 cups a day receives half the RDA; the other half comes from sun exposure and other food sources. Older adults need half this amount. Children who drink 2 cups or more will have a head start toward meeting their vitamin D needs for growth. Strict vegetarians, and especially their children, may have low vitamin D intakes because no fortified plant source exists. In the United States breakfast cereals may be fortified with vitamin D, as their labels indicate.

The RDA for vitamin D is 5 micrograms per day for adults older than 24 years and is higher during growth or bone formation—in pregnancy, lactation, childhood, adolescence, and in early adult life while bones continue to gain density. People who are housebound or institutionalized or who work at night may incur (over years) a vitamin D deficiency that leads to deficiency of calcium severe enough to damage their bones. Adults who can tolerate milk receive a source of both calcium and vitamin D; those who experience sensitivities to milk must seek alternative calcium sources and should make it a point to spend time outdoors.

❚❚▶ *Vitamin D increases the blood level of minerals, notably calcium and phosphorus, permitting bone formation and maintenance. A deficiency in childhood can cause rickets and in later life osteomalacia. People exposed to the sun make vitamin D from cholesterol; fortified milk is an important food source. Vitamin D is the most toxic of all the vitamins, and excesses are dangerous or deadly.*

Vitamin E

Vitamin E, because it can be oxidized, is like a bodyguard for other substances; it serves as an antioxidant. By being destroyed itself, vitamin E protects the polyunsaturated fats and other fat-soluble substances such as vitamin A from destruction by oxygen. Vitamin E exerts an especially important antioxidant effect in the lungs, where the cells are exposed to high oxygen concentrations that can destroy their membranes. As the red blood cells carry oxygen from the lungs to other tissues, vitamin E protects their cell membranes too. Vitamin E also protects the white blood cells that defend the body against disease. Indeed, deficiency of vitamin E suppresses the immune system, and large doses of the vitamin stimulate it in several species of animals. Normal nerve development also depends on vitamin E.

A deficiency of vitamin E produces a wide variety of symptoms in laboratory animals, but most of these symptoms have not been reproduced in human beings, despite many attempts. Three reasons have been given for this. First, the vitamin is so widespread in food that it is almost impossible to create a vitamin E-deficient diet. Second, the body stores so much vitamin E in its fatty tissues that a person could not keep on eating a vitamin E-free diet for long enough to deplete these stores and to produce a deficiency. Third, the cells may recycle their working supply of vitamin E, using the same molecules over and over.[15] It may be, however, that rare vitamin E deficiencies are seen in people without diseases. People in whom they are most likely are those who for years eat diets extremely low in fat, or who use fat substitutes such as diet margarines and salad dressings as their only sources of fat, or who consume diets composed largely of highly processed or "convenience" foods—since vitamin E is destroyed by extensive heating at high temperatures.

A number of disease conditions do cause vitamin E deficiencies—notably, conditions that cause malabsorption of fat. These include disease or injury of the liver (which makes bile, necessary for digestion of fat), the gallbladder (which delivers bile into the intestine), and the pancreas (which makes fat-digesting enzymes), as well as a number of hereditary diseases involving digestion and use of nutrients. In children with these diseases, supplements given in time can prevent damage to the developing nervous system, and to the retina of the eye. In adults, vitamin E supplements also prevent neurological disorders caused by vitamin E deficiency due to disease.[16]

Although vitamin E deficiency is rare, many horror stories have been told about vitamin E deficiency diseases in human beings. Extravagant claims have been made that it cures all sorts of things because it has effects on animals' hearts, muscles, and reproductive systems that it does not have in the organs of human beings. While research has revealed possible roles for vitamin E, it has also clearly discredited claims that vitamin E prolongs the life of the heart, improves athletic endurance and skill, enhances sexual performance, or cures sexual dysfunction in males. Some of this research gave the vitamin E family of compounds their name, the **tocopherols**. *Tokos* is a Greek word meaning "offspring."

One proven vitamin E deficiency symptom in human beings occurs in premature babies because they are born before the transfer of the vitamin from the mother to the infant that takes place in the very last weeks of pregnancy. Without vitamin E, the red blood cells rupture (**erythrocyte hemolysis**), and the infant becomes anemic. Two other conditions are apparently caused sometimes by vitamin E deficiency in human beings. One is a painful but nonmalignant disease characterized by painful lumps in the breasts (**fibrocystic breast disease**). This can also be worsened by caffeine toxicity, so it sometimes responds to vitamin E supplements and sometimes to abstinence from caffeine. The other is a leg disorder that involves pain on walking and cramps in the calves at night.†

tocopherols (tuh-KOFF-er-alls): a kind of alchohol. The active form of vitamin E is *alpha*-tocopherol.

erythrocyte (eh-REETH-ro-sight) **hemolysis** (he-MOLL-ih-sis): rupture of the red blood cells, caused by vitamin E deficiency (*erythro* means "red"; *cyte* means "cell"; *hemo* means "blood"; *lysis* means "breaking").

fibrocystic breast disease: a harmless disease in which the breasts become lumpy and painful, caused sometimes by vitamin E deficiency and sometimes associated with caffeine toxicity (*fibro* means "fibrous tissue"; *cyst* means "closed sac").

†The leg disorder is known as intermittent claudication (*claudicare* means "to limp").

The RDA for vitamin E is based on body size—8 milligrams a day for women, 10 for men.* The need for vitamin E rises as polyunsaturated oil intake rises. People who need vitamin E supplements are, as mentioned, people with very low fat intakes as well as people with diseases impairing fat absorption, which cause vitamin E deficiency.

Cases of vitamin E toxicity are rare. The medical literature contains isolated reports of adverse effects on laboratory animals and of nausea, intestinal distress, and other vague complaints in human beings. Large doses may augment the effects of anticoagulant medication used to oppose unwanted blood clotting; people taking such drugs risk uncontrollable bleeding when they also take large doses of vitamin E. However, the impression remains that for most individuals, daily doses below 300 milligrams are harmless.

Wheat germ oil is rich in vitamin E, as are whole grains, wheat germ, green plants, nuts, and seeds. Animal fats, such as milk fat or the fat of meats, have negligible vitamin E. Many plant foods provide generous amounts of vitamin E, as long as they are whole rather than highly processed foods. Oil that has been heated to frying temperatures as well as food fried in it retains little intact vitamin E.

▐▐▶ *Vitamin E acts as an antioxidant in cell membranes and is especially important for the integrity of cells that are constantly exposed to high levels of oxygen— the lungs and blood cells, both red and white. Vitamin E deficiency is rare in human beings, but it does occur in newborn premature infants. The vitamin is widely distributed among plant foods; toxicity is rare.*

Vitamin K

Vitamin K is the fat-soluble vitamin necessary for the synthesis of at least two proteins involved in blood clotting. It also works with vitamin D in helping to regulate blood calcium levels (calcium is also needed for blood to clot). If blood cannot clot, then wounds may bleed for a dangerously long time; this is why people's blood is drawn to measure clotting time before they go into surgery. Vitamin K is sometimes administered before operations to reduce bleeding in surgery but is of value at this time only if a vitamin K deficiency exists. Vitamin K does not improve clotting in those with other bleeding disorders, such as the genetic disease hemophilia.

In some heart problems there is a need to *prevent* the formation of clots within the circulatory system. This is popularly referred to as "thinning" the blood. One of the best-known medicines for this purpose is dicumarol, which interferes with the action of vitamin K in permitting clotting. Vitamin K therapy is necessary for people taking dicumarol if uncontrolled bleeding occurs.

Like vitamin D, vitamin K can be obtained from a nonfood source—in this case, the intestinal bacteria. Billions of bacteria normally reside in the intestines, and some of them synthesize vitamin K. The extent to which the body uses the vitamin K synthesized by these bacteria is not known, but it is possible that people obtain about half of their daily needs from them. Vitamin K's richest plant food source is dark-green leafy vegetables, which provide from 50 to 800 micrograms per 3-ounce serving, and there is one rich animal food

K stands for the Danish word koagulation (clotting).

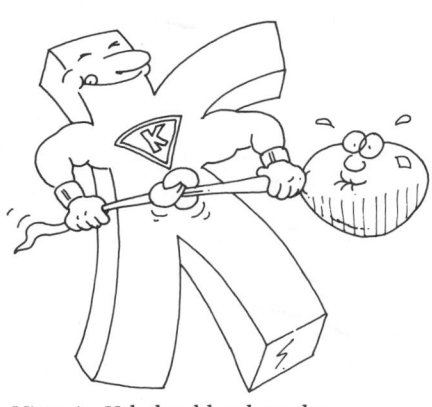

Vitamin K helps blood to clot.

*The RDA gives values for vitamin E in α TE (alpha tocopherol equivalents). 1 α TE = 1 mg of alpha tocopherol. Appendix C provides other conversion factors..

source—liver. Food tables do not include vitamin K contents of foods because they are not known with sufficient precision.

An RDA for vitamin K was published for the first time in 1989 (see the RDA tables on the inside front cover). It seems likely that few U.S. adults experience vitamin K deficiency, even if they do not often eat green leafy vegetables or liver.[17] Newborn infants whose intestinal tracts are not yet inhabited by bacteria and people who have taken antibiotics that have killed the intestinal bacteria may develop vitamin K deficiencies. Supplements of the vitamin are needed in these cases.

Vitamin K is not toxic in the range of amounts commonly consumed from natural sources, but toxicity can result when supplements of a synthetic version of vitamin K are given, especially to infants or to pregnant women. Toxicity symptoms include breakage of the red blood cells, causing the release of their pigment that colors the skin yellow, and also causing brain damage.‡ Because amounts of the vitamin contained in supplements can easily reach toxic levels, it is available as a single vitamin only by prescription.

▌▌▶ *Vitamin K is necessary for blood to clot; deficiency causes uncontrolled bleeding. The bacterial inhabitants of the digestive tract produce vitamin K, and most people derive about half their requirement from them and half from food. Excesses are toxic.*

> **coenzyme** (co-EN-zime): a small molecule that works with an enzyme to promote the enzyme's activity. Many coenzymes have B vitamins as part of their structure (*co* means "with").

▐▐▐ The Water-Soluble Vitamins

All of the other vitamins—the B vitamins and vitamin C—are water soluble. They can be leached out of foods into cooking or washing water by incorrect preparation. They are easily absorbed into the bloodstream and are just as easily excreted out of the body in the urine. Under ordinary circumstances, you need not be concerned about consuming small excesses. Some of the water-soluble vitamins can remain in the lean tissues for periods of a month or more, but these tissues are actively exchanging materials with the body fluids at all times, and so these vitamins are likely to be picked up by the extracellular fluids, carried away by the blood, and excreted in the urine. Generally, the RDA committee suggests that you make sure your three-day intake average meets the RDA by choosing foods that are rich in water-soluble vitamins.[18] Foods never deliver toxic doses. The large doses provided by vitamin supplements can reach toxic levels, but the most likely hazard to the taker is that, as one person aptly noted, "If you take supplements of the water-soluble vitamins, you may have the most expensive urine in town."

The water-soluble vitamins require special measures in food preparation to avoid losing or destroying them—see the Food Feature of Chapter 14.

The B Vitamins and Their Relatives

The B vitamins act as part of coenzymes. A **coenzyme** is a small molecule that combines with an enzyme to make it active. (Recall that enzymes are large proteins that do the body's building, dismantling, transporting, and other work; see pages 162–163.) Sometimes the vitamin part of the enzyme is the

---

‡A toxic dose of a vitamin K compound such as *menadione* causes the liver to release the blood cell pigment (*bilirubin*) into the blood (instead of excreting it into the bile) and leads to *jaundice*; when bilirubin invades the brain of an infant, the condition, called *kernicterus*, is often fatal.

■■■ Figure 7–5

Coenzyme Action.

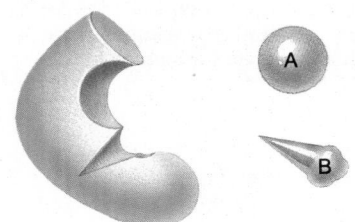

Without the coenzyme, compounds A and B don't respond to the enzyme.

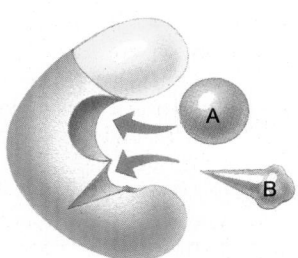

With the coenzyme in place, A and B are attracted to the active site on the enzyme, and they react.

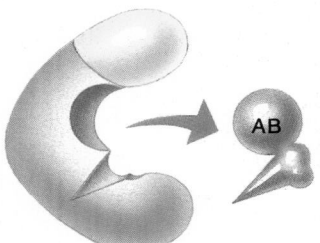

The reaction is completed.

active site, where the chemical reaction takes place. The substance to be worked on is attracted to the active site and snaps into place, and the reaction proceeds instantaneously. The architecture of each enzyme is designed to accomplish just one kind of job. Without its coenzyme, however, the enzyme is as useless as a padlock without its key. Figure 7–5 shows how a coenzyme enables an enzyme to do its job.

Each B vitamin has its own special character, and the amount of detail known about each one is overwhelming. To simplify their introduction, this section describes some of the ways in which the B vitamins work together in the body and emphasizes the consequences of deficiencies. The Food Feature at the end of this chapter shows how to select foods that will provide adequate amounts of all of the B vitamins.

B Vitamin Roles in Metabolism

Figure 7–6 shows some ways in which carbohydrates, lipids, and amino acids participate in tissue metabolism. It is not presented to teach details; that is best left to graduate courses in biochemistry. The purpose of the figure is to give an impression of how the B vitamins work together in the metabolism of energy nutrients and in the making of new cells. A few details are presented in the figure legend.

The amounts of B vitamins people need are determined differently for each vitamin. For three of the B vitamins, thiamin, riboflavin, and niacin, the amounts needed are proportional to energy expenditure. For vitamin B_6, which is tied closely to amino acid metabolism, the amount is proportional to protein intake. The recommended intakes are summarized in the RDA tables (inside front cover).

■■▶ *The B vitamins facilitate the work of every cell. Some help generate energy, others help make DNA, RNA, protein, and new cells.*

B Vitamin Deficiencies and Toxicities

As long as B vitamins are present, their presence is not felt. Only when they are missing does their absence manifest itself in a lack of energy and a multitude of other symptoms, as you can imagine after looking at Figure 7–6. The reactions by which B vitamins facilitate energy release take place in every cell, and no cell can do its work without energy. Thus in a B-vitamin deficiency, every cell is affected. Among the symptoms of B-vitamin deficiencies are nausea, severe exhaustion, irritability, depression, forgetfulness, loss of appetite and weight, pain in muscles, impairment of the immune response, loss of control of the limbs, abnormal heart action, severe skin problems, teary or bloodshot eyes, and many more. Because cell renewal depends on energy, protein, and DNA/RNA availability, and because all of these depend on the B vitamins, tissues in which the cells' life spans are shortest are most readily damaged by B vitamin deficiency. Thus the digestive tract (whose cells replace themselves every three days) and the blood (whose cells live an average of six weeks) are invariably damaged. In children, full recovery may be impossible; in the case of a thiamin deficiency, for example, permanent brain damage can result.

In academic discussions of the vitamins, clearly different deficiency symptoms are given for each one. Actually such clear-cut symptoms are found only

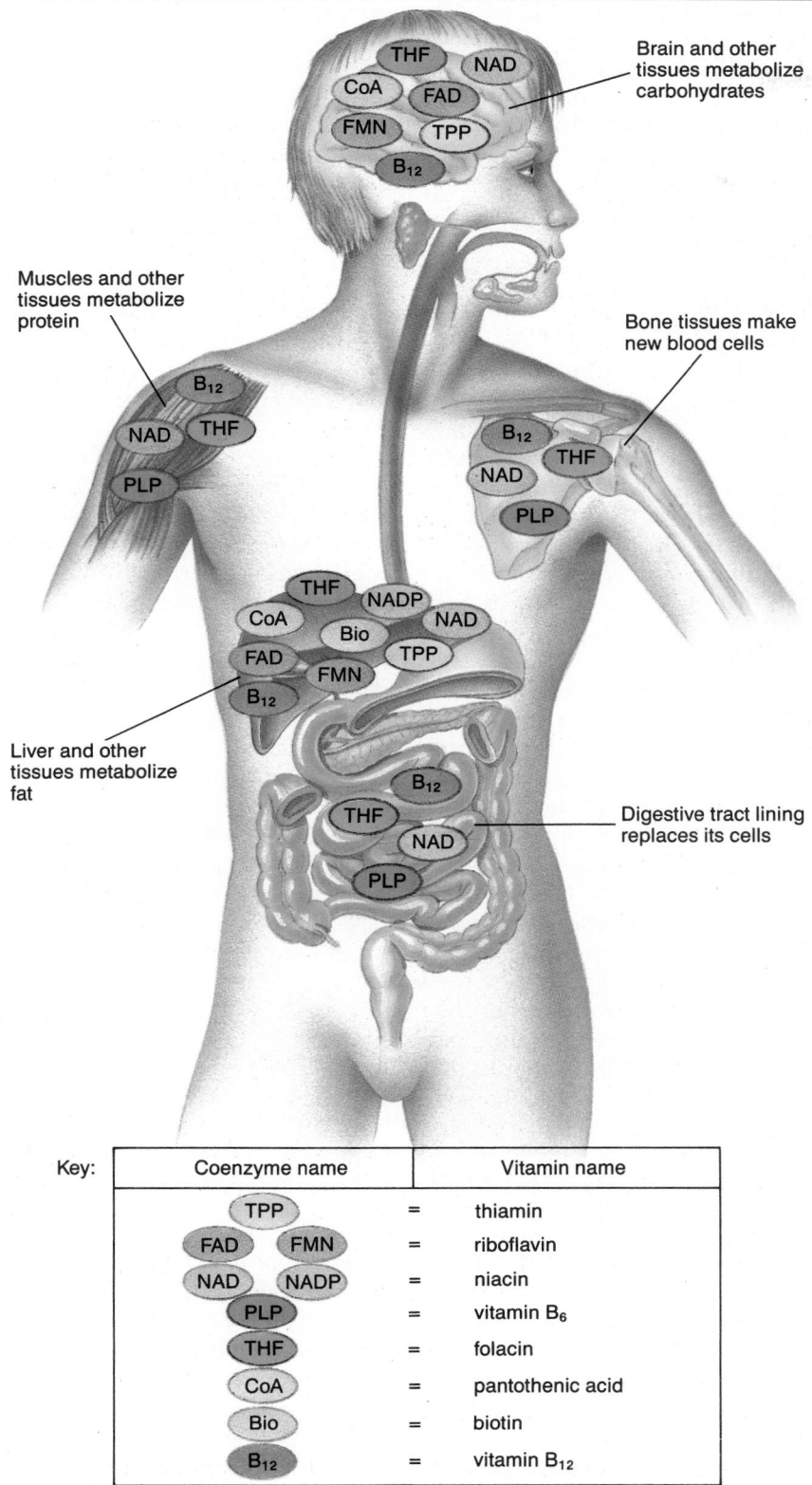

Brain and other tissues metabolize carbohydrates

Muscles and other tissues metabolize protein

Bone tissues make new blood cells

Liver and other tissues metabolize fat

Digestive tract lining replaces its cells

Key:

Coenzyme name			Vitamin name
TPP		=	thiamin
FAD	FMN	=	riboflavin
NAD	NADP	=	niacin
PLP		=	vitamin B₆
THF		=	folacin
CoA		=	pantothenic acid
Bio		=	biotin
B₁₂		=	vitamin B₁₂

■■■ **Figure 7–6**

Some Roles of the B Vitamins in Metabolism: Examples. This figure does not attempt to teach intricate biochemical pathways or names of B vitamin-containing enzymes. Its sole purpose is to show a few of the many tissue functions that depend on B vitamin-containing enzymes. The B vitamins work in every cell, and this displays less than 1/1000ᵗʰ of what they actually do. Every B vitamin is part of one or more coenzymes that make possible the body's chemical work. For example, the niacin coenzymes are necessary for most of the energy pathways. The thiamin and riboflavin coenzymes are also important in the energy pathways. The folate and vitamin B₁₂ coenzymes are necessary for the making of RNA and DNA and thus new cells. The vitamin B₆ coenzyme is necessary for the processing of amino acids, and therefore, of protein. Many other relationships are also critical to metabolism.

thiamin (THIGH-uh-min): a B vitamin.

beriberi: the thiamin-deficiency disease, characterized by loss of sensation in the hands and feet, muscular weakness, advanced paralysis, and abnormal heart action that can cause death.

riboflavin (RIBE-o-flay-vin): a B vitamin.

niacin, nicotinic acid, niacinamide, nicotinamide: four names for the same B vitamin. Niacin can be eaten preformed or can be made in the body from tryptophan, one of the amino acids.

pellagra (pell-AY-gra): the niacin-deficiency disease (*pellis* means "skin"; *agra* means "rough"). Symptoms include the "4 D's"—diarrhea, dermatitis, dementia, and, ultimately, death.

in laboratory animals that have been fed contrived diets that lack just one ingredient. In real life, a deficiency of any one B vitamin seldom shows up by itself because people don't eat nutrients singly; they eat foods that contain mixtures of nutrients. Still the deficiency of one B vitamin may appear predominant in a cluster of deficiencies, and often, if it is corrected by giving wholesome food rather than single supplements, the subtler deficiencies will be corrected along with it. Table 7–3 at the end of the chapter summarizes the symptoms of B-vitamin deficiencies and toxicities, and the next few sections treat each B vitamin separately.

THIAMIN AND RIBOFLAVIN. The **thiamin** deficiency disease **beriberi** was first observed in the Far East, where rice provided about 90 percent of the total calories most people consumed and therefore was their principal source of thiamin. When the custom of polishing rice (removing its brown coat, which contained the thiamin) became widespread, beriberi swept through the population like an epidemic. Most other vitamins can be obtained by taking a helping of this or that (if you choose the right food), but small amounts of thiamin are so evenly distributed in foods that its removal from such a major staple food effectively removes it from the diet altogether. Scientists wasted years of time and effort hunting for a microbial cause of beriberi before they realized that the cause of beriberi was not something present in the environment but something absent from it.

Just before the year 1900, an observant physician working in a prison in the East Indies discovered that beriberi could be cured with proper diet. The physician noticed that the chickens at the prison developed a stiffness and weakness similar to that of the prisoners who had beriberi. The chickens were being fed the rice left on the plates of prisoners. When the rice bran, which had been discarded in the kitchen, was given to the chickens, their paralysis was cured. As might be expected, the doctor met resistance when he tried to feed the rice bran—the "garbage"—to the prisoners. Later, extracts of rice bran were used to prevent infantile beriberi; still later, thiamin was synthesized.

People living in developed countries today who consume almost any reasonable diet are safe from thiamin deficiency as long as they consume mostly whole foods to meet their energy needs. People addicted to alcohol, though, may develop a deficiency because they obtain energy from alcohol, which carries almost no nutrients with it and often displaces food. In addition, alcohol causes excretion of thiamin in the urine, doubling the risk of deficiency.

When thiamin is deficient, **riboflavin** may be lacking too, but the deficiency symptoms (listed in Table 7–3) may be unseen because those of thiamin deficiency are more severe. When foods remedy the thiamin deficiency, because they invariably also contain some riboflavin, both deficiencies clear up.

NIACIN. The **niacin**-deficiency disease **pellagra** appeared in Europe in the 1700s when corn from the New World came into wide acceptance as a staple food. At about the turn of this century in the United States, pellagra was wreaking havoc throughout the South and Midwest. Hundreds of thousands of pellagra victims were thought to be suffering from a contagious disease until this dietary deficiency was pinned down.

Early workers seeking to find the cause of pellagra observed that well-fed people *never* got it. From there they defined a diet that reliably produced the

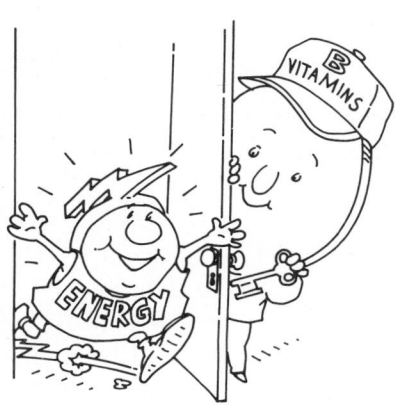

Niacin, thiamin, and riboflavin are important in pathways that release energy from energy-yielding nutrients.

disease—one of cornmeal, pork fat, and molasses. The disease still occurs in poorly nourished people of today's urban slums and particularly in those with alcohol addiction. Pellagra is also still common in parts of Africa and Asia. Figure 7–7 shows the skin disorder associated with pellagra. For comparison, Figure 7–8 (page 210) shows a skin disorder associated with vitamin B_6 deficiency—a reminder that any nutrient deficiency affects the skin and all other cells. The skin just happens to be the organ you can see.

The key nutrient that prevents pellagra is niacin, but any protein containing sufficient amounts of the amino acid tryptophan will serve in its place. Tryptophan, which is abundant in almost all proteins (but is lacking from the protein of corn), is converted to niacin in the body. In fact, it is possible to cure pellagra by administering tryptophan alone. Thus a person eating more than adequate protein (as most people do) will not be deficient in niacin. The amount of niacin in a diet is therefore stated in terms of **niacin equivalents**, a measure that takes available tryptophan into account. Self-Study exercise 1, on p. 230, shows how to estimate niacin equivalents.

Certain forms of niacin supplements in amounts 10 times or more the RDA cause "niacin flush," a dilation of the capillaries of the skin with perceptible tingling that, if intense, can be painful. Physicians administer large niacin doses as part of the arsenal of drugs against atherosclerosis. When used this way, niacin leaves the realm of nutrition to become a pharmacological agent, a drug. As with any drug, self dosing with niacin is ill advised; large doses may injure the liver, cause ulcers, and produce some symptoms of diabetes.

FOLATE AND VITAMIN B_{12}. The vitamin **folate** is required to make all new cells. Deficiencies may result from an inadequate intake, impaired absorption, increased excretion, or increased metabolic need for the vitamin. Many medications can impair folate status; ten major groups of drugs have been shown to interfere with the body's use of folate, including aspirin and its relatives, anticonvulsants, and oral contraceptives.[19] Deficiencies cause anemia and abnormal digestive function (recall that the blood cells and digestive tract cells divide most rapidly and so are most vulnerable to deficiency). In the United States a significant number of cases of folate-deficiency anemia occur yearly, especially among pregnant women and people with alcoholism.

Folate, with the help of **vitamin B_{12}**, works to make red blood cells. Vitamin B_{12} also serves the body alone in helping maintain the sheaths that surround and protect nerve fibers. It also may influence the cells that build bone tissue.[20] A deficiency of vitamin B_{12} often expresses itself in the blood as an anemia identical to that caused by folate deficiency. This is because without sufficient vitamin B_{12}, folate fails to do its blood-building work. Giving extra folate will clear up this blood condition, but it is a poor choice, for the deficiency of vitamin B_{12} can continue, undetected. Vitamin B_{12}'s other functions then become compromised and the results can be devastating—damaged nerve sheaths, creeping paralysis, and general malfunctioning of nerves and muscles. The name **pernicious anemia** is given to the condition of anemia caused by vitamin B_{12} malabsorption because of the hidden, sneaky, and frightening way in which vitamin B_{12} deficiency damages the nerves, even after extra folate has normalized the blood.

The blood symptoms of deficiencies of either folate or vitamin B_{12} include the presence of large, immature red blood cells. However, if the anemia of

niacin equivalents: the amount of niacin present in food, including the niacin that can theoretically be made from its precursor tryptophan present in the food.

folate (FOH-late), **folacin,** or **folic acid:** a B vitamin that acts as part of a coenzyme important in the manufacture of new cells.

vitamin B_{12}: a B vitamin that enables folate to get into cells and also helps maintain the sheath around nerve cells. Vitamin B_{12}'s scientific name is cyanocobalamin.

pernicious (per-NISH-us) **anemia:** vitamin B_{12} deficiency disease, caused by B_{12} malabsorption and characterized by large, immature red blood cells and damage to the nervous system undetectable by blood tests.

■■■ Figure 7–7

Pellagra. The typical dermatitis of pellagra develops on skin that is exposed to light.

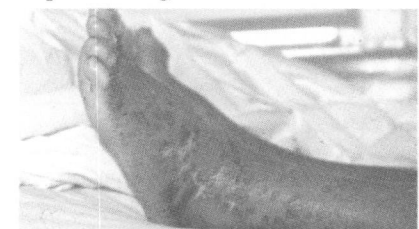

intrinsic factor: a factor found inside a system. The intrinsic factor necessary to prevent pernicious anemia is now known to be a compound that helps in the absorption of vitamin B_{12}.

vitamin B_6: a B vitamin. Its three active forms are *pyridoxine*, *pyridoxal*, and *pyridoxamine*.

vitamin B_{12} deficiency has been treated, mistakenly, by administering folate, the blood cells may appear normal. Then only the nerve damage caused by vitamin B_{12} deficiency might cue the physician to the problem, but it is hard to diagnose correctly. More likely, the damage will proceed unchecked.[21] Because of the danger of its masking vitamin B_{12} deficiency, the amount of folate in over-the counter vitamin preparations is limited by law.[22] In some cases, even without high folate intakes, vitamin B_{12} deficiency may not produce blood symptoms. Especially in people suffering from psychiatric disorders, nerve damage from vitamin B_{12} deficiency may be difficult to diagnose, and effective treatment can be tragically delayed.

Vitamin B_{12} is present only in animal tissues, not in plants. This places the uninformed, strict vegetarian at special risk. People who give up all foods of animal origin may not show signs of deficiency right away because up to five years' worth of vitamin B_{12} can be stored in the body; but eventually signs develop.[24] Additionally, vegetarians are most likely to be well supplied with folate because, as its name, derived from the word *foliage*, implies, folate is abundant in vegetables and fruits. A pregnant or lactating woman who is eating such a diet should be aware that her infant can develop a vitamin B_{12} deficiency, even if the mother remains healthy. A deficiency of this vitamin can cause irreversible nervous system damage in the infant, and this may be the first sign of the deficiency. All strict vegetarian mothers must be sure to use B_{12}-fortified products or to take the appropriate supplements. The Food Feature mentions some vitamin B_{12} sources for the vegetarian.

The absorption of vitamin B_{12} requires an **intrinsic factor**—a compound made inside the body. The design for this factor is carried in the genes. The intrinsic factor is synthesized in the stomach, where it attaches to the vitamin; the complex then passes to the small intestine and is absorbed into the bloodstream. A few people have an inherited abnormality of the gene for intrinsic factor, usually first observed in midlife. Without normal intrinsic factor for absorption of vitamin B_{12} in food, they develop deficiency symptoms. In this case or in the case of stomach injury that limits production of intrinsic factor, vitamin B_{12} must be supplied by injection to bypass the defective digestive system.

The way folate masks the anemia of vitamin B_{12} deficiency underlines a point already made several times. It takes a skilled professional to make a correct diagnosis, and the risk you take when you diagnose yourself or listen to would-be experts is clearly serious. A second point should also be underlined here. Since vitamin B_{12} deficiency in the body may be caused either by a lack of the vitamin in the diet or by a lack of intrinsic factor necessary to absorb it, a change in diet alone may not correct it—another reason for seeking professional diagnosis of physical symptoms.

VITAMIN B_6, BIOTIN, AND PANTOTHENIC ACID. Most of the B vitamins are toxic in excess. A particularly notable example—that of **vitamin B_6**—is described in the accompanying Consumer Caution, "Vitamin B_6 Supplements." Others are in the summary tables at the end of the chapter, and safe doses are listed in Controversy 7.

In the cells, vitamin B_6 helps to change one kind of amino acid, of which cells have an abundance, to others that the cells need more of. It also aids in the conversion of tryptophan to niacin and plays important roles in the synthesis of hemoglobin. It also assists in releasing stored glucose from glycogen and is thus important in regulating blood glucose.

■■■ **Figure 7–8**

Vitamin B_6 Deficiency. In this dermatitis, the skin is greasy and flaky, unlike the skin affected by the dermatitis of pellagra.

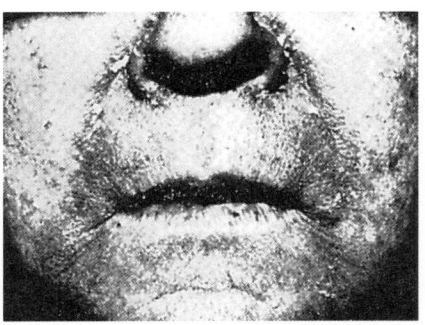

Because of these diverse functions, vitamin B_6 deficiency is expressed in general symptoms, such as depression, nausea, and vomiting. Other symptoms include the greasy skin rash shown earler, and irritation of the nerves. A shortage of vitamin B_6 also impairs the immune response.

Two other B vitamins, **biotin** and **pantothenic acid**, are important in metabolism. Biotin is a cofactor for several enzymes in the metabolism of carbohydrate, fat, and protein. Pantothenic acid is a component of a key coenzyme that makes possible the release of energy from the energy nutrients. Although rare diseases may precipitate deficiencies of biotin and pantothenic acid, both vitamins are widespread in foods, and healthy people eating ordinary diets are not at risk for deficiencies.

❚❚▶ *Historically famous vitamin B deficiency diseases are beriberi (thiamin), pellagra (niacin), and pernicious anemia (vitamin B_{12}). Pellagra can be prevented by adequate protein because the amino acid tryptophan can be converted to niacin in the body. A high intake of folate can mask the blood symptom of pernicious anemia but will not prevent the associated nerve damage. Vitamin B_6 is currently promoted for many questionable uses. Biotin and pantothenic acid are important to the body and are abundant in food.*

---

biotin (BY-o-tin): a B vitamin; a coenzyme necessary for fat synthesis and other metabolic reactions.

pantothenic (PAN-to-THEN-ic) **acid:** a B vitamin.

Chinese restaurant syndrome: an intolerance reaction that may occur in one out of several hundred people 20 minutes after the ingestion of the additive MSG (monosodium glutamate, or Accent). Symptoms include burning sensations, chest and facial flushing and pain, and throbbing headache. A *syndrome* is a cluster of symptoms.

CONSUMER CAUTION❚❙❙ Vitamin B_6 Supplements

Juanita gets sick in Chinese restaurants; Joann has pain in her left hand. Harriet is taking oral contraceptives, and James has had a heart attack and fears another. George has sores in his mouth, Angela is becoming senile, and Margie feels miserable before her menstrual period. What do all these people have in common? All are taking 1 gram/day of vitamin B_6 supplements. Some of them are getting better, and some are getting sicker because they are beginning to overdose.

Chinese restaurant syndrome is a sensitivity to the flavor enhancer monosodium glutamate (MSG) used in Asian cookery. The symptoms are warmth, stiffness, weakness, and tingling in the limbs; chest and facial flushing; headaches; light headedness; and stomachaches or sensations like heartburn. In 1981 a group of researchers, speculating that Chinese restaurant syndrome might be caused by vitamin B_6 deficiency, tested 27 students with poor vitamin B_6 status who proved sensitive to MSG. The researchers gave vitamin B_6 (50-milligram doses each day for three months) to nine of the students and an inert placebo (see pages 10, 12) to the other three without telling them which was which. At the end of that time, eight of the nine who had received the vitamin were no longer sensitive to MSG, while all three of the untreated subjects still reacted adversely to it.

People have concluded that Chinese restaurant syndrome was caused by vitamin B_6 deficiency, and it seems possible that some cases are. But the experiment shows clearly that some also are not. Although eight out of nine people improved with vitamin B_6 treatment, one subject's reaction didn't change. The dose that relieved deficiency was 50 milligrams a day. Juanita

continued on the next page

carpal tunnel syndrome: tingling and numbness in part of the hand and wrist and shooting pains up the arm caused by swelling of tissue surrounding a nerve that passes through the wrist bones. Possible causes include fluid accumulation and hormone imbalances as well as vitamin B_6 deficiency.

should not be taking a gram a day of vitamin B_6—that's 1000 milligrams, 20 times more than the therapeutic dose, and it isn't even clear that she has a deficiency. Any responsible clinician would test her directly to see.

In **carpal tunnel syndrome**, a tendon in the wrist tightens on the nerves of the hand, causing excruciating pain. Surgery is often needed to relieve it. However, in 1978 a case was reported in which a 40-year-old man with carpal tunnel syndrome gained relief by taking supplements of 100 milligrams/day of vitamin B_6 for ten weeks. At the same time a vitamin B_6-dependent enzyme in his red blood cells went from abnormal to normal in its action. When he was given a placebo for nine weeks, both his physical state and the enzyme activity deteriorated; when he was given the real vitamin again, both became normal.

The researchers who reported this case also reviewed evidence that other people with carpal tunnel syndrome might have vitamin B_6 deficiencies. They also found clearly that there were other causes of the syndrome in other cases. Joann should not blindly self-prescribe vitamin B_6 without first receiving testing and a diagnosis.

Harriet began taking vitamin B_6 supplements when she learned that hormones in oral contraceptives alter the body's handling of the amino acid tryptophan and that vitamin B_6 assists in its metabolism. When women on oral contraceptives take an added 5 milligrams of vitamin B_6, normal tryptophan handling resumes. This suggests but does not prove that women on oral contraceptives have a vitamin B_6 requirement greater than the RDA of 1.6 milligrams/day, although not greater than 5 milligrams. Larger doses can bring on altered hormone action that could interfere with the oral contraceptive's effectiveness as well as produce toxic effects. Like the other enthusiasts in this story, Harriet should be tested for a B_6 need, and she is way out on a limb in taking 1000 rather than 5 milligrams a day.

With respect to heart disease, vitamin B_6 deficiencies have been linked to injuries in the arteries of animals. Occasional reports surface of low vitamin B_6 status in heart attack victims, but researchers must still determine whether the low levels were caused *by* the heart attack, caused it, or just coincided with it. High doses of the vitamin (perhaps 40 milligrams/day) may modify a blood protein that acts in blood clotting. The tests showing this effect were performed on blood samples in test tubes, however, not in human beings, so many more experiments are needed to determine safety or effectiveness of vitamin B_6 supplements in preventing clotting. James needs a test to see if his vitamin B_6 status is normal. Only if he had blood enzyme levels consistent with a deficiency would he be justified in taking supplements—and then not megadoses, just therapeutic doses.

Oral lesions can also be a manifestation of vitamin B_6 deficiency. However, practically every nutrient deficiency and many other conditions also cause oral lesions. Their presence indicates George's need for a diagnosis, not a need for vitamin B_6.

As for vitamin B_6 and senility, a deficiency has been shown to change the brain cells of rats in ways that suggest premature aging; and it is known that older people have an increased likelihood of vitamin B_6 deficiency. But to demonstrate degenerative brain changes in animals, the researchers had to

continued on the next page

deprive them almost totally of the vitamin; total absence of the vitamin is *not* seen in human populations and is surely not the case for Angela. (On the other hand, people live much longer than rats, so time is available for the effects of slight vitamin deficiency to accumulate.) Angela should certainly be checked for vitamin B$_6$ deficiency—but then, her entire nutrition profile should be studied, and she should also be questioned about fluid intake, chest infections, urinary tract infections, depression, use of medications, alcohol use, exercise habits, and other possibilities.

What about vitamin B$_6$ and Margie's premenstrual syndrome (PMS)? No one, as of this writing, knows what causes PMS. Chapter 13 devotes a section to PMS and nutrition from which you might conclude that Margie needs no supplements but just good food.

Taking excess vitamin B$_6$ may be dangerous. Women who took more than 2 grams/day of vitamin B$_6$ for two months or more attempting to cure the edema of PMS developed numb feet, then lost sensation in their hands, then became unable to work. Later, in some cases, their mouths became numb. At the last report, although their symptoms had been improving after withdrawal of the supplements, it was unknown whether they had incurred irreversible nerve damage.

From other studies doses as low as 200 milligrams, taken for a long time, have caused "pins and needles," numbness of the hands, difficulty walking, and other symptoms, and some do not completely disappear when the supplements are withdrawn. Sometimes symptoms associated with PMS improve or disappear on *stopping* ingestion of the vitamin: depression, headaches, tiredness, bloatedness, irritability, and nerve malfunction.

Deficiencies of vitamin B$_6$ do exist in our population, but if you or anyone you know suspects a vitamin B$_6$ deficiency, consult a registered dietitian (RD) and a physician. If they have reason to believe you have a vitamin B$_6$ deficiency, *and once they have excluded other diagnoses*, they will recommend a therapeutic dose supplement for a time—probably 50 to 200 milligrams for not more than six to ten weeks. Meanwhile they will counsel you on improving your diet so that continued supplementation will not be necessary.

SOURCES: Possible vitamin B$_6$ deficiency uncovered in persons with the "Chinese restaurant syndrome," *Nutrition Reviews* 40 (1982): 15–16; K. Folkers, Biochemical evidence for a deficiency of vitamin B$_6$ in the carpal tunnel syndrome based on a crossover clinical study, *Proceedings of the National Academy of Sciences USA* 75 (1978): 3410–3412; The vitamin B$_6$ requirement in oral contraceptive users, *Nutrition Reviews* 37 (1979): 344–345; Does pyridoxal phosphate have a non-coenzymatic role in steroid hormone action? *Nutrition Reviews* 38 (1980): 93–95; J. E. Leklem and R. D. Reynolds, eds., *Clinical and Physiological Applications of Vitamin B-6. Current Topics in Nutrition and Disease* (abstract). *Journal of the American Dietetic Association* 89 (1989): 586,589; Inhibition of platelet aggregation and clotting by pyridoxal-5'-phosphate, *Nutrition Reviews* 40 (1982): 55–57; S. Bapurao, L. Raman, and P. G. Tulpule, Biochemical assessment of vitamin B$_6$ nutritional status in pregnant women with orolingual manifestations, *American Journal of Clinical Nutrition* 36 (1982): 581–586; E. J. Root and J. B. Longenecker, Brain cell alterations suggesting premature aging induced by dietary deficiency of vitamin B$_6$ and/or copper, *American Journal of Clinical Nutrition* 37 (1983): 540–552; S. C. Vir and A. H. G. Love, Vitamin B$_6$ status of the hospitalized aged, *American Journal of Clinical Nutrition* 31 (1978): 1383–1391; H. Schaumberg and coauthors, Sensory neuropathy from pyridoxine abuse, *New England Journal of Medicine* 309 (1983): 445–448; More B$_6$ toxicity reported, *Nutrition Forum*, November 1985, p. 84; K. Dalton, Pyridoxine overdose in premenstrual syndrome, *Lancet*, 18 (1985): 1168–1169.

inositol (in-OSS-ih-tall): a nonessential nutrient.

lipoic (lip-OH-ic) acid: a nonessential nutrient.

choline (KOH-leen): a nonessential nutrient.

nonvitamins: compounds that have known functions in the body, but that are not essential nutrients. Nonvitamins are often misrepresented by quacks and sold as essential nutrients.

acetylcholine (ASS-uh-teel-KOH-leen): a transmitter of nerve-to-nerve messages within the brain, a substance that can be made from dietary choline.

Non-B Vitamins

The section on the B vitamins has left a few compounds unrecognized that are sometimes *called* B vitamins. These are **inositol**, **lipoic acid**, and **choline**. They might more appropriately be called **nonvitamins** because they are not essential nutrients for human beings. Deficiencies can be induced in laboratory animals for experimental purposes, however. Like the B vitamins described above, they serve as coenzymes in metabolism. Even if they were essential in human nutrition, supplements would be unnecessary because they are abundant in foods. Choline has an interesting role with respect to a special kind of memory defect in the elderly, however, that is worth a moment of attention.

The nerves that are responsible for the storage and retrieval of information in the brain rely on chemicals to transmit their signals. One of these transmitter chemicals is **acetylcholine**, which is made from choline. Normally the brain has to make all such substances for itself because it is shielded from the rest of the body by a protective barrier that won't allow changed concentrations of chemicals in the blood to affect the brain. There are only a few exceptions, among them, a few drugs such as alcohol and narcotics, and choline. High doses of choline given to animals raise the blood concentration, and this raises the brain concentration higher than normal, stimulating the brain to synthesize more acetylcholine as a result. Other neurotransmitters that respond this way to diet were described in Controversy 6.

Some elderly people develop Alzheimer's disease, a progressive impairment of memory that can lead over several years' time to total incapacity to care for themselves. Some work suggests that the progress of this disease may be slowed or halted by large doses of choline. The researchers working with it emphasize that this is not a deficiency disease but that they are simply taking advantage of a curiosity of the brain to treat nonnutritional diseases. Poor memory from poor circulation, brain damage, social isolation, or other causes would not be helped by choline.

Another specific use of choline is for clients with mental disorders who have been treated for a long time with the major psychoactive drugs. In reaction to the drugs they develop bizarre movements of the facial muscles, and this side effect seems to be countered by choline. Both of these uses of choline are instances of nonnutrition therapies developed out of the discovery that large doses of a normal substance may sometimes have unexpected, beneficial, drug-like effects. It is still too early to say, however, whether these treatments may also incur some risk.

In addition to choline, inositol, and lipoic acid, other substances have been mistaken for essential nutrients for people because they are needed for growth by bacteria or other life forms. These substances include PABA (para-aminobenzoic acid), bioflavonoids ("vitamin P" or hesperidin), and ubiquinone (coenzyme Q). Other names you may hear are "vitamin B_{15}," or pangamic acid (a hoax); "vitamin B_{17}" (laetrile or amygdalin, not a cancer cure and not a vitamin by any stretch of the imagination); "vitamin B_T" (carnitine, an important piece of cell machinery but not a vitamin); and more.

▌▌▶ *Many substances people claim are B vitamins are not, although some may have nonnutrient effects or be useful as drugs. Among them are inositol, lipoic acid, and choline.*

Vitamin C

Two hundred-odd years ago, any man who joined the crew of a seagoing ship knew he had only half a chance of returning alive—not because he might be slain by pirates or die in a storm but because he might contract **scurvy**, a dread disease that might kill as many as two-thirds of a ship's men on a long voyage. Only ships that sailed on short voyages, especially around the Mediterranean Sea, were safe from this disease. It was not known at the time that the special hazard of long ocean voyages was that the ship's cook used up his fresh fruits and vegetables early and relied for the duration of the voyage on cereals and live animals.

The first nutrition experiment to be conducted on human beings was devised nearly 250 years ago to find a cure for scurvy. A British physician divided some sailors with scurvy into groups. Each group received a different test substance: vinegar, sulfuric acid, seawater, oranges, or lemons. The ones receiving the citrus fruits were cured within a short time. Sadly, it was 50 years before the British Navy made use of the information and required all its vessels to provide lime juice to every sailor daily. The term *limey* was applied to the British sailors in mockery because of this requirement. The name later given to the vitamin, **ascorbic acid**, literally means "no scurvy."

Vitamin C is required for the production and maintenance of **collagen**, a protein substance that forms the base for all connective tissues in the body— bones, teeth, skin, and tendons. Collagen forms the scar tissue that heals wounds, the reinforcing structure that mends fractures, and the supporting material of capillaries that prevents bruises. Besides helping to produce and to maintain collagen, adequate vitamin C is necessary to protect against infections and to promote the absorption of iron.

Many substances found in foods and important in the body can be destroyed by oxidation. Remember the role of vitamin E in protecting fat-soluble substances. Vitamin C works in much the same way with water-soluble substances, protecting them from oxidation by being oxidized itself instead. The vitamin is also important to the production of thyroxin, the hormone that regulates basal metabolic rate and body temperature.

In times of stress, the supply of vitamin C is depleted because it is involved in the release of the stress hormones from the adrenal gland. Vitamin makers have used this fact to sell "stress-formula" supplements that are largely vitamin C with B vitamins added. In truth, the amount of extra vitamin C used up during stress is so small that it is well within the safety margin of the RDA. If you are under stress (and who isn't?), generous servings of vitamin C-rich fruits and vegetables will more than cover your needs.

Most of the symptoms of scurvy can be attributed to the breakdown of collagen in the absence of vitamin C: loss of appetite, growth cessation, tenderness to touch, weakness, bleeding gums (shown here in Figure 7–9), loose teeth, swollen ankles and wrists, and tiny red spots in the skin where blood has leaked out of capillaries. One symptom, anemia, reflects an important role already mentioned—that vitamin C helps the body to absorb and to use iron (see Chapter 8).

In the United States scurvy is seldom seen today except in some bottle-fed infants, in elderly men, and in people addicted to alcohol. Breast milk supplies enough vitamin C, but infants who receive no vitamin C in formula, fruit juice,

scurvy: the vitamin C deficiency disease.

ascorbic acid: one of the active forms of vitamin C (the other is dehydroascorbic acid). Many people refer incorrectly to all vitamin C by the name *ascorbic acid*.

collagen (COLL-a-jen): the chief protein of most connective tissues, including scars, ligaments, and tendons, and the underlying matrix on which bones and teeth are built.

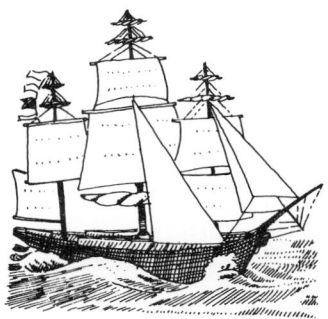

Long voyages without fresh fruits and vegetables spelled death by scurvy for the crew.

■■■ **Figure 7–9**

Scurvy. Vitamin C deficiency causes breakdown of collagen, which supports the teeth.

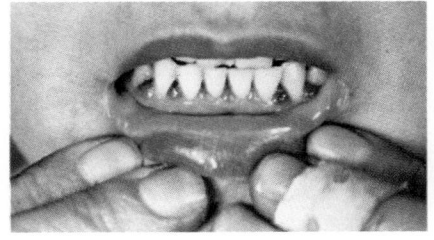

■■■ **Figure 7–10**

Vitamin C Recommendations from Several Sources

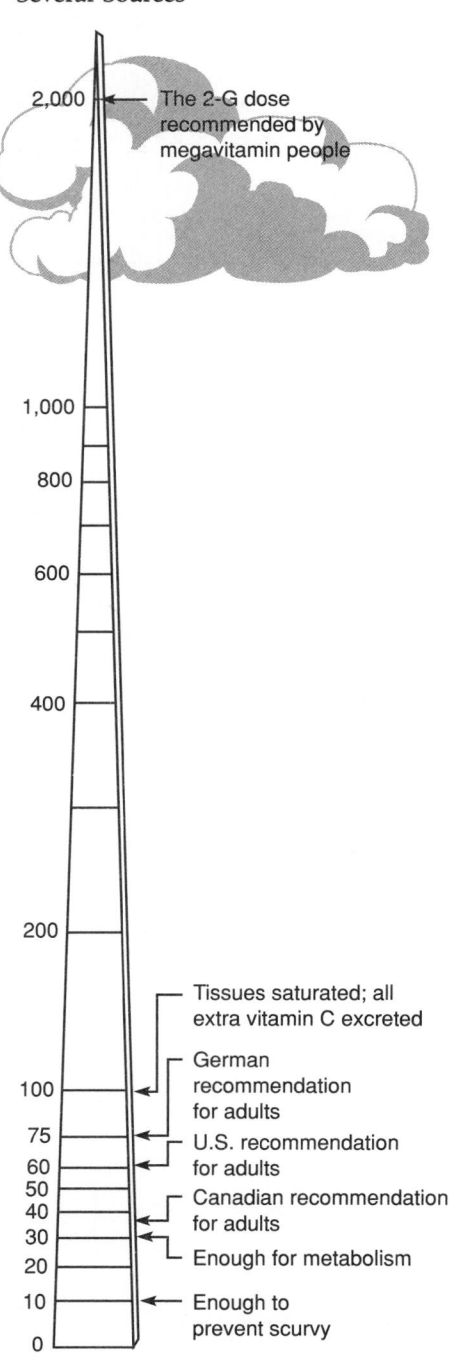

or other outside sources are at risk. By six months of age, babies should be guaranteed enough vitamin C by also having some fruits and vegetables in their diets. Elderly people may develop an aversion to "acid foods" that bring on heartburn and thus restrict their intakes of vitamin C. What appears to be age-related confusion or walking problems may in fact be the onset of scurvy and would be easily reversed with vitamin C therapy.[25] People addicted to alcohol rarely eat enough food to meet their needs and thus may suffer from a number of nutrient deficiencies, including scurvy.

Researchers find evidence of subclinical vitamin C deficiency in some groups of people, particularly teenage boys who do not eat fruits, vegetables, or salads and elderly men who cook for themselves. Smoking cigarettes, among its many harmful effects, interferes with the use of vitamin C. Taking extra vitamin C can normalize blood levels but cannot protect against the damage caused by smoking.

The adult RDA for vitamin C of 60 milligrams is midway between two extremes. At one extreme is the requirement, 10 milligrams per day, which is all you need to prevent the symptoms of scurvy from appearing. At the other extreme is the amount at which the body's pool of vitamin C is full to overflowing: about 100 milligrams per day. The RDA for smokers is set at the high end, 100 milligrams, because this amount is needed to maintain blood levels comparable to those of nonsmokers.[26] Other authorities have set different standards; for example, Canada recommends 30 milligrams per day and Germany 75. The differences between these recommendations may seem large, but when you consider that vitamin C intakes from foods can easily vary from below 10 to over 1000 milligrams (1 gram) a day, you can see that the official recommendations are all within the same rather narrow range (Figure 7–10).

An advocate of the taking of large doses of vitamin C is Dr Linus Pauling, whose first popular book, *Vitamin C and the Common Cold*, came out in 1970. According to Pauling, much larger quantities than the RDA enable the vitamin to protect cells from attack by cold viruses. Pauling advocates taking 1 or 2 grams (1000 to 2000 milligrams) of vitamin C per day, about 20 to 40 times the RDA.

Many controlled, double-blind studies on vitamin C and colds have been performed since Dr Pauling's controversial first book came out. Taken together, they show that the effects of vitamin C, if any, are statistically very small. This does not exclude the possibility that the effects on a few individuals might be considerable, especially if their vitamin C intakes have been low. Research on such effects is difficult to perform because people tend to be influenced by what they expect from their medicine. In one now classic study, a questionnaire given at the end revealed that the subjects who received **placebos** who thought they were receiving vitamin C had fewer colds than the group receiving vitamin C who thought they were receiving placebos.[27] The **placebo effect** can sometimes be a more effective cure than any medicine.

Pauling and others have also suggested that vitamin C megadoses might be effective against cancer, but careful research using 10-gram/day doses of the vitamin on people with advanced cancer has shown no difference in either symptoms or survival time. Vitamin C as a cancer cure thus seems hopeless. However, no one questions the need for adequate amounts of vitamin C to defend the body against the onset of cancer.

The widespread use of megadoses of vitamin C has enabled researchers to study their toxic effects. Effects that are theoretically possible (but that have not been seen with intakes as high as 3 grams a day) include formation of kidney stones, upset of the acid-base balance, destruction of vitamin B_{12}, and interference with the action of vitamin E.

Other toxic effects, however, have been seen often enough to warrant concern. Nausea, abdominal cramps, and diarrhea are often reported. Several instances of interference with medical regimens are known. The large amounts of vitamin C excreted in the urine can obscure the results of tests used to detect diabetes, giving a false-positive result in some instances and a false-negative result in others. People taking medications to prevent blood clotting may unwittingly abolish their effect if they also take massive doses of vitamin C.

People of certain racial groups are more likely to be harmed by vitamin C megadoses than others. Some black Americans, Sephardic Jews, Asians, and members of other groups have an inherited enzyme deficiency that makes them susceptible to high doses of vitamin C, which can make their red blood cells burst, causing hemolytic anemia. Those with sickle-cell anemia may also be more vulnerable to megadoses of vitamin C. In sickle-cell anemia (see p. 157), red cells clump and clog capillaries. Those who have a tendency toward gout and those who break down vitamin C abnormally are more prone to forming stones if they take megadoses.

The published research on large doses of vitamin C reveals few instances in which taking more than 100 to 300 milligrams a day is beneficial. Adults may not be taking major risks if they dose themselves with 1 to 2 grams a day, but doses approaching 10 grams are clearly unsafe. In short, the range of safe vitamin C intakes seems to be broad. Between the absolute minimum of 10 milligrams a day and the reasonable maximum of 1000 milligrams, nearly everyone should be able to find a suitable intake. People who venture outside these limits do so at their own risk. Food sources such as those shown in the margin are always appropriate. The Food Feature offers suggestions on making the diet rich in vitamin C.

This chapter has treated all 13 of the vitamins. Tables 7–2 and 7–3 sum up the basic facts about each one.

▣▷ *Vitamin C, an antioxidant, is needed for proper maintenance of the connective tissue protein collagen, protects against infection, and helps in iron absorption. The theory that vitamin C prevents or cures colds or cancer is not well supported by research. Vitamin C megadoses may be hazardous; ample vitamin C can be obtained from foods.*

> **placebos** (plah-SEE-bows): inert, harmless substances that resemble medicine, used in research to distinguish the effects of faith and hope from the effects of the medicine.
>
> **placebo effect:** the healing effect that faith in medicine, even inert medicine, often has.

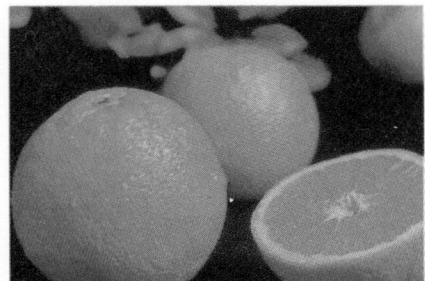

When nutritionists say "vitamin C," people think "oranges". . .

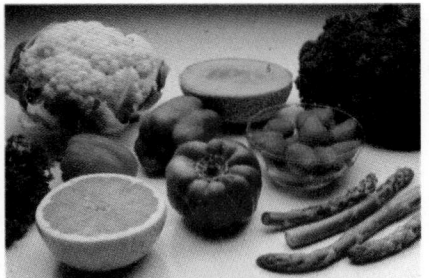

But these foods are richer in vitamin C for their calorie cost.

■■■ **Table 7-2 The Fat-Soluble Vitamins—A Summary**

VITAMIN NAMES	CHIEF FUNCTIONS IN THE BODY	DEFICIENCY DISEASE NAME	DEFICIENCY SYMPTOMS	TOXICITY SYMPTOMS	SIGNIFICANT SOURCES
Vitamin A (retinol, retinal, retinoic acid); precursor is provitamin A carotenoids such as beta carotene	Vision; maintenance of cornea, epithelial cells, mucous membranes, skin; bone and tooth growth; reproduction; hormone synthesis and regulation; immunity; cancer protection	Hypovitaminosis A	*Blood/Circulatory System*		Retinol: fortified milk, cheese, cream, butter, fortified margarine, eggs, liver
			Anemia (small-cell type)[a]	Red blood cell breakage, nosebleeds	
			Digestive System		Beta carotene: Spinach and other dark, leafy greens; broccoli; deep orange fruits (apricots, cantaloupe) and vegetables (squash, carrots, sweet potatoes, pumpkin)
			Diarrhea, general discomfort	Abdominal cramps and pain, nausea, vomiting, diarrhea, weight loss	
			Immune System		
			Depression; frequent respiratory, digestive, bladder, vaginal, and other infections	Overreactivity	
			Mouth, Gums, Teeth		
			Abnormal tooth and jaw alignment		
			Nervous/Muscular Systems		
			Night blindness (retinal)	Blurred vision, pain in calves, fatigue, irritability, loss of appetite, bone pain	
			Skin and Cornea		
			Keratinization, corneal degeneration leading to blindness,[b] rashes	Dry skin, rashes, loss of hair	
			Other		
			Kidney stones, impaired growth	Cessation of menstuation, growth retardation, liver and spleen enlargement	

[a]Small-cell anemia is termed *microcytic anemia;* large-cell type is *macrocytic* or *megaloblastic anemia.*
[b]Corneal degeneration progresses from *keratinization* (hardening) to *xerosis* (drying) to *xerophthalomia* (thickening, opacity, and irreversible blindness).

■■■ **Table 7–2** (continued)

VITAMIN NAMES	CHIEF FUNCTIONS IN THE BODY	DEFICIENCY DISEASE NAME	DEFICIENCY SYMPTOMS		TOXICITY SYMPTOMS	SIGNIFICANT SOURCES
Vitamin D (calciferol, cholecalciferol, dihydroxy-vitamin D); precursor is the body's' own cholesterol	Mineralization of bones (raises calcium and phosphorus blood levels by increasing absorption from digestive tract, withdrawing calcium from bones, stimulating retention by kidneys)	Rickets osteomalacia	*Blood/Circulatory System*		Raised blood calcium	Self-synthesis with sunlight; fortified milk, fortified margarine, eggs, liver, small fish (sardines)
			Digestive System		Constipation, weight loss	
			Nervous System		Excessive thirst, headaches, irritability, loss of appetite, weakness, nausea	
			Other			
			Abnormal growth, joint pain, soft bones		Kidney stones, stones in arteries, mental and physical retardation	
E (alpha-tocopherol, tocopherol)	Antioxidant (detoxification of strong oxidants), stabilization of cell membranes, regulation of oxidation reactions, protection of PUFA and vitamin A	(No name)	*Blood/Circulatory System*			Polyunsaturated plant oils (margarine, salad dressings, shortenings), green and leafy vegetables, wheat germ, whole-grain products, nuts, seeds
			Red blood cell breakage, anemia		Augments the effects of anticlotting medication	
			Digestive System		General discomfort	
			Nervous/Muscular Systems			
			Degeneration, weakness, difficulty walking, leg cramps			
			Other			
			Fibrocystic breast disease			
Vitamin K (phylloquinone, naphthoquinone)	Synthesis of blood-clotting proteins and a blood protein that regulates blood calcium	(No name)	*Blood/Circulatory System*			Bacterial synthesis in the digestive tract; liver, green leafy vegetables, cabbage-type vegetables, milk
			Hemorrhaging		Interference with anticlotting medication; vitamin K analogues may cause jaundice	

■■■ Table 7–3 The Water-Soluble Vitamins—A Summary

VITAMIN NAMES	CHIEF FUNCTIONS IN THE BODY	DEFICIENCY DISEASE NAME	DEFICIENCY SYMPTOMS	TOXICITY SYMPTOMS	SIGNIFICANT SOURCES
Thiamin (vitamin B₁)	Part of a coenzyme used in energy metabolism, supports normal appetite and nervous system function	Beriberi	*Blood/Circulatory System* Edema, enlarged heart, abnormal heart rhythms, heart failure	Rapid pulse	Occurs in all nutritious foods in moderate amounts; pork, ham, bacon, liver, whole grains, legumes, nuts
			Nervous/Muscular Systems Degeneration, wasting, weakness, pain, low morale, difficulty walking, loss of reflexes, mental confusion, paralysis	Weakness, headaches, insomnia, irritability	
Riboflavin (vitamin B₂)	Part of a coenzyme used in energy metabolism, supports normal vision and skin health	Ariboflavinosis	*Mouth, Gums, Tongue* Cracks at corners of mouth,ᶜ magenta tongue	(No symptoms reported)	Milk, yogurt, cottage cheese, meat, leafy green vegetables, whole-grain or enriched breads and cereals
			Nervous System and Eyes Hypersensitivity to light,ᵈ reddening of cornea		
			Other Skin rash	Interference with anticancer medication	
Niacin (nicotinic acid, nicotinamide, niacinamide, vitamin B₃; precursor is dietary tryptophan)	Part of a coenzyme used in energy metabolism; supports health of skin, nervous system, and digestive system	Pellagra	*Digestive System* Diarrhea	Diarrhea, heartburn, nausea, ulcer irritation, vomiting	Milk, eggs, meat, poultry, fish, whole grain and enriched breads and cereals, nuts, and all protein-containing foods
			Mouth, Gums, Tongue Black, smooth tongueᵉ		
			Nervous System Irritability, loss of appetite, weakness, dizziness, mental confusion progressing to psychosis or delirium	Fainting, dizziness	
			Skin Flaky skin rash on areas exposed to sun	Painful flush and rash ("niacin rush"), sweating	
			Other	Abnormal liver function, low blood pressure	

ᶜCracks at the corners of the mouth are termed *cheilosis* (kee-cOH-sis).
ᵈHypersensitivity to light is *photophobia*.
ᵉSmoothness of the tongue is caused by loss of its surface structures and is termed *glossitis* (gloss-EYE-tis).

■■■ Table 7–3 (continued)

VITAMIN NAMES	CHIEF FUNCTIONS IN THE BODY	DEFICIENCY DISEASE NAME	DEFICIENCY SYMPTOMS	TOXICITY SYMPTOMS	SIGNIFICANT SOURCES
Vitamin B_6 (pyridoxine, pyridoxal, pyridoxamine)	Part of a coenzyme used in amino acid and fatty acid metabolism, helps convert tryptophan to niacin, helps make red blood cells	(No name)	*Blood/Circulatory System*		Green and leafy vegetables, meats, fish, poultry, shellfish, legumes, fruits, whole grains
			Anemia (small-cell type)[a]	Bloating	
			Digestive System		
			Mouth, Gums, Tongue		
			Smooth tongue[e]		
			Nervous/Muscular Systems		
			Abnormal brain wave pattern, irritability, muscle twitching, convulsions	Depression, fatigue, impaired memory, irritability, headaches, numbness, damage to nerves, difficulty walking, loss of reflexes, weakness restlessness	
			Skin		
			Irritation of sweat glands, rashes, greasy dermatitis	"Pins and needles" sensation	
			Other		
			Kidney stones	Bone pain	
Folate (folic acid, folacin, pteroylglutamic acid)	Part of a coenzyme used in new cell synthesis	(No name)	*Blood Circulatory System*		Leafy green vegetables, legumes, seeds, liver
			Anemia (large-cell type)[a]		
			Digestive System		
			Heartburn, diarrhea, constipation	Diarrhea	
			Immune System		
			Depression, frequent infections		
			Mouth, Gums, Tongue		
			Smooth red tongue[e]		
			Nervous System		
			Depression, mental confusion, fainting	Insomnia, irritability	
			Other		
				Masking of vitamin B_{12} deficiency symptoms	

[a]Small-cell anemia is termed *microcytic anemia*; large-cell type is *macrocytic* or *megaloblastic anemia*.
[e]Smoothness of the tongue is caused by loss of its surface structures and is termed *glossitis* (gloss-EYE-tis).

VITAMIN NAMES	CHIEF FUNCTIONS IN THE BODY	DEFICIENCY DISEASE NAME	DEFICIENCY SYMPTOMS	TOXICITY SYMPTOMS	SIGNIFICANT SOURCES
Vitamin B_{12} (cyanocobalamin)	Part of a coenzyme used in new cell synthesis, helps maintain nerve cells	(No name[f])	*Blood/Circulatory System* Anemia (large-cell type)[a]	(No toxicity symptoms known)	Animal products (meat, fish, poultry, shellfish, milk, cheese, eggs)
			Mouth, Gums, Tongue Smooth tongue[e]		
			Nervous System Fatigue, degeneration progressing to paralysis		
			Skin Hypersensitivity		
Pantothenic acid	Part of a coenzyme used in energy metabolism	(No name)	*Digestive System* Vomiting, intestinal distress	Occasional diarrhea	Widespread in foods
			Nervous System Insomnia, fatigue		
			Other	Water retention (infrequent)	
Biotin	Part of a coenzyme used in energy metabolism, fat synthesis, amino acid metabolism, and glycogen synthesis	(No name)	*Blood/Circulatory System* Abnormal heart action	(No toxicity symptoms reported)	Widespread in foods
			Digestive System Loss of appetite, nausea		
			Nervous/Muscular Systems Depression, muscle pain, weakness, fatigue		
			Skin Drying, rash, loss of hair		
Vitamin C (ascorbic acid)	Collagen synthesis (strengthens blood vessel walls, forms scar tissue, matrix for bone growth), antioxidant, thyroxine synthesis, amino acid metabolism, strengthens resistance to infection, helps in absorption of iron	Scurvy	*Blood/Circulatory System* Anemia (small-cell type),[a] atherosclerotic plaques, pinpoint hemorrhages	Blood cell breakage in certain racial groups[g]	Citrus fruits, cabbage-type vegetables, dark green vegetables, cantaloupe, strawberries, peppers, lettuce, tomatoes, potatoes, papayas, mangos
			Digestive System	Nausea, abdominal cramps diarrhea, excessive urination	
			Immune System Depression, frequent infections		

[a] Small-cell anemia is termed *microcytic anemia;* large-cell type is *macrocytic* or *megaloblastic anemia.*
[e] Smoothness of the tongue is caused by loss of its surface structures and is termed *glossitis* (gloss-EYE-tis).
[f] The name *pernicious anemia* refers to the vitamin$_{12}$ deficiency caused by lack of intrinsic factor, but not to that caused by inadequate dietary intake.
[g] Groups susceptible to vitamin C toxicity are Sephardic Jews, Africans, and Asians.

■■■ Table 7–3 (continued)

VITAMIN NAMES	CHIEF FUNCTIONS IN THE BODY	DEFICIENCY DISEASE NAME	DEFICIENCY SYMPTOMS	TOXICITY SYMPTOMS	SIGNIFICANT SOURCES
Vitamin C (continued)			*Mouth, Gums, Tongue*		
			Bleeding gums, loosened teeth		
			Muscular/Nervous Systems		
			Muscle degeneration and pain, hysteria, depression	Headache, fatigue, insomnia	
			Skeletal System		
			Bone fragility, joint pain		
			Skin		
			Rough skin, blotchy bruises	Rashes	
			Other		
			Failure of wounds to heal	Interference with medical tests; aggravation of gout symptoms; deficiency symptoms may appear at first on withdrawal of high doses	

Food Feature

Choosing Foods Rich in Vitamins

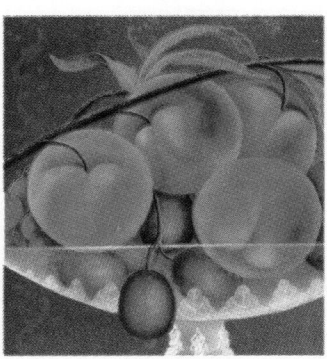

Most people, on learning of the importance of obtaining adequate vitamins, want to know if they are getting enough of them from their food. One way to tell is to look at the vitamins in a serving of some foods. This method is shown in Figure 7–11. (Another new way is to compare foods for vitamin richness on a per calorie basis; this method is shown later.) Overall, Figure 7–11 teaches that servings of a few foods stand out as excellent providers of certain nutrients, and most foods contribute to nutrient needs in a general way. Vitamin needs are generally best met by including a wide variety of foods in the context of the whole diet and not by single foods.

The colored bars on the right-hand side of Figure 7–11 show how much of a nutrient is in a serving of food as compared to the U.S. RDA. The colors represent the various food groups: blue is for the milks and milk products, green for vegetables, purple for fruits, brown for legumes, gold for breads and cereals, and red for meat, fish, and poultry. Except for liver, few foods consistently appear at the tops of the charts. For example, while orange juice ranks high on the vitamin C list, you would not want to rely on oranges for riboflavin. Variety in food choices remains a key to diet planning (Chapter 2).

For the most part, the serving sizes in these figures are those that people might realistically eat. For example, 3 ounces is used for most meats, and people wishing to compare these portions to exchanges in Appendix D can easily convert this to three lean meat exchanges. Similarly, the vegetable serving size is 1 cup instead of the one-half cup portions of the exchange lists.

Some people, after viewing a table such as this, are led to believe that to meet their vitamin needs, they must memorize the richest sources of each vitamin and include those foods daily. This is a false notion and can lead people to limit the variety of foods they choose while overemphasizing the components of a few foods. While it is reassuring to know that your carrot-raisin salad at lunch provided more than the entire U.S. RDA for vitamin A, it is a mistake to think that you must then go on to select equally rich sources of all the other vitamins. For one thing, such rich sources do not exist for many vitamins. For another, foods work in harmony to provide nutrients. For example, a baked potato, while not a star performer among vitamin C providers, contributes substantially to a day's need for this nutrient and contributes some thiamin too. By the end of the day, assuming that your food choices were made with reasonable care, the bits of thiamin, vitamin B$_6$, and vitamin C from each serving of food have built one on the other to construct a total, adequate diet.

About half of the vitamin A in foods consumed in the United States comes from vegetables and fruits, and half of this comes from the dark leafy greens (like spinach—not celery or cabbage) and the rich yellow or deep orange vegetables and fruit (such as winter squash, cantaloupe, carrots, and sweet potatoes—not corn or bananas). The other half of the vitamin A comes from milk, cheese, butter, and other dairy products, eggs, and liver. Since vitamin A is fat soluble, it is lost when milk is skimmed of its cream. To compensate, nonfat milk is often fortified with vitamin A.

The next two nutrients, thiamin and riboflavin, are among those added to refined grain foods in the enrichment process (see pages 93–95). While this does not make enriched foods rich sources of the vitamins, it does ensure that the thiamin and riboflavin in a serving of refined grain foods will equal those in whole-grain foods. For this reason, almost any bread would fall at about the same place on some of these graphs as does whole-grain bread.

With a few exceptions, nutritious foods generally provide small quantities of thiamin, as shown by Figure 7–11. A few meats are exceptionally good thiamin sources; these are members of the pork family. As you can see in the graph, one small pork chop (275 calories) provides over one-half the U.S. RDA for thiamin, but this should not suggest that you include pork with its accompanying saturated fat and cholesterol in your diet each day. Legumes and grains are also good, low-fat sources, and they provide beneficial fiber and nutrients often lacking in meat-rich diets. On the other hand, beans lack vitamin B_{12} provided by meats. Lean pork is nutritious, but, as with all meats, it provides maximum benefits when used in moderation within a diet built of a variety of foods. Peanut butter is a good source of thiamin, as it is of most B vitamins, but use it in moderation if you have to control calories.

As for riboflavin, certain meats, all milk products, and some vegetables make sizable contributions to the daily requirement. Like thiamin, most other foods donate at least some riboflavin, so that most days most people meet their needs without a special effort.

The vitamin B_6 data provide another twig to fuel the argument for variety. From just the few foods listed here, you can see that no one source can provide the whole day's requirement but that a variety of meats, fish, and poultry; potatoes; and a few vegetables and fruits can work together to supply it.

Folate and vitamin C are represented in foods in the last two graphs of Figure 7–11. These nutrients are both richly supplied by fruits and vegetables. The richest source of either may be only a moderate source of the other, but the recommended servings of fruits and vegetables in food group plans cover both needs amply. Note that the U.S. RDA for folate is twice most people's RDA. This is because the U.S. RDA were derived from the RDA tables of over 20 years ago when human needs were less precisely known. If you receive even half the U.S. RDA for this nutrient, most likely your need will be met.

The beginning of this Food Feature promised a new way to compare foods and the nutrients they contain. This way is especially meaningful to those who must limit their energy intakes. Table 7–4 compares how much of a vitamin foods contribute per calorie, or per 100 calories. When you compare foods on this basis, the vegetables suddenly assume considerably greater prominence as rich sources of all of the vitamins—especially useful if you like to consume large quantities of them.

This table is designed to reveal several things, but it is also intended to make you laugh. It shows how ridiculous it is to try to use any one food to meet a nutrient need—with the notable exceptions of vitamins A, folate, and vitamin C, which are concentrated in a few foods.

Just for fun, then, the right-hand side of each section shows how much of a serving of each food would deliver your entire need of the nutrient for the day—and for what calorie cost. Thus, for example, to get your vitamin A for the day, you could eat about a cup of almost any kind of dark green, leafy vegetables—but you could also eat half a carrot or 1 bite of fried beef liver. Vitamin A is clearly a nutrient that is easy to get in adequate amounts. Notice, though, that all the apples in Washington can't meet your need for vitamin A. Poor food sources of every vitamin have been included in every table to remind you to keep your diet balanced.

Thiamin presents a contrast. Again, this table shows that to meet your thiamin need, you have to do it by eating reasonable portions of several nutritious foods. A rule of thumb is that ten portions of nutritious foods will deliver a day's worth of thiamin. Inspection of the other tables will reveal other patterns of distribution of the vitamins in foods.

(Food Feature Continued)

Figure 7–11 Food Sources of Vitamins Selected to Show a Range of Values—Commonly Eaten Portions Ranked Richest to Poorest

Vitamin A

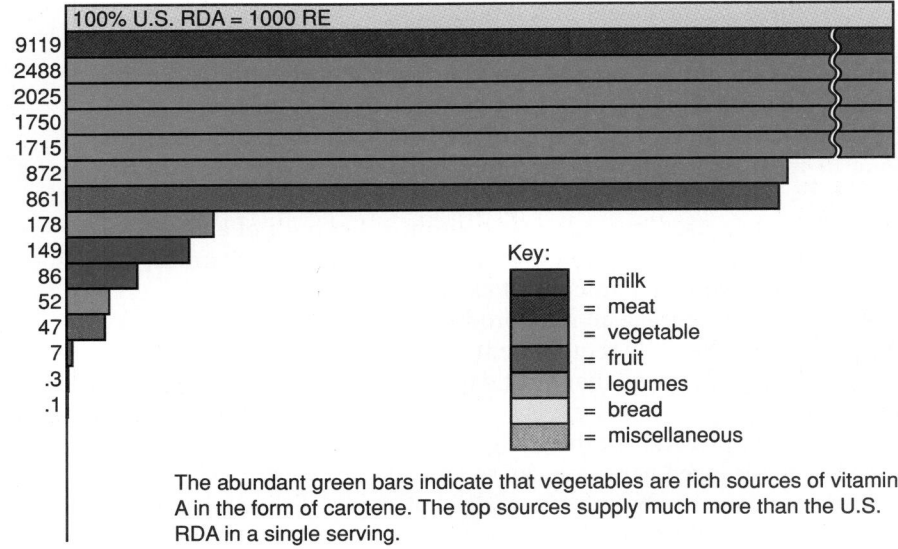

100% U.S. RDA = 1000 RE

Food, serving size (energy)	
Beef liver, 3 oz fried (185 cal)	9119
Sweet potato, 1 baked (118 cal)	2488
Carrot, 1 whole fresh (31 cal)	2025
Spinach, 1 c fresh cooked (41 cal)	1750
Butternut squash, 1 c baked (83 cal)	1715
Winter squash, 1 c mashed (96 cal)	872
Cantaloupe, 1/2 (94 cal)	861
Tomatoes, 1 c cooked (60 cal)	178
Milk or yogurt, 1 c nonfat (86 cal)	149
Cheddar cheese, 1 oz (114 cal)	86
Summer squash, 1 c cooked (36 cal)	52
Peach, 1 fresh medium (37 cal)	47
Apple, 1 fresh medium (80 cal)	7
Sirloin steak, 3 oz lean (180 cal)	.3
Whole-wheat bread, 1 slice (70 cal)	.1

Key:
= milk
= meat
= vegetable
= fruit
= legumes
= bread
= miscellaneous

The abundant green bars indicate that vegetables are rich sources of vitamin A in the form of carotene. The top sources supply much more than the U.S. RDA in a single serving.

Thiamin

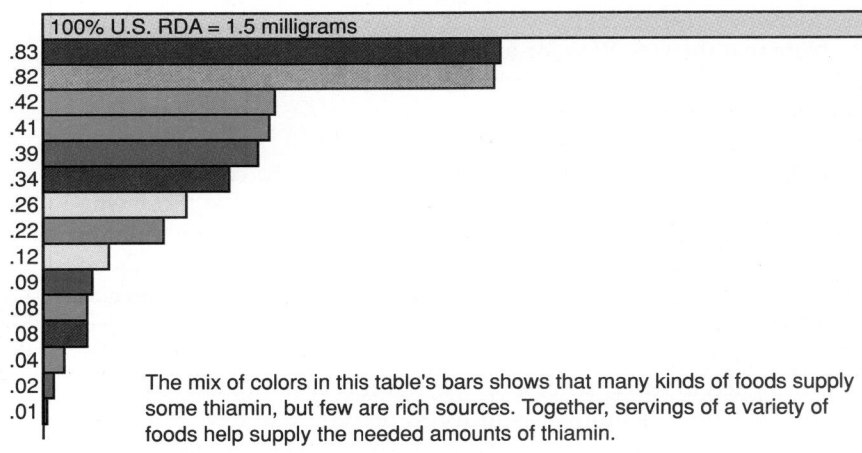

100% U.S. RDA = 1.5 milligrams

Food, serving size (energy)	
Pork chop, 3.1 oz broiled (275 cal)	.83
Sunflower seeds, 1/4 c dry (205 cal)	.82
Black beans, 1 c cooked (225 cal)	.42
Green peas, 1 c cooked (146 cal)	.41
Watermelon, 1 slice (152 cal)	.39
Oysters, 1 c raw (160 cal)	.34
Oatmeal, 1 c cooked (145 cal)	.26
Baked potato, 1 whole (220 cal)	.22
Whole-wheat bread, 1 slice (70 cal)	.12
Nonfat milk or yogurt, 1 c (86 cal)	.09
Summer squash, 1 c cooked (36 cal)	.08
Sirloin steak, 3 oz lean (180 cal)	.08
Cabbage, 1 c raw shredded (16 cal)	.04
Apple, 1 fresh medium (80 cal)	.02
Cheddar cheese, 1 oz (114 cal)	.01

The mix of colors in this table's bars shows that many kinds of foods supply some thiamin, but few are rich sources. Together, servings of a variety of foods help supply the needed amounts of thiamin.

Riboflavin

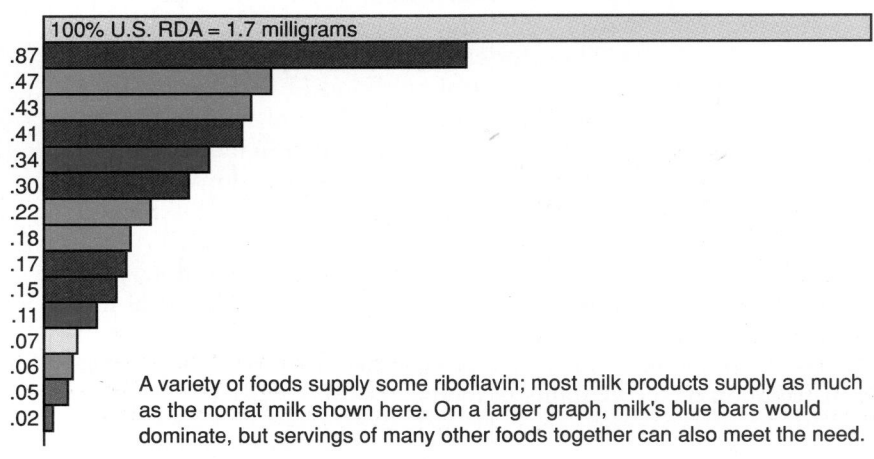

100% U.S. RDA = 1.7 milligrams

Food, serving size (energy)	
Liver sausage, 2 pieces (205 cal)	.87
Mushroom pieces, 1 c cooked (42 cal)	.47
Spinach, 1 c cooked (41 cal)	.43
Oysters, 1 c raw (160 cal)	.41
Milk or yogurt, 1 c nonfat (86 cal)	.34
Pork roast, 3 oz (187 cal)	.30
Asparagus, 1 c cooked (44 cal)	.22
Broccoli, 1 c cooked (46 cal)	.18
Sirloin steak, 3 oz lean (180 cal)	.17
Salmon, 3 oz smoked (150 cal)	.15
Cheddar cheese, 1 oz (114 cal)	.11
Whole-wheat bread, 1 slice (70 cal)	.07
Romaine lettuce, 1 c chopped (9 cal)	.06
Orange, 1 fresh medium (60 cal)	.05
Apple, 1 fresh medium (80 cal)	.02

A variety of foods supply some riboflavin; most milk products supply as much as the nonfat milk shown here. On a larger graph, milk's blue bars would dominate, but servings of many other foods together can also meet the need.

Vitamin B₆

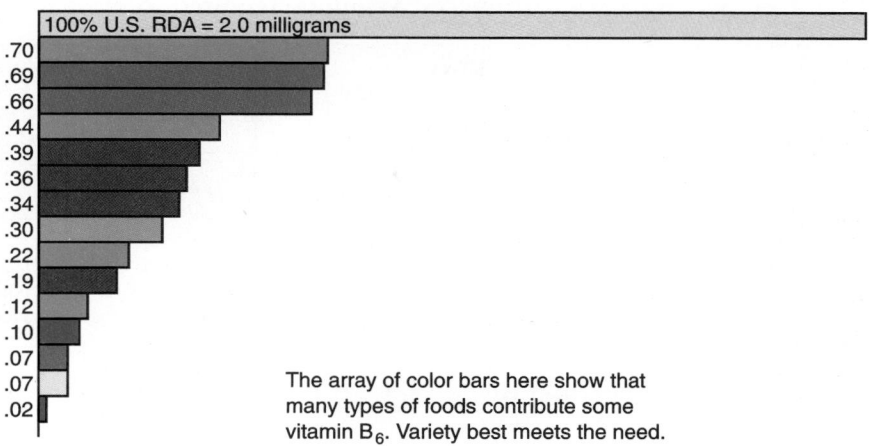

Food, serving size (energy)

Food	Value
Baked potato, 1 whole (220 cal)	.70
Watermelon, 1 slice (152 cal)	.69
Banana, 1 peeled (105 cal)	.66
Spinach, 1 c cooked (41 cal)	.44
Turkey, 3 oz (145 cal)	.39
Sirloin steak, 3 oz lean (180 cal)	.36
Pork chop, 3.1 oz broiled (275 cal)	.34
Navy beans, 1 c cooked (225 cal)	.30
Broccoli, 1 c cooked (46 cal)	.22
Salmon, 3 oz broiled/baked (140 cal)	.19
Summer squash, 1 c cooked (36 cal)	.12
Milk or yogurt, 1 c nonfat (86 cal)	.10
Apple, 1 fresh medium (80 cal)	.07
Whole-wheat bread, 1 slice (70 cal)	.07
Cheddar cheese, 1 oz (114 cal)	.02

100% U.S. RDA = 2.0 milligrams

The array of color bars here show that many types of foods contribute some vitamin B₆. Variety best meets the need.

Folate

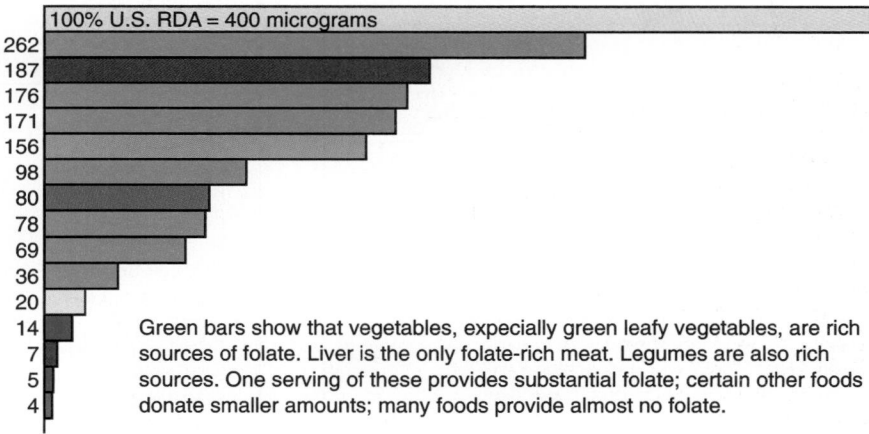

Food, serving size (energy)

Food	Value
Spinach, 1 c cooked (41 cal)	262
Beef liver, 3 oz fried (185 cal)	187
Asparagus, 1 c cooked (44 cal)	176
Turnip greens, 1 c cooked (29 cal)	171
Lima beans, 1 c cooked (217 cal)	156
Beets, 1 c cooked (52 cal)	98
Cantaloupe, 1/2 (94 cal)	80
Broccoli, 1 c cooked (46cal)	78
Winter squash, 1 c baked (96 cal)	69
Summer squash, 1 c baked (36 cal)	36
Whole-wheat bread, 1 slice (70 cal)	20
Milk or yogurt, 1 c nonfat (86 cal)	14
Sirloin steak, 3 oz lean (180 cal)	7
Cheddar cheese, 1 oz (114 cal)	5
Apple, 1 fresh medium (80 cal)	4

100% U.S. RDA = 400 micrograms

Green bars show that vegetables, expecially green leafy vegetables, are rich sources of folate. Liver is the only folate-rich meat. Legumes are also rich sources. One serving of these provides substantial folate; certain other foods donate smaller amounts; many foods provide almost no folate.

Vitamin C

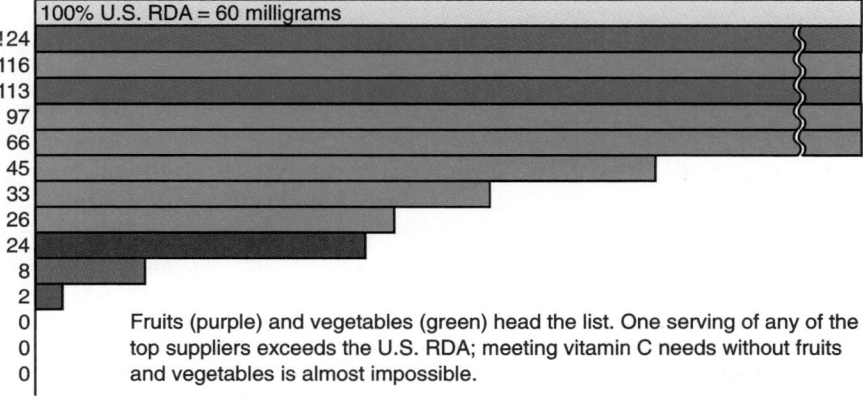

Food, serving size (energy)

Food	Value
Orange juice, 1 c fresh (111 cal)	124
Broccoli, 1 c cooked (46 cal)	116
Cantaloupe, 1/2 (94 cal)	113
Brussels sprouts, 1 c cooked (60 cal)	97
Green pepper, 1 whole (18 cal)	66
Tomato juice, 1 c canned (42 cal)	45
Cabbage, 1 c raw shredded (16 cal)	33
Baked potato, 1 whole (220 cal)	26
Oysters, 1 c raw (160 cal)	24
Apple, 1 fresh medium (80 cal)	8
Milk or yogurt, 1 c nonfat (86 cal)	2
Whole-wheat bread, 1 slice (70 cal)	0
Sirloin steak, 3 oz lean (180 cal)	0
Cheddar cheese, 1 oz (114 cal)	0

100% U.S. RDA = 60 milligrams

Fruits (purple) and vegetables (green) head the list. One serving of any of the top suppliers exceeds the U.S. RDA; meeting vitamin C needs without fruits and vegetables is almost impossible.

■■■ TABLE 7–4 Serving Sizes and Energy Amounts Required to meet the U.S. RDA from Single Sources

IF YOU WANTED 100% OF THE U.S. RDA OF VITAMIN A FROM THIS FOOD:	YOU WOULD HAVE TO EAT THIS SIZE SERVING:
Carrot, whole fresh	0.5 carrot (16 cal)
Beef liver, fried	0.3 oz (19 cal)
Dandelion green, cooked	0.8 c (28 cal)
Spinach, cooked	0.7 c (29 cal)
Turnip greens, cooked	1.3 c (38 cal)
Sweet potato, baked	0.4 potato (47 cal)
Butternut squash, baked	0.7 c (58 cal)
Cantaloupe melon	0.6 melon (113 cal)
Broccoli, cooked	4.5 c (207 cal)
Nonfat milk	6.7 c (576 cal)
Oysters, raw	4.5 c (720 cal)
Cheddar cheese	11 oz (1254 cal)
Apple, fresh medium	too much (too many cal)
Sirloin steak, lean	too much (too many cal)
Sole/flounder, baked	too much (too many cal)
Whole wheat bread	too much (too many cal)

IF YOU WANTED 100% OF THE U.S. RDA OF THIAMIN FROM THIS FOOD:	YOU WOULD HAVE TO EAT THIS SIZE SERVING:
Mushrooms, raw sliced	20 c (360 cal)
Green peas, cooked	3.2 c (403 cal)
Sunflower seeds, dry	0.5 c (410 cal)
Pork chop	5.3 oz (468 cal)
Broccoli, cooked	11c (506 cal)
Watermelon	3.8 sl (578 cal)
Turnip greens, cooked	20 c (580 cal)
Oysters, raw	5.3 c (848 cal)
Whole wheat bread	14 sl (980 cal)
Nonfat milk	17 c (1462 cal)
Sole/flounder, baked	100 oz (3960 cal)
Sirloin steak, lean	42 oz (2544 cal)
Apple, fresh medium	100 apples (8000 cal)
Cheddar cheese	too much (too many cal)

IF YOU WANTED 100% OF THE U.S. RDA OF RIBOFLAVIN FROM THIS FOOD:	YOU WOULD HAVE TO EAT THIS SIZE SERVING:
Beef liver, fried	1.4 oz (93 cal)
Mushroom pieces, cooked	3.7 c (155 cal)
Spinach, cooked	4 c (164 cal)
Broccoli, cooked	5.3 c (244 cal)
Dandelion greens, cooked	9 c (319 cal)
Braunschweiger sausage	4 (410 cal)
Nonfat milk	5 c (430 cal)
Oysters, raw	4 c (640 cal)
Cheddar cheese	9 oz (1026 cal)
Sirloin steak, lean	19.5 oz (1152 cal)
Ricotta cheese, part skim	3.7 c (1258 cal)
Whole wheat bread	25 sl (1750 cal)
Sole/flounder, baked	60 oz (2400 cal)
Apple, fresh medium	100 apples (8000 cal)

IF YOU WANTED 100% OF THE U.S. RDA OF VITAMIN B_6 FROM THIS FOOD:	YOU WOULD HAVE TO EAT THIS SIZE SERVING:
Spinach, cooked	4.5 c (185 cal)
Mustard greens, cooked	11 c (231 cal)
Cauliflower, cooked	8 c (240 cal)
Broccoli, cooked	6.3 c (290 cal)
Banana, peeled	3 banana (315 cal)
Watermelon	2.9 sl (441 cal)
Chicken breast, roasted	4 halves (568 cal)
Navy beans, cooked dry	2.8 c (630 cal)
Tuna, canned	14 oz (635 cal)
Baked potato, whole	2.9 potato (638 cal)
Sunflower seeds, dry	1 c (820 cal)
Sole/flounder, baked	21 oz (840 cal)
Sirloin steak, lean	20.5 oz (1248 cal)
Nonfat milk	20 c (1720 cal)
Apple, fresh medium	25 apples (2000 cal)
Whole wheat bread	33 sl (2310 cal)
Cheddar cheese	100 oz (11,400 cal)

The riboflavin part of the table illustrates another point. In Figure 7–11, meats and dairy products rank high on the list. In this table four of the top six are vegetables. The point is that while you *could* eat sirloin steak to meet your need for riboflavin, you would have to eat more than a pound to do so—together with more than 1000 calories. On the other hand, you could eat mushrooms (if you could wolf down 4 cups of them), and the accompanying calories would amount to only 155. Clearly vegetables (especially dark green vegetables) are a richer source of riboflavin *per calorie* than meats are, and a day's meals that included generous servings of several vegetables would make it unnecessary to include so much meat.

■■■ TABLE 7−4 continued

IF YOU WANTED 100% OF THE U.S. RDA OF FOLATE FROM THIS FOOD:	YOU WOULD HAVE TO EAT THIS SIZE SERVING:
Romaine lettuce, chopped	5.3 c (48 cal)
Spinach, cooked	1.5 c (62 cal)
Turnip greens, cooked	2.3 c (67 cal)
Parsley, chopped fresh	3.6 c (72 cal)
Asparagus, cooked	2.3 c (101 cal)
Broccoli, cooked	3.7 c (170 cal)
Mushrooms, raw sliced	25 c (450 cal)
Beef liver, fried	7.9 oz (481 cal)
Lima beans, cooked	2.3 c (598 cal)
Whole wheat bread	25 sl (1750 cal)
Nonfat milk	25 c (2150 cal)
Oysters, raw	17 c (2720 cal)
Apple, fresh medium	100 apples (8000 cal)
Sirloin steak, lean	10 lb (9600 cal)
Cheddar cheese	100 oz (11,400 cal)

IF YOU WANTED 100% OF THE U.S. RDA OF VITAMIN C FROM THIS FOOD:	YOU WOULD HAVE TO EAT THIS SIZE SERVING:
Green peppers, whole	0.6 pepper (11 cal)
Parsley, chopped fresh	1.2 c (24 cal)
Cauliflower, cooked	0.9 c (27 cal)
Broccoli, cooked	0.6 c (28 cal)
Strawberries, fresh	0.7 c (32 cal)
Papaya, whole fresh	0.3 papaya (35 cal)
Brussels sprouts, cooked	0.6 c (36 cal)
Mustard greens, cooked	1.8 c (38 cal)
Cantaloupe melon	¼ melon (47 cal)
Orange, fresh medium	0.9 orange (54 cal)
Grapefruit juice, fresh	0.6 c (58 cal)
Oysters, raw	0.8 c (128 cal)
Apple, fresh medium	7.7 apples (616 cal)
Nonfat milk	33 c (2838 cal)
Sole/flounder, baked	150 oz (6000 cal)
Cheddar cheese	too much (too many cal)
Whole wheat bread	too much (too many cal)

As for folate and vitamin C, any way you look at them, vegetables and fruits are the richest sources. Such analyses are enough to make even the most dedicated meat eater resolve to eat more vegetables and to illustrate that variety is needed to obtain such vitamins as B_6 that are more widely distributed.

Many people couldn't imagine eating large plates of vegetables, but from a nutrition standpoint, it makes sense. The calorie cost is almost nil; the nutrient contributions are highly significant; and the nutrients that are still needed can be obtained from economical portions of milk products, meats, and related foods. The pleasures of sweet or fat-containing foods can then be fitted in, within a reasonable calorie allowance, without incurring the price of obesity.

It also makes sense *not* to leave meats and animal products out of the diet altogether. Vitamin B_{12} is unique among the nutrients in being found almost exclusively in meats and animal products. Anyone who eats meat is guaranteed an adequate intake, and lacto-ovo vegetarians (who use milk, cheese, and eggs) are also protected from deficiency. But vegans must use vitamin B_{12}-fortified soy milk, some fermented foods, or other such products or take vitamin B_{12} supplements.

There is no limit to the amount that you can learn about the nutrient contents of foods from studying tables like these. People who enjoy that sort of thing continue picking up new bits of information throughout their lives ("Oh, mushrooms are the richest in thiamin per 100 calories?"). Table 7−4 shown here can only whet your appetite for more information (and vegetables); Appendix A shows the complete nutrient contents of more than 1000 foods.

▋▋▋ SELF-STUDY

Evaluate Your Vitamin Intakes

Several of these exercises make use of the information you recorded on Forms 1 to 3 in Appendix F.

1. Start with vitamin A. Compare your average intake with the standard (RDA or Recommended Nutrient Intakes [RNI]); you recorded these earlier on Form 3. What percentage of your recommended intake did you consume? Was this enough? What foods contribute the greatest amount of vitamin A to your diet? If you consumed more than the recommendation, was this too much? Why or why not? In what ways would you change your diet to improve vitamin A intake? Answer these same questions for thiamin, riboflavin, niacin, vitamin B_6, folate, and vitamin C.

Note on niacin: Remember that preformed dietary niacin is not the only source your body uses; it also uses the amino acid tryptophan, if there is extra available after protein needs are met. If your niacin intake seems low, perform the following calculation. Record the total protein you consumed (in grams). Subtract your recommended protein intake to obtain an estimate of "leftover" protein available to make niacin (in grams). Divide this number by 100 to obtain the total tryptophan you might have had available from which to make niacin (tryptophan represents about 1/100 of the weight of most dietary proteins). Multiply this number by 1000 to convert grams to milligrams.

Now, about 60 milligrams of tryptophan can be converted to about 1 milligram of niacin in the body, so divide by 60 to get "niacin equivalents." Finally, add to the equivalents the amount of niacin you obtained preformed in your diet, and compare this total with the recommended intake. This is only a rough estimate of the amount of niacin you might have derived from your diet but perhaps better than none. If your niacin and protein intakes are both low, you should do something about it—probably increase your protein intake, for a start.

2. Appendix A does not show vitamins D, E, and K, but you can guess at the adequacy of your intakes. For vitamin D, answer the following questions. Do you drink fortified milk (read the label)? Eat eggs? Fortified breakfast cereal? Liver? Are you in the sun enough to promote vitamin D synthesis? (Remember to use sunscreen to reduce the risk of skin cancer—see the chapter discussion.)

3. For vitamin E, consider the foods you ate in 24 hours. Vitamin E often accompanies linoleic acid in foods. Did you consume enough linoleic acid? (See Self-Study 4.)

4. For vitamin K, does your diet include 2 cups of milk or the equivalent in milk products every day? Does it include leafy vegetables frequently (every other day)? Do you take antibiotics regularly (which inhibit the production of vitamin K by your intestinal bacteria)?

Notes

1. Food and Nutrition Board, *Recommended Dietary Allowances*, 10th ed. (Washington, D.C.: National Academy of Sciences, 1989), p. 20.

2. K. P. West, G. R. Howard, and A. Sommer, Vitamin A and infection: Public health implications, *Annual Reviews of Nutrition* 9 (1989): 63–86.

3. West, 1989.

4. K. P. West and coauthors, Vitamin A supplementation and growth: A randomized community trial, *American Journal of Clinical Nutrition* 48 (1988): 1257–1264; Muhilal and coauthors, Vitamin A-fortified monosodium glutamate and health, growth, and survival of children: A controlled field study, *American Journal of Clinical Nutrition* 48 (1988): 1271–1276.

5. West, 1989.

6. J. E. Olson, Vitamin A and cancer (a letter to the editor), *Journal of the American Dietetic Association* 86 (1986): 1730, 1732.

7. T. O. Carpenter and coauthors, Severe hypervitaminosis A in siblings: Evidence of variable tolerance to retinol intake, *Journal of Pediatrics* 111 (1987): 507–512.

8. Masked hypervitaminosis A and liver injury, *Nutrition Reviews* 40 (1982): 303–305.

9. H. Reichel, H. P. Koeffler, and A. W. Norman, The role of the vitamin D endocrine system in health and disease, *New England Journal of Medicine* 320 (1989): 980–991; Ca^{2+} priming and differentiation induced by 1,25-dihydroxyvitamin D_3, *Nutrition Reviews* 47 (1989): 91–93.

10. Study sheds light on TB resistance, *Science News* 133 (1988): 60.

11. T. Ziporyn, Possible link probed, deafness and vitamin D, *Journal of the American Medical Association* 250 (1983): 1951-1952.

12. A. R. Webb and M. F. Holick, Role of sunlight in the cutaneous production of vitamin D_3, *Annual Reviews of Nutrition* 8 (1988): 375–399.

13. D. Farley, Tanning salon sees the light, *FDA Consumer*, December 86/January 87, pp. 37–38.

14. M. Rudolf, K. Arulanantham, and R. M. Greenstein, Unsuspected nutritional rickets, *Pediatrics* 66 (1980): 72–76;

Vitamin D deficiency rickets, revisited, *Nutrition Reviews* 38 (1980): 116–118.

15. J. Raloff, Vitamin E fights radicals—again and again, *Science News* 27 (1989): 327.

16. M. A. Guggenheim, *Vitamin E deficiency diseases*, a booklet available from the Vitamin Nutrition Information Service, Hofmann-La Roche, Inc., Nutley, NJ 07110; D. P. R. Muller, J. K. Lloyd, and O. H. Wolff, Vitamin E and neurological function, *Lancet*, 29 January 1983, pp. 225–228.

17. Food and Nutrition Board, 1989, p. 109.

18. Food and Nutrition Board, 1989, p. 20.

19. D. A. Roe, *Drug-Induced Nutritional Deficiencies* (Westport, Conn.: AVI, 1976), pp. 3, 16–17.

20. R. Carmel and coauthors, Cobalamin and osteoblast-specific proteins, *New England Journal of Medicine* 319 (1988): 70–75.

21. J. Lindenbaum and coauthors, Neuropsychiatric disorders caused by cobalamin deficiency in the absence of anemia or macrocytosis, *New England Journal of Medicine* 318 (1988): 1720-1728.

22. Over-the-counter preparations in doses greater than 0.4 milligrams per day are marketed only for pregnant and lactating women. Federal Regulation 21, *Code of Federal Regulations*, Section 172, 345, cited by L. Alhadeff and coauthors (letter), *Nutrition Reviews* 42 (1984): 265–267.

23. Anon, Unrecognized cobalamin-responsive neuropsychiatric disorders, *Nutrition Reviews* 47 (1989): 208–210.

24. V. Herbert, Vitamin B_{12}: Plant sources, requirements, and assay, *American Journal of Clinical Nutrition* 48 (1988): 852-858.

25. J. B. Reuler, V. C. Broudy, and T. G. Cooney, Adult scurvy, *Journal of the American Medical Association* 25 (1985): 805–807.

26. Food and Nutrition Board, 1989, p. 119.

27. T. C. Chalmers, Effects of ascorbic acid on the common cold, *American Journal of Medicine* 58 (1975): 532–536.

▥ C O N T R O V E R S Y   7 ▰▰▰▰▰▰▰ ▥▥▥

Vitamin Supplements

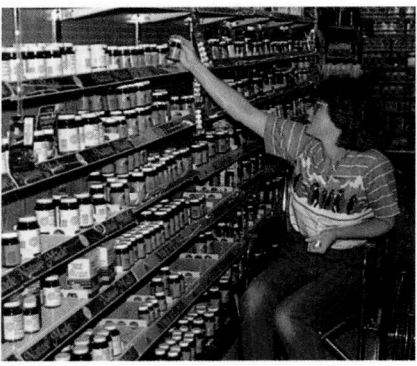

Does the woman depicted above really need the supplement she is choosing? Many people are not sure that they meet their nutrient needs using foods alone. Fully half the population uses nutrient **supplements** regularly, collectively spending billions of dollars on them each year.[1] Many take a single daily pill; others take huge quantities of single nutrients. Most people self-prescribe them on the advice of friends or magazines that may or may not be reliable. This Controversy examines the arguments for and against taking supplements. Should a person decide to take one, it goes on to tell how to go about choosing it.

▥▥▥ Arguments for Supplements

Nutrition surveys of the U.S. populations do detect deficiencies of pro-tein, vitamins, and minerals. The incidence of these deficiencies is low, but they do exist, and they fuel the argument that most people may need to take supplements. The logic states that if deficiency symptoms exist, then **marginal** or **subclinical deficiencies** must also exist, causing vague symptoms that are probably not always recognized even by skilled health care providers. Perhaps many individuals, even if outwardly healthy, may be subtly impaired by nutrient deficiencies.

The newsletter *Nutrition and the M.D.* describes marginal deficiencies as states of unwellness shy of classical deficiencies:

■ When people are becoming deficient in thiamin, classic signs of beriberi don't appear until the sixth week. But as the deficiency develops, loss of appetite and weight, irritability, insomnia, and discomfort appear within three to four weeks, together with a fall in a blood enzyme (transketolase, detectable only by laboratory test).

■ No clinical signs of a developing riboflavin deficiency appear until the eighth week, but behavioral symptoms can be detected by the sixth week.

■ As vitamin B_6 deficiency develops, clients complain of fatigue and headache; only later does one see the classic, small red blood cells of anemia.

In other words, somewhere between the adequate levels of a nutrient and the classic signs of deficiency, there is an area in which people neither feel nor function well. Since some people with classic deficiencies are seen in North America, there may be even more people in the in-between area.

In some cases there are predisposing conditions (people are not healthy; are addicted to alcohol or other drugs; have kidney diseases; or use medications that interfere with nutrient action). But *Nutrition and the M.D.* adds: "There is probably a large additional group of people at risk of developing marginal vitamin deficiencies. These include young and older women consuming diets that are marginally adequate for energy and those patients with chronic debilitative illnesses who are often anorexic and have poor food intake."[2] As an example of a slight and subtle nutrient deficiency, the authors of a hospital study on surgery clients reported that a slight thiamin deficit resulted in poor wound healing. They were impressed: "The data served to emphasize once more the invaluable benefits of **optimal nutrition** in preventive and post-operative medicine."[3]

For people who are at risk of marginal deficiencies, supplements may be a rational and beneficial choice. It has been suggested that all of the following adults are on that list:[4]

■ People with low energy intakes, such as habitual dieters.*
■ The elderly, especially if they are malnourished.
■ People with illnesses that take away the appetite.*

*The taking of supplements by groups tagged with an asterisk is endorsed by the societies mentioned in note 10 (p. 238).

■ People with illnesses that impair absorption of nutrients, including diseases of the liver, gallbladder, pancreas, and digestive system.*
■ People taking medications that interfere with the body's use of specific nutrients.
■ People who have diseases, infections, or injuries or who have undergone surgery resulting in increased metabolic needs.
■ Women who are pregnant or lactating, whose metabolic needs are therefore increased. *
■ Strict vegetarians.*
■ Women who bleed excessively during menstruation.*
■ People whose calcium intakes are too low to forestall osteoporosis.

Most of those people would benefit from a multivitamin-mineral supplement that supplied approximately the RDA amount of every nutrient. Those taking drugs that interfered with specific nutrients would need individual advice. Pregnancy and lactation incur increased needs for iron, calcium, and folate in particular; strict vegetarians may not receive enough calcium, vitamin B_{12}, iron, and zinc from fruits, vegetables, and grains; and women who lose much blood during menstruation need iron supplements. In addition, newborns routinely need a single dose of vitamin K at birth,* and infants may need supplements depending on whether they are receiving formula or not and on whether their water is fluoridated or not (see Chapter 12).

These special cases are discussed in later chapters. Iron supplements receive attention in Chapter 8; Cal-cium supplements in Controversy 8; supplements for pregnancy and infancy in Chapter 12, and for people taking medications, Controversy 12. The end of this Controversy comes back to the question of how to choose a general multivitamin-mineral supplement, but first there are arguments against doing so.

■■■ Arguments against Supplements

One argument is not so much against supplements in general as against high-dose supplements. High doses of almost every nutrient are dangerous. People's tolerances for high doses of nutrients vary, just as their risks of deficiencies vary. Thus amounts that some can tolerate may not be safe for others, and no one knows who falls into which category.

Toxic overdoses of vitamins and minerals may be more common than we realize. One physician, reporting several cases of harm from vitamin overdoses, warns that the known cases are just the tip of the iceberg.[5] Only a few alert health care providers recognize the signs of short-term acute toxic doses; and no doubt many cases of chronic, low-level nutrient toxicity, in which the effects develop more subtly and slowly, go unrecognized. In the United States supplements are treated by law as foods rather than as drugs, so manufacturers are not required to prove their safety or effectiveness or even their ability to be absorbed by the body. In view of the hazards they present, many authorities believe they should be required to bear warning labels.

Knowledge of nutrient toxicity is limited, and it is impossible to say just how much of a nutrient is too much. Assuming, however, that it is best to err on the conservative side, Table C7–1 presents upper limits for vitamin and mineral doses to be obtained from supplements. Still to be published is a set of **safety indexes** for nutrients—indexes of the safety of doses higher than the RDA. The safety index for calcium is 10, for example (up to 10 times the U.S. RDA is a safe dose for an adult); that for selenium is only 5.[6]

Another argument against the use of supplements is that no one knows exactly how to formulate the "ideal" supplement. What nutrients should be included? How much of each? And how should an individual choose a supplement, since no one's needs are exactly like anyone else's?

Another argument against supplements is that they may lull the takers into a false sense of security. A person might eat irresponsibly, thinking, "My supplement will cover my needs." Or, experiencing the warning sign of a disease, a person might postpone seeking a diagnosis, thinking, "I probably need a nutrient supplement to make this go away." Such self-diagnosis is always dangerous.

Other invalid reasons why people may take supplements include:

■ Their feelings of insecurity about the nutrient content of the food supply.

■■■ Table C7–1 Vitamin and Mineral Doses for Supplements

SUBSTANCE	AMOUNT RECOMMENDED FOR PREVENTION[a]
Vitamins	
Vitamin A (IU)[b]	250 to 2500
Vitamin D (IU)[b]	400 (up to age 18)
	200 (adults)
Vitamin E (IU)[b]	6 to 30
Thiamin (mg)	1 to 2
Riboflavin (mg)	1 to 2
Niacin (as niacinamide, mg)	10 to 20
Vitamin B_6 (mg)	1.5 to 2.5
Folate (mg)	0.1 to 0.4
	(pregnancy, lactation see RDA)
Vitamin B_{12} (μg)	3 to 10
Pantothenic acid (mg)[c]	5 to 20
Biotin (mg)	Not recommended in supplement form
Vitamin C (mg)	50 to 100
Minerals	
Calcium (mg)	400 to 800
Phosphorus (mg)	No need to supplement
Magnesium (mg)	No need to supplement
Iron (Mg)	10 to 30 (women)
	30 to 60 (pregnancy, lactation see RDA)
Zinc (mg)	10 to 25 (adults)
	25 (pregnancy, lactation see RDA)
Iodine (mg)	Not recommended in supplement form.

[a]The FDA and the Committee on RDA do not recommend that these nutrients be used to attempt to correct deficiencies, because deficiencies often arise from nonnutritional causes such as disease or interference by drugs. In these cases the underlying causes of the deficiencies must be correctly diagnosed and treated; supplements may mask, but will not correct, the problems.
[b]Some supplements are measured in International Units (IU). To convert to RDA-compatible units, see the conversion factors in Appendix C.
[c]Use only in multivitamin form.

SOURCE: Parts adapted from The American Medical Association's Council on Scientific Affairs, Vitamin preparations as dietary supplements and as therapeutic agents, *Journal of the American Medical Association* 257 (1987): 1929–1936; A. Hecht, Vitamins over the counter: Take only when needed, *FDA Consumer*, April 1979, pp. 17–19; Food and Nutrition Board, *Recommended Dietary Allowances*, 10th ed. (Washington, D.C.: National Academy of Sciences, 1989).

■ Their desire for additional energy or strength.
■ Their belief that supplements will help them cope with stress.
■ Their desire to prevent, treat, or cure symptoms or diseases from the common cold to cancer.

Ironically, one study found that supplement users eat diets of more nutrient-dense foods than nonusers and therefore need the supplements even less.[7] In addition, little relationship exists between the nutrients individuals need and the ones they take in pills.[8]

Another problem is that of **bioavailability**. In general, nutrients are absorbed best from foods, in which they are dispersed among other ingredients that may facilitate their absorption. Taken in pure, concentrated form, they are more likely to interfere with each other's absorption or with the absorption of the nutrients in foods eaten at the same time. Minerals provide examples: zinc hinders copper and calcium absorption, iron hinders zinc absorption, calcium hinders magnesium and iron absorption, and magnesium hinders the absorption of calcium and iron. The same interference takes place when people use foods that are fortified with added minerals, another reason to rely on ordinary whole foods for optimal absorption of nutrients.[9]

In view of all the negatives associated with supplement taking, several nutrition societies have indicated that most people should *not* use them:

Healthy children and adults should obtain adequate nutrient intakes from dietary sources. Meeting nutrient needs by choosing a variety of foods in moderation, rather than by supplementation, reduces the potential risk for both nutrient deficiencies and nutrient excesses. Individual recommendations regarding supplements and diets should come from physicians and registered dietitians... . There are no demonstrated benefits of self-supplementation beyond [the RDA] allowances.[10]

From the perspective of the experts, then, it seems that supplementation is not the wisest course for most people. They urge that whenever a person's diet is inadequate, the action to take is not supplementation but improvement of the person's food choices and eating patterns.[11] Still, when a supplement is needed, some pointers can assist in its selection.

▇▇▇ Selection of Supplements

People often think in terms of "vitamin pills." However, when vitamins are needed, minerals will be needed too. A single, balanced vitamin-mineral supplement should do the job for all of the people listed earlier.[12]

If you decide to take a vitamin-mineral supplement, you may find yourself bewildered in front of a drugstore counter, reading the clever, and usually deceptive, ads on labels—"For vitality!" "Infants only!" "For those with active lives!" "What you need for stress!" or "Be more fun, sexier, smarter, and healthier!"—the key to each quality to be found, of course, in *that* particular supplement. The first step in escaping the clutches of the health hustlers is to imagine that you have a bottle of white paint and can simply white out the picture of the sexy people on the beach and the meaningless, glittering generalities like "new and improved." No matter how lovely the container, you are shopping for a nutrient supplement. (If a pretty container is what you need, you can get one for less in housewares.) After you have whited out the label claims, all you have left is the list of ingredients, what form they are in, and the price. From here you can make a rational decision based on facts.

You have two basic questions to answer. The first question: What form do you want—chewable, liquid, or pills? If you'd rather drink your vitamins and minerals than chew them, fine. (Remember, you whited out *infant* on the labels, so now those bottles are just liquid supplements.) The second question: Who are you? What vitamins and minerals do *you* need? The RDA table on the inside front cover and the table for Canadians (Appendix B) are the standards appropriate for virtually all reasonably healthy people (if you aren't healthy, see your health care provider).

Generally an appropriate supplement provides all the RDA nutrients in amounts smaller than, equal to, or very close to the RDA.[13] Avoid any preparation that, in a daily dose, provides more than the RDA of vitamin A, D, or any mineral or more than ten times the RDA for *any* nutrient. A warning: Expect to reject about 80 percent of available preparations when you choose according to these criteria; be choosy where your health is concerned. Other warnings follow.

Avoid preparations with high levels of iron (more than 10 milligrams per dose) except for menstruating women. People who menstruate need more iron, but people who don't, don't. Iron is hard to get rid of once it's in the body, so an excess of iron can cause problems, just as a deficiency can (Chapter 8).

Avoid "organic" or "natural" preparations. They are no better than standard types, but they cost much more. The word *synthetic* may sound like "fake," but to synthesize just means to put together, and such supplements are identical to vitamins synthesized by plants and animals. Your body can't tell the difference, but your wallet can.

Avoid products that make "high-potency" claims. More is not better. The RDA is more than enough. You do eat foods, too, after all, so you get well over RDA amounts of vitamins and minerals.

Avoid therapeutic doses (or higher) unless they are prescribed by a physician. Nutrients can build up and cause unexpected problems. (For example, a man who takes vitamins and begins to lose his hair may think it means he needs *more* vitamins, when in fact hair loss may be an early sign of vitamin A overdose.)

Avoid preparations that contain items not needed in human nutrition, such as choline and inositol. It's not that those particular items will harm you, but they reveal a marketing strategy that makes the whole mix suspect. The manufacturer may want you to believe that its brand of pills contains the latest "new" nutrient that the takers of all other brands have left out, but, in fact, for every valid discovery of this kind, there are 999,999 frauds.

Avoid "stress formulas." Although the stress response depends on certain B vitamins and vitamin C, the RDA amount provides all that is needed of these, even during examinations.

Avoid pills containing ground parsley, alfalfa, and other vegetable components. They may deliver a few of the same nutrients as a plate of salad or broccoli, but salad and broccoli are much more nutritious—and cheaper.

Avoid geriatric "tonics." They are generally poor in vitamins and minerals and yet so high in alcohol as to threaten inebriation. The liquids designed for infants are more complete.

Local or store brands are just as good as national brands. If they are less expensive, it is not because they are inferior but because the price does not have to cover the cost of national advertising. (One full-page color ad in a national magazine costs upwards of $60,000.) The less expensive pills may be from the same batch as the higher priced ones but without the price tag of the brand name.

Steer clear of doses that are too high. Think of the original Stone Age person, who had to depend only on foods for life and health. If the foods available to Stone Age people *could* have supplied the amount of a nutrient being advocated, then perhaps it is not unsafe for us, their descendants, to ingest that amount ourselves.

By this standard, the doses some people take are clearly excessive. To obtain 840 milligrams of vitamin E from its best food source, **wheat germ**, for example, you would have to eat 15 pounds of wheat germ, yet some people take supplements containing more than 840 milligrams of vitamin E every day. To obtain 5 grams of vitamin C, you would have to eat 19 pounds of oranges, yet some people consume more than that much vitamin C daily from supplements.

Our ancestors survived for centuries without nutrient supplements and arrived successfully at the point of producing us. On this basis alone, it can be argued that we must need no more vitamins or minerals than what *we* can obtain from food. That much, but not more, would be reasonable to look for in a supplement.

But, come to think of it, if all the nutrients we need can come from food, why not just get them from food? Foods have much more to recommend them than do supplements. Nutrients in foods come in an infinite variety of combinations with a multitude of different carriers, absorption facilitators, antioxidation protectors, and other benefits. They come with water, fiber, and a host of beneficial and interesting nonnutrients (see Controversy 14). They come with calories (you have to eat some calories each day; why not ask nutritious foods to deliver them?) They offer pleasure, satiety, and opportunities for socializing while eating. In no way can nutrient supplements hold a candle to foods as a means of meeting human health needs.

Sharing Nutrition Knowledge

A problem that remains for the reader who is persuaded of the view presented here is, "How do I tell my friends?" Trying to convince a pill-popping friend not to take pills and powders can easily turn into the unfortunate experience of losing the friend. Dr Alfred E. Harper, PhD, professor of nutritional sciences, University of Wisconsin, has put it like this: "Isn't it amazing how, when you explain to someone that what they have accepted as fact is not so, they become angry with *you* rather than with the person who gave them the inaccurate information in the first place."[14] Yes, it is amazing and painful. But the response is not surprising when you recall that the person who has paid his or her own money as the price for believing a bogus fact has a personal stake in having the fact be true.

To avoid alienating people, we can adopt several strategies. For one thing, we can always acknowledge the validity of the feelings and values that underlie the practices. Then we can learn the true facts as thoroughly as we can, getting them all in perspective, and then communicate them clearly. Finally, we can confront only those practices that are dangerous and learn to ignore those that are merely neutral.

▓▓▓ Miniglossary

bioavailability: absorbability, the individual differences in nutrients' ease of absorption.

bone meal: a nutrient supplement made from bone, intended to supply calcium and other bone minerals.

desiccated liver: dehydrated liver powder sold in health-food stores, supposed to contain in concentrated form all the nutrients found in liver. *Desiccated* means "totally dried."

garlic oil: an extract of garlic.

granola: a cereal mixed from rolled oats and other grains.

kelp: a kind of seaweed used by the Japanese as a foodstuff.

marginal deficiency: see *subclinical deficiency*.

nutritional yeast: a preparation of yeast cells, often praised as a concentrated source of B vitamins. This is brewer's, not baker's, yeast; see items 992 and 993 in Appendix A.

optimal nutrition: the best possible nutrition, more than just freedom from overt deficiency signs. This term describes people free of risk of marginal deficiencies, free of imbalances, and at zero risk of toxicities.

powdered bone: a supplement made from bone, intended to supply calcium and other bone minerals.

safety index: a numerical statement of the safety of high doses of nutrients. A safety index of 5, for example, means that doses up to five times the U.S. RDA are safe.

spirulina: a kind of algae ("blue-green manna") said to contain large amounts of vitamin B_{12} and to suppress appetite. It does neither.

subclinical deficiency (also called a *marginal deficiency*): a nutrient deficiency that has no detectable (clinical) symptoms. The term is often used to scare consumers into buying unneeded nutrient supplements.

super blue-green algae: an aquatic plant said to have special health-promoting powers; such claims have not been verified by science; and the product probably amounts to "just freeze-dried pond scum," as one realistic reporter put it.

supplements: preparations (such as pills, powders, or liquids) containing nutrients; not foods. Breakfast cereals that contain "100 percent of the U.S. RDA" for certain nutrients are defined by law as dietary supplements, not foods. See also Chapter 14.

wheat germ: the oily embryo of the wheat kernel, rich in nutrients.

To demonstrate this skill, let us rank some items selected by a friend who, with great enthusiasm for nutrition, takes huge stockpiles of nutrient supplements. Let's say that at breakfast this person takes 500 milligrams of vitamin C, 1000 units of vitamin E, several tablespoons of **nutritional yeast**, some **kelp** tablets, several different pills containing vitamins A and D, a **spirulina** tablet, **super blue-green algae**, and assorted other pills containing trace minerals. This person sprinkles **desiccated liver**, **powdered bone**, **bone meal**, **garlic oil**, and wheat germ on a bowl of **granola**, then pours powdered nonfat milk over it all. Where would you begin?

Most risky: the A and D capsule and the minerals because overdoses are likely and have serious ill effects.

Next: the nutritional yeast (it is not needed and may contribute to B vitamin overdose); the powdered bone (the calcium from such a source is very poorly absorbed, and some bone meal has been found to contain high levels of lead); the kelp tablets (which may contain too much iodine and even arsenic, a poison and a possible cancer-causing agent); and super blue-green algae, which has no proven benefits and carries with it unknown side effects.

Next: the vitamin C and the vitamin E. These are not the highest doses people take and get away with, but they are high enough to be toxic in some individuals. (See Chapter 7 for more about vitamin toxicity.)

Next: the desiccated liver. Using it may be a neutral practice (although it is high in cholesterol, and the liver is an organ that concentrates toxins); the biggest harm in this may be to the wallet.

Last: the wheat germ, the granola, and the powdered nonfat milk. These are nutritious foods, they can be bought in the grocery store, and the nonfat milk in particular is an economical source of valuable nutrients.

In counseling the user of mega-supplements, you might offer a caution about the use of the potent supplements listed first and keep your own counsel about the remaining ones unless you are asked. This way you may preserve your friendship, and you may provide a substantial boost to exactly what the person treasures most—good health.

Notes

1. $ 2.9 billion for vitamins, *FDA Consumer*, April 1987, p. 4.

2. Marginal vitamin deficiency, *Nutrition and the M.D.*, July 1983.

3. Thiamin and wound repair, *Nutrition Reviews* 40 (1982); 316-318.

4. D. Heber and W. Mertz, Food versus pills versus fortified foods, *Dairy Council Digest*, March-April 1987; R. E. Schucker, Food versus pills versus fortified foods, *Dairy Council Digest*, March-April 1987; A. E. Harper, Nutrition Insurance—A skeptical view, *Nutrition Forum*, May 1987, pp. 33–37.

5. Santa Barbara physician warns of vitamin overdosing, *California Council Against Health Fraud Newsletter*, March/April 1983, p. 2.

6. Heber and Mertz, 1987.

7. N. Kurinij; M. A. Klebanoff, and B. I. Graubard, Dietary supplement and food intake in women of child-bearing age, *Journal of the American Dietetic Association* 86 (1986): 1536–1540.

8. S. J. A. Bowerman and I. Harrell, Nutrient consumption of individuals taking or not taking nutrient supplements, *Journal of the American Dietetic Association* 83 (1983): 298–305.

9. Heber and Mertz, 1987.

10. The societies that joined to make this statement were the American Dietetic Association, the American Society for Clinical Nutrition, and the American Institute of Nutrition. The American Medical Association reviewed it and endorsed it. Heber and Mertz, 1987.

11. Heber and Mertz, 1987.

12. This discussion is adapted with permission from L. K. DeBruyne and S. R. Rolfes, *Selection of supplements* (a monograph in the *Nutrition Clinics* Series available from Stickley Publishing Co., 210 Washington Square, Philadelphia, PA 19106).

13. L. S. Bell and M. Fairchild, Evaluation of commercial multivitamin supplements, *Journal of the American Dietetic Association* 87 (1987): 341–343.

14. A. E. Harper, Science and the consumer, *Journal of Nutrition Education* 11 (1979): 171.

Water and Minerals

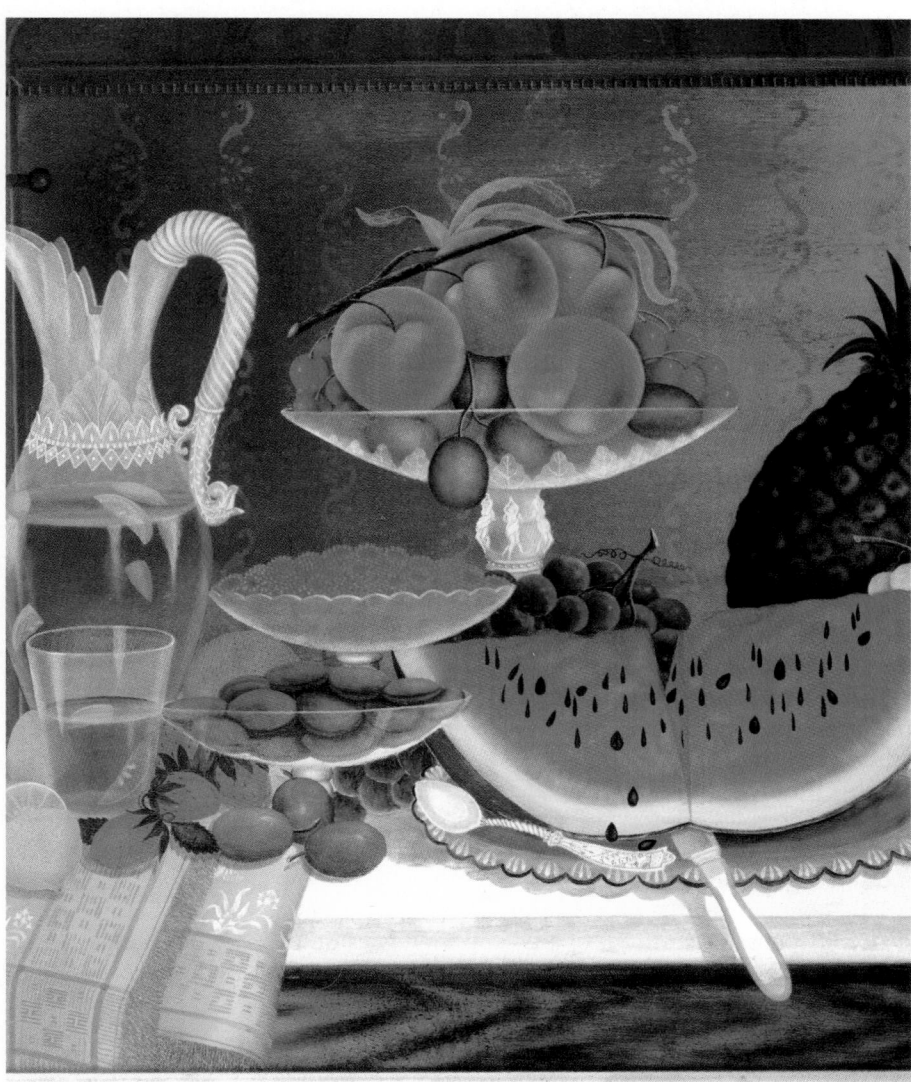

Still Life by Henri Church. The Collection of Frances O. Stem Babinsky.

minerals: naturally occurring, inorganic, homogeneous substances; chemical elements.

major minerals: essential mineral nutrients found in the human body in amounts larger than 5 grams.

trace minerals: essential mineral nutrients found in the human body in amounts less than 5 grams.

Elements that are essential to life:

- Carbon.
- Hydrogen.
- Oxygen.
- Nitrogen.
- Major minerals:
    - Calcium.
    - Chloride.
    - Magnesium.
    - Phosphorus.
    - Potassium.
    - Sodium.
    - Sulfur.
- Trace minerals:
    - Arsenic.
    - Boron.
    - Chromium.
    - Cobalt.
    - Copper.
    - Fluoride.
    - Iodine.
    - Iron.
    - Manganese.
    - Molybdenum.
    - Nickel.
    - Selenium.
    - Silicon.
    - Zinc.

"Ashes to ashes and dust to dust." This familiar quotation reminds us of our mortality. Perhaps we need this reminder to put our own importance into perspective, and it is true that when the life force leaves the body, what is left behind ultimately becomes nothing but a small pile of ashes. Carbohydrates, proteins, fats, vitamins, and water are present at first, but they soon disappear.

The carbon atoms in all the carbohydrates, fats, proteins, and vitamins combine with oxygen to produce carbon dioxide, which vanishes into the air; the hydrogens and oxygens of those compounds unite to form water; and this water, along with the water that was a large part of the body weight, evaporates. The ashes that are left behind are the **minerals**, a small pile that weighs only about 5 pounds. The pile is not impressive in size, but when you consider the tasks these minerals perform, you may realize their great importance in living tissue.

Consider calcium and phosphorus. If you could separate these two minerals from the rest of the pile, you would take away about three-fourths of the total. Crystals made of these two minerals, plus a few others, form the structure of the bones and so provide the architecture of the skeleton.

Run a magnet through the one-fourth of the pile that remains, and pick up the iron. It would not fill a teaspoon, but it is billions of billions of iron atoms. As part of hemoglobin, these iron atoms have the special property of being able to attach to oxygen and to make it available at the sites where metabolic work is taking place, inside the cells.

If you were able to extract all the other minerals, leaving only copper and iodine in the pile of ashes, you would want to close the windows before you did it. A slight breeze would blow these remaining bits of dust away. Yet the copper in the dust is the catalyst necessary for iron to hold and to release oxygen, and iodine is the critical mineral in the hormone thyroxin. Figure 8–1 shows the amounts of **major minerals** and a few of the **trace minerals** in the human body. Other minerals such as gold and aluminum, while present in the body, are not known to be nutrients.

That a distinction is made between the major and the trace minerals doesn't mean that one group is more important in the body than the other. A daily deficiency of a few micrograms of iodine is just as serious as a deficiency of the several hundred milligrams of calcium. Major minerals and trace minerals all play specific roles. However, because the major minerals are present in larger total quantities, they influence the body fluids, thereby affecting the whole body in a general way.

This chapter begins with a discussion of the characteristics of water—the most indispensable nutrient of all—and then goes on to show how some of the major minerals affect it. Then the chapter discusses the specialized roles of the minerals.

Water

You began as a single cell bathed in a nourishing fluid. Ever since you became a beautifully organized, air-breathing body of billions of cells, each of your cells has had to remain next to water to remain alive. Water brings to each cell the exact ingredients it requires and carries away the end products of the life-sustaining reactions that take place within its boundaries.

Water in the body is not simply a river coursing through the arteries, capillaries, and veins. Some of the water is part of the chemical structure of

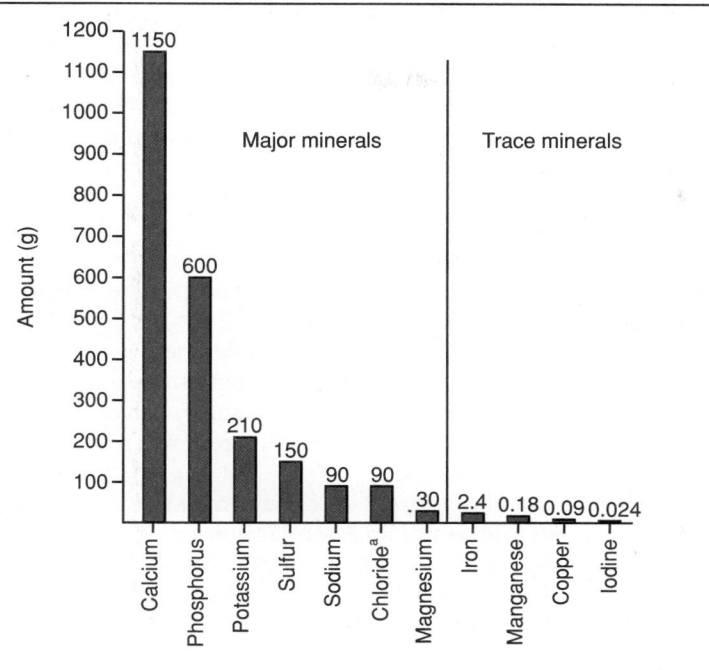

■■■ **Figure 8–1**

Minerals in a 60-Kilogram Person.
The major minerals are those present in amounts larger than 5 grams (a teaspoon). The trace minerals number a dozen or more; only four are shown. A pound is about 454 grams; thus only calcium and phosphorus appear in amounts larger than a pound.
ᵃChlorine appears in the body as the ion chloride.

compounds that form the cells, tissues, and organs of the body. For example, proteins hold water molecules within them. This water is locked in and is not readily available for any other use. Water also participates actively in many chemical reactions.

As the medium for the body's traffic of nutrients and waste products, water is nearly a universal solvent. Luckily for our physical integrity, this is not quite the case, but water does dissolve amino acids, glucose, minerals, and many other substances needed by the cells. Fatty substances are specially packaged with water-soluble proteins so that they too can travel freely in the blood and lymph. Water is thus the transport vehicle for all the nutrients.

Another important characteristic of water is its incompressibility. Its molecules resist being crowded together. Thanks to this characteristic, water can act as a lubricant and a cushion for the joints. For the same reason it can protect a sensitive tissue such as the spinal cord from shock. The fluid that fills the eye serves in a similar way to keep optimal pressure on the retina and lens. The unborn infant is cushioned against shock by the bag of amniotic fluid in which it develops. Water also lubricates the digestive tract and all tissues moistened with mucus.

Still another of water's special features is its heat-holding capacity. This characteristic of water is familiar to coastal dwellers who know that land surrounded by water is protected from wide variations in temperature from day to night. Water itself changes temperature slowly; at night, when the land cools, the water gives up its heat gradually to the air, moderating the coolness of the night. In contrast, the desert varies widely in temperature from day to night because it is dry. Similarly, water helps to maintain body temperature. A great deal of heat is required to change water from a liquid to a gas, so when we sweat, the evaporating water carries off large quantities of body heat.

Boasting scientist: I'm working on discovering the universal solvent.

Skeptical backwoodsman: Is that so? Well, when you've got it, what are you going to keep it in?

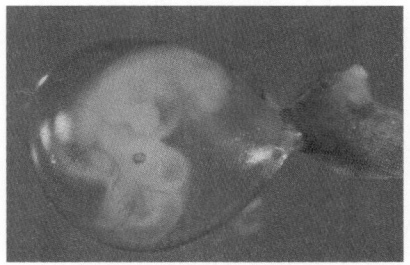

Life begins in water.

hard water: water with a high calcium and magnesium concentration.

soft water: water containing a high sodium concentration.

bottled water: Water bought for drinking in the hope that it may provide some benefit beyond those of local tap water. Bottled water must meet the same minimum federal standards for sanitation and purity as do all municipal water supplies. No additional standards apply.

dehydration: loss of water. The symptoms progress rapidly from thirst through weakness to exhaustion and delirium and end in death.

water intoxication: the condition in which body water content is too high. Symptoms are headache, muscular weakness, lack of concentration, poor memory, and loss of appetite.

water balance: the balance between water intake and water excretion, which keeps the body's water content constant.

Water supplies can affect people's health, and many people are concerned about the availability of safe water supplies. Population, industry, and agriculture all tap available water, reducing its quantity, and they add pollutants, degrading its quality. To read about the quantity and safety of the water supply, see Chapter 15. Beyond these concerns there are a few things to consider about water and its content of minerals.

Water naturally occurs as **hard water** or **soft water**, a distinction that affects health with regard to three minerals. Hard water has high concentrations of calcium and magnesium. Soft water's principal mineral is sodium. In practical terms, soft water makes more bubbles with less soap; hard water leaves a ring on the tub, a jumble of rocklike crystals in the teakettle, and a gray residue in the wash. Soft water may seem the more desirable, then, and homeowners may even purchase water softeners that remove magnesium and calcium and replace them with sodium. However, soft water appears to contribute to a higher incidence of hypertension and heart disease in areas where it is used, and hard water may have the opposite effect.

Soft water also more easily dissolves certain metals, such as cadmium and lead, from pipes. Cadmium is not an essential nutrient. In fact, it can harm the body, affecting at least some enzymes by displacing zinc from its normal sites of action. Cadmium is also suspected of promoting hypertension. Lead is another toxic metal, and the body seems to absorb it more readily from soft than from hard water, possibly because the calcium in hard water protects against its absorption. People who live in old buildings should run the tap a minute before drawing water for use at breakfast because old plumbing may contain cadmium or lead. Running the tap will flush out the water that spent the night collecting metals from the pipes.

Softening water in your home may be unwise, then, especially if your family is prone to heart disease. One person we know solves the problem by connecting the water softener only to the hot-water line, then using hot water for washing and bathing and only cold water for cooking and drinking. Another idea is to drink only **bottled water**. Bottled water may or may not contain less undesirable material (including sodium) than does ordinary tap water. Read more about water in Chapter 15.

❚❚▶ *Water provides the medium for transportation, chemical reactions, shock protection, lubrication, and temperature regulation in the human body. Hard water is high in calcium and magnesium; soft water is high in sodium, and it dissolves cadmium and lead from pipes.*

❚❚❚ The Body Fluids

Water makes up about 60 percent of the body's weight. It is such an integral part of us that people seldom are conscious of its importance—unless they are deprived of it. You can survive a deficiency of any of the other nutrients for long times, some of them even for months or years, but you can survive only a few days without water. Since the body's self-purification process requires that it excrete at least a quart of water a day, a person must drink that much each day to avoid life-threatening losses.

The total amount of fluid in the body is kept constant by delicate balancing mechanisms. Imbalances can occur—**dehydration** and **water intoxication**—

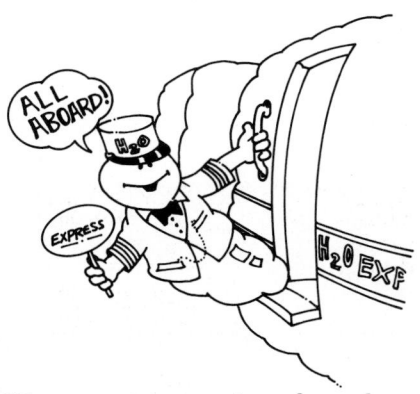

Water transports nutrients from place to place in the body.

but the balances are restored to normal as promptly as the body can manage it. Both intake and excretion are controlled to maintain **water balance**.

WATER INTAKE. Nearly all foods contain some water, and some are over 90 percent water. The energy-yielding nutrients in them give rise to additional water as the body breaks them down. The remainder of the water that you need comes from beverages. The committee on the Recommended Dietary Allowance (RDA) recommends that people consume between 1 and 1 1/2 milliliters of water for each calorie spent in the day. For the person who expends about 2000 calories a day, this works out to 2 or 3 liters, or about 6 to 8 cups. Besides this water from beverages, 2 to 4 cups of fluids come from foods. Sweating increases water needs.

Thirst and satiety govern water intake. When the blood is too concentrated (having lost water but not salt and other dissolved substances) the molecules and particles in the blood attract water out of the salivary glands. The mouth becomes dry as a result, and you drink to wet your mouth. The brain center known as the hypothalamus (described in Chapter 3) also monitors the concentration of the blood. When it finds it is too high, it initiates impulses that stimulate drinking behavior. The volume of the blood also plays a role: thirsty animals drink until nerves in their hearts, known as stretch receptors, are stimulated enough to turn off the drinking.[1] Thus thirst adjusts to provide a water intake that exactly meets the need.

Thirst lags behind water lack, though. A water deficiency that develops slowly can switch on drinking behavior in time to prevent serious dehydration, but one that develops fast may not. Also, thirst itself does not remedy a water deficiency; drinking does. You have to notice that you are thirsty, pay attention, and take the time to get a drink. The athlete, the long-distance casual runner, the gardener in hot weather, and the elderly person whose attention wanders can experience serious dehydration; they need to be alert to their thirst signals and to drink promptly in response to them. (Chapter 10 offers more on the fluid needs of active people.)

WATER EXCRETION. Water excretion is governed by the brain and the kidneys. The hypothalamus senses when the body's salt concentration is too high and calls forth a hormone from the pituitary gland that directs the kidneys to shift water back into the bloodstream from the pool destined for excretion. The kidneys themselves also respond to the salt concentration in the blood passing through them and secrete regulatory substances of their own. The net result is that the more water the body needs, the less it excretes. Still, there is a minimum amount of water that the body must excrete to carry off waste materials in the urine and feces, to generate sweat, and to evaporate from the lungs, and a minimum must be drunk each day to replace that water. Figure 8–2 shows how intake and excretion naturally balance out.

BODY FLUIDS AND MINERALS. It is never a bad idea to drink extra water. Water never accumulates in the body of a healthy person; the urine simply becomes more dilute. The only conceivable hazard is that in excreting the water, the body can lose too much salt. But this would be an extreme case, and

■■■ **Figure 8–2**

Water Balance.

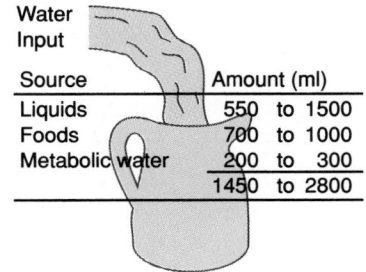

Water Input		
Source	Amount (ml)	
Liquids	550	to 1500
Foods	700	to 1000
Metabolic water	200	to 300
	1450	to 2800

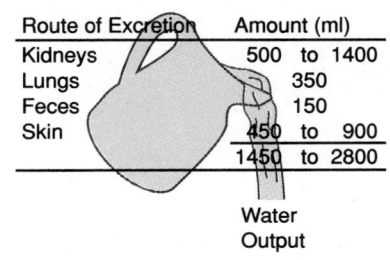

Water Output		
Route of Excretion	Amount (ml)	
Kidneys	500	to 1400
Lungs	350	
Feces	150	
Skin	450	to 900
	1450	to 2800

Water Output

ions (EYE-ons): electrically charged particles, such as sodium (positively charged) or chloride (negatively charged).

electrolytes: compounds that partly dissociate in water to form ions.

fluid and electrolyte balance: maintenance of the proper amount and kind of fluid in each compartment of the body.

fluid and electrolyte imbalance: failure to maintain the proper amount and kind of fluid in every body compartment; a medical emergency.

acid-base balance: maintenance of the proper degree of acidity in each of the body's fluids.

buffers: compounds that can help to keep the acidity of a solution from changing by neutralizing acids and bases.

normally food intake ensures proper salt balance. The section on sodium later describes the need for salt and also the need to limit its intake.

About 40 percent of the body's water weight is inside the cells, and about 15 percent bathes the outsides of the cells. The remainder is in the blood vessels. Special provisions ensure that the cells do not collapse when water leaves them or swell up when too much water enters them. The cells cannot manage this by pumping water across their membranes because water slips in and out freely. However, they can pump minerals across their membranes, and these minerals attract the water to come along with them. The cells use minerals for this purpose in a special form: as **ions** or **electrolytes**—single, electrically charged particles.

Figure 8–3 shows how the body uses electrolytes to move its fluids around, and Figure 6–9 of Chapter 6 showed that proteins form the pumps that move minerals across cell membranes. The successful result is **fluid and electrolyte balance**—the proper amount and kind of fluid in every compartment of the body.

If something happens to overwhelm the system, severe illness can result quickly, since fluid can shift rapidly from one compartment to another. For example, in vomiting or diarrhea, the loss of water from the intestinal tract pulls fluid from between the cells in every part of the body. Fluid then leaves the inside of the cells to restore balance. Meanwhile the kidneys detect the water loss and attempt to retrieve water from the pool destined for excretion. To do this they raise the sodium concentration outside the cells, and this pulls still more water out of them. When this happens the very serious condition of **fluid and electrolyte imbalance** occurs. Water and minerals lost in vomiting or diarrhea ultimately come from every body cell.

The minerals help manage still another balancing act—the **acid-base balance**, or pH, already mentioned in Chapter 6. Among the major minerals, when dissolved in water, some give rise to acids, some to bases. A small percentage of water molecules (H_2O) also exist as positive and negative ions—H (positive) and OH (negative). Excess H ions in a solution make it an acid—they lower the pH; excess OH ions make it a base—they raise pH.

The body's proteins and some of its minerals (as salts) help prevent changes in the acid-base balance of its fluids by serving as **buffers**—molecules that gather up or release H ions as needed to maintain a neutral pH. The kidneys help to control the balance by excreting more or less acid, and the lungs help also by excreting more or less carbon dioxide (in solution in the blood, carbon dioxide forms an acid, carbonic acid). The maintenance of the acid-base balance by means of these tight controls permits all other life processes to take place.

▮▮▶ *Water makes up about 60 percent of the body's weight. Obligatory water losses amounting to over a quart a day necessitate the consumption of the same amount. Electrolytes in the body fluid help keep fluids in their proper compartments and help buffer the environment in which all life processes take place.*

▮▮▮ The Major Minerals

While all the major minerals help to maintain the balances just described, each also plays some special roles of its own. These roles are described in the following sections and all are summarized in Table 8–2 at the end of the chapter. The order does not imply that the first are the most important.

■■■ Figure 8–3

Fluids and Electrolytes.

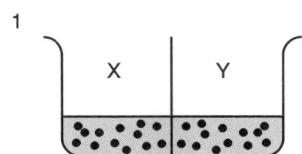

1. With equal numbers of solute particles on both sides, there are equal amounts of water.

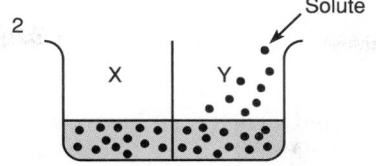

2. Now additional solute is added to side Y. Solute cannot flow across the divider.

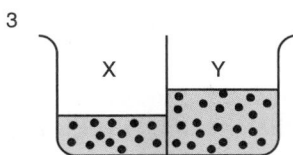

3. Water does flow across the divider, and it tends to remain on side Y, where there is more solute. The *volume* of water becomes greater on side Y, and the *concentrations* on sides X and Y become equal.

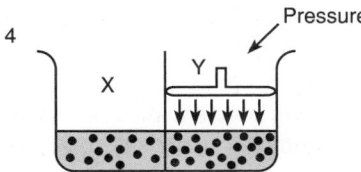

4. Now suppose that pressure (such as a pump) compresses the fluid on side Y. The amount of pressure just sufficient to restore the original volume would equal the *osmotic pressure* exerted by the added particles.

> **diffusion:** the process by which a substance tends to distribute itself evenly throughout the available space.
>
> **osmotic** (os-MOT-ic) **pressure, osmosis** (os-MOH-sis): the force that moves water into a space where a dissolved substance such as sodium chloride is more concentrated (*osmos* means "pushing").

Water goes where the dissolved particles are because it is attracted to them. The body therefore regulates its water distribution by distributing its particles into the spaces where it "wants" water.

All matter is in constant motion, that is, the atoms and molecules of matter are in constant motion. This motion is not visible to the eye but is no less real. Because of it, the molecules of two adjacent liquids or solids mingle with each other. The direction of the **diffusion** of a substance is toward the place of lower concentration of the substance. For example, a person far from the kitchen can detect the frying of breakfast bacon. The molecules of the odor diffuse from the kitchen to the bedroom. Eventually the bacon smell will be the same in both rooms, and although back-and-forth diffusion will continue, the odor will not again become concentrated in either room.

This movement of an odor in air is an example of a gas diffusing in a gas. You have seen a liquid diffuse in a liquid when you poured cream into a cup of coffee. Even without stirring, you could watch the cream molecules diffuse into the coffee. Two substances separated by a membrane can even diffuse through the membrane until their concentrations on both sides are equal.

Sometimes a membrane will allow water to pass through it but will hold back certain particles. Then a force is created. The force is **osmotic pressure.** For example, if concentrated salt particles cannot flow out of a cell (because they cannot penetrate its membrane), then water will flow into the cell to dilute them. Water will move from a dilute solution to a strong solution until the *concentration* of particles is the same in both. There will then be more water where there are more particles and less water where there are fewer particles. The simplest way to state how osmotic pressure moves water from one side of a membrane to the other is to say that "water follows salt."

You have seen this force at work if you have ever salted a lettuce salad and let it stand a half hour before eating it. When you returned to it, the lettuce was wilted, and the salad bowl had water in it. The water had shifted out of the cells toward the higher concentration of salt. The lettuce cells collapsed when they lost their fluid contents.

Water can flow freely across the membranes of most cells inside the body, but minerals cannot. Therefore the cells use minerals to keep the water in the needed amounts in different places. The sodium ion is the main positive ion used for this purpose outside of cells, and the potassium ion is the main one used inside of cells. The negative chloride ion is used in association with both. Proteins in the cell membranes act as pumps to keep each ion in its proper compartment. As long as the body stays healthy, the cells' fluid contents will be maintained this way.

hydroxyapatite: the chief crystal of bone, formed from calcium and phosphorus. (See also *fluorapatite*, p. 263.)

osteoporosis (OSS-tee-oh-pore-OH-sis), also known as **adult bone loss**: a condition of older persons in which the bones become porous and fragile (*osteo* means "bones"; *poros* means "porous"). See this Chapter's Controversy section.

A note about spelling: phosphorus is the noun, phosphorous is the adjective.

Calcium and Phosphorus

Many people have the idea that calcium and phosphorus, once deposited in bone, stay there forever—that once a bone is built, it is inert, like a rock. Not so. Bones are in a state of constant flux, with formation and dissolution taking place every minute of the day and night.

FORMING BONES. Calcium and phosphorus are essential to the formation of bone (Figure 8-4). As bones begin to form, calcium phosphate salts, along with some other minerals, particularly fluoride, lay down crystals on a foundation material composed of the protein collagen. These crystals, called **hydroxyapatite**, invade the collagen and gradually lend more and more rigidity to the maturing bones until they are able to support the weight they will have to carry. Thus the long leg bones of children can support their weight by the time they have learned to walk. (Chapter 7 showed that the increase in length of the long bones involves a dismantling step for which vitamin A is essential, that vitamin C is needed for collagen to form, and that vitamin D helps make calcium available for the assembly process.)

The formation of teeth follows a pattern similar to that of bones: hydroxyapatite crystals form on a collagen matrix to create the dentin that gives strength to the teeth (Figure 8-5). Calcification of the "baby" teeth occurs in

---

■■■ **Figure 8-4**

A Bone.

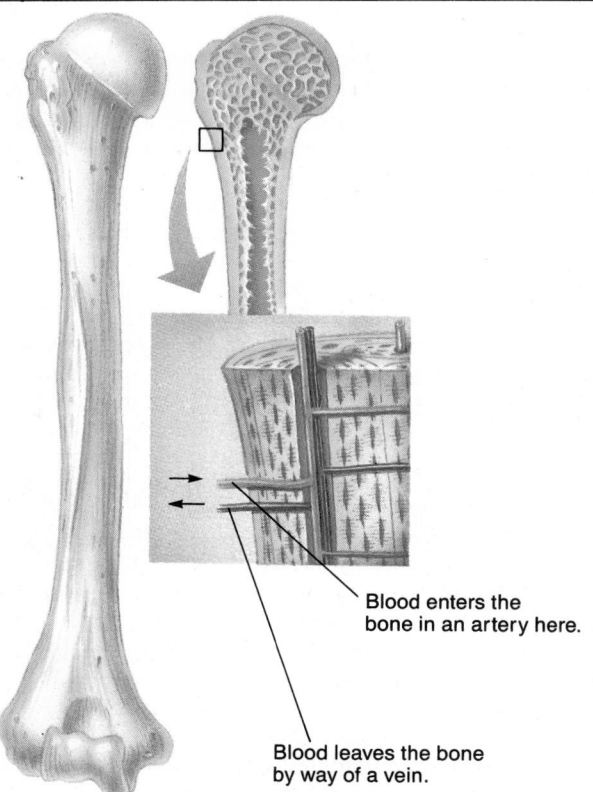

Blood travels in capillaries throughout the bone. It brings nutrients to the cells that maintain the bone's structure, and carries away waste materials from those cells. It picks up and deposits minerals as instructed by hormones.

This bone derives its structural strength from the lacy network of crystals that lie along the bone's lines of stress. If minerals are withdrawn to cover deficits elsewhere in the body, the bone will grow weak, and ultimately will crumble.

Blood enters the bone in an artery here.

Blood leaves the bone by way of a vein.

the gums during the latter half of the infant's time in the womb. The calcification of the permanent teeth takes place during early childhood, up to about the age of three; that of the "wisdom" teeth begins at about the age of ten. The turnover of minerals in teeth is not as rapid as in bone, but some withdrawal and redepositing does take place throughout life. Fluoride hardens and stabilizes the crystals of both bones and teeth, opposing the withdrawal of minerals from them.

OTHER FUNCTIONS. Calcium and phosphorus are also indispensable to the body outside the structures of bones and teeth. The functions of phosphorus are critical to life. Phosphorous salts buffer the acid-base balance of cellular fluids. Each cell also depends on phosphorus as part of its genetic material, thus making phosphorus essential for growth and renewal of tissues. In cells' metabolism of energy nutrients, phosphorous compounds handle energy and work with many enzymes and vitamins to extract the energy from nutrients. Recall from Chapter 5 that phosphorus is part of certain lipids—phospholipids—that form the membranes that surround each cell and its parts. Luckily, needs for phosphorus are easily met by almost any diet, and deficiencies are unknown. For this reason, this discussion turns its attention to calcium.

As for calcium, about 99 percent of the body's calcium is in the bones and teeth; less than 1 percent is in the fluid that bathes the cells; and an even smaller amount is inside the cells. These minute amounts play major roles, however. In addition to its structural roles, calcium:

◼ Regulates the transport of ions across cell membranes and is particularly important in nerve transmission.
◼ Helps maintain normal blood pressure (see Chapter 11).
◼ Is essential for muscle contraction and therefore for the maintenance of the heartbeat.
◼ Plays an essential role in the clotting of blood.
◼ Maintains the "glue" that holds cells together.

CALCIUM BALANCE. Cells need continuous access to calcium, so the body maintains calcium concentration in the blood. The skeleton serves as a bank from which the blood can borrow and return calcium as needed. Withdrawals and deposits of calcium are not at the mercy of the amount taken in food but are regulated by hormones sensitive to blood levels of calcium.* This means that you can go without dietary calcium for years and never suffer a noticeable symptom. Only late in life will you suddenly discover that your savings account has dwindled to the point at which the integrity of your skeleton can no longer be maintained—that throughout your adult years you have been developing **osteoporosis**, or **adult bone loss**. Osteoporosis constitutes a major health problem for many older people. The problem and its possible causes and preventions are the topic of this chapter's Controversy. (Remember from the previous chapter that a vitamin D deficiency causes the diseases rickets in children and osteomalacia in adults. Rickets and osteomalacia involve

◼◼◼ **Figure 8–5**

A Tooth. The inner layer of dentin is bonelike material that forms on a collagen matrix. The outer layer of enamel, which is harder than bone, forms on a keratin matrix. Both dentin and enamel contain hydroxyapatite crystals (made of calcium and phosphorus); those of enamel may harden with fluoride to become fluorapatite.

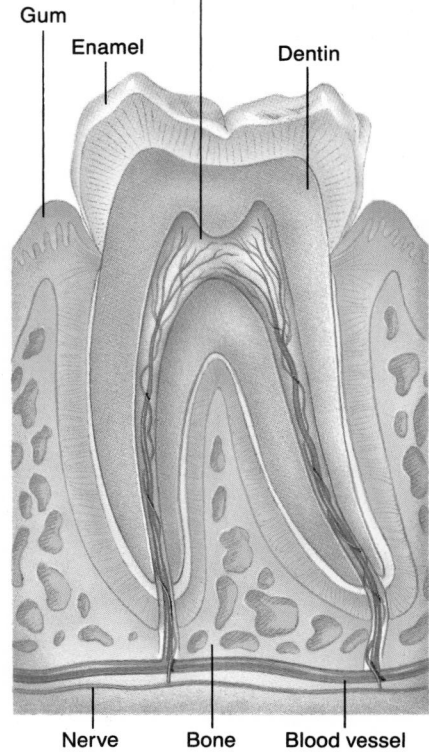

Pulp (blood vessels, nerves)
Gum
Enamel
Dentin
Nerve   Bone   Blood vessel

---

*Calcitonin, made in the thyroid gland, is secreted whenever the calcium concentration in the blood rises too high. It acts to stop withdrawal from bone and to slow absorption from the intestine. Parathormone, from the parathyroid glands, has the opposite effect.

peak bone mass: the highest attainable bone density for an individual, developed during the first three decades of life.

kefir: a yogurt-based beverage.

nori: a type of seaweed popular in Asian, particularly Japanese, cooking.

softening and bending of the bones. Osteoporosis involves the bones' becoming fragile and shattering.)

Not everyone agrees that the amount of calcium stored in the skeleton is affected by calcium intake; it may be determined by heredity or other lifestyle factors such as exercise or smoking.[2] However, it does seem to be true that the amount of calcium stored in the skeleton early in life is one of the primary determinants of susceptibility to osteoporosis later. Factors that influence osteoporosis development are further discussed in Controversy 8.

The body is sensitive to an increased need for calcium, although it sends no signals to the conscious brain indicating calcium need. Instead it adjusts its absorption of the mineral in the intestine and conserves it in the kidneys. During periods of growth, the intestinal absorption of calcium increases. Infants and children absorb up to 60 percent of ingested calcium; pregnant women, about 50 percent; and other adults, about 30 percent. The body also absorbs a higher percentage of calcium when less total mineral is provided in the diet. Deprived of calcium for months or years, an adult may absorb as much as 60 percent of that available; when supplied for years with abundant calcium, the same person may absorb only 10 percent. It takes time to adjust to changing intakes, though, and it is impossible to rectify a calcium deficiency that has occurred over many years by taking massive supplements for only a few days or weeks.

MEETING THE CALCIUM RDA. Because the human body can adjust its calcium absorption to varying levels of intake, setting recommended allowances is difficult. The U.S. and Canadian recommendations for calcium intake are high, especially for young people up to the age of 24 years, but are perhaps rightly so because people develop their **peak bone mass** during this time. After 25 years of age or so, the skeleton no longer adds to bone density, and after about 40 years of age, regardless of calcium intake, it begins to lose density.[3] Thus it is critical to obtain enough calcium during the young years of life so that the skeleton starts out with maximal mass. Then when the inevitable bone loss of aging begins, the skeleton stays stronger throughout the rest of life. Based on the hope that a high calcium intake would maximize bone density during the growing years, the RDA for calcium has been set at 1200 milligrams daily for young adults up to the age of 24 years. After 24 years, the RDA is set at 800 milligrams a day throughout life.

Milk and milk products are traditional sources of calcium for people who can tolerate them. Table 8–1 shows the current milk recommendations that help to meet the RDA for various age groups. People who do not use milk because of lactose intolerance, preference, or allergy must obtain calcium from other sources. Care is needed, though—*wise* substitutions must be made. Most of milk's many sisters are recommended choices: yogurt, **kefir**, buttermilk, cheese (especially the low-fat or nonfat varieties), and, for people who can afford the calories, ice milk. Some highly reputed milk products are less-than-ideal sources. Cottage cheese is only fair, 2 cups being equivalent in calcium to 1 cup of milk. Butter, cream, and cream cheese contain negligible calcium, being almost pure fat. Figure 8–6 compares the calcium values of a variety of foods, and Figure 8–7 on page 250 shows rich calcium sources.

If no milk product is acceptable as is, consider tinkering with it to make it work. Add chocolate to milk; fruit to yogurt; or nonfat milk powder to *any*

■■■ Table 8–1 Recommended Fluid Milk Intakes

AGE	RECOMMENDED INTAKE
Children under 9	2 to 3 c
Children 9 to 12	3 + c
Teenagers	4 + c
Adults	2 c
Pregnant women	3 + c
Lactating women	4 + c
Older women	3 to 5 c

■■■ Figure 8—6

Food Sources of Calcium Selected to Show a Range of Values.
Commonly Eaten Portions Ranked Richest to Poorest.

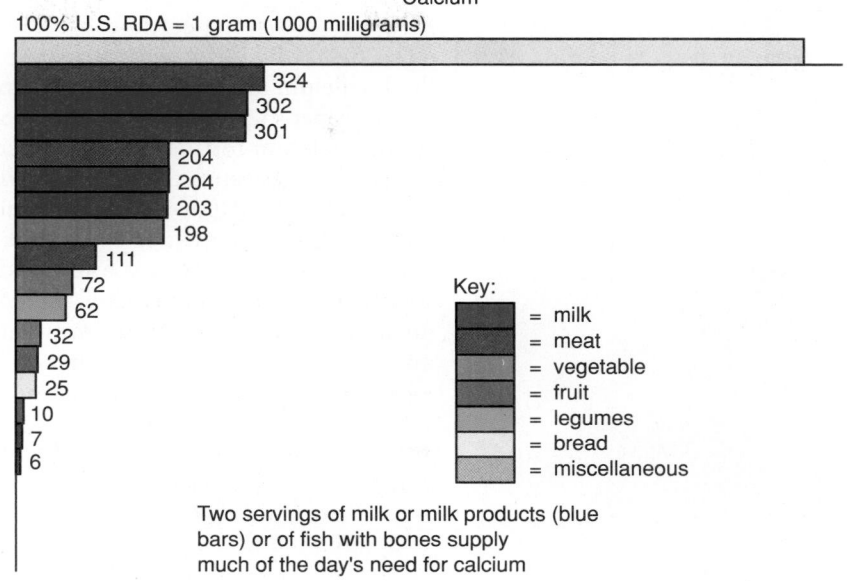

Food, serving size (energy)	Calcium 100% U.S. RDA = 1 gram (1000 milligrams)
Sardines, 3 oz canned with bones (175 cal)	324
Milk or yogurt, 1 c nonfat (86 cal)	302
Romano cheese, 1 oz (110 cal)	301
Salmon, 3 oz canned with bones (130 cal)	204
Cheddar cheese, 1 oz (114 cal)	204
Muenster cheese, 1 oz (104 cal)	203
Turnip greens, 1 c cooked (29 cal)	198
Oysters, 1 c raw (160 cal)	111
Broccoli, 1 c cooked (46 cal)	72
Kidney beans, 1 c canned (230 cal)	62
Cabbage, 1 c raw shredded (14 cal)	32
Cantaloupe, 1/2 (94 cal)	29
Whole-wheat bread, 1 slice (70 cal)	25
Apple, 1 fresh medium (80 cal)	10
Sirloin steak, 3 oz lean (180 cal)	7
Salmon, 3 oz meat only (120 cal)	6

Key:
= milk
= meat
= vegetable
= fruit
= legumes
= bread
= miscellaneous

Two servings of milk or milk products (blue bars) or of fish with bones supply much of the day's need for calcium

dish—meatloaf, cookies, hamburgers, gravies, soups, casseroles, puddings, even beverages such as coffee or tea, hot or iced. Only 5 heaping tablespoons are the equivalent of a cup of fresh milk.

For the many people who cannot use milk and milk products, small fish such as canned sardines or other canned fishes prepared with their bones, as well as oysters, are rich in calcium. Another rich source is extracts made from bones. (Witches are said to make magic with such brews, but actually wise food preparers of all cultures favor them too. The Vietnamese people's tradition of making such stock helps account for their adequate calcium intake without the use of milk.) To make the extract, soak cracked bones from chicken, turkey, pork, or fish in vinegar, and then slowly boil them. The bones release calcium into the acid medium, and most of the vinegar taste boils off. Then use the stock in place of water to cook soup, vegetables, rice, or stew. One *tablespoon* of such stock may contain over 100 milligrams of calcium.

Among vegetables, broccoli, beet greens, and kale are good sources of available calcium.[4] So are collard and mustard greens, watercress and parsley, and probably some seaweeds, such as the **nori** popular in Japanese cookery. Certain other foods, including spinach, swiss chard, and rhubarb, appear equal to milk in calcium contents but actually provide no calcium or very little calcium to the body because they contain binders that prevent calcium's absorption. (The presence of calcium binders does not make greens inferior foods from other standpoints. Dark greens are a superb source of riboflavin, virtually indispensable for the vegan or anyone else who does not drink milk. Greens also are rich in iron and dozens of other essential nutrients.)

■■■ **Figure 8–7**

Calcium in Foods.

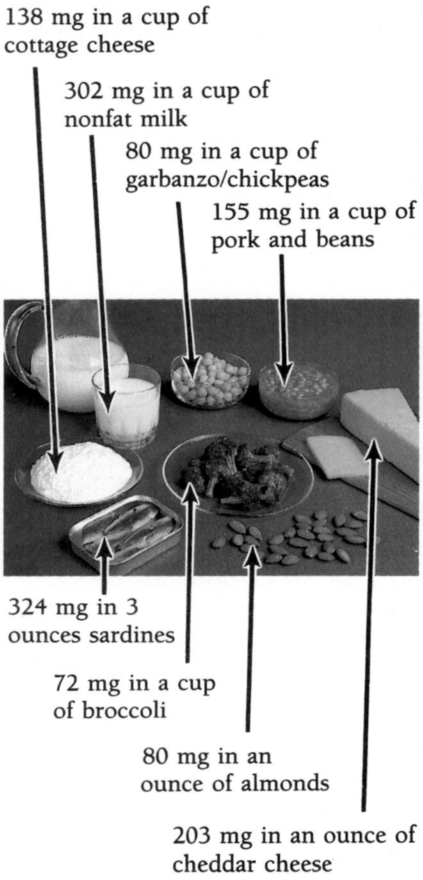

138 mg in a cup of
cottage cheese

302 mg in a cup of
nonfat milk

80 mg in a cup of
garbanzo/chickpeas

155 mg in a cup of
pork and beans

324 mg in 3
ounces sardines

72 mg in a cup
of broccoli

80 mg in an
ounce of almonds

203 mg in an ounce of
cheddar cheese

Next in order of preference among nonmilk sources of calcium are foods that contain large amounts of calcium salts by an accident of processing or by intentional fortification. In the processed category are bean curd (tofu—a calcium salt is often used to coagulate it); canned tomatoes (firming agents donate 63 milligrams per cup); stone-ground or self-rising flour; stone-ground whole or self-rising cornmeal; and blackstrap molasses. Among food products specially fortified to add calcium to people's diets, the richest in calcium is high-calcium milk itself (milk with extra calcium added), which provides more calcium per cup than any natural milk—500 milligrams per 8 ounces. Then comes calcium-fortified orange juice, with 300 milligrams per 8 ounces—a good choice because the bioavailability of its calcium compares favorably with that of milk. Calcium-fortified soy milk can also be prepared so that it contains more calcium than whole cow's milk. Infant formula, based on soy, is fortified with calcium, and no law forbids adults to use it in cooking for themselves. Finally, there are supplements intended to meet calcium needs without regard to needs for energy or other nutrients. Most people who take calcium supplements do so in hopes of warding off osteoporosis, but as Controversy 8 points out, supplements are not magic bullets against the condition.

■■▷ *Calcium makes up bone and tooth structure and plays roles in nerve transmission, muscle contraction, and blood clotting. Calcium absorption increases when there is a dietary deficiency or an increased need such as during growth. Milk and milk products are rich calcium sources, as are fish with bones, certain green vegetables, and calcium-fortified foods.*

Sodium

Salt has been known throughout recorded history. The Bible's saying "You are the salt of the earth" means that a person is valuable. If, on the other hand, "you are not worth your salt," you are worthless. Even the word *salary* comes from the word *salt*.† Sodium is the positive ion in the compound sodium chloride (table salt) and other salts and contributes 40 percent of its weight. Thus if a person consumes a gram of salt, that person consumes 400 milligrams of sodium. As already mentioned, sodium is the chief ion used to maintain the volume of fluid outside cells.

A deficiency of sodium would be harmful, but there is seldom a sodium shortage in the diet. Foods usually include more salt than is needed, and the body absorbs it freely. The kidneys filter the surplus out of the blood into the urine. They can also sensitively conserve salt. In the rare event of a deficiency, they can return to the bloodstream the exact amount needed.‡ Normally the amount of sodium you excrete in a day equals the amount you have ingested

---

†To the chemist, a salt results from neutralization of an acid and a base. Sodium chloride—table salt—results from the reaction between hydrochloric acid and the base sodium hydroxide. The positive sodium ion unites with the negative chloride ion to form the salt, and the positive hydrogen ion unites with the negative hydroxide ion to form water.

Base + acid = salt + water.

Sodium hydroxide + hydrochloric acid = sodium chloride + water.

‡The amount of sodium to be returned by the kidneys to the blood is under the control of an adrenal gland hormone, aldosterone.

that day. About 30 to 40 percent of the body's sodium is thought to be stored on the surface of the bone crystals, where the body can easily draw upon it to replenish the blood concentration, if necessary.

If the blood level of sodium rises, as it will after a person eats salted foods, thirst ensures that the person will drink water until the sodium-to-water ratio is restored. Then the kidneys can excrete the extra fluid along with the extra sodium.

For a brief summary of the kidneys' action, see Chapter 3.

Dieters sometimes think that eating too much salt or drinking too much water will make them gain weight, but they do not gain fat, of course. They gain water, but they excrete excess water immediately. Excess salt is excreted as soon as enough water is drunk to carry the salt out of the body. From this perspective, then, the way to keep body salt (and "water weight") under control is to drink more, not less, water.

The connection of salt with high blood pressure in salt-sensitive people is well known, and most people have learned that they should not consume too much sodium. Some question has arisen recently, however, about whether the culprit in relation to high blood pressure is sodium alone, the particular combination of sodium and chloride, or even the chloride ion alone. Chapter 11 describes the relationships of these and other factors to blood pressure.

If the blood level of sodium drops, both water and sodium must be replenished to avert emergency. Overly strict use of low-sodium diets in the treatment of hypertension, kidney disease, or heart disease can deplete the body of needed sodium; so can vomiting, diarrhea, or heavy sweating. Under normal conditions of sweating due to exercise, salt losses may easily be replaced later in the day with ordinary foods. Guidelines for replacement of both salt and water after heavy sweating are given in Chapter 10.

Pregnant women used to be told to restrict their sodium intakes to prevent pregnancy-induced hypertension (see Chapter 12). Now it is clear that they need not make special efforts to do so but should eat well-rounded diets of ordinary foods and should avoid consuming salt in excess.

Diets rarely lack sodium. For this reason no RDA has been set; instead, the RDA committee estimated the *minimum* sodium requirement for adults to be 500 milligrams.[5] The National Research Council (NRC) recommendations emphasize moderation, not adequacy, and thus set a maximum intake of *salt* at 6 grams (2400 milligrams sodium). Most people in the United States average about 6 to 18 grams of salt per day. Cultures vary in their use of salt. Asian people, whose staple sauces and flavorings are based on soy sauce and monosodium glutamate (MSG or Accent), consume about 30 to 40 grams of salt per day.

One of the most important favors you can do yourself, especially if you have heart disease in your family, is to learn to control your salt intake. An obvious step is to control your use of the saltshaker, but this source may account for as little as 15 percent of your total salt intake. A more productive step may be to limit intakes of processed foods, the source of up to 75 percent of the salt in most people's diets.[6] (The other 10 percent occurs naturally in foods.) This chapter's Food Feature shows how to cut down on salt, and Table 8–3 of that section shows how processing adds sodium to foods while depleting another mineral of interest, potassium.

▐▌▶ *Sodium is the main positively charged ion outside the body's cells. Sodium attracts water, and thus too much sodium (or salt) may aggravate hypertension. Diets rarely lack sodium.*

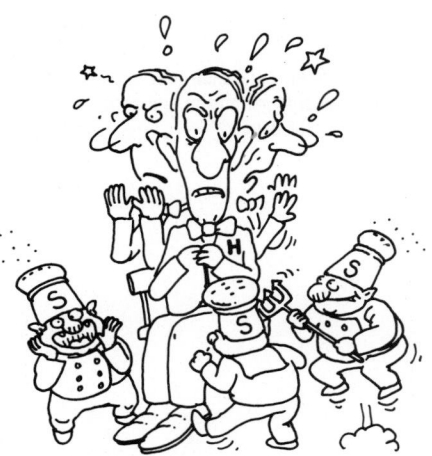

Salt may aggravate hypertension.

■■■ **Figure 8–8**

Food Sources of Potassium Selected to Show a Range of Values.
Commonly Eaten Portions Ranked Richest to Poorest

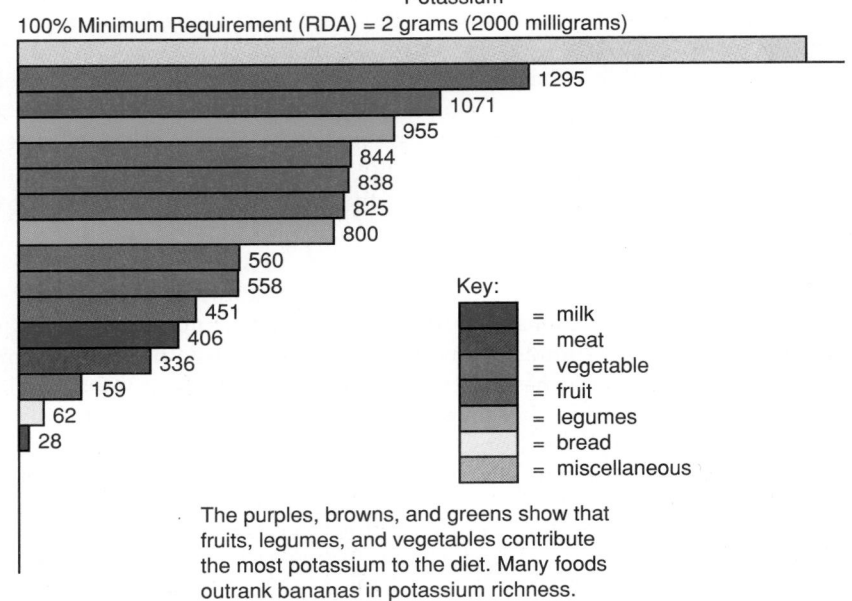

Food, serving size (energy)

Potassium
100% Minimum Requirement (RDA) = 2 grams (2000 milligrams)

Peach halves, 10 dried (311 cal) — 1295
Winter squash, 1 c baked (96 cal) — 1071
Lima beans, 1 c cooked (260 cal) — 955
Baked potato, 1 whole (220 cal) — 844
Spinach, 1 c cooked (41 cal) — 838
Cantaloupe, 1/2 (94 cal) — 825
Pinto beans, 1 c cooked (265 cal) — 800
Watermelon, 1 slice (152 cal) — 560
Asparagus, 1 c cooked (44 cal) — 558
Banana, 1 peeled (105 cal) — 451
Milk or yogurt, 1 c nonfat (86 cal) — 406
Sirloin steak, 3 oz lean (180 cal) — 336
Apple, 1 fresh medium (80 cal) — 159
Whole-wheat bread, 1 slice (70 cal) — 62
Cheddar cheese, 1 oz (114 cal) — 28

Key:
= milk
= meat
= vegetable
= fruit
= legumes
= bread
= miscellaneous

The purples, browns, and greens show that fruits, legumes, and vegetables contribute the most potassium to the diet. Many foods outrank bananas in potassium richness.

Potassium

Potassium is the principal, positively charged ion inside body cells. It plays a major role in maintaining fluid and electrolyte balance and cell integrity. It is also critical to maintaining the heartbeat; the sudden deaths that occur during fasting or severe diarrhea and in kwashiorkor children are thought to be due to heart failure caused by potassium loss.

Dehydration leads to potassium loss from inside cells. It is especially dangerous because potassium loss from brain cells makes the victim unaware of the need for water. Because of this adults are warned not to take **diuretics** (water pills) that cause potassium loss, except under the direction of a physician. When taking such diuretics, a person should alert all other health care providers to their use. Any physician prescribing such diuretics will tell the client to eat potassium-rich foods to compensate for the losses and, depending on the diuretic, may advise a lower sodium intake, too.

If a person should sweat profusely day after day and fail to replenish potassium stores, gradual potassium depletion might occur. However, even four days of sweating while eating a low-potassium diet did not deplete people's plasma or muscle potassium in one study.[7] Furthermore, any food made of unbroken cells that have not been exposed to too much processing is rich in potassium. Thus potassium needs are easily met. Bananas, despite their fame as a rich potassium source, are just moderate. Bananas, however, are available everywhere, are easy to chew, and have a sweet taste that almost everyone likes. As Figure 8–8 shows, foods of all kinds offer abundant potassium, and most whole vegetables and fruits are outstanding.

Unlike sodium, potassium may exert a positive effect against hypertension and related ills—see Chapter 11 for details.

Potassium chloride pills are available over the counter and are sold in health food stores without a warning label, but they should not be used except on a physician's advice. People's lives are not normally threatened by potassium overdoses as long as they are taken by mouth because the presence of excess potassium in the stomach triggers a vomiting reflex that expels the unwanted substance. A person with a weak heart should not be put through this trauma, however, and a baby may not be able to withstand it.

❚❚▷ *Potassium is the major, positive ion inside cells, important in many metabolic and structural functions. Diuretics can deplete potassium and so can be dangerous; potassium excess can also be dangerous.*

Other Major Minerals

Magnesium, chloride, and sulfur are grouped together, not to indicate that they are less important than others but only because space here is limited. Indeed, much more is known about these critical elements, and each is unique in its ability to perform its specific functions in the body.

MAGNESIUM. Magnesium barely qualifies as a major mineral: only about 1 ¾ ounces are present in the body of a 130-pound person. In the body, magnesium is critical to the operation of hundreds of enzymes and directly affects the metabolism of potassium, calcium, and vitamin D. Most magnesium is in the bones, and the supply can be tapped to maintain a constant blood level whenever dietary intake falls too low. The kidney can also act to conserve magnesium. Deficiency of magnesium may occur as a result of inadequate intake, vomiting, diarrhea, alcoholism or protein malnutrition; in hospital clients who have been fed incomplete fluids into a vein for too long; or in persons using diuretics.

People whose drinking water has a high magnesium content experience a lower incidence of sudden death from heart failure than other people. It seems likely that magnesium deficiency makes the heart unable to stop itself from going into spasms once it starts.[8] Such a deficiency can cause hallucinations that can be mistaken for mental illness or drunkenness.

Survey results show that the RDA is seldom met, but the development of overt deficiency symptoms in the absence of some other predisposing factor is unlikely.[9] Figure 8–9 (next page) shows which foods rank high in magnesium. It is easily lost from foods during processing, so slightly processed or unprocessed foods are the best choices.

CHLORIDE. The chloride ion is a major negative ion in the body. In the fluids outside the cells, it accompanies sodium; inside the cells it occurs primarily in association with potassium. Thus it helps to maintain the crucial fluid balances (acid-base and electrolyte balances) mentioned in the earlier discussion of water. The chloride ion also plays a special role as part of the hydrochloric acid that maintains the strong acidity of the stomach. Its principal food source is salt, both added and naturally occurring in foods. In its chlorine form, the mineral is deadly poison and is thus useful as a disinfectant, so long as it is handled carefully.

diuretics (dye-you-RET-ics): medications causing increased water excretion (*dia* means "through"; *ouron* means "urine").

Chapter 10 comes back to discuss magnesium in relation to the exercising body.

■■■ Figure 8–9

Food Sources of Magnesium Selected to Show a Range of Values.
Commonly Eaten Portions Ranked Richest to Poorest.

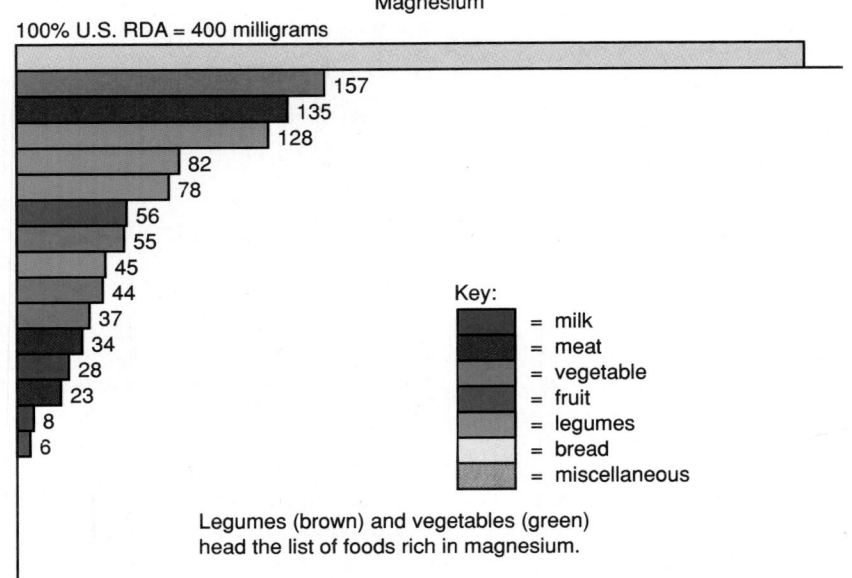

Food, serving size (energy)	Magnesium
	100% U.S. RDA = 400 milligrams
Spinach, 1 c cooked (41 cal)	157
Oysters, 1 c raw (160 cal)	135
Sunflower seeds, 1/4 c dry (205 cal)	128
Lima beans, 1 c cooked (260 cal)	82
Garbanzo beans, 1 c cooked (270 cal)	78
Figs, 5 dried (239 cal)	56
Baked potato, 1 whole (220 cal)	55
Cashew nuts, 1 oz roasted (163 cal)	45
Summer squash, 1 c cooked (36 cal)	44
Broccoli, 1 c cooked (46 cal)	37
Shrimp, 3.5 oz boiled (109 cal)	34
Milk or yogurt, 1 c nonfat (86 cal)	28
Sirloin steak, 3 oz lean (180 cal)	23
Cheddar cheese, 1 oz (114 cal)	8
Apple, 1 fresh medium (80 cal)	6

Key:
= milk
= meat
= vegetable
= fruit
= legumes
= bread
= miscellaneous

Legumes (brown) and vegetables (green)
head the list of foods rich in magnesium.

SULFUR. Sulfur plays no roles of its own but forms part of proteins and other compounds; deficiencies are unknown. The summary table at the end of this chapter presents the main facts on the major minerals.

■■▶ *Magnesium is essential for cellular reactions; deficiencies can result from vomiting, diarrhea, alcoholism, or protein malnutrition. Chloride is the body's major negative ion inside and outside of cells. It is essential to the acid-base balance and is part of the stomach's hydrochloric acid. Sulfur is also considered a major mineral, although it occurs only as part of other compounds such as protein.*

■■■ The Trace Minerals

Laboratory techniques developed in the last two decades have enabled scientists to detect minerals in smaller and smaller quantities in living cells. Knowledge of the "new" trace elements is coming out of this research. An obstacle to determining their precise roles lies in the difficult task of providing an experimental diet lacking in the one element under study. Thus research in this area is limited to study of laboratory animals, which can be fed highly refined, purified diets in environments that are free of all contamination. Whole books have been published on the trace minerals alone, and research is still rapidly expanding knowledge about them.

Iodine

Iodine is needed by the body in an infinitesimally small quantity, but its principal role in human nutrition makes obtaining this amount critical. Iodine is a part of thyroxin, the hormone responsible for regulating the basal metabolic rate. Iodine must be available for thyroxin to be synthesized.

The amount in the diet is variable and generally reflects the soil in which plants are grown or on which animals graze. Iodine is plentiful in the ocean, so seafood is a completely dependable source. In parts of the United States in areas that were never under the ocean (most notably the Great Plains states and Oregon's Willamette valley), the soil is poor in iodine. In those areas the use of iodized salt and the consumption of foods shipped in from other, iodine-rich areas have been necessary to wipe out the iodine deficiency that once was widespread. Surprisingly, sea salt delivers little iodine to the eater because iodine becomes a gas and escapes off the salt during the drying process.

When the iodine level of the blood is low, the cells of the thyroid gland enlarge in an attempt to trap as many particles of iodine as possible. Sometimes the gland enlarges until it is visible, forming a **goiter**. People with the condition suffer sluggishness and weight gain, and in a pregnant woman, severe iodine deficiency causes the extreme and irreversible mental and physical retardation of the infant known as **cretinism.** Much of the mental retardation can be averted if the pregnant woman's deficiency is detected and treated in time, but if it goes uncorrected, the child may live out its life with an IQ as low as 20 (100 is average).

In most regions the need for iodine is easily met by consuming seafood and vegetables grown in iodine-rich soil. In developed countries food is shipped from place to place to such an extent that some iodine-rich food is likely to be available everywhere. In iodine-poor regions the iodization of salt has all but eliminated the widespread misery caused there earlier by goiter and cretinism. However, goiter is still prevalent in developing nations. In the United States salt-box labels state whether salt is iodized; in Canada all table salt is iodized.

Excessive intakes of iodine can also cause an enlargement of the thyroid gland resembling goiter, which in infants can be so severe as to block the airways and to cause suffocation. A dramatic increase in iodine intakes in the United States concerns some observers. Intakes reached an all-time high of 800 micrograms per day in 1974; it has since declined somewhat but is still several times the RDA of 150 micrograms. The toxic level at which detectable harm results is thought to be over 2000 micrograms per day for an adult, an amount only a few times higher than the amount most people receive daily. Like chlorine and fluorine, iodine is a deadly poison in large amounts.

Most of the excess iodine in U.S. diets today comes from bakery products—iodates (dough conditioners) are used by the baking industry—and from milk (most dairies feed cows iodine-containing medications and use iodine to disinfect milking equipment). One cup of milk supplies nearly the RDA of iodine, and so does less than a half teaspoon of iodized salt.[10] Both the dairy and bakery industries have been reducing their use of iodine compounds, but the sudden emergence of this problem points to a need for continued surveillance of the food supply.

⁐▶ *Iodine is part of the hormone thyroxin, which influences energy metabolism. The deficiency diseases are goiter and cretinism. Iodine occurs naturally in seafood*

goiter (GOY-ter): enlargement of the thyroid gland due to iodine deficiency.

cretinism (CREE-tin-ism): severe mental and physical retardation of an infant caused by iodine deficiency during pregnancy.

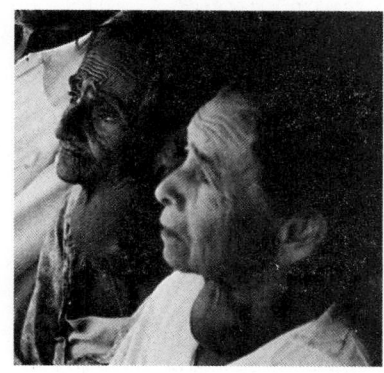

These people have goiter, enlargement of the thyroid gland due to iodine deficiency.

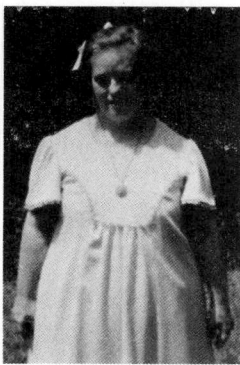

An adult with cretinism—her mother was iodine deficient while pregnant with her.

and in foods grown on land that was once covered by oceans; it is an additive in milk and bakery products. Large amounts are poisonous.

Iron

Iron is probably the most widely known of all the essential minerals. Television viewers, particularly, hear that the woman who "takes good care of herself" takes iron supplements every day and that "you should, too."

Most of the iron in the body is a component of the proteins **hemoglobin** and **myoglobin.** Both these compounds use iron to help carry or hold oxygen. Hemoglobin is the oxygen carrier in the red blood cells, and myoglobin is the oxygen reservoir in the muscle cells.

All the cells need oxygen to combine with the carbon and hydrogen atoms they release as they break down energy nutrients. The body then excretes the carbon dioxide and water; thus it constantly needs fresh oxygen and nutrients to keep the cells going. As cells use up and excrete their oxygen (as carbon dioxide and water), the red blood cells shuttle between metabolizing tissues and lungs to bring in fresh oxygen supplies. Besides helping hemoglobin to carry oxygen around and myoglobin to hold it in muscles, iron helps many enzymes in energy pathways to use oxygen.

IRON-DEFICIENCY ANEMIA. In **iron-deficiency anemia** the red blood cells contain too little hemoglobin and thus deliver too little oxygen to the tissues. This limits cells' energy metabolism. Symptoms of iron-deficiency anemia include some that actually reflect energy deficiency—tiredness, apathy, and a tendency to feel cold. Others reflect impairment of brain functions, such as the ability to concentrate, that depend on adequate iron in the brain.

A curious symptom seen in some people with iron deficiency is an appetite for ice, clay, paste, and other nonnutritious substances. Some people have been known to eat as many as eight trays of ice in a day, for example. This behavior has been observed in women and children of low-income groups who are deficient in either iron or zinc, and has been given the name **pica.** When caused by iron deficiency, pica clears up dramatically within days after iron is given, even if anemia is present and the red blood cells haven't yet responded. The mental symptoms of anemia are also among the first to improve with iron therapy.

A sample of iron-deficient blood examined under the microscope shows small red blood cells that are unusually light in color. To diagnose iron deficiency, the physician usually measures the blood hemoglobin level. Iron supplements will correct anemia—provided, of course, that iron deficiency has caused it (see the Consumer Caution entitled "Iron-Fortified Foods and Iron Supplements" later in this chapter).

Millions of people the world over suffer from iron deficiency without the benefit of a diagnosis. Even in the United States and Canada, about 20 percent of all women and 3 percent of men have no iron in their body stores; some 8 percent of women and 1 percent of men have anemia, along with its associated ills. Long before the red blood cells are affected, physical work capacity and productivity are impaired. Children deprived of iron become irritable, unable to concentrate, and restless. These symptoms are among the first to appear when the body's iron level begins to fall and are among the first to disappear when iron intake is increased again.[11]

Feeling fatigued, weak, and apathetic is a sign that something is wrong, but it is not a sign that you necessarily need iron or other supplements. Two actions are called for: first, get your diet in order; then, if symptoms persist, consult a physician for a diagnosis.

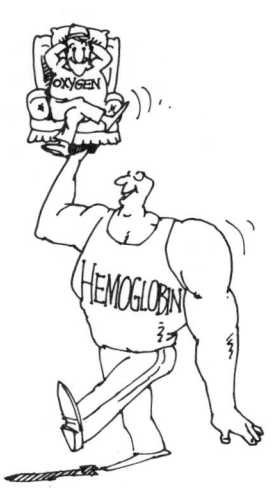

Hemoglobin in red blood cells uses iron to carry oxygen to the body's cells.

The worldwide impact of full-blown anemia and of iron deficiency milder than anemia can hardly be overstated. Iron deficiency occurs in as many as *half* of all persons in some settings, even in developed countries—most predictably among inner-city dwellers and rural poor. With reduced energy available to work, plan, think, or learn, people simply do these things less, and they may appear to others to be lazy or apathetic. Because they work and play less, they become less physically fit. To alleviate just this one form of malnutrition worldwide would be to dramatically improve the quality of a *billion* lives.

In most developed countries, incidence of full-blown iron-deficiency anemia ranges from 10 to 20 percent, and the incidence of less severe iron deficiency must be higher still.[12] In the United States, evidence suggests that anemia rates among one group—low-income children—may be falling, and this is welcome news indeed.[13]

CAUSES OF IRON DEFICIENCY. The cause of iron deficiency is usually malnutrition, that is, inadequate iron intake, either from sheer lack of food or from high consumption of the wrong foods. In the western world the cause is often that we choose too few iron-rich foods, and too many foods high in sugar and fat. Even vegetarians who design their own meal plans without following traditional patterns often shortchange themselves on iron and are prone to anemia.

Among nonnutritional causes of anemia, blood loss is the primary one. About 80 percent of the iron in the body is in the blood, so iron losses are great whenever blood is lost. Menstruation causes iron losses that make a woman's need for iron half again as great as a man's. In many countries parasitic infections of the digestive tract cause people to lose blood daily; for their entire lives they may feel tired and unenergetic but never know why. Ulcers can also cause blood loss leading to anemia.

People of certain groups need more iron than others. Growth involves enlargement of the blood volume, so infants, children, adolescents, and pregnant women need extra iron. Absorption increases, to be sure, but still, these people must be sure to eat iron-rich foods. Also, as mentioned, menstruating women need extra iron.

A key difference between women and men is a difference in their body stores of iron; women are often at the borderline of deficiency. Should a woman lose blood for any reason, even by donating to a blood bank, she would need to make a special effort to replenish her iron stores.

IRON ABSORPTION AND STORAGE. Iron deficiency may also be caused by poor absorption of the iron that is in food. Factors that impair iron availability are tea, coffee, soy protein, wheat bran, calcium supplements, and fiber. Also, stomach acid aids iron absorption; if acid secretion is sluggish, as it often is in older people, iron absorption declines. Even without these influences, though, a normal, healthy person absorbs only about 10 percent of the iron from a mixed diet—about 2 to 10 percent from vegetables and eggs and about 10 to 30 percent from red meats. Figure 8–10 shows iron amounts in food regarded as rich iron sources.

Much of the iron in meat, fish, and poultry is bound into molecules of heme, the iron-containing part of hemoglobin and myoglobin. Heme iron is much

hemoglobin (HEEM-oh-globe-in): the oxygen-carrying protein of the blood; found in the red blood cells (*hemo* means "blood"; *globin* means "spherical protein").

myoglobin (MYE-o-globe-in): the oxygen-holding protein of the muscles (*myo* means "muscle").

iron-deficiency anemia: one of the anemias characterized by red blood cell shrinkage and color loss caused by iron deficiency. Accompanying symptoms are weakness, apathy, headaches, pallor, intolerance to cold, and inability to pay attention. (For other anemias see index.)

pica (PIE-ka): a craving for nonfood substances. Also known as **geophagia** (gee-oh-FAY-gee-uh) when referring to clay eating, **pagophagia** (pag-oh-FAY-gee-uh) when referring to ice craving. (*picus* means "woodpecker"; *geo* means "earth"; *pago* means "frost"; *phagia* means "to eat".)

heme (HEEM): the iron-containing portion of the hemoglobin and myoglobin molecules.

Factors that hinder iron absorption:

- Tea.
- Coffee.
- Soy protein.
- Wheat bran.
- Calcium supplements.
- Fiber.

MFP factor: a factor (identity unknown) present in Meat, Fish, and Poultry that enhances the absorption of nonheme iron present in the same foods or in other foods eaten at the same time.

iron overload: the state of having more iron in the body than it needs or can handle. Iron can become toxic and damage the liver.

Factors that increase iron absorption:

■ Vitamin C.
■ MFP factor.
■ Normal stomach acidity.

■■■ Figure 8–10

Iron in Foods.

2.34 mg in half a liverwurst, whole-wheat sandwich

6.30 mg in 5 steamed clams

1.80 mg in a half cup black beans

3.21 mg in a half cup spinach

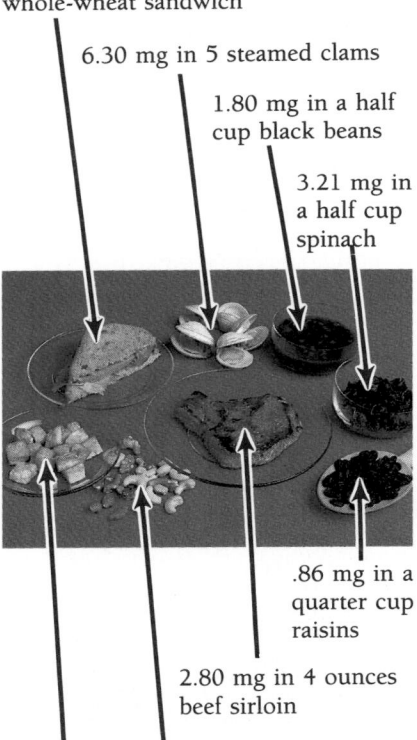

.86 mg in a quarter cup raisins

2.80 mg in 4 ounces beef sirloin

1.05 mg in an ounce of nuts

6.65 mg in a half cup tofu

more absorbable than nonheme iron. Meat, fish, and poultry also contain a factor (**MFP factor**) other than heme that increases by four times the absorption of nonheme iron from other foods eaten with it. Vitamin C taken with nonheme iron can triple its absorption. A system has been devised, based on all these factors, to calculate the amount of iron absorbed from a meal (see the Self-Study at the end of this chapter).

Knowing how important adequate iron is to good health, you may think that a "wise" body would absorb *all* the iron in foods. But iron is toxic in large amounts, and once inside, it is difficult to excrete. The body's defense against iron poisoning is a control system: the intestinal cells trap some of the iron and hold it within their boundaries. When they are shed, these cells carry out of the intestinal tract the excess iron that they collected during their brief lives. When the intestinal lining is damaged (by alcohol abuse, for example), the body is vulnerable to poisoning by excess iron. Table 8–2 summarizes the effects of iron toxicity. Be forewarned against unnecessarily taking supplements that contain high doses of iron and keep such pills safely out of children's reach.

Once inside the body, iron is treated like gold; the body hoards it. The liver packs iron that has been kept in the bone marrow into new red blood cells and ships them out to the blood, where they live for about three to four months. When they die, the liver breaks them down and saves their iron, and sends it back to the bone marrow to be kept for reuse. Only tiny losses of iron occur in the clipping of nails, the cutting of hair, and the shedding of skin cells.

The iron RDA is 10 milligrams a day for men and older women. For women of childbearing age, the RDA is 15 milligrams to replace menstrual losses; during pregnancy a woman's need doubles to 30 mg of iron. Adult men experience iron-deficiency anemia rarely, but some men inherit a tendency to develop the toxicity condition known as **iron overload**. Should a man have a *low* hemoglobin concentration, this alerts his care provider to examine him for a blood-loss site.

To be sure to meet iron needs, it is best to rely on foods (the Consumer Caution on Iron-Fortified Foods and Iron Supplements shows why). However, the usual Western mixed diet provides only about 5 to 6 milligrams of iron in each 1000 calories, not enough for some people. An adult male who eats upwards of 2500 calories a day has no trouble meeting his RDA of 10 milligrams, but a woman who eats fewer calories and needs *more* iron understandably does have trouble meeting her 15-milligram RDA. A woman must double her diet's average iron-to-calorie ratio. To do this, she must select high-iron, low-calorie foods from each food group. Figure 8–11 (page 260) shows how iron is distributed in foods. Although you might expect meats to dominate the top of the graph (iron per serving), notice that legumes and spinach rank higher. However, remember that the iron from meat is more absorbable, so both meats and legumes are good sources. When you eat meat with legumes (franks and beans, chili con carne), MFP factor enhances iron absorption from both. The vitamin C from a slice of tomato and a leaf of lettuce in a sandwich will enhance iron absorption from the bread. The meat and tomato in spaghetti sauce help the eater to absorb the iron from the spaghetti. (A sauce cooked in an iron pan draws iron from this source, too.) Meat iron is always well absorbed, but iron from vegetables, legumes, and grains needs help.

■■▶ *Most iron in the body is contained in hemoglobin and myoglobin or occurs as a part of enzymes in the energy-yielding pathways. Iron-deficiency anemia is a problem worldwide. Iron is lost through menstruation and other bleeding; the shedding of intestinal cells protects against overload. Too much iron is toxic. For optimal iron intake, use meat, other iron sources, and vitamin C together.*

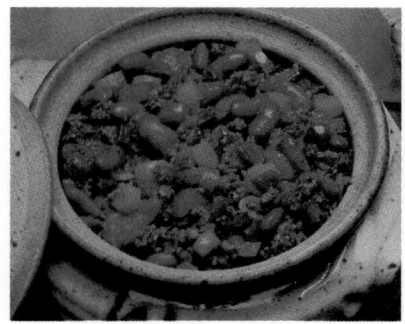

The meat and tomatoes in this chili help the eater to absorb iron from the beans.

CONSUMER CAUTION▮▮▮	**Iron-Fortified Foods and Iron Supplements**

Some people need iron in supplement form. The Committee on RDA acknowledges that pregnant women may need it, and the Canadian Recommended Nutrient Intakes (RNI) also includes this statement. However, the iron from supplements is far less well absorbed than that from food, so the doses have to be as high as 50 milligrams per day. A person can improve the absorption of the iron from supplements by taking meat or vitamin C-rich foods or juices along with them. The supplement taker should look for the word "ferrous" on the label; the ferrous form is better absorbed than the ferric form.

Cooking foods in iron pans is somewhat like taking supplements—ferric iron from the metal pan contaminates the food. The iron content of 100 grams of spaghetti sauce simmered in a glass dish is 3 milligrams, but it is 87 milligrams when the sauce is cooked in a black iron skillet. Even in the short time it takes to scramble eggs, their iron content can be tripled by cooking them in an iron pan. Similarly, the reason why dried peaches or raisins contain more iron than the fresh fruit is because they are dried in iron pans. This iron is in the form of inorganic salts and is not as well absorbed as that from meat, but some does get into the body.

The use of enriched or fortified foods is another option. Iron added to foods is "reduced iron," that is, it is in the ferrous form, which is well-absorbed. In the right food carrier, absorption of iron from enriched foods can be significant. At present, 25 percent of all the iron consumed in the United States is in foods to which iron has been added, including the familiar enriched breads and cereals and fortified breakfast cereals. These food sources are important because people eat so much of them as to derive significant iron from the total.

A number of proposals have been made for further fortification—of milk, fish, rice, infant foods, coffee, junk foods, salt, sugar, and soy sauce. Worldwide fortification of soy sauce could improve the iron status of a third of the world's people. A proposal to increase the iron level in enriched bread above that now enforced has been defeated; that level of fortification is used in Sweden and is believed to account for the people's better iron status there than in the United States. However, some people are genetically prone to iron overload conditions, and even the current levels of enrichment place them at risk of toxicity. Even for healthy men, the safety of high iron intakes is questioned. In this country it is extremely difficult to obtain a balanced, nutritious diet that meets women's iron needs while keeping men's iron intakes to a minimum.

In any case, foods are a better source of iron than are fortification or supplements. Two stories illustrate this point—one set in the United States, the other in West Java. The first was a study of over 200 adults in Boston who had hemoglobin levels below normal. Two-thirds were given iron-fortified foods

continued on next page

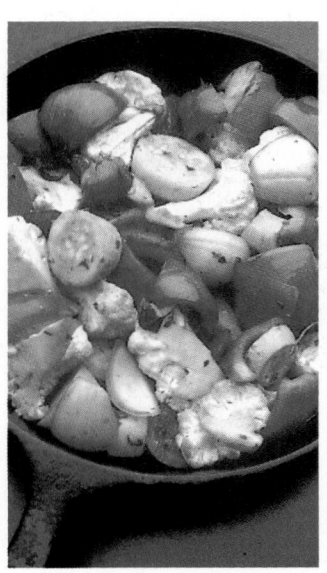

The old-fashioned iron skillet adds supplemental iron to foods.

for six to eight months; the others were given the same foods without added iron. At the end of the study *all* had higher hemoglobin levels. Food made the difference, with or without added iron.[14]

The study in West Java involved rubber plantation workers with iron-deficiency anemia. The more anemic they were, the less work they could do, and the more often they got sick with infections. Half were given an iron supplement, the other half a placebo—but *both* improved in work output. Apparently the placebo effect enabled both groups to work better; this led to increased pay; and the workers spent the extra money on food. The extra food supplied 3 to 5 extra milligrams of iron a day, together with vitamin C![15]

Zinc

Zinc occurs in a very small quantity in the body but works with proteins in every organ as a helper for some 70 enzymes. The summary table at the end of the chapter enumerates some of its many vital activities.

No nationwide survey has yet undertaken to assess the extent of zinc deficiency in the United States or Canada, but indications are that it does occur, especially where certain predisposing factors are present. A deficiency of zinc

■■■ **Figure 8–11**

Food Sources of Iron Selected to Show a Range of Values.
Commonly Eaten Portions Ranked Richest to Poorest

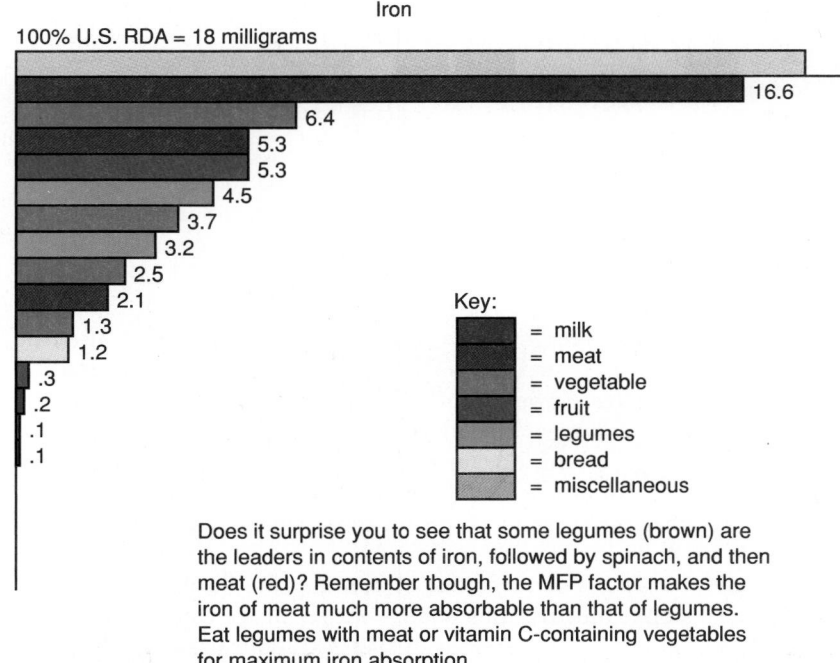

Food, serving size (energy)	Iron (mg)
Oysters, 1 c raw (160 cal)	16.6
Spinach, 1 c cooked (41 cal)	6.4
Beef liver, 3 oz fried (185 cal)	5.3
Peach halves, 10 dried (311 cal)	5.3
Lima beans, 1 c cooked (260 cal)	4.5
Parsley, 1 c chopped fresh (20 cal)	3.7
Kidney beans, 1 c canned (230 cal)	3.2
Green peas, 1 c cooked (67 cal)	2.5
Sirloin steak, 3 oz lean (180 cal)	2.1
Broccoli, 1 c cooked (46 cal)	1.3
Whole-wheat bread, 1 slice (70 cal)	1.2
Apple, 1 fresh medium (80 cal)	.3
Cheddar cheese, 1 oz (114 cal)	.2
Orange, 1 fresh medium (80 cal)	.1
Milk or yogurt, 1 c nonfat (86 cal)	.1

100% U.S. RDA = 18 milligrams

Key:
= milk
= meat
= vegetable
= fruit
= legumes
= bread
= miscellaneous

Does it surprise you to see that some legumes (brown) are the leaders in contents of iron, followed by spinach, and then meat (red)? Remember though, the MFP factor makes the iron of meat much more absorbable than that of legumes. Eat legumes with meat or vitamin C-containing vegetables for maximum iron absorption.

in human beings was first reported in the 1960s from studies with growing children and adolescent boys in the Middle East. The native diets were typically low in animal protein and high in whole grains and beans; consequently they were high in fiber and other zinc-binding factors known as **phytates.** Furthermore, the bread they ate was unleavened; the phytates had not been broken down by yeast as normally occurs in leavened bread. The zinc deficiency was marked by severe growth retardation and arrested sexual maturation—symptoms that were at least partly reversed by zinc supplementation.

In the United States, too, poor growth, poor appetite, and impaired taste sensitivity may indicate zinc deficiency. When pediatricians or other health workers evaluating children's health note poor growth accompanied by poor appetite, they should think zinc.

Since the first reports, zinc deficiency has been recognized elsewhere, and it is known to affect much more than just growth. It alters digestive function profoundly and causes diarrhea, which worsens the malnutrition already present, with respect not only to zinc but to all nutrients. It drastically impairs the immune response, making infections likely—including infections in the intestinal tract, which worsen malnutrition, including zinc malnutrition. Normal vitamin metabolism depends on zinc, so zinc-deficiency symptoms often include vitamin-deficiency symptoms. Zinc deficiency disturbs thyroid function and slows the body's energy metabolism. It alters taste, causes loss of appetite, slows wound healing—in fact, its symptoms are so all-pervasive that generalized malnutrition and sickness are more likely to be the diagnosis than zinc deficiency alone.

Zinc is toxic in large quantities, and toxicity can occur from use of zinc supplements. Doses of zinc only a few milligrams above the RDA lower the body's copper content—an effect that, in animals, leads to degeneration of the heart muscle. High doses of zinc alter cholesterol metabolism and appear to accelerate the development of atherosclerosis (Table 8–2 lists other symptoms). Zinc poisoning can be fatal. Unlike iron, some excess zinc can escape from the body; the pancreas secretes zinc-rich juices into the digestive tract, some of which pass unabsorbed out of the body.

Meats, shellfish, and poultry are top providers of zinc (Figures 8–12 and 8–13). Among plant sources, some legumes and whole grains are rich in zinc, but it is not so well absorbed from them as from meat. The RDA of 15 milligrams per day for men and 12 milligrams per day for women is probably not met by most people; the average intake is probably closer to 10 milligrams. Vegetarians are advised to eat varied diets that include whole-grain breads well leavened with yeast, which improves the availability of zinc.

▐▐ ▷ *Zinc assists enzymes in all cells. Deficiency in children causes growth retardation with sexual immaturity. Zinc is toxic in large amounts. Animal foods are the best sources.*

Selenium

Selenium works with vitamin E to protect vulnerable body chemicals from oxidation. A deficiency of selenium in people can open the way for a specific

---

phytates: compounds present in plant foods (particularly whole grains and beans) that bind zinc and prevent its absorption.

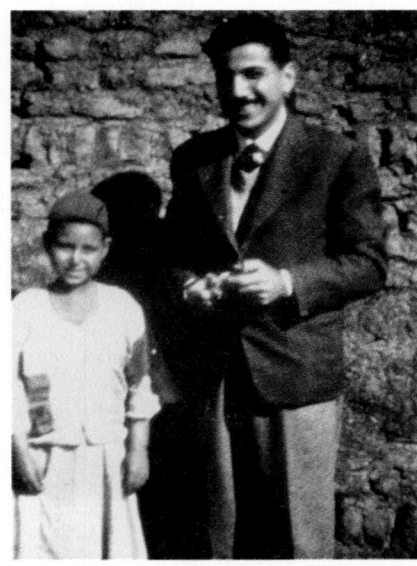

The Egyptian boy in the picture is 17 years old but is only 4 feet tall, like a 7-year-old in the United States. His genitalia are like those of a 6-year-old. The retardation is rightly ascribed to zinc deficiency because it is partially reversible when zinc is restored to the diet.

Controversy 7 presented a table of safe mineral intakes.

■■■ Figure 8–12

**Food Sources of Zinc Selected to Show a Range of Values.
Commonly Eaten Portions Ranked Richest to Poorest.**

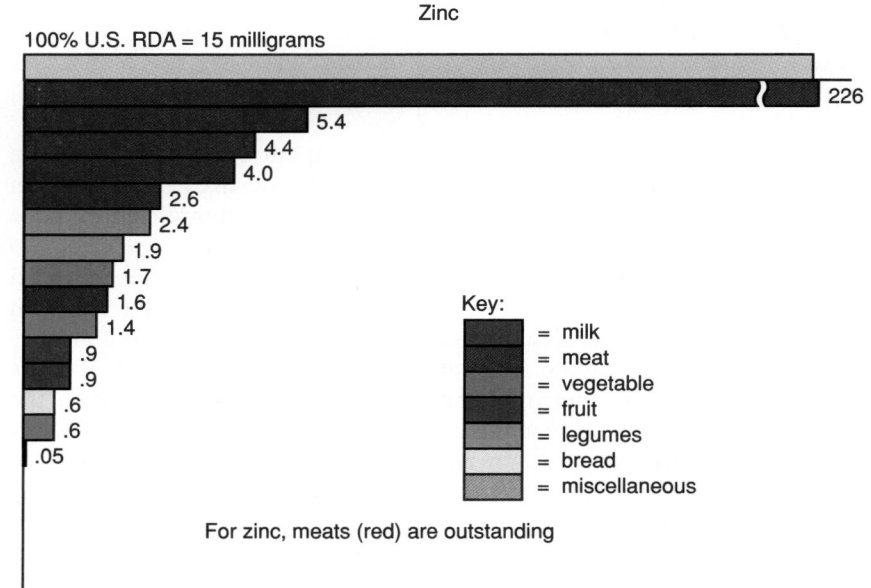

Zinc

100% U.S. RDA = 15 milligrams

Food, serving size (energy)	
Oysters, 1 c raw (160 cal)	226
Crabmeat, 1 c canned (135 cal)	5.4
Sirloin steak, 3 oz lean (180 cal)	4.4
Lamb chop, 3 oz braised (238 cal)	4.0
Turkey, 3 oz (145 cal)	2.6
Black-eyed peas, 1 c cooked (190 cal)	2.4
Pinto beans, 1 c cooked (265 cal)	1.9
Green peas, 1 c cooked (67 cal)	1.7
Shrimp, 3.5 oz broiled (109 cal)	1.6
Spinach, 1 c cooked (41 cal)	1.4
Milk or yogurt, 1 c nonfat (86 cal)	.9
Cheddar cheese, 1 oz (114 cal)	.9
Whole-wheat bread, 1 slice (70 cal)	.6
Broccoli, 1 c cooked, (46 cal)	.6
Apple, 1 fresh medium (80 cal)	.05

Key:
= milk
= meat
= vegetable
= fruit
= legumes
= bread
= miscellaneous

For zinc, meats (red) are outstanding

■■■ Figure 8–13

Zinc in Foods.

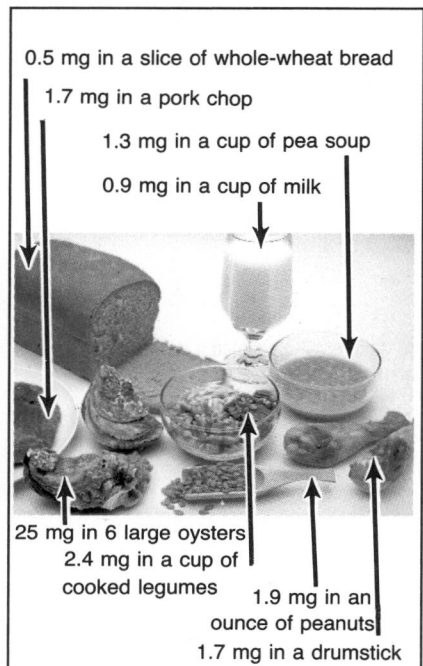

0.5 mg in a slice of whole-wheat bread
1.7 mg in a pork chop
1.3 mg in a cup of pea soup
0.9 mg in a cup of milk
25 mg in 6 large oysters
2.4 mg in a cup of cooked legumes
1.9 mg in an ounce of peanuts
1.7 mg in a drumstick

type of heart disease (unrelated to the heart disease discussed in Chapters 5 and 11). The condition, first identified in China among people from areas with selenium-deficient soils, led researchers to connect selenium deficiency to disease, thus elevating the mineral to its rightful place among the essential nutrients (see the inside front cover). The soils in the United States and Canadá grow foods that supply enough but not too much selenium.

In laboratory animals, selenium deficiency is hard to produce—it takes feeding selenium-free diets to two generations to induce it. Among people, selenium deficiency has been reported in those too ill to eat and who were fed formulas through a vein for a long time. (These formulas used to be selenium deficient; today's formulas supply selenium.) Anyone who eats a normal diet composed of mostly unprocessed foods need not worry about selenium—it is widely distributed in foods such as meats and shellfish, and in vegetables and grains grown on selenium-rich soil. From current indications it is likely that most people in the United States receive well over the RDA amount.[16] Toxicity is possible, especially when people take selenium supplements over a long period. It brings on symptoms such as hair loss, diarrhea, and nerve abnormalities.

▌▌▷ *Selenium works with vitamin E to protect body compounds from oxidation. A deficiency induces a disease of the heart; deficiency in developed countries is rare.*

Fluoride

Fluoride has not been proven to be an essential nutrient.[17] Only a trace of fluoride occurs in the human body, but studies have demonstrated that with this amount, the crystalline deposits in bones and teeth are larger and more perfectly formed. Fluoride replaces the hydroxy portion of hydroxyapatite, forming **fluorapatite,** a crystal that is more resistant to decay.

Drinking water is the usual source of fluoride. In communities in which the water contains too much— 2 to 8 parts per million—discoloration of the teeth, **fluorosis,** may occur. Where fluoride is lacking, the incidence of dental decay is very high. Fluoridation of water to raise its fluoride concentration to 1 part per million is recommended as an important public health measure. (Twenty to eighty times this amount is required over many years to discolor teeth, and while unsightly, fluorosis is harmless to health.) An intake of fluoride during childhood protects teeth from decay throughout life, especially if begun before age 16[18]. It also may make the bone crystals of older people more resistant to the mineral loss of osteoporosis. (Once osteoporosis sets in, fluoride is useless in reversing it, however.) Figure 8–14 on the next page shows the extent of fluoridation nationwide; states that have adopted fluoridation in more than half of their counties are shown in color.

Despite fluoride's value, violent disagreement often surrounds the fluoridation of community water at first. Proponents argue that fluoridation is an obvious, safe, and cost-effective measure to reduce the incidence of dental caries in the young. Opponents argue that altering the community water supply is "unnatural" and deprives its consumers of the freedom to choose not to take fluoride. They fear accidental overdoses, perhaps mistaking the relatively nontoxic salt sodium *fluoride* for the highly volatile gas *fluorine,* which is deadly in excess. They may claim that fluoridated communities have an increased cancer rate, but studies on this do not show a connection.

On the basis of the accumulated evidence of its beneficial effects, fluoridation has been endorsed by the National Institute of Dental Health, the American Medical Association, the National Cancer Institute, and the National Nutrition Consortium. The allegation that it causes cancer has no basis in fact and has been refuted by the National Cancer Institute, the American Cancer Society, and the National Institute of Dental Research.

Now that fluoride has been added to many water supplies, the amounts in foods processed with use of that water are increasing, so that the total fluoride consumed by certain populations may be greater than expected. No hazard exists at present levels of fluoride consumption, but continued monitoring is important.

❚❚▷ *Fluoride stabilizes bones and makes teeth resistant to decay. Excess fluoride discolors teeth; massive doses are toxic.*

Other Trace Minerals

Several other trace minerals are now recognized as important to health. Experiments on animals have suggested that *chromium* works closely with the hormone insulin, facilitating the uptake of glucose into cells and the release of its energy. Chromium occurs in foods in association with several different complexes; the one that is best absorbed and most active is a small organic compound, the **glucose tolerance factor (GTF).** When chromium is lacking, insulin action is impaired and a diabetes-like condition results. Chromium deficiency is unlikely in healthy people eating varied diets composed mostly of whole foods because the mineral is supplied by many foods.[19] However,

fluorapatite (FLOOR-app-uh-tight): a crystal of bones and teeth, formed when fluoride displaces the hydroxy portion of hydroxyapatite (see p. 246). Fluorapatite resists being dissolved back into body fluid.

fluorosis (floor-OH-sis): discoloration of the teeth due to ingestion of too much fluoride during tooth development.

glucose tolerance factor (GTF): an organic compound containing chromium found in foods.

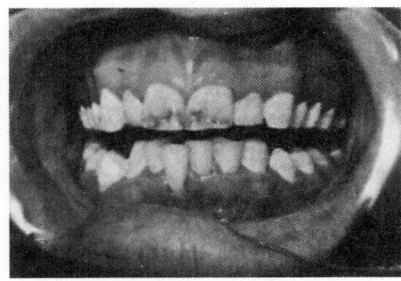

Fluorosis

■■■ Figure 8–14

Fluoridation in the United States.

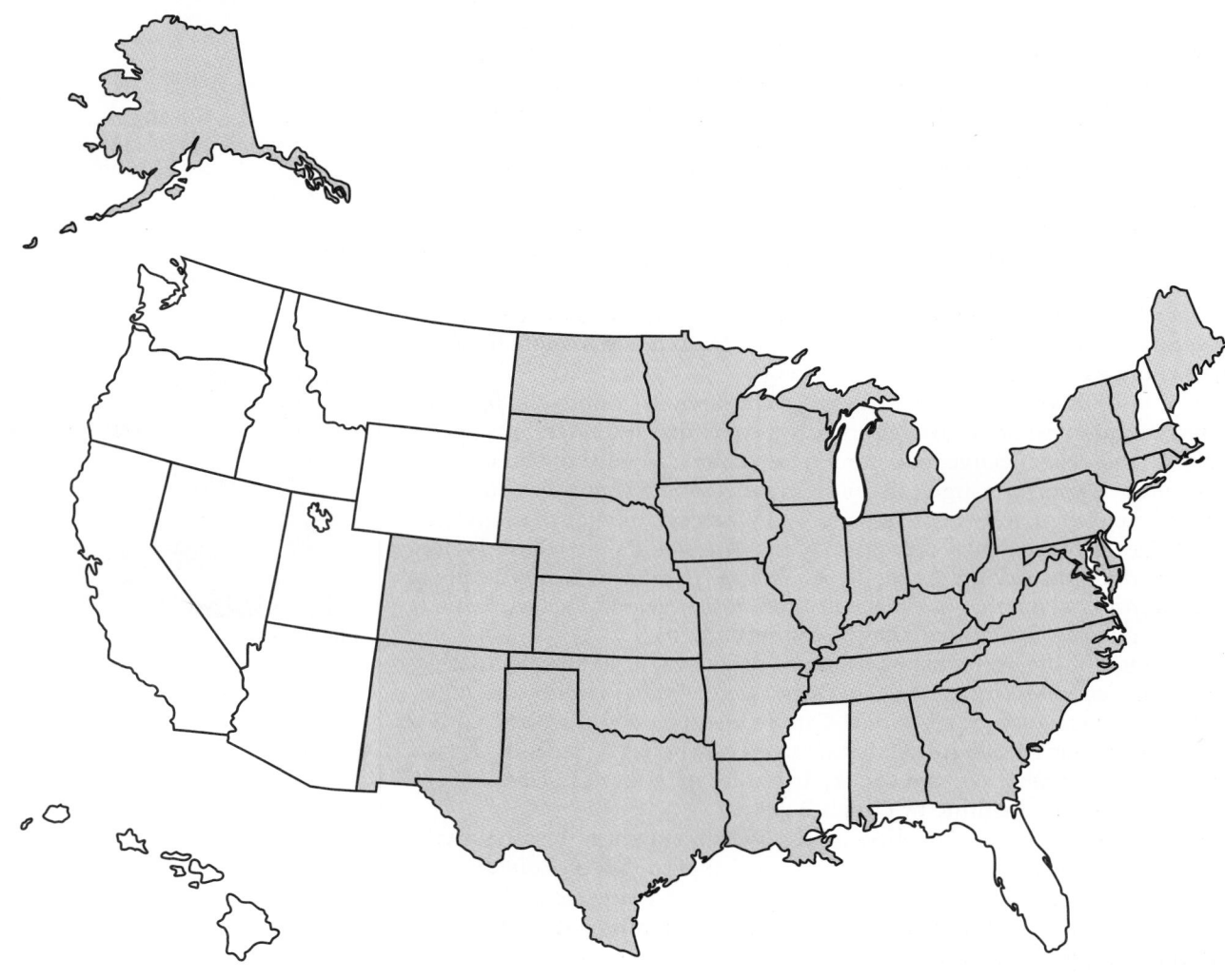

More than half the population
using public water in these states
is drinking fluoridated water.

SOURCE: Fluoridation Census—1985, U.S. Department of Health and   Center for Prevention Services, Dental Disease Prevention Activity,
Human Services, Public Health Service, Centers for Disease Control,   Atlanta, Georgia 30333, July 1988.

chromium is easily lost during food processing, as are other trace minerals and heavy dependence on refined foods makes deficiencies likely.

Boron, now recognized as active in the maintenance of human bone tissue, may also play roles in brain areas related to alertness and motor activity.[20] *Cobalt* is recognized as the mineral in the large vitamin B_{12} molecule; the alternative name for vitamin B_{12}, cobalamin, reflects its presence. *Copper* helps form hemoglobin and collagen and is needed in many enzymes. *Nickel* is important for the health of many body tissues; deficiencies harm the liver and other organs.[21] *Silicon* is known to be involved in bone calcification, at least in animals.[22] The future may reveal that many other trace minerals also play key roles: barium, cadmium, lead, lithium, mercury, silver, tin, vanadium. Even arsenic—known to be a poison and a carcinogen—may turn out to be essential in tiny quantities.

As research on the trace minerals continues, many interactions among them are also coming to light. An excess of one may cause a deficiency of another. (A slight manganese overload, for example, may aggravate an iron deficiency.) A deficiency of one may open the way for another to cause a toxic reaction. (Iron deficiency, for example, makes the body much more susceptible than normal to lead poisoning.) Good food sources of one are poor food sources of another, and factors that cooperate with some trace elements oppose others. (Vitamin C, for example, enhances the absorption of iron and depresses that of copper.) The continuous outpouring of new information about the trace minerals is a sign that we have much more to learn.

All of the trace minerals are toxic in excess. The hazards of overdoses are among the chief risks faced by people who take multiple nutrient supplements. The way to obtain the trace minerals is from food—not hard to do, as long as you eat whole foods. Some claim that organically grown foods contain more trace minerals than those grown on chemical fertilizers. Organic fertilizers do contain more trace minerals than do refined chemical fertilizers, and plants do take up some of the minerals they are given, so this claim may turn out to be valid.

Table 8–2 sums up what this chapter has said about the minerals and fills in some additional information.

▐▌▷ *Chromium may work with the hormone insulin to control blood glucose concentration. Copper helps make hemoglobin. Many other trace elements also play important roles in the body.*

◼◼◻ Table 8–2 The Minerals—A Summary

MINERAL NAME	CHIEF FUNCTIONS IN THE BODY	DEFICIENCY SYMPTOMS	TOXICITY SYMPTOMS	SIGNIFICANT SOURCES
Major Minerals				
Calcium, phosphorus	The principal minerals of bones and teeth. Calcium also acts in normal muscle contraction and relaxation, nerve functioning, blood clotting, blood pressure, and immune defenses. Phosphorus is important in cells' genetic material, in cell membranes as phospholipids, in energy transfer, and in buffering systems.	Calcium: stunted growth in children; adult bone loss (osteoporosis). Phosphorus deficiency unknown.	Excess calcium is excreted except in hormonal imbalance states (not caused by nutritional deficiency). Excess phosphorus may cause calcium excretion.	Calcium: milk and milk products, small fish (with bones), tofu (bean curd), greens, legumes. Phosphorus: all animal tissues.
Magnesium	Another factor involved in bone mineralization, the building of protein, enzyme action, normal muscular contraction, transmission of nerve impulses, and maintenance of teeth.	Weakness; confusion; depressed pancreatic hormone secretion; if extreme, convulsions, bizarre movements (especially of eyes and face), hallucinations, and difficulty in swallowing. In children, growth failure.[a]	Not known; large doses have been taken in the form of the laxative Epsom salts, without ill effects except diarrhea.	Nuts, legumes, whole grains, dark green vegetables, seafoods, chocolate, cocoa.
Sodium	Sodium, chloride, and potassium (electrolytes) maintain cells' normal fluid balance and acid-base balance in the body. Sodium is critical to nerve impulse transmission.	Muscle cramps, mental apathy, loss of appetite.	Hypertension.	Salt, soy sauce, processed foods.
Chloride	Chloride is also part of the hydrochloric acid found in the stomach, necessary for proper digestion.	Growth failure in children; muscle cramps, mental apathy, loss of appetite; can cause death (uncommon).	Normally harmless (the gas chlorine is a poison but evaporates from water); can cause vomiting.	Salt, soy sauce; moderate quantities in whole, unprocessed foods, large amounts in processed foods.
Potassium	Potassium facilitates reactions, including the making of protein; the maintenance of fluid and electrolyte balance; the support of cell integrity; the transmission of nerve impulses; and the contraction of muscles, including the heart.	Deficiency accompanies dehydration; causes muscular weakness, paralysis, and confusion; can cause death.	Causes muscular weakness; triggers vomiting; if given into a vein, can stop the heart.	All whole foods: meats, milk, fruits, vegetables, grains, legumes.

[a]A still more severe deficiency causes tetany, an extreme, prolonged contraction of the muscles similar to that caused by low blood calcium.

■■■ Table 8–2 continued

MINERAL NAME	CHIEF FUNCTIONS IN THE BODY	DEFICIENCY SYMPTOMS	TOXICITY SYMPTOMS	SIGNIFICANT SOURCES
Sulfur	A component of certain amino acids; part of the vitamins biotin and thiamin and the hormone insulin; combines with toxic substances to form harmless compounds; also as part of proteins, stabilizes their shape by forming sulfur-sulfur bridges (see Figure 6–8 in Chapter 6).	None known; protein deficiency would occur first.	Would occur only if sulfur amino acids were eaten in excess; this (in animals) depresses growth.	All protein-containing foods.
Iodine	A component of the thyroid hormone thyroxin, which helps to regulate growth, development, and metabolic rate.	Goiter, cretinism.	Depressed thyroid activity; goiter-like thyroid enlargement.	Iodized salt; seafood; plants grown in most parts of the country and animals fed those plants.
Iron	Part of the protein hemoglobin, which carries oxygen in the blood; part of the protein myoglobin in muscles, which makes oxygen available for muscle contraction; necessary for the utilization of energy.	Anemia: weakness, pallor, headaches, reduced resistance to infection, inability to concentrate, lowered cold tolerance.	Iron overload: infections, liver injury, acidosis, bloody stools, shock.	Red meats, fish, poultry, shellfish, eggs, legumes, dried fruits.
Selenium	Part of an enzyme that breaks down reactive chemicals that harm cells; works with vitamin E.	Muscle discomfort, weakness, pancreas damage, heart disease (cardiomyopathy).	Nausea, abdominal pain, nail and hair changes, nerve damage, fatigue, irritability, diarrhea.	Seafoods, organ meats; other meats, grains and vegetables depending on soil conditions.
Zinc	Part of the hormone insulin and many enzymes; involved in making genetic material and proteins, immune reactions, transport of vitamin A, taste perception, wound healing, the making of sperm, and normal fetal development.	Growth failure in children, sexual retardation, loss of taste, poor wound healing.	Fever, nausea, vomiting, diarrhea, muscle incoordination, dizziness, anemia, accelerated atherosclerosis, kidney failure.	Protein-containing foods: meats, fish, poultry, grains, vegetables.

▓▓▓ Food Feature

Controlling Salt Intake

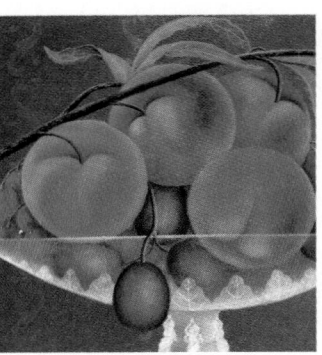

The role of diet, and specifically sodium, in the *prevention* of hypertension has been debated. The evidence is inconclusive. The value of a low-sodium diet in the treatment of *established* hypertension is unquestioned, however. Studies have shown that even mild restriction of sodium can produce a modest but definite fall in blood pressure in many people.

One of the problems that has plagued researchers investigating the links between salt and hypertension is that heretofore they have not distinguished between *sodium* and *sodium chloride,* or salt. That distinction is just now being recognized, and its implications have not yet found their way into practical advice on food choices. Salt alone may be what people need to limit, but most advice is still phrased in terms of sodium. Fortunately most guidelines to reduce dietary sodium intake also reduce salt intake, so here are some recommendations for those who wish to reduce their salt *and* sodium intakes.

First, remember from the chapter that what you pour from the salt shaker may only contribute 10 or 15 percent of the total salt you consume. Processed foods may contribute up to 75 percent of your total salt, added during processing. All the rest of the foods you consume—all the whole, unprocessed foods—contain only small amounts of sodium naturally, and these foods plus the water you drink contribute the remainder of the day's intake. Use many more whole foods, and you will have accomplished a tremendous reduction in your salt and sodium intake. Notice, too, from Table 8–3, that in each food group the least processed

▓▓▓ Table 8–3 Processing Reduces Potassium, Raises Sodium in Foods

FOOD	POTASSIUM (mg)[a]	SODIUM (mg)[a]	RATIO
Milk Foods			
Milk (whole), 1 c	370	120	3:1
Chocolate pudding, 1 c (homecooked)	445	146	3:1
Chocolate pudding, 1 c (instant)	352	880	1:2
Meats			
Beef roast (cooked), 3 oz	254	54	5:1
Corned beef (canned), 3 oz	116	855	1:7
Chipped beef, 3 oz	377	2946	1:8
Vegetables			
Corn (cooked), 1 c	408	28	15:1
Creamed corn (canned), 1 c	344	730	1:2
Sugar-coated cornflakes, 1 c	17	103	1:6
Fruits			
Peaches (fresh), 1	171	1	171:1
Peaches (canned), 1	150	10	15:1
Peach pie, 1 piece	235	423	1:2
Grains			
Whole-wheat flour, 1 c	486	6	81:1
Whole-wheat bread, 1 slice	62	222	1:4
Wheat crackers, 4	62	118	1:2

[a]Data are taken from Appendix A.

foods are not only lowest in sodium but also highest in potassium, an added benefit. No recommendation has been made for the potassium-to-sodium ratio of the diet, but the RDA tables indicate that a 2-to-1 ratio or higher is acceptable; lower might not be.

In reducing your intakes of processed foods, pay particular attention to those listed in Table 8−4. Also, notice that processed foods don't always taste salty. Most people are surprised to learn that a serving of cornflakes contains more sodium than a serving of cocktail peanuts—and that a serving of instant chocolate pudding contains still more. In the case of the peanuts, they may *taste* saltier than cornflakes because the salt sits on the surface, allowing faster contact with the salt-sensing taste buds. The sodium of instant pudding originates as sodium-containing thickeners, not from salt itself.

If you add no salt during cooking, you may find that just a tiny shake of salt at the table will sit atop your food (remember the peanuts) to provide a salty flavor, and you won't even miss the salt normally added in cooking. Soon you may learn to skip the salt entirely and enjoy the unsalted flavors of foods, or you may learn to enhance them with salt-free spices such as cinnamon, curry, garlic, ginger, lemon, mustard powder, nutmeg, paprika, parsley, and thyme. Sour flavors, such as lemon juice and vinegar, are especially useful in replacing salt because they enhance whatever natural salty flavor a food may have. As salt intake decreases, the taste buds adjust, and the taste of food with less salt becomes the preferred taste, so cut down on salt gradually while your taste buds adjust. Many cookbooks with helpful tips are available.

Make substitutions too. In particular, use low-salt canned bouillon and broth and homemade, salt-free stocks. Choose salt-free or low-sodium products whenever they are offered. Many other low-sodium products are available, but in general you can make a low-sodium diet attractive without using these products. Some people, however, like to use them to add variety.

When soft water is used in food products, it may contribute significantly to salt intake, so learn whether your water is hard or soft, and adjust your use accordingly. Be aware that medications, toothpastes, mouthwashes, and other nonfood products may also contain salt.

In salt substitutes the sodium is generally replaced by potassium. Some people don't like the taste of salt substitutes but may find them acceptable if used sparingly. (Don't heat them, though, because they turn bitter.) Often people

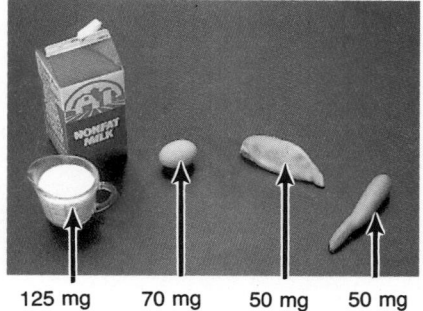

125 mg   70 mg   50 mg   50 mg
(1 c)   (1 egg) (3 oz)   (100 g)

Unprocessed foods are low in sodium.

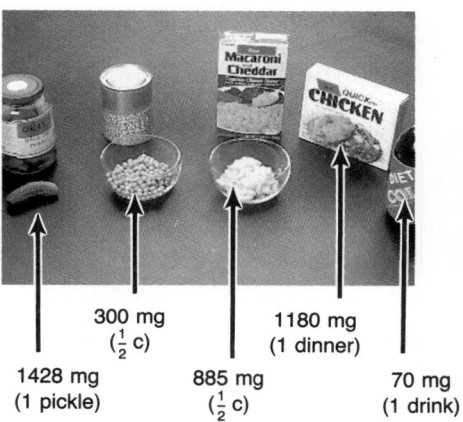

                300 mg   1180 mg
                (½ c)   (1 dinner)

1428 mg   885 mg   70 mg
(1 pickle)   (½ c)   (1 drink)

Many processed foods are high in sodium,

■■■ Table 8−4 Foods That Are High in Salt or Sodium

Foods prepared in brine, such as pickles, olives, and sauerkraut.
Salty or smoked meat, such as bologna, corned or chipped beef, frankfurters, ham, luncheon meats, salt pork, sausage, and smoked tongue.
Salty or smoked fish, such as anchovies, caviar, salted and dried cod, herring, sardines, and smoked salmon.
Snack items such as potato chips, pretzels, salted popcorn, and salted nuts and crackers.
Bouillon cubes; seasoned salts (including sea salt); soy, Worcestershire, and barbecue sauces.
Cheeses, especially processed types.
Canned and instant soups.
Prepared horseradish, catsup, and mustard.

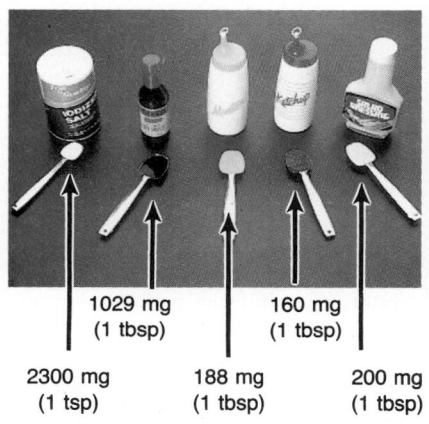

                1029 mg   160 mg
                (1 tbsp)   (1 tbsp)

2300 mg   188 mg   200 mg
(1 tsp)   (1 tbsp)   (1 tbsp)

as are many condiments.

The box of terms on p. 47 of Chapter 2 defined some sodium terms used on food labels.

find foods more acceptable without any salt at all. The use of a potassium-containing salt substitute serves the dual purpose of increasing potassium intake while reducing sodium intake.[§] Some products contain a combination of regular table salt and salt substitute. Although these products may be more palatable, they also can contribute a significant amount of salt to the diet.

Besides all these considerations, many positive choices are possible. The person who wishes to use diet to prevent or to reduce high blood pressure should limit alcohol intake and should also eat plenty of fresh fruits, vegetables, milk products, legumes, and meats for potassium, calcium, and magnesium. Also it is important for the person to maintain appropriate weight and engage in regular, enjoyable, vigorous physical activity, topics emphasized in the next two chapters.

§ People with renal insufficiency should not use salt substitutes containing potassium.

SELF-STUDY

Evaluate Your Mineral Intakes

To make these evaluations, use the information you recorded on Form 3 in Appendix F.

1. Start with calcium. What percentage of your recommended intake did you consume? Was this enough? What foods contribute the greatest amount of calcium to your diet? If you consumed more than the recommendations, was this too much? Why or why not? In what ways would you change your diet to improve it in this respect?
2. NRC recommendations are in terms of *salt*, but Appendix A and food labels list only sodium. "Salt" refers to the salt added to processed foods and the salt you shake onto foods when you cook them or when you help yourself to them at the table. (It excludes the salt present in the *unprocessed* foods you eat; this is considered to be negligible.) To compare your sodium or salt intake to recommendations in a meaningful way, you must account for salt from two sources: processed foods and the salt shaker.

First consider the processed foods you eat. Go over the foods you listed on Form 1 and decide which ones were processed in some way. The sodium values listed in

Appendix A are averages of many brands. Read your food labels to help you compare actual sodium values of the brands you regularly eat to the Appendix's average values for foods of the same type. Translate milligrams of sodium listed on labels into grams of salt by dividing the number of milligrams of sodium by 400. Example: if you ate 1200 milligrams of sodium, that would translate to 3 grams of salt.

Now consider your use of the salt shaker. You can roughly estimate the amount of salt you add to foods if you are willing to weigh your salt shaker on a sensitive balance at the start of the day, use only that salt shaker all day and only for yourself, and weigh it again at the end of the day. Example: you might have used 2 grams of salt this way.

Total the salt you took in from processed foods and from the salt shaker. Compare your estimated intake with the recommendation that you should have not more than 6 grams of added salt per day. How does your intake compare with the recommendation? Example: the two examples just offered add up to 5 grams, within the suggested limits.

3. Now think in terms of *sodium*. The 6-gram salt limit is equivalent to a 2400-milligram sodium limit. Six grams of salt contains 2400 milligrams of sodium. Heighten your awareness of the sodium contents of processed foods. Look up the following foods in Appendix A and list their sodium contents: dill pickle, corn flakes, cottage cheese, hot dog, chicken pot pie, canned soup (your choice), margarine, potato chips, peanuts, chocolate pudding. Also look at the sodium column in your own food records. Which foods that *you* eat are high in sodium? Were any of the brands of processed foods you chose out of line with the average values of Appendix A? Is there another way you could enjoy these foods without too much sodium? Would you substitute a lower-sodium food or brand for the high-sodium varieties?
4. Calculate your intakes of magnesium, phosphorus, and potassium, and compare them with the recommended intakes. If you need to improve your diet with respect to these minerals, how will you go about doing so?
5. Go on to iron. What percentage of your recommended intake did you con-

continued on the next page

▌▌▌ SELF-STUDY *continued*

sume? Was this enough? Which of the foods you eat supply the most iron? Rank your top five iron contributors. How many were meats? Legumes? Greens? Other? Are enriched or whole-grain products important to your iron intake?

6. Compute your iron absorption from a meal of your choosing, following the instructions in Form 6 in Appendix F. How could you eat differently to improve your iron absorption?

7. Now turn to zinc. What percentage of the recommendation did you consume? What were your best food sources of zinc? What guidelines do you need to follow to be sure of obtaining enough zinc from the foods you eat?

8. Iodine, fluoride, and other trace elements are not listed in Appendix A, but you can evaluate your intakes as follows. For iodine, answer these questions: Are you in an area of the country where the soil is iodine poor? If so, do you use iodized salt? Do you consume milk and bakery products? Do you think you obtain too little, too much, or just enough iodine?

9. For fluoride, answer these questions: Is the water in your county naturally high in fluoride, or fluoridated? (Call the county health department.) If not, how do you and your family ensure that your intakes of fluoride are optimal?

10. For trace elements, try to get a sense of where your typical diet falls on the spectrum between unprocessed,

natural (whole) foods, and processed foods. List, with their calorie amounts, the foods you ate in three days that were whole, unprocessed foods like those on the exchange lists. List separately those that were highly processed foods, such as TV dinners, pastries, and instant gravies. What percentage of the calories you consume comes from whole, natural foods? What percentage from processed foods? Since processed foods tend to lack trace elements, do you suppose you get enough trace elements in your diet?

Notes

1. T. Vokes, Water homeostasis, *Annual Review of Nutrition* 7 (1987): 383–406.

2. L. W. Turner and E. N. Whitney, Nature versus nurture: The calcium controversy, *Nutrition Clinics*, September/October 1989.

3. Food and Nutrition Board, *Recommended Dietary Allowances*, 10th ed. (Washington, D.C.: National Academy of Sciences, 1989), p. 176.

4. L. H. Allen, Calcium bioavailability and absorption: A review, *American Journal of Clinical Nutrition* 35 (1982): 798–808.

5. Food and Nutrition Board, 1989, p. 253.

6. Food and Nutrition Board, 1989, p. 251.

7. D. L. Costill, R. Cote, and W. J. Fink, Dietary potassium and heavy exercise: Effects on muscle water and electrolytes, *American Journal of Clinical Nutrition* 36 (1982): 266–271.

8. Magnesium deficiency and ischemic heart disease, *Nutrition Reviews* 46 (1988): 311–312.

9. P. O. Webster, Magnesium, *American Journal of Clinical Nutrition* 45 (1987): 1305–1312; Food and Nutrition Board, 1989, pp. 190–191.

10. H. C. Holt, B. J. Demott, and J. A. Bacon, The iodine concentration of market milk in Tennessee, 1981–1986, *Journal of Food Protection* 52 (1989): 115–118.

11. L. Hallberg, Iron, Chapter 32 in *Present Knowledge in Nutrition*, 5th ed. (New York: Nutrition Foundation, 1984), pp. 459–478.

12. N. S. Scrimshaw, Functional consequences of iron deficiency in human populations, *Journal of Nutrition Science and Vitaminology* 30 (1984): 47–63.

13. R. Yip and N. J. Binkin, Declining childhood anemia prevalence in the U.S.: Evidence of improving iron nutrition (abstract), *American Journal of Clinical Nutrition* 45 (1987): 849 P. R. Dallman, Iron in *Present Knowledge in Nutrition* 6th ed., M. L. Brown, ed. (Washington, D.C.: International Life Sciences Institute, 1990), pp. 241–260.

14. S. N. Gershoff and coauthors, Studies of the elderly in Boston: 1. The effects of iron fortification on moderately anemic people, *American Journal of Clinical Nutrition* 30 (1978): 134–141.

15. Scrimshaw, 1984.

16. Food and Nutrition Board, 1989, p. 219.

17. Food and Nutrition Board, 1989, p. 235.

18. E. R. Schlesinger and coauthors, Newburgh-Kingston caries-fluorine study, 12: Pediatric findings after 10 years, *Journal of the American Dental Association* 52 (1956): 296–306.

19. E. G. Offenbacher and F. X. Pi-Sunyer, Chromium in human nutrition, *Annual Review of Nutrition* 8 (1988): 543–563.

20. F. H. Nielsen and coauthors, Effect of dietary boron on mineral, estrogen, and testosterone metabolism in postmenopausal women, *FASEB Journal* 1 (1987): 394–397; J. G. Penland, Effects of low dietary boron and magnesium on the brain function of healthy adults (abstract), *FASEB Journal* 3(1989): A 1242.

21. Nielson, 1985.

22. Nielson, 1985.

23. E. R. Monsen and coauthors, Estimation of available dietary iron, *American Journal of Clinical Nutrition* 31 (1987): 134–141. Moderate iron stores assumed.

CONTROVERSY 8

Osteoporosis and Calcium

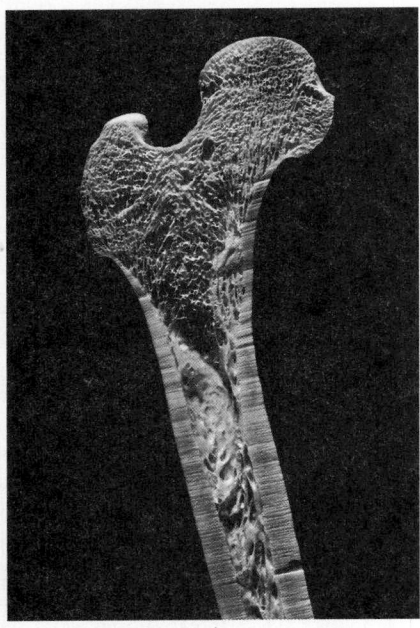

Last year well over a million people in the United States suffered bone breaks attributable to osteoporosis, making it one of the most prevalent of the degenerative diseases. Similarly, of all women over 65 years of age, one-third will suffer fractures of the spine during their lives.[1]

Osteoporosis sets in silently, producing no symptoms until late in life. You cannot tell if you are losing bone tissue, but if you are, you may later pay a high price in pain and disability. The causes are tangled, and it is not yet clear whether calcium nutrition can prevent osteoporosis or help to slow it down. This Controversy addresses several questions about osteoporosis: What is it and who gets it? What factors increase a person's risk of developing it? What, if anything, can people do to lessen their risks? And where does calcium fit into the picture?

The Problem of Osteoporosis

Osteoporosis often first becomes apparent when someone's hip suddenly gives way. People say, "She fell and broke her hip," but the fact of the matter may be that the hip was so fragile that it broke *before* she fell. Even the slight jarring from stepping down off a curb may be enough to shatter a bone made porous by loss of minerals. The break is not clean; it is an explosion into fragments so numerous and scattered that they cannot be reassembled. To remove them is a struggle, and to replace them with an artificial joint requires major surgery. Such a fracture condemns many older people to wheelchairs for the rest of their lives. About a third die of complications within a year.

To understand how bones lose minerals in later years, you must first know a few things about bones. The opening photograph shows a human leg bone sliced lengthwise, exposing the lacy network of calcium-containing crystals (the **trabecular bone**) inside. These lacy crystals, part of the body's calcium bank, can be tapped to raise blood levels when the supply from the day's diet runs short and are redeposited in bone when dietary cal-cium is plentiful. Invested in savings during the milk-drinking years of childhood and young adulthood, these calcium deposits provide a nearly inexhaustible fund of calcium.

In contrast to trabecular bone, **cortical bone** is a dense, ivorylike bone that forms an exterior shell that surrounds and protects trabecular bone. Cortical bone also composes the shafts of the long bones, as you can easily see in the photograph; if you look closely at the ball at the top of the bone, you can also see the thin cortical shell surrounding the trabeculae. Both types of bone are crucial to overall bone strength, since cortical bone provides the outer wall, while trabecular bone provides support along the lines of stress.

The differences between the two types of bone are meaningful with regard to osteoporosis. Trabecular bone is generously supplied with blood vessels and is more metabolically active than is cortical bone. Trabecular bone is also more sensitive to hormones that govern withdrawal of calcium from day to day. Cortical bone's calcium can be withdrawn, but slowly and at a steady pace. Trabecular bone, on the other hand, readily gives up some of its mineral content whenever blood calcium needs replenishing. Losses of trabecular bone become significant for men and women in the third decade of life, although losses can occur any time calcium's withdrawal exceeds its deposit. Cortical bone losses, not as variable from day to day, begin at about 40 years of age; bone tissue recedes slowly but surely thereafter.

Menopause imposes special perils on women's bones. Bone losses surge as hormone levels change and menstruation ceases. This surge lasts for a few years following menopause, then tapers off so that, once again, women's losses equal those sustained by men of the same ages. Losses of bone minerals continue throughout the remainder of a woman's lifetime, but not at the free-fall pace of the menopause years.

Adult bone losses are symptomless as they occur, but later symptoms of osteoporosis can be dramatic. Researchers have associated the loss of the two types of bone, trabecular and cortical, with two types of osteoporosis, type I and type II, identified by their symptoms—the types of bone breaks they most often produce.[2] Type I osteoporosis is characterized by losses of trabecular bone, sometimes exceeding three times the expected rate, and bone breaks may come on suddenly when the victim passes the age of 65 years. In this condition trabecular bones become so fragile that even the body's own weight can overburden the spine—vertebrae may suddenly disintegrate and crush down, painfully pinching major nerves. Wrists may break as trabecula-rich bone ends weaken, and teeth may loosen or fall out as the trabecular bone of the jaw recedes. Women are most often the victims of this type of osteoporosis, six to one over men.

In type II osteoporosis, the calcium of both cortical and trabecular bone is drawn out of storage, but slowly over the years. As old age approaches, the vertebrae may compress into wedge shapes, usually painlessly, forming what is often called "dowager's hump," the posture many older people assume as they "grow shorter." Figure C8-1 shows the effect of the compression of spinal bone on a woman's height and posture. Because the cortical shell as well as the trabecular interior weaken, breaks most often occur in the hip, as in the opening example. A woman is twice as likely as a man to suffer this form of osteoporosis, and it is likely that her condition was predestined years before, during the postmenopausal period of heavy calcium losses sustained by her bones.

Scientists are working to discover factors that contribute to osteoporosis and ultimately to find ways to prevent it. So far, many findings seem to conflict with each other, and others simply lead to more questions. However, at least some areas of agreement have been reached concerning factors that influence osteoporosis. Whether a person develops osteoporosis seems to depend partly on heredity and partly on the environment. (In this sense nutrition counts as part of the environment, along with every other component of life not dictated by genetic inheritance.) The strongest predictor of bone density is age, followed by gender. Others, not necessarily in this order, are racial inheritance, nutrition, hormonal health, physical activity, body weight, smoking, alcohol, and drugs.

■■■ Age

The bones are at their strongest and most dense in young adulthood. They lose strength and density as they age, due to changes in the body's bone-dismantling and bone-building equipment. Up to about the mid-20s, bone-building activities are dominant, and more bone is deposited than is withdrawn. Then the balance changes as a person approaches the age of 30 years. Bones stop growing, and withdrawal tends to equal losses for awhile. As years pass, bone building equipment is lost, and bone dismantling dominates.

Other factors weigh in the balance of bone withdrawal and deposition with age. One may be calcium nutrition. In the older years women tend to eat fewer calcium-rich foods than in youth. Another is calcium absorption, which declines after about the age of 70 years, probably because the kidneys do not activate vitamin D as well as they used to (active vitamin D promotes calcium absorption).[3] Also, sunlight is needed to form vitamin D, and many older people fail to go outdoors into the sunshine. Some of the hormones that regulate bone maintenance and calcium metabolism also change with age and accelerate bone mineral withdrawal.† In summary, these age-related factors probably combine to push bone loss: loss of bone-building equipment, reduced calcium intakes,

---

†Among the hormones suggested as influential are immunoreactive parathyroid hormone and calcitonin.

▪▪▪ Figure C8–1

Loss of Height in a Woman Caused by Adult Bone Loss. The woman on the left is about 50 years old. On the right, she is 80 years old. Her legs have not grown shorter; only her back has lost length, due to collapse of her spinal bones (vertebrae). Collapsed vertebrae cannot protect the spinal nerves from pressure that causes excruciating pain.

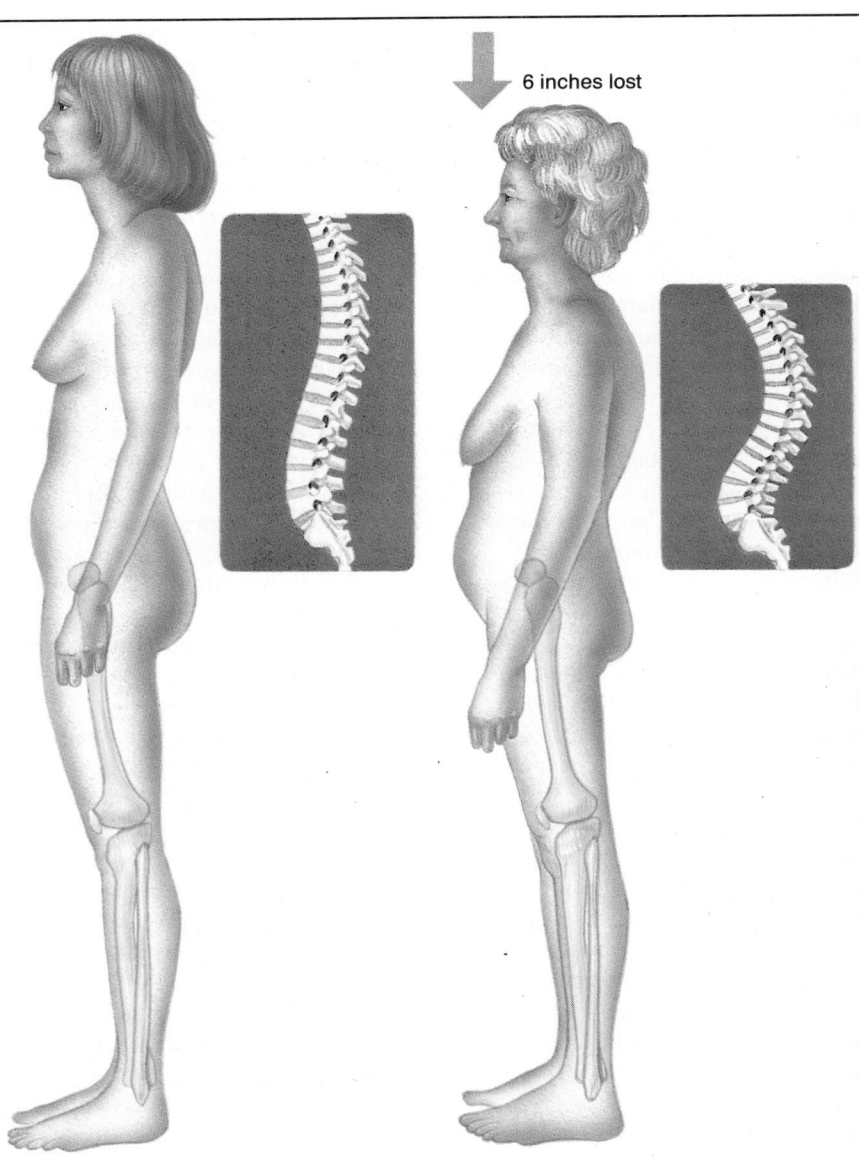

6 inches lost

Effects of osteoporosis on a woman's height. On the left is a woman at menopause and on the right, the same woman 30 years later. Notice that collapse of her vertebrae has shortened her back; the length of her legs has not changed.

impaired absorption, reduced vitamin D status, and a hormonal climate that favors bone mineral withdrawal.

Scientists agree completely on some points concerning the strength of bones in later years: bone strength later depends to at least some degree on how well bone strength was developed during youth. Afterward, throughout life, other factors, some of them under personal control, can either hasten the normal bone loss that occurs in everyone or slow it down. However, once a person reaches the bone-losing years of middle age, those who formed dense bones during youth have the advantage. They simply have more bone tissue starting out and can lose more before beginning to suffer ill effects. After bone loss has begun, there are still a few things you can do to save your bones, and these will be discussed later.

■■■ Gender and Hormones

After age, being male or female is the next strongest predictor of loss of bone density with aging. Losses occur in both sexes, but are more substantial in older women than in older men. As mentioned earlier, the years following menopause are costly in terms of both cortical and trabecular bone. Many researchers feel that postmenopausal bone losses occur because the ovaries reduce their estrogen output. Actually, when young women cease menstruating, they undergo rapid bone losses too. This happens in diseases when ovaries must be removed[4] or

when, as long-distance runners, women have developed athletic amenorrhea (see Chapter 10). Estrogen replacement therapy can help non-menstruating women to prevent further bone loss but may carry slight medical risks. For those who take them, the drugs do indeed reduce the incidence of fractures.[5]

Evidence concerning menopause and bone loss would seem to clinch the case in favor of estrogen deficiency as a cause of osteoporosis in women, but a complication arises when researchers consider cases of men with bone loss. While men do not produce significant estrogens, they do suffer more fractures after removal of the testes (in cases of disease) or when their testes lose functional ability with aging.[6] This would seem to imply that both male and female sex hormones may play a role in osteoporosis.

One more complication to the estrogen theory is that some women may lose bone tissue in middle age before menopause, as though they were predisposed to do so. In these women hormones must be only one of several factors acting around the middle of life to deplete bones. Still, being female and experiencing menopause remain prime risk factors for the development of osteoporosis.

■■■ Race and Inheritance

Ethnic inheritance and race determine some of a person's biochemical and physiological characteristics. Many inherited diseases follow racial lines—for example, sickle-cell

anemia among blacks, cystic fibrosis in Europeans, or Tay-Sachs disease among Jews. Not all people belonging to these groups have the genetic potential to develop such diseases, but group members run higher risks than nonmembers.

Racial traits accompany risks of osteoporosis. Black people have denser bones than do white people, and the differences are evident even before birth.[7] This holds true for both sexes of all ages and expresses itself in a lower rate of osteoporosis among blacks. Hip fractures, for example, are reported to be about three times more likely in 80-year old white women than in black women of the same age.

Other ethnic groups have lower bone densities than do white people. Asians from China and Japan, Mexican-Americans, hispanic people from Central and South America, and Inuit people from St. Lawrence Island all have lower bone density than do white people from the United States with Northern European background. Knowing this might lead to the prediction that these groups would suffer more bone fractures, but the picture is not that tidy. Chinese people living in Singapore have low bone density, but have hip fracture rates among the lowest in the world. In Yugoslavia, bone fracture rates are tied to locations—lower rates in high-calcium–intake areas, higher rates in low-calcium-intake areas—despite racial similarities. This demonstrates that although a person's genes may lay the groundwork for a likely outcome, environmental factors, most times under the control of the individual, influence the genes' ultimate expression. We'll get back to calcium nutrition later, but two other factors modify the expression of genetics in this regard—physical activity and body weight.

■■■ Physical Activity and Body Weight

While you can't do much about your genetic inheritance, physical activity and body weight are more under personal control. It has long been known that when people lie idle, such as when they are confined to bed, the bones lose strength just as the muscles do. (Astronauts who must live with reduced gravity also face these problems.)

The correlation between muscle strength and bone strength holds true for most people.[8] To keep the bones healthy, weight-bearing exercises, such as walking, dancing, jogging, sports, gardening, or calisthenics, are especially effective. Recently even swimming has been added to the list of activities that build bone strength, although how exactly it does so is not yet known.[9] When muscles work they pull on the bones, thus stressing them and signalling that strong bone tissue is needed. Additionally, the hormones that promote synthesis of new muscle tissue also favor the building of bone.

Activities that stress the bones challenge them and demand that they strengthen their structures. To

be effective in preventing bone loss the activity must include a warm-up lasting 10 or more minutes, aerobic activity (see Chapter 10) lasting 30 to 60 minutes, and must be performed at least three times each week.

As for body weight, osteoporosis is most often associated with underweight. Slender women run a greater risk of suffering from osteoporosis than do heavier women. Bone loss is a well-known side effect of a too-low body weight in women. This holds true even for black women, who are normally more resistant to osteoporosis than are women of other races.[10]

■■■ Smoking and Alcohol

Smokers experience more fractures from slight injury than do nonsmokers, and so do people who are addicted to alcohol. Researchers speculate that the lower body weight of smokers may be one factor; early menopause in female smokers may be another.[11]

People with addictions to alcohol often suffer from osteoporosis, and even men who are addicted suffer more bone breaks than others. It may be that because alcohol (a diuretic) causes fluid excretion, it induces excessive calcium losses through the urine. Also, women's ovaries are sensitive to the effects of alcohol, and drinking may upset the hormonal balance required for healthy bones.

Table C8–1 summarizes the risk factors covered so far and includes some others, among them, low calcium intake, discussed next. The more risk factors that apply to you, the greater your chances of developing osteoporosis in the future and the more seriously you should take the advice offered in the last section of this Controversy.

■■■ Calcium Nutrition

As mentioned, adequate calcium nutrition in the early years may protect the bones in later life. When calcium nutrition is inadequate during childhood and youth, whether due to vitamin D deficiency or to calcium deficiency, the result is poor calcification of the bones.

In addition to calcium and vitamin D, other minerals and vitamins are required to form and to stabilize the bones. Taken during the bone-building years, fluoride may increase bone density. However, fluoride does not prevent bone fractures, as was once hoped, and thus fluoride supplementation as part of therapy for osteoporosis has been called into question.[12]

While a chronically low calcium intake throughout life has been implicated as a risk factor, osteoporosis is not a calcium-deficiency disease comparable to iron-deficiency anemia.[13] In iron-deficiency anemia, high iron intakes reliably reverse the condition; in osteoporosis, though, high calcium intakes alone during adult life do little or nothing to reverse bone loss. One study of over a

■■■ Table C8–1 Risk Factors for Osteoporosis

Age.
Gender.
Race.
Family history of osteoporosis.
Low calcium intake.
Exessive caffeine use.
Excessive fiber in the diet (see Chapter 4).
Menopause.
Never having given birth.
Inactivity or extreme activity with cessation of menstruation.
Low body weight.
Lean body composition.
Short stature, small frame size.
Heavy alcohol use.
Stomach or intestine surgery (surgery can reduce calcium absorption).
Disease states or long-term medications (consult a physician).

SOURCE: Adapted from B. L. Riggs and L. J. Melton, Involutional osteoporosis, *The New England Journal of Medicine* 314 (1986): 1676-1686; L. W. Turner and E. N. Whitney, Nature versus nurture: The calcium controversy, *Nutrition Clinics,* September/October, 1989.

hundred women aged 23 to 88 years demonstrated this. Each woman's daily calcium intake was essentially the same from day to day, but between individuals the average daily consumptions ranged from as little as one-third the RDA to almost three times the RDA. Despite the dramatic differences in intakes of calcium, the rates of loss of bone minerals were similar for all the women of the study.[14] An early report also found no correlation between calcium intakes in adults (between 500 and 1500 milligrams daily) and incidence of osteoporosis.[15]

These and similar findings seem to provide proof that adding calcium to the diets of adults does not protect against osteoporosis, but some research suggests otherwise. In one study, women who had attained menopause, who had begun drinking three cups of milk a day, and who had continued drinking this amount for two years showed marked improvement in calcium balance.[16] Researchers in another study found that women who took in less than about 400 milligrams of calcium a day lost spinal bone tissue faster than women whose intakes were close to 800 milligrams (the RDA amount for older women).[17] Still another study found low dietary calcium to be associated with increased hip fractures in men and women, even taking into account other factors such as smoking, alcohol intake, and exercise.[18]

Although evidence concerning calcium intake conflicts, most experts agree that there must certainly exist a low threshold for calcium intakes, below which bone loss accelerates. It is important to obtain at least the minimum needed to pro-

tect the bones, and the RDA and Canadian RNI for adults are set well above this minimum.

Exactly what level of calcium constitutes the minimum is a point of disagreement. Some cultures seemingly maintain calcium balance on small intakes, and these countries set their calcium recommendations much lower than does the United States or Canada. For example, the World Health Organization (WHO) recommends between 400 and 500 milligrams of calcium per day.

Calcium's absorption into the body complicates the matter of setting an exact minimum because people who consume less calcium absorb more, and vice versa. It might seem, then, that people could switch to calcium-poor diets and allow their bodies to adjust and to absorb more, but the adjustment takes months or years, and, as mentioned, there seems to be a minimum intake threshold not yet established beneath which bone loss accelerates. Irreplaceable bone tissue would be lost rapidly should a person suddenly reduce calcium intake. Even if the body did adapt, the increase in absorption that would follow might not fully make up for the reduced calcium intake and might not support calcium balance and bone mineral retention.[19]

■■■ Calcium Recommendations

Unfortunately few girls and women meet the RDA for calcium during their bone-forming years.[20] (Boys and men obtain levels close to those recommended because they eat more food.) This may mean that most girls start their adult lives with less than optimal bone density.

Unlike magnesium or potassium, calcium is not widespread in the diet. To obtain it, you must learn its sources and make an effort to include them. It is worthwhile to look over the calcium column of Appendix A as well as the calcium section of the last chapter to see which foods are rich or poor sources. Notice, especially, the consistent performance by the milk group. Without these foods, obtaining calcium is difficult.

In the past, experts have recommended that postmenopausal women obtain 1500 milligrams of calcium a day—almost twice the current RDA. Women rarely meet even the RDA of 800 to 1200 milligrams from food within their energy allowances. Not enough firm evidence exists to justify making a recommendation to everyone, but some evidence suggests that women within ten years after menopause may benefit from taking extra calcium.[21] Most importantly, for young people in the bone-building years, it seems a wise course to obtain the amount recommended in the RDA or RNI. But how? A bit of hard-won advice: use foods if at all possible, not supplements.

People in the young, bone-building years of life would best serve their bone health by following the recommendations of Table C8-2. Calcium supplements cannot equal any of the items listed in the table, and no one should be led to think that popping pills can take the place of sound food choices and other healthy habits. For those who desire complete details on supplements, however, a discussion follows.

▪▪▪ A Perspective on Supplements

People who are unwilling, or unable, to consume milk products or other calcium-rich foods in amounts that provide the recommended calcium may choose calcium supplements instead. For some, such as people in treatment for established osteoporosis or those with milk allergies or lactose intolerance, supplements may be of benefit. Supplements are also part of standard therapy for osteoporosis, along with gentle exercise and, for women, estrogen replacement.

Taking calcium supplements entails problems though. For example, calcium carbonate and calcium hydroxyapatite interfere with iron absorption. People who take these pills with foods absorb less iron from those foods and could develop iron deficiencies. Other risks associated with excessive calcium intakes are listed in Table C8-3. Take heed and use supplements with care. About 2500 milligrams is thought to be the maximum safe dose for calcium, so supplements should provide less than this amount, since some calcium is present in foods.

Regular vitamin-mineral pills contain no significant calcium at all, as you can tell from the label. The label may list some number of milligrams of calcium, but remember

▪▪▪ Table C8–2 A Lifetime Plan for Healthy Bones

AGE, YEARS	ACTION
0–18	Use milk as the primary beverage to meet the RDA for calcium within a balanced diet that provides all nutrients; play actively, in sports or other activities; limit television; do not start smoking or drinking alcohol; drink fluoridated water.
19–25	Choose milk as the primary beverage, or if milk causes distress, include other calcium sources to meet the RDA; commit to a lifelong program of physical activity; do not smoke or drink alcohol—if you have started, quit; drink fluoridated water.
26–50	Continue as for 19-to-25 year olds; at menopause, women should be evaluated for possible estrogen replacement therapy. Obtain the RDA for calcium from food. Take calcium and fluoride supplements only if prescribed by physician.
51 and above	Continue as for 19-to-25 year olds; continue following physician's advice concerning estrogen and supplements. Continue striving to meet the calcium RDA from diet, and continue bone-strengthening exercises.

■■■ Table C8–3 Problems Arising from Calcium Supplementation

People who take calcium supplements risk:

Exposure to contaminants. (Some preparations of bone meal and dolomites are contaminated with hazardous amounts of arsenic, cadmium, mercury, and lead.)

Accelerated calcium loss. (Calcium-containing antacids that also contain aluminum and magnesium hydroxide, such as Rolaids, cause a net calcium loss.)

Urinary tract stones or kidney damage in susceptible individuals. (This is seen in those who have a history of kidney stones.)

Vitamin D toxicity. (Vitamin D is needed to enhance calcium absorption, but continued high intakes of vitamin D, which is present in many calcium supplements, can be toxic.)

Excess blood calcium. (This complication is seen only with doses of calcium that are fourfold or more greater than those doses customarily prescribed.)

Milk alkali syndrome. (This alkalosis is also only seen with doses of calcium of 4 to 10 grams/day. This condition disappears when supplementation is discontinued.)

Impaired iron status. (This is due to the change in stomach pH caused by calcium, which results in decreased iron bioavailability.)

Other nutrient interactions. (Calcium phosphate dibasic inhibits magnesium absorption.)

Drug interactions. (An example is toxicity from digoxin.)

Constipation or confusion. (Older people are especially prone to these conditions.)

SOURCES: Lead in bonemeal supplements still of concern, *National Council Against Health Fraud,* September 1987; B. G. Shah, Calcium supplementation with antacids, *Journal of the American Medical Association* 257 (1987): 541; Should you take a calcium supplement? *FDA Consumer,* October 1986, p. 35; Complications of excess calcium intake, *Nutrition and the MD,* October 1987; Adverse effects of calcium supplements, *Nutrition and the MD,* January 1987; N. M. Resnick and S. L. Greenspan, "Senile" osteoporosis reconsidered, *Journal of the American Medical Association* 261 (1989): 1025–1029.

that the U.S. RDA for calcium is a gram—a thousand milligrams.

Calcium supplements are available in three forms. Simplest are the purified calcium compounds, such as calcium carbonate, citrate, gluconate, lactate, malate, phosphate or the like, and compounds of calcium with amino acids (called **amino acid chelates**). Then there are mixtures of calcium with other compounds, such as mixtures of calcium carbonate with magnesium carbonate, with aluminum salts (as in some **antacids**), or with vitamin D. Then there are powdered forms of calcium-rich materials, such as **bone meal, powdered bone, oyster shell,** or **dolomite** (limestone).

If you wanted a calcium supplement, which of these should you choose? Before comparing on any other basis, you should eliminate some right away as unsafe. Some preparations of bone meal and dolomite, for example, have been found to be contaminated with high enough levels of arsenic, cadmium, mercury, and lead to pose a hazard to the health of the person who takes them routinely.

The next question to ask is how well the body absorbs and uses the calcium from various supplements. Based on limited research to date, it seems that most healthy people absorb calcium equally well—and as well as from milk—from any of these supplements: amino acids chelated with calcium, calcium acetate, calcium carbonate, calcium citrate, calcium gluconate, calcium lactate, and calcium phosphate dibasic. People absorb calcium less well from a mixture of calcium carbonate and magnesium carbonate, from oyster-shell calcium fortified with inorganic magnesium, from a chelated calcium-magnesium combination, or from calcium carbonate fortified with vitamins and iron. A way to get around the problem with nutrient interactions may be to take calcium supplements between, not with, meals. But for anyone with reduced stomach acid secretion, this is not a satisfactory solution, since only a meal stimulates the secretion of enough stomach acid to permit the absorption of the calcium. (Score another point here for food sources of calcium.)

Consider another point for food. *Some* people absorb calcium better from milk and milk products than from even the most absorbable supplements named above.[22] Still

---

■■■ Miniglossary of Bone Terms

cortical bone: the ivory-like outer bone layer that forms a shell over trabecular bone and comprises the shaft of a long bone.

trabecular (tra-BECK-you-lar) **bone:** the lacy inner bone that supports the bone's structure.

---

another: After absorption, the source affects the body's internal use of the nutrient. Only one study has shown this to be true of calcium, but that study shows that the body makes better use of calcium from milk than from calcium carbonate.[23]

Supposing that you can absorb the supplement taken between meals and that your body will use it well, then the next question to ask is, "Which contains the most calcium per pill?" The more calcium in a single pill, the fewer pills you have to take. Read the label to find out. Calcium carbonate is 40 percent calcium; calcium gluconate only 9 percent. They vary.

Finally, consider the cost, and choose a supplement. Establish a routine so that you will not forget to take it; remember, you will have to do this every day for the rest of your life. Take it several times a day in divided doses rather than all at once; divided doses can improve a day's total absorption by up to 20 percent.[24]

■■■ Some Closing Thoughts

Think one more time before you commit yourself to taking supplements for calcium. The RDA is 800 milligrams of calcium for adults over 25 years, and people with risk factors for osteoporosis (Table C8-1) are urged to strive toward their RDA amount daily. Are you absolutely sure you cannot adjust your food and beverage intakes to provide it? Everyone seems to prefer that you use foods, and it is much easier, more pleasant, and less expensive than taking supplements. The Consensus Conference on Osteoporosis recommended milk. The American Society for Bone and Mineral Research recommends foods as a source of calcium in preference to supplements.[25] Nutrition authorities Mayer and Goldberg, whose syndicated column on nutrition reaches newspaper readers nationwide, state, "We stand firmly in favor of dietary measures to meet the RDA . . . of calcium."[26] The writers of this book are so impressed with the importance of using abundant, calcium-rich foods that they have worked out a way to do so at every meal. Seldom is such a consensus seen among nutritionists.

Just as important as calcium intake is exercise. Dr Robert Heaney of Omaha's Creighton University stated the case for exercise informally but accurately in *Time* magazine (February 23, 1987). "Osteoporosis is a total life-style problem. You can't cure a bad life-style with a pill, and it's a terrible strategic mistake to encourage people to think you can. If I'm sitting all day, don't walk to work, don't carry loads or work in the garden on the weekend, I'm going to lose bone. You can give me all the calcium in the world, and it's not going to stop it." Cells do not helplessly accept what is given to them, but they do respond with the help of the necessary regulators to the demands put upon them, and then they select the nutrients they need from what is offered. The way to make bone density increase is to put a demand on the bones, to make them work, and then to provide the raw materials from which they can grow strong: calcium, other minerals, all the nutrients in the right balance. In addition, take the steps suggested in Table C8-2 at each stage of life. That way you have the best possible chance of preserving bone health throughout life.

Notes

1. B. L. Riggs and L. J. Melton, Involutional osteoporosis, *New England Journal of Medicine* 314 (1986): 1676–1686.
2. C. Niewoehner, Calcium and osteoporosis *Cereal Foods World* 33 (1988): 784–787.
3. Riggs, 1986.
4. H. K. Genant and coauthors, Quantitative computed tomography of vertebral spongiosa: A sensitive method for detecting early bone loss after oophorectomy, *Annals of Internal Medicine* 97 (1982): 699–705.
5. B. Ettinger, H. K. Genant, and

▓▓▓ Miniglossary of Calcium Supplement Terms

amino acid chelates: compounds of minerals (such as calcium) combined with amino acids in a form that favors their absorption. (A *chelating agent* is a molecule that surrounds another molecule and therefore is useful for either promoting or preventing its movement from place to place.)

antacids: acid-buffering agents used to counter excess acidity in the stomach. Calcium-containing preparations (such as Tums) contain available calcium. Antacids with aluminum or magnesium hydroxides (such as Rolaids) can accelerate calcium losses.

bone meal, powdered bone: crushed or ground bone preparations intended to supply calcium to the diet. Calcium from bone is not well absorbed and is often contaminated with toxic materials.

dolomite: a compound of minerals (calcium magnesium carbonate) found in limestone and marble. Dolomite is powdered and is sold as a calcium-magnesium supplement but may be contaminated with toxic minerals, is not well absorbed, and interacts adversely with absorption of other essential minerals.

oyster shell: a product made from the powdered shells of oysters, sold as a calcium supplement, but not well absorbed by the digestive system.

C. E. Cann, Long-term estrogen replacement therapy prevents bone loss and fractures, *Annals of Internal Medicine* 102 (1985): 319–324.

6. C. Foresta and coauthors, Osteoporosis and decline of gonadal function in the elderly male, *Hormone Research* 19 (1984): 18–22.

7. A history of racial and ethnic differences in regard to bone health is found in W. S. Pollitzer and J. J. B. Anderson, Ethnic and genetic differences in bone mass: A review with a hereditary vs environmental perspective, *American Journal of Clinical Nutrition* 50 (1989): 1244–1259.

8. M. Sinake and coauthors, Relationship between bone mineral density of spine and strength of back extensors in healthy postmenopausal women, *Mayo Clinic Proceedings* 61 (1986): 116–122; J. McBride, No bone loss when seniors work out, *Journal of the American Dietetic Association* 89 (1989): 73.

9. E. S. Orwoll and coauthors, The relationship of swimming exercise to bone mass in men and women, *Archives of Internal Medicine* 149 (1989): 2197–2200.

10. O. Walden and J. DeWorth, Body size of black women who suffered a hip fracture, *Journal of Nutrition for the Elderly*, April 1988, pp. 3–8.

11. G. Wardlaw, The effects of diet and life-style on bone mass in women, *Journal of the American Dietetic Association* 88 (1988): 17–25.

12. Fluoride's promise fractured, *Consumer Reports Health Letter*, June 1990, pp. 45–56.

13. R. P. Heaney and coauthors, Calcium nutrition and bone health in the elderly, *American Journal of Clinical Nutrition* 36 (1982): 986–1013.

14. B. L. Riggs and coauthors, Dietary calcium intakes and rates of bone loss in women, *Journal of Clinical Investigation* 80 (1987): 979–982.

15. R. W. Smith and B. Frame, Concurrent axial and appendicular osteoporosis: Its relation to calcium consumption, *New England Journal of Medicine* 273 (1965): 73–78.

16. R. R. Recker and R. P. Heaney, The effect of milk supplements on calcium metabolism, bone metabolism, and calcium balance, *American Journal of Clinical Nutrition* 41 (1985): 254–263.

17. B. Dawson-Hughes, J. Jacques, and C. Shipp, Dietary calcium intake and bone loss from the spine in healthy postmenopausal women, *American Journal of Clinical Nutrition* 46 (1987): 685–687.

18. T. L. Holbrook, E. Barrett-Connor, and D. L. Wingard, Dietary calcium and risk of hip fracture: 14-year prospective population study, *Lancet* 12 (1988): 1046–1049.

19. L. H. Allen, Calcium bioavailability and absorption: A review, *American Journal of Clinical Nutrition* 35 (1982): 783.

20. J. A. T. Pennington, B. E. Young, and D. B. Wilson, Nutritional elements in U.S. diets: Results from the Total Diet Study, 1982 to 1986, *Journal of the American Dietetic Association* 89 (1989): 659–664; Dietary calcium and the prevention of postmenopausal osteoporosis: Review from the National Nutrition Institute in Canada, *Nutrition Today*, May/June 1988, pp. 33–35.

21. K. J. Polley and coauthors, Effect of calcium supplementation on forearm bone mineral content in postmenopausal women: A prospective, sequential controlled study, *Journal of Nutrition* 117 (1987): 1929–1935.

22. M. S. Sheikh and coauthors, Gastrointestinal absorption of calcium from milk and calcium salts, *New England Journal of Medicine* 317 (1987): 532–536.

23. L. D. McBean, Food versus pills versus fortified foods, *Dairy Council Digest*, March-April 1987.

24. More on supplementation: Calcium redux, *Nutrition Action*, December 1984, pp. 12–13.

25. McBean, 1987.

26. J. Mayer and J. Goldberg, Sufficient calcium intake still a major problem, *Tallahassee Democrat*, 5 November 1987.

Energy Balance and Weight Control

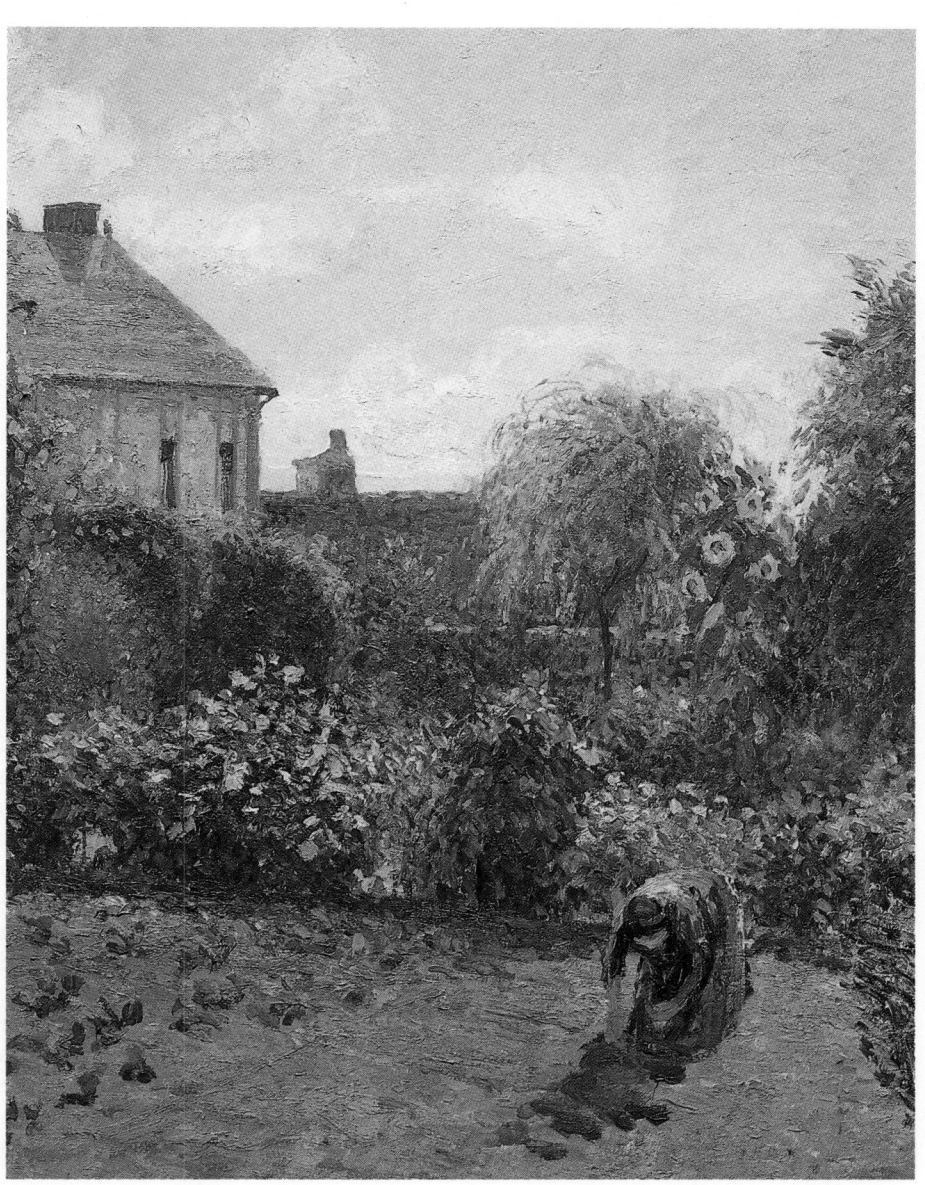

The Artist's Garden at Eragny; (detail) Camille Pissarro; National Gallery of Art, Washington; Ailsa Mellon Bruce Collection.

CONTENTS

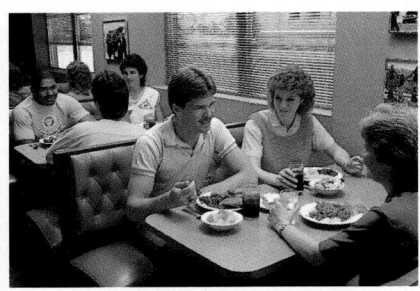

While you cannot control your weight directly, you can control your eating behavior.

Are you pleased with your body weight? If you answered yes, you are a rare individual. Nearly all people in our society think they should weigh more or less (mostly less) than they do. Usually their primary reason is appearance, but they often perceive, correctly, that physical health is also somehow related to weight.[1]

People also think of their weight as something they should control. They are right, but a pair of misconceptions makes their task difficult. The first is to focus on *weight*; the second is to focus on *controlling* weight. To put it simply, it isn't your weight you need to control; it's the fat in your body in proportion to the lean. And it isn't possible to control either one, directly; it is possible only to control your *behavior*. In other words, the words "Weight Control" in this chapter's title are wrong; they should be replaced with the words "Behavior to Promote Appropriate Body Composition." If the chapter bore that name, though, hardly anyone would read it.

This chapter's missions are to present the problems associated with deficient and excessive body fatness; to present strategies for solving these problems; and to show how to maintain appropriate body proportions of body components, once achieved.

The Problems of Underweight and Overweight

Both deficient and excessive body fat present health risks. It has long been known that thin people will die first during a siege or in a famine. A fact not always recognized, even by health care providers, is that overly thin people are also at a disadvantage in the hospital, where they may have to go for days without food so that they can undergo tests or surgery. Underweight also increases the risk for any person fighting a wasting disease. In fact, people with cancer often die from starvation, not from the cancer itself. Thus underweight people are urged to gain body fat as an energy reserve and to acquire protective amounts of all the nutrients that can be stored.

As for excess body fat, for one thing, it can precipitate hypertension and thus increase the risk of stroke. Often weight loss alone can normalize the blood pressure of an overfat person; some people with hypertension can tell you exactly at what weight their blood pressure begins to rise. Weight gain can also precipitate diabetes in genetically susceptible people and thus bring on its associated ills (Chapter 4). If hypertension or diabetes runs in your family, you urgently need to take steps toward weight control. Excess body fatness (especially in the central abdominal area of the body) also increases the risk of heart disease by worsening atherosclerosis. Excess fat demands to be fed by miles of extra capillaries, increasing the heart's work load to the point of damaging it. A recent study of middle-aged women indicated that being even mildly or moderately overweight increases the risk of heart disease.[2] Other conditions associated with overfatness include abdominal hernias, some cancers, varicose veins, gout, gallbladder disease, arthritis, respiratory problems, liver malfunction,[3] complications in pregnancy and surgery, flat feet, and even a high accident rate.

Some obese people can escape at least some of the health problems mentioned, but no one who is fat in our society quite escapes the social and economic handicaps. Fat people are less sought after for romance, less often hired, and less often admitted to college. They pay higher insurance premiums, and they pay more for clothing. Psychologically, too, a body size that embarrasses a person diminishes self-esteem.

The health risks of overfatness are so many that it has been declared a disease: **obesity**.[4] People who are obese are urged to reduce their weight. Their health risks are expected to normalize as they do.

A warning about weight reduction is in order, though: some people are able to lose weight, but few are able to maintain the new desirable weight. Repeated cycles of weight loss and weight regain are common and can be more hazardous to health than obesity itself.[5] Weight maintenance, the steady state in which weight varies little over the years, is as important to health as weight loss.

❚❚▶ *Both deficient and excessive body fatness present health risks, and overfatness presents social and economic handicaps as well.*

❚❚❚ Definition of Appropriate Weight

Once upon a time the definition of appropriate weight was simple. A person's weight could be compared with that in the "ideal weight" tables. If the actual weight were 20 percent or more above the table weight, then the person was obese; if it was 10 percent under, the person was underweight. Now (to tell a long story in a few words), the term *ideal weight* is no longer in use, and the definition of obesity is no longer simple.

Among the problems were these. Weight depends on a person's **frame size**—but how do you measure frame size? Weight doesn't matter as much as body composition, and especially body fat content, but how do you measure body fat content? How much body fat there is doesn't matter as much as where it is located on the body, but how do you tie this to ideal weight and the definition of obesity? In addition, the weight tables on which standards are based were designed for insurance purposes and not as guides for nutrition status.[6]

The problem of using weight as an indicator of health or risk status is that body weight says so little about body composition. A person who doesn't seem to weigh too much may be too fat; a person who does seem to weigh too much may not be. A dancer or an athlete, whose muscles are well developed and whose bones have become well mineralized by responding to constant stress, may weigh the same as a sedentary person, yet the dancer or athlete may be at a healthy weight, and the sedentary person may be too fat. An example of incorrectly relying on height-weight tables to determine obesity occurred with a group of football players. They were rejected from the armed forces for being obese according to the table, but their *muscle* weight was actually responsible for the elevated scale weights.[7] There is no easy way to look inside a person and see the bones and muscles. Nevertheless, you need at least an approximation to work with, so, imperfect as they are, Table 9−1 provides standards to determine frame size and the inside back cover, page X, provides the standard height and weight tables.

Nutritionists today often use a more sensitive indicator of body composition than weight, the **body mass index (BMI)**:

$$BMI = \frac{weight\ (kilograms)}{height^2\ (meters)}$$

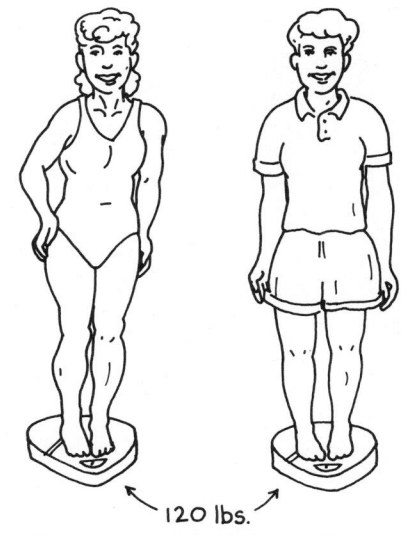

Both women weigh 120 pounds. One has more muscle and bone; the other, more fat.

■■■ Table 9–1 How to Determine Your Frame Size by Elbow Breadth

To make a simple approximation of your frame size:

Extend your arm, and bend the forearm upwards at a 90-degree angle. Keep the fingers straight, and turn the inside of your wrist away from your body. Place the thumb and index finger of your other hand on the two prominent bones on *either side* of your elbow. Measure the space between your fingers against a ruler or a tape measure.[a] Compare the measurements with the following standards.

These standards represent the elbow measurements for medium-framed men and women of various heights. Measurements smaller than those listed indicate you have a small frame, and larger measurements indicate a large frame.

Men

Height in 1-Inch Heels	Elbow Breadth of Medium-Frame Man
5 ft 2 inches to 5 ft 3 inches	2 1/2 to 2 7/8 inches
5 ft 4 inches to 5 ft 7 inches	2 5/8 to 2 7/8 inches
5 ft 8 inches to 5 ft 11 inches	2 3/4 to 3 inches
6 ft 0 inches to 6 ft 3 inches	2 3/4 to 3 1/8 inches
6 ft 4 inches and over	2 7/8 to 3 1/4 inches

Women

Height in 1-Inch Heels	Elbow Breadth of Medium-Frame Woman
4 ft 10 inches to 4 ft 11 inches	2 1/4 to 2 1/2 inches
5 ft 0 inches to 5 ft 3 inches	2 1/4 to 2 1/2 inches
5 ft 4 inches to 5 ft 7 inches	2 3/8 to 2 5/8 inches
5 ft 8 inches to 5 ft 11 inches	2 3/8 to 2 5/8 inches
6 ft 0 inches and over	2 1/2 to 2 3/4 inches

[a]For a more accurate measurement, have your health care provider measure your elbow breadth with a caliper.

SOURCE: Courtesy Metropolitan Life Insurance Company.

A BMI of greater than 27.2 in men or 26.9 in women indicates the need for weight reduction. No lower limit is set to indicate the need for weight gain. Figure 9–1 (pages 287–288) shows you how to use both the traditional tables and the body mass index and guides you to develop a safe range of weights as one tentative answer to the question, "What is an appropriate weight for you?"

As the struggle continues, the height-weight tables have two undeniable advantages in assessing obesity—they are available and easy to use. If you choose to use them, be sure to add an inch to your barefoot height (you are assumed to be wearing shoes with 1-inch heels), and adjust for clothing (the tables assume three to five pounds for clothes).

If the weight tables cause frustration in would-be users, perhaps that reaction brings with it a benefit—it leads them to ask deeper questions about the state of the body most compatible with good health and long life. When answers finally come to the asker, they will doubtless have to do with body composition.

■■▶ *The definition of appropriate weight based on frame size, weight, and standard tables is beset with problems. The currently preferred definition is based on body mass index (BMI).*

When physical health alone is considered, a wide range of weights is acceptable for a person of a given height. Within the safe range, the definition of appropriate weight is up to the individual, depending on factors such as family history, occupation, physical and recreational activities, and personal preferences.

1. Determine the safe range for a person your height and sex.

☐ Record your height: _____ft, _____inches.

☐ Determine your frame size, using Table 9–1. Record whether you have a small, medium, or large frame: _____frame.

☐ Look up the appropriate weight for a person your height, sex, and frame size in the table on the inside back cover, page X. (*Note:* The heights listed assume you were measured in shoes with 1-inch heels. If you wore no shoes to be measured, add an inch; if you wore shoes with heels higher or lower than an inch, adjust accordingly.) Record the entire range: _____to _____lb.

Example: For a man 5 ft 7 inches tall (in shoes) with a small frame, the range of weights is 138 to 145 lb.

☐ Determine the bottom end of the safe range. A person who is more than 10% below the lowest indicated weight for height is considered underweight to a degree that might compromise health. Take 10% off the bottom end of your range: _____lb.

Example: 10% of 138 lb is 13.8 lb (rounded off to 14 lb). Bottom end of range is 138 minus 14 or 124 lb.

☐ Determine the top end of the safe range. A person who is more than 20% above the highest indicated weight for height is considered obese. Add 20% to the top end of your range: _____lb.

Example: 20% of 145 lb is 29 lb. The top end of the range is 145 plus 29, or 174 lb.

☐ Record your safe range here: _____to _____lb.

Example: 124 to 174 lb.

Note: For a second opinion about your weight range, consult the BMI grid on the inside back cover.

2. If your weight is below the bottom end of this safe range, you need to gain weight for your health's sake. If your weight is above the top end of the range, determine your body mass index to obtain confirmation that you need to lose weight. (Refer to the nomogram on the next page. Use your weight without clothing and your height without shoes.) A body mass index greater than 27.2 in men or 26.9 in women indicates the need for weight loss.

Example: A man 5 ft 6 inches tall (without shoes), according to this figure, would have a body mass index of 27.2 if he weighed 169 lb. This would be a more accurate upper limit of his safe weight range; he should not exceed this weight, unless advised by a health professional to do so. Revise the top end of your safe range if necessary.

3. Check your health history for further confirmation. A family or personal medical history of diabetes (noninsulin-dependent type), hypertension, or high blood cholesterol signifies a high priority for weight control.

4. Choose a goal weight within the safe range. Answering the following questions should help you to determine where, within the safe range, your personal appropriate weight may be:

☐ Does your occupation demand that you have a certain body shape? Record the weight, within the safe range, that would most nearly approximate this body shape: _____ lb.

☐ Do you engage in a sport or other physical activity that requires a particular body weight for optimal performance? Consult your instructor or other expert in that sport or activity, and record the weight recommended on that basis: _____lb.

☐ Do you hope to start a pregnancy soon? If so, consult your health care provider about the ideal weight with which to begin a pregnancy: _____lb.

☐ Undress and stand before a mirror. Do you think you need to gain or to lose weight? Add or subtract pounds to arrive at a personal goal weight (but be sure to stay within the safe range): _____lb.

Based on all of these considerations, choose a final goal weight. No formula exists for this estimate, but don't choose a weight outside the safe range without a professional assessment.

Your goal weight: _____lb.

■■■ **Figure 9–1**

What Is an Appropriate Weight for You?

■■■ Figure 9–1 continued.

Nomogram for Body Mass Index (BMI). Weights and heights are without clothing. With clothes, add 5 pounds for men or 3 pounds for women, and 1 inch in height for shoes. Draw a straight line or place a ruler from your height (left) to your weight (right). At the point where it crosses the BMI line, read your BMI. A BMI greater than 27.2 for men or 26.9 for women indicates obesity.

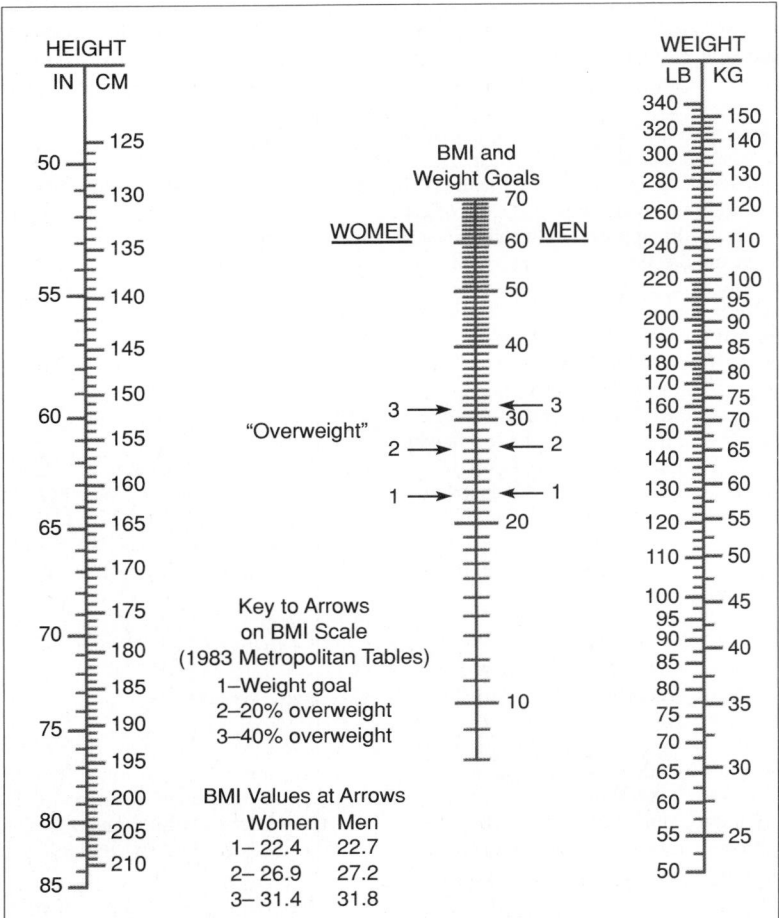

SOURCE: From the 1983 Metropolitan Life Insurance Company tables, designed by B. T. Burton and W. R. Foster, Health implications of obesity, an NIH Consensus Development Conference, *Journal of the American Dietetic Association* 85 (1985): 1117-1121.

■■■ Body Composition

Several laboratory techniques for estimating body fatness have been developed and used for more than ten years. These include:

■ Anthropometry: measurements of height and weight, **fatfold** thickness (see opposite margin), body circumferences, and body breadths.
■ Density (the measurement of body weight compared with volume): Lean tissue is denser than fat tissue, so the denser a person's body is, the more lean tissue it must contain. From the density, an estimate of the percentage of body fat can be derived.

Sophisticated techniques are available to determine these measures, and some can not only estimate lean versus fat tissue but also determine where the fat is located.*[8]

*Techniques include underwater weighing, isotope dilution, ultrasound, bioelectrical impedance, computed tomography, magnetic resonance imaging, and neutron activation.

The distribution of fat on the body is important because fat around the middle—**central obesity**—may represent a greater risk to health than fat elsewhere. Abdominal fat, when mobilized, goes directly to the liver, where it is made into cholesterol-carrying low-density lipoprotein (LDL); and it has been shown to correlate more closely than fat located elsewhere on the body with an increased incidence of diabetes and coronary artery disease.[9] Fatfold measurements do not take this fat distribution difference into account. A simple comparison of waist and hip measurements may become a standard part of the assessment of body fatness in years to come.[10]

Even after you have a body fatness estimate, problems arise. For example, how do you interpret it? What is the "ideal" amount of fat for a body to have? The question—ideal for what?—has to be answered first.

The ideal depends partly on who you are. A man of normal weight may have, on the average, 15 percent and a woman 20 percent of the body weight as fat. Special needs exist. For example, competitive endurance athletes need a certain minimum of body fat to provide fuel, to insulate the body, and to permit normal fat-soluble hormone activity, but not so much as to weigh them down. An Alaskan fisherman, on the other hand, needs a blanket of insulating fat to prevent excessive loss of body heat. For a woman starting pregnancy, the ideal percentage of body fat may be different again; the outcome of pregnancy is compromised if the woman begins it with too little body fat. Below a threshold for body fat content set by heredity, some individuals become infertile, develop depression or abnormal hunger regulation, or become unable to keep warm. These thresholds are not the same for each function or in all individuals, and much remains to be learned about them. Beyond these basic needs for body fat, you should probably strive to keep body fat content as low as possible so as to minimize health risks associated with overfatness.

Just as there is a minimum percentage of body fat that is ideal for a given individual, there is also a maximum, and this too may differ from person to person. Blood pressure and other disease-risk indicators also rise and fall with body fatness—blood glucose and blood cholesterol, for example. For those in whom these signs appear with added fat, weight reduction is most critical. The most useful definition of obesity might be, "*body fatness in excess of that consistent with optimal health, as determined by a reliable measure.*" But for now the measures to pinpoint such a level of fatness are still to be worked out.

The person seeking a single, authoritative answer to the question "How much should I weigh?" is bound to be disappointed. No one can tell you *exactly* how much you should weigh; but with health as a value, at least you have a starting framework. Your weight should fall within the range that supports your health. Within the range, the weight to pick is up to you. Your own standards are important.

▐▌▶ *The assessor can determine the percentage of fat in a person's body by measuring fatfold thickness, by determining body density, or by other means. The assessor should also note distribution of fat in obese people, since central obesity is more hazardous to health than other forms of obesity.*

▐▐▐ The Mystery of Obesity

Why do some people get fat? Why do some get thin? And most amazingly, how do some people stay at the same weight year after year? Is obesity due to

> **fatfold:** the thickness of a fold of skin on the back of the arm (over the triceps muscle), below the shoulder blade (subscapular), or in other places, as measured with a caliper (depicted below). Also called *skinfold*.
>
> **central obesity:** excess fat on the abdomen and around the trunk.

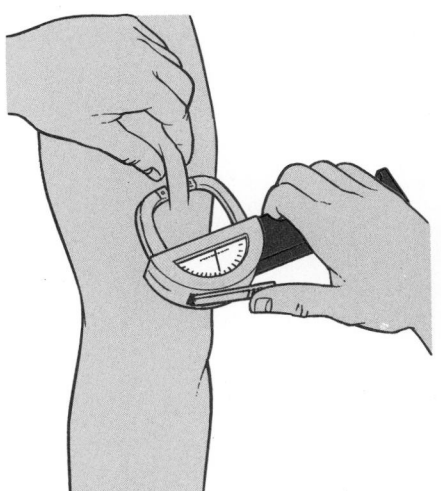

In a fatfold test, a clinician lifts a fold of skin from the back of the arm or other area and measures its thickness with a caliper that applies a fixed amount of pressure.

set-point theory: the theory that the body tends to maintain a certain weight by means of its own internal controls.

brown fat: adipose tissue abundant in hibernating animals and human infants. Brown fat cells are packed with pigmented, energy-burning enzymes that give brown fat its characteristic color.

external cue theory: the theory that some people eat in response to such external factors as the presence of food or the time of day rather than in response to such internal factors as hunger.

hunger: defined in Chapter 3, the physiological need to eat, experienced as a drive for obtaining food; an unpleasant sensation.

appetite: also defined in Chapter 3, the psychological desire to eat, a learned motivation and a positive sensation.

satiety: the feeling of fullness or satisfaction at the end of a meal that prompts a person to stop eating.

arousal: heightened activity of certain brain centers associated with excitement and anxiety.

stress eating: eating in response to stress, an inappropriate response.

genetics or to environmental influences? For a person who has one parent with a weight problem, the chance of becoming obese is 60 percent; if both parents have weight problems, the probability rises to 90 percent.[11] In general, two schools of thought attempt to explain this effect. One attributes it to inherited metabolic causes, the other to behavioral factors. The two views are not mutually exclusive, and both are usually operating, even in the same person. Furthermore, even behavioral tendencies can have a genetic basis.

One popular metabolic theory of obesity is the **set-point theory**. Researchers have noted that many people who lose weight on reducing diets subsequently return to their original weight.[12] This theory states that somehow the body chooses a weight that it wants to be and defends that weight by regulating eating behaviors and hormonal actions. The causes are thought to lie in hunger-regulating mechanisms or in their systems of burning fuels.

A tissue that specializes in generating heat is **brown fat**. Heredity may influence the development of brown fat cells.[13] Regular white fat cells store energy in fat's chemical bonds and have a slow metabolic rate; brown fat cells break those bonds and actively release their stored energy as heat. Brown fat is more abundant and more active in lean animals than in fat ones. It is theorized that a person whose brown fat burns off too little energy or a person who has less than the normal amount of brown fat would thus store more white fat than another person with the same energy intake. So far no one has suggested ways of increasing brown fat's activity or abundance to affect weight control.

A different point of view contends that obesity is determined by behavioral responses to environmental stimuli.[14] Proponents of this view hold that people overeat as a response to their surroundings—foremost among them, the availability of a multitude of delectable foods. People who eat at mealtimes even though they aren't hungry, who clean their plates even though they are satisfied sooner, and who partake of food "because it is there" are responding to environmental influences. This is the so called **external cue theory**—the theory that, at least in some people, outside-the-body factors override internal regulatory systems.

One way researchers have attempted to study what makes people overeat is to investigate **hunger**, **appetite**, and **satiety**. Hunger is a drive programmed into us by our heredity. Appetite, which is learned, can teach us to ignore hunger or to overrespond to it. Hunger is physiological, while appetite is psychological, and the two do not always coincide. Satiety (feeling of fullness) signals that it is time to stop eating, most likely the result of communication between the stomach and small intestine and the brain's hypothalamus (see Chapter 3). Some overeaters claim they never feel full.

Eating behavior may be a response not only to hunger and appetite but also to complex human sensations such as yearning, craving, addiction, or compulsion. For an emotionally insecure person, eating when lonely may be less threatening than calling a friend and risking rejection. Often people eat to relieve boredom or depression. Any kind of **arousal** can cause overeating, perhaps because aroused feelings are mistaken for hunger. The eating done in response to arousal is **stress eating**. However, while some people overeat in response to stress, others cannot eat at all. It is not known why people react differently, but research continues.

Another promising area of study concerns the effect on body weight of the energy-nutrient distribution of the diet. Evidence is building to support the theory that dietary fat is stored virtually unchanged in the body, thus preserving a maximum of its original energy. Carbohydrate, on the other hand, must be dismantled and reassembled into fat before storage in the body, processes that cost energy to perform. Thus the total stored energy from excess carbohydrate, its "fattening power," may be far less than researchers once believed. It could be that people who store too much body fat while eating a reasonable amount of food consistently choose foods with too much fat. Controversy 10 delves into the details of this emerging topic.

One other cause of obesity stands out—lack of exercise. The control of hunger/appetite appears to work well in most healthy, active people; few athletes are obese. But appetite control often fails when activity falls below a certain minimum level. Some obese people eat less than lean people, but they are so extraordinarily inactive that they still manage to have an energy surplus.

Although we may have been born with the instinct to eat, we are not helpless when confronted with food. We also have the ability to override the instinct to eat. Later sections of this chapter show how people can modify their behavior by changing their responses to cues to action and by arranging for consequences after the behavior.

❚❚▷ *Some of the causes of obesity may include a genetically set body weight (set point) or abnormal brown fat. Among theories of behavioral causes are inappropriate responses to the sight, smell, and taste of foods; to stress; or to the fat content of meals. A major contributor to obesity is underactivity.*

❚❚❚ Energy Balance

Regardless of theories of metabolism and behavior, people in the real world gain and lose weight. Suppose you decide that you are too fat or too thin. How did you get that way? By having an unbalanced energy budget, that is, by eating either more or less food energy than you spent.

Energy In

A day's energy balance can be stated like this:

Change in energy (fat and glycogen) stores equals food energy taken in minus energy spent on metabolism and muscle activities.

More simply:

$$\text{Change in energy stores} = \text{energy in} - \text{energy out.}$$

Food energy consumed in a day is the only contributor to the "energy-in" side of the energy-balance equation. Before you can decide how much food energy you need in a day, you must first become familiar with the amounts of energy in foods.

Scientists use laboratory methods (notably, burning under controlled conditions) to release and to measure the energy in foods; they state the energy in calories. (You can look up the calorie amounts associated with several hundred foods obtained in this way in Appendix A.) In addition to looking up food energy values in a table, you can also estimate them using the exchange system, which classes foods by their protein, fat, and carbohydrate contents expressed in grams. (You also have to add calories from alcohol if it is present.) A later section shows you how to use the exchange system to estimate calories quickly.

Remember these average values of the energy-yielding nutrients:

1 g carbohydrate = 4 cal.
1 g fat = 9 cal.
1 g protein = 4 cal.

Also remember:
1 g alcohol = 7 cal.

basal metabolism: the sum total of all the involuntary activities that are necessary to sustain life, including respiration, circulation, and new tissue synthesis and excluding digestion and voluntary activities. Basal metabolism accounts for the largest component of the average person's daily energy expenditure. It is measured while lying down, while awake, and at least 12 hours after eating.

voluntary activities: activities (such as walking, sitting, running) conducted by voluntary muscles.

basal metabolic rate (BMR): the rate at which the body uses energy to support its basal metabolism.

1 lb body fat = 3500 cal.

Light activity, for both women and men, means sleeping or lying down for eight hours a day, sitting for seven hours, standing for five, walking for two, and spending two hours a day in light physical activity.

The energy RDA are presented in the inside front cover, page C; examples of Canadian energy allowances are presented in Appendix B.

As examples of the numbers of calories associated with energy intakes and expenditures, an apple provides you with 125 calories; an average candy bar with 425 calories. For a 150-pound person, brisk walking for 20 minutes costs about 100 calories; jogging for 20 minutes costs about 200 calories. You may already know that for each 3500 calories you eat in excess of expenditures, you store approximately 1 pound of body fat.†

Energy Out

While it is easy to estimate the energy present in a meal or in a day's meals, it is not easy to determine the energy an individual spends or needs. The U.S. Committee on Recommended Dietary Allowances (RDA) and the Canadian Department of National Health and Welfare have published recommended energy intakes for various age-sex groups in their populations. These are useful for population studies, but among individuals in a group, the range of energy needs is so broad that it is impossible to guess a person's need without knowing something about the person's lifestyle. The RDA, for example, assumes that a 20-year-old woman stands 5 feet 5 inches tall, weighs about 128 pounds, is of average body fatness, engages in light activity, and needs 2200 calories of energy a day. A healthy 20-year-old man is assumed to stand 5 feet 10 inches tall, to weigh 160 pounds, to be lightly active, and to need 2900 calories a day. Taller people, because of their greater surface area, need proportionately more energy and shorter people proportionately less energy to balance their energy budgets. Older people generally need less due to both slowed metabolism and reduced activity, with the number of calories diminishing by about 5 percent per decade beyond the age of 30 years.

People vary in their energy needs. In any group of 20 similar people with similar activity levels, one may expend twice as much energy per day as another.[15] Clearly it is impossible to pinpoint any person's energy need within such a wide range without studying that person.

One way to obtain an estimate of your energy needs is to monitor your food intake and body weight over a period of time in which your activities are typical of your lifestyle. If you keep a strictly accurate record of all the foods and beverages you consume for a week or two and if your weight has not changed during the past few months, you can conclude that your energy budget is balanced. At least a week of record keeping is necessary, though, because intakes fluctuate from day to day. (On about half the days you eat less food energy than the average; on the other half more.)

An alternative method of determining energy output is to compute two components of energy expenditure and then to add them together.‡ The body spends energy in two major ways: (1) to fuel its **basal metabolism** and (2) to fuel its **voluntary activities**. You can change the latter of these now, to spend more or less energy in a day, and you can also change the first category of energy expenditure but indirectly and over time, as explained later.

The basal metabolism supports the body's work that goes on all the time, without conscious awareness. The beating of the heart, the inhaling and ex-

---

†Pure fat is worth 9 calories per gram. A pound of it (450 grams), then, would store 4050 calories. A pound of body fat is not pure fat, though; it contains water, protein, and other materials, hence the lower calorie value.

‡Another energy component is the body's heat production, *thermogenesis*. This energy is thought to have four components: heat from basal metabolism, from physical activity, from processing food, and from adapting to environmental changes. For the purpose of roughly estimating energy expenditure, thermogenesis can be ignored.

■■■ Table 9–2 Factors that Affect the BMR

FACTOR	EFFECT ON BMR
Age	In youth, the BMR is higher; age brings less lean body mass and slows the BMR.
Height	Tall, thin people have higher BMRs.
Growth	Children and pregnant women have higher BMRs.
Body composition	The more lean tissue, the higher the BMR. The more fat tissue, the lower the BMR.
Fever	Fever raises the BMR.
Stress	Stress hormones raise the BMR.
Environmental temperature	Both heat and cold raise the BMR.
Fasting/starvation	Fasting/starvation hormones lower the BMR.
Malnutrition	Malnutrition lowers the BMR.
Thyroxin	The thyroid hormone thyroxin is a key BMR regulator; the more thyroxin produced, the higher is the BMR.

haling of air, the maintenance of body temperature, and the sending of nerve and hormonal messages to direct these activities are the basal processes that maintain life. The **basal metabolic rate (BMR)** is surprisingly fast. A person whose total energy needs are 2000 calories a day spends as many as 1200 to 1400 of them to support basal metabolism. The hormone thyroxin directly controls basal metabolism—the less secreted the lower the energy requirements for basal functions. Many other factors affect the BMR (Table 9–2).

You cannot change your BMR much today. You can, however, change the second component—voluntary activities—and so spend more calories today. If you keep doing this day after day, it will ultimately change your BMR. A way to increase your BMR to the maximum possible is to make exercise a daily habit, so that your body composition will change toward the lean. Lean tissue is more metabolically active than fat tissue, so your basal energy output will pick up the pace as well.

As for fuel for voluntary activities, the amount of energy you spend in exercise depends somewhat on your personal style. For example, the heavier the weight of the body parts you move in your activity and the longer the time you invest, the more calories you spend. Are you well trained or a novice? (The streamlined moves of an expert swimmer, for example, cost less than the movements of the untrained.) These and other factors bear on how much fuel an activity will require. Table 9–3 (next page) shows the approximate number of calories people of various weights spend on activities. (For fun, Table 9–4 translates some activity values into food-energy terms.)

Long periods of vigorous activity, engaged in frequently, can place great demands on energy supplies. A football or basketball player may need 5000 calories a day during the season, and on some days the player may need even more to play well and to maintain weight. (To avoid gaining unwanted fat after the season, it is equally important for an athlete to cut back to an energy intake that suits the off-season activity.) The next section shows how to calculate an approximation of your daily energy output.

❚❚▷ *The balance between food energy taken in and energy expended determines how much fat a person's body stores or uses up. Food energy (calories) taken in can be estimated from the exchange system or published tables. Two major components of energy expenditure are basal metabolism and voluntary activities.*

■■■ Table 9–3 Energy Demands of Activities

ACTIVITY	cal/lb/min[a]	BODY WEIGHT (lb)				
		110	125	150	175	200
		CALORIES PER MINUTE				
Aerobic dance (vigorous)	.062	6.8	7.8	9.3	10.9	12.4
Basketball (vigorous, full court)	.097	10.7	12.1	14.6	17.0	19.4
Bicycling						
13 miles per hour	.045	5.0	5.6	6.8	7.9	9.0
15 miles per hour	.049	5.4	6.1	7.4	8.6	9.8
17 miles per hour	.057	6.3	7.1	8.6	10.0	11.4
19 miles per hour	.076	8.4	9.5	11.4	13.3	15.2
21 miles per hour	.090	9.9	11.3	13.5	15.8	18.0
23 miles per hour	.109	12.0	13.6	16.4	19.0	21.8
25 miles per hour	.139	15.3	17.4	20.9	24.3	27.8
Canoeing (flat water, moderate pace)	.045	5.0	5.6	6.8	7.9	9.0
Cross-country skiing (8 miles per hour)	.104	11.4	13.0	15.6	18.2	20.8
Golf (carrying clubs)	.045	5.0	5.6	6.8	7.9	9.0
Handball	.078	8.6	9.8	11.7	13.7	15.6
Horseback riding (trot)	.052	5.7	6.5	7.8	9.1	10.4
Rowing (vigorous)	.097	10.7	12.1	14.6	17.0	19.4
Running						
5 miles per hour	.061	6.7	7.6	9.2	10.7	12.2
6 miles per hour	.074	8.1	9.2	11.1	13.0	14.8
7.5 miles per hour	.094	10.3	11.8	14.1	16.4	18.8
9 miles per hour	.103	11.3	12.9	15.5	18.0	20.6
10 miles per hour	.114	12.5	14.3	17.1	20.0	22.9
11 miles per hour	.131	14.4	16.4	19.7	22.9	26.2
Studying	.011	1.2	1.4	1.7	1.9	2.2
Soccer (vigorous)	.097	10.7	12.1	14.6	17.0	19.4
Swimming						
20 yards per minute	.032	3.5	4.0	4.8	5.6	6.4
45 yards per minute	.058	6.4	7.3	8.7	10.2	11.6
50 yards per minute	.070	7.7	8.8	10.5	12.3	14.0
Table tennis (skilled)	.045	5.0	5.6	6.8	7.9	9.0
Tennis (beginner)	.032	3.5	4.0	4.8	5.6	6.4
Walking (brisk pace)						
3.5 miles per hour	.035	3.9	4.4	5.2	6.1	7.0
4.5 miles per hour	.048	5.3	6.0	7.2	8.4	9.6

[a]To calculate calories spent per minute of activity for your own body weight, multiply cal/lb/min by your exact weight and then multiply that number by the number of minutes spent in the activity. For example, if you weigh 142 pounds, and you want to know how many calories you spent doing 30 minutes of vigorous aerobic dance: .062 × 142 = 8.8 calories per minute. 8.8 × 30 (minutes) = 264 total calories spent.

SOURCE: Adapted in part with permission from The Consumers Union of the United States, *Physical Fitness for Practically Everybody: The Consumers Union Report on Exercise* (Mt. Vernon, N.Y.: Consumers Union, 1983), and from G. P. Town and K. B. Wheeler, Nutritional concerns for the endurance athlete, *Dietetic Currents* 13 (1986): 7–12.

■■■ Table 9–4 Activity Equivalents of Food Energy Values

FOOD	CALORIES	ACTIVITY EQUIVALENT FOR A 150-POUND PERSON TO WORK OFF THE CALORIES (MINUTES)		
		WALK[a]	RUN[b]	WAIT[c]
Apple, large	125	24	8	75
Regular beer, 1 glass (8 oz)	100	19	6	61
Cookie, chocolate chip	50	10	3	30
Ice cream, 1/2 cup	175	34	11	106
Steak, T-bone (6 oz)	475	91	31	288

[a]Energy cost of walking at 3.5 mph—5.2 calories per minute.
[b]Energy cost of running at 9 miles per hour—15.5 calories per minute.
[c]Energy cost of sitting—1.65 calories per minute.

Estimation of Energy Output

To estimate total energy expenditure, first estimate the two major components separately, then add them together. The first component is the energy spent in basal metabolism. Follow these steps. Use the BMR factor 1.0 calorie per kilogram of body weight per hour for men or 0.9 for women (men usually have more muscles than do women). Example (for a 150-pound man):

1. Change pounds to kilograms:

150 pounds divided by 2.2 pounds per kilogram = 68 kilograms.

2. Multiply weight in kilograms by the BMR factor:

68 kilograms times 1 calorie per kilogram per hour = 68 calories per hour.

3. Multiply the calories used in one hour by the hours in a day:

68 calories per hour times 24 hours per day = 1632 calories per day.

The second major component of energy expenditure is the energy spent on voluntary muscular activity. The following figures are crude approximations based on the amount of muscular work a person typically performs in a day. To select the one appropriate for you, remember to think in terms of the amount of *muscular* work performed; don't confuse being *busy* with being *active*. If you sit down most of the day and drive or ride whenever possible, use the value for a sedentary person. If you move around some of the time, as a teacher might during working hours, use the light activity values. If you do some amount of exercise, such as an hour of jogging four or five times a week, or if your occupation calls for some physical work, consider yourself moderately active. A person whose job requires much physical labor, such as a roofer or a carpenter, would be in the heavy activity range. The exceptional category is reserved for those few who spend many hours a day in intense physical training, such as professional or college athletes during their season. Perform calculations for both percentages given for your gender and activity level to provide a range of energy intakes appropriate for people similar to you:[§]

§Percentages derived from the RDA (1989) formula for energy expenditure within about 20% of total calories.

■ Sedentary: Men 25 to 40%; women 25 to 35%.
■ Light activity: Men 50 to 70%; women 40 to 60%.
■ Moderate activity: Men 65 to 80%; women 50 to 70%.
■ Heavy activity: Men 90 to 120%; women 80 to 100%.
■ Exceptional activity: Men 130 to 145%; women 110 to 130%.

If the 150-pound man we used for an example were a student who biked about ten minutes a day and walked to classes but otherwise sat and studied, we could estimate the range of energy he needed for light activity by multiplying his BMR calories per day by both 50 and 70 percent:

1632 calories per day times 50 percent = 816 calories per day.
1632 calories per day times 70 percent = 1142 calories per day.

The man needs from 816 to 1142 calories per day for his activities. Now total the two components. The man in our example spends, in a day:

1632 calories per day + 816 calories per day = 2448 calories per day.
1632 calories per day + 1142 calories per day = 2774 calories per day.

Express the man's needs as a range: 2448 to 2774 calories/day.

■■▷ *To estimate the energy spent on basal metabolism, use the factor (for men) 1.0 cal/kg/hr (or for women, 0.9 cal/kg/hr) for a 24-hour period. Then add an increment of this amount depending on the extent of daily muscular activity.*

■■■ Weight Gain and Loss

The balance between the energy you take in and the energy you spend determines whether you will gain, lose, or maintain body fat. However, when you step on the scale and note that you weigh a pound or two more or less than you did the last time you weighed, this may not indicate that you have gained or lost body fat. A change in body weight may reflect shifts in body fluid content, in bone minerals, or in lean tissues such as muscles. It may also reflect the time of day. People generally weigh the least before breakfast. It is important for people concerned with weight control to realize that quick, large changes in weight are usually not changes in fat alone, or even at all.

A person who stands about 5 feet 10 inches tall and who weighs 150 pounds carries about 90 of those pounds as water and 30 as fat. The other 30 pounds are the so-called lean tissues—muscles; organs such as the heart, brain, and liver; and the bones of the skeleton.‖ Stripped of water and fat, then, the person weighs only 30 pounds! This lean tissue is vital to health. The person who seeks to lose weight wants, of course, to lose fat, not this precious lean tissue. And for someone who wants to gain weight, it is desirable to gain lean and fat in proportion, not just fat.

The type of tissue gained or lost depends on how the person goes about gaining or losing it. To lose fluid, for example, one can take a "water pill" (diuretic), causing the kidneys to siphon extra water from the blood into the urine. Or one can engage in heavy exercise while wearing thick clothing in the

The balance between energy in and energy out determines whether a person stores or uses body fat.

‖For a healthy 5-foot tall person who weighs 100 pounds, the comparable figures would be 60 pounds of water, 20 pounds of fat, 20 pounds of lean.

heat, losing abundant fluid in sweat. (Both practices are dangerous, incidentally, and are not being recommended here.) To gain water weight, a person can overconsume salt and water; for a few hours the body will then retain water until it manages to excrete the salt. (This, too, is not recommended.) Most quick weight-loss diets promote large fluid losses that register temporary, dramatic changes on the scale but that accomplish little loss of body fat. Worse, they also promote breakdown of lean tissue. A later section on strategy stresses physical activity as a means of maintaining lean tissue during weight loss.

Weight Gain

Weight gain comes from eating more food energy than you spend. What does your body do with it? Previous chapters have already provided the answer; the energy-yielding nutrients contribute to body stores as follows:

◼ Carbohydrate (other than fiber) is broken down to sugars for absorption. In the body tissues, these may be built up to *glycogen* or converted to *fat* and stored.
◼ Fat is broken down to glycerol and fatty acids for absorption. Inside the body, these are especially easy for the body to convert to *fat* for storage.
◼ Protein is broken down to amino acids for absorption. (Inside the body, these may be used to replace lost body *protein* and, in a person who is exercising, to build new muscle and other lean tissue. But this protein is not counted as excess; the eater needed to put it to use). Any excess amino acids have their nitrogen removed and are converted to *fat*.

Note that although three kinds of energy-yielding nutrients enter the body, they become energy stores only as glycogen and fat. Alcohol also becomes fat if it isn't burned off. Glycogen stores amount to about three-fourths of a pound; fat stores can, of course, amount to many pounds. Note, too, that when excess protein is converted to fat, it cannot be recovered later as protein because the nitrogen is stripped from the amino acids and is excreted in the urine. No matter whether you are eating steak, brownies, or baked beans, then, if you eat enough of them, any excess protein will be turned to fat within hours.

It is worth emphasizing these points by repeating them:

◼ Any food can make you fat if you eat enough of it. A net excess of energy is stored in the body as fat in fat tissue.
◼ Fat from food is especially easy for the body to store as fat tissue.
◼ Protein is not stored in the body except in response to exercise; it is present only as working tissue.[¶] Some working protein tissue is lost each day and can be replaced only by protein eaten that day. Excess protein becomes body fat.

◼◼▷ *When energy balance is positive, the three energy-yielding nutrients are converted to glycogen or fat and are stored. Dietary fat is especially easy for the body to store. Protein cannot later be recovered as amino acids; only its energy value is recovered.*

Moderate Weight Loss

When you eat less food energy than you need, the body has to draw on its stored energy fuel to keep going. It is a great advantage to us that we can eat

¶Amino acids are present in all body fluids, performing such functions as maintaining the acid-base balance there, and the liver is considered by some to be an amino acid storage site.

periodically, store fuel, and then use up that fuel between meals. The between-meal interval is normally about four to six hours—about the length of time it takes to use up most of the available liver glycogen—or 12 to 14 hours at night, when body systems are slowed down and the need is less.

When you moderately restrict your calories and consume an otherwise balanced diet that meets your protein needs, your body will be forced to use up its stored fat for energy. Gradual weight loss will occur. This is preferred to rapid weight loss because lean body mass is spared and fat is lost.

Rapid Weight Loss

If a person doesn't eat for, say, three whole days or a week, then the body makes one adjustment after another. After about a day, the liver's glycogen is essentially exhausted. Where, then, can the body obtain glucose to keep its nervous system going? Not from the muscles' glycogen because that is reserved for the muscles' own use. The underfed body must turn to the protein in its own lean tissues.

An alternative source of energy might be the abundant fat stores most people carry, but at this stage these are of no use to the nervous system. The muscles and other organs use fat as fuel, but the nervous system ordinarily cannot. Most importantly, the body's major fuel, fat, cannot be converted to glucose—the body possesses no enzymes to carry out this conversion.[#] The body does, however, possess enzymes that can convert protein to glucose.

If the body were to continue to consume its lean tissue unchecked, death would ensue within about ten days. After all, not only skeletal muscle but also the liver, the heart muscle, the lung tissue, the blood cells—all vital tissues—are being burned as fuel. (In fact, fasting or starving people remain alive only until their stores of fat are gone or until half their lean tissue is gone, whichever comes first.) To prevent this, the body plays its last ace: it begins converting fat into compounds that the nervous system can adapt to use and so forestall the end. This is ketosis, which was first mentioned in Chapter 4 as an adaptation to prolonged fasting or carbohydrate deprivation.

In ketosis, instead of breaking down fat molecules to carbon dioxide and water, as it normally does, the body takes partially broken-down fat fragments and combines them to make ketone bodies, compounds that are normally rare in the blood.[**] These ketone bodies circulate in the bloodstream and help to feed the brain, since about half of the brain's cells can make the enzymes needed to use them for energy. Within a few weeks the brain can meet most of its energy needs using ketone bodies. Thus indirectly the nervous system begins to feed on the body's fat stores. This reduces the nervous system's need for glucose, it spares the muscle and other lean tissue from being devoured quickly, and it prolongs the starving person's life. Thanks to ketosis, a healthy person starting with average body-fat content can live totally deprived of food for as long as six to eight weeks. Figure 9–2 reviews how energy is used during both feasting and fasting and in ketosis.

Fasting has been practiced as a periodic discipline by respected, wise people in many cultures. Clearly the body tolerates short-term fasting, although there is no evidence that it becomes "cleansed," as some believe. Ketosis may harm

In early food deprivation:

- The nervous system cannot use fat as fuel; it can use only glucose.
- Body fat cannot be converted to glucose.
- Body protein can be converted to glucose.

#Glycerol, 5 percent of fat, can yield glucose but is a negligible source.
**Ketone bodies are energy-containing compounds made by joining two or more fragments of fatty acids together. Ketone bodies were defined in Chapter 4.

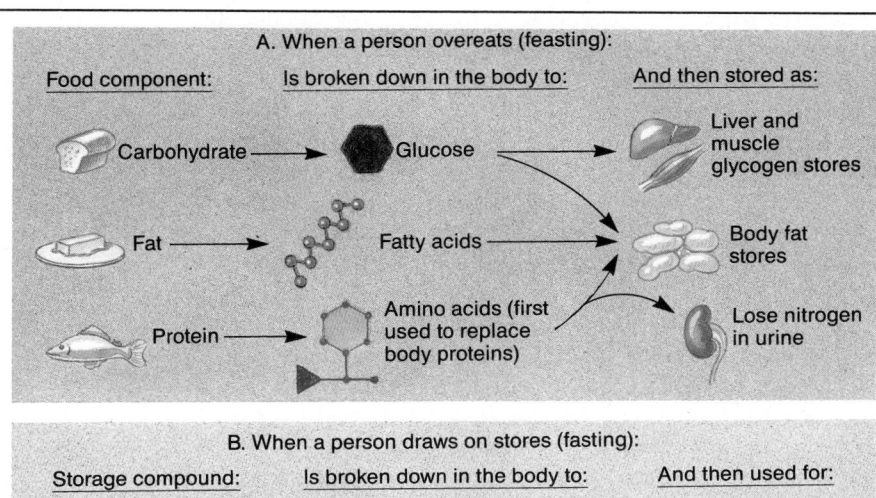

A. When a person overeats (feasting):

Food component: — Is broken down in the body to: — And then stored as:

Carbohydrate → Glucose → Liver and muscle glycogen stores

Fat → Fatty acids → Body fat stores

Protein → Amino acids (first used to replace body proteins) → Lose nitrogen in urine

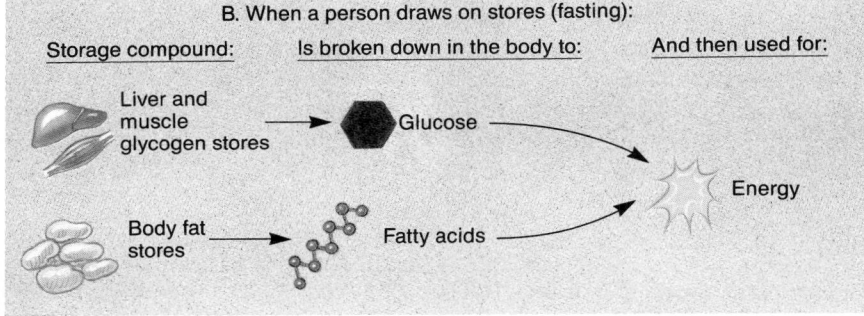

B. When a person draws on stores (fasting):

Storage compound: — Is broken down in the body to: — And then used for:

Liver and muscle glycogen stores → Glucose → Energy

Body fat stores → Fatty acids → Energy

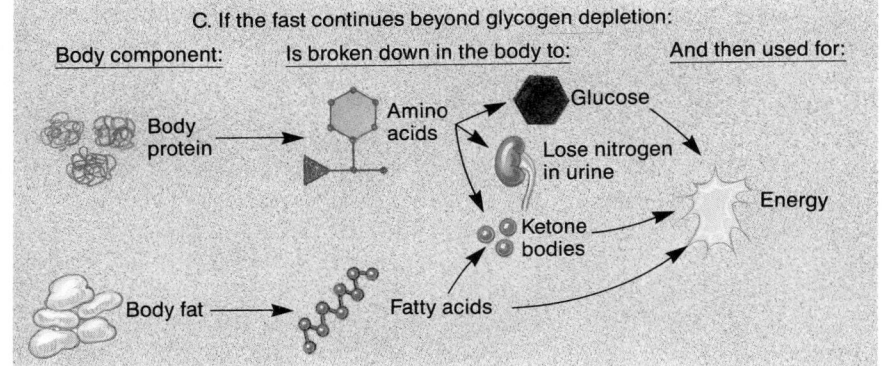

C. If the fast continues beyond glycogen depletion:

Body component: — Is broken down in the body to: — And then used for:

Body protein → Amino acids → Glucose → Energy

Lose nitrogen in urine

Ketone bodies → Energy

Body fat → Fatty acids → Energy

■■■ **Figure 9—2**

Feasting and Fasting. In A, the person is storing energy. In B, the person is drawing on stored energy. In C, the person is in ketosis.

the body by upsetting the acid-base balance of the blood and by promoting mineral losses in the urine. In addition, people with eating disorders (see this chapter's Controversy section) often report that a fast or a bout of severely restricted dieting heralded the beginning of their loss of control over eating.

For the person who merely wants to lose weight, fasting is usually not the best way. The body's lean tissue continues to be degraded to supply glucose to those nervous system cells that cannot use ketone bodies as fuel. The body is deprived of nutrients it needs to assemble new enzymes, red and white blood cells, and other vital components. The body also slows its metabolism during a fast to conserve energy. A low-calorie diet has actually been observed to promote the same rate of *weight* loss over the long run and a faster rate of *fat* loss than a total fast.[16] Just how to design a low-calorie diet is the subject of a later section, but it should be mentioned that any diet too low in carbohydrate will bring about responses that are similar to fasting. They are examples of how *not* to design a diet and are described in the Consumer Caution that follows the next section.

▮▮▶ *When energy balance is negative, glycogen returns glucose to the body; when glycogen runs out, body protein is called upon to do so. Fat also supplies fuel as fatty acids. In a fast, after glycogen runs out, fat supplies fuel as ketone bodies.*

▮▮▮ Weight-Loss Strategies

Whether a person wants to lose 10 pounds or 50 pounds, the techniques of diet, physical activity, and behavior modification discussed here apply equally. The following sections are written in terms of advice to "you," not to put you under pressure to take it personally but to give you the illusion of listening in on a conversation in which an obese person (with say 50 pounds to lose) is being competently counseled by someone familiar with the techniques known to be safe and effective.

Diet

No particular food plan is magical, and no particular food must be either included or avoided. You are the one who will have to live with the plan, so you had better be involved in designing it. Don't think of yourself as going "on" a *diet* because then you may be tempted to go "off." Think of yourself as adopting an eating *plan* for life. It must consist of foods that you like or can learn to like, that are available to you, and that are within your means.

Choose an energy level you can live with. For the person wanting to lose weight, a deficit of 500 calories a day for seven days (3500 calories a week) is enough to lose a pound a week of body fat. It is easiest to do this by both increasing activity (see next section, "Physical Activity") and reducing food intake, since it is urgent not to try to cut calories too far for all the reasons already mentioned. A rule of thumb is that you need to eat at least 10 calories per pound of current body weight each day to lose fat efficiently while retaining lean tissue.

Anyway, there is no point in hurrying because you will never go off the plan; you will only modify it slightly when you have reached your goal. Nutritional adequacy is hard to achieve on a low-calorie diet; even a small person should not try to get by on fewer than 1200 calories (1000 at the very least). A larger person should adjust the calories upwards; some people can lose weight steadily on diets of 1600 calories or more. (For the lower calorie ranges, it is appropriate to use a balanced vitamin-mineral supplement; see Controversy 7 for how to choose one.) Table 9–5 presents a sample, balanced 1250-calorie weight-loss plan.

Counting the calories in foods is time consuming, and only the most motivated will persist at it for long. For the rest of us, some acquaintance with the exchange system (introduced in Chapter 2) provides a simpler method. The foods depicted in Figure 9–3 could be found one by one in Appendix A, but

Strategies for diet planning:

1. Get involved personally.

2. Adopt a realistic plan.

■■■ Table 9–5 A Sample Day's Balanced Weight-Loss Plan

EXCHANGE ITEM	NUMBER OF EXCHANGES	CARBOHYDRATE (g)	PROTEIN (g)	FAT (g)	ENERGY (cal)
Starch/bread	4	60	12	Trace	320
Meat (lean)	5	0	35	15	275
Vegetables	4	20	8	0	100
Fruit	4	60	0	0	240
Milk (nonfat)	2	24	16	Trace	180
Fat	3	0	0	15	135
Total		164 g	71 g	30 g	1250 cal

ªThis 1250-cal diet typifies the balance recommended for a weight-loss diet: approximately 50% of the calories are from protein, carbohydrate, 25% from protein, and 25% from fat. (Carbohydrate supplies 656 cal; protein, 284 cal; and fat, 270 cal.) When the dieter returns to a maintenance plan by adding mostly carbohydrate foods, the ratio will resemble the 15% protein, 30% fat, and 55% carbohydrate recommended for a maintenance diet.

it is quicker to translate them into exchanges and to add up the energy values to get a rough idea of the total. With some practice you can look at any plate of food and "sense" the number of calories it represents. The energy amounts to remember are:

■ One nonfat milk exchange— 90 calories (for low-fat milk, 120 calories; for whole milk, 150).
■ One vegetable exchange— 25 calories.
■ One fruit exchange— 60 calories.
■ One starchy vegetable/bread exchange— 80 calories.
■ One lean meat exchange— 55 calories (for medium-fat meat, 75 calories; for high-fat meat, 100 calories). Remember, one exchange of meat is 1 *ounce*.
■ One fat exchange— 45 calories.
■ One teaspoon sugar— 20 calories.

So how many calories are in the meal in Figure 9–3? The answer is at the end of this chapter.

Along with calories, put nutritional adequacy high on your list of priorities. This is a way of putting yourself first. "I like me, and I'm going to take good care of me" is the attitude to adopt. A plan that uses the minimum servings suggested in the Four Food Group Plan (Chapter 2) without frills and that allows a teaspoon of fat at each meal provides less than 1200 calories; most people could lose weight at a satisfactory rate following such a plan and meet most of their nutrient needs too. Women, however, might need an iron supplement. Within each category, search the exchange lists for a number of foods on each list that you like, and use them often. If you plan resolutely to include a certain number of servings of food from each food group each day, you may be so busy making sure you get what you need that you will have little time or appetite left for high-fat or empty-calorie foods. Foods such as vegetables and whole grains take a lot of eating too—crunchy, wholesome foods offer bulk and satiety for far fewer calories than smooth, refined foods. Limit your meats: an ounce of ham contains more calories than an ounce of bread, and many of them are from fat. Especially don't lose track of the fat you add. Remember, fat calories probably contribute more to body fat stores than do carbohydrate calories, and fat has so many calories per bite that it is easy to overload quickly.

3. Keep track of calories and especially those from fat.

■■■ **Figure 9–3**

Calorie Quiz. In case you'd like to try guessing how many calories are in the meal depicted here, the answer is provided in Figure 9–12.

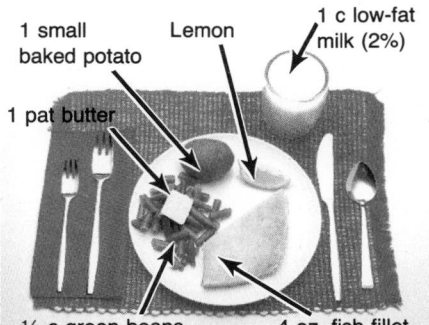

4. Make the diet adequate.
5. Emphasize high nutrient density.
6. Individualize. Use foods you like.
7. Stress dos, not don'ts.

8. Eat regular meals with no skipping—at least three a day.

Just a few bites of fatty food can provide the whole allowance of calories for a meal before the diner has eaten enough food for satiety.

Three meals a day is standard for our society, but your lifestyle may not facilitate eating three meals. No law says you shouldn't have four or five meals—only be sure they are smaller, of course. What is important is to eat regularly and, if at all possible, to eat before you are very hungry. Make sure it is hunger, not appetite, urging you to eat. When you do decide to eat, eat the entire meal you have planned for yourself. Then don't eat again until the next meal. Save "free" or favorite foods or beverages for a planned snack at the end of the day if you need insurance against late-evening hunger.

❚❚▶ *People should be involved in planning their own weight-loss diets. Diet plans should be adequate, should control calories, and should be as personally pleasing as possible.*

CONSUMER CAUTION ❚❚❚ Low-Carbohydrate and Very-Low-Calorie Diets

Many low-carbohydrate diets have been promoted to the public in many different guises. Each diet has enjoyed a surge of popularity thanks largely to a sizable initial weight loss. These diets are designed to make a person go into ketosis. The sales pitch is that "you'll never feel hungry" and that "you'll lose weight fast—faster than you would on any ordinary diet." Both claims are true, but both are misleading. Loss of appetite accompanies any low-calorie diet. Fast weight loss means loss of water and lean tissue, and the water is rapidly regained when people begin eating normally again. But most importantly, these diets, undertaken without medical supervision, are dangerous.

Names of some low-carbohydrate diets include Air Force Diet, Atkins Diet, Calories Don't Count Diet, Drinking Man's Diet, Herbalife Diet, Mayo Diet, Protein-sparing Fast, Scarsdale Diet, Simeons HCG Diet, Ski Team Diet, and Stillman Diet. New ones keep coming out under new names.

Many physiological hazards accompany low-carbohydrate diets: high blood cholesterol, hypoglycemia, mineral imbalances, and other metabolic abnormalities. Some low-carbohydrate diets, particularly the protein-sparing fast type, have caused heart failure. These diets are never recommended by legitimate practitioners, although some very-low-calorie diets (VLCDs) may be appropriate for some people under close medical supervision.

In an effort to find a diet that will provide rapid weight loss and that is medically safe, many commercially prepared VLCD formulas have been devised and tested on thousands of people. Since 1980 some success has been legitimately claimed within limits that are important to acknowledge.

Most VLCD formulas contain about 400 calories and are available by prescription only. They provide the Recommended Dietary Allowance (RDA) of all vitamins and minerals.

Studies indicate high rates of short-term success with VLCDs. Typically people adhere to them only for a short time, lose weight rapidly, and fail to maintain. In an attempt to increase the programs' long-term effectiveness and

continued on next page

safety, the better programs provide medical supervision and also retrain clients to change their lifestyles. The valid programs include regimens of exercise, nutrition education, and support groups to increase their long-term effectiveness. The programs that are professionally recommended to provide effective and safe weight loss include Health Management Resources, Medibase (Advanced Health Care), Medifast, and Optifast. Table 9–6 provides details regarding each program.

It is encouraging that progress is being made toward designing plans that meet the demand for quick weight loss with a minimum of hazards because some people will always demand such plans. Still, it is preferable to undertake the kind of plan that changes eating habits permanently.

SOURCES: Very-low-calorie diets, *Berkeley Wellness Letter*, published in association with the School of Public Health, University of California, January 1989; J. S. Garrow, Are liquid diets safe or necessary? *Recent Advances in Obesity Research V* (Westport, Conn.: Food and Nutrition Press, 1987), pp. 327–331; W. H. Dietz, Jr. and I. Greenberg, Clinical experience with the use of a multifaceted program including very low calorie diets, in *Management of Obesity by Severe Caloric Restriction*, eds. G. L. Blackburn and G. A. Bray (Littleton, Mass.: PSG Publishing, 1985), pp. 335–348.

Physical Activity

The second component of a successful weight-control program is physical activity. Some people hate the very idea of exercise, but a formal exercise program isn't necessary. Obese people often, understandably, do not enjoy moving their bodies. They feel heavy, clumsy, even ridiculous. A word to reassure them: weight loss, at least to a point, is possible without exercise, but even if you choose not to alter your habits at first, let your mind be open to the

■■■ **Table 9–6 Medically Supervised VLCDs**

PROGRAM	DOCTOR REFERRAL REQUIRED	WEIGHT REQUIREMENT	PROCEDURE
Health Management Resources	No	Must be at least 20% above ideal weight or at medical risk	500 cal/day of formula for 12 weeks, 4–6 weeks of refeeding, 18 months of maintenance
Medibase (Advanced Health Care)	Yes	Must be 25% above ideal body weight	420–800 cal/day of formula for 12 weeks, 16 weeks of refeeding, 40 weeks of maintenance
Medifast	Yes	Must be 25% above ideal body weight	450 cal/day of formula for 12 weeks, 6 weeks of refeeding, 12 weeks of maintenance
Optifast	Yes	Must be 30% above ideal body weight	420–800 cal/day of formula for 12 weeks, 6 weeks of refeeding, 7 weeks of required maintenance, more is optional

SOURCE: Adapted from Very-low-calorie diets, *Berkeley Wellness Letter,* published in association with the School of Public Health, University of California, January 1989.

ratchet effect or yoyo effect (of dieting): the effect of repeated rounds of dieting; the person rebounds to a higher weight (and higher body fat content) at the end of each round.

behavior modification: a theory in psychology that holds that a behavior can be controlled by controlling the environmental factors that cue, or trigger, the behavior.

Thinness is not the same as fitness. For a definition of fitness, see the next chapter.

Strategies for using exercise for weight control:

1. Choose active exercise; move large muscle groups.
2. Think in terms of time, not speed.
3. Exercise informally, in daily routines.

■■■ Figure 9–4

The Ratchet Effect. Each round of dieting, without physical activity, is followed by a rebound of weight to a higher level than before. The body fat content increases, and caloric needs fall after each round, making the next round of weight loss harder.

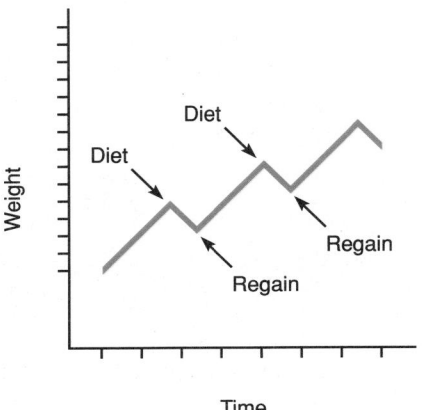

possibility that you will want to take up some activity later on. You can start by simply walking instead of driving. As the pounds come off, moving your body will become a pleasure.

Weight loss without physical activity can have a negative effect on body composition, especially if the weight is regained. A person who diets without being active loses both lean and fat tissue. If the person then gains weight without physical activity, more fat than lean is gained. Fat tissue is less active metabolically than lean tissue, and so the person's daily energy expenditure is less. Each time a person loses weight and regains it while remaining inactive, that person's metabolism requires fewer calories. If the person eats the same amount as before the last diet, the person will not maintain but will gain weight. This is one explanation for the so-called **ratchet effect**, or **yoyo effect** of dieting (Figure 9–4) and underlines the importance of physical activity as part of a weight-loss plan. Exercise is especially useful in weight maintenance, as a later section shows.

Loss of metabolically active muscle tissue due to inactivity does not account completely for the ratchet effect.[17] Other effects must also be operating; perhaps obese people who have dieted repeatedly are metabolically different to begin with. In any case, it must be clear by now that physical activity provides many benefits for as long as you keep your body conditioned. Among the benefits that relate to body weight are:

■ Increased expenditure of energy.
■ Long-term increase in resting metabolic rate.
■ Promotion of weight loss, particularly loss of body fat.[18]
■ Appetite control.
■ Control of stress and stress-induced overeating or undereating.
■ Increased self-esteem.

Chapter 10 provides much more information on fat and energy use during activity, but a few strategies are in order here. For one thing, you must keep in mind that if exercise is to help you with weight control, it must be active exercise—voluntary moving of muscles. Being moved passively, as by a machine at a health spa or by a massage, neither increases energy expenditure nor builds muscles. The more muscles you move, the more muscle tissue you build, and the more calories you spend.

People sometimes think that workouts have to be fast paced. This is not true. For example, whether you choose to walk or to run a given distance, you will use up about the same amount of energy; walking will just take you longer.†† For burning up fat, the longer (not the faster) the better.

Another strategy is to incorporate more physical activity into your daily schedule in many simple, small-scale ways. Park the car at the far end of the parking lot; use the stairs instead of the elevator; work your abdominal muscles while you stand in line; tighten your buttocks each time you get up from your chair. These activities add up to only a few calories each, but over a year's time they become significant.

■■▷ *Physical activity is important in weight control: it favors a lean body composition. To be effective, exercise needs to be active, not passive.*

††Runners use about 10% more energy because they push their weight up as well as forward with each step.

Supporting both diet and exercise is the third component of weight control—**behavior modification**. Behavior modification works to cement into place behaviors that lead to and perpetuate the desired body weight. This chapter's Food Feature applies behavior modification principles mostly to weight loss and shows how some apply also to weight gain.

The six elements of behavior modification are as follows:

1. Eliminate inappropriate eating cues.
2. Suppress the cues you cannot eliminate.
3. Strengthen cues to appropriate eating and exercise.
4. Repeat the desired eating and exercise behaviors.
5. Arrange or emphasize negative consequences of inappropriate eating.
6. Arrange or emphasize positive consequences of appropriate eating and exercise behaviors.

Before you begin to apply strategies that employ the six principles above, establish a baseline, a record of your present eating behaviors against which to measure future progress. Keep a diary so that you can learn what your particular eating stimuli, or cues, are.

To begin, set about eliminating or suppressing the cues that prompt you to eat inappropriately. There may be many such cues in the overeater's life: watching television, talking on the telephone, entering a convenience store, being offered food, and many more. Resolve to respond no longer to such cues by eating. Respond only to one set of cues designed by you: one particular place in one particular room. Also:

- Don't buy problem foods (shop when you aren't hungry).
- Serve only low-calorie sauces and toppings (avoid rich ones).
- Let spouse and children buy, store, and serve their own sweets (monitor children's total intake).
- Change channels or look away when the television shows food commercials.
- Shop only from a list.
- Carry appropriate snacks, and avoid vending machines.
- Prepare only as much food as you have planned to eat.

If some cues to inappropriate eating behavior can't be eliminated, suppress them:

- Minimize contact with excessive food (serve individual plates, don't put serving dishes on the table, leave the table when finished).
- Clear plates directly into the garbage.
- Create obstacles to the eating of problem foods (for example, make it necessary to unwrap, cook, and serve each one separately).
- Make small portions of food look large (spread food out, serve on small plates).
- Control deprivation so that you will not overeat to compensate (plan and eat regular meals, don't skip meals, avoid getting overtired, avoid boredom by keeping cues to interesting activities in plain sight).

Next, to strengthen the cues to appropriate eating and activity:

- Encourage others to eat appropriate foods with you.
- Keep your favorite appropriate foods in the front of the refrigerator.
- Learn appropriate portion sizes.

Food Feature

Behavior Modification for Weight Control

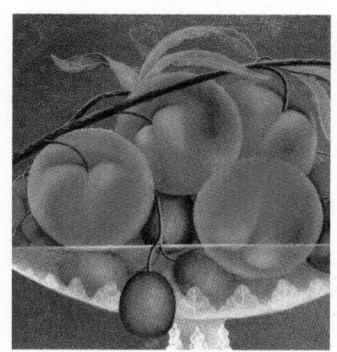

Strategies to modify behavior:

1. Establish a baseline and keep records.
2. Eliminate or suppress cues to inappropriate eating.
3. Strengthen cues to appropriate behaviors.

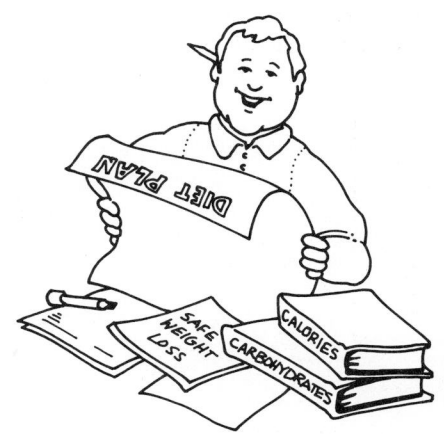

It's up to you to design a diet you can live with.

■ Save permitted foods from meals for snacks (and these should be your only snacks).
■ Prepare permitted foods attractively.
■ Keep your ski poles (hiking boots, tennis racket) by the door.

A way to alter the response itself is to repeat the desired behavior:

■ Slow down (pause for two to three minutes, put down utensils, swallow before reloading the fork, always use utensils).
■ Leave some food on the plate.
■ Move more (shake a leg, pace, fidget, flex your muscles).
■ Join in and cultivate fitness with a group of active people.

4. Slow down eating; move more.

Arrange to have negative consequences follow inappropriate eating behavior and activity. Scolding is *not* a negative consequence (it is a form of attention-giving, which is positive), so don't ask to be scolded:

■ Have others nearby when you eat.
■ Ask that others respond neutrally to your deviations (make no comment). This is a negative consequence because it withholds attention.
■ If you slip, don't punish yourself.

5. Arrange negative consequences for negative behaviors.

Consider the last item. If you ate an extra 1000 calories yesterday, don't try to eat 1000 fewer calories today. Just go back to your plan. On the other hand, you can plan ahead and budget for special occasions. If you want to celebrate your birthday with cake and ice cream, cut a few calories from your bread and milk allowance each day for several days *beforehand*. Your weight loss will be as smooth as if you had stayed with the daily plan.

Make sure, also, that positive consequences, including material rewards, follow the desired behaviors. Rewards should be personal—they should give *you* pleasure; and they should be immediate (see Table 9–7 for specific suggestions):

■ Update records of food intake, exercise, and weight change regularly.
■ Arrange for material reinforcement—rewards (other than food) for each unit of behavior change or weight loss.
■ Provide social reinforcement (ask to be encouraged).
■ Take well-spaced weighings to avoid discouragement.

6. Reward yourself. Make rewards personal and immediate.

■■■ **Table 9–7 Activities and Rewards to Substitute for Eating**

Exercise or sports	Shopping
Attending sporting events	Naps
Reading	Relaxation exercises
Telephoning	New clothes
Hobbies and crafts	Weekend trips
Listening to music	Movie or theater trips
Gardening or yardwork	Saving money for future use
Recreation	Self-praise
Household chores	Praise by significant others
Bathing	Token rewards (stars, stickers)

Adapted from: B. B. Hollie, Using behavior modification in nutrition counseling, *Journal of the American Dietetic Association,* December 1988, pp. 1530–1538.

■■■ Table 9–8 Weight-Loss Programs Compared

PROGRAM	CLIENT INTERACTION	EATING PLAN	EXERCISE PROMOTION	BEHAVIOR MODIFICATION	MAINTENANCE PLAN	COST
Diet Center	Individual and Group	900 and 1000 cal sheets	Yes	Yes	Yes	Initial fee averages $700 for 9-week program
Nutri/System	Individual	800 to 1000 cal diets, food provided	Yes	Yes	Yes	Ranges from $100 to $1000 plus $48 to $58 per week for food
Overeaters Anonymous*	Group	Self-selected or physician prescribed	No	No	No	None
Slender Center	Individual	ADA exchange plans	Yes	Yes	Yes	Weekly dues
TOPS	Group	Physician-prescribed ADA exchange plans	Yes	Yes	Yes	$12 annual fee
Jenny Craig International	Group	1000 cal diets, food provided	Yes	Yes	Yes	$185 to $235 plus $65 to $70 weekly for food
Weight Watchers	Group	ADA exchange plans	Yes	Yes	Yes	Start-up cost averages $26 plus weekly dues of $8

*Focuses on emotional and spiritual aspects of compulsive eating, uses a 12-step program patterned after Alcoholics Anonymous, views compulsive eating as an addiction.

Adapted from: E. Rosenblatt, Weight-loss programs, *Postgraduate Medicine*, May 1988, pp. 137–148.

If you stop making progress, you may have to get tough with yourself. Ask yourself honestly, "What am I doing wrong?" (no one is listening in). Seldom does an unpredicted weight plateau of any duration have no explanation in the dieter's own choices.

Also, if you stop making progress, be aware that this may be a good time to stop. Your weight may be at a point that you are willing to accept, at least for the present. In fact, you may have come to realize that your original goal weight was unrealistic or not worth the effort it would take to get there.

People who believe that if only they were thin or muscular they would be happy are bound for disappointment. Many benefits follow physical fitness, improved mental attitude among them, but many other health components come into play as well—emotional, spiritual, interpersonal. You may decide to join the ranks of people who have rejected the magazine-cover physical ideal and opt to work on other facets of your life leading to self-acceptance. Hold your head high and take the attitude, "This is the way I am choosing to be right now."

7. Maintain self-esteem.

If you feel you are unable to progress further in your weight control efforts on your own, you may find help in a group such as TOPS or Weight Watchers. These programs are compared in Table 9–8. Or you may benefit from individual nutrition counseling with a registered dietitian (RD). RDs are trained to assist with food-behavior change. It may also help to obtain some assertiveness

8. Learn and practice assertiveness.

training. Learning to say "No, thank you" might be one of your first objectives. Learning not to "clean your plate" might be another.

From all the available behavior changes, you choose the ones to begin with. Don't try to master them all at once. No one who attempts too many changes at one time is successful. Set your own priorities. Pick one behavior you can handle, start with that, and practice it until it is habitual and automatic. Then select another.

9. Use small-step modification.

As you progress in physical activity and behavior modification, enjoy your new, emerging self. Inside every fat person is a fit person struggling to be freed. Get in touch with—reach out your hand to—your fit self, and help that self to feel welcome in the light of day.

On learning of the effort and will demanded for weight loss, many people wonder if there might be a program to ease their task. Some are sound and can assist a person who needs guidance and support in following the steps outlined in this section. Others are ineffective or even unsafe. Table 9-9 spells out clues for detecting unsound weight loss programs. Table 9-10 cautions against some wrong ways to lose weight.

■■■ Table 9-9 Clues to Unsound Weight-Loss Promotions

1. Promises of dramatic, rapid weight loss (ie, substantially more than 1 percent of total body weight per week).
2. Promotion of diets that are extremely low in calories (ie, below 800 calories per day; 1200 calories per day diets are preferred) unless under the supervision of competent medical experts.
3. Attempt to make clients dependent upon special products rather than teaching how to make good choices from the conventional food supply (this does not condemn the marketing of low-calorie convenience foods that may be chosen by consumers).
4. Failure to encourage permanent, realistic lifestyle changes, including regular exercise and the behavioral aspects of eating wherein food may be used as a coping device (ie, programs should focus upon changing the causes of overweight rather than simply the effects, which is the overweight itself).
5. Misrepresentation of salespeople as "counselors" supposedly qualified to give guidance in nutrition and/or general health. Even if adequately trained, such "counselors" would still be objectionable because of the obvious conflict of interest that exists when providers profit directly from products they recommend and sell.
6. Collection of large sums of money at the start or requirement that clients sign contracts for expensive, long-term programs. Such practices too often have been abused as salespeople focus attention upon signing up new people rather than delivering continuing, satisfactory service to consumers. Programs should be on a pay-as-you-go basis.
7. Failure to inform clients about the risks associated with weight loss in general or the specific program being promoted.
8. Promotion of unproven or spurious weight-loss aids such as human chorionic gonadotrophin hormone (HCG), starch blockers, diuretics, sauna belts, body wraps, passive exercise, ear stapling; acupuncture, electric muscle stimulating (EMS) devices, spirulina, amino acid supplements (eg, arginine, ornithine), glucomannan, and so forth.
9. Claims that "cellulite" exists in the body.
10. Claims that use of an appetite suppressant or methylcellulose (a "bulking agent") enables a person to lose body fat without restricting accustomed caloric intake.
11. Claims that a weight-control product contains a unique ingredient or component unless it is unavailable in other weight-control products.

SOURCE: Reprinted with permission from *National Council Against Health Fraud Newsletter,* March/April 1987, National Council Against Health Fraud, Inc.

■■■ Table 9–10 Wrong Ways to Lose Weight

METHOD	WHY IT IS NOT RECOMMENDED
Low-carbohydrate diets	Promote loss of lean tissue, medically unsafe
Water pills	Promote loss of body water, not fat
Diet pills[a]	Usually ineffective, sometimes have short-term effectiveness only, medically unsafe for some people
Expanding pills	Designed to give feeling of fullness; have caused many cases of illness requiring surgery and at least one death
Spa belts and rollers	Do not melt or jiggle fat away, only massage body parts
Spa saunas and whirlpools	Promote loss of body water, not fat
Massages	Do not rub away fat, only rub body parts
Muscle stimulators	Temporarily reduce body measurements, do not reduce fat content
Hormones	Ineffective for weight loss, medically unsafe
Glucomannon	Ineffective for weight loss
Laxatives	Ineffective for weight loss, cause dehydration, unsafe
Bee pollen	Ineffective for weight loss
Spirulina	Ineffective for weight loss
Lipectomy and suctioning	Cosmetic only, not effective for obesity, entail surgical risks, many unqualified physicians performing these
Bypass surgery	Ineffective for weight loss and dangerous
Stomach stapling	Negative side effects, damaged stomach tissue, ineffective for long-term change
Gastric balloon	Ineffective for long term, pain and ulcers in some

[a]Including over-the-counter preparations such as phenylpropanolamine and prescriptions such as amphetamines.

Finally, be aware that it can be harder to maintain a new weight than to achieve it. On arriving at the goal weight after months of self-discipline and new habit formation, the victor must at all costs avoid "celebrating" by resuming old eating habits. The section on weight maintenance will help you to maintain your new weight once you have achieved it.

■■■ Weight-Gain Strategies

It is as hard for a person who tends to be underweight to gain a pound as it is for a person who tends to be overweight to lose one. Like the weight loser, the person who wants to gain must learn new habits and learn to like new foods.

The person who is underweight has a special problem—deciding whether, and how, to try to gain. The first question to ask is whether the underweight affects health. If you are healthy at your present weight, stay there; if you are at risk of illness, try to gain. Medical advice can help you make the distinction.

People who wish to gain weight for appearance's sake or to improve athletic performance should be aware that a healthful weight gain can only be achieved through physical conditioning combined with eating a high-calorie diet. Eating more calories of food can bring about weight gain, but it will be mostly fat, and this can be more detrimental to health than the underweight. In an athlete, such a weight gain can impair performance. Therefore in weight gain, as in weight loss, physical activity is an essential component of a sound plan.

The best activities for weight gain are those that build strength, such as workouts with weights or machines, or calisthenics. These activities build muscle bulk. Other types of physical activity also improve appearance by firming and defining the muscles and by lending a grace of movement characteristic of a fit body. For this reason anyone taking on an exercise program should learn more about the components of fitness and strive for a balanced program.[19]

Weight gain is an individual matter. In deciding whether to undertake it, be as aware as you can be of what your body will permit and tolerate, and be willing to accept what you cannot change. Some people are unalterably thin by reasons of heredity or early physical influences.

As important to weight gain as activity are the calories to support that activity—otherwise you will lose weight (body fat). If you eat just enough to support the activity, you will build muscle, but at the expense of body fat, that is, fat will be burned to support the muscle building. If you eat more, you will gain both muscle and fat.

It takes an excess of about 2000 to 2500 calories, in theory, to support the gain of a pound of pure lean tissue.[20] The rate at which a person can build muscle tissue also depends on the person. Both men and women have a mixture of both male and female hormones; those with more male hormones build muscle more easily than others, but it is not known what the limits are. (Chapter 10 provides cautions on the use of steroid hormone drugs.) Conventional advice on diet to the person building muscle is to eat about 700 to 1000 calories a day above normal energy needs; this is enough to support both the added activity and the formation of new muscle.

If you want to gain weight, you may need to learn to eat different foods. No matter how many sticks of celery you consume, you won't gain weight very fast because celery simply doesn't offer enough calories. The person who cannot eat much volume is encouraged to use calorie-dense foods in meals (the very ones the dieter is trying to stay away from). These foods are high in fat, but if they are contributing energy that will be spent sparing protein, they will not contribute to heart disease. They will help you build a stronger body. Choose nutritious foods, but choose milkshakes instead of milk, peanut butter instead of lean meat, avocado instead of cucumber, whole-wheat muffins instead of whole-wheat bread. When you do eat celery, put cream cheese on it; add cream and sugar to coffee; use creamy dressings on salads, whipped toppings on fruit, margarine on potatoes, and the like. Because fat contains twice as many calories per teaspoon as sugar, it adds calories without adding much bulk, and its energy is in a form that is easy for the body to store.

Expect to feel full, sometimes even uncomfortably so. Most underweight individuals are accustomed to small quantities of food. When they begin eating significantly more food, they complain of uncomfortable fullness. This is normal, and it passes over time.

Eat more frequently. Make three sandwiches in the morning and eat them between classes in addition to the day's three regular meals. Spend more time eating each meal: if you fill up fast, eat the highest calorie items first. Start with the main course. Drink between meals, not with them, to save space for higher calorie foods. Make milkshakes to drink between meals. Always finish with dessert. Many an underweight person has simply been too busy (for months) to eat or to exercise enough to gain or to maintain weight. These strategies will help you to change this behavior pattern.

Behavior modification principles can work to change the behaviors of undereating as well as overeating. The person who needs to gain weight must, like the person who needs to lose weight, strengthen cues to appropriate eating and exercise (review the Food Feature, "Behavior Modification for Weight Control"). The undereater might identify and select the cues that the overeater is trying to eliminate. For example, *do* snack while watching television; make large portions of food look small; relax more.

▶▶ *The person who wants to gain weight, like the one who wants to lose, is most likely to succeed by tailoring diet, activity, and behavior modification to personal preferences.*

▌▌▌ Weight Maintenance

"I have lost 200 pounds, but I was never more than 20 pounds overweight." This statement expresses the frustration that thousands of dieters experience and that you may have experienced as well—the struggle to *lose* weight and the even greater struggle to *maintain* the desirable weight. Equally frustrating is the realization that hard work invested in gaining weight is visibly slipping away. For many, alternating weight loss and weight gain becomes a lifelong pattern. What makes the difference between a successful, long-term weight loss and a temporary one?

Characteristics of Those Who Succeed

Researchers discovered some predictors of success for weight maintenance when they studied 26 women who had lost a minimum of 40 pounds and maintained their weight losses for at least a year.[21] The researchers focused particularly on the women's eating habits, thought changes, body images, families, and friends. One factor was *social support*:

■ The women attended support groups regularly.
■ They had supportive relationships with others or learned to create such relationships.

Another factor was *physical activity*:

■ Exercise appeared to be vital to their weight maintenance.

Still another was *behavioral self-control*. The successful women:

■ Followed written diet plans, planned meals, and kept records.
■ Ate three meals a day at planned times.
■ Followed a rule of no eating after a certain time in the evening (usually about 6:00 to 8:00 pm).
■ Greatly reduced their sugar and salt intakes.
■ Used high-fiber foods as staple foods.
■ Usually drank 8 glasses or more of water a day.
■ Reduced their eating speed.

They also showed that they possessed the ability to cope by cultivating positive attitudes and beliefs:

■ They used positive self-talk: "You can do it," "You're a success."
■ They believed they could succeed in spite of past diet failures.
■ They dealt successfully with feelings of envy or discomfort from family members or friends.

Also important were *realistic expectations*:

■ The women had reasonable expectations regarding body size and shape.
■ The women had reasonable expectations of how long the weight-loss process would take.

These, then, are five characteristics that people can cultivate: social support, physical activity, behavioral self-control, coping abilities, and realistic expectations. In addition to these, key traits are an attitude of ownership and responsibility, self-efficacy, self-acceptance, and self-actualization.

Regarding ownership, researchers observed this trait among 50 people who were able to maintain weight loss. All 50 people had come to a full understanding that they alone were ultimately responsible for their weight control.[22] They realized that no person other than themselves could control their weight for them. In contrast, many unsuccessful dieters place the responsibility for their weight control outside of themselves, on weight-loss programs, on health care professionals, or on pills and potions. This attitude weakens people's self-confidence and predicts failure.

Ownership is learnable. All 50 successful dieters claimed to have experienced previous failures at maintaining appropriate body weight but then came to a turning point—the point at which they accepted responsibility for their own body weight. Only then were they able to develop workable solutions to maintain desirable weights.

Related to ownership is self-efficacy—a person's belief that he or she has the ability to respond effectively to a situation by using available skills. A study of Weight Watchers members found self-efficacy to be important to success in weight loss.[23] Self-efficacy is also a trait in those who are successful in maintaining their weight. Those who succeed have greater confidence in their ability to control eating urges than those who regain their lost weight.[24] Expectation of success also has strong positive effects on behavior change.[25]

Another characteristic essential for successful weight maintenance is self-acceptance. Self-hate predicts failure. Some people want to lose weight because they are disgusted with their appearance and hate themselves when they get on the scale, but, ironically, they will likely regain any weight that they lose. Honesty in facing the need to make changes is crucial, of course, but self-hate and self-criticism create a spiral of negative, self-defeating behaviors, including inappropriate eating behaviors. The paradox of behavior change is that self-acceptance (loving the overweight self) is the basis for self-change. Letting go of negative feelings frees the person from the self-hate spiral, enabling him or her to change. Another benefit of self-acceptance is unshakable self-worth that does not depend on body weight. Self-discipline is most easily sustained when self-acceptance supports it.

Still another characteristic of successful weight maintenance is self-actualization. Self-actualizing individuals are those who have met their basic physical and emotional needs and who seek to realize their full potential.[26] Basic needs that must be met before people can maintain weight begin at a primitive level: needs for food, clothing, and shelter. Next is the need to feel physically safe and secure. If safe and secure, people are free to notice their need to be loved, to feel emotionally secure. If these emotional needs are met, they can seek to achieve the ultimate—self actualization, or the realization of their full potential. In fact, self-actualization training for weight-loss clients can greatly improve their chances of maintaining the loss. This makes them less likely to experience **lapse** or **relapse**.

▮▮▶ *Many traits characterize people who succeed at maintaining lost weight. The more of these a person possesses or cultivates, the more likely that person will succeed.*

> **lapse:** a falling back into a former condition. In weight maintenance, a temporary, expected backslide into old habits.
>
> **relapse:** the outcome of an uncontrolled series of lapses, such as regaining of weight after successful loss and returning to old patterns of eating.

Lapse Management and Relapse Prevention

"I did it again," a chronic dieter confided. "I binged again after five years of dieting." Some dieters are forever frustrated by their backsliding behavior. "I feel angry, depressed, and ashamed. All of those meetings! All that therapy! All that work! Why do I still go back to old behaviors?" Disappointment, frustration and self-condemnation are common in dieters who find themselves in a relapse.[27]

The term *relapse* describes the end result of a loss of control that results in defeat for dieters, and it doesn't have to happen. Many a relapse begins with just a *lapse,* and dieters need to understand the differences in kind and degree. Lapses can happen to people who have been dieting for ten months or ten years. They are a normal part of the behavior-change process and do not indicate lack of will power. A dieter in a lapse can take corrective action and can thus regain control. However, a lapse can lead to relapse: weight gain due to total abandonment of the weight-control program. The dieter's responses to individual lapses determine if relapse will occur; if the dieter *perceives* a total loss of control, then relapse is likely.[28]

The way people view the habit-change process can influence whether they will ultimately succeed at behavior change or slide into chronic problem behavior.[29] A perfectionistic, "all or nothing" attitude is destructive and can lead people to think that a mistake means that control is totally and forever lost. Examples of this erroneous thinking and of right thinking to counteract it are found in Table 9–11 on page 314. If any of the myths in the table sound familiar, it could be that erroneous thinking is blocking your progress in weight maintenance. Arm yourself with the truth to combat false thoughts.

When faced with a lapse into old behaviors, cope with it. Review the behavior modification strategies in the weight-loss section of this chapter. Identify those that apply to the circumstances surrounding your lapse, and redouble your attention to them. For example, if after a party you find that you unexpectedly overate, you might benefit from first adopting an attitude of compassion and forgiving yourself. Then get tough with yourself and commit to specific actions to control your intake at the next party. Vow to say "no" to food when you're not hungry (to fortify against social pressure), to eat a balanced meal beforehand (to defend against hunger), and to position yourself well away from party buffets (to reduce temptation).

It helps to monitor your behavior with regard to your plan for weight maintenance. For example, set specific tolerance ranges for lapses, and take action if you should exceed them. Look for any of the following:

■■■ Table 9–11 Myths and Truths Regarding Lapses

Myths contribute to negative thinking that can turn lapses into full-blown relapses. Dieters must be aware of these myths so that they can change them in their own thinking.

Myth: I've been working on this for so long that I shouldn't be making mistakes.
Truth: Even experts make mistakes.
Myth: If I was really doing well, I wouldn't be having these slips.
Truth: Having slips is a normal part of the behavior-change process. I am doing well even though I have slips.
Myth: People wouldn't respect me if they knew I was backsliding like this.
Truth: The important people respect me for my effort to change and know that slips are not reflective of my character.
Myth: Once changed, a behavior is gone forever.
Truth: Old behaviors try to creep back in, even those that were long gone.
Myth: I couldn't possibly be doing this again; I know better.
Truth: Yes, I know better, but even superior knowledge cannot prevent lapses.
Myth: Oh, no! I'm back to square one.
Truth: I may have slipped, but not all the way back to square one. I have made progress and now I can vault ahead of where I stopped.

■ A weight gain of from 3 to 5 pounds.
■ A lack of physical activity for more than four days in a row.
■ A second repetition of any old destructive behavior.
■ Withdrawal from support system for a period lasting more than a week.
■ Failure to participate in nonfood-oriented leisure activities for more than a week.

Take action. Review the appropriate steps to behavior modification, and apply them.

Improving behavior is rarely a straight-line progress; it more often follows a path of two steps forward, one step back. For people to succeed in weight control, they must accept lapses as inevitable. One way to do this is to view lapses as helpful: they help people acquire information about their behaviors. One study shows that for many people, success comes after several lapses have revealed to them their behaviors of concern.[30] Facing problem behaviors and learning how to cope with them is a necessary step on the path to success.[31]

In weight maintenance, as in life, self-acceptance and compassion create a positive, energizing cycle. Self-care, the fruit of self-acceptance, leads to better

■■■ Figure 9–5

Calorie Quiz Answers. We figure about 490 calories for the meal.

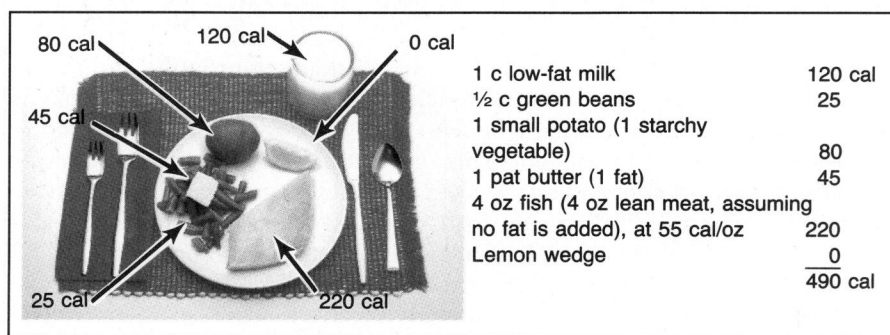

1 c low-fat milk	120 cal
½ c green beans	25
1 small potato (1 starchy vegetable)	80
1 pat butter (1 fat)	45
4 oz fish (4 oz lean meat, assuming no fat is added), at 55 cal/oz	220
Lemon wedge	0
	490 cal

NOTE: Appendix A values yield a total of about 439 cal, lower because these foods are low-calorie choices within the exchange groups. Any answer within about 50 to 100 cal of this is a good estimate.

feelings and to more self-care; emotional, physical, and nutritional health are built on this positive cycle. When the normal lapses occur, the healthy person can cope by saying, "Oops! I'm doing it again, but, it's okay, I do it less often now, and I'm making progress."

▌▌▶ *After achieving a weight goal, many people find maintenance a challenge. A key to maintaining desired weight is distinguishing lapses from relapse. Lapses offer opportunities to practice needed recovery skills; they are part of success, not of failure.*

▐▐▐ SELF-STUDY

Practice Diet Planning.

Diets can be planned using the exchange system to gain weight, to lose weight, or to stay the same. (Chapter 2 explained the exchange system, and Appendix D presents lists of exchanges.) For practice in the use of this convenient system, try planning two diets, one for weight maintenance or gain, the other for weight loss.

Diet for Weight Maintenance or Gain

1. Determine your daily energy output following the example on pages 295–296. If you choose to maintain weight, your diet should provide energy equal to a middle value of your daily energy output range. If you wish to gain weight, it should be about 500 calories above the midpoint of this range.
2. Decide on the proportions in which protein, fat, and carbohydrate calories will be represented in the diet. A suggested ratio is about 10 to 15 percent of the energy from protein, not more than 30 percent from fat, and the rest from carbohydrate. Given the daily calorie level you chose, how many calories will you allot to each nutrient?
3. Translate these calorie amounts into grams. (Remember, 1 gram of protein or carbohydrate = 4 calories; 1 gram of fat = 9 calories.) Enter these gram amounts and your intended calorie total at the top of Form 7 (Appendix F).

4. Now decide how many exchanges of milk, vegetables, and fruit you'd like to have each day; enter these numbers in the form; and compute the number of grams of carbohydrate, protein, and fat they will deliver (don't compute calories yet). See Appendix D for the exchange system values. (Caution: use pencil. You'll want to change these numbers several times before you finalize your plan.)

Only one more set of foods—the starch/bread exchanges—contribute any carbohydrate to the diet. Select the number of starch/bread exchanges that will bring your total carbohydrate intake close to the amount you want. Adjust the numbers of these four exchanges until they seem reasonable to you.

Suggestions: Plans for adults should include two to three milk exchanges daily, two or more vegetable exchanges, and at least two, and preferably more, fruit exchanges. The number of starch/bread exchanges is variable, but the list includes many nutritious foods containing complex carbohydrates. It is not unusual for women's diets to include four to six starch/bread exchanges and for men's to include twice as many or even more. High-calorie diets can have many more of all of these carbohydrate-containing exchanges.

If you have a special fondness for sugar or sugar-containing foods, add a line to Form 7 under "Starch/bread", and allow yourself some "sugar exchanges". At the end of this step, you should have a carbohydrate gram total within about 10 percent of the number you planned in step 3.
5. Subtotal the protein grams delivered by these four types of foods. Only one more list of foods—the meat exchanges—will contribute any protein to the diet. Select the number of meat exchanges you need to bring your total protein intake close to what you planned in step 3.

Note: The recommended intake of carbohydrate is high compared with what many people are used to. Planners often find that once they have completed step 4 of this procedure, they have almost used up their protein allowance and must therefore drastically limit their consumption of meat exchanges. If it works out this way for you, you have two choices. You can accept the dictates of this pattern and resolve to limit your intake of meats and meat alternates accordingly. Or you can increase the number of protein grams you will allow yourself (step 3) and reduce carbohydrate and/or fat to keep the calorie level within bounds.

At the end of this step you should have a protein gram total that agrees (within 10 percent) with your plan of step 3 and that falls between your protein RDA and twice that amount.

continued on the next page

▐▐▐ SELF-STUDY continued

6. Subtotal the fat grams delivered by these five categories of foods. Now use the fat exchanges to bring your total fat intake up to the level planned in step 3.

7. Fill in the far right column of Form 7 with the calorie amounts contributed by the exchanges you have selected, and check to see that the total agrees (within 10 percent) with the calorie level you set in step 1. The completed form now indicates the total exchanges of each type that you will consume on each day of your diet.

8. Distribute the exchanges you have selected into a meal pattern like that on Form 8 in Appendix F. You may want to plan four to six meals a day or to have only one snack; if so, or if you have other preferences, make your own form.

9. Finally, to see how your diet plan might work out on an actual day, make a sample menu. Look over the exchange lists, and choose foods you would like to eat that fit the pattern you worked out in step 8. For example, your meal pattern for breakfast might specify:

■ 1 fruit exchange.
■ 2 starch/bread exchanges.
■ 1 milk exchange.
■ 1 sugar exchange.
■ 1 fat exchange.

So you might choose:

■ 1/2 cup orange juice.
■ 3/4 ounce dry cereal and 1 slice toast.
■ 1/2 cup milk on the cereal and 1/2 cup milk in a glass.
■ 1 teaspoon sugar on the cereal.
■ 1 pat margarine on the toast.

Once you've completed your diet plan, make a form for monitoring your weight-loss progress and maintenance of your goal weight (see step 10 of the next section for how to do this).

Diet for Weight Loss

1. Set your daily calorie intake level. If you wish to lose a pound a week, set it 500 calories per day below the midpoint of your range of energy needs. You could set it higher or lower than this, but on no account should you set it below 1000 calories per day, unless you are under 5 feet tall.

2. Decide on the proportions in which protein, fat, and carbohydrate calories will be represented in the diet. A suggested ratio is that offered in Table 9–5: about 50 percent of the calories from carbohydrate and 25 percent each from protein and fat.

3. Translate these calorie amounts into grams, as in the previous diet plan, and enter them and your energy level into Form 7.

4. Now, using pencil on Form 7, decide on the number of carbohydrate-containing exchanges you'll have, as in step 4 of the first plan. Try to include two milk, two vegetable, and at least two fruit exchanges, and make up the rest of your carbohydrate intake with starch/bread exchanges. Allow no sugar unless you really can't do without it. At the end of this step you should have a carbohydrate gram total within about 10 percent of the number you planned in step 3.

5. Now subtotal the protein grams you have so far, and bring your total protein intake up to the level of your plan by adding meat exchanges until you have

arrived at the protein gram total that agrees (within 10 percent) with your plan of step 3.

6. Now subtotal the fat grams you have so far, and add fat exchanges to bring your total fat intake up to the level planned in step 3.

7. Fill in the calorie amounts contributed by the exchanges you have selected, and check to see that the total agrees (within 10 percent) with the calorie level you set in step 1.

8. Distribute the exchanges into a meal pattern using Form 8 or your own form based on your own preferences.

9. Make a day's sample menu, as in step 9 of the first plan.

10. Using a monitoring system can greatly increase the odds for success in weight maintenance. To monitor, make a form to track your performance. Some people like detailed lists to monitor every aspect of their changed behavior, but some people (the authors of this book, for example) find most useful a simple grid with the days of the week indicated across the top of the form and behaviors to be monitored listed down the left column. Include such items as morning weight, water intake, adherence to a diet plan at all the day's meals, proper exercise, support-group attendance, and any other predictors of success that apply to you (check the bullet lists on pages 311–312 for ideas). Remember to allow for lapses and to set tolerances beyond which you take corrective action.

Notes

1. Parts of this discussion are adapted from Chapter 6, Weight Control, in *Life Choices: Health Concepts and Strategies*, by F. S. Sizer and E. N. Whitney (St. Paul, Minn.: West, 1988).

2. J. E. Manson and coauthors, A prospective study of obesity and risk of coronary heart disease in women, *New England Journal of Medicine* 322 (1990): 882–889.

3. K. Fackelmann, Weight loss builds a healthy liver, *Science News*, May 1989, p. 135.

4. G. Kolata, Obesity declared a disease (Research News), *Science* 227 (1985): 1019–1020.

5. C. L. Roch and A. Coulster, Effects of weight cycling, *Nutrition and the MD*, March 1989, p. 7.

6. A. Frisancho, Nutritional anthropometry, *Journal of the American Dietetic Association* 88 (1988): 553–555.

7. Frisancho, 1988.

8. M. D. Van Loan and coauthors, Use of total-body electrical conductivity for monitoring body composition changes during weight reduction, *American Journal of Clinical Nutrition* 46 (1987): 5–8; M. D. Van Loan and coauthors, TOBEC methodology for body composition assessment: A cross-validation study, *American Journal of Clinical Nutrition* 46 (1987): 9–12.

9. R. P. Donahue and coauthors, Central obesity and coronary heart disease in men, *Lancet*, 11 April 1987, pp. 821–824.

10. M. Ashwell, T. J. Cole, and A. K. Dixon, Obesity: New insight into the anthropometric classification of fat distribution showed by computed tomography, *British Medical Journal* 290 (1985): 1692–1694.

11. A. Forse, P. N. Benotti, and G. L. Blackburn, Morbid obesity: Weighing the treatment options—surgical intervention, *Nutrition Today*, September/October 1989, pp. 10–16.

12. Failure to maintain weight loss: Permissive role of lipoprotein lipase, *Nutrition Reviews*, October 1989, pp. 328–331.

13. For a perspective on theories of obesity, including heredity and the brown fat theory, see J. D. Nash, Eating behavior and body weight: physiological influences, *American Journal of Health Promotion*, Winter 1987, pp. 5–15.

14. This discussion of causes of obesity is adapted from Chapter 8, Energy balance and weight control, in *Understanding Nutrition*, 5th ed., by E. N. Whitney; E. M. N. Hamilton; and S. R. Rolfes (St. Paul, Minn.: West, 1990).

15. Refractory obesity and energy homeostasis, *Nutrition Reviews*, November 1983, pp. 349–351.

16. T. B. Van Itallie and M. U. Yang, Current concepts in nutrition and diet and weight loss, *New England Journal of Medicine* 297 (1977): 1158–1161; Evaluation of 3 weight-reducing diets, *Nutrition and the MD*, March 1978; M. F. Ball, J. J. Canary, and L. H. Kyle, Comparative effects of caloric restriction and total starvation on body composition in obesity, *Annals of Internal Medicine* 67 (1967): 60–67.

17. C. A. Geissler and coauthors, The daily metabolic rate of the post-obese and the lean, *American Journal of Clinical Nutrition* 45 (1987): 914–920.

18. K. N. Pavlou and coauthors, Physical activity as a supplement to a weight-loss dietary regimen, *American Journal of Clinical Nutrition* 49 (1989): 1110–1114.

19. L. K. DeBruyne, F. S. Sizer, and E. N. Whitney, *The Fitness Triad: Motivation, Training, and Nutrition* (St. Paul, Minn.: West, 1991).

20. W. D. McArdle, F. I. Katch, and V. L. Katch, *Exercise Physiology: Energy, Nutrition, and Human Performance*, 2nd. ed. (Philadelphia: Lea & Febiger, 1986), pp. 527–528.

21. L. Pauley and W. J. Wyatt, Big losers: A compilation of success characteristics, *The Bariatrician*, Fall 1987, pp. 23–27.

22. You can lose weight and keep it off, *Tufts University Diet and Nutrition Letter*, March 1989, pp. 1–2.

23. C. Mitchell and R. B. Stuart, Effect of self-efficacy on dropout from obesity treatment, *Journal of Consulting and Clinical Psychology* 52 (1984): 1100–1101.

24. G. Colletti, J. A. Supnick, and T. J. Payne, 1985 as cited in Brownell and coauthors, Understanding and preventing relapse, *American Journal of Psychology* 41 (1986): 765.

25. Mitchell and Stuart, 1984.

26. A. Maslow, *Toward a Psychology of Being* (Princeton, N.J.: Van Nostrand, 1968).

27. L. W. Turner, Weight maintenance and relapse prevention, *Nutrition Clinics,* January/February 1990.

28. C. L. Rock and A. Coulston, Preventing relapse in dieters, *Nutrition and the MD*, January 1989, p. 7.

29. B. Sternberg, Relapse in weight control: Definitions, processes, and prevention strategies, in *Relapse Prevention: Maintenance Strategies in the Treatment of Addictive Behaviors*, ed. G. A. Marlatt and J. R. Gordon (New York: Guilford Press, 1985), pp. 521–545.

30. S. Schachter, Recidivism and self-cure from smoking and obesity, *American Psychologist* 37 (1982): 436–444.

31. Brownell and coauthors, 1986.

▩▩▩ C O N T R O V E R S Y   9

Eating Disorders

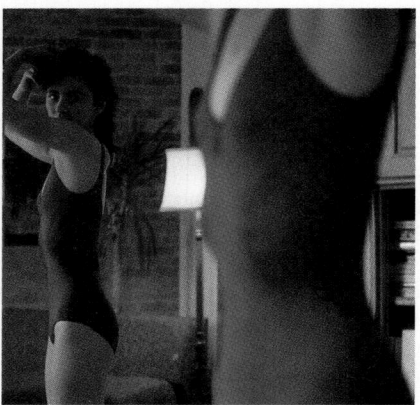

An estimated 2 million people in the United States, primarily girls and women, suffer from some form of the eating disorders **anorexia nervosa** and **bulimia**.[1] Most of these have bulimia, and many more still may not receive a diagnosis, but they "diet" to the point of incurring nutritional consequences.[2] Researchers suspect that hereditary and environmental factors combine to cause eating disorders. Societal beliefs, psychological processes, neurological problems, and addictive processes in the brain may all play roles. Although no treatment is foolproof, an approach that includes medical, psychological, nutritional, and educational components seems to work best.[3] For help in bolstering victims' self-esteem and inner strength, some treatment teams include addiction-recovery techniques in their programs.[4]

▩▩ Anorexia Nervosa

Julie is 18 years old. She is a superachiever in school and a fine dancer. She watches her diet with great care, and she exercises and practices ballet daily, maintaining a heroic schedule of self-discipline. She is thin, but she is not satisfied with her weight and is determined to lose more. She is 5 feet 6 inches tall and weighs 85 pounds. She has anorexia nervosa.

Julie is unaware that she is undernourished, and she sees no need to obtain treatment. She stopped menstruating (developed amenorrhea) several months ago and has become moody. She insists that she is too fat, although her eyes lie in deep hollows in her face. She denies that she is ever tired, although she is close to physical exhaustion, and she no longer sleeps easily. Her family is concerned, and although reluctant to push her, they have finally insisted that she see a psychiatrist. The psychiatrist has prescribed group therapy as a start but warns that if she does not begin to gain weight soon she may need hospitalization to save her life.

Women and girls from middle- or upper-class families are the most likely victims of anorexia nervosa, although there are many exceptions to this generalization. Men account for fewer than one out of ten cases.[5] Typical victims suffer bouts of depression, and as children, victims may have failed to develop on a normal timetable. The family unit may have problems, such as substance abuse or other addictions, and is

likely to overvalue outward appearances while undervaluing inner self-esteem. Julie is a perfectionist, and her parents expect perfection, so the intermeshing of their needs is tight.

Julie identifies so strongly with her parents' ideals and goals that she cannot get in touch with her own identity. She feels like a robot, and she may act that way, too—polite but controlled, rigid, and unspontaneous. Food intake, however, is something she can control. For the anorexia victim, the rejection of food may signify rejection of disturbed relationships.

You may wonder how a person as thin as Julie could continue to starve herself. Julie uses tremendous discipline against her hunger to strictly limit her portions of low-calorie foods. She can recite the calorie counts of dozens of foods and the calorie costs of as many exercises. If she feels that she has gained an ounce of weight, she runs or jumps rope until she is sure she has exercised it off. If she fears that the food she has eaten outweighs the exercise she has done, she takes laxatives promptly to remove the food from her system. She is unaware that this has no effect on body fat because her other ways of staying thin are so effective. She is starving; she is desperately hungry; she doesn't eat because her need for self-control is even more fierce than her need for food. On learning of the disorder, other people say they wish they had "a touch" of it to get thin. They think that people with anorexia feel no hunger.

Central to the diagnosis of anorexia is a distorted body image that overestimates body fatness.[6] The psychiatrist tested Julie's self-image: when asked, she drew a picture of herself that was grossly distorted. When asked to draw her best friend, Julie rendered an accurate image. The psychiatrist knew that the more she overestimated her body size, the more resistant she would be to the treatment and the more unwilling to examine her faulty values and misconceptions.[7] Table C9–1 shows the criteria professionals look for when diagnosing anorexia nervosa.

Some women *without* weight loss meet all the criteria for the condition based on their attitudes and behaviors, as if they had just the beginnings of the disorder. This seems to be particularly true among women whose activities make them highly visible: fashion models, long-distance runners, and dancers. It is not known whether such women may later develop the clinical, full-blown condition.

Anorexia nervosa damages the body in many of the same ways as starvation. Victims suffer many hormonal aberrations. The heart pumps less efficiently, the heart muscle becomes weak and thin, the chambers diminish in size, and the blood pressure falls. In young people, growth ceases. Sudden stopping of the heart, perhaps due to magnesium deficiency and related electrolyte imbalances, accounts for many deaths by heart failure.[8]

Starvation also brings other physical deterioration: impaired immune response, anemia, a loss of digestive functions that worsens malnutrition, altered blood lipids, too much vitamin A and too little protein in the blood, dry skin, low body temperature, painful nerve endings and abnormal nerve functioning, and the development of a cover of fine body hair as a means of keeping warm.

The electrical activity of the brain becomes abnormal, and fitful sleep with bad dreams is common. Women with anorexia always have amenorrhea.[9] In both sexes sexual response may fail.

Teams of physicians, nurses, psychiatrists, family psychologists, and dietitians work together to treat people with anorexia nervosa. The goal of treatment is to initiate and to sustain weight gain as well as to reverse underlying psychological, personal, and family problems. Concerning food, the person may be able to accept only small quantities at first— 800 to 1200 calories or so—until the impaired digestive tract has recovered. Thereafter a balanced high-calorie diet with supplemental vitamins and minerals may be of benefit. Certain severe cases may require that the starving person be force fed through tubes, but this step is extreme and has serious physical and psychological consequences for the victim.[10] Few of those who seek treatment make a full recovery. Only about half resume normal menstrual cycles; most relapse back into at least some form of abnormal eating when treatment ceases. About 6 percent die, 1 percent by suicide.†

■■■ Table C9–1 Diagnosis of Anorexia Nervosa

Refusal to maintain body weight over a minimal normal weight for age and height, eg, weight loss leading to maintenance of body weight 15% below that expected; or failure to make expected weight gain during period of growth, leading to body weight 15% below that expected.

Intense fear of gaining weight or becoming fat, even though underweight.

Disturbance in the way in which one's body weight, size, or shape is experienced; eg, the person claims to "feel fat" even when emaciated or believes that one area of the body is "too fat" even when obviously underweight.

In females, absence of at least three consecutive menstrual cycles when otherwise expected to occur (primary or secondary amenorrhea). (A woman is considered to have amenorrhea if her periods occur only following hormone, eg, estrogen, administration.)

SOURCE: American Psychiatric Association, *Diagnostic and Statistical Manual of Mental Disorders,* 4th ed. (Washington, D.C.: American Psychiatric Association, 1987), p. 67, with permission.

†This is from a review of 19 studies on about 1000 clients over a five-year period. Other deaths are from infection; heart disease; lung disease; and iatrogenic causes including aspiration, electrolyte imbalance from intravenous therapy, and vitamin D poisoning. M. A. Balaa and D. A. Drossman, *Anorexia Nervosa and Bulimia: The Eating Disorders, Disease-a-Month* (Chicago: Year Book Medical Publishers, June 1985), p. 34.

Almost everyone in our society is engaged in the pursuit of thinness. The criteria for diagnosis identify those with *clinical* cases of anorexia nervosa, but many people who meet only some of these criteria also avoid food and thus suffer weight loss and malnutrition. Many things can cause a person to stop eating. Depression, for example, can lead to loss of appetite, as can reaction to grief or trauma.

Some people, on learning of anorexia nervosa, assume that some of their thin friends who have trouble maintaining their weight must have the condition; most times this is not the case. A professional diagnosis is required to identify cases, and even then the process is difficult. However, if you are concerned about a friend whom you may fear has an eating disorder, you help most by clearly organizing your thoughts on why you suspect it may be so. Be specific: "Casy has been skipping lunch and exercising two hours each day," rather than, "she looks thin." Then, discuss your suspicions with others who are concerned to verify your perception. Finally, in a gentle, caring way, present your suspicions to your friend, and give the friend the National Anorexic Aid Society hotline number* at the bottom of this page. Then relax, knowing you've done what you could.

*The NAAS hotline number is 614–436–1112.

■■■ Bulimia

Sophie is a charming, intelligent, 20-year-old woman of normal weight who thinks constantly about food. She starves herself and then secretly binges; when she has eaten too much, she vomits. Few people would fail to recognize these symptoms as characteristics of bulimia.

Bulimia is distinct from anorexia nervosa, and it is more prevalent. Bulimia is most common in women, although more men suffer from bulimia than from anorexia nervosa. The secretiveness of bulimic behaviors makes recognition of the problem difficult, but once recognized, the diagnosis is based on the symptoms listed in Table C9–2.

Like the typical person with bulimia, Sophie is single, female, and white. She is well educated and close to her ideal body weight, although her weight fluctuates 10 or more pounds up and down over a few weeks. Sophie seldom lets bulimia interfere with her work or other activities, although a third of all bingers do. From early childhood she has been a high achiever with strong dependence on her parents. When Sophie was a young teen, she cycled on and off of crash diets but could never maintain an appropriate weight. Sophie feels anxious at social events and cannot easily establish close relationships. She is sometimes depressed and is often impulsive. Some people with bulimia abuse drugs, steal compulsively (kleptomania), or are sexually promiscuous.

A bulimic binge itself is not like normal eating, and the food is not consumed for its nutritional value. During a binge, Sophie's eating is accelerated by her hunger from previous calorie restriction, and she may eat anywhere from 1000 to many thousands of calories of easy-to-eat, low-fiber, smooth-textured, high-fat, and, especially, high-carbohydrate foods. After the binge she pays the price of having swollen hands and feet, bloating, fatigue, headache, nausea, and pain. It is a compulsion and usually occurs in several stages: "anticipation and planning, anxiety, urgency to begin, rapid and uncontrollable consumption of food, relief and relaxation,

■■■ Table C9–2 Diagnosis of Bulimia

Recurrent episodes of binge eating (rapid consumption of a large amount of food in a discrete period of time).
A feeling of lack of control over eating behavior during the eating binges.
Regular practice of either self-induced vomiting, use of laxatives or diuretics, strict dieting or fasting, or vigorous exercise to prevent weight gain.
A minimum average of two binge eating episodes a week for at least three months.
Persistant overconcern with body shape and weight.

SOURCE: American Psychiatric Association, *Diagnostic and Statistical Manual of Mental Disorders*, 4th ed. (Washington, D.C.: American Psychiatric Association, 1987), pp. 68–69, with permission.

EAT EVERYTHING!

NEVER EAT!

The person with bulimia alternately binges and starves.

disappointment, and finally shame or disgust."[11] To purge the food from their bodies, some people use **cathartics**—strong laxatives that can injure the lower intestinal tract. Others use **emetics**—drugs that induce vomiting and are intended as first aid for poisoning. It was emetic abuse that caused the death of popular singer Karen Carpenter in 1983.

Unlike Julie, Sophie is aware that her behavior is abnormal, and she is deeply ashamed of it. She feels inadequate ("I can't even control my eating"), and so she tends to be passive and to look to others, primarily men, for confirmation of her sense of worth. When she experiences rejection, either in reality or in her imagination, her bulimia becomes worse. Then Sophie's depression may deepen, and she may seek solace in drug or alcohol abuse.

Binging and purging bring other consequences. Fluid and electrolyte imbalances caused by vomiting or diarrhea can lead to abnormal heart rhythms and can injure the kidneys, which have to cope with the altered balance. Urinary tract infections can lead to kidney failure. Vomiting causes irritation and infection of the voice box, esophagus, and salivary glands, and erosion of the teeth and dental caries. The esophagus may rupture or tear, as may the stomach. The hands may be bruised and lacerated from scraping on the teeth while inducing vomiting. Overuse of emetics can lead to heart failure.

Bulimia is in many respects easier to treat than anorexia nervosa because people who experience it recognize that their behavior is abnormal, and they seek change. The dietary goals of treatment are to help clients gain control over food and establish regular eating patterns.[12] This requires adherence to a rigid eating plan. Weight-loss dieting itself is a strong trigger to binging, and so weight maintenance, rather than cyclic gains and losses, is a must for the person who has recovered from bulimia. Once the person gains control, planning and consuming adequate, regular meals becomes a lifelong task to prevent relapse.

▮▮▮ Eating Disorders as Addictions

What could drive a person to voluntarily starve to death or continue to eat beyond the point of pain? This question has led researchers to link eating disorders with another self-destructive force—substance addictions.

Anorexia nervosa and substance addiction are both obsessive, compulsive behaviors. Relapse after treatment for anorexia is as likely as relapse after treatment for drug addiction, and many times the same people suffer from both.

Bulimia sufferers score high when tested on scales of addictive personality traits.[13] Indeed, the rates of alcohol, marijuana, and cigarette abuse are high among people with eating disorders.[14] Especially connected to eating disorders is cocaine addiction. In one study approximately 25 percent of those seeking help with cocaine addiction were found to be bulimic, 7 percent to be bulimic and anorexic, and 2 percent to meet the criteria for anorexia nervosa alone.[15] Of the general population, in contrast, 5 percent of all college and high school-aged females have bulimia and 0.5 percent of female adolescents have anorexia.[16] Even a very young bulimic girl may be more prone to abuse substances than her nonbulimic peers.[17]

Researchers believe that anorexia nervosa may be linked to addiction through the chemical workings of the brain. Evidence exists that anorexia improves when treated with naloxone, a drug that controls heroin addiction. Given to an addict, the drug can block the craving for heroin; given to people with anorexia nervosa, it can abolish their compulsive drive to starve.[18] Naloxone also blocks people's feelings of thrill that arise when they listen to well-loved music. These seemingly unrelated effects may not be so unrelated—it is likely that feelings of thrill associated with drug use, self-starvation, or music arise from the same set of brain chemicals, namely the **endogenous opiates**, or **endorphins**, neurotransmitters that kill pain and induce feelings of pleasure (neurotransmitters were introduced in Controversy 6).[19] Any chemical use or other behavior that stimulates the site of origin of these chemicals (the **limbic system** of the brain) is likely to be repeated, sometimes irresistibly.[20] Naloxone interferes with this system, thus eliminating the craving.

Some of the brain's endorphins have also been implicated for direct roles in appetite regulation.[21] Such endorphin concentrations of women with bulimia may differ from those of women who eat normally.[22] Researchers found that the plasma concentration of one of the endorphins was depressed in the bulimic women and that the relationship was linear—the lower the endorphin, the worse the bulimia. This was taken to imply that when endorphin levels drop too low, this may trigger bulimia. However, the opposite case could as easily be true—that bulimic binging somehow depresses certain brain endorphins.

The purging of bulimia also stimulates the brain's addiction centers. ("Purging the soul" by intense crying—catharsis—may do the same thing.) A study produced these findings—that vomiting itself increased the blood concentrations of chemicals that indicate endorphin release.[23] In addition, pain sensitivity was reduced after vomiting, a feeling of peacefulness and relief ensued, and depression reportedly lifts, suggesting that vomit-

ing stimulates the release of endorphins. Obviously, the endorphin question with regard to eating disorders is far from settled.

Another neurotransmitter, serotonin, is also implicated in bulimia. (Serotonin was discussed in Controversy 6.) Almost 90 percent of people who first seek help for bulimia are subsequently found to be clinically depressed.[24] Feelings of depression can result from low serotonin in the brain, and serotonin plays roles in the regulation of food intake, particularly carbohydrate-rich food. Antidepressant medications given to depressed bulimia sufferers have been found to lift depression, to reduce bulimic tendencies, and to restore normal appetite.[25] Today many drugs used to treat psychological disorders are being tried in the treatment of bulimia.

A word of caution: although science has hinted at connections between addictions and eating disorders, this theory is most tentative, and no one should believe for a moment that individual foods might be addicting. Claims that sugar, flour, fat, or other food components can lead to addiction are false, and can mislead victims of eating disorders down a path of quackery, and thus delay their recovery. People with eating disorders need treatment from a team of true professionals as mentioned at the start of this Controversy, including a psychologist and a dietitian. Even excellent treatment does not ensure recovery, but without it the chances for recovery are slim.

While relief from compulsive overeating is attainable for some by way of psychological and other ap-

proaches, a common-sense nutritional approach seems helpful as well. The compulsive overeater must at some point learn not to compulsively *undereat*, since clearly, excessive dietary restriction triggers binges. Many a former bulimia victim has taken a major step toward recovery by learning to eat enough food to satisfy hunger needs. In many cases this may mean eating not less than 1600 calories a day.[26]

■■■ Eating Disorders in Society

Eating disorders are probably as complex in their development as are the addictions. Both probably have a genetic component—some people are predisposed to becoming addicted or to developing an eating disorder through their inheritance. Both probably have psychological components, and both develop within the context of society. Proof that society plays a role in eating disorders is found in their demographic distribution—they are known only in developed nations, and they become more prevalent as wealth increases.

A food-centered society that favors thinness in women puts a woman in a bind. Families may encourage hearty eating with socializing around the dinner table. Party hosts take trouble to provide delicacies, and guests are obliged to indulge. A child raised in such a setting and also made to aspire to a thin ideal may see little alternative but to celebrate with the family; to indulge in vast quantities of food;

■■■ Miniglossary of Eating Disorder Terms

anorexia nervosa: a disorder seen (usually) in teenage girls involving self-starvation to the extreme (*an* means "without"; *orex* means "mouth"; *nervos* means "of nervous origin").

bulimia (alternative spelling **bulemia**) (byoo-LEEM-ee-uh): recurring binge eating combined with a morbid fear of becoming fat, sometimes followed by self-induced vomiting or purging; other terms used to describe this eating behavior include **compulsive eating** and **bulimia nervosa** (*buli* means "ox").

cathartic: a strong laxative.

emetic (em-ETT-ic): an agent that causes vomiting.

endogenous opiates, endorphins: compounds made in the brain whose actions mimic that of opiate drugs (morphine, heroin) in reducing pain and stimulating pleasure.

limbic system: a group of tissues at the center of the brain responsible for feelings of pleasure and involved in the addiction process.

---

and then to vomit, crash diet, or fast to "undo" her possible weight gain. Then, starving and guilty, she may begin binging in secret so as not to appear to be a glutton.

There is no doubt that our society sets unrealistic ideals for body weight in women and devalues those who do not conform to them. At so tender an age as 12 years, beautifully growing, normal-weight girls are already worried that they are too fat. Most are "on diets," and many are poorly nourished. Some eat too little food to support normal growth; thus they miss out on their adolescent growth spurt and may never catch up.[27] Many eat so little that they are propelled by hunger into binge-purge cycles. Magazines, newspapers, and television all present the message that to be thin is to be beautiful and happy. People with eating disorders attempt to conform to these unreasonable ex-pectations, even to the detriment of their health. Perhaps a young women's best defense against these disorders is to learn to appreciate her own uniqueness, to discover and honor her body's real needs, and to become unwilling to sacrifice health for conformity. The author Eda Le-Shan, once a slave to bulimic behavior, achieved this inner ideal and described her recovery from overeating: "Deep inside there had always been a small child begging for my attention . . . . All I gave her was food. Now I give her love."[28]

Notes

1. D. Farley, Eating disorders: When thinness becomes an obsession, *FDA Consumer*, May 1986, pp. 20–23.

2. F. Lifshitz and N. Moses, Nutritional dwarfing: Growth, dieting, and fear of obesity, *Journal of the American College of Nutrition* 7 (1988): 367–376.

3. Position of the American Dietetic Association: Nutrition intervention in the treatment of anorexia nervosa and bulimia, *Journal of the American Dietetic Association* 88 (1988): 68.

4. B. McCormick, Alcohol centers now treating "food addicts" (abstract), *Journal of the American Dietetic Association* 86 (1986): 1758.

5. Farley, 1986.

6. J. B. Murray, Psychological aspects of anorexia nervosa, *Genetic, Social, and General Psychology Monographs* 112 (1986): 5–40; A. E. Andersen, Anorexia nervosa: Who are you? Where are you? (editorial), *Mayo Clinic Proceedings* 63 (1988): 511–513.

7. H. Bruch, Anorexia nervosa, *Nutrition Today,* September-October 1978, pp. 14–18.

8. V. Fonseca and C. W. H. Havard, Electrolyte disturbances and cardiac failure with hypomagnesaemia in anorexia nervosa, *British Medical Journal* 291 (1985): 1680–1682.

9. M. A. Balaa and D. A. Drossman, *Anorexia Nervosa and Bulimia: The Eating Disorders*, *Disease a Month* (Chicago: Year Book Medical Publishers, June 1985), pp. 1–52.

10. B. R. Carruth, adolescence in *Present Knowledge in Nutrition,* ed. M. L. Brown (Washington, D.C.: International Life Sciences Institute, 1990), pp. 325–332.

11. Balaa and Drossman, 1985.

12. M. Story, Nutrition management and dietary treatment of bulimia, *Journal of the American Dietetic Association* 86 (1986): 517–519.

13. P. De Silva and S. Eysenck, Personality and addictiveness in anorexia and bulimic patients, *Personality and Individual Differences* 8 (1987): 749–751.

14. J. D. Killen and coauthors, Depressive symptoms and substance use among adolescent binge eaters and purgers: A defined population study, *American Journal of Public Health* 77 (1987): 1539–1541; Health and Public Policy Committee, American College of Physicians, Eating disorders: Anorexia nervosa and bulimia, *Annals of Internal Medicine* 105 (1986): 790–794.

15. M. Jonas and M. S. Gold, Cocaine abuse and eating disorders, Letters, *Lancet*, 15 February 1986, pp. 390–391.

16. Farley, 1986.

17. Jonas and Gold, 1986.

18. J. E. Mitchell and coauthors, Naloxone but not CCK-8 may attenuate binge-eating behavior in patients with the bulimia syndrome, *Biological Psychiatry* 21 (1986): 1399–1406; I. H. Mills, The neuronal basis of compulsive behaviour in anorexia nervosa, *Journal of Psychiatric Research* 19 (1985): 231–235.

19. A. Goldstein, Brain chemistry and the addictions, *Journal of Substance Abuse Treatment* 3 (1986): 157–161.

20. N. Bejerot, *Addiction, an Artificially Induced Drive* (Springfield, Ill.: Charles C. Thomas, 1972).

21. M. S. Gold and H. A. Sternbach, Endorphins in obesity and in the regulation of appetite and weight, *Integrative Psychiatry* 2 (1984): 203–207.

22. D. A. Waller and coauthors, Eating behavior and plasma beta-endorphin in bulimia, *American Journal of Clinical Nutrition* 44 (1986): 20–23.

23. H. D. Abraham and A. B. Joseph, Bulimic vomiting alters pain tolerance and mood, *International Journal of Psychiatry in Medicine* 16 (1986): 311–316.

24. Killen and coauthors, 1987.

25. D. B. Herzog and P. M. Copeland, Bulimia nervosa—psyche and satiety, *New England Journal of Medicine* 319 (1988): 716–718; L. G. Tolstoi, The role of pharmacotherapy in anorexia nervosa and bulimia, *Journal of the American Dietetic Association* 89 (1989): 1640–1646.

26. S. Dalvit-McPhillips, A dietary approach to bulimia treatment, *Physiology and Behavior* 33 (1984): 769–775.

27. Lifshitz and Moses, 1988.

28. E. LeShan, *Winning the Losing Game: Why I Will Never Be Fat Again* (New York: Crowell, 1979).

Nutrition and Physical Activity

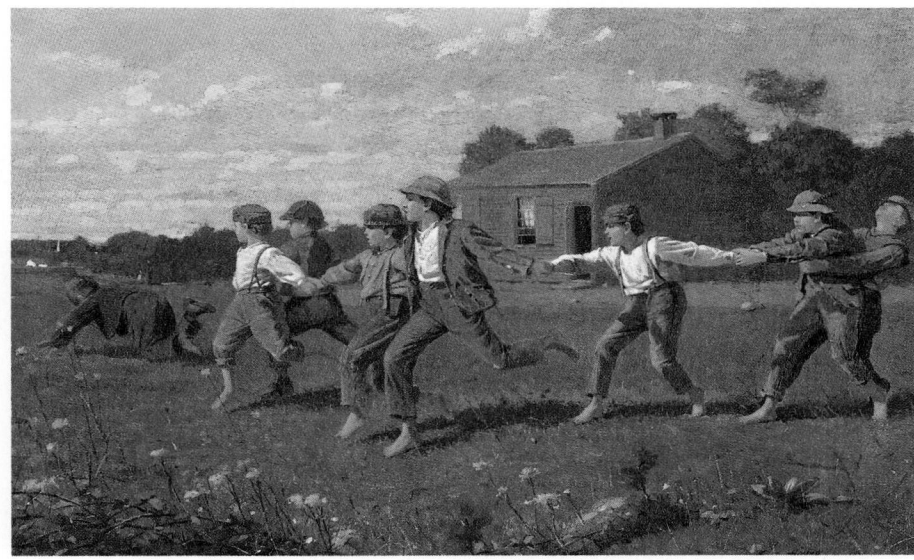

Winslow Homer, *Snap the Whip,* The Metropolitan Museum of Art, Gift of Christian A. Zabriskie, 1950 (50.41).

▦▦▦ In the body, nutrition and physical activity go hand in hand. The working body demands energy-yielding nutrients to fuel activity, and it needs
protein and a host of supporting nutrients with which to build lean tissue. In
addition, exercise requires the body to dip into its stores of fuel—fat and
glycogen. By using up fat and depositing lean tissue, exercise pushes body
composition toward the lean and thus raises the body's rate of energy output
(the basal metabolic rate or BMR, explained in Chapter 9).

The notion that a minimum daily average amount of physical activity is
indispensable to health has just recently gained agreement among health professionals. There is no RDA for exercise, but there probably should be one.
Stretching the point, we can even speak of "exercise deficiency" just as we
speak of nutrient deficiencies. Such a deficiency would lead to accelerated
development of the diseases associated with sedentary life—cardiovascular
disease, obesity, intestinal disorders, apathy, insomnia, accelerated bone loss,
and many more. Researchers who conducted an extensive study on fitness and
mortality concluded that "moderate levels of physical fitness that are attainable
by most adults appear to be protective against early mortality."[1] People who
engage in regular physical activity can receive many of these benefits:

- More enjoyable, perhaps even longer, life.
- Improved mental outlook.[2]
- Improved mental capacity.
- Feeling of vigor.
- Feeling of belonging—the fun and companionship of sports.
- Improved self-image and self-confidence.
- Reduced incidence and severity of personality disorders.[3]
- Reduced fatness and increased lean body tissue.[4]
- Greater bone density (protection against osteoporosis).[5]
- Improved circulation, heart capacity, and lung function.[6]
- Sound, beneficial sleep.
- A youthful appearance; healthy skin; improved muscle tone.
- Reduced risk of cardiovascular disease.[7]
- Slowed cardiovascular aging.[8]
- Reduced low-density lipoprotein (LDL) cholesterol; raised high-density li-
poprotein (HDL), indicators of low heart disease risk.
- Normalized blood pressure and slower resting pulse rate, indicators of a
healthy cardiovascular system.[9]
- Reduced risk of stroke (even in oral contraceptive users, who have an
increased risk).
- Improvement of symptoms in some people with diabetes.[10]
- Reduced risk of constipation and colon disorders, including cancer.[11]
- Faster wound healing.
- Improvement or elimination of menstrual cramps.
- Improved resistance to colds and infections.[12]

Science cannot promise that you will receive all of these benefits if you
exercise, but almost everyone who is physically active reaps at least some of
them. If even half of these rewards were yours for the asking, wouldn't you step
up to claim them? Despite evidence of the benefits, not even half of the

population of the United States exercises regularly.* Perhaps this is because they think of exercise as work, another task to add to their already work-filled days. We'd like them to think, instead, in terms of physical activities—that is, fun and leisure activities that meet people's needs for both relaxation and the maintenance of a fit body. This chapter uses the terms *physical activity* and *exercise* to mean the same thing; you call it whichever has the pleasanter associations for you.

Physical activity, or its lack, affects everyone's nutrition and overall health, so this chapter is written for "you," whoever you are—the athlete, the health seeker, the sports player, the weight-loss seeker, or the person who has yet to begin exercising. To understand the interactions between physical activity and nutrition, you must first know a few things about **conditioning**.

▋▋▋ The Essentials of Conditioning

For the person seeking health, physical activity is as important as nutrition or sleep.[13] It promotes **fitness**, and since a fit body looks healthy and attractive, it enhances appearance. Fitness doesn't require that you develop a Ms. Olympia or Mr. Universe body; rather, you need to develop your own potential along several lines. You need to achieve enough of the four components of fitness—**flexibility, strength, muscle endurance,** and **cardiovascular endurance**—to allow you to meet the everyday demands of life, plus some to spare. Nutrition alone cannot endow you with fitness or athletic ability, but it can complement the effort you put forth to obtain them. Conversely, unwise food selections can stand in your way.

Researchers have yet to discover how little physical activity is too little and how much might be too much. Standard advice is that a minimum of 20 minutes of the kind of activity that produces cardiovascular endurance three times or more each week is necessary for a strong heart. Other experts recommend that people spend 3500 calories in any sort of physical activity each week to benefit heart health. Activities that raise the heart rate for more than 20 minutes, **aerobic** activities, use most of the large muscle groups of the body (legs, buttocks, and abdomen). Examples are swimming, cross-country skiing, rowing, fast walking, jogging, fast bicycling, soccer, hockey, basketball, water polo, lacrosse, and rugby. Still others say that for weight control purposes, you have a "three-mile body": as long as you obtain the equivalent of three miles of walking a day, your appetite and energy output will tend to balance without much effort on your part

Heart and artery disease kills more people in the United States than anything else. Of the actions you can take to prevent or to forestall this disease, regular aerobic activity is among the most powerful because it builds cardiovascular endurance. In **cardiovascular conditioning,** the total blood volume and number of red blood cells increase, so that the blood can carry more oxygen. The heart muscle becomes stronger and larger, and each beat empties the heart's chambers more completely, so that the heart pumps more blood per beat. This

*In 1983, the proportion of adults aged 18 to 65 years exercising regularly was estimated at just over 35%, with children participating in daily physical education programs at 33%, and adults over 65 taking regular walks at 36%. Public Health Service implementation plans for attaining the objectives for the nation, *Public Health Reports Supplement,* September-October 1983, p. 155.

conditioning: the physical effect of **training**, improved flexibility, strength, and endurance.

training: practicing an activity, which leads to conditioning. Training is what you do, conditioning is what you get.

fitness: the body's ability to meet physical demands, composed of four components: flexibility, strength, muscle endurance, cardiovascular endurance.

flexibility: the ability to bend without injury; flexibility depends on the elasticity of muscles, tendons, and ligaments and on the condition of the joints.

strength: the ability of muscles to work against resistance.

endurance: the ability to sustain an effort for a long time. One type, **muscle endurance**, is the ability of a muscle to contract repeatedly within a given time without becoming exhausted. Another type, **cardiovascular endurance**, is the ability of the cardiovascular system to sustain effort over a period of time.

aerobic (air-ROE-bic): requiring oxygen.

cardiovascular conditioning: the effect of regular exercise on the cardiovascular system—including improvements in heart, artery, and lung function and increased blood volume.

stroke volume: the amount of blood ejected by the heart toward the tissues at each beat.

Cardiovascular conditioning is characterized by:

- Increased blood volume and oxygen delivery.
- Increased heart strength and **stroke volume.**
- Slowed resting pulse.
- Increased breathing efficiency.
- Improved circulation.
- Reduced blood pressure.

anaerobic (AN-air-ROE-bic): not requiring oxygen.

hypertrophy (high-PURR-tro-fee): an increase in size (for example, of a muscle) in response to use.

atrophy (AT-tro-fee): a decrease in size because of disuse.

overload: an extra physical demand placed on the body; an increase in the frequency, duration, or intensity of an exercise. A principle of training is that for a body system to improve, it must be worked at frequencies, durations, or intensities that increase by increments.

myoglobin: the muscles' red iron-containing protein that is associated with energy pathways involving oxygen. Also called myohemoglobin.

makes fewer beats necessary, so the pulse rate falls. The muscles that inflate and deflate the lungs gain strength and endurance, allowing breathing to become more efficient. Blood moves easily through the blood vessels because the muscles of the arteries contract powerfully, and movement of the skeletal muscles pushes the blood through the veins. This keeps blood pressure normal because vessel resistance diminishes. Figure 10–1 shows the major relationships between the heart, lungs, and muscles.

An informal pulse check can give you some indication of how conditioned your heart is. The average resting pulse rate for adults is around 70 beats per minute, but the rate can be higher or lower. Active people can have resting pulse rates of 50 or even lower. To take your pulse, place your finger over a pulse point (the side of the throat for instance) and count the number of beats in 30 seconds; multiply by two to get beats per minute.

In contrast to aerobic activity, **anaerobic** activity generally does not bring about cardiovascular conditioning but develops strength and bulk of muscles. It involves sudden, all-out exertions of muscles that last less than 90 seconds. Examples include sprinting (100 meter dash), serving a tennis ball, jumping a fence, doing pushups, or lifting a weight.

As important as cardiovascular conditioning is, it is only one facet of conditioning. All fitness components are important to health and appearance. For balanced fitness, stretching enhances flexibility, weight training or calisthenics develops muscle strength and endurance, while aerobic activity improves cardiovascular fitness.

People shape their bodies by what they do and by what they choose not to do. Muscle cells and tissues respond to the **overload** of exercise by gaining strength and size, a response called **hypertrophy.** The converse is also true: if not called on to perform, muscles **atrophy.** Thus cyclists often have well-developed legs but little arm or chest strength; a tennis player may have one arm that is superbly strong, while the other is just average. A swimmer usually develops in a balanced way—arms, legs, back, and chest all perform and so develop uniformly. This doesn't mean that everyone should give up tennis and cycling for swimming but only that a variety of kinds of physical activities will produce the most uniform overall fitness. This is one of the reasons why people are told to work different muscle groups from day to day. It makes sense to give muscles a rest anyway because it takes a day or two to restore muscle fuel supplies and to repair any slight damage incurred through exercise.

Muscle tissues adapt to the type of activity performed. The muscle cells of a superbly trained weightlifter store extra granules of glycogen and have built up their associated connective tissue and thickened their contractile proteins, thereby increasing their work capacity.† This athlete's muscle cells, although superbly suited for work that requires strength and quickness, are not well suited to endurance competition. In the same way, the muscle cells of a distance swimmer have expanded stocks of **myoglobin,** the muscle's version of hemoglobin, and other equipment needed to burn fat and to sustain prolonged exertion; muscles thus adapted are not suited to power competition. This means that people who wish to play a sport should train mainly by playing that sport, so as to develop in their muscle fibers the specific metabolic equipment most needed in the game.[14] However, keep in mind that to some degree

†All muscles contain a variety of muscle cells (fibers), but there are two main types—slow-twitch (also called *red fibers*) and fast-twitch (also called *white fibers*). Slow-twitch cells are most suited to perform fat-burning aerobic work, while fast-twitch store extra glycogen for anaerobic work. Muscle fibers of one type can take on some of the characteristics of the other as the body adapts to exercise.

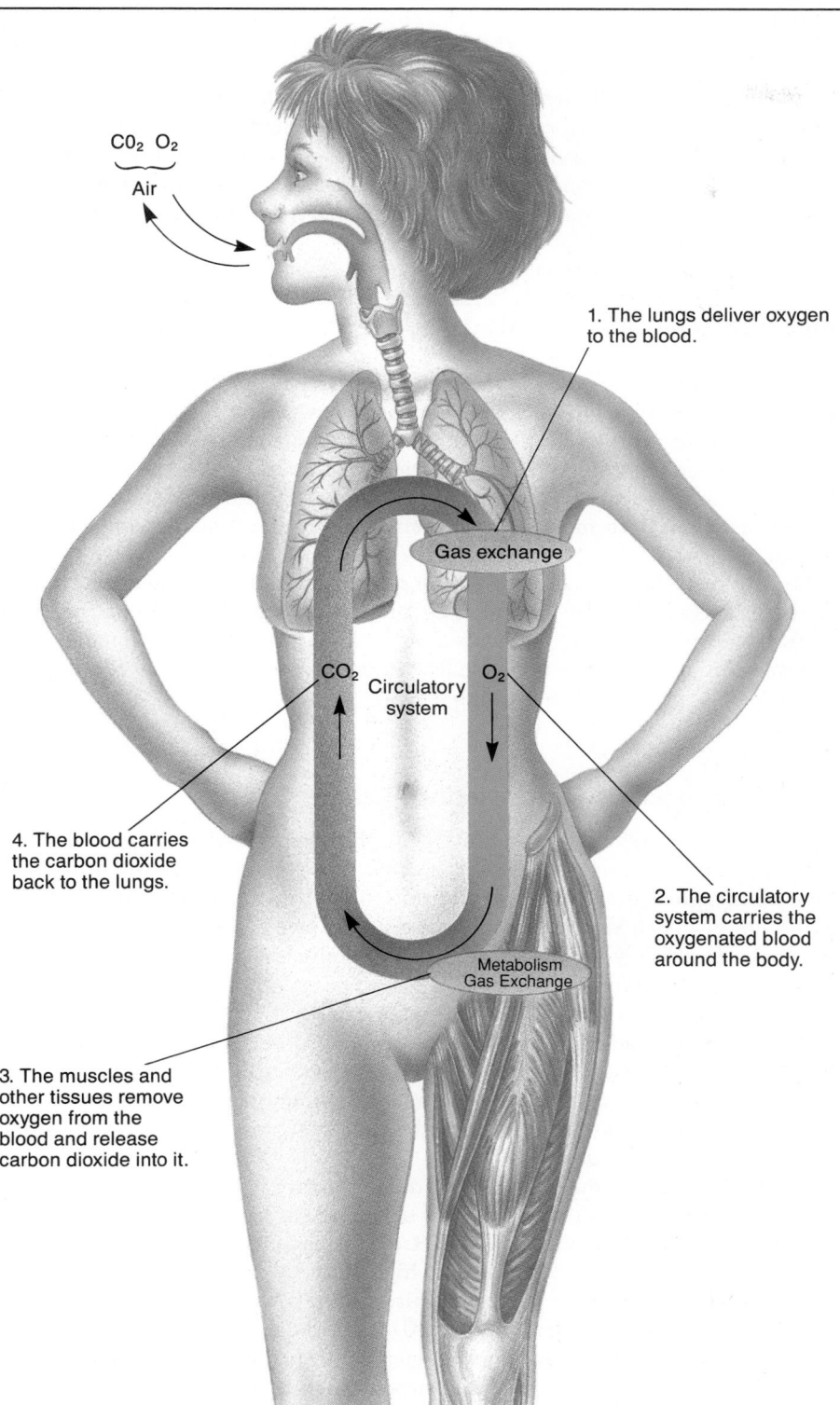

CO$_2$ O$_2$
Air

1. The lungs deliver oxygen to the blood.

Gas exchange

CO$_2$ Circulatory system O$_2$

4. The blood carries the carbon dioxide back to the lungs.

2. The circulatory system carries the oxygenated blood around the body.

Metabolism
Gas Exchange

3. The muscles and other tissues remove oxygen from the blood and release carbon dioxide into it.

■■■ **Figure 10–1**

Delivery of Oxygen by the Heart and Lungs to the Muscles.
The more fit a muscle is, the more oxygen it draws from the blood. That oxygen is drawn from the lungs, so the person with more fit muscles extracts from the inhaled air more oxygen than a person with less fit muscles. The cardiovascular system responds to the demand for oxygen by building up its capacity to deliver oxygen. Researchers can measure cardiovascular fitness by measuring the amount of oxygen a person consumes per minute while working out, a measure called **VO$_2$ max**.

VO$_2$ max: the maximum volume of oxygen consumed per minute.

champions are born with the right genetic potential to excel, and that fact cannot be changed even through hard work.[15]

▌▌▶ *Physical activity benefits people's physical, psychological, and social well-being and improves their resistance to disease. A certain minimum amount of physical activity is indispensable to health. To build fitness—whose components are flexibility, strength, and muscle and cardiovascular endurance—a person must apply overload. Muscles adapt to activities they are called upon to perform.*

▌▌▌ Exercise and the Body's Use of Fuels

The exercising body responds to physical activity by adjusting its fuel metabolism. When you begin to exercise, hormones, including epinephrine and norepinephrine, are released into the bloodstream and signal the liver and fat cells to liberate their stored energy nutrients, primarily glucose and fatty acids, with a few amino acids mixed in. Thus hormones set the table for the muscles' energy feast, and the muscles help themselves to the fuels passing by in the blood.

During rest, the body derives a little more than half of its energy from fatty acids and most of the rest from glucose, along with a small percentage of amino acids from protein. The next few sections explain that fuel use depends on an interplay among the fuels available, the intensity and duration of the exercise, and the body's prior conditioning.

Using Glycogen and Glucose for Fuel

Glucose, stored in the liver and muscles as glycogen, is vital to physical activity. During exercise, the liver releases its glucose into the bloodstream. The muscles pick up this glucose and use it in addition to their own private glycogen stores. Although glycogen stores are ample to support everyday activity, they are not as abundant as body fat stores; glycogen is limited. A person with 30 pounds of body fat to spare may have only a pound or so of glycogen to draw on.

The body constantly uses and replenishes its glycogen. How much glycogen a body stores depends partly on the amount of carbohydrate in the diet. Exercise also affects the amount of glycogen that muscles store—muscles that deplete their glycogen through work adapt to store greater amounts of glycogen to support that work. The more glycogen you store, the longer the stores will last during exercise.

A classic study compared fuel use during exercise among three groups of runners, each on a different diet. For several days before testing, one of the groups consumed a normal mixed diet (55 percent of calories from carbohydrate), a second group consumed a high-carbohydrate diet (83 percent of calories from carbohydrate), and the third group consumed a high-fat diet (94 percent of calories from fat). Figure 10–2 shows that the high-carbohydrate diet allowed the athletes to work longer before exhaustion. This study and many others that followed suggest that a high-carbohydrate diet enhances an athlete's endurance by ensuring ample glycogen stores. The last section of this chapter describes how to choose a performance diet, paying special attention to carbohydrate.

■■■ **Figure 10−2**

The Effect of Diet on Physical Endurance. A high-carbohydrate diet can triple an athlete's endurance.

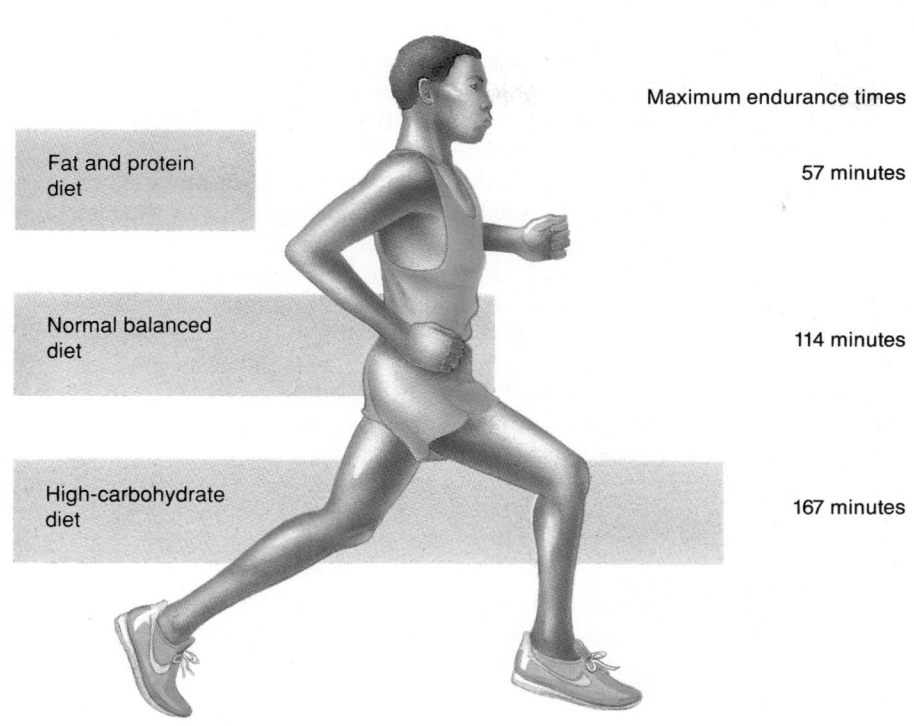

Maximum endurance times

Fat and protein diet — 57 minutes

Normal balanced diet — 114 minutes

High-carbohydrate diet — 167 minutes

Source: Data from P. Astrand, Something old and something new . . . very new, *Nutrition Today,* June 1968, pp. 9−11.

How long an exercising person's glycogen will last depends not only on diet but also partly on the intensity of the exercise. The most intense activities, such as sprinting, quickly use up glycogen.[16] Other, less intense activities, such as jogging, are more conservative of glycogen, but joggers still use it, and eventually they will run out of it. Glycogen depletion usually occurs in less than two hours of vigorous exercise.

The relationship between the intensity of exercise and the amount of glucose used as fuel depends on the availability of oxygen. Oxygen plays a key role in the workings of the muscles' metabolic engines. With ample oxygen, muscles can extract all available energy from glucose, and during *moderate* exercise, the lungs and circulatory system have no trouble keeping up with the muscles' need for oxygen. The exerciser breathes deeply and easily, and the heart beats steadily—the exercise is aerobic. Figure 10−3 (next page) shows that with oxygen, aerobic metabolism extracts all the energy it can from both glucose and fatty acids. Thus moderate aerobic exercise conserves glycogen.

Intense exercise presents a different picture. The heart and lungs can provide only so much oxygen only so fast. When muscle exertion is so great that the demand for energy outstrips the oxygen supply, aerobic metabolism cannot sufficiently meet energy needs. Muscles must instead draw more heavily on their limited supply of glucose because glucose can be partially broken down *anaerobically*. The upper portion of Figure 10−3 shows that glucose can take an anaerobic path to yield some energy during oxygen deficit.

oxygen debt: a deficit of oxygen built up by a body's performing exercise so demanding that the cardiovascular system cannot deliver oxygen fast enough to the muscles to support aerobic metabolism; the debt must be repaid by rapid breathing after the activity slows down or stops.

lactic acid: an acid produced from glucose during anaerobic metabolism. When oxygen becomes available, lactic acid can be completely broken down or converted back to glucose.

Figure 10–4 shows that during low-intensity aerobic activity, energy demands do not exceed the available oxygen, and fat can supply much of the energy, permitting glycogen to be conserved. In contrast, during high-intensity anaerobic activity, energy demands do exceed the available oxygen, fat cannot be used to meet the increased energy needs, and more glucose must be broken down, depleting glycogen more rapidly.

In anaerobic metabolism the exerciser's body builds up an **oxygen debt**. Glucose is spent rapidly during oxygen debt, and fragments of glucose molecules accumulate in the muscle tissue. This is why if you exercise intensely, you may have to slow down or even stop to "catch your breath" (replenish your oxygen supply). When you do, your body begins relying on aerobic metabolism once more. (That's why this physiological state is called a *debt;* oxygen can be "repaid" later.) The nervous and hormonal systems respond to glucose fragments generated by anaerobic activity by speeding up the heart and lungs, but a point comes at which they can't keep up. At this point the fragments are converted to **lactic acid.**

■■■ **Figure 10–3**

Glucose and Fatty Acids in Their Energy-releasing Pathways. Glucose is partially broken down to yield some energy without the help of oxygen. Later the partially broken down glucose molecules encounter oxygen and are then carried through a complete breakdown cycle that yields carbon dioxide, water, and energy. Fat can be broken down only in the presence of oxygen.

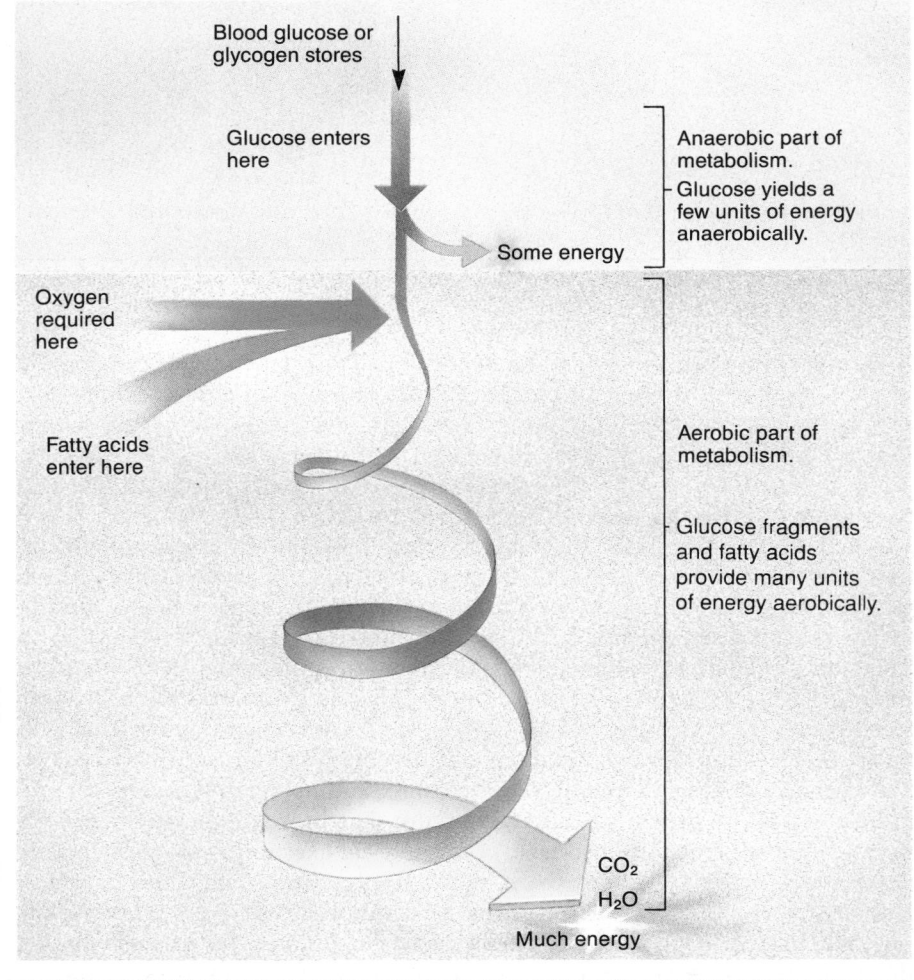

Blood glucose or glycogen stores

Glucose enters here

Anaerobic part of metabolism.
Glucose yields a few units of energy anaerobically.

Some energy

Oxygen required here

Fatty acids enter here

Aerobic part of metabolism.

Glucose fragments and fatty acids provide many units of energy aerobically.

CO_2
H_2O

Much energy

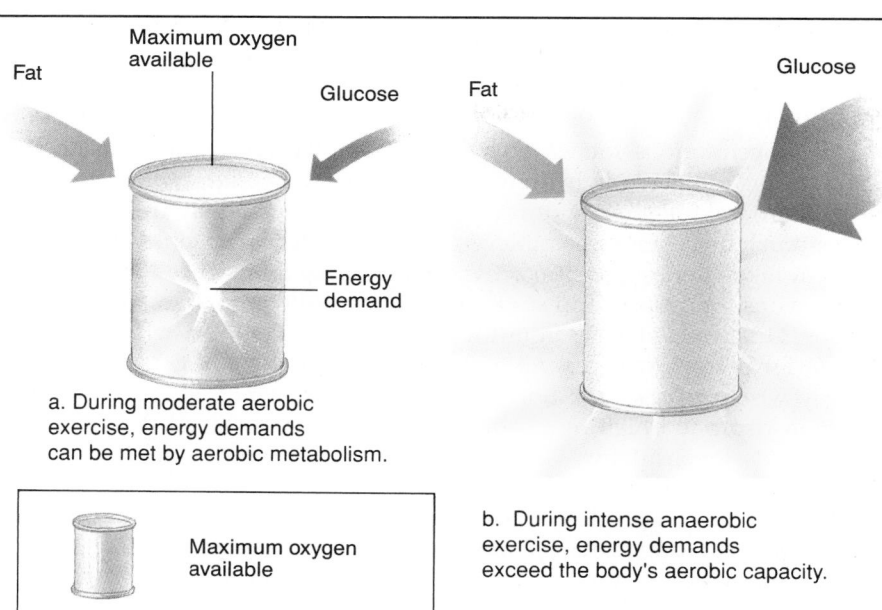

a. During moderate aerobic exercise, energy demands can be met by aerobic metabolism.

Maximum oxygen available

Energy demands of exercise

b. During intense anaerobic exercise, energy demands exceed the body's aerobic capacity.

■■■ Figure 10–4

Fuels, Oxygen, and Exercise Intensity.[†]   The cylinders represent the body's oxygen capacity. As long as energy demands do not exceed the body's available oxygen, as shown here in **part a**, energy is supplied through aerobic metabolism using mostly fat for fuel. When energy demands exceed the body's oxygen supply (**part b**), anaerobic metabolism must meet the extra demand by partially breaking down large quantities of glucose.

[†]This figure shows only the two main fuels, glucose and fat. Protein also contributes some fuel and can stand in for glucose to some degree.

Lactic acid buildup causes burning pain and brings on muscle fatigue within seconds if the blood cannot clear it away. A strategy for dealing with lactic acid buildup is to relax the muscles at every opportunity so that the circulating blood can carry it away and bring oxygen to support aerobic metabolism. This is what mountaineers are doing when they relax their leg muscles at each step (the "mountain rest step"). When exercise diminishes or ceases, oxygen is restored to the tissues, and much of the lactic acid is routed to the liver, where it is converted back into glucose.

Glycogen use during exercise depends not only on the *intensity* but also on the *duration* of the exercise—how long it continues. Within the first 20 minutes or so of moderate exercise, a person uses up about one-fifth of the available glycogen.[17] As the muscles devour their own glycogen, they become ravenous for more glucose and increase their uptake of blood glucose 20-fold or more.[18] If you tested the person's blood glucose during exercise, you would see it rise for a while, signaling that the liver is pouring out its stored carbohydrate for use by muscles. The muscles' increased uptake of blood glucose would keep the blood glucose concentration from rising too high, and indeed you would soon see it begin to decline.

A person who continues exercising moderately (mostly aerobically) for longer than 20 minutes begins to use less and less glycogen and more and more fat for fuel. Still, glycogen use continues, and if the exercise goes on for long enough and at high enough intensity, muscle and liver glycogen stores will run out almost completely. Physical activity can continue for a short time thereafter only because the liver scrambles to produce from available lactic acid and certain amino acids the minimum amount of glucose needed to briefly forestall

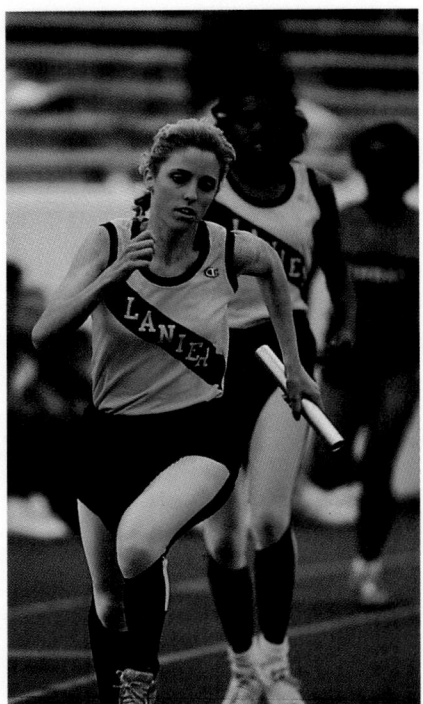

Short-duration, high-intensity exercise draws heavily on glycogen reserves.

Factors that affect glucose use in exercise:

■ Amount of carbohydrate in the diet.
■ Intensity and duration of the exercise.
■ Degree of training to perform the exercise.

Chapter 4 described the action of insulin on blood sugar.

hypoglycemia. When hypoglycemia hits, it brings nervous system function almost to a halt, making exercise difficult, if not impossible. This is "hitting the wall" in a marathon, another type of fatigue.

To avoid hypoglycemia, endurance athletes must try to maintain their blood glucose concentrations for as long as they can. Three strategies to do this include eating a high-carbohydrate diet beforehand (see the Food Feature for a discussion), taking glucose during the exercise, and training the muscles to store as much glycogen as possible. As for taking glucose, people used to fear that sugar taken during physical activity might bring on reactive hypoglycemia due to the insulin response to sugar. Normally insulin stimulates all tissues of the body to take up glucose from the blood and to stow it away—the wrong response for performance. Exercise is a special case, though. During exercise, the body wisely releases the hormone epinephrine, which keeps the insulin level from rising too high in response to glucose in the blood. Exercise also increases muscle sensitivity to insulin so that muscle tissue is singled out as the main recipient of blood glucose.

At the end of a competition, when glycogen is running low, glucose taken in during the event can make its way slowly from the digestive tract to the muscles. The glucose from dilute sugared drinks can augment the body's supply of glucose just enough to forestall exhaustion.[19]

Before concluding that sugar might be good for your own performance, consider first whether you engage in *endurance* activity, that is, do you run, swim, bike, or ski nonstop at a rapid pace for more than 1 1/2 hours at a time? If not, the sugar picture changes. For an everyday jog or swim, sugar won't help performance, and, unless the timing is right, it may actually be a hindrance. If an exerciser makes the mistake of taking sugar within the three hours *before* exercise, the sugar will stimulate insulin to pour forth, causing blood glucose to drain away, and hypoglycemia during exercise then becomes likely. Research on runners shows that a sugar drink taken directly before exercise can reduce athletic performance by 25 percent.

The third factor that enables athletes to maintain adequate blood-glucose levels during exercise is training of muscles. A person trained to do the exercise at hand can work at high intensities longer than a less-trained person; trained muscles can burn more fat and thus require less glucose, even during strenuous exercise. When you first attempt an activity, you use much more glucose than an athlete who is trained to perform it. Oxygen delivery to the muscles by the heart and lungs plays a role in this effect, but equally important, untrained muscles have a smaller capacity to use their oxygen and so depend heavily on the anaerobic breakdown of glucose, even when the exercise is just moderate. In conclusion, to maintain blood glucose for as long as possible in endurance competition, attend to diet and especially to carbohydrate intake, take dilute sugar-containing fluids if your activity lasts longer than 1 1/2 hours, and train your muscles by practicing the activity.

People with diabetes should know that the enhancing effect of exercise on insulin activity described in this section may have implications for them. The effect lasts beyond the exercise period and makes exercise helpful in the defense against the disease. Those who must take insulin or insulin-eliciting drugs sometimes find that they can reduce their daily drug requirements through the effects of regular exercise. (Another benefit to those with diabetes: exercise helps in weight loss, and excess body fatness is a key risk factor for type II diabetes.)

❚❚▷ *Glucose is essential to exercise. Long-duration, low-intensity (aerobic) exercise conserves glycogen; short-duration, high-intensity (anaerobic) exercise draws heavily on glycogen. A high-carbohydrate diet replenishes glycogen stores and best facilitates exercise.*

Using Fat and Fatty Acids for Fuel

If a person should eat nothing but fat and protein with no measurable carbohydrate, that person would burn more fat than normal during exercise. However, that person would also sacrifice athletic performance, as Figure 10–2 showed, and would needlessly degrade tissue proteins as the body struggled to produce the glucose it needed from amino acids. When you add to these facts that a high-fat diet is a major risk factor for cardiovascular disease and that even those who exercise are not immune to heart attacks and strokes, it is no wonder that every reliable source speaks out against high-fat diets for athletes.

Body fat stores are more important to fat use in exercise than is fat in the diet. Unlike the glycogen stores, which are limited, fat stores can fuel hours of exercise without running out; body fat is (theoretically) an unlimited source of energy. Early in exercise the blood fatty-acid concentration falls as the muscles begin to draw on the available fatty acids, but then if exercise continues for more than a few minutes, the hormone epinephrine is called into play. Epinephrine signals the fat cells to break apart their stored triglycerides and to liberate more fatty acids into the blood. After about 20 minutes of exercise, the blood fatty-acid concentration rises and surpasses the normal resting concentration. It is during this phase of sustained, submaximal exercise—beyond the first 20 minutes—that the fat cells begin to shrink in size as they empty out their lipid stores.

Intensity and duration of exercise affect fat use. In general, the percentage of energy contributed by fat diminishes as the *intensity* of exercise increases. Figure 10–3 showed that fat can be broken down for energy in only one way—by aerobic metabolism. When intensity of exercise is so great as to incur oxygen debt, the body cannot burn more fat—it burns more glucose instead.

In general, the longer the *duration* of exercise, the greater the percentage of energy contributed by fat. The person who wishes to burn fat by exercising should know that patient, persistent, consistent, low-intensity training, such as fast walking, is the road to maximum use of fat and conservation of glycogen. An old rule of thumb states that to burn fat the fastest, you should exercise at an intensity at which you can talk normally but not sing. If you can sing, speed up; if you can't talk you are incurring oxygen debt and should slow down.

After physical activity has ceased, fat use may continue at an accelerated rate for some time thereafter. Although not all sources agree, one study suggests that metabolism remains elevated for at least six hours after walking on a treadmill for 10 minutes.[20] Another reports increased fat use 24 hours after a one-hour aerobic exercise session.[21] It takes energy to link glucose molecules back into glycogen and to build new muscle tissue; fat supplies some of this energy. Exercise favors the continued liberation of stored fat too.[22] The body adapted to strenuous and prolonged aerobic exercise burns more fat all day long, not just during the exercise. In other words, intense exercise of more than an hour's duration probably raises a person's BMR.

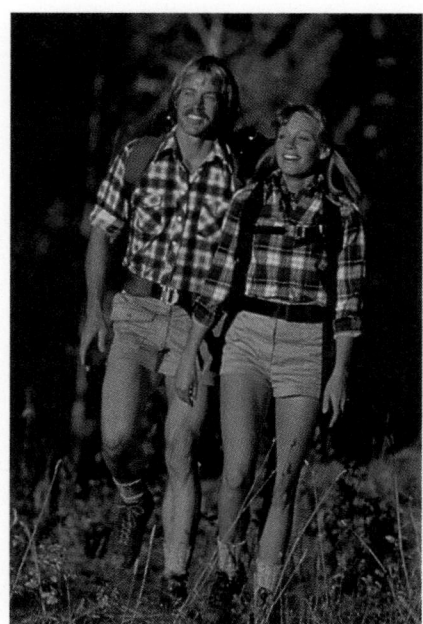

The key to burning fat is this: slow, steady, long-duration exercise works best.

■■■ Table 10–1 Characteristics of the Body's Energy Systems in Exercise

ENERGY SYSTEM	OXYGEN NEEDED?	EXERCISE DURATION	EXERCISE INTENSITY	ACTIVITY EXAMPLE
Stored high-energy compounds[a] (immediate availability)	No	Less than 30 sec	All initial movements; extremely intense exercise	100-yd dash, shot put
Carbohydrate (incomplete breakdown to lactic acid)	No (anaerobic)	30 sec to 3 min	Very high	1/4-mi run at maximal speed
Carbohydrate (complete breakdown)	Yes (aerobic)	3 min to 20 min	High	Cross-country skiing, distance swimming or running
Fat	Yes (aerobic)	More than 20 min	Moderate	Distance running or jogging

[a]ATP (adenosine triphosphate) and PC (phosphocreatine).

SOURCE: Adapted from M. H. Williams, Human energy; in *Nutritional Aspects of Human Physical and Athletic Performance*, 2nd ed. (Springfield, Ill.: Charles C. Thomas, 1985), pp. 21–57; E. L. Fox, Sports activities and the energy continuum, in *Sports Physiology*, 2nd ed. (New York: W. B. Saunders Company, 1984), pp. 26–39.

The fat used in physical activity is liberated as fatty acids from the internal fat pads and from the fat under the skin. Areas that have the most fat to spare donate the greatest amounts of fatty acids to the blood (although they may not be the areas that appear to you as the most fatty). This is why "spot reducing" doesn't work—muscles do not own the fat that surrounds them. Fat cells release fatty acids not into the underlying muscles but into the blood, and all the muscles share it. Proof of this is found in a tennis player's arms—the fatfolds measure the same in both arms, even though the muscles of one arm are better developed than those of the other. A balanced exercise program will, however, tighten muscles underneath the fat in trouble spots to improve the overall appearance. Keep in mind that some body fat is essential to good health, and a later section describes the problems of young women who exercise away too much of their body fat.

Table 10–1 summarizes the energy systems that work together to supply energy in exercise, as discussed so far. The next section describes the roles of protein in exercise. Protein is not a major source of energy for exercise, but it still provides some; more importantly, it provides the structural material of muscle tissue.

Factors that affect fat use in exercise:

■ Amount of fat in the diet.
■ Intensity and duration of the exercise.
■ Degree of training to perform the exercise.

■■▷ *In exercise, the body draws on its vast stores of fat from all over the body. Sustained, moderate exercise uses up fat most efficiently and accelerates metabolism. Persistent training increases the muscles' use of fat over glycogen.*

Using Protein and Amino Acids for Building Muscles and for Fuel

If a high-fat diet is ill advised for athletes, what about a high-protein diet? Athletes' needs for protein may be just slightly higher than the needs of others, but these needs are well covered by a nutritious diet of ordinary foods. People who exercise use protein in the same ways other people do—to build muscle and other lean tissue structures and, to some extent, to fuel activity. This discussion focuses on both these needs for protein, beginning with building muscles.

The making of body proteins accelerates in the hours of rest that follow physical activity.[23] This is when the body remodels the tissues it needs for performance. Additionally, whenever the body rebuilds a part of itself, it must tear down the old structures to make way for the new ones. Exercise, with just a slight overload, triggers the protein-dismantling and protein-synthesizing equipment of each muscle cell to begin working.

Physical work signals muscle cells' genetic material to begin producing the kinds of proteins that will best support that work.[24] Take jogging, for example. In the first difficult sessions, the body is not yet equipped to perform aerobic work easily. The cells' genetic material gets the message that an overhaul is needed. The muscles don't change appreciably in just one or two occasions of exercise, but within a few weeks, remodeling occurs and jogging becomes easier.[25]

Protein is critical to the synthesis of new muscle tissue, but it still plays only a supportive role. Beyond this, much is still unknown about exactly how muscles build the tissues they need for exercise, and what is known deserves a moment's attention.

Scientists are trying to elucidate the ways by which the genetic protein-making equipment inside the nuclei of muscle cells might "know" that proteins are needed, and further, which proteins to build in response to physical activity of the body. Researchers now know that muscle contractions initiate controlling signals that communicate directly with muscles' genetic material. Information about the intensity and the pattern of muscular contractions conveys that proteins are needed to support physical activity. Thus, exercise itself delivers information to the muscles' genetic material.

The genes of muscle cells respond specifically to the type of signals they receive.[26] For example, a cell of someone working with weights might receive information that muscle fibers need added bulk for strength and more enzymes for anaerobic glucose breakdown. In this case, the training prompts the muscle cells to begin making those proteins while breaking down unneeded ones. Likewise, on receiving a signal that aerobic exercise is taking place, the muscle cells would begin building the fatburning equipment of aerobic metabolism and breaking down others. Muscle cells are exquisitely responsive to the need for proteins, but they are also conservative in building them. They tailor their work to meet the demand exactly.

Finally, after all the decisions of how to build are made, nutrition comes into play. On the mandate from exercise, the muscles draw on the amino acids and other nutrients present in their fluids to build the needed structures. This bears on the athlete's need to obtain protein from the diet. During active muscle-building phases of training, a weight lifter might add to existing muscle mass between 1/4 ounce and 1 ounce (between 7 and 28 grams) of protein each day.[27] This only happens during periods of *building* muscle, and not during times of maintenance.

Not only do athletes retain more protein, but they also burn a little more protein as fuel too. Studies of nitrogen balance show that muscles speed up their use of amino acids for energy during exercise, just as they speed up their use of glucose and fatty acids.[28] Still, protein is not a major source of energy—it is estimated to contribute an average of about 10 percent of the total fuel used, both during exercise and during rest.[29] Endurance athletes use up branched-chain amino acids: amino acids that, unlike the others, can directly provide energy to muscle tissue: leucine, isoleucine, and valine.

Factors that affect protein use in exercise:

■ Amount of *carbohydrate* in the diet.
■ Intensity and duration of exercise.
■ Degree of training.

enormous amounts of all energy fuels during performance, so they break down a proportionately larger amount of protein than do people who exercise moderately. (However, they eat more total food to supply energy and thus they also consume more protein.)

The factors that modify how much protein is used during activity seem to be the same three that modify the use of glucose and fat—for one, diet. Athletes who consume diets rich in carbohydrate burn less protein than those who eat protein- and fat-rich diets.[30] This could be related to the protein-sparing effect of carbohydrate first discussed in Chapter 6. Some amino acids can be converted into glucose. Others, the **branched-chain amino acids** take its place in energy pathways. Exercise requires glucose, and if the diet is lacking carbohydrate, much more protein will be used for fuel in place of glucose.

A second factor, the intensity and duration of the exercise, also modifies protein use.[31] Low- to moderate-intensity exercise of long duration demands large quantities of fuel, including some protein. Short-duration, high-intensity anaerobic exercise demands less total protein fuel.[32]

A third factor also modifies use of protein—the degree of training. The better trained the athlete, the less protein used during exercise.

As mentioned earlier, all athletes probably need just a little more protein than do sedentary people. Endurance athletes burn greater quantities of protein for fuel than power athletes do, and they retain some, especially in the muscles used for their sport. Power athletes use less protein for fuel than do endurance athletes but still spend some, and they retain much more. Therefore *any* athlete in training should attend to protein needs but should not neglect carbohydrate needs in the process. Otherwise they will burn off as fuel the very protein that they wish to retain in muscle.

How much protein should an athlete consume? The American Dietetic Association (ADA) recommends 1 gram protein per kilogram of body weight each day (1 g/kg/day), an amount somewhat higher than the 0.8 g/kg/day recommended for sedentary people.[33] The association acknowledges a study of young men who ate diets containing 1 g/kg/day of protein and then began training. At first these men developed negative nitrogen balance—they lost body protein, at least at first. Later in the study as training progressed the men's nitrogen balance gradually became positive—they built up body protein while still eating the diet containing 1 g/kg/day of protein.[34] This shift from negative to positive nitrogen balance with no change in diet supports the ADA protein recommendation. The initial protein losses in the study could have been caused by something other than insufficient dietary protein, such as the training itself.

Other experts disagree with the ADA and recommend higher protein intakes. For example, one group of researchers found that 2 g/kg/day of protein during the early stages of training effectively maintained positive nitrogen balance during that time and prevented a drop in the levels of certain blood proteins, including hemoglobin, observed at lower protein intakes.[35] Still another authority suggests different protein intakes for different sports in increments between 1 and 1.6 g/kg/day. Table 10–2 lists some recommendations and translates them into daily intakes for an athlete who weighs 70 kilograms (154 pounds), but after considering them, an athlete might still wonder what level is best and how the recommendations translate into diet. Before drawing conclusions, read the Food Feature, where questions about choosing a performance diet are answered.

■■■ Table 10–2 Total Daily Protein Needs of a 70-Kilogram Athlete

AUTHORITY	RECOMMENDATION (g/kg/day)	PROTEIN/DAY (g)
Food and Nutrition Board (RDA)	0.8	56
American Dietetic Association	1.0	70
Brotherhood (endurance athletes)	1.0 to 1.2	70 to 84
Brotherhood (power athletes)	1.3 to 1.6	91 to 112
Yoshimura (early training)	2.0	140

SOURCE: Data from Food and Nutrition Board, *Recommended Dietary Allowances,* 10th ed. (Washington, D.C.: National Academy of Sciences, 1989); Position of the American Dietetic Association: Nutrition for physical fitness and athletic performance for adults, *Journal of the American Dietetic Association* 87 (1987): 933–939; J. R. Brotherhood, Nutrition and sports performance, *Sports Medicine* 1 (1984): 350–389; H. Yoshimura and coauthors, Anaemia during hard physical training (sports anaemia) and its causal mechanism with special reference to protein nutrition, *World Review of Nutrition and Dietetics* 35 (1980): 1–86.

■■▶ *Athletes use a little more protein both for energy and for building muscle tissue than do other people but need not strive to consume more than the amount in an average U.S. diet.*

■■■ Vitamins and Minerals—Keys to Energy Use

Popular belief has it that athletes need to take supplements of vitamins and minerals to perform well. Do active people need more of these nutrients? The following sections attempt to answer this question for several B vitamins; for vitamins C, A, D, and E; and for a few of the minerals.

Vitamins and Performance

According to one survey, 84 percent of world-class athletes use vitamin supplements.[36] It goes without saying that athletes need adequate vitamins and minerals to do what they do, and Table 10–3 on the next page shows just a few reasons why. But do athletes or active people need more nutrients than sedentary people? If so, which nutrients do they need more of? You might guess that since athletes spend more energy than average, they might need more of the B vitamins that are involved in the breakdown of energy-yielding nutrients—thiamin, riboflavin, niacin, and vitamin B_6—or possibly B_{12} to build blood, or vitamin C for strong tissues. The sections that follow explore what is known about how the metabolic work of exercise affects requirements of these vitamins.

Scientists have studied the effects of thiamin supplements in athletes. They gave supplements to one group of athletes and compared the physical performance of that group to that of athletes eating only a regular adequate diet.[37] They found that extra thiamin did not benefit performance. They concluded that an *adequate* diet supplies all the thiamin a person needs, even an athlete doing heavy work. This is because almost any kind of nutrient-dense food supplies thiamin, and athletes with greater energy needs eat larger amounts of food. Most diets are adequate in thiamin, and even athletes do not need more than that provided by food.

This does not mean that thiamin or any of the other vitamins is not important. The words *adequate diet* are weighty in this regard. To be adequately

■■■ **Table 10–3 Some Roles of Vitamins and Minerals in Exercise**

VITAMIN OR MINERAL	FUNCTION
Thiamin, riboflavin, niacin	Energy-releasing reactions
Vitamin B$_6$, zinc	Building of muscle protein
Folate, vitamin B$_{12}$	Building of red blood cells to carry oxygen
Vitamin C	Collagen formation for joint and other tissue integrity; hormone synthesis
Iron	Transport of oxygen in blood and in muscle; energy transformation reactions
Calcium, vitamin D, vitamin A, phosphorus	Building of bone structure; muscle contractions; nerve transmissions; component of high-energy molecules
Sodium, potassium, chloride	Maintenance of fluid balance; transmission of nerve impulses for muscle contraction
Chromium	Assistance in insulin's energy-storage function
Magnesium	Cardiac and other muscle contraction; energy-releasing reactions

Note: This is just a sampling. Other vitamins and minerals play equally indispensable roles in exercise.

nourished, most of the athletes' extra energy needs must be met with nutrient-dense foods, not fats, sweets, or highly refined foods. Even sedentary people who consume a "junk" diet, that is, a diet of foods relatively empty of nutrients, can become thiamin deficient. This effect is magnified for the exerciser who spends many more calories of energy each day than do others.

Riboflavin, another B vitamin, also plays a role in energy release. The link between riboflavin and physical performance arises from its role in the cells' chemical reactions that release energy in aerobic metabolism. To try to answer the question of whether extra riboflavin assists in athletic performance, researchers studied groups of overweight, sedentary women who began an exercise regimen in addition to weight-loss dieting.[38] One group of women consumed 1.2 milligrams per day of riboflavin (the RDA is 1.3 milligrams) while the other group consumed slightly more (1.4 milligrams). Blood tests to evaluate riboflavin activity seemed to indicate a deficiency in the group that consumed the lower amount. However, aerobic capacity of both groups increased similarly. Riboflavin in amounts greater than the RDA did not improve this aspect of physical performance. To fully answer questions about riboflavin requirements during exercise will require more research.

Unlike the two other B vitamins just discussed, niacin may affect performance more directly, especially when taken as a supplement. Excess niacin suppresses the release of fatty acids and thus forces muscle to use extra glycogen during exercise. Whether this impairs performance is unknown, but it probably shortens the time to glycogen depletion and makes the work seem more difficult to the exerciser.[39] A nutrient-dense diet supplies abundant niacin even for athletes, and people who take niacin supplements before exercise probably hinder their training through niacin's suppressing action on fatty acid release.

Vitamin B_6 plays key roles in the release of energy from nutrients, in the liberation of glucose from glycogen, and in the formation of hemoglobin. Thus sellers of supplements claim that vitamin B_6 in amounts greater than the RDA promotes extra aerobic endurance. However, research does not support these assertions. Experimentally, supplemental vitamin B_6 does not improve aerobic performance.[40] To ensure that the diet is adequate in vitamin B_6, a person need only include some green leafy vegetables, meats, fish, legumes, fruits, and whole grains. Pills, even of megadoses of vitamin B_6, can't improve on the nutrients in a performance diet.

The belief that vitamin B_{12} supplementation will enhance performance stems from its role in the production of red blood cells. Anemias of all kinds diminish the number and function of circulating red blood cells, and they rob the blood of its oxygen-carrying capacity. This starves the cells for oxygen and restricts aerobic energy metabolism. Vitamin B_{12} deficiency causes anemia, but so do iron and folate deficiencies (and others, see margin). Chances are, a diet low enough in vitamin B_{12} to bring on anemia will be low in other nutrients as well. A person with so poor a diet does not need to take pills; more important, eat right.

Some athletes take supplements or shots of vitamin B_{12} prior to competition because they believe that this can enhance endurance and oxygen delivery. The limited research thus far does not support this concept. For a well-nourished athlete, any perceived benefits from vitamin B_{12} supplements or shots are based on psychology, not physiology.[41] In fact, taking *any* vitamin directly before competition runs contrary to science. Vitamins function only as small parts of larger working units, enzymes. A molecule of a vitamin floating around in the blood is simply waiting for the tissues to combine it with its appropriate other parts so that it can do its work. This takes time—hours or days. A vitamin taken right before competition is still in the blood during the event and could not improve performance, even if the person were clinically deficient in that vitamin.

Years ago evidence that exercise caused increased excretion of vitamin C seemed to indicate that vitamin C in amounts two to three times the RDA might best serve the needs of the athlete. Since that time the great bulk of work designed to explore this theory has disproved it. Most experiments show that athletes perform no better when taking vitamin C supplements than when they receive the RDA amount from food. Even so, athletes are often told by "advisors" in health food stores to ingest huge quantities of vitamin C, measured in multiples of a gram. These amounts are clearly beyond those first suspected to be useful, and could be harmful.

For people who eat a reasonable diet, it is almost impossible *not* to receive two to three times the RDA for vitamin C. A person who drinks a small glass of orange juice and eats a baked potato and a serving of broccoli in a day receives about five times the RDA for vitamin C from these foods alone. When shown the full array of values for vitamins and minerals, including vitamin C, in foods such as these, people have been known to throw away their pills and to learn to cook broccoli.

Of the fat-soluble vitamins, supplemental A and D have been shown not to benefit athletic performance, and they are toxic in excess. One other fat-soluble vitamin, vitamin E, has been promoted for athletes. In its role as an antioxidant of polyunsaturated fatty acids, it is as important to athletes as to anyone else.

Nutrients necessary to ward off anemias include vitamins A, B_{12}, B_6, folate, and the minerals zinc, copper, and magnesium along with protein—in short, the perfect mix of nutrients that occurs naturally in whole foods.

stress fracture: bone damage or break caused by stress on bone surfaces during exercise.

athletic amenorrhea: cessation of menstruation associated with strenuous athletic training.

Vitamin E protects delicate cell membranes against destruction by oxygen. Vitamin E may similarly protect a part of the aerobic metabolic equipment that transforms energy nutrients into the energy of work, of obvious importance to athletes.‡

Researchers are only beginning to explore the effects of training on vitamin E. In one study researchers found that even though trained muscles contain much of the aerobic metabolic equipment that requires vitamin E's protection from oxygen, trained muscles contain no more vitamin E than do untrained muscles.[42] As the oxygen carriers for the body, red blood cells need the protection that vitamin E has to offer. Too little vitamin E causes red blood cell membranes to weaken and to break open, spilling out their hemoglobin. The result is anemia. Without a doubt, the anemia of vitamin E deficiency would hinder athletic performance should it occur in people, but that is unlikely. As Chapter 7 described, vitamin E is widespread in foods, and its deficiency is practically never seen. It is too early to say how any of this can be applied to the diets of athletes. Many facts are still unknown, but the evidence indicates that extra vitamin E in supplement form does not enhance athletic performance.

This section has mentioned only a few of the 15 vitamins, but the story is the same for the others: active people do not need supplements of vitamins—they need food of the right kinds, in the right amounts.

Like the vitamins, minerals are essential to exercise. Calcium and iron stand out as minerals of importance because many people fail to meet their needs for these minerals; the next sections focus on them.

❚❚▷ *Vitamins are essential for releasing the energy trapped in energy-yielding nutrients and for other functions that support exercise. Most active people can meet their vitamin needs with an ordinary diet of nutrient-dense foods sufficient to meet their energy needs.*

Exercise and Bone Loss

Osteoporosis, the condition of reduced bone mass, increases susceptibility to fractures, including **stress fractures**, and bone breaks that are due to exercise. Controversy 8 points out that moderate exercise protects against bone loss, but extremes in exercise may be detrimental to bone health, at least in some young women.[43] A side effect of the extremely low body-fat content that sometimes occurs with overzealous endurance training in women is **athletic amenorrhea,** characterized by low estrogen concentrations, infertility, and possibly increased calcium losses. A recent study of ballet dancers found those with extremely low body-fat content and who suffered from amenorrhea incurred more bone injuries than did those with more normal body fatness.[44] Amenorrheic athletes with low body fatness may be at much greater risk for osteoporosis than other women.[45] All women, especially athletes, need to eat enough food to maintain reasonable body weights.

Some disturbing results of a recent survey, indicated that a full third of female athletes questioned practiced some sort of pathological eating behaviors, mostly of the types that characterize anorexia nervosa and bulimia.[46] These behaviors are harmful to bone health and general health, and they impair physical performance. It has been suggested that at least part of the reason so

Anorexia and bulimia were discussed in Controversy 9.

‡The molecule believed to be protected is coenzyme Q.

many athletic women engage in self-destructive behaviors related to their body weights is because they have adopted weight standards that are invalid for athletes. Women athletes are heavier for their heights (they have more healthy muscle and bone tissue), and they are taller than other women. When the athletes consult weight standards designed for sedentary women, they can easily be led to believe, wrongly, that they are too fat. Many resort to bulimic techniques in an attempt to lose weight and to solve an imaginary problem.[47] Standard height and weight charts should never be applied to athletes. Underwater weighing and other body composition measures are more appropriate for them. Women with eating disorders must receive treatment for their conditions before they can hope to compete with well-nourished athletes in sports.

◼◼▷ *Weakened bones can fracture under the stress of exercise. Women who have too little body fatness and amenorrhea are especially susceptible to stress fractures and osteoporosis. For others, moderate exercise strengthens the bones.*

> **runner's anemia:** a true iron-deficiency anemia that develops in many high-mileage runners.
>
> **sports anemia:** a transient condition of low hemoglobin in the blood, associated with the early stages of sports training or other strenuous activity.

Iron and Performance

Endurance athletes, and especially women athletes, are prone to iron deficiency. Iron status might be affected by exercise in any of several ways. One possibility is that iron lost in sweat creates the deficiency, although the sweat of trained athletes contains less iron than the sweat of others (an adaptation to conditioning). Another possible route to iron loss is red blood cell destruction; blood cells are squashed when body tissues (such as the soles of the feet) make high-impact contact with an unyielding surface (such as the ground). Perhaps more significant than losses is reduced iron absorption in some athletes and increased iron demands by muscles to make the iron-containing molecules of aerobic metabolism. In addition, exercise may cause small blood losses through the digestive tract, at least in some athletes.

Vegetarian women athletes may be especially at risk for low iron status.[48] A nutrition survey found more than one-third of the women runners studied had depleted iron stores.[49] Of adolescent girl gymnasts, a study found 95 percent to have iron intakes below the RDA.[50] Habitually low intakes of iron-rich foods and high iron losses through menstruation and those causes mentioned above may cause iron deficiency in young women athletes.

Iron deficiency impairs performance because iron is crucial to the body's handling of oxygen. The symptoms of iron-deficiency anemia include impaired oxygen transport. This reduces aerobic work capacity and the person tires easily. Even marginal iron deficiency without clinical signs of anemia can impair physical performance to some extent in some people.[51]

On the other hand, low iron indicators in the blood do not always accompany decrements in performance. In a study of male marathon runners, blood iron measures indicated that the men suffered from marginal anemia. Even so, their running speeds remained unchanged.[52] The below-normal blood iron measures observed in these men are not unusual for distance runners and may indicate a particular type of iron-deficiency anemia, **runner's anemia.**

The condition known as **sports anemia** is not a true iron-deficiency condition. Sports anemia is characterized by a temporary decrease in hemoglobin concentration after a sudden increase in aerobic exercise. Its exact cause remains controversial, but marginal iron intakes may contribute to it. In addition, strenuous aerobic exercise promotes destruction of fragile, older, red blood cells and increases the plasma volume of the blood, thereby reducing red blood cell count in a measured amount of blood. Sports anemia appears to be an adaptive, temporary response to endurance training. Iron-deficiency anemia requires iron-supplementation therapy; sports anemia goes away by itself.

The best strategy concerning iron may be to try to determine your individual needs. Many menstruating women probably border on iron deficiency even without the additional iron losses incurred through exercise.[53] Teens of both sexes, because they are growing, have high iron needs too. Especially for women and teens, then, prescribed supplements may be needed to correct a deficiency of iron as determined by medical testing. (Medical testing is needed to eliminate nondietary causes of anemia, such as internal bleeding or cancer.)

Other Minerals

Other minerals are also affected by training. Three trace minerals—chromium, zinc, and copper—are of current scientific interest. These minerals have been found to be excreted in larger amounts when people exercise than when they are sedentary.[54] So far it is too early to say whether the excretion is meaningful in terms of people's nutrition, but studies of runners have shown that even with low zinc levels in their blood, running performance is not hindered.[55]

Electrolytes, the charged minerals sodium, potassium, chloride, and magnesium, are lost from the body in sweat. People who are just beginning an exercise regimen lose electrolytes to a much greater extent than do trained people; as the body adapts to exercise, it becomes better at conserving most electrolytes.

An exception is magnesium; its losses in sweat are about the same for trained and untrained individuals. One study found magnesium levels in the blood serum to be lower in exercising people than in others; the effect remained even three months after the exercise program began.[56] This could mean that a magnesium deficiency was coming on, or it could mean that the magnesium had moved out of the blood and into the tissues in response to training.

As for potassium, it usually remains safely inside the cells where it does its work. However, in prolonged dehydration from profuse sweating, it may migrate outside of cells, and it may be lost by excretion in the urine. Even so, it is easily replaced with just a few servings of fresh fruits and vegetables. Avoid potassium supplements unless prescribed by a physician because while they better some conditions, they worsen others. Most times athletes need not make a special effort to replenish lost electrolytes; a regular diet that meets their energy and nutrient needs also supplies all the electrolytes they need.

Overwhelmingly, studies indicate that athletes who take supplements gain no competitive advantage.[57] Despite this, athletes constitute a huge market and a favorite target of the supplement industry. Athletes stand out as one of the groups most often victimized by frauds. The following Consumer Caution touches on a few of the most common schemes aimed at athletes, and warns of the dangers faced by athletes who use steroid and other drugs.

⚀▷ *Adequate mineral intake is critical to exercise. Stress fractures are associated with the risk factors of osteoporosis, and especially with a too-low body weight. Runner's anemia is a true iron-deficiency anemia; sports anemia is probably a normal effect of training.*

> **ergogenic:** the term implies "energy giving," but, in fact, no products impart such a quality; *ergo* = work, *genic* = gives rise to.

CONSUMER CAUTION ⫞⫞⫞   **Athletes as Consumers: Pills, Powders, and Potions**

    Athletes can be sitting ducks for quacks who sell a tide of products—steroid drugs or steroid-drug substitutes, protein supplements, vitamin or mineral supplements, carbohydrate or "complete" drinks, "muscle-building" powders, electrolyte pills, and many other so-called **ergogenic** products (see the list of definitions on page 349). Some home recipes are also well-known—raw eggs, caffeine, or others. The term *ergogenic* implies that such products have special work-enhancing powers. Actually no food or supplement is ergogenic. Do any home or commercial potions have merits?

    Advertisements for commercial products may read as these do: "SWINDLE amino acids deposit slabs of muscle bulk," "HOODWINK enzymes ram the body into turbo charge," "Ultrapotent TECHNOHYPE vitamins and minerals blast carbs through your system." Fortunately ads like these are easy to see through—they are transparent in their purpose of trying to extract money from readers.

    However, some advertising, though just as false, creates the illusion of credibility to gain readers' trust and thus boost sales. Such an ad might have graphs, tables, and a professional-looking "review of the literature" citing such credible sources as the *American Journal of Clinical Nutrition* and *Journal of the American Medical Association.*

    This sounds scientific, and it may be, but don't forget that advertisements are written not to teach, but to sell. A careful reading might reveal that the company has taken the facts out of context. In one such case, ad writers cited an article to support an invalid conclusion: that healthy athletes should use supplements. However, researchers reporting in the cited article had found only that supplements were useful in treating a disease—a true fact. However, the ad writers had twisted the facts to support sales of their products.§

    Products and gimmicks advertised this way (and others available through other sources) vary in their effects from useless to dangerous. Among the most dangerous are steroid drugs and blood doping. Anabolic steroids, normally present in men, trigger muscle bulking in response to exercise in both men and women. Injections of these hormones have been shown to augment the effects of weight training in at least some athletes, but the price is high. In all steroid users, the blood lipid profile sharply changes to the type associated with a high risk of heart disease. Steroids can cause liver damage that often leads to cancer, rupture, or hemorrhage. Men who use steroids suffer permanent shrinkage of their testicles, while women are permanently masculinized. Mood swings, aggressive behavior, and sex drive changes are likely.

§If you have questions about a fitness product, book, or program, write to the American College of Sports Medicine at their address in Appendix E.

continued on next page

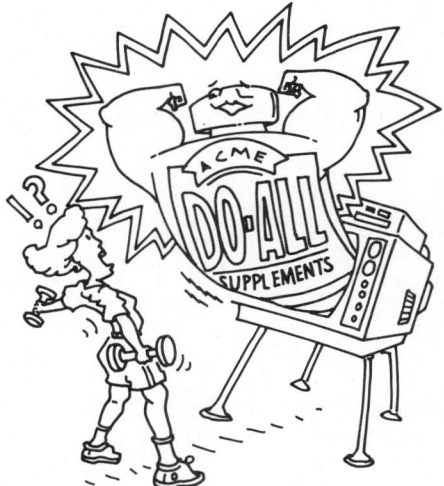

Advertisements for supplements can overpower common sense.

Growth hormone, often offered with steroids, can induce huge body size, a widened jawline, a widened nose, protruding brow and teeth, weakened heart walls, and an increased likelihood of death before the age of 50 years—a condition known as acromegaly. Athletes facing these consequences, even those for whom the drugs made careers in sports possible, try to warn young athletes away—the price of using drugs is too dear, even for the benefit of success in sports.

Blood doping is injecting not drugs but red blood cells to enhance blood's oxygen-carrying (aerobic) capacity before a competition. Some studies confirm an aerobic benefit from the practice but also point out that it may carry negative health consequence. One possible outcome is excess blood clotting, especially in athletes who become dehydrated.

Herbs are hawked as legal substitutes for steroid drugs. Sellers falsely claim that these herbs contain hormones, enhance the body's natural hormones, or both. In some cases, an herb may contain some amount of a plant steroid but not of the type that functions anabolically. The body cannot convert herbal compounds to anabolic steroids. In short, none of these products has any proven anabolic steroid activity nor can they increase muscle strength, but they may contain toxins (see Controversy 14). Don't make the mistake of equating "natural" with "harmless."

Vitamin and mineral supplements can be more toxic than herbs if overdone, and they are offered to athletes in abundance. As should be clear, supplements do not enhance the performance of well-nourished people. However, an ordinary multivitamin and mineral supplement might be prudent when an athlete's need for energy outstrips the ability to eat the quantity of food required to supply it. Choose one on the basis of the information in Controversy 7, and don't be led astray by the words "athlete" or "fitness" on a label. People with nutrient deficiencies need a diagnosis and a nutrient dosage prescribed by a physician.

Protein powders can supply amino acids to the body. Many athletes take these powders with the false hope of stimulating muscle growth. However, purified protein preparations are stripped of other needed nutrients to support the building of muscle. Nature's protein sources—lean meat, milk, and legumes—supply them all and more. Protein taken in excess of the body's need is burned off as energy or is stored as body fat and places an extra burden on the kidneys to excrete the nitrogen generated from its breakdown or conversion.

Amino acid supplements can be especially dangerous, and are never needed by healthy athletes. Advertisers point to research that identifies the branched-chain amino acids as the main ones used as fuel by exercising muscles. What the ads leave out is that compared to glucose and fatty acids, branched-chain amino acids provide minuscule amounts of fuel and that when they are needed, the liver liberates exactly the right amounts of branched-chain amino acids with precise timing. Ordinary foods provide abundant branched-chain amino acids, and the liver holds onto them until they are needed. Pills of tryptophan were banned from sales after many people sickened and at least one person died after taking tryptophan sup-

continued on next page

More about amino acid supplements in the Consumer Caution of Chapter 6.

plements. Replacements for tryptophan soon appeared on the shelves of health-food stores, but some of these, too, have proved dangerous and have been banned.

What about drinks or candylike bars claiming to provide "complete" nutrition? These mixtures of carbohydrate, protein (usually amino acids), fat, and certain vitamins and minerals usually taste good and provide additional food energy for those who need it. However, they fall short of providing "complete" nutrition, since they lack fiber, many nutrients, and the nonnutrients of real food. Beyond energy, they provide nothing special for active people.

A nutritionally "complete" drink could be of use to the nervous athlete who cannot tolerate solid food the day of an event. A liquid meal taken three or four hours before competition can supply some of the fluid and carbohydrate needed to replace a pregame meal of solid food. A milkshake of nonfat milk and ice milk blended with flavorings could do the same thing and less expensively.

Among home recipes for performance, raw eggs are famous. Did raw egg drinks account for movie boxer Rocky's performance and help him win matches? Probably not more than scrambled eggs might have. Raw and cooked eggs are chemically almost identical, both providing high-quality protein and other nutrients. However, raw eggs do contain the nonnutrient avidin that is destroyed by cooking. Avidin binds the vitamin biotin and is used in experiments to induce the symptoms of biotin deficiency (skin rashes, leg paralysis, and hair loss). Raw yolks do not contain avidin, but they do contain as much cholesterol as cooked yolks and thus may contribute to the risk of heart disease if eaten in excess of 3 or 4 per week (see Chapter 11).

More immediate a threat than either biotin deficiency or heart disease is a foodborne bacterial infection (*Salmonella*) that produces fever, vomiting, diarrhea, and abdominal pain. Even fresh, Grade A, grocery-store eggs have been identified as the transmitters of such bacteria. To be safe, cook your eggs; in fact, avoid all raw animal and seafood products, and follow the other food safety rules of Chapter 14, as well.

Moderate doses of the mild stimulant **caffeine** (2 milligrams per pound of body weight or 2 to 3 cups of coffee) one hour prior to exercise seem to assist many people's athletic performance. Caffeine stimulates the body's release of fatty acids into the blood early in exercise, thus conserving glycogen. (Controversy 12 provides a list of common caffeine-containing beverages, foods, and medicines.) Better than caffeine for this purpose is a warm-up activity. Light exercise before a workout stimulates fat release, as does caffeine, but also warms the muscles and connective tissues, making them flexible and resistant to injury while caffeine does not.

Caffeine also has adverse effects—stomach upset, nervousness, sleeplessness, irritability, headaches, and diarrhea. Its diuretic effect is potentially hazardous for exercisers in a hot environment. Caffeine-containing beverages should be used, if at all, in moderation and *in addition* to other fluids, not as a substitute for them. In college, national, and international athletic competitions, the use of caffeine is forbidden in amounts greater than the equivalent of 5 or 6 cups of coffee drunk within an hour or two, and urine tests that detect caffeine in excess of this amount disqualify athletes from competition.

continued on next page

caffeine: a natural stimulant found in many common beverages and foods including coffee, tea, and chocolate. Controversy 12 provides a full discussion of caffeine's effects and sources.

heat stroke: an acute and dangerous reaction to heat buildup in the body.

The overwhelming majority of potions touted as for athletes are frauds. The placebo effect is strong at work in athletes, so even if a reliable source reports a performance boost from a newly tried concoction, give it time. Chances are that the effect was simply the power of the mind over the body. Incidentally, don't discount that power, since it is formidable. You can use it by imagining yourself as a winner and by visualizing yourself as capable in your sport. You don't have to rely on magic for an extra edge because you already have a real one—your mind.

SOURCES: P. G. Dyment and B. Goldberg, Anabolic steroids and the adolescent athletes, *Pediatrics* 83 (1989): 127–128; M. Alen and P. Rahkila, Reduced high-density lipoprotein-cholesterol in power athletes: Use of male sex hormone derivatives, an atherogenic factor, *International Journal of Sports Medicine* 5 (1984): 341–342; O. L. Webb, P. M. Laskarzewski, and C. J. Glueck, Severe depression of high-density lipoprotein cholesterol levels in weight lifters and body builders by self-administered exogenous testosterone and anabolic-androgenic steroids, *Metabolism* 33 (1984): 971–975; H. Haupt and G. D. Rovere, Anabolic steroids: A review of the literature, *American Journal of Sports Medicine* 12 (1984): 469–484; D. R. Lamb, Anabolic steroids in athletics: How well do they work and how dangerous are they? *American Journal of Sports Medicine* 12 (1984): 31–38; M. H. Williams, Introduction, in *Nutritional Aspects of Human Physical and Athletic Performance* (Springfield, Ill.: Charles C. Thomas, 1985), pp. 3–19; Controversial blood doping revisited, *Science News,* May 1987, p. 344; V. E. Tyler, "Bodybuilding" herbs, *Nutrition Forum* ,Stickley, Philadelphia, PA, March 1988, p. 23; M. St. Louis and coauthors, The emergence of grade A eggs as a major source of *Salmonella enteritidis* infections, *Journal of the American Medical Association* 259 (1988): 2103–2107; D. L. Costill, G. P. Dalsky, and W. J. Fink, Effects of caffeine ingestion on metabolism and exercise performance, *Medicine and Science in Sports* 10 (1978): 155–158; F. T. O'Neil, M. T. Hynak-Hankinson, and J. Gorman, Research and application of current topics in sports nutrition, *Journal of the American Dietetic Association* 86 (1986): 1007–1015.

▌▌▌ Temperature Regulation and Fluid Intake

The body's need for water far surpasses that for any other nutrient. Should the body lose too much water, as in dehydration, its life-supporting chemistry would become compromised. Exercisers can be prone to dehydration.

The body loses water primarily via sweat; second to that, breathing costs water, exhaled as vapor. In exercise, both routes can be significant, and dehydration is a real threat. The first symptom of dehydration is fatigue. A rapid water loss equal to 5 percent of the body weight can reduce muscular work capacity by 20 to 30 percent.[58] The athlete who arrives at an event even slightly dehydrated arrives with a disadvantage.

Sweat is the body's coolant. Working muscles produce heat as a by-product of energy release. To rid itself of the excessive heat that builds up during exercise, the body routes its blood supply through the capillaries just under the skin. At the same time the skin secretes sweat, and this evaporates, cooling the skin and the underlying blood. Cooled blood then flows back to cool the body's core.

In humid, hot weather, sweat doesn't evaporate well because the surrounding air is already laden with water. Body heat builds up and triggers maximum sweating—the body's only defense against excess heat. Still, without sweat evaporation, little cooling takes place. In such conditions active people must take precautions to prevent **heat stroke**, the dangerous accumulation of body

▊▊▊ Some "Ergogenic" Aids

bee pollen: a product consisting of bee saliva, plant nectar, and pollen that confers no benefit on athletes and may cause an allergic reaction in individuals sensitive to it.

bioflavonoids: substances in foods that meet no nutritional need. Some are called "vitamin P" (erroneously) by faddists.

branched-chain amino acids: see text page 338.

cell salts: a mineral preparation supposedly prepared from living cells.

DNA (deoxyribonucleic acid): one of the genetic materials of cells, falsely promoted as an ergogenic aid.

gelatin: a soluble form of the protein collagen, used to thicken foods, and sometimes falsely promoted as an ergogenic aid.

glycine: a nonessential amino acid, promoted as an ergogenic aid because it is a precursor of the high-energy compound phosphocreatine. Other amino acids commonly packaged for athletes and that are equally useless include branched-chain amino acids, ornithine, arginine, and lysine.

growth hormone releasers: herbs or pills falsely promoted for enhancing athletic performance.

herbal steroids: a mixture of herbs, falsely referred to as "adaptogens" or "aphrodisiacs," marketed with false claims that they contain hormones or enhance hormonal activity.

octacosanol: an alcohol isolate extracted from wheat germ, often falsely promoted to enhance athletic performance.

phosphate pills: pills of a salt that has been demonstrated to increase the levels in red blood cells of a metabolically important phosphate compound (diphosphoglycerate) and the potential of the cells to deliver oxygen to the body's muscle cells; but then the pills do not improve the ability to perform endurance exercise or increase the efficiency of aerobic metabolism.

RNA (ribonucleic acid): one of the genetic materials of cells, necessary in protein synthesis, falsely claimed to enhance athletic performance.

royal jelly: a substance produced by worker bees and fed to the queen bee, often falsely promoted as capable of enhancing athletic performance.

spirulina: a microscopic blue-green alga inappropriately used as a supplement by athletes; potentially toxic.

superoxide dismutase (SOD): an enzyme made in cells that protects them from oxidative damage. When taken orally, the body digests and inactivates this protein enzyme; it is useless to athletes.

wheat germ oil: oil extracted from wheat kernels, often falsely promoted as an energy booster.

heat with accompanying loss of body fluid. The only way to prevent heat stroke is to drink enough fluid before and during the activity, to rest in the shade when tired, and to wear lightweight clothing that encourages evaporation. (Hence the danger of rubber or heavy suits sold supposedly to promote weight loss during exercise—they promote profuse sweating, prevent sweat evaporation, and invite heat stroke.) If you experience any of the symptoms of heat

Symptoms of heat stroke: headache, nausea, dizziness, clumsiness, stumbling, sudden cessation of sweating or increased sweating, and confusion or other mental changes.

stroke listed in the margin, stop your activity, sip fluids, seek shade, and ask for help—the condition can be fatal and demands medical attention.

In cold weather, **hypothermia**, or loss of body heat, can pose as serious a threat as heat stroke. During exercise in cold weather, the body still sweats and needs fluids. But the fluids should be warm or at room temperature, not cold.

Athletes can lose 2 to 4 quarts of fluid in *every hour* of heavy exercise. The digestive system can absorb only about a quart an hour. Hence the athlete must hydrate before and rehydrate during and after exercise to replace it all. Even then, in hot weather the digestive tract may not be able to absorb enough water fast enough to keep up with an athlete's sweating losses, and some degree of dehydration becomes inevitable. Athletes who are preparing for competition are often advised to drink extra fluids in the few days before the event, especially if they are in training. The extra water is not stored in the body, but drinking extra water ensures maximum tissue hydration at the start of the event. Some coaches and athletes who withhold water during practice take a great risk because they believe the body adapts to use less water. This false and dangerous idea has cost some athletes their health, and some have even died. Drinking a few extra glasses of water causes no harm, and it can be protective.

Casual exercisers should be aware that exercise blunts the thirst mechanism, especially in cold weather. During exercise, thirst signals too late, after fluid stores are depleted, so don't wait to feel thirsty before drinking. Table 10–4 presents one schedule of hydration for exercise. To find out how much water you need to replenish exercise losses, weigh yourself before and after the activity—the difference is all water. One pound equals roughly 2 cups fluid (a quart equals 2 pounds).

What is the best fluid for an exercising body? Surprisingly, just plain cool water, especially in warm weather, for two reasons—(1) because it rapidly leaves the digestive tract to enter the tissues, and (2) because it cools the body. Many good-tasting drinks are marketed for active people. Manufacturers reason that if a drink tastes good, people will drink more, thereby ensuring adequate hydration. The drinks can also provide a psychological edge to people who equate the drinks with success in sports. Manufacturers also claim that the drinks attempt to duplicate the mineral composition of sweat (most fall short with respect to magnesium) and so can facilitate performance. They also claim that glucose in the drinks supplies energy from carbohydrate—another supposed edge over plain water. Do sports drinks provide advantages over plain, cool water? Here are some current lines of thought.

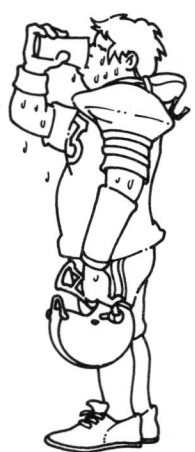

Exercisers must plan to drink fluids before, during, and after physical activity.

■■■ Table 10–4 Schedule of Hydration Before and During Exercise

WHEN TO DRINK	TOTAL AMOUNT OF FLUID (CONSUME IN 1C SERVINGS)
2 hr before exercise	About 3 c
10 to 15 min before exercise	About 2 c
Every 60 to 90 min during exercise	About 1 qt (or one l)
After exercise	Replace each pound of body weight lost with 2 c (1/2 l) fluid

SOURCE: Adapted from J. B. Marcus, ed., *Sports Nutrition* (Chicago: American Dietetic Association, 1986), p. 57; American College of Sports Medicine position stand on the prevention of thermal injuries during distance running, *Medicine and Science in Sports and Exercise* 19 (1987): 529–533.

As for minerals, when water is lost, electrolytes are also lost, of course; but the athlete normally need not try to replace them except to resume eating normal food after the event. In rare cases of the most strenuous competition at the world-class level, many days of heavy sweating and drinking plain water has been reported to dilute the blood concentration of sodium, and in these few cases, sodium repletion was needed. Only if the athlete works up a drenching sweat, exceeding 5 to 10 pounds a day (or 3 percent of body weight) for several consecutive days is electrolyte replacement advised. Under such exertion, drinking a commercial "sweat replacer" beverage diluted by half with water may be prudent. Equally effective is a homemade mixture of one-third teaspoon of salt (sodium chloride) and 1 cup of fruit juice (to provide potassium and carbohydrate) added to each quart of water. Avoid electrolyte or salt tablets; they increase potassium losses, can irritate the stomach, cause vomiting, and always cause water to flow out of the tissues into the digestive tract at first, thereby temporarily worsening dehydration and impairing performance.

A beverage that supplies glucose in some form might be useful during endurance activity lasting longer than 2 hours. It used to be thought that the sugar in the drinks slowed fluid absorption, but recent research indicates that fluid transport to the tissues is equally rapid from beverages containing up to 6 percent glucose, as from plain water.[59] Some drinks contain glucose in the form of starchlike **glucose polymers** in hopes of improving fluid availability, but the effect is not proven.

Athletes, like others, sometimes drink beverages that contain alcohol but these are inappropriate for activity. Like caffeine, alcohol is a diuretic, and both promote the excretion of water and of vitamins such as thiamin, riboflavin, and folate, and of minerals such as calcium, magnesium, and potassium—exactly the wrong effect for fluid balance and nutrition. It is hard to overstate alcohol's detrimental effects on physical activity. Its diuretic effect impairs temperature regulation, making hypothermia or heat stroke much more likely, it alters perceptions, slows reaction time, it decreases strength and endurance, and deprives people of their judgment, thereby compromising their safety in sports. Many sports-related fatalities and injuries each year involve alcohol or other drugs.

❚❚▶ *Fluid is crucial to exercise performance and must be provided before, during, and after activity. Heat stroke is a dangerous condition caused by fluid loss that inhibits the body's cooling system. Electrolytes are lost during exercise but do not require replacement during activity.*

hypothermia: a below-normal body temperature.

glucose polymers: compounds that supply glucose, not as single molecules but linked in chains somewhat like starch. The object is to attract less water from the body into the digestive tract.

Read about alcohol's effects on the brain in Controversy 11.

Choosing a Performance Diet

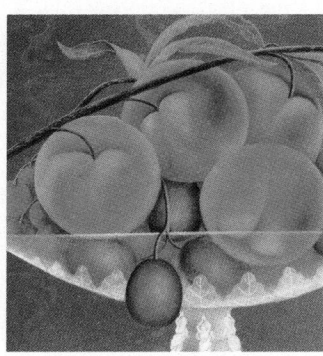

Compare and decide which best meets your needs:

■ 1 sandwich of:
  2 slices bologna, 2 slices white bread,
  2 tbsp mayonnaise — 525 calories
  (9 percent protein, 23 percent carbohydrate,
    68 percent fat)
OR
■ 2 sandwiches of:
  2 slices lean ham, 4 slices whole-wheat bread,
  2 tsp mayonnaise — 503 calories
  (20 percent protein, 51 percent carbohydrate,
    29 percent fat)

No particular diet supports an athlete's performance perfectly; many different diets can be excellent for athletes. However, food choices must be made within the framework of rules for diet planning presented in Chapter 2.

First, athletes need a diet composed mostly of nutrient-dense foods, the kind that supply a maximum of vitamins and minerals for the energy they provide. When athletes eat mostly refined, processed foods that have suffered nutrient losses and that contain added sugar and fat, nutrient status suffers.[60] Even if these foods are fortified or enriched, manufacturers cannot replace the whole range of nutrients and nonnutrients lost in refining processes. Consider, for example, that manufacturers mill out food's trace minerals magnesium and chromium but do not replace them. This doesn't mean that athletes can *never* choose a white bread, bologna, and mayonnaise sandwich but only that later they should eat a large, fresh salad or big portions of vegetables and whole-grain breads and drink a glass of milk to compensate. That way the nutrient-dense foods provide most of the needed nutrients, including magnesium and chromium; the bologna sandwich provided extra energy, mostly from fat.

Athletes must eat for energy, and energy needs may be immense. However, wise athletes want full glycogen stores, and they strive to reduce the risks of heart disease and cancer and so must limit fats. Simply stated, a diet that is high in carbohydrate (65 percent of total calories or more), low in fat (20 percent or less), and adequate in protein (12 to 15 percent) ensures full glycogen and other nutrient stores while meeting the athlete's energy needs. Even if the athlete does not compete in glycogen-depleting events, such a diet will help to control weight (thus reducing diabetes and other disease risks) and to provide adequate fiber while supplying abundant nutrients and energy. With these principles in mind, compare the two 500-calorie sandwich meals in the margin. The trick to getting enough carbohydrate energy is easy at least the theory — just reduce the amount of fat and meat in a meal and let carbohydrate-rich foods fill in for them.

Athletes whose sport exhausts their glycogen stores sometimes use a technique called **carbohydrate loading** to trick their muscles into storing extra glycogen before a competition. In the early days athletes were taught to restrict carbohydrates and to exercise heavily to empty their muscles of glycogen. Before the event they cut back on exercise and switched abruptly to an extremely high-carbohydrate diet. Muscle glycogen rebounded to as high as three to four times the normal amount.

Carbohydrate loading practiced this way can have negative side effects that outweigh any performance advantage, including abnormal heartbeat, swollen and painful muscles (glycogen attracts and holds water), and weight gain immediately before competition. Today athletes use a safer plan. First, the athlete increases exercise intensity *without* restricting carbohydrates. Next, during the week before competition, the athlete gradually cuts back on exercise, rests completely the day before, and eats a very high-carbohydrate diet for a few days before competition. In this plan athletes never restrict carbohydrate intake; they only manipulate exercise levels and pack extra carbohydrate in at the end. Extra glycogen gained this way can benefit an athlete who must keep going 90 minutes or longer at a stretch. Those whose work is of shorter duration need only eat a regular high-carbohydrate diet. In a hot climate, extra glycogen confers an additional advantage on the endurance athlete; as glycogen breaks down, it releases water, which helps to meet the athlete's fluid needs.

There is some good news for people who would not go to the extreme of carbohydrate loading but who still wish to have full glycogen stores. It appears that a high-carbohydrate meal within two hours after physical activity accelerates the rate of glycogen storage by 300 percent.[61] Eating the meal after two hours has passed reduces the glycogen synthesis rate by almost half. So after your workout, you might want to relax with a glass of orange juice and some crackers or some other carbohydrate-rich snack, just for your glycogen's sake.

Adding carbohydrate-rich foods is a sound and reasonable option for increasing energy intake, up to a point. The point at which it becomes unreasonable is when the person's energy needs outstrip the capacity to eat enough food to provide them. At that point the person must find ways of adding food energy to the diet, mostly through the addition of refined sugars and fats. Still, this energy-rich diet must be superimposed on the nutrient-rich choices for adequacy. Energy alone is not enough.

In addition to carbohydrate, athletes need protein. How much of what kinds of foods supply enough protein to meet the needs of athletes? The exchange lists, of course, point out rich protein sources, and meats and milk head the list. To suggest that athletes eat more than the recommended servings of meat would be narrow advice for many reasons. For one thing, athletes must protect themselves from heart disease, and even lean meats contain fat, much of it saturated fat.

Earlier in this chapter Table 10–2 showed some possible protein intakes for a 70-kilogram athlete based on recommendations of various authorities. It is likely that an athlete weighing 70 kilograms who exercises vigorously on a daily basis could require 3000 calories per day. To meet such an energy requirement, an athlete could select from a variety of nutrient-dense foods. Figure 10–5 on the next page provides one example; it itemizes the foods added to the Monday's meal selections pictured in Chapter 2 to attain a 3000-calorie diet. In addition to the items listed, 2 percent lowfat milk replaced the nonfat milk. These meals supply 124 grams of protein, an amount greater than all but the highest recommended level of 2 g/kg/day (140 g/day) for such a person. Obviously the more energy an athlete requires, the more protein that athlete will receive, assuming the foods chosen are nutrient dense. The meals provide 61 percent of their calories from carbohydrate. Athletes who train exhaustively and who train for endurance events may want to aim for somewhat higher carbohydrate levels—from 65 to 70 percent. Beyond these specific concerns of total energy, protein, and carbohydrate, the diet most beneficial to athletic performance is remarkably similar to the diet of most people.

Table 10–5 shows some sample diet plans for athletes who wish to increase their energy and carbohydrate intakes. These plans are effective only if the user chooses foods to provide nutrients as well as energy—extra milk for calcium and riboflavin, many fruits and vegetables for folate and vitamin C, modest portions of lean meat, and especially red meat for iron[62] and other vitamins and minerals, and whole grains for B vitamins, magnesium, zinc, and chromium. In addition, these foods provide plenty of sodium, potassium, and chloride.

Athletes may eat particular foods or practice rituals before competition that convey psychological advantages. One eats steak the night before; another spoons up honey at the start of the event. As long as these foods or rituals remain harmless, they should be respected. Still, science has recommendations for the **pregame meal.** Generally it should be light (300 to 1000 calories) and

carbohydrate loading: a regimen of exhaustive exercise followed by consuming a high-carbohydrate diet that enables muscles to store glycogen beyond their normal capacity; also called glycogen loading or glycogen supercompensation.

pregame meal: a light meal eaten three to four hours before athletic competition.

To make glycogen, muscles need carbohydrate, but they also need rest, so vary daily exercise routines to work different muscles on different days.

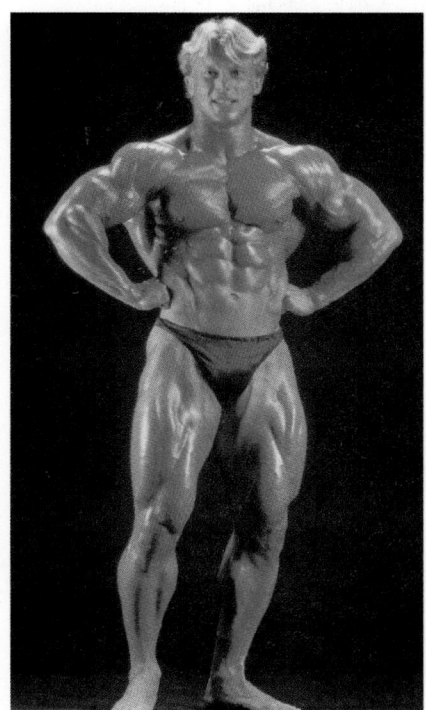

This is a body that vegetables built: Andreas Cahling, a vegetarian.

■■■ Figure 10–5

An Athlete's Meals. This figure shows how to modify Monday's Meal selections of Chapter 2 (pp. 52–53) to meet an athlete's needs.

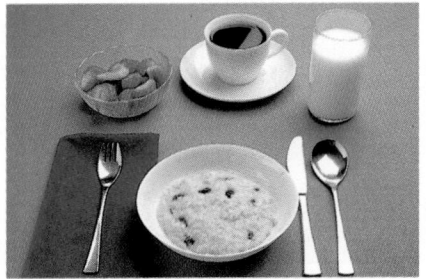

The original breakfast *plus:*
  2 pieces whole-wheat toast
  4 tsp jelly
  1/2 c orange juice
  2 tsp brown sugar on the oatmeal
  2% fat milk instead of nonfat

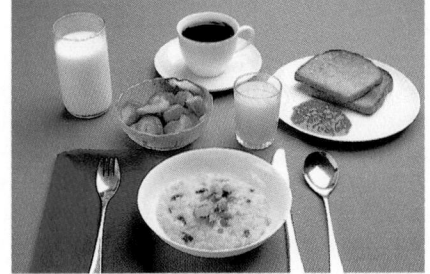
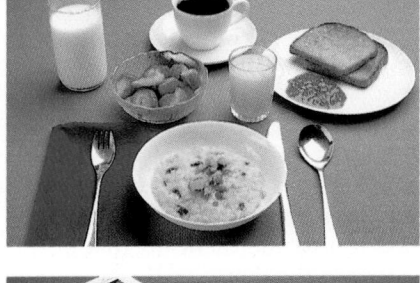

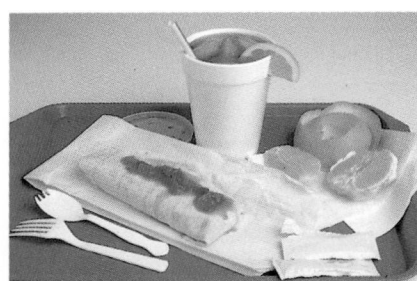

The original morning snack

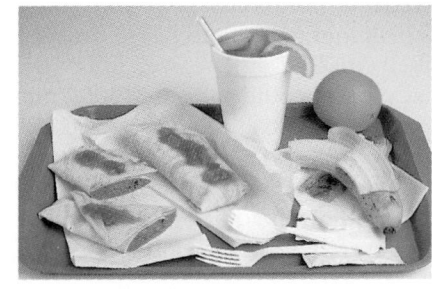

The original lunch *plus:*
  1 beef and bean burrito
  1 banana

Plus an afternoon snack:
  1 c 2% fat milk
  1 piece angel food cake

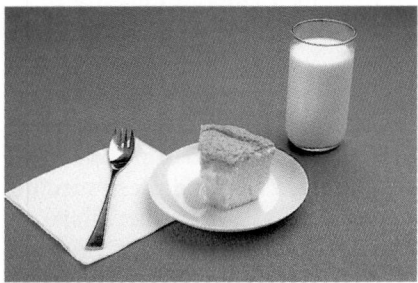

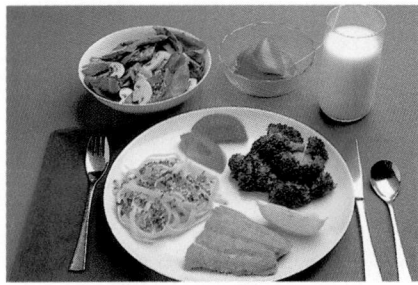

The original dinner *plus:*
  1 dinner roll
  2 tsp butter
  1/4 c noodles
  1/2 c sherbet
  2% fat milk instead of nonfat

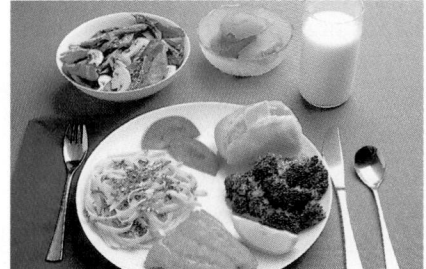

Total cal: 1759
57% cal from carbohydrate
24% cal from fat
19% cal from protein

Total cal: 3119
61% cal from carbohydrate
24% cal from fat
15% cal from protein

easy to digest and should contain fluids. The competitor should finish eating three to four hours before competition to allow time for the stomach to empty before exertion because digestion interferes with muscle work.[63]

Breads, potatoes, pasta, and fruit juices—carbohydrate-rich foods low in fat, protein, and fiber—are the basis of the pregame meal. Fiber-rich, bulky foods such as raw vegetables or whole grains, while usually desirable, are best avoided at the pregame meal. Fiber in the digestive tract attracts water out of the blood and can cause stomach discomfort during performance. Some athletes prefer liquid meals that are commercially available and easy to digest.

The person who wants to excel physically will apply the most accurate nutrition knowledge along with dedication to rigorous training. A diet that provides ample fluid and consists of a variety of nutrient-dense foods in quantities to meet energy needs will not only enhance athletic performance but overall health as well. Training and genetics being equal, who would win a competition—the person who habitually consumes less than the amounts of nutrients needed or one who arrives at the event with a long history of full nutrient stores and well-met metabolic needs?

Good ideas for a pregame meal:
Apricot nectar, pineapple juice, grape juice, jello, sherbet, popsicles, jams, jellies, honey toast, pancakes with syrup, baked white or sweet potatoes, pasta with steamed vegetables, raisins, figs, dates, frozen yogurt, graham crackers, sponge cake, angel-food cake.

Not recommended:
Stuffing, muffins, biscuits, croissants, french fries, onion rings, potato chips, meats, cheese, pasta with meat and cheese, pies, ice cream, eggnog, creams, nuts, butter, gravy, mayonnaise, salad dressing, frosted cakes.

■■■ Table 10–5 Examples of High-Carbohydrate Food Patterns for Various Energy Levels

CALORIES PROVIDED		1200[a]	1500[b]	2000	2500	3000	4000	5000
TYPE OF FOOD	REPRESENTATIVE SERVING SIZE				NUMBER OF SERVINGS			
Lowfat milk (2%)	1 cup (1 exchange)	2	2	3	3	4	6	8
Vegetable	1/2 cup (1 exchange)	2	5	6	7	10	12	14
Fruit	1/2 cup (1 exchange)	2	5	7	10	11	14	20
Starchy vegetable or grain	1/2 cup or 1 slice (1 exchange)	4	6	7	9	10	14	18
Meat[c] or meat alternate	2 1/2 ounces (2 1/2 exchanges)	2	2	2	2	4	4	4
Fat	1 teaspoon (1 exchange)	2	2	3	4	5	6	8

[a]The servings presented in this column represent only a core plan to provide adequate protein and to supply most of the vitamins and minerals people need daily. This basic plan provides about 50% of its energy as carbohydrate, 20% as protein, and 30% as fat.
[b]Plans 2 through 7 provide 55% to 61% of total energy as carbohydrate, 17% to 22% as protein, and 21% to 25% as fat.
[c]This table differs from Table 2–7 of Chapter 2 in that it suggests numbers of servings, not single exchanges. It also gives values for medium-fat meats, but try to choose mostly low-fat meats. (See Appendix D for meats and other food exchanges.)
SOURCE: L. K. Debruyne, F. S. Sizer, E. N. Whitney, The Fitness Triad: Motivation, Training, and Nutrition (St. Paul, Minn.: West, 1991).

▌▌▌ SELF-STUDY

Evaluate Your Food Choices

1. The preceding Self-Studies have revealed the strengths and weaknesses of your nutrient intakes and energy balance. By now you may be looking at foods in a new light. Knowing what nutrients your diet tends to lack, you may be interested in finding foods that are especially rich in those nutrients. If you need to limit calories, you may need to find foods that supply those nutrients for the lowest possible calorie cost. You will recognize this description as the definition of a *nutrient-dense food* (Chapter 2).

Review your food records and select three nutrients that your diet supplies in the smallest quantities relative to your need. (For many young women, these nutrients might be vitamin A, calcium, and iron.) Enter the names of these nutrients in the spaces provided at the tops of columns A, B, and C in Form 9 (Appendix F). Now make a list of ten foods you like and would be willing to eat frequently that might supply these nutrients in significant quantities. List these foods in the first column of Form 8. List the size of the serving of each food that you would eat, and look up the amounts of nutrients 1, 2, and 3 and the calories that each serving would supply. Express the amount of nutrient 1 as a percentage of your RDA, round it off to the nearest whole number, and enter it in column A of the form. (For example, suppose you

selected vitamin A as a nutrient of importance to you and your RDA was 800 RE. Suppose you choose one peach as a food you might like to eat. Appendix A reveals that one peach offers 47 RE of vitamin A. That's 5.875 percent of your RDA—the calculation is 47 divided by 800 times 100. Round off to 6, and enter that number in column A of the form.) Perform a similar calculation for nutrients 2 and 3, and enter the results in columns B and C of the form.

Now express the amount of calories the food would supply as a percentage of your recommended intake of energy, and enter the result in column D of the form. (Example: Suppose your recommended intake of energy is 2000 calories. A peach supplies 37 calories. That's about 2 percent of your energy need for the day.)

Divide A by D and enter the result in column E. This number represents the amount of nutrient 1 the food supplies relative to your need, compared with the amount of energy the food supplies relative to your need. (Example: A peach offers 6 percent of your need for vitamin A and only 2 percent of the calories you can eat, so it gets a 3 for this nutrient.) Divide B by D and enter in column F; and divide C by D and enter in column G to obtain similar scores for the next two nutrients. Now add columns E, F, and G to obtain a nutrient score for the

food. This score, which is arbitrary (created by us), serves as a basis for comparing this food with other foods as a source of the nutrients you most need. The higher this score is, the more of that food you can eat without running through your calorie allowance before you have met your nutrient needs.

Don't stop at ten foods if this exercise interests you. Don't stop at three nutrients either. (We did only because we ran out of horizontal space on the page.) You have much to learn about the virtues of food for meeting your particular nutrient needs by making comparisons of this kind.

2. Finally, you are prepared to make a judgment about supplements, as suggested at the very end of the first Self-Study: Record what you eat. Review your records once again. In light of the food choices you are now making, is there any nutrient in which your diet falls short of the RDA? If so, describe the supplement you would need, and set about obtaining it.

Notes

1. S. N. Blair and coauthors, Physical fitness and all-cause mortality, *Journal of the American Medical Association* 262 (1989): 2395–2401.

2. V. Gurley, A. Neuringer, and J. Massee, Dance and sports compared: Effects on psychological well-being, *Journal of Sports Medicine* 24 (1984): 58–68.

3. K. T. Francis and R. Carter, Psychological characteristics of joggers, *Journal of Sports Medicine* 22 (1982): 386–391; R. M. Hayden and G. J. Allen, Relationship between aerobic exercise,

anxiety, and depression: Convergent validation by knowledgeable informants, *Journal of Sports Medicine* 24 (1984): 69–74.

4. Quantity and quality of exercise for developing and maintaining fitness in healthy adults, a position paper of The American College of Sports Medicine, *The Physician and Sportsmedicine,* October 1978, pp. 39–41.

5. N. E. Lane, D. A. Block, and H. H. Jones, Long distance running, bone density, and osteoarthritis, *Journal of the American Medical Association* 255 (1986): 1147–1151.

6. Quantity and quality of exercise, 1978.

7. S. Rainville and P. Vaccaro, Lipoprotein cholesterol levels, coronary artery disease and regular exercise: A review, *American Corrective Therapy Journal* 37 (1983): 161–165; B. Stamford, Improving coronary circulation, *The Physician and Sportsmedicine* 11, November 1983, p. 163.

8. N. B. Belloc and L. Breslow, Relationship of physical health status and health practices, *Preventive Medicine* 1 (1972): 409–421.

9. C. M. Tipton, Exercise, training, and hypertension, *Exercise and Sports Sciences Review* 12 (1984): 245–306.

10. K. Jung, Physical exercise therapy in juvenile diabetes mellitus, *Journal of Sports Medicine* 22 (1982): 23–31.

11. D. H. Garabrant and coauthors, Job activity and colon cancer risk, *American Journal of Epidemiology* 119 (1984): 1005–1014.

12. A. Viti and coauthors, Effect of exercise on plasma interferon levels, *Journal of Applied Physiology,* August 1985, pp. 426–428; H. B. Simon, The immunology of exercise, *Journal of the American Medical Association* 252 (1984): 2735–2738; J. G. Cannon and M. J. Kluger, Exercise enhances survival rate in mice infected with *Salmonella typhimurium, Proceedings of the Society for Experimental Biology and Medicine* 175 (1984): 518–521.

13. Much of this discussion about fitness is derived from Chapter 7, Fitness, F. S. Sizer and E. N. Whitney, *Life Choices: Health Concepts and Strategies* (St. Paul, Minn.: West, 1988).

14. B. Saltin and P. Gollnick, Skeletal muscle adaptability: Significance for metabolism and performance, in *Handbook of Physiology: Skeletal Muscle,* eds. L. D. Peachey, R. H. Adrian, and S. R. Geiger (Bethesda, Md.: American Physiological Society, 1983), pp. 555–631.

15. Saltin and Gollnick, 1983.

16. E. H. Christensen and O. Hansen, Arbeitsfahigkeit und ehrnahrung, *Skandinavisches Archiv fuer Physiologie* 8 (1939): 160–175, as cited in E. L. Fox, *Sports Physiology,* 2nd ed. (New York: Saunders, 1984), pp. 40–57.

17. E. Jequier, Carbohydrates: Energetics and performance, *Nutrition Reviews* 44 (1986): 55–59.

18. R. C. Hickson, Carbohydrate metabolism in exercise, *Report of the Ross Symposium on Nutrient Utilization during Exercise* (Columbus, Ohio: Ross Laboratories, 1983), pp. 1–8.

19. J. M. Davis and coauthors, Carbohydrate-electrolyte drinks: Effects on endurance cycling in the heat, *American Journal of Clinical Nutrition* 48 (1988): 1023–1030.

20. F. Dolgener and C. Larsen, Effect of acute exercise on resting metabolic rate in obese and non-obese females (abstract), *Medicine and Science in Sports and Exercise* 16 (1984): 161.

21. G. Holm and coauthors, Effects of submaximal physical exercise on adipose tissue metabolism in man, *International Journal of Obesity* 1 (1977): 249–257.

22. R. Bielinski, Y. Schutz, and E. Jequier, Energy metabolism during the postexercise recovery in man, *American Journal of Clinical Nutrition* 42 (1985): 69–82.

23. P. W. R. Lemon, K. E. Yarasheski, and D. Dolny, The importance of protein for athletes, *Sports Medicine* 1 (1984): 474–484.

24. P. Babij and F. W. Booth, Biochemistry of exercise: Advances in molecular biology relevant to adaptation of muscle to exercise, *Sports Medicine* 5 (1988): 137–143.

25. J. F. Hickson and coauthors, Failure of weight training to affect urinary indices of protein metabolism in men, *Medicine and Science in Sports and Exercise* 18 (1986): 563–567.

26. Babij and Booth, 1988.

27. J. R. Brotherhood, Nutrition and sports performance, *Sports Medicine* 1 (1984): 350–389.

28. Lemon, Yarasheski, and Dolny, 1984.

29. Brotherhood, 1984.

30. P. W. R. Lemon, Protein and exercise: Update 1987, *Medicine and Science in Sports and Exercise* 19 (1987): S179–S188.

31. Lemon, 1987.

32. G. J. Kasperek and R. D. Snider, Effect of exercise intensity and starvation on activation of branched-chain keto acid dehydrogenase by exercise, *American Journal of Physiology* 252 (1987): E33–E37, as cited by Lemon, 1987.

33. Position of the American Dietetic Association: Nutrition for physical fitness and athletic performance for adults, *Journal of the American Dietetic Association* 87 (1987): 933–939.

34. I. Gontzea, R. Sutzescu, and S. Dumitrache, The influence of adaptation to physical effort on nitrogen balance in man, *Nutrition Reports International* 11 (1975): 231–236.

35. H. Yoshimura and coauthors, Anaemia during hard physical training (sports anaemia) and its causal mechanism with special reference to protein nutrition, *World Review of Nutrition and Dietetics* 35 (1980): 1–86.

36. Use of nutritional supplements by athletes, in *Nutrition and Athletic Performance,* eds. W. Haskell, J. Scala, and J. Whitman (Palo Alto, Calif.: Bull Publishing, 1982), pp. 106–155.

37. M. H. Williams, The role of vitamins in physical activity, in *Nutritional Aspects of Human Physical and Athletic Performance,* 2nd ed. (Springfield, Ill.: Charles C. Thomas, 1985), pp. 147–185.

38. A. Belko and coauthors, Effects of exercise on riboflavin requirements: Biological validation in weight reducing women, *American Journal of Clinical Nutrition* 41 (1985): 270–277.

39. Williams, 1985.

40. Williams, 1985.

41. V. Herbert, N. Colman, and E. Jacob, Folic acid and vitamin B_{12}, in *Modern Nutrition in Health and Disease,* 6th ed., eds. R. S. Goodhart and M. E. Shils (Philadelphia, Pa.: Lea and Febiger, 1980), pp. 229–259.

42. K. Gohil and coauthors, Effect of exercise training on tissue vitamin E and ubiquinone content, *Journal of Applied Physiology* 63 (1987): 1638–1641.

43. M. E. Nelson and coauthors, Diet and bone status in amenorrheic runners, *American Journal of Clinical Nutrition* 43 (1986): 910–916.

44. J. E. Benson and coauthors, Relationship between nutrient intake, body mass index, menstrual function, and ballet injury, *Journal of the American Dietetic Association* 89 (1989): 58–63.

45. B. B. Peterkin, Women's diets: 1977 and 1985, *Journal of Nutrition Education* 18 (1986): 251–257.

46. L. W. Rosen, Pathogenic weight-control behavior in female athletes, *Physician and Sportsmedicine,* January 1986, pp. 79–86.

47. P. K. Welch and coauthors, Nutrition education, body composition, and dietary intake of female college athletes, *Physician and Sportsmedicine,* January 1987, pp. 63–64, 67–69, 73–74.

48. A. C. Snyder, L. L. Dvorak, and J. B. Roepke, Influence of dietary iron source on measures of iron status among female runners, *Medicine and Science in Sports and Exercise* 21 (1989): 7–10.

49. P. A. Deuster and coauthors, Nutritional survey of highly trained women runners, *American Journal of Clinical Nutrition* 44 (1986): 954–962.

50. D. Benardot, M. Schwartz, and D. Heller, Nutrient intake in young, highly competitive gymnasts, *Journal of the American Dietetic Association,* 89 (1989): 401–403.

51. W. B. Strong and coauthors, The effect of iron therapy on the exercise capacity of nonanemic iron-deficient adolescent runners, *American Journal of Diseases of Children* 142 (1988): 165–169.

52. R. H. Dressendorfer, C. E. Wade, and E. A. Amsterdam, Development of pseudoanemia in marathon runners during a 20-day road race, *Journal of the American Medical Association* 246 (1981): 1215–1218.

53. Food and Nutrition Board, *Recommended Dietary Allowances,* 10th ed. (Washington, D.C.: National Academy of Sciences, 1989), p. 200.

54. W. W. Campbell and R. A. Anderson, Effects of aerobic exercise and training on the trace minerals chromium, zinc, and copper, *Sports Medicine* 4 (1987): 9–18.

55. Williams, 1985, p. 213.

56. G. Stendig-Lindberg, Changes in serum magnesium concentration after strenuous exercise, *Journal of the American College of Nutrition* 6 (1987): 35–40.

57. M. H. Williams, Vitamin supplementation and physical performance, *Report of the Ross Symposium on Nutrient Utilization During Exercise* (Columbus, Ohio: Ross Laboratories, 1983), pp. 26–30.

58. J. E. Greenleaf and coauthors, Drinking and water balance during exercise and heat acclimation, *Journal of Applied Physiology: Respiratory, Environmental and Exercise Physiology* 54 (1983): 414–419.

59. J. M. Davis and coauthors, Carbohydrate-electrolyte drinks: Effects on endurance cycling in the heat, *American Journal of Clinical Nutrition* 48 (1988): 1023–1030.

60. S. A. Tilgner and M. R. Schiller, Dietary intakes of female college athletes: The need for nutrition education, *Journal of the American Dietetic Association* 89 (1989): 967–969; D. R. Green and coauthors, An evaluation of dietary intakes of triathletes: are RDA's being met? *Journal of the American Dietetic Association* 89 (1989): 1653–1654.

61. J. L. Ivy and coauthors, Muscle glycogen synthesis after exercise: Effect of time of carbohydrate ingestion, *Journal of Applied Physiology* 64 (1988): 1480–1485.

62. Snyder, 1989.

63. American Dietetic Association, 1987.

▐▐▐ C O N T R O V E R S Y   1 0 ▐▐▐

Are Fat Calories More Fattening?

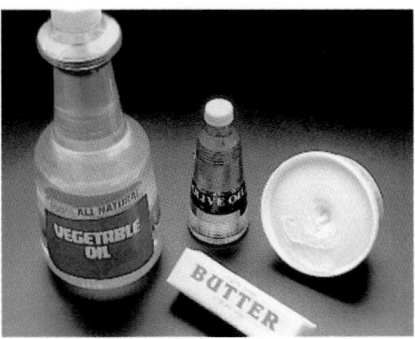

Chapter 9 taught that body weight depends on the balance between "calories in" and "calories out." Simple enough. That is the traditional way of thinking. But this tidy mathematical formula has always posed problems for real people who try to use it. Some people's bodies do not seem to obey the rule that 3500 extra calories of either butter or potatoes puts on a pound of body fat. When such people limit calories, they fail to lose weight. Why?

Genetics may hold a part of the answer to that question. Some people's bodies probably are inherently more conservative with their fuels and thus tend to store more fat than others. Another partial answer might be that people who fail to lose weight lead sedentary lives. Even if they eat reasonable quantities of food, they may be exercising so little that they cannot lose weight. This Controversy explores a new possibility originating from new, exciting research showing that the composition of the diet with regard to fat may influence body fatness more than the diet's total calorie count. In other words, it may make a world of difference to body fatness whether you choose extra butter or extra potatoes. This Controversy explores the new avenues of research that seem to indicate that calories of fat are more fattening than those of carbohydrate or protein.[1]

How did this line of thinking come to light?
As often happens in science, researchers were testing an unrelated theory when they stumbled onto some interesting clues. A study designed to determine whether a fat-rich diet can lead rats to overeat proceeded normally.[2] Rats were fed a high-fat diet (42 percent of the calories from fat), and they voluntarily ate a smaller quantity of food than rats given a control diet, so that they received the same number of calories as the controls. It was as if the rats had internal calorie counters that determined just how much food energy they needed to eat to match the amount of energy they expended.

Then the researchers noticed something strange—even though both groups ate the same number of calories of food energy, the rats eating the fat-rich diet became severely obese. The rats' body composition changed to over 50 percent body fat, whereas the control rats remained at 30 percent body fat. Thus it appears, for rats, anyway, that a high-fat diet may induce obesity even with a moderate food-energy intake. In rats, then, food energy alone cannot explain obesity; the fat content of the diet seems to play a role too.

So the researchers discovered that rats don't eat more total food energy when their food contains a lot of fat. Is the same true of people?
When researchers decided to study people instead of rats in this way, the findings were slightly different. One study allowed women to eat freely from three different diet plans: a low-fat diet (15 to 20 percent of calories from fat), a medium-fat diet (30 to 35 percent), and a high-fat diet (45 to 50 percent).[3] The women followed each plan for two weeks. The foods in each diet plan were similar in taste and appearance; they differed only in the percentages of calories contributed by fat (and therefore by carbohydrate as well). Unlike rats, the women did eat more food energy from the high-fat diet than from the other diets, although they compensated a little for the diet's fat content. One factor—the percentage of calories from fat—influenced total calorie intakes the most: the more fat in the diet, the more calories of food energy the women consumed. But they compensated as best they could: the more fat in the diet, the less total bulk of food the women consumed.

The reason why the women failed to compensate fully is that fat occupies so little bulk. For example, only 2 teaspoons of fat in an 80-calorie glass of nonfat milk more than doubles the calories to 170. Therefore, to successfully replace nonfat milk with whole milk while keeping calories constant, one would have to reduce the total milk portion drunk by more than half. The women in this study tended to cut down on total food when its fat content was high but did not do so to the extent necessary to keep calories constant. *I would guess that the womens' weight went up.*

Yes, their body weight changed, as you guessed. Women eating low-fat diets lost weight, while women on high-fat diets gained. Whether the total calories, the total fat, or both were responsible for the weight changes was unclear.

The above experiment asked the question whether people given a high-fat diet tend to overeat. The answer seems to be yes, although they compensate somewhat. When food is fat-rich, people consume more calories than they need. This may help to account for the obesity seen in Americans eating a fat-rich diet today. *Chapter 5 stated that fat in food lends a feeling of satiety. Why wouldn't people stop eating after getting enough calories from fat to meet their energy needs?*

Chapter 5 is correct—meals with fat do lend satiety, and the feeling of fullness lasts longer than after eating meals low in fat. However, satiety is complex, and another finding suggests that people also need to eat carbohydrate for satiety. An experiment was designed to study intakes of fat and energy when men were allowed to eat freely first from a high-fat diet and then from a normal diet.[4] In this study the men overate when they consumed the high-fat diet, taking in over 1000 calories per day more than when they were eating the normal diet. The researchers suspected that the

men ate until they had obtained a certain amount of *carbohydrate,* that is, that the men were deriving their satiety from carbohydrate, regardless of the amount of fat accompanying that carbohydrate. It could be that the body's satiety mechanism is geared to a certain threshold intake of carbohydrate and that only after that amount is eaten does the person feel satisfied.

If people do, indeed, eat to obtain a certain amount of carbohydrate, then the higher the diet is in fat relative to carbohydrate, the more fat and total food energy (calories) they will have to eat before they are satisfied. Thus restricting dietary carbohydrate may lead to obesity by way of inducing people to eat too much total fat.

I know that total food energy (calories) affects body fatness. Does food fat do more than just contribute calories?

Because dietary fat contributes to energy intake so dramatically, researchers have difficulty distinguishing whether total energy or fat itself has a greater influence on obesity development. One group of scientists studied 155 obese men who were eating a "typical American diet"—about 15 percent of total calories from protein, 38 percent from carbohydrate, 41 percent from fat, and 6 percent from alcohol.[5] Their total average food-energy intakes (2570 calories per day) fell short of current recommendations (2900 calories per day).[6] Researchers found no correlation between total food-energy intakes and the men's body fat measurements. They did, however, find that the more *fat* a

man ate, the fatter was his body and, conversely, that the more carbohydrate a man took in, the lower his body fat. These findings suggest that when people eat diets high in fat, they tend to preserve their body fat efficiently, even with moderate food-energy intakes.

Another study showed the same relationship to hold true in women: those who ate higher fat diets had higher body-fat contents than total energy intake alone would predict.[7] Once again the data suggested that dietary fat plays a role in the development of obesity independently of total energy intake.

In still another study, researchers compared 244 adults with respect to their body composition and the composition of their diets and found that those people who ate the highest fat foods had the highest percentages of body fat.[8] When researchers provided either high-fat or moderate diets to men who were attempting to gain weight, they found that to achieve the same amount of weight gain required less time and fewer calories for those eating the high-fat diets than for those eating the moderate diets.[9]

So high-fat diets really do push body composition toward increased fatness?

Yes, these experiments all seem to show that they do. Apparently even with moderate food-energy intakes, people convert large percentages of their dietary fat to body fat.[10] The picture that comes to mind is that immediately after a meal, when fat levels in the blood are high, fat storage cells take up that fat and store it. The remainder of this Controversy explores possible underlying reasons for fat's being more fattening than the other energy-yielding nutrients.

Chapter 1 first explained that dietary proteins and carbohydrates offer the body 4 calories of energy per gram, whereas dietary fats offer 9 calories per gram. Chapter 5 mentioned that these values are derived from laboratory experiments in which foods are burned and that the body may differ from the laboratory. One of those differences is that, unlike laboratory experiments, the body is not perfect in its conservation of fuel. The body loses a small percentage of the food energy in a meal over the several hours that follow. The energy escapes as heat in the **thermic effect of food (TEF)**—the energy required to digest food and to absorb, transport, metabolize, and store nutrients. The remaining energy is all that is available to the body.

How does TEF relate to the question of the fattening power of fat?
A person spends about 10 percent of a meal's total energy on TEF, but this varies considerably, depending on the composition of the meal.[11] A high-carbohydrate meal uses more energy in TEF than does a high-fat meal.[12] As dietary carbohydrate increases, the TEF of the meal increases. Not only that, but a high-carbohydrate meal enhances the TEF of the next meal consumed.[13] The body tends to be inefficient in using food energy from a high-carbohydrate diet. In contrast, as the percentage of fat in the diet increases, TEF heat production declines.[14]

Thus while the amount of energy available from foods (as measured in calories) may be the same in diets of different composition, the *efficiency* with which the body uses or stores that energy may vary considerably, depending on the diet's composition.
Does this mean that the numbers of calories assigned to a gram of fat or carbohydrate are wrong?
No, the numbers are correct—for the number of calories of energy contained by a food. But scientists may need to assign new values for the calories the body actually derives from that food. To that end, researchers again studied rats to compare the efficiency of sucrose, protein sources, and fat in providing the body with energy. When compared with sucrose (whose energy factor was assumed, as usual, to be 4 calories per gram), fat was so much more efficient that it appeared to provide the equivalent of 11 calories per gram.[15] These researchers suggest that the commonly accepted values of 9 calories per gram for fat and 4 for carbohydrate may not always correspond perfectly to the amounts of calories the body uses or stores.[16] Of course, fat cannot provide more calories than it contains, so researchers now are questioning the assumption that carbohydrate yields 4 calories per gram. Perhaps, from the body's standpoint, the factor 9 for fat is accurate enough, but for the less-efficient carbohydrate, the factor should be only 3 calories per gram.
Why is the body so efficient at storing dietary fat as body fat?
To convert a molecule of food fat to body fat, the body need only disassemble triglycerides to fatty acids and glycerol, absorb the parts, and put them back together again. To convert a molecule of sucrose to fat, however, the body has to split the glucose from fructose, absorb them, dismantle them into small fragments, then assemble the fragments into fatty acid chains, and finally attach them to a glycerol backbone to make a triglyceride. This work demands many calories of energy. Thus the costs of converting dietary fat to body fat are far less than those of converting dietary carbohydrate to body fat. In general, the converting dietary fat to body fat requires only 3 percent of the ingested calories; but the shift from dietary carbohydrate to body fat requires 23 percent of ingested energy.[17]

Clearly, from all of the experiments reported here, a diet's total calories are not the only variable that predicts whether fat will be stored or not. The total fat, the total carbohydrate, and the fat-to-carbohydrate ratio of the diet also matter.
Okay. So a high-fat diet leads to obesity. That's not surprising. But a diet low in fat is usually high in carbohydrate. Doesn't excess carbohydrate also lead to obesity?
Carbohydrates and fats each contribute large shares to both a person's energy intake and output. Recall from Chapter 4 that the body handles some excess carbohydrate by storing it as glycogen. Just as dietary fat efficiently converts to body fat, dietary carbohydrate efficiently becomes glycogen at the cost of only 7 percent of ingested calories.[18] The body does not

---

▮▮▮ Miniglossary

thermic effect of foods (TEF): energy required to digest food and to absorb, transport, metabolize, and store nutrients.

---

convert glucose to fat until after glycogen stores have filled, and then that fat made from carbohydrate does not seem to contribute much to the body's fat stores.[19]

Thus a high-carbohydrate diet, regardless of its total food-energy content in calories, increases body fat stores very little, if at all.[20] As was apparent in Chapter 10, large intakes of carbohydrates encourage glycogen storage, not fat deposition.[21] For carbohydrate to contribute significantly to body fat requires a carbohydrate intake that exceeds by far the body's total energy need for several consecutive days. The sheer bulk of carbohydrate-rich, low-fat foods sufficient to supply this much energy would discourage even people with the largest appetites from eating too much. Thus dietary carbohydrate unaccompanied by excess fat poses little threat to energy balance and weight control.

Chapter 10 taught that the mix of fuels used by the body depends partly on the composition of the diet. Does this affect body fatness?
Yes. Energy balance and body weight require that the body burn a mix of fuels in similar proportions to the mix of fuels in the diet.[22] The composition of the diet partly determines body fat and glycogen stores, and it also affects how much of each fuel is burned for energy.

The body maintains its carbohydrate stores by adjusting the balance between fuel intake and fuel use.[23] In other words, when carbohydrate intake rises or falls, the body uses more or less glucose for fuel.[24] The body's change of fuel mix in response to changing dietary carbohydrate intakes occurs with much more precision than it does for changing fat intakes, most likely because it must: glycogen stores are small and run out quickly, so glucose is used conservatively when the diet supplies only small amounts. Also, glycogen storage space is limited, so when stores are full to overflowing, the body uses *more* glucose. Fat reserves, in contrast, exceed glycogen reserves by about 100-fold, and the body has no need to conserve fat should the diet be low in fat. Conversely, fat storage space is unlimited, so if you eat more fat, the body doesn't bother to burn it off.

A full explanation for why people gain and lose weight remains open. This Controversy has focused narrowly on the body's efficiency in handling various fuels from the diet. Besides diet composition and the extent to which the body is conditioned, other factors such as genetics, age, smoking, and alcohol intake also influence the body's metabolic efficiency.[25] As research continues, people can begin

to apply what is known. And from what we now know about food fat, it is clearly wise to habitually select low-fat, high-carbohydrate whole foods. This is the way a person can control body weight most easily. The person who wants to lose weight, and calculates only calories and makes no distinctions about their sources, must fight an uphill battle.

Notes

1. This Controversy is adapted from S. R. Rolfes, *A Matter of Fat: Emerging Insights into Obesity Development* (a 1990 monograph in the *Nutrition Clinics* series available from J. B. Lippincott Company, East Washington Square, Philadelphia, PA 19105).
2. L. B. Oscai, M. M. Brown, and W. C. Miller, Effect of dietary fat on food intake, growth and body composition in rats, *Growth* 48 (1984): 415–424.
3. L. Lissner, Dietary fat and the regulation of energy intake in human subjects, *American Journal of Clinical Nutrition* 46 (1987): 886–892.
4. A. Tremblay and coauthors, Impact of dietary fat content and fat oxidation on energy intake in humans, *American Journal of Clinical Nutrition* 49 (1989): 799–805.
5. D. M. Dreon and coauthors, Dietary fat:carbohydrate ratio and obesity in middle-aged men, *American Journal of Clinical Nutrition* 47 (1988): 995–1000.
6. Food and Nutrition Board, *Recommended Dietary Allowances,* 10th ed. (Washington, D.C.: National Academy Press, 1989), p. 33.

7. I. Romieu, Energy intake and other determinants of relative weight, *American Journal of Clinical Nutrition* 47 (1988): 406–412.

8. Tremblay, 1989.

9. E. Danforth, Diet and obesity, *American Journal of Clinical Nutrition* 41 (1985): 1132–1145.

10. K. A. Donato and D. M. Hegsted, Efficiency of utilization of various sources of energy for growth, *Proceedings of the National Academy of Sciences* 82 (1985): 4866–4870.

11. Danforth, 1985.

12. R. S. Schwartz and coauthors, The thermic effect of carbohydrate versus fat feeding in man, *Metabolism* 34 (1985): 285–293.

13. Danforth, 1985.

14. G. A. Leveille and P. F. Cloutier, Isocaloric diets: Effects of dietary changes, *American Journal of Clinical Nutrition* 45 (1987): 158–163.

15. Donato, 1985.

16. K. A. Donato, Efficiency and utilization of various energy sources for growth, *American Journal of Clinical Nutrition* 45 (1987): 164–167; Role of fat and fatty acids in modulation of energy exchange, *Nutrition Reviews* 46 (1988): 382–388.

17. Leveille, 1987; Danforth, 1985.

18. Danforth, 1985.

19. K. J. Acheson and coauthors, Glycogen storage capacity and de novo lipogenesis during massive carbohydrate overfeeding in man, *American Journal of Clinical Nutrition* 48 (1988): 240–247.

20. Danforth, 1985.

21. Acheson, 1988.

22. J. P. Flatt, Dietary fat, carbohydrate balance, and weight maintenance: Effects of exercise, *American Journal of Clinical Nutrition* 45 (1987): 296–306.

23. W. G. H. Abbott and coauthors, Short-term energy balance: Relationship with protein, carbohydrate, and fat balances, *American Journal of Physiology* 255 (1988): E332–E337.

24. J. P. Flatt, Effect of carbohydrate and fat intake on postprandial substrate oxidation and storage, *Topics in Clinical Nutrition* 2 (1987): 15–27.

25. Romieu, 1988.

CHAPTER 11

Nutrition and Disease Prevention

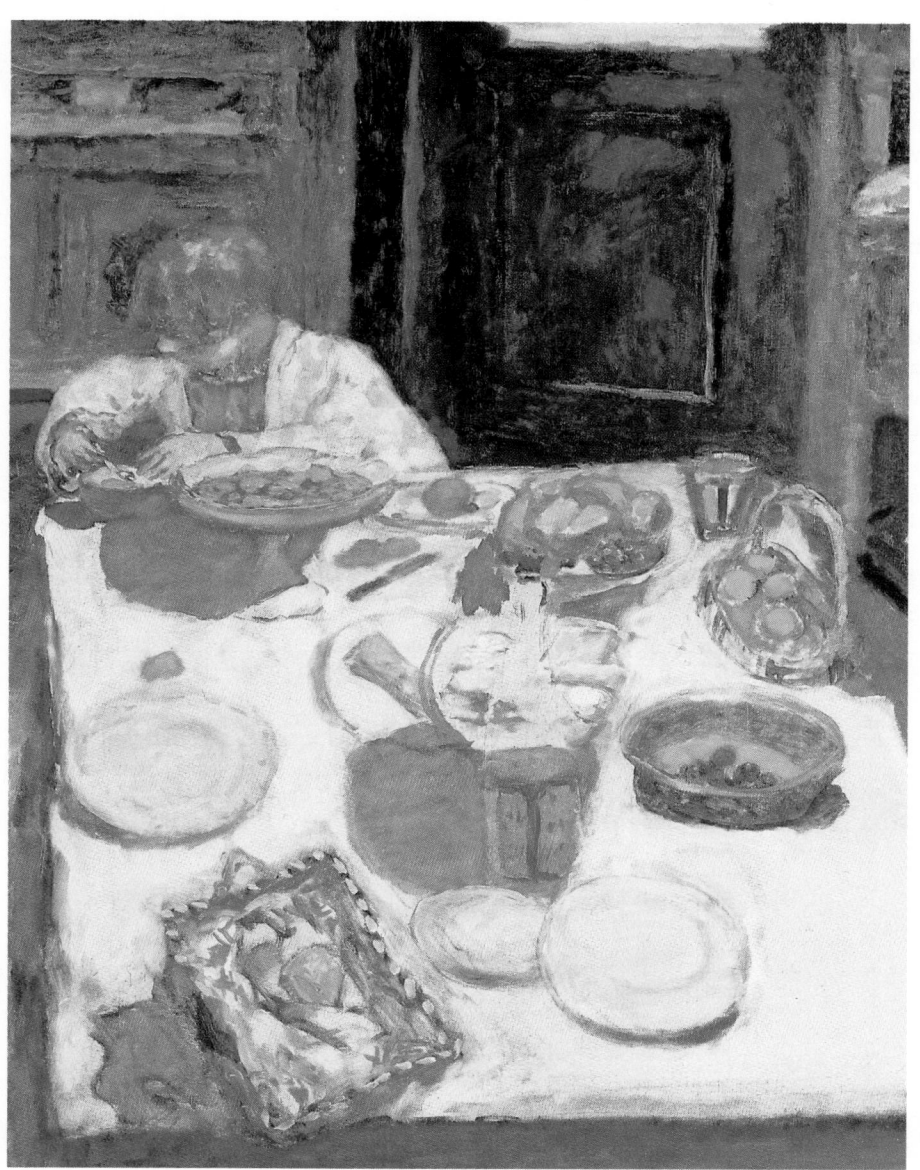

Pierre Bonnard, *The Table,* Tate Gallery/Art Resource, N.Y.

CONTENTS

▌▌▌ Throughout history our ancestors feared infectious diseases, such as tuberculosis, smallpox, and polio, that claimed many lives and curtailed the average life expectancy. Today medical research has bestowed upon us both prevention and cure for many of the infectious diseases. At least in developed nations, today's average life expectancy is considerably longer than that of 100 years ago. Our water supply is disinfected to prevent the spread of infection, and immunizations protect us individually; consequently most children live well into their later years. Despite these advances, though, infectious diseases can still make people sick, and even with medical treatments, they can kill or lead to consequences that last a lifetime (hepatitis, a liver infection, is associated with increased risk of liver cancer, for example). We are also faced with a fatal, incurable viral infection—AIDS.* While it is too much to claim that adequate nutrition can prevent infectious diseases, it is true that a healthy, well-nourished immune system fights daily to prevent minor infections from becoming major problems. It is also true that strict attention to the food safety rules presented in Chapter 14 can prevent many cases of infections, including hepatitis, from occurring.

While a few infectious diseases remain serious threats, the diseases we face most often are of a different nature. Table 11–1 shows today's top ten killer diseases, as identified by the *Surgeon General's Report*, 1988. Of the ten, five are associated directly with nutrition and three with excessive alcohol intake, which of course affects nutrition adversely (see table notes). Taken together, these eight conditions account for about three-fourths of the nation's 2 million

*AIDS is Acquired Immune Deficiency Syndrome, caused by infection with the HIV virus, which is transmitted primarily by sexual contact, by contact with infected blood, or by needles shared among drug users.

■■■ Table 11–1 The Ten Leading Causes of Illness and Death, United States, 1987

RANK	CAUSE OF DEATH	NUMBER	PERCENT OF TOTAL DEATHS
1[a]	Heart diseases	759,400	35.7
	(Coronary heart disease)	(511,700)	(24.1)
	(Other heart disease)	(247,700)	(11.6)
2[a]	Cancers	476,700	22.4
3[a]	Strokes	148,700	7.0
4[b]	Unintentional injuries	92,500	4.4
	(Motor vehicle)	(46,500)	(2.2)
	(All others)	(45,700)	(2.2)
5	Chronic obstructive lung disease	78,000	3.7
6	Pneumonia and influenza	68,600	3.2
7[a]	Diabetes mellitus	37,800	1.8
8[b]	Suicide	29,600	1.4
9[b]	Chronic liver disease and cirrhosis	26,000	1.2
10[a]	Atherosclerosis	23,100	1.1
	Total	2,125,100	100.0

[a]Causes of death in which diet plays a part.
[b]Causes of death in which excessive alcohol consumption plays a part.
SOURCE: National Center for Health Statistics, *Monthly Vital Statistics Report,* 37, no. 1 (1988), as cited in *The Surgeon General's Report on Nutrition and Health, Summary and Recommendations,* DHHS (PHS) publication no. 88-50211, (Washington, D.C.: Government Printing Office, 1988), Table 2, p. 4.

deaths each year. (The other two are chronic obstructive lung disease, which is most often related to smoking, and pneumonia/influenza, which strikes old people and infants whose defenses are weak.)

Poor nutrition is preventable, and the surgeon general urges that the nation's people make whatever dietary changes they can in the effort to improve their health status and outlook. Nutrition is important enough in disease prevention to warrant an entire chapter on the relationship between the two—mostly covering nutrition's role against degenerative diseases before they set in, its preventive role. First, however, this chapter takes a brief look at how nutrition helps to support the immune system and strengthens the body during disease. Even people who already have AIDS can benefit from proper nutrition.

▌▌▌ Nutrition and Immunity

Your immune system is your bodyguard. It accompanies you everywhere you go. It defends you so alertly and silently that you are not even aware of the thousands of enemy attacks mounted against you by microbes (germs) every day. If your immune system falters, though, you become vulnerable to disease-causing agents that you encounter, and infectious disease invariably follows.

Nutrients and the Immune System

Of all the body's systems, the immune system responds most sensitively to subtle changes in nutrition status. When people become ill and are unable to eat well, malnutrition often sets in, compromising immunity. Impaired immunity increases disease risk, disease states reduce food intake, and nutrition status suffers further. Thus disease and poor nutrition together form a downward spiral that must be broken for recovery to occur (Figure 11–1, next page).

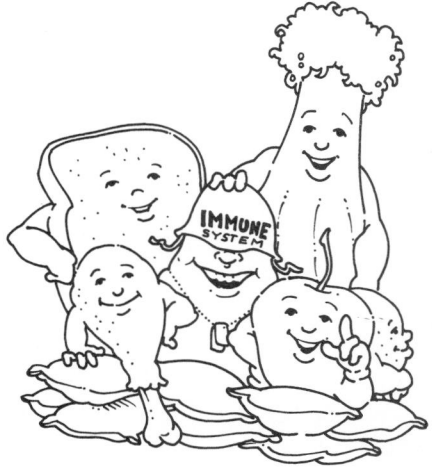

An optimal diet best protects and supports the immune system.

Chapter 3 said that an overdose or deficiency of any nutrient is likely to weaken the immune system. The chapters on vitamins and minerals listed toxicity symptoms from nutrient overdoses, and many of these can damage immunity. People who suffer from malnutrition develop more infections than well-nourished people, and it has been shown that nutrition therapy can improve their resistance to infection.[1] Table 11–2 on page 369 shows the effects of malnutrition on various immune-system organs and tissues. Listed first on the table are the first barriers a foreign material encounters when trying to enter the body—the skin and the mucous membranes. During malnutrition the skin becomes thinner, with less connective tissue, and the absorptive microvilli of the mucous membranes become flattened. One type of antibody normally present in mucous membrane secretions (including those of the lungs and digestive tract) is depressed in malnutrition, and this may help explain why malnourished children have repeated lung and digestive tract infections. Invaders (antigens) that would normally be barred from the body are allowed to enter, and the attack against them, once they are inside, is weak.

Special Section: Nutrition in the Treatment of AIDS

While nutrition has no powers to prevent infection with the AIDS virus, the American Dietetic Association holds that "nutrition intervention and education for those individuals [infected] should be a primary concern."[2] The reason is

■■■ Figure 11-1

Nutrition and Immunity.

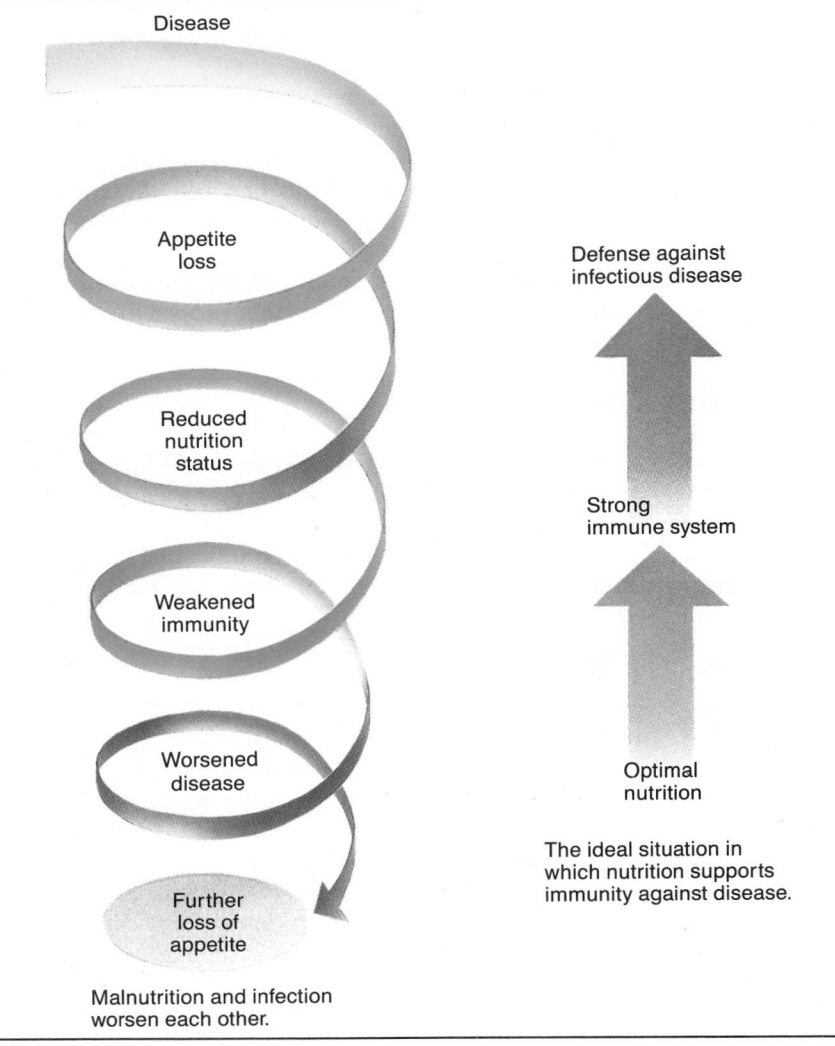

Malnutrition and infection worsen each other.

The ideal situation in which nutrition supports immunity against disease.

clear—malnutrition injures the immune system; adequate nutrition supports it. Severe malnutrition with wasting of lean body tissue is common in people with AIDS and appears to be related to poor food intake, increased nutrient requirements, poor nutrient absorption, and losses of fluids and nutrients associated with persistent diarrhea.[3] AIDS kills by stripping its victims of their immune defenses; malnutrition may render victims doubly vulnerable to recurrent secondary infections that often are the cause of death in AIDS patients.[4]

AIDS is becoming more prevalent. More and more people are finding that someone they know has been diagnosed with it. Adequate nutrition, while offering nothing in the way of cure, can enhance strength, provide comfort, and generally improve life's quality.[5] People who wish to offer help to someone with AIDS can do no better than to tend intelligently to the person's nutrition, often overlooked in treatment. People with AIDS suffer aggressive anorexia and so may refuse food. Often, they are more likely to eat small frequent meals,

■■■ Table 11-2 Effects of Malnutrition on the Body's Defense System

SYSTEM COMPONENT	EFFECTS OF MALNUTRITION
Skin	Thinned, with less connective tissue
Digestive tract and other body linings	Microvilli flattened; antibody secretions reduced
Lymph tissues	Thymus gland, lymph nodes, and spleen reduced in size; cells of immune defense depleted
General response	Invader kill time delayed; circulating immune cells reduced; antibody response may be impaired

degenerative diseases: chronic, irreversible diseases characterized by degeneration of the body organs due in part to such personal lifestyle choices as nutrition, smoking, alcohol use, and lack of physical activity. Examples are diabetes, cancer, heart disease, and osteoporosis.

risk factors: factors known to be related to (or correlated with) a disease but not proven to be causal.

such as an assortment of nutritious snacks and juices rather than three large meals. A valid goal for those with AIDS is to ensure that the total diet is in keeping with National Research Council (NRC) recommendations, since such a diet is superbly supportive of nutrition status. In addition to food, a supplement containing the Recommended Dietary Allowance (RDA) amounts of vitamins and minerals can be helpful and will not cause harm. Some liquid meal supplements are fortified with vitamins and minerals, and they provide energy-yielding nutrients. They also taste good.

Whatever foods are served, primary attention must be paid to food safety. A foodborne organism such as *Salmonella* can cause a deadly infection in people with compromised immunity. Should AIDS complications progress, the person's diet may become more prescriptive, dictated by therapy, and a dietitian's advice may be necessary.[6] Still, the caring attitude shown through attention to nutrition can lend emotional support to the sick person—a powerful medicine in itself.

Family, friends, and victims may, out of desperation, try special diet regimens or supplements in hopes of finding a cure or adding days to life. In the case of AIDS, no diet or nutrient regimen has been shown helpful beyond providing the nutrients needed for a fight. However, to extinguish hope would serve no purpose, and unproved dietary "remedies" might best be allowed as long as they do no harm.

AIDS is most times a preventable tragedy. The authors urge you to seek out information about AIDS prevention and to heed it.*

■■▶ *Adequate nutrition is a key player in maintaining a healthy immune system to guard against infectious diseases.*

■■■ People's Choices and Their Risks of Disease

In contrast to the infectious diseases, each of which has a distinct microbial cause such as the tuberculosis bacterium or the AIDS virus, the **degenerative diseases** of adulthood tend to have clusters of suspected causes known as **risk factors**. Among them are environmental, behavioral, social, and genetic factors, and combinations of these interacting with each other. In many cases one disease or condition intensifies the risk of another.

*An excellent free pamphlet is *Nutrition & Aids* available from Task Force at Wang Associates, Inc., 19 West 21st St., New York, NY 10010.

■■■ Table 11–3 Priorities in Nutrition—Lifestyle Risk Factors—Surgeon General's Report, 1988

NUTRITION CHANGES RECOMMENDED FOR ALL PEOPLE	THIS IS ESPECIALLY IMPORTANT IF YOUR FAMILY HISTORY INDICATES:	AND/OR IF YOUR MEDICAL HISTORY INDICATES:
Fats and cholesterol: Reduce consumption of fat (especially saturated fat) and cholesterol.[a]	Diabetes, obesity, cancer, or any form of cardiovascular disease (atherosclerosis, hypertension, heart attacks, strokes)	Glucose intolerance, high blood cholesterol or triglycerides, hypertension
Energy and weight control: Achieve and maintain a desirable body weight.[b]	Diabetes, obesity, cancer, or any form of cardiovascular disease (atherosclerosis, hypertension, heart attacks, strokes)	Glucose intolerance, high blood cholesterol or triglycerides, hypertension
Carbohydrate: Increase consumption of complex carbohydrates and fiber.[c]	Diabetes, obesity, cancer, or any form of cardiovascular disease (atherosclerosis, hypertension, heart attacks, strokes)	Glucose intolerance, high blood cholesterol or triglycerides, hypertension
Salt/sodium: Reduce intake of salt/sodium.[d]	Hypertension, diabetes, or any form of cardiovascular disease (atherosclerosis, hypertension, heart attacks, strokes)	Hypertension
Alcohol: To reduce the risk for chronic disease, take alcohol only in moderation (no more than two drinks a day), if at all.[e]	Liver disease (cirrhosis), cancer, any form of cardiovascular disease (atherosclerosis, hypertension, heart attacks, strokes), osteoporosis	Glucose intolerance, high blood cholesterol or triglycerides, hypertension, any sign of adult bone loss
OTHER ISSUES FOR SOME PEOPLE		**RECOMMENDED DIET ESPECIALLY FOR:**
Fluoride: Community water systems should contain fluoride at optimal levels for prevention of tooth decay. If such water is not available, use other appropriate sources of fluoride.	Osteoporosis, dental problems	Girls and women
Sugars: Limit the consumption and frequency of use of foods high in sugars.	Susceptibility to dental caries	Children
Calcium: Increase consumption of foods high in calcium, including low-fat dairy products.	Osteoporosis, cancer	Girls and women
Iron: Be sure to consume good sources of iron.[f]	Iron deficiency anemia	Low-income families, children, teens, girls, women

[a]Choose foods relatively low in fats and cholesterol, such as vegetables, fruits, whole-grain foods, fish, poultry, lean meats, and low-fat dairy products. Use food preparation methods that add little or no fat.

[b]To achieve and to maintain desirable body weight, choose a dietary pattern in which energy (calorie) intake is consistent with energy expenditure. To reduce energy intake, limit consumption of foods relatively high in calories, fats, and sugars, and minimize alcohol consumption. Increase energy expenditure through regular and sustained physical activity.

[c]To increase consumption of complex carbohydrates and fiber, eat more whole-grain foods and cereal products, vegetables (including dried beans and peas), and fruits.

[d] To reduce intake of salt/sodium, choose foods relatively low in sodium, and limit the amount of salt added in food preparation and at the table.

[e] To exercise moderation in the use of alcohol, take no more than two drinks a day. Avoid drinking any alcohol before or while driving, operating machinery, taking medications, or engaging in any other activity requiring judgment. Avoid drinking alcohol while pregnant.

[f]Foods that are good sources of iron include lean meats, fish, certain beans, and iron-enriched cereals and whole-grain products. This issue is of special concern for low-income families.

SOURCE: Adapted from *The Surgeon General's Report on Nutrition and Health: Summary and Recommendations,* DHHS (PHS) publication no. 88-50211, (Washington, D.C.: Government Printing Office, 1988), Table 1, p. 3.

One pivotal risk factor is obesity, which aggravates the risk of almost every other disease. Consider just one possible chain of causes and effects: obesity contributes to impaired glucose tolerance and diabetes (see Chapter 4), these problems contribute to hypertension (and obesity aggravates it), and hypertension worsens the risk of stroke, especially in people with diabetes. Obesity and the urgency of successful weight control therefore pervade this discussion, whatever disease may be under consideration.

People's behaviors, including food behaviors, are interwoven with all of these conditions. The choice to eat high-fat foods, for example, is a choice to increase the probabilities of becoming obese and thereby of contracting any of several diseases: cancer, hypertension, diabetes, atherosclerosis, diverticulosis, or others. Figure 11–2 (next page) shows the interrelationships of some of the risk factors of today's major degenerative diseases and highlights the food-related behaviors that contribute to them.

The exact contribution diet makes to each disease is hard to estimate. Many experts believe that diet accounts for about a third of all cases of coronary heart disease, but they argue that it may cause from one-tenth to nine-tenths of all cases of cancer. Evidence is indirect and cannot be quantified but strongly implicates an important role of diet. Moreover, diet advocates insist that diet is largely under people's own control. If a dietary change can't hurt and might help, why not make it?

To make such choices is doubtless more important for some people than for others, since some people are genetically predisposed to certain diseases. A way to begin deciding whether the diet recommendations presented here are important to you is to examine your own family history to see which diseases are common to your forebears. Another way to decide what lifestyle changes to make is to notice, on your next physical examination, which test results are out of line. Table 11–3 presents a summary of the signs to watch for in both categories.

Table 11–3 points to the places where you can make the personal investments that will bring the greatest probable rewards. Accepting that you have certain unchangeable "givens," you can look to the things you can change and choose the most influential among them. For example, a person with diabetes and heart disease in the immediate family is urgently advised to avoid becoming obese. For another example, a person with hypertension is urged to control weight, to exercise regularly, to eat a nutritious diet, and to not smoke.

The 1988 *Surgeon General's Report* makes clear the points just mentioned. Its major concern is our high intake of foods rich in fat, which often crowd more beneficial foods out of the diet—foods rich in complex carbohydrates and fiber. You will notice that the surgeon general's recommendations for the improvement of our nutrition closely parallel those of the *NRC Report* presented in Chapter 2. As the following details about each disease unfold, watch for the reasons why each of the surgeon general's recommendations is important.

The major killer diseases are atherosclerosis, hypertension, and cancer, but first a word about diabetes is in order. Diabetes is related to the major killer diseases, as shown in Figure 11–2. The progression of degenerative diseases is hastened by both diabetes and obesity, and each of these two conditions worsens the other.[7] It is important to know that the incidence of diabetes increases with age, since in all people the pancreas gradually loses some of its ability to produce insulin.[8] Thus although other diseases may appear to be more critical, diabetes and the obesity it engenders may have contributed to the development of those conditions.

■■▶ *Diet and lifestyle risk factors associated with one degenerative disease may contribute to others as well; some degenerative diseases themselves contribute to some of the others.*

■■■ Figure 11–2

Diet/Lifestyle Risk Factors and
Degenerative Diseases.

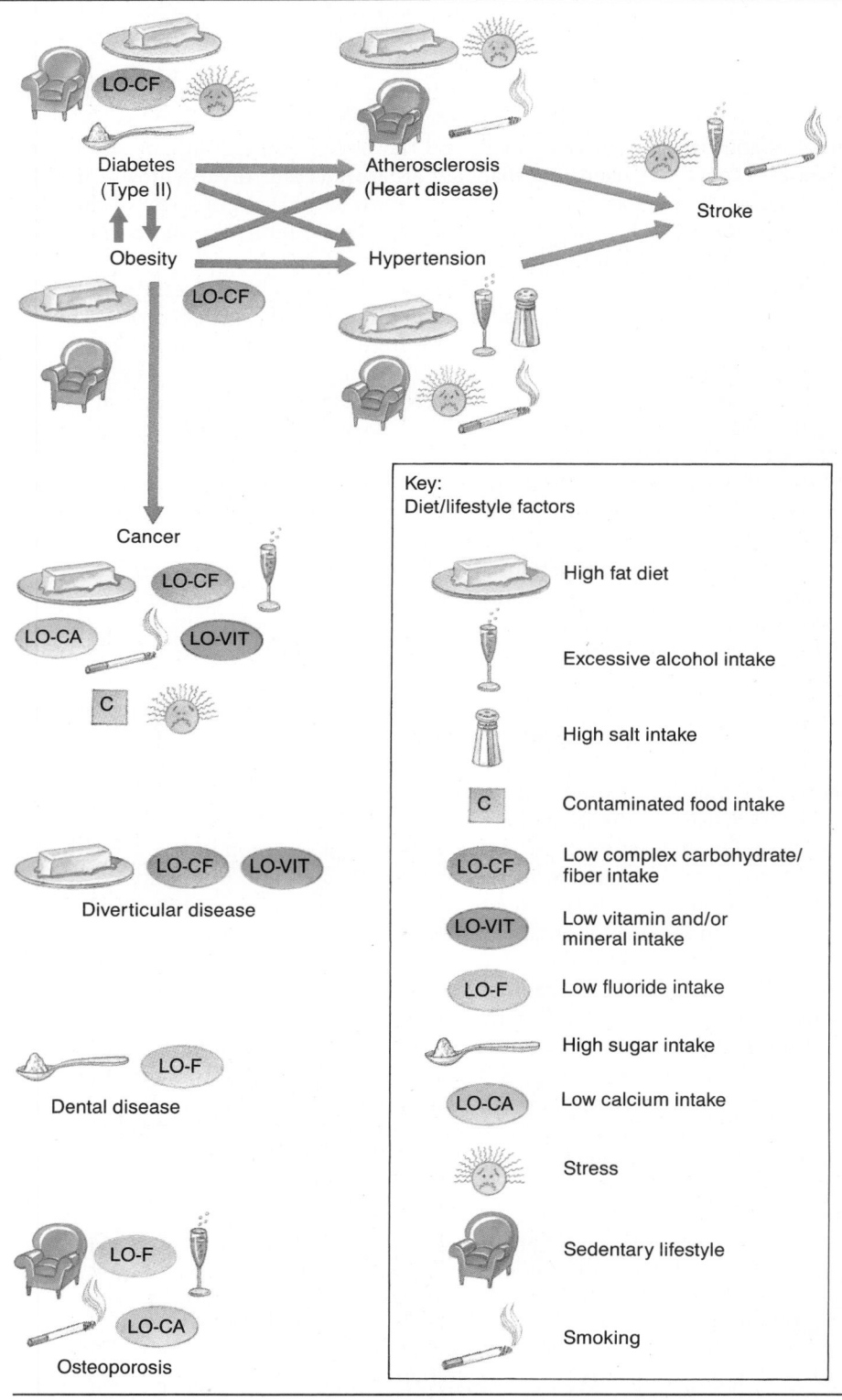

▓▓▓ Nutrition and Atherosclerosis

For decades our major causes of death have been diseases of the heart and blood vessels (**cardiovascular diseases**, or **CVD**). CVD accounts for more than any other single cause of the nation's deaths each year, mostly by way of heart attacks and strokes.[9] Efforts to fight CVD have led to valuable discoveries and public education. We now know that smoking, high blood pressure, and high blood cholesterol are the three major risk factors for CVD, and many people have changed their lifestyles accordingly. Many have quit smoking or have refrained from beginning. Many have been willing to change their diets, consuming less food energy, less fat, less cholesterol, less salt, and more fiber. Many are exercising more. The rate of CVD has fallen steadily since 1950 for some or all of these reasons; still, it is high. Can we lower it further? In particular, what factors can we control to increase our chances of leading long and healthy lives?

The twin demons that lead to most CVD are **atherosclerosis** and **hypertension**. Atherosclerosis is the common form of hardening of the arteries; hypertension is high blood pressure; and each makes the other worse.

How Atherosclerosis Develops

No one is free of atherosclerosis. The question is not whether you have it but how far advanced it is and what you can do to retard or to reverse it. It usually begins with the accumulation of soft, fatty streaks along the inner walls of the arteries, especially at branch points (Figure 11−3, next page). These gradually enlarge and become hardened **plaques**, making the artery walls lose their elasticity and narrowing the passage through them. Most people have well-developed plaques by the time they are 30 years old.

Normally the arteries expand with each heartbeat to accommodate the pulses of blood that flow through them. Arteries hardened and narrowed by plaques cannot expand, and so the blood pressure rises. The increased pressure puts a strain on the heart and damages the artery walls further. At damaged points, plaques are especially likely to form; thus the development of atherosclerosis is a self-accelerating process.

As pressure builds up in an artery, the arterial wall may become weakened and balloon out, forming an **aneurysm**. An aneurysm can burst, and when this happens in a major artery such as the **aorta**, it leads to massive bleeding and death.

Abnormal blood clotting also contributes to life-threatening events. Clots form and dissolve in the blood all the time, and the balance between these processes ensures that they do no harm. That balance is disturbed in atherosclerosis. Small, cell-like bodies in the blood, known as **platelets**, normally cause clots to form whenever they encounter injuries in blood vessels; but in atherosclerosis they respond in the same way to plaques and form clots when none are needed. Omega-6 and omega-3 fatty acids (see Consumer Caution I on pages 378−379) help control the action of the platelets, and an imbalance among these compounds may contribute to the formation of clots. Substances released by platelets also may aggravate the growth of plaques.

A clot, once formed, may remain attached to a plaque in an artery and gradually grow until it shuts off the blood supply of that portion of the tissue supplied by the artery. That tissue may die slowly and be replaced by scar tissue. The stationary clot is called a **thrombus**, and when it has grown large

---

CVD (cardiovascular disease): a general term for all diseases of the heart and blood vessels. Atherosclerosis is the main form of CVD.

atherosclerosis (ath-er-oh-scler-OH-sis): the commonest form of artery disease characterized by plaques along the inner walls of the arteries. (The related term **arteriosclerosis** means *all* forms of hardening of the arteries and includes some rare diseases.)
  athero = porridge or soft
  scleros = hard
  osis = too much

hypertension: high blood pressure (see the next major section of this chapter).

plaques (PLACKS): mounds of lipid material mixed with smooth muscle cells and calcium, that develop in the artery walls in atherosclerosis. (The same word is also used to describe an entirely different kind of accumulation of material on teeth, which promotes dental caries.)
  placken = patch

aneurysm (AN-you-rism): the ballooning out of an artery wall at a point where it has been weakened by deterioration.

aorta (ay-OR-tuh): the large, primary artery that conducts blood from the heart to the body's smaller arteries.

platelets: tiny, disc-shaped bodies in the blood, important in blood clot formation.
  platelet = little plate

thrombus: a stationary clot. When it has grown enough to close off a blood vessel, it is a **thrombosis**. A **coronary thrombosis** is the closing off of a vessel that feeds the heart muscle. A **cerebral thrombosis** is the closing off of a vessel that feeds the brain.
  coronary = crowning (the heart)
  thrombo = clot
  cerebrum is part of the brain

Omega-6 and omega-3 fatty acids were described in Chapter 5.

■■■ Figure 11–3

The Formation of Plaques in Atherosclerosis.
When plaques have covered 60 percent of the coronary artery walls, the critical
phase of heart disease begins.

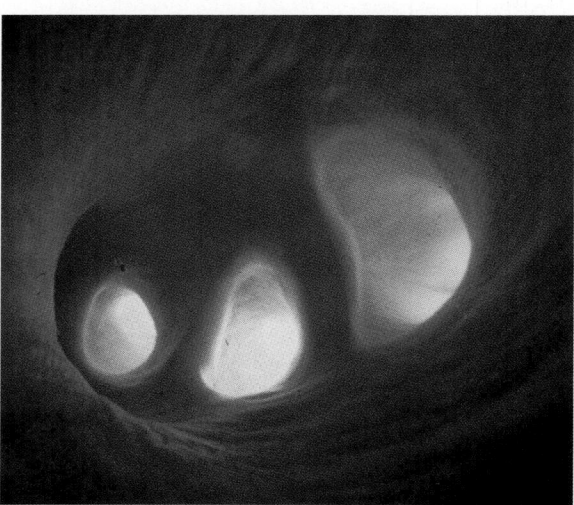

A. A healthy artery provides an open passage for the
   flow of blood.

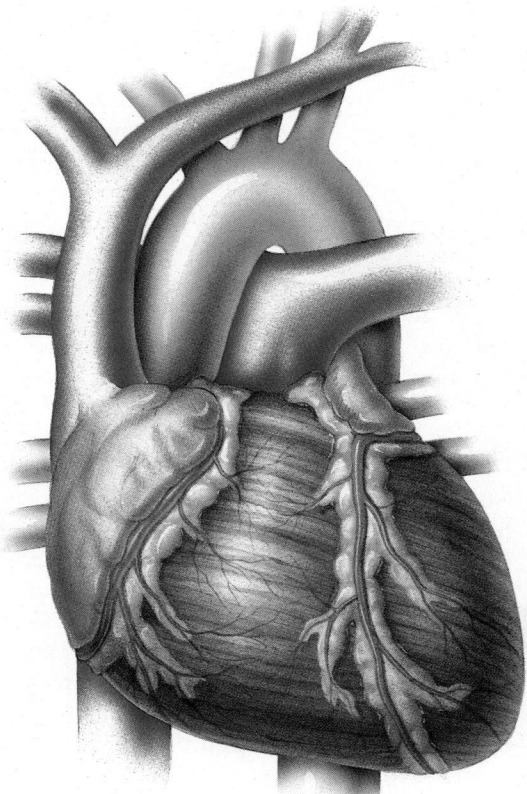

C. These are the coronary arteries, which bring
   nourishment to the heart muscle. If one of these
   arteries becomes blocked by plaque, the part of
   the heart muscle that it feeds will die.

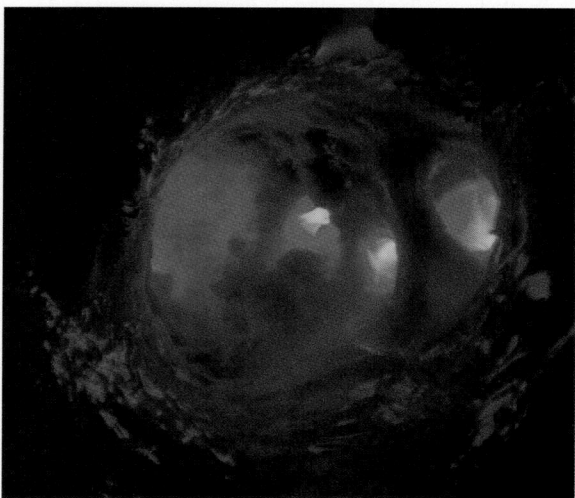

B. Plaques form along the artery's diameter, reducing
   blood flow. Clots can form, aggravating the
   problem.

enough to close off a blood vessel, it is a thrombosis. A coronary thrombosis
is the closing off of a vessel that feeds the heart muscle. A cerebral thrombosis
is the closing off of a vessel that feeds the brain.

A clot can also break loose, becoming an **embolus**, and travel along the
system until it reaches an artery too small to allow its passage. Then the tissues
fed by this artery will be robbed of oxygen and nutrients and will die suddenly

(embolism). Such a clot can lodge in an artery of the heart, causing sudden death of part of the heart muscle; we say that the person has had a **heart attack**. When the clot lodges in an artery of the brain, killing a portion of brain tissue, we call the event a **stroke**.

On many occasions it is not clear what has caused a heart attack or stroke. An artery appears to go into spasms, and the blood supply to a portion of the heart muscle or brain is cut off, but examination reveals no visible cause.[10] Much research today is devoted to finding out what causes plaques to form, what causes arteries to go into spasms, what governs the activities of platelets, and why the body allows clots to form unopposed by clot-dissolving cleanup activity.

Hypertension makes atherosclerosis worse. A stiffened artery, already strained by each pulse of blood surging through it, is more greatly stressed if the internal pressure is high. Lesions (injured places) develop more frequently, plaques grow faster, and weakened vessels are more likely to burst, causing hemorrhage.

Atherosclerosis also makes hypertension worse. By hardening the arteries, it makes them unable to expand with each beat of the heart, so the internal pressure rises. This leads to further hardening of the arteries, as already explained. Hardened arteries also fail to let blood flow freely through the body's blood pressure-controlling organs, the kidneys; the kidneys sense the reduced flow of blood and respond as if the blood pressure were too low—they raise it further (see "Hypertension," later).

▌▌▶ *Plaques of atherosclerosis worsen hypertension and trigger abnormal blood clotting, leading to heart attack or stroke. Heart attacks and strokes can also be caused by abnormal vessel spasms.*

> **embolus** (EM-boh-luss): a thrombus that breaks loose. When it causes sudden closure of a blood vessel, it is an **embolism**.
> *embol* = to insert
>
> **heart attack**: the event in which an embolus lodges in vessels that feed the heart muscle, causing sudden tissue death. Also called *myocardial infarction*.
> *myo* = muscle
> *cardial* = of the heart
> *infarct* = tissue death
>
> **stroke**: the sudden shutting off of the blood flow to the brain by a thrombus or embolism or by the bursting of a vessel (hemorrhage).

Risk Factors for CVD

The risk factors for atherosclerosis are listed in Table 11–4. It befits a nutrition book to focus on dietary strategies to reduce them. It should be noted, though, that diet is not the only, and perhaps not even the most important, factor in the causation of CVD. In fact, among the many controversies over diet and nutrition in recent years, one of the noisiest ones has been over the questions of how important diet is in heart disease; whether changes in diet can reduce the risk; and if so, whether such changes should be advocated for everyone or just for selected high-risk individuals.

The big *diet-related* risk factors for CVD are glucose intolerance and obesity (already mentioned), hypertension (the subject of the next section), and high

■■■ **Table 11–4 Risk Factors for Atherosclerosis**

Smoking
Hypertension
High blood cholesterol, high LDL and/or low HDL
Obesity (30% or more overweight)
Glucose intolerance (diabetes)
Lack of exercise
Stress
Heredity (history of CVD in family members younger than 55 years of age)
Gender (being male)

■■■ **Table 11−5 Standards for Atherosclerosis Risk Factors**

HYPERTENSION	OBESITY

Diastolic[a] pressure:
  90−104 = mild
  105−114 = moderate
  115+   = severe
Blood cholesterol[b]
  Below 200 mg/dL = desirable
  200−239 mg/dL = borderline high
  240 + mg/dL = high
	Body mass index greater than 27.2 for men or 26.9 for women (see Chapter 9, Figure 9−1).
	Lipid profile
	  LDL > 140 mg/dL indicates risk
	  HDL < 35 mg/dL indicates risk
	
	Triglycerides (fasting):[c]
	  > 250 mg/dL may indicate risk.

[a]The diastolic pressure is the lower of the two numbers in the blood pressure reading—for example, the 70 in 105/70.

[b]Consult a physician, who will consult this reference and weigh all factors in deciding what to recommend.

[c]High triglycerides are not normally indicative of direct risk but may reflect carbohydrate sensitivity, impaired glucose tolerance, or diabetes, and these conditions are risk factors for CVD.

SOURCE: National Cholesterol Education Program, Report of the Expert Panel on Detection, Evaluation, and Treatment of High Blood Cholesterol in Adults, *Annals of Internal Medicine*, December 1987.

blood cholesterol (to be discussed here). The standards by which each of these risk factors is labeled "high" are shown in Table 11−5.

Controversy surrounds the question of how cholesterol is linked to CVD. No one disputes that high *blood* cholesterol, particularly high low-density lipoprotein (LDL), predicts CVD, but people do dispute the hypothesis that links *diet* to CVD. The hypothesis has two parts: (1) that high blood cholesterol (LDL) is at least partly caused by a diet high in saturated fat and cholesterol; and (2) that reducing the amounts of saturated fat and cholesterol in the diet, by lowering blood cholesterol, will reduce the rate of CVD.

Both parts of this hypothesis have some strong support, but pieces are missing. With respect to the first part (whether a high-fat diet elevates blood cholesterol), blood cholesterol can be raised in both animals and people by raising the amounts of saturated fat and cholesterol in their diets—but whether the high blood cholesterol we see among so many people in the real world is *caused* by that aspect of their diets has been impossible to demonstrate. With respect to the second part (reducing fat and cholesterol intakes will reduce the risk of CVD), it is possible to lower blood cholesterol in both animals and people by reducing the amounts of saturated fat and cholesterol in their diets— but whether this reduces their risks of heart disease has been impossible to demonstrate.

Most investigators and organizations, including the American Heart Association, however, see links between our high-fat, high-cholesterol diet and heart disease, and they hold out the hope that continued research will confirm and clarify these relationships. The consensus seems to be that while experimental work continues, everyone over two years of age should be screened for high blood cholesterol and that those at high risk should be treated first with diet and then, if necessary, with drugs to bring it down.[11] Most agree that the first treatment should be diet.[12] Most agree that the percentage of calories from fat in the diet should be no more than 30 percent and perhaps even lower.

As mentioned, the blood cholesterol of concern in atherosclerosis risk is LDL cholesterol. (Recall from Chapter 5 that cholesterol is carried in several lipoproteins, chief among them LDL and HDL.) The HDL also carry cholesterol, but raised HDL concentrations relative to LDL represent cholesterol on its way out of the arteries back to the liver, a reduced risk of developing atherosclerosis, and a reduced risk of heart attack (Figure 11–4). Cholesterol carried in LDL correlates *directly* with heart disease, whereas HDL cholesterol correlates *inversely* with risk.

Some people have abnormal lipid profiles (high in LDL and low in HDL) for genetic reasons, but some may have them due to such poor health habits as overeating, overconsumption of fat, or underactivity. To normalize their blood lipid profiles, these people may need to change their lifestyles.

▮▮▶ *Although research has yet to prove that a diet high in saturated fat and cholesterol causes high blood cholesterol, most experts agree that almost everyone should be screened for high blood cholesterol and be treated if necessary.*

Diet and Exercise Recommendations to Reverse High Blood Cholesterol

The goal of dietary measures to slow the advance of atherosclerosis is to reduce total blood cholesterol and, particularly, LDL cholesterol. The measures recommended by a review panel of experts in 1987 to 1988 involve a two-step plan, shown in Table 11–6. Step one of the plan also reflects recommendations of Canadian experts for reducing elevated cholesterol. If step one brings high blood cholesterol down, good; if not, the therapy goes on to step two. Step one involves a total fat intake of fewer than 30 percent of calories, with saturated fatty acids only one third of that and dietary cholesterol less than 300 milligrams a day. Step two reduces saturated fat and cholesterol further, as shown. (To accomplish this degree of fat restriction may require guidance from a registered dietitian). Atherosclerotic disease is so common in the United States that many experts advocate this plan for everyone, even those without abnormal blood lipids.[13]

In addition to diet, some types of exercise are particularly effective in lowering LDL and in raising HDL concentrations. Frequent and sustained *aerobic* exercise may help to reverse atherosclerosis. There is some evidence to suggest that weight training can raise HDL somewhat, if undertaken regularly.[14] Even

▮▮▮ **Figure 11–4**

HDL and LDL and Risk of Heart Disease.

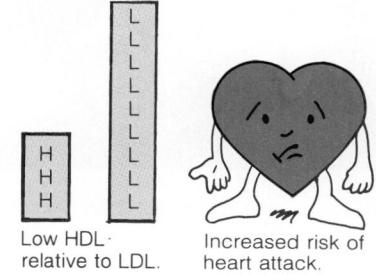

Low HDL relative to LDL.   Increased risk of heart attack.

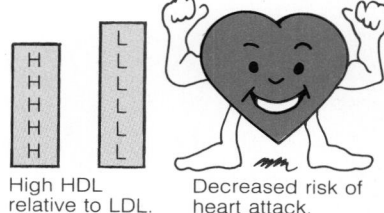

High HDL relative to LDL.   Decreased risk of heart attack.

A minimum of 20 minutes of aerobic activity three times a week is necessary to build cardiovascular endurance, reduce blood pressure, and slow the pulse.

▮▮▮ **Table 11–6 Energy Nutrient Balance to Reduce Blood Cholesterol**

	TOTAL FAT[a]	SATURATED FATTY ACIDS[ab]	Carbohydrates[a]	Protein[a]	CHOLESTEROL
Step One	<30%	<10%	50%–60%	10%–20%	<300 mg/dL
Step Two	<30%	<7%	50%–60%	10%–20%	<200 mg/dL

[a]All but cholesterol are expressed as percentages of total food energy. Total food energy intake should be such as to achieve and to maintain desirable weight.
[b]Polyunsaturated fatty acids can contribute up to 10% of food energy intake; monounsaturated fatty acids, 10% to 15%.
SOURCE: Adapted from N. D. Einst and J. C. LaRosa, Recommendations for treatment of high blood cholesterol, The National Cholesterol Education Program Adult Treatment Panel, *Contemporary Nutrition* 13(1), 1988 and Canadian Consensus Conference on Cholesterol: Final report, *Canadian Medical Association Journal* 139, supplement (1988): 4–8.

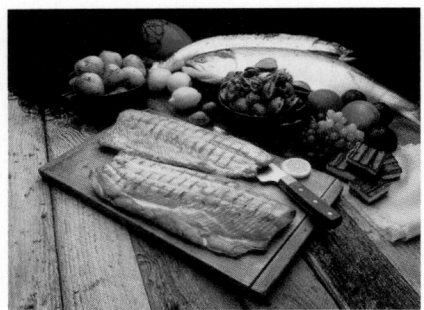

Salmon is rich in omega-3 fatty acids.

light exercise, such as walking, may lower LDL and raise HDL if consistently pursued. Some researchers wonder if exercise is really the factor that raises blood HDL or if the weight loss that often accompanies exercise is the real cause. The answer seems to be yes, that exercise alone is responsible for raised HDL concentrations, and yes, that weight loss helps. Both factors not only raise HDL concentrations independently of one another, but their effects are *additive*.[15]

Thus correcting diet and exercise will do more than help ward off heart disease. Body weight has proven, in some studies, to be the most important single determinant of blood cholesterol level,[16] but even if weight control does not reduce blood cholesterol, it will help by reducing blood pressure (see next section). So will exercise (and this, too, is explained further in the next section). So will eating a low-fat diet. Even if the high-fiber, high-complex-carbohydrate aspect does not help by way of cholesterol, it will help by normalizing glucose tolerance (diabetes, remember, is a major risk factor for CVD). Even if the monounsaturated oils and the oils from the fish do not help by way of lowering blood cholesterol, they may help by favoring the right fatty acid balance so that clot formation is unlikely. (Before you conclude that fish oil capsules might be appropriate, read this chapter's Consumer Caution I.) An adequate diet will protect the health of the heart muscle itself; mineral deficiencies may bring on disease of the heart muscle and arteries.[17] While you are at it, exercise. Don't smoke. Relax. Meditate or pray. Play. Happy people have lower blood cholesterol levels.[18]

▌▌▶ *Dietary measures to reduce fat, saturated fat, and cholesterol intakes are the first line of treatment for high blood cholesterol.*

These fish provide at least 1 gram omega-3 acids in 100 grams of fish (100 grams equals about 3.5 ounces):
  Anchovy, European.
  Bluefish.
  Capelin conch.
  Herring: Atlantic or Pacific.
  Mackerel: Atlantic, chub, Japanese horse or king.
  Mullet.
  Sablefish.
  Salmon, all varieties.
  Saury.
  Scad, Muroaji.
  Sprat.
  Sturgeon: Atlantic or common.
  Trout, lake.
  Tuna: albacore or bluefin.
  Whitefish, lake.

CONSUMER CAUTION ▐▐▐   **I. Fish Oil Supplements**

In contrast to the negative impacts of fats on heart health are those of moderate intakes of the omega-3 fatty acids found in fish oils. Chapter 5 described some beneficial effects of omega-3 fatty acids. Important to CVD are three effects: lowering blood cholesterol and triglyceride concentrations, and reducing the tendency of the blood to clot.† Products the body makes from the omega-3 fatty acids also regulate blood pressure, the immune response, and the inflammatory response to injury and infection.

How much fish do we need to eat to receive the beneficial effects of omega-3 fatty acids? Sources do not agree. The American Heart Association currently recommends two to three fish meals a week. The Canadian Recommended Nutrient Intakes (RNI) recommends 1 to 1 1/2 grams of omega-3 fatty acids a day. Among fresh fish, choose the fatty varieties—salmon, herring, sardines, mackerel. To receive the most omega-3 acids from canned fish, choose the water-packed variety because omega-3 acids disperse in packing oils to be drained away before consumption of the fish. For tuna, choose white albacore, which provides a gram of omega-3 acids per 5 ounces. Cheaper, light tuna varieties may contain only a sixth as much.

continued on next page

Fish oil supplements are not recommended for a numbers of reasons. Their effectiveness is unproven, and the Food and Drug Administration (FDA) disallows advertisements and labels to claim they are effective in preventing or treating diseases. Omega-3 fatty acids may react with oxygen during processing, thus destroying their protective properties.[19] Concentrated supplements make it easy to take too much fish oil, and an overdose can cause excessive bleeding, interfere with wound healing, or worsen Type II diabetes.[20] Fish oil supplements are made from fish livers, which may have accumulated toxic concentrations of pesticides, heavy metals, and other environmental contaminants that can be concentrated in the pills. They also contain large amounts of vitamins A and D, which can have toxic effects. Lastly, they are expensive.

In addition to being excellent sources of omega-3 fatty acids, fish contain many valuable nutrients. They are leaner than many other animal-protein sources and are rich in minerals (with the exception of iron) and vitamins. Fish-based imitation seafood products, while tasty, do not contain the same levels of nutrients or omega-3 fatty acids as do unprocessed fish. These beneficial components are washed away in processing, and in their place lurks many times the sodium of fresh fish.[21] Many experts recommend that people eat fish periodically for its nutrients. Now there's another reason to eat fish— it could help forestall heart disease.

†Among the effects on blood cholesterol is a shift in the ratio between lipoproteins HDL_2 and HDL_3 that is associated with lower heart disease risk. M. Abbey, Effect of fish oil on lipoproteins, lecithin: cholesterol acyltransferase, and lipid transfer protein activity in humans, *Arteriosclerosis* 10 (1990): 85–94.

These foods also supply over 1 gram per 100 grams:
- Beechnuts, dried.
- Butternuts, dried.
- Chia seeds, dried.
- Hickory nuts, dried.
- Soybean kernels, roasted.
- Soybeans, green, raw.
- Soybean sprouts, cooked.
- Walnuts, black, English, Persian.

Most other whole foods add at least some omega-3 fatty acids to the diet.

CONSUMER CAUTION ▌▌▌ II. Niacin Megadoses

Periodically, the media repopularize the idea that the vitamin niacin can lower blood cholesterol. While it is true that under controlled conditions, pharmaceutical doses of a particular form of niacin act like a drug in lowering blood cholesterol somewhat, this effect is beyond that of a nutrient. Like drugs, nutrients are chemicals and, in large doses, they may affect the body in ways unrelated to nutrition. Regular niacin supplements are useless in lowering blood cholesterol, and high doses of niacin can cause side effects such as skin flushing ("niacin flush"), abnormal liver function, and some symptoms of diabetes.

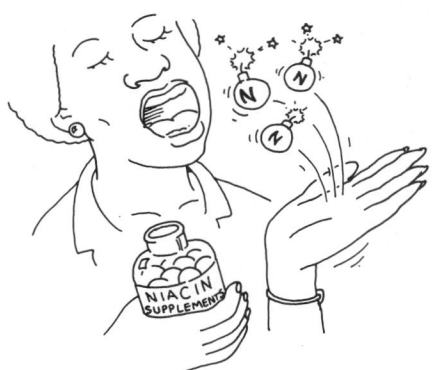

High doses of niacin may cause unexpected side effects.

▌▌▌ Nutrition and Hypertension

Anyone concerned with the risk of cardiovascular disease that atherosclerosis presents must also be concerned about high blood pressure. The two together are a threatening combination. You cannot tell if you have high blood pressure; it presents no symptoms you can feel. But if you do have it, it threatens to impair the quality of your life and even strike you down before your time. Chronic elevated blood pressure, or hypertension, is the most prevalent form of cardiovascular disease, believed to affect some 60 million people in the

systolic (sis-TOL-ik) **pressure**: the first figure in a blood pressure reading (the "dub" of the heartbeat), which represents arterial pressure caused by the contraction of the left ventricle of the heart.

diastolic (dye-as-TOL-ik) **pressure**: the second figure in a blood pressure reading (the "lub" of the heartbeat), which represents the arterial pressure when the heart is between beats.

United States—more than a third of the entire adult population.[22] It contributes to half a million strokes and to over a million heart attacks each year.[23] The higher the blood pressure above normal, the greater the risk of heart disease. (Except in extreme cases, low blood pressure is generally a sign of long life expectancy and low heart disease risk.)

The most effective single step you can take toward protecting yourself from hypertension is to find out whether you have it. At checkup time, a health care professional can give you an accurate resting blood pressure reading. (Self-test machines in drugstores and other places are often inaccurate.) If your resting blood pressure is above normal, the reading should be repeated before confirming the diagnosis of hypertension. Thereafter it should be checked at regular intervals. When blood pressure is measured, two numbers are important: the pressure during contraction of the heart's ventricles (large pumping chambers) and the pressure during ventricular relaxation. The numbers are given as a fraction, with the top number representing the **systolic pressure** (ventricle contraction) and the bottom number the **diastolic pressure** (ventricular relaxation). Return to Table 11–5 on page 376 to see how to interpret your resting blood pressure.

Resting blood pressure should ideally be 120 over 80 or lower. However, it is generally considered normal if it is less than 140 over 90. Above this level the risks of heart attacks and strokes increase in direct proportion to increasing blood pressure, especially diastolic pressure.

▌▌▶ *Hypertension is silent, progressively worsens atherosclerosis, and makes heart attacks and strokes more likely. All adults should know their blood pressure.*

How Hypertension Develops

Blood pressure is vital to life. It pushes the blood through the major arteries into smaller arteries and finally into tiny capillaries whose thin walls permit exchange of fluids between the blood and the tissues (Figure 11–5). When the pressure is right, the cells receive a constant supply of nutrients and oxygen and are relieved of their wastes.

The pressure the blood exerts on the inner walls of the arteries is the result of two forces acting together: the heart's pushing the blood into the arteries and the smallest arteries and capillaries resisting its flow. The heart's push ensures that the blood circulates through the whole system; the resistance and resulting pressure ensure that some of the blood's components, including nutrients, are pushed through the capillary walls to feed the tissues. One other factor contributes to blood pressure: the volume of fluid in the vascular system—and that, in turn, is affected by the number of dissolved particles it contains. By the rule that "water follows salt," the more salt in the blood, the more water there will be.

The kidneys depend on the blood pressure to help them filter waste materials out of the blood into the urine. (The pressure has to be high enough to force the blood's fluid out of the capillaries into the kidney's filtering networks.) If the blood pressure is too low, the kidneys set in motion actions to increase it; they release hormones into the bloodstream to constrict the peripheral blood vessels and to lead to the retention of water and salt in the body.

When dehydration sets these actions in motion, they are beneficial because when the blood volume is low, higher blood pressure is needed to deliver

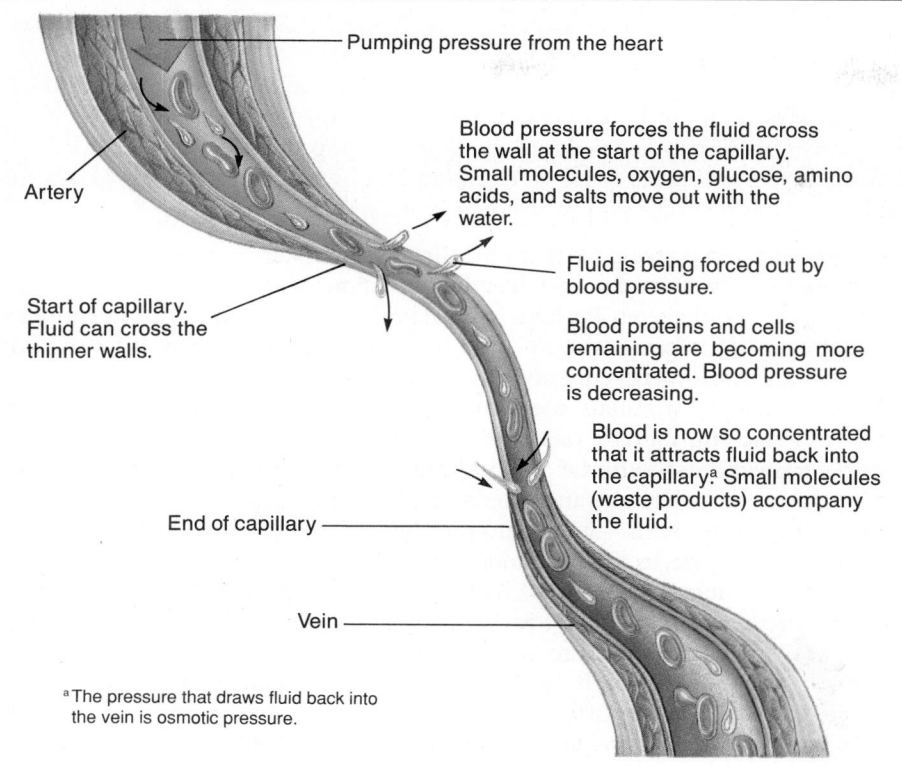

Pumping pressure from the heart

Blood pressure forces the fluid across the wall at the start of the capillary. Small molecules, oxygen, glucose, amino acids, and salts move out with the water.

Artery

Fluid is being forced out by blood pressure.

Blood proteins and cells remaining are becoming more concentrated. Blood pressure is decreasing.

Start of capillary. Fluid can cross the thinner walls.

Blood is now so concentrated that it attracts fluid back into the capillary[a] Small molecules (waste products) accompany the fluid.

End of capillary

Vein

[a] The pressure that draws fluid back into the vein is osmotic pressure.

■■■ Figure 11–5

The Blood Pressure. Two major contributors to the pressure inside an artery are the heart's pushing blood into it and the small-diameter arteries and capillaries at its other end resisting the blood's flow (peripheral resistance). Another determining factor is the volume of fluid in the circulatory system, which depends in turn on the number of dissolved particles in that fluid.

substances to the tissues. By constricting the blood vessels and conserving water and sodium, the kidneys ensure that normal blood pressure is maintained until the dehydrated person can drink water. Atherosclerosis also sets this process in motion, however, and this is not beneficial. Atherosclerosis, by obstructing blood vessels, fools the kidneys: they react as if there were a water deficiency. Actually the blood pressure may be normal initially, and the kidneys raise it too high, with harmful effects on the heart which has to pump blood against this pressure. Only when the blood pressure is high, straining the heart, do the kidneys obtain enough pressure to filter the blood properly. As mentioned earlier, hypertension aggravates atherosclerosis by mechanically injuring the artery linings, making plaques likely to form; this may raise the blood pressure further, and so the problem intensifies.

Obesity makes hypertension still worse. Added adipose tissue means miles of extra capillaries through which the blood must be pumped. The combination of hypertension, atherosclerosis, and obesity puts a severe strain on the heart and arteries, leading to many forms of cardiovascular disease and death. Strain on the heart's pump, the left ventricle, can enlarge and weaken it, until finally it fails (heart failure). Pressure in the aorta may cause it to balloon out and burst (aneurysm). Pressure in the small arteries of the brain may make them burst and bleed (a form of stroke). The kidneys can be damaged when the heart is unable to adequately pump blood through them (kidney failure).

Epidemiological studies have identified several risk factors to predict the development of hypertension, including:

☐ *Age.* Blood pressure levels increase with age; most people who develop hypertension do so in their 50s and 60s.

☐ *Family background.* A family history of hypertension and heart disease raises the risk of developing hypertension two to five times.

☐ *Obesity.* Obese people are more likely to develop hypertension.

☐ *Race.* Hypertension is twice as common among blacks as among whites; it tends to develop earlier and to become more severe.

Also hypertension appears to be an insulin-resistant state. This is true even in the absence of obesity and may reflect the operation of a factor common to both hypertension and diabetes. Perhaps insulin itself is, in some way, at some times, a causal agent of hypertension.[24] A tantalizing bit of supporting information suggests that insulin may enhance the kidney's reabsorption of sodium.[25] Another is that it may stimulate the activity of the hormones associated with the stress response and thereby raise the blood pressure.[26]

While researchers continue looking for the cause or causes, clearly it is urgent that we do what we can to detect and to treat hypertension wherever it presents its deadly threat—or better still, that we prevent it. A major national effort has been made to identify and to treat hypertension. Even mild hypertension can be dangerous; individuals who have it benefit from treatment, showing a reduced incidence of early death and illness.[27] Diet changes alone, even without the drugs used to reduce blood pressure, can bring about these benefits in some people without the undesirable side effects of the drugs.

◗◗▶ *Atherosclerosis, obesity, and possibly insulin contribute to hypertension.*

Weight Control, Diet, and Hypertension

What are the diet-related factors that affect blood pressure? Most people might respond "salt" (thinking sodium), but research into sodium's role has disappointed investigators who hoped they were on the track to a single answer. Many other factors are suspect, and among them, two are as weighty as salt— obesity and alcohol intake.

WEIGHT CONTROL. Evidence supports the positive link between obesity and hypertension already mentioned. This is not to say that every obese person becomes hypertensive or that all people with hypertension are overweight but that those who are obese and hypertensive should sit up and take notice. Weight reduction in most overweight people with hypertension significantly lowers blood pressure. This is so even if the person does not go all the way to achieve ideal body weight. Those who are using drugs to control their blood pressure can often reduce or discontinue use of them if they lose weight.[28] Even a 10-pound weight loss in people who have been maintained on aggressive hypertensive drug therapy for five years more than doubles the chance that they can normalize their blood pressure without drugs.[29] Weight loss alone may be one of the most effective nondrug treatments for hypertension.[30]

Physical activity, of course, is part of the energy balance equation. The more active you are, the more energy you spend, and the less fat you accumulate (or the more you burn off). But moderate activity of the right kind also helps to reduce hypertension directly. Although blood pressure rises temporarily at each bout of exercise, the effect in the long run is to lower the resting blood pressure significantly.[31]

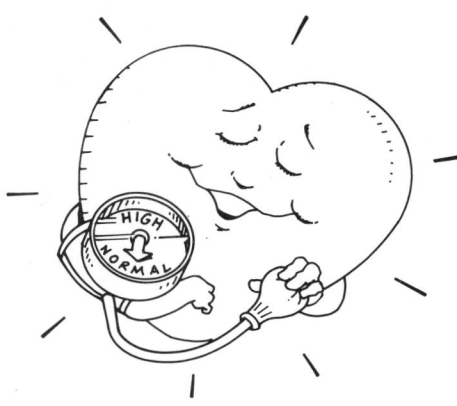

A first step against hypertension: know your blood pressure.

The "right kind" of activity is the aerobic, endurance type that conditions the heart, increasing its stroke volume, and reducing its work load. Such activity also changes the hormonal climate in which the body does its work. It alters stress hormone secretion and lowers blood pressure. It brings about a redistribution of body water, and it eases transit of the blood through the peripheral arteries.[32] If heart and artery disease has already set in, a monitored exercise program may actually help to reverse it.[33] Physical activity may stimulate development of new arteries to nourish the heart muscle, and this may be a factor in the excellent recovery seen in some heart attack victims who exercise.[34]

Stroke volume and other heart characteristics were discussed in Chapter 10.

SODIUM/SODIUM CHLORIDE. Salt clearly has something to do with blood pressure. In fact, for years research on populations has seemed to indicate that high sodium intakes were "the" factor responsible for people's high blood pressure; but recently that notion has been falling into disfavor. Much of the early research that implicated sodium in hypertension's causation may have unwittingly uncovered the effects of sodium's silent partner, chloride; so now we talk in terms of salt.[35]

Most people can safely consume more salt than they need and rely on the body's system of checks and control mechanisms to regulate its excretion and retention as needed. "Sodium-sensitive" individuals, however, experience high blood pressure from excesses in sodium or salt intake. People with chronic renal disease, those whose parents (one or both) have hypertension, blacks, and persons over 50 years of age are most likely to be sodium or salt sensitive.[36]

Salt avoidance prevents hypertension in "salt-sensitive" individuals, but for others—the majority of people with hypertension—it may be ineffective. Salt restriction does not lower the blood pressure in half of the hypertensive people in whom it is tried.[37] It is important to look further to see what other dietary factors might be relevant.

POTASSIUM. Some authorities believe that potassium might both prevent and treat hypertension.‡ Even in people without high blood pressure, potassium added to the diet in amounts equivalent to that in a serving or two of fruits and vegetables has been associated with reduced risk of stroke; so potassium in the diet seems worthy of attention.[38] People who eat many foods high in salt often happen to be eating fewer potassium-containing foods at the same time.[39] Table 8–3 in Chapter 8 showed that as the *same* food goes through several processing steps, it loses potassium and gains sodium, so that its potassium-sodium ratio falls dramatically. Sodium avoidance may help in two ways, then —by reducing blood pressure in salt-sensitive individuals and by indirectly raising potassium intakes in people who replace processed foods with whole foods. A similar thing can be said of calcium, as the next paragraphs show.

CALCIUM. Several surveys report that people with hypertension consume less calcium than those with normal blood pressure.[40] Researchers estimate that people with the lowest calcium intakes (below 300 milligrams per day) have a

---

‡People using diuretics to control hypertension should know that some cause potassium excretion and can induce a deficiency. Those using these drugs must be particularly careful to include rich sources of potassium in their daily diets.

two to three times greater risk of developing hypertension than people with the highest calcium intakes (1200 milligrams per day).[41]

Calcium may be important in both prevention and treatment of hypertension. One study showed that a calcium-rich diet reduced blood pressure, even in some people with normal blood pressure. It is recommended, therefore, that people with hypertension and those who are or at risk of developing it *at least* meet the current RDA for calcium— 800 to 1200 milligrams a day for adults. Milk products are recommended because they provide not only calcium, but also potassium and magnesium, which may also help keep blood pressure normal. Low-fat or nonfat milk products are especially beneficial because fat contributes to hypertension too.

FAT. Fat is well known as a dietary factor contributing to atherosclerosis, but few people realize that it plays an independent role in relation to blood pressure. Diets high in saturated fat are associated with hypertension. Populations that consume small quantities of animal products—vegetarians, for example— have a low incidence of hypertension. When people restrict their total dietary fat and increase the ratio of polyunsaturated to saturated fatty acids, their blood pressure falls.[42] The recommendations on dietary fat made earlier for atherosclerosis thus apply to hypertension too: limit total fat; of the fat allowed, use mostly monounsaturated and polyunsaturated fats, including fish oils; limit saturated fat.

ALCOHOL. Alcohol has several roles in relation to heart disease. In moderate doses, alcohol initially reduces pressure in the peripheral arteries and so reduces blood pressure, but high doses clearly raise blood pressure.[43] Hypertension is common in people with alcoholism.[44] The hypertension is apparently caused directly by the alcohol,[45] and it leads to cardiovascular disease, the same as hypertension caused by any other factor.[46] Furthermore, alcohol causes strokes—even *without* hypertension.[47] The surgeon general's advice on alcohol use is straightforward: if you drink, do so in moderation. *Moderation* means 1 to 2 drinks a day, not more.[48] The NRC Report does not recommend the use of alcohol at all; for those who do drink, the NRC recommends limiting daily intake to 1 ounce pure alcohol, the equivalent of 2 drinks. (For more on alcohol and nutrition, see this chapter's Controversy.)

OTHER FACTORS. Research is continuing to reveal relationships of other factors to hypertension. For example, adequate (but not excessive) magnesium seems to protect against it. Magnesium deficiency makes the walls of arteries and capillaries more likely to constrict, thus raising blood pressure.[49] Since hypertension may also be an insulin-resistant state, it is possible that measures to prevent diabetes can also protect against hypertension. Other substances may affect blood pressure in one way or another: roles for cadmium, selenium, lead, caffeine, and protein are currently under study.[50]

The role of diet in *treatment* of hypertension is not questioned. The single most effective dietary measure the person with hypertension can take is to reduce weight if overweight. For the salt-sensitive person, it is also effective to reduce sodium, or at least salt, intake. As for diet in *prevention* of hypertension, there is less agreement, but many professionals and agencies believe that enough evidence is available to warrant a recommendation to the general public to moderately restrict salt intake. They reason that, at worst, such a diet cannot be harmful. The Food Feature of this chapter provides more detail on dietary measures that help support normal blood pressure.

◫▷ *For most people, weight reduction, aerobic exercise, and a diet that provides adequate nutrients works to keep blood pressure normal. For some, salt restriction is also required.*

▮▮▮ Nutrition and Cancer

One out of every four people will eventually contract **cancer**. Dietary fat is thought to be especially important in relation to cancer, but diet relates to cancer in several ways. It is important to get them all in perspective. Constituents in foods may be cancer causing, cancer promoting, or protective against cancer. Also, for the person who has cancer, diet can make a crucial difference in recovery.

Of course nondiet factors are important in relation to cancer too. A few cancers are genetic and will appear regardless. For other cancers, environmental factors other than diet are involved—smoking, for example, and water and air pollution. The emphasis here is on diet, of course.

How Cancer Develops

The steps in cancer development are thought to be:

1. Exposure to a **carcinogen**.
2. Entry of the carcinogen into a cell.
3. **Initiation**, probably by the carcinogen's somehow altering the cellular genetic material.
4. Enhancement of cancer development by **promoters**, probably involving several more steps before the cell begins to multiply out of control; tumor formation.

Researchers think that the first three steps, which culminate with initiation, are the key ones, and people have the idea that they should therefore learn to avoid eating foods that contain carcinogens. In particular, many people have learned to fear food additives. However, food additives probably have little to do with the causation of cancer. Contaminants of food—chemicals that get into foods by accident—may be powerful carcinogens, but the additives permitted in foods are not. Additives are not discussed in this section but receive attention in Chapter 14.

Findings on Diet and Cancer

Epidemiological studies have shown that the incidence of certain cancers varies both by geographical area and by racial group. For example, Japanese people living in Japan develop more stomach cancers and fewer colon cancers than people in the United States. However, when Japanese people come to the United States, their children develop both stomach and colon cancers at a rate like that of U.S. citizens. Japan and the United States are both industrial

---

cancer: a disease in which cells multiply out of control, forming masses (**tumors**) that disrupt normal functioning of one or more organs.

carcinogen (car-SIN-oh-jen): a cancer-causing substance.
carcin = cancer
gen = gives rise to

initiation: an event, probably in the cell's genetic equipment, caused by radiation or by a chemical carcinogen that can give rise to cancer.

promoters: factors that do not initiate cancer but that favor its development once the initiating event has taken place. Other factors, **antipromoters**, oppose the development of cancer.

trans-fatty acids: fatty acids with unusual shapes that can arise when polyunsaturated oils are hydrogenated

countries, and their environmental pollution rates are similar. However, something in the environment must account for the changed cancer pattern in immigrants, and an obvious candidate is diet.

Another finding is that vegetarians have lower mortality rates from cancer than the rest of the population, even when cancers linked to smoking and alcohol are taken out of the picture. In general, studies of populations have suggested that low cancer rates correlate with high vegetable and grain intakes. Case-control studies, in which researchers can control some of the variables, have supported the population studies, and they implicate fat in cancer causation.

Laboratory studies using animals confirm suspicions that fat, of all dietary components, is uniquely correlated with cancer. Fat does not initiate the cancers, however. To get the tumors started, an experimenter has to expose the animals to a known carcinogen. After that exposure, the high-fat diet makes more cancers develop and makes them develop earlier than do low-fat diets. Thus fat appears to be a cancer promoter rather than an initiator. A high-fat diet may promote cancer in any of a number of ways:

■ By causing the body to secrete more of certain hormones (for example, estrogen), thus creating a climate favorable to the development of certain cancers (for example, breast cancer).

■ By promoting the secretion of bile into the intestine; bile may then be converted by organisms in the colon into compounds that cause cancer.

■ By being incorporated into cell membranes and changing them so that they offer less defense against cancer-causing invaders.

It may not be fat in general but certain forms of fat that have these effects. Some findings point to linoleic acid, the essential omega-6 fatty acid of vegetable oils, as particularly implicated in causation of cancer. Polyunsaturated fats, in general, are more often positively associated with tumor growth than are saturated fats. Importantly, it seems that omega-3 fatty acids and monounsaturated fatty acids may not promote cancer, and some preliminary evidence suggests that omega-3 acids may oppose the cancer-promoting effects of linoleic acid.[51] It would do no harm to reduce consumption of most forms of fat and also to ensure adequate intake of omega-3 fatty acids.

Another concern about fat and cancer centers around a chemical accident that occurs when polyunsaturated oils are hardened by hydrogenation processing. The fatty acids in the oils change in shape, creating unusual products that are not made by the body and that occur only rarely in foods. These unfamiliar fatty acids, or **trans-fatty acids**, can be taken up into cell membranes, where some researchers suspect they can alter functions, making people more prone to certain kinds of cancers. Recent evidence also suggests that in terms of the health of the heart and arteries *trans*-fatty acids are more similar to saturated fats than to the oils from which they were made.[52] Undoubtedly total fat consumption has more bearing on cancer susceptibility than consumption of *trans*-fatty acids.

There would appear to be no harm in reducing total fat intake to the point at which it contributes a maximum of 30 percent of total calories, as recommended for CVD prevention, and some cancer researchers suggest an even stricter limit: 20 percent of total calories. For the "average American" to accomplish this degree of fat restriction in practice means reducing the amount of fat used in food preparation and finding substitutes for many traditional foods: replace butter and margarine with butter flavorings; choose low-fat or fat-free mayonnaise and salad dressings; use broth instead of gravy. Of the fats used, olive oil and fish oils would seem to be the most desirable—just as for prevention of cardiovascular disease. For fat indispensable to cooking, canola oil may provide some benefit—it contains about 10 percent omega-3 fatty acids, almost as much monounsaturated fat as olive oil, and the least saturated fat of any cooking oil. However, foods fried in canola oil tend to absorb more total fat than foods fried in other oils.

At the same time, it seems desirable to increase plant fiber intakes. Fiber might help protect against some cancer, for example, by promoting the excretion of bile from the body or by speeding up the transit time of all materials through the colon so that the colon walls are not exposed for long to cancer-causing substances. That fiber does have an independent, protective effect of some kind is supported by evidence from Finland. The Finns eat a high-fat diet, but unlike other such diets, theirs is high in fiber as well. Their colon cancer rate is low, suggesting that fiber has a protective effect even in the presence of a high-fat diet.[53]

It seems apparent from all of these studies that foods contain two kinds of substances that affect people's susceptibility to cancer: promoters and antipromoters. Dietary fats act as promoters; fiber may act as an antipromoter, and indications are that many other factors in foods also act as antipromoters. If a fat-rich diet is implicated in causation of certain cancers and if fiber and/or a vegetable-rich diet are associated with prevention, then vegetarians should have a lower incidence of those cancers. They do, as many studies have shown.

A number of studies have supported special roles for plant foods in cancer resistance. One study found less frequent use of vegetables in people with colon cancer; another found, specifically, less use of cabbage, broccoli, and brussels sprouts in colon cancer victims. Stomach cancer, too, correlates with low vegetable intakes—in one study, vegetables in general; in another, fresh vegetables; in others, lettuce and other fresh greens or vegetables containing vitamin C.

Cancers of the head and neck seem to correlate best not with diet but with the combination of alcohol and tobacco consumption. Alcohol intake alone is associated with cancers of the mouth and throat, and alcoholism often damages the liver and increases the risk of liver cancer. Some evidence links alcohol intake with breast cancer, but these results have been challenged by later studies. Cancer of the rectum occurs more often in people who drink more than 15 ounces of beer each day.[54] It is unknown whether cancer's association with alcohol intake results from alcohol itself or from other compounds in alcoholic beverages.

Some dietary factors are implicated as protective against cancers of the head and neck, particularly fruits and raw vegetables and specifically the fruits and vegetables that contribute carotene (the vitamin A precursor) and the B vitamin riboflavin. Carotene and its relatives, the retinoids, are also important in preventing cancers of epithelial origin, including skin cancer.[55]

Vitamin A regulates aspects of cellular division that go awry in cancer. It also helps to maintain the immune system. Immunity can work against cancer even after a tumor has begun to form. Lung cancer incidence can be as much as 60 to 80 percent lower in people with high vitamin A intakes than in those with low intakes. In Japan, a study of about three hundred thousand people showed lung cancer rates to be 20 to 30 percent lower in smokers who ate yellow or green vegetables daily than in those who did not. In ex-smokers who ingested

Chapter 5's Food Feature presents details of cutting fat from the diet, and Figure 5–8 showed the fatty acid and cholesterol contents of common fats.

cruciferous vegetables: a group of vegetables named for their cross-shaped blossoms. They have been shown to protect against cancer in laboratory animals. Examples are cauliflower, cabbage, brussels sprouts, broccoli, turnips, and rutabagas.

indoles: a family of compounds with a structure resembling that of the amino acid tryptophan, mentioned here because they have anticancer activity.

dithiolthiones: a class of compounds, important in connection with diet and cancer because some are found in plant foods and seem to exhibit anticancer activity.

protease inhibitors: compounds that inhibit the action of protein-digesting enzymes.

■■■ Table 11–7 Cruciferous Vegetables and Carotene-rich Fruits and Vegetables

CRUCIFEROUS VEGETABLES	CAROTENE-RICH FRUITS AND VEGETABLES
Broccoli	Apricots
Brussels sprouts	Asparagus
Cabbage (all varieties)	Broccoli
Cauliflower	Cantaloupe
Greens (collards, mustards, turnips)	Carrots
Kale	Green onions
Kohlrabi	Greens (all varieties)
Rutabaga	Lettuce (dark green)
Turnip roots	Mango
	Oriental cabbages
	Papaya
	Parsley
	Spinach
	Squash (hard, winter)
	Sweet potato

yellow or green vegetables daily, the reduction was much greater, as if the *repair* of damage done by smoking after the initiation of cancer was enhanced by something in the vegetables.[56]

For anyone who might be tempted to think that pills containing vitamin A or carotene might provide the same benefit as green vegetables, it should be pointed out immediately that green vegetables have also been seen to have a protective effect beyond those already discussed for vitamin A, vitamin C, and fiber. Selenium is also potentially important in the fight against cancer.[57] Other nutrients are also cited as possible antipromoters: vitamin B_6, folate, pantothenic acid, vitamin B_{12}, vitamin E, iron, zinc, and more. Besides, nonnutrient substances in vegetables may also act to inhibit cancer promoters, and these would not be found in vitamin pills.

Some nonnutrient compounds that affect cancer vulnerability occur in foods. Best-known are those in vegetables of the cabbage family—the so-called **cruciferous vegetables**. These compounds, known as **indoles, dithiolthiones**, and other chemicals, activate enzymes that destroy carcinogens. Table 11–7 lists cruciferous vegetables and carotene-rich fruits and vegetables. Another class of possible anticancer compounds occurs in soybeans, chick peas, lima beans, and potatoes. These are **protease inhibitors**, and they are thought to inhibit enzymes associated with the spreading of tumors. Another still unidentified, nonnutrient in soybeans may act as an inhibitor of hormones that stimulate growth of breast cancer. Nonnutrients are discussed further in Controversy 14.

Other vegetables and fruits contain other constituents that may activate the enzyme system that degrades carcinogens.[58] These constituents are so widespread among plants that the single-most valuable application of the information obtained to date is *not* to eat cabbages or soybeans in particular but to eat a wide variety of vegetables and fruits in generous quantities.

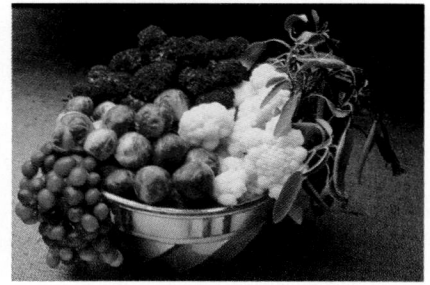

These foods contain nutrients and nonnutrients that may protect against cancer.

◫◫▶ *A high-fat diet is associated with the development of cancer. Fiber; vitamin C; the vitamin A precursor carotene; many other vitamins and minerals; and the nonnutrients found in cruciferous vegetables, potatoes, and certain legumes are thought to be protective.*

 Food Feature

Diet for Disease Prevention

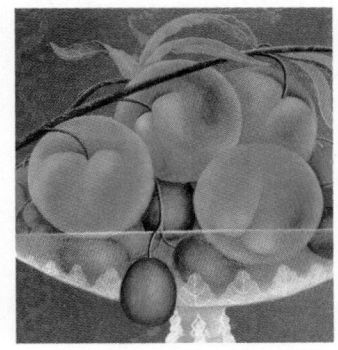

This chapter began with infectious diseases, went on to the major diseases affecting the heart and blood vessels, and concluded with cancer—three apparently dissimilar conditions with apparently distinct sets of causes. Yet all are responsive to diet, and in some ways the responses are similar. Dietary excesses increase the likelihood of all of them; overdoses of vitamins and minerals diminish immune function, invite infection; and excess food energy and fat intakes set the stage for heart disease and cancer. Dietary deficiencies increase the likelihood of all of them, particularly deficiencies in vitamin, mineral, and fiber intakes. Not all diet recommendations apply equally to all of the diseases (salt has a special relationship with hypertension, for example), but fortunately for the consumer, the dietary recommendations to help prevent individual diseases do not contradict each other.

For those who choose to change their diets, the pointers relevant to atherosclerosis in the *NRC Report* cited in Chapter 2 are repeated here:

■ Reduce total fat intake to 30 percent or less of calories. Reduce saturated fat intake to less than 10 percent of calories and the intake of cholesterol to less than 300 milligrams daily.

■ Every day eat five or more one-half cup servings of a combination of vegetables and fruits, especially green and yellow vegetables and citrus fruits. Also increase intake of starches and other complex carbohydrates by eating six or more daily servings of a combination of breads, cereals, and legumes. Carbohydrates should total more than 55 percent of calories.

■ Maintain protein intake at moderate levels, that is, approximately the current RDA for protein but not exceeding twice that amount or 1.6 grams per kilograms of body weight for adults.

■ Balance food intake and physical activity to maintain appropriate body weight.

To keep total fat down, select low-fat foods. If the percentage of calories from fat is to be less than 30 percent, then it is especially important to limit foods such as sour cream, butter, margarine, mayonnaise, cheese and cream cheese; foods high in hidden fat such as processed, convenience foods with sauces, fried foods, fat-marbled meat cuts, sausages, or ground beef, whole milk, and the many others identified in Chapter 5. For each 1000 calories of food, 33 grams of fat should be the maximum allowed. Shop for foods whose labels indicate no more than 3 grams of fat per 100 calories.

When you must add fat, use olive oil or canola oil, since these are high in monounsaturated fatty acids; but use them, like all fat, sparingly. Eat periodic meals of fish, especially fatty fish, to balance your intakes of omega-6 fatty acids with the omega-3 type. Consult Appendix A, the columns showing fat breakdown, for further details on the fatty acid contents of your favorite foods.

As far as cholesterol is concerned, use eggs in moderation (three to four per week); but unless medically advised to do so, do not shun them altogether. They are an inexpensive source of high-quality protein, and while high in cholesterol, they are not as high as was once thought, and they are not high in saturated fat. Feel free to use shellfish; they are not as high in cholesterol as has

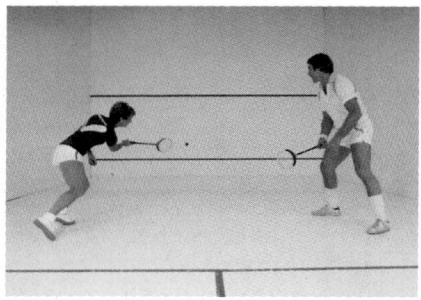

Exercise regularly, all your life.

been believed, and they do contain beneficial fatty acids. And to help lower blood cholesterol, choose foods high in soluble fiber—oats, oat bran, barley, and legumes—as well as fruits and vegetables.

Standard advice to those who wish to correct high blood pressure through diet is to eat less salt. Probably, though, the person wishing to avoid hypertension would benefit from all the recommendations relevant to atherosclerosis and from a serious program of weight control. Expend energy so as to earn the right to eat more nutrient-dense foods. In other words, be physically active. (If that benefit doesn't motivate you, then exercise to improve your circulation, to reduce your weight, to improve your morale, or to make friends—but do exercise.) Eat foods high in potassium (whole foods), high in calcium and magnesium (milk products and appropriate substitutes), low in fat, and high in fiber (whole grains, legumes, vegetables, fruits). Vary your diet because not all the factors that affect blood pressure have been studied yet. Use moderation with respect to alcohol too.

Many of the dietary guidelines for cancer prevention are identical to those given for CVD prevention in that they recommend controlling energy and fat, increasing intakes of fruits and vegetables, and limiting intakes of salt-cured products. Some, though, are unique to cancer prevention—notably those listed below numbered 4, 5, 6, and 8:

1. Control total food energy intake.
2. Reduce the consumption of both saturated and unsaturated fats.
3. Include fruits (especially citrus fruits), vegetables (particularly carotene-rich and cruciferous vegetables), and whole-grain products in the daily diet.
4. Avoid possible carcinogens by limiting consumption of foods preserved by salt curing, salt packing, or smoking.
5. Do not eat spoiled food or food that smells or appears old.
6. Continue to evaluate food additives for carcinogenic activity.§
7. Consume only moderate amounts of alcohol, if any.
8. Monitor drinking water for toxic substances.

To the recommendations made in these guidelines, we would add one other already mentioned for hypertension: vary your choices. Don't let your diet become monotonous. This last suggestion is based on an important concept in the prevention of cancer initiation—dilution. Whenever you switch from food to food, you are diluting whatever is in one food with what is in the others. It is safe to eat *some* salt-cured or smoked meats, but don't eat them all the time. Eat many green, yellow, and orange vegetables; they are all needed in the diet for many good reasons. If you include high-fiber foods and reduce your fat intake as well, you have every reason to feel confident that you are providing your body with the best nutrition at the lowest possible risk.

It is worth repeating the surgeon general's remark, first quoted in Chapter 1 of this book, that for the two out of three Americans who do not smoke or drink excessively, "your choice of diet can influence your long-term health prospects more than any other action you might take."[59] Indeed, healthy adults are privileged to have the fruits of recent research on the preventive effects of a nutritious diet: they are the first generation in history with the opportunity

§The Committee on Diet, Nutrition, and Cancer of the National Research Council, which published these guidelines, specifically stated, however, that additives legally permitted in foods were not implicated in cancer causation. *Executive Summary: Diet, Nutrition, and Cancer* (Washington, D.C.: National Academy Press, 1982).

to know how to lay the foundation for healthy later years through a lifetime of proper nutrition.

Notes

1. J. W. Alexander, Immunity, nutrition and trauma: An overview, *Acta Chirurgica Scandinavica* 522 (1985): 141–150.

2. Position of The American Dietetic Association: Nutrition intervention in the treatment of human immunodeficiency virus infection, *Journal of the American Dietetic Association* 89 (1989): 839–841.

3. P. O'Sullivan, R. A. Linke, and S. Dalton, Evaluation of body weight and nutritional status among AIDS patients, *Journal of the American Dietetic Association* 85 (1985): 1483–1484.

4. B. M. Dworkin and coauthors, Selenium deficiency in the acquired immunodeficiency syndrome, *Journal of Parenteral and Enteral Nutrition* 10 (1986): 405–407.

5. S. S. Resler, Nutrition care of AIDS patients, *Journal of the American Dietetic Association* 88 (1988): 828–832.

6. J. T. Dwyer and coauthors, Unproven nutrition therapies for AIDS: What is the evidence? *Nutrition Today* March/April 1988, pp. 25–33.

7. S. Lillioja and coauthors, Impaired glucose tolerance as a disorder of insulin action, *New England Journal of Medicine* 318 (1988): 1217–1225.

8. G. F. Cahill, Beta-cell deficiency, insulin resistance, or both? *New England Journal of Medicine* 318 (1988): 1268–1270.

9. *America's Health: A Century of Progress But a Time of Despair*, a booklet (1983) from the American Council on Science and Health, 47 Maple Street, Summit, NJ 07901.

10. H. Sheldon, *Boyd's Introduction to the Study of Disease*, 9th ed. (Philadelphia: Lea and Febiger, 1984), Chapter 13, The Heart, pp. 347–348.

11. Lowering blood cholesterol to prevent heart disease, NIH Consensus Conference, *Journal of the American Medical Association* 253 (1985): 2080–2086.

12. A. M. Gotto, Hypercholesterolemia: An assessment of screening and diagnostic techniques, *Modern Medicine*, April 1987, pp. 28–32.

13. The Canadian consensus conference on cholesterol: Final report, *Canadian Medical Association Journal*, supplement, 139 (1988).

14. I. H. Ullrich, C. M. Reid, and R. A. Yeater, Increased HDL-cholesterol levels with a weight lifting program, *Southern Medical Journal* 80 (1987): 328–331.

15. G. Sopko and coauthors, The effects of exercise and weight loss on plasma lipids in young obese men, *Metabolism* 34 (1985): 227–236.

16. Body weight and serum cholesterol, *Nutrition Reviews* 43 (1985): 43–44.

17. Diet, metals, and hidden heart disease, *Science News*, 27 September 1986, p. 201.

18. Try a little TLC, *Science 80*, January-February 1980, p. 15.

19. G. Fernandez at the 1988 American Chemical Society national meeting, as reported by J. Raloff, No-fault fat: More praise for fish oil, *Science News* 134 (1988): 228.

20. H. Glauber and coauthors, Adverse metabolic effect of omega-3 fatty acids in non-insulin–dependent diabetes mellitus, *Annals of Internal Medicine* 108 (1988): 663–668.

21. A. Toufexis, A fishy deal in the freezer, *Time,* 16 January 1989, p. 80.

22. E. D. Frohlich, Physiological observations in essential hypertension, *Journal of the American Dietetic Association* 80 (1982): 18–20.

23. W. B. Kannel and T. J. Thom, Incidence, prevalence, and mortality of cardiovascular diseases, in *The Heart,* 6th ed., ed. J. W. Hurst (New York: McGraw-Hill, 1986), pp. 557–565.

24. E. Ferrannini and coauthors, Insulin resistance in essential hypertension, *New England Journal of Medicine* 317 (1987): 350-357; L. Landsberg, Insulin and hypertension: Lessons from obesity (editorial), *New England Journal of Medicine* 317 (1987): 378–379.

25. Ferrannini and coauthors, 1987; Landsberg, 1987.

26. J. W. Rowe and coauthors, Effect of insulin and glucose infusions on sympathetic nervous system activity in normal man, *Diabetes* 30 (1981): 219–225, as cited by Landsberg, 1987.

27. Hypertension Detection and Follow-up Program Cooperative Group, The effect of treatment on mortality in "mild" hypertension, *New England Journal of Medicine* 307 (1982): 976-980.

28. E. Reisin and coauthors, Effect of weight loss without salt restriction on the reduction of blood pressure in overweight hypertensive patients, *New England Journal of Medicine* 298 (1978): 1–6.

29. H. G. Langford and coauthors, Dietary therapy slows the return of hypertension after stopping prolonged medication, *Journal of the American Medical Association* 253 (1985): 657–664.

30. S. Wassertheil and coauthors, Effective dietary intervention in hypertensives: Sodium restriction and weight reduction, *Journal of the American Dietetic Association* 85 (1985): 423–430.

31. C. M. Tipton, Exercise, training, and hypertension, *Exercise and Sports Sciences Reviews* 12 (1984): 245–306; R. S. Williams, R. A. McKinnis, and F. R. Cobb, Effects of physical conditioning on left ventricular ejection fraction in patients with coronary artery disease, *Circulation,* July 1984, pp. 69–75.

32. G. Nomura, Physical training in essential hypertension: Alone and in combination with dietary salt restriction, *Journal of Cardiac Rehabilitation* 4 (1984): 469–475.

33. Tipton, 1984.

34. K. Przyklenk and A. C. Groom, Effects of exercise frequency, intensity, and duration on revascularization in the transition zone of infarcted rat hearts, *Canadian Journal of Physiology and Pharmacology* 63 (1985): 273–278.

35. T. W. Kurtz, H. A. Al-Bander, and C. Morris, "Salt-sensitive" essential hypertension in men: Is the sodium ion alone important? *New England Journal of Medicine* 317 (1987): 1043–1048.

36. A. M. Altschul and J. K. Grommet, Sodium intake and sodium sensitivity, *Nutrition Reviews* 38 (1980): 393–402.

37. J. K. Huttunen and coauthors, Dietary factors and hypertension, *Acta Medica Scandinavica* (Supplement) 701 (1985): 72–82.

38. K. T. Khaw and E. Barrett-Connor, Dietary potassium and stroke-associated mortality: A 12-year prospective population study, *New England Journal of Medicine* 316 (1987): 235–240.

39. H. G. Langford, Dietary potassium and hypertension: Epidemiologic data, *Annals of Internal Medicine* 98 (1983): 770-772.

40. H. Henry and coauthors, Increasing calcium intake lowers blood pressure: The literature reviewed, *Journal of the American Dietetic Association* 85 (1985): 182–185.

41. D. A. McCarron and coauthors, Blood pressure and nutrient intake in the United States, *Science* 224 (1984): 1392–1398.

42. R. Weinsier, Recent developments in the etiology and treatment of hypertension: Dietary calcium, fat, and magnesium, *American Journal of Clinical Nutrition* 42 (1985): 1331–1338.

43. J. P. Knochel, Cardiovascular effects of alcohol, *Annals of Internal Medicine* 98 (1983): 849–854.

44. Knochel, 1983.

45. A. L. Klatsky, G. D. Friedman, and M. A. Armstrong, The relationships between alcoholic beverage use and other traits to blood pressure: A new Kaiser Permanente study, *Circulation* 73 (1986): 628–636.

46. G. D. Friedman, A. L. Klatsky, and A. B. Siegelaub, Alcohol intake and hypertension, *Annals of Internal Medicine* 98 (1983): 846–849.

47. J. S. Gill and coauthors, Stroke and alcohol consumption, *New England Journal of Medicine* 315 (1986): 1041–1046.

48. A. L. Klatsky, M. A. Armstrong, and G. D. Friedman, Relationship of alcoholic beverage use to subsequent coronary artery disease hospitalization, *American Journal of Cardiology* 58 (1986): 710–714.

49. M. R. Joffres, D. M. Reed, and K. Yano, Relationship of magnesium intake and other dietary factors to blood pressure: The Honolulu heart study, *American Journal of Clinical Nutrition* 45 (1987): 469–475.

50. J. Tuomilehto and coauthors, Nutrition-related determinants of blood pressure, *Preventive Medicine* 14 (1985): 413–427.

51. L. A. Sauer, R. T. Cauchy, and A. S. Hurtubise, Effects of omega-6 and omega-3 fatty acids on the rate of 3H-thymidine incorporation (^{3}H-TI) in hepatoma 7288CTC perfused in situ, *FASEB Journal* 43 (1990): A508.

52. R. P. Mensink and M. B. Katan, Effect of dietary *trans*-fatty acids on high density and low density lipoprotein cholesterol levels in healthy subjects, *New England Journal of Medicine* 323 (1990): 439–445.

53. E. L. Wynder, Dietary habits and cancer epidemiology, *Cancer* 43 (1979): 1955–1961, as cited by S. H. Brammer and R. L. DeFelice, Dietary advice in regard to risk for colon and breast cancer, *Preventive Medicine* 9 (1980): 544–549.

54. H. K. Seitz and U. A. Simoonowski, Alcohol and carcinogenesis, *Annual Review of Nutrition* 8 (1988): 99–119.

55. J. L. Werther, Food and cancer, *New York State Journal of Medicine*, August 1980, pp. 1401–1408.

56. Werther, 1980.

57. P. Knekt and coauthors, Serum selenium and subsequent risk of cancer among Finnish men and women, *Journal of the National Cancer Institute* 82 (1990): 864–868.

58. L. W. Wattenberg and W. D. Loub, Inhibition of polycyclic aromatic hydrocarbon-induced neoplasia by naturally occurring indoles, *Cancer Research* 38 (1978): 1410–1413.

59. *The Surgeon General's report on Nutrition and Health, Summary and Recommendations* (Washington, D. C.: DHHS [PHS] publication no. 88–50211, 1988).

CONTROVERSY 11

Alcohol and Nutrition

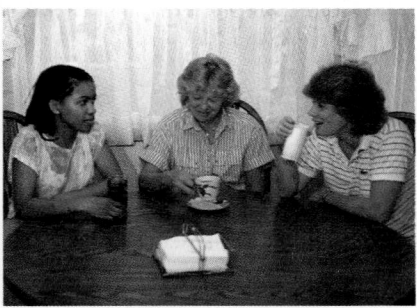

People naturally congregate to enjoy conversation and companionship, and it is natural, too, to offer beverages to companions. All beverages ease conversation whether or not they contain alcohol. Still, some people choose alcohol over cola, milk, or coffee, and they should know a few things about alcohol's short term and long term effects on health. One consideration is energy—alcohol yields energy to the body, and many alcoholic drinks are much more fattening than their non-alcoholic counterparts. Additionally, alcohol has a tremendous impact on the overall well-being of the body, as the rest of the Controversy makes clear.

People consume alcohol in servings they call "a drink." However, the serving that some people consider one drink may not be the same as the standard drink that delivers 1/2 ounce pure ethanol:

■ 3 to 4 ounces wine.
■ 10 ounces wine cooler.
■ 12 ounces beer.

■ 1 ounce hard liquor (whiskey, gin, brandy, rum, vodka).

The percentage of alcohol in distilled liquor is stated as *proof*: 100-proof liquor is 50 percent alcohol; 90-proof is 45 percent, and so forth. Compared with hard liquor, beer and wine have a relatively low percentage of alcohol.

Alcohol Enters the Body

From the moment an alcoholic beverage is swallowed, the body confers special status on it. Unlike foods, which require digestion, the tiny alcohol molecules are all ready to be absorbed; they can diffuse right through the walls of an empty stomach and reach the brain within a minute. A person can become intoxicated almost immediately when drinking, especially if the person's stomach is empty. When the stomach is full of food, molecules of alcohol have less chance of touching the walls and diffusing through, so alcohol affects the brain a little less immediately. (By the time the stomach contents are emptied into the small intestine, it doesn't matter that food is mixed with the alcohol. The alcohol is absorbed rapidly anyway.)

A practical pointer derives from this information. If a person wants to drink socially and not become intoxicated, the person should eat the snacks provided by the host (avoid the salty ones; they make you thirstier). Carbohydrate snacks are best suited for slowing alcohol absorption. High-fat snacks help too because they slow peristalsis, keep-

ing the alcohol in the stomach longer.[1]

If one drinks slowly enough, the alcohol, after absorption, will be collected into the liver and processed without much affecting other parts of the body. If one drinks more rapidly, however, some of the alcohol bypasses the liver and flows for a while through the rest of the body and the brain.

Alcohol Arrives in the Brain

People use alcohol today as a kind of social anesthetic to help them relax or to relieve anxiety. One **drink** relieves inhibitions, and this gives people the impression that alcohol is a stimulant. Actually the way it does this is by sedating *inhibitory* nerves, allowing excitatory nerves to take over. This is temporary. Ultimately alcohol acts as a depressant and sedates all the nerve cells. Figure C11−1 on page 395 describes alcohol's effects on the brain.

It is lucky that the brain centers respond to elevating blood alcohol in the order described in Figure C11−1 because a person usually passes out before managing to drink a lethal dose. It is possible, though, for a person to drink fast enough so that the effects of alcohol continue to accelerate after the person has gone to sleep. The occasional death that takes place during a drinking contest is attributed to this effect. The drinker drinks fast enough, before passing out, to receive a lethal dose. Table C11−1 (page 396) shows the

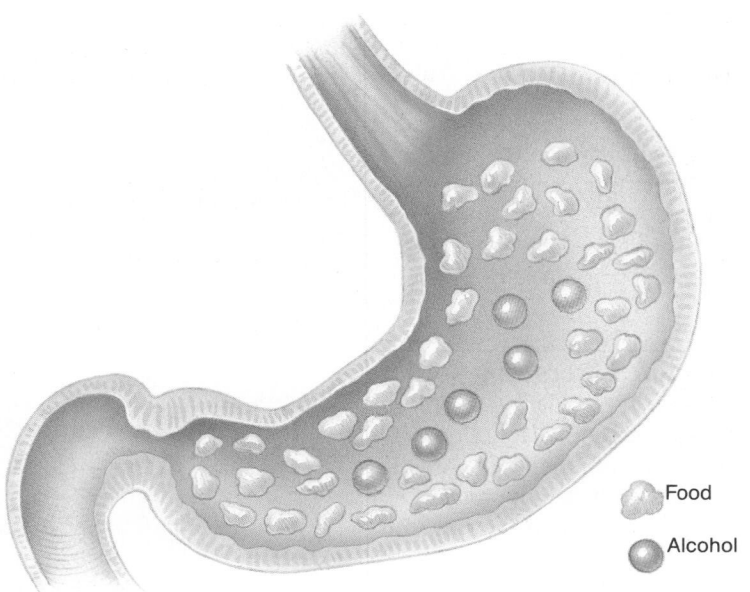

Food

Alcohol

The alcohol in a stomach filled with food has a low probability of touching the walls and diffusing through. Food also keeps alcohol in the stomach longer.

blood alcohol levels that correspond with progressively greater intoxication and Table C11−2 (page 396) shows the brain responses that occur at these blood levels.

Brain cells are particularly sensitive to excessive exposure to alcohol. The brain shrinks, even in people who drink only moderately.[2] The extent of the shrinkage is proportional to the amount drunk.[3] Abstinence, together with good nutrition, reverses some of the brain damage—possibly all of it if heavy drinking has not continued for more than a few years—but prolonged drinking beyond an individual's capacity to recover can cause severe and irreversible effects on vision, memory, learning ability, and other functions.[4]

Anyone who has had an alcoholic drink knows that alcohol increases

urine output. This is because alcohol depresses the brain's production of **antidiuretic hormone**. Loss of body water leads to thirst. The only fluid that will relieve dehydration is water, but if alcohol is the only drink available, the thirsty person may choose another alcoholic beverage and worsen the problem. The smart drinker, then, alternates alcoholic beverages with nonalcoholic choices and when thirsty chooses the latter.

The water loss caused by hormone depression involves loss of more than just water. The water takes with it important minerals, such as magnesium, potassium, calcium, and zinc, depleting the body's reserves. These minerals are vital to the maintenance of fluid balance and to nerve and muscle action and coordination, as Chapter 8 made clear.

■■■ Alcohol Arrives in the Liver

The capillaries that surround the digestive tract merge into veins that carry the alcohol-laden blood to the liver. Here the veins branch and re-branch into capillaries that touch every liver cell. The liver cells make nearly all of the body's alcohol-processing machinery, and the routing of blood through the liver allows the cells to go right to work on the alcohol. The liver's location at this point along the circulatory system guarantees that it gets the chance to remove toxic substances before they reach other body organs such as the heart and brain.

The liver makes and maintains two sets of equipment for metabolizing alcohol. One is an enzyme that removes hydrogens from alcohol to break it down; the name almost says what it does—**alcohol dehydrogenase** (**ADH**).* This handles about 80 percent or more of body alcohol. The other alcohol-metabolizing equipment is a chain of enzymes (known as the **MEOS**) thought to handle about 10 to 20 percent of body alcohol.[5] With high blood alcohol concentrations, the MEOS activity is enhanced, as will be shown later. But let us look at the ADH system first.

*There are actually two ADH enzymes, each for a specific task in alcohol breakdown. Enzyme 1, alcohol dehydrogenase, converts alcohol to acetaldehyde. Enzyme 2, acetaldehyde dehydrogenase, converts acetaldehyde to a common body compound, acetyl CoA, identical to that derived from carbohydrate and fat during their breakdown.

■■■ **Figure C11–1**

Alcohol's Effects on the Brain.
When alcohol flows to the brain, it first sedates the frontal lobe, the reasoning part. As the alcohol molecules diffuse into the cells of this lobe, they interfere with reasoning and judgment. If the drinker drinks faster than the rate at which the liver can oxidize the alcohol, then the speech and vision centers of the brain become sedated, and the area that governs reasoning becomes more incapacitated. Later the cells of the brain responsible for large-muscle control are affected; at this point people under the influence stagger or weave when they try to walk. Finally, the conscious brain is completely subdued, and the person passes out. Now the person can drink no more; this is fortunate because a higher dose's anesthetic effect could reach the deepest brain centers that control breathing and heartbeat, and the person could die.

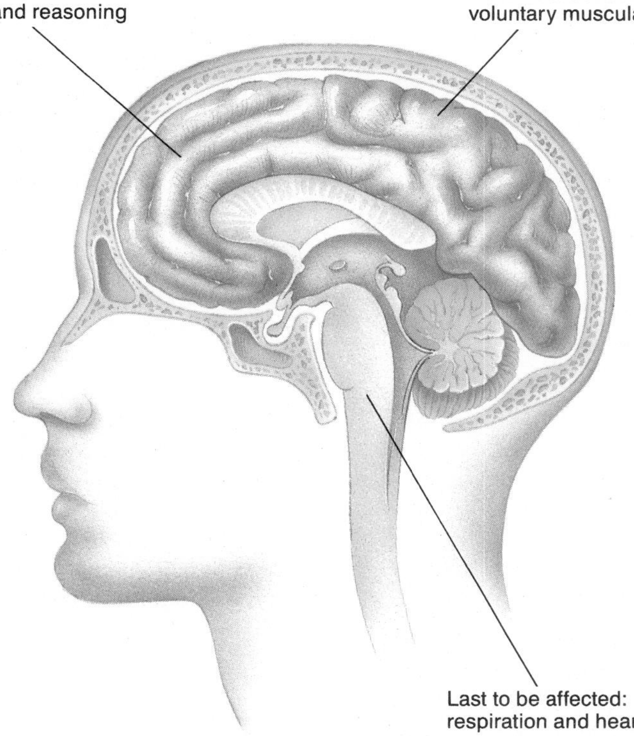

Most sensitive: judgement and reasoning

Next most sensitive: voluntary muscular control

Last to be affected: respiration and heart action

The amount of alcohol a person's body can process in a given time is limited by the number of ADH enzymes that reside in the liver.† If more molecules of alcohol arrive at the liver cells than the enzymes can handle, the extra alcohol must wait. It enters the general circulation and is carried to all parts of the body, circulating again and again through the liver until enzymes are available to degrade it.

The number of ADH enzymes present is affected by whether or not a person eats. Fasting for as little as a day causes degradation of body proteins, including the ADH enzymes in the liver, and this can reduce the rate of alcohol metabolism by half. Prudent drinkers drink slowly, with food in their stomachs, to allow the alcohol molecules to move to the liver cells gradually enough for the enzymes to handle the load. It takes about an hour and a half to metabolize one drink, depending on a person's body size, on previous drinking experience, on how recently the person has eaten, and on general health at the time. The liver is the only organ that can dispose of significant quantities of alcohol, and its maximum rate of alcohol clearance is fixed. This explains why only time will restore sobriety. Walking will not; muscles cannot metabolize alcohol. Nor will it help to drink a cup of coffee. Caffeine is a stimulant, but it won't speed up the metabolism of alcohol. The police say ruefully that a cup of

†Some ADH enzymes reside in the stomach, offering a protective barrier against alcohol entering the blood. Research shows that alcoholics make less stomach ADH, and so do women. Women may absorb about one-third more alcohol than men, even when they are the same size and drink the same amount of alcoholic beverage.

■■■ Table C11–1 Alcohol Doses and Blood Levels

Number of Drinks[a]	PERCENT BLOOD ALCOHOL BY BODY WEIGHT				
	100 lb	120 lb	150 lb	180 lb	200 lb
2	0.08	0.06	0.05	0.04	0.04
4	0.15	0.13	0.10	0.08	0.08
6	0.23	0.19	0.15	0.13	0.11
8	0.30	0.25	0.20	0.17	0.15
12	0.45	0.36	0.30	0.25	0.23
14	0.52	0.42	0.35	0.34	0.27

[a]Taken within an hour or so.

coffee will only make a sleepy drunk into a wide-awake drunk.

As the ADH enzymes break alcohol down, they produce hydrogen ions (acid), which must be picked up by a compound that contains the B vitamin niacin as part of its structure. Normally this acid is disposed of through a metabolic pathway, but when alcohol is present in the system, this pathway shuts down. The niacin-containing compound remains loaded with hydrogens that it cannot get rid of and so becomes unavailable for a multitude of other vital body processes for which it is required.

The synthesis of fatty acids also accelerates as a result of the liver's exposure to alcohol. Fat accumulation can be seen in the liver after a single night of heavy drinking. **Fatty liver**, the first stage of liver deterioration seen in heavy drinkers, interferes with the distribution of nutrients and oxygen to the liver cells. If the condition lasts long enough, the liver cells die, and fibrous scar tissue invades the area—the second stage of liver deterioration called **fibrosis**. Fibrosis is reversible with good nutrition and abstinence from alcohol, but the next (last) stage—**cirrhosis**—is not. All of this points to the importance of moderation in the use of alcohol.

The presence of alcohol alters amino acid metabolism in the liver cells. Synthesis of some proteins important in the immune system slows down, weakening the body's defenses against infection. Synthesis of lipoproteins speeds up, increasing blood triglyceride levels. In addition, excessive alcohol increases the body's acid burden and interferes with normal uric acid metabolism, causing symptoms like those of **gout**.

Liver metabolism clears most of the alcohol from the blood. However, about 10 percent is excreted through the breath and in the urine. This fact is the basis for the breathalyzer test that law enforcement officers administer when they suspect someone of driving under the influence of alcohol.

■■■ Benefits of Moderate Alcohol Use

The effects of wine, beer, and other fermented beverages have been known to human societies for more than 5000 years. Taken in moderation, alcohol relaxes people, reduces their inhibitions, and encourages social interactions.

The term *moderation* is important in the statement just made. Just what is moderation in the use of alcohol? No single amount of alcohol per day is appropriate for everyone because people differ in their tolerance levels. But authorities have attempted to set a limit that is appropriate for most healthy people: not more than 3 drinks a day for the average-sized, healthy man; not more than 2 drinks a day for the average-sized, healthy woman. This amount is

■■■ Table C11–2 Alcohol Blood Levels and Brain Responses

BLOOD LEVEL (%)	BRAIN RESPONSE
0.05	Judgment impaired
0.10	Emotional control impaired
0.15	Muscle coordination and reflexes impaired
0.20	Vision impaired
0.30	Drunk, totally out of control
0.35	Stupor
0.50–0.60	Total loss of consciousness, finally death

supposed to be enough to produce an elevation of mood without incurring any long-term harm to health. Doubtless some people could consume slightly more; others could definitely not handle nearly so much without significant risk. If you think your own drinking might not be moderate or normal or has caused problems in your life, or if you feel guilty about your drinking, you may want to seek a professional evaluation.

Alcohol in any beverage has the same mood effects. In addition, wine in particular is credited with some special effects. The high potassium content of grape juice is beneficial to people with high blood pressure; when the grape juice is made into wine, the potassium remains in the wine, so this effect carries over. In fact, since alcohol raises blood pressure, the grape juice is more suitable than wine for people with hypertension. Dealcoholized wine also increases the absorption of potassium, calcium, phosphorus, magnesium, and zinc; so does wine, but the alcohol in it promotes the *excretion* of these minerals, so the dealcoholized version is preferred.[6]

Alcoholic beverages affect the appetite. Usually they reduce it, making people unaware that they are hungry. But in people who are tense and unable to eat, small doses of wine taken 20 minutes before meals improve the appetite. Certain acid compounds in the wine, known as congeners, are credited with this effect. For undernourished people and for people with severely depressed appetites, wine may facilitate eating even when psychotherapy fails to do so.

Limited research shows an association between moderate alcohol consumption and a reduced risk of heart disease, especially for women.[7] A study of more than 87,000 women found that, compared with nondrinkers, women who consumed 3 to 15 drinks per week had less of a risk of coronary heart disease.[8]

The mechanism by which moderate alcohol consumption seems to be protective against heart disease remains to be proved. Some research suggests that alcohol elevates the concentration of high-density lipoproteins (HDL) in people's blood. However, other research has shown that of two types of HDL, only one (HDL_3) is affected by alcohol. HDL_2 is the type known to be protective against heart disease, and this type is thought to remain unaffected by alcohol.[9] The association between moderate alcohol consumption and stroke is less clear. Moderate alcohol consumption in the study just mentioned lowered the risk of one type of stroke but increased the risk of a different type. Some researchers argue that the concept that moderate alcohol consumption is protective against heart disease ignores the abundant evidence showing a relationship between alcohol consumption and poor health.[10]

Another example of the beneficial use of alcohol is provided by research showing that moderate use of wine in later life improves morale, stimulates social interaction, and promotes more restful sleep.[11] In nursing homes, improved patient and staff relations were attributed to greater self-esteem among elderly patients who drank moderate

amounts of wine. Researchers hypothesize that chronic fatigue may be responsible for some behaviors associated with old age. The positive effects of wine on sleep may alleviate the fatigue, permitting more social interactions. Clearly, more research is needed to confirm the risks and benefits of moderate drinking.

◼◼◼ Alcohol's Long-Term Effects

By far the longest term effects of alcohol are those felt by the child of a woman who drinks during pregnancy. This is a topic so important that it is given a space of its own in Chapter 12, and the recommendation is made that pregnant women should not drink at all. For nonpregnant adults, however, what are the effects of alcohol over the long term?

A couple of drinks set in motion many destructive processes in the body, but the next day's abstinence reverses them. As long as the doses taken are moderate, time between them is ample, and nutrition is adequate meanwhile, recovery is probably complete.

If the doses of alcohol are heavy and the time between them is short, complete recovery cannot take place, and repeated onslaughts of alcohol gradually take a toll on the body. For example, alcohol is directly toxic to skeletal and cardiac muscle, causing weakness and deterioration in a dose-related manner.[12] Alcoholism makes heart disease more likely probably because alcohol in high doses raises the blood pressure, as Chapter 11 made clear. Cirrhosis can develop after 10 to 20 years from the additive effects of frequent heavy drinking episodes. Alcohol abuse also increases a person's risk of cancer of the mouth, throat, esophagus, rectum, and lungs.[13] Women who drink even moderately may run an increased risk of developing breast cancer.[14] Although some dispute these findings, a reliable source tentatively ranks daily human exposure to ethanol as high in relation to other possible carcinogenic hazards.[15] Other long-term effects of alcohol abuse include[16]:

■ Ulcers of the stomach and intestines.
■ Psychological depression.
■ Kidney damage, bladder damage, prostate gland damage, pancreas damage.
■ Skin rashes and sores.
■ Impaired immune response.
■ Deterioration in the testicles and adrenal glands, leading to feminization and sexual impotence in men.
■ Central nervous system damage.
■ Malnutrition.
■ Increased risk of violent death.

This list is by no means all inclusive. Alcohol has direct toxic effects, independent of the effect of malnutrition, on all body organs.

The more alcohol a person drinks, the less likely that he or she will eat enough food to obtain adequate nutrients. Alcohol is empty calories, like pure sugar and pure fat; it displaces nutrients. In a sense, each time you drink 150 calories of alcohol, you are spending those calories on a luxury item and getting no nutritional value in return. The more calories you spend this way, the fewer you have left to spend on nutritious foods. Table C11–3 shows the calorie amounts of typical alcoholic beverages.

Alcohol abuse not only displaces nutrients from the diet but also affects every tissue's metabolism of nutrients. Alcohol causes stomach cells to oversecrete both acid and an agent of the immune system, histamine, that produces inflammation. These changes make the stomach and esophagus linings vulnerable to ulcer formation. Intestinal cells fail to absorb thiamin, folate, and vitamin B_{12} (Figure C11–2, next page). Liver cells lose efficiency in activating vitamin D and alter their production and excretion of bile. Rod cells in the retina, which normally process vitamin A alcohol (retinol) to the form needed in vision, find themselves processing drinking alcohol instead. The kidneys excrete magnesium, calcium, potassium, and zinc.

Alcohol's intermediate products interfere with metabolism too. They dislodge vitamin B_6 from its protective binding protein so that it is destroyed, causing a vitamin B_6 deficiency and thereby lowered production of red blood cells.

Most dramatic is alcohol's effect on folate. When alcohol is present, it is as though the body were actively trying to expel folate from all its sites of action and storage. The liver, which normally contains enough folate to meet all needs, leaks folate into the blood. As the blood folate concentration rises, the kidneys are deceived into excreting it, as though it were in excess. The intestine normally releases and retrieves folate continuously, but it becomes damaged by folate deficiency and alcohol toxicity, so it fails to retrieve its own folate and misses out on any that may trickle in from food as well. Alcohol also interferes with the action of what little folate is left, and this inhibits the production of new cells, especially the rapidly dividing cells of the intestine and the blood. Alcohol abuse causes a folate deficiency that devastates digestive system function.

■■■ Table C11–3 Calories in Alcoholic Beverages and Mixers

BEVERAGE	AMOUNT (OZ)	ENERGY (CAL)
Beer	12	150
Light beer	12	100
Gin, rum, vodka, whiskey (86 proof)	1 1/2	105
Dessert wine	3 1/2	140
Table wine	3 1/2	85
Tonic, ginger ale, other sweetened carbonated waters	8	80
Cola, root beer	8	100
Fruit-flavored soda, Tom Collins mix	8	115
Club soda, plain seltzer, diet drinks	8	1

▦ Figure C11–2

Alcohol's Effect on Vitamin Absorption (Example).
In the presence of alcohol, intestinal cells fail to absorb thiamin, except at very high concentrations.

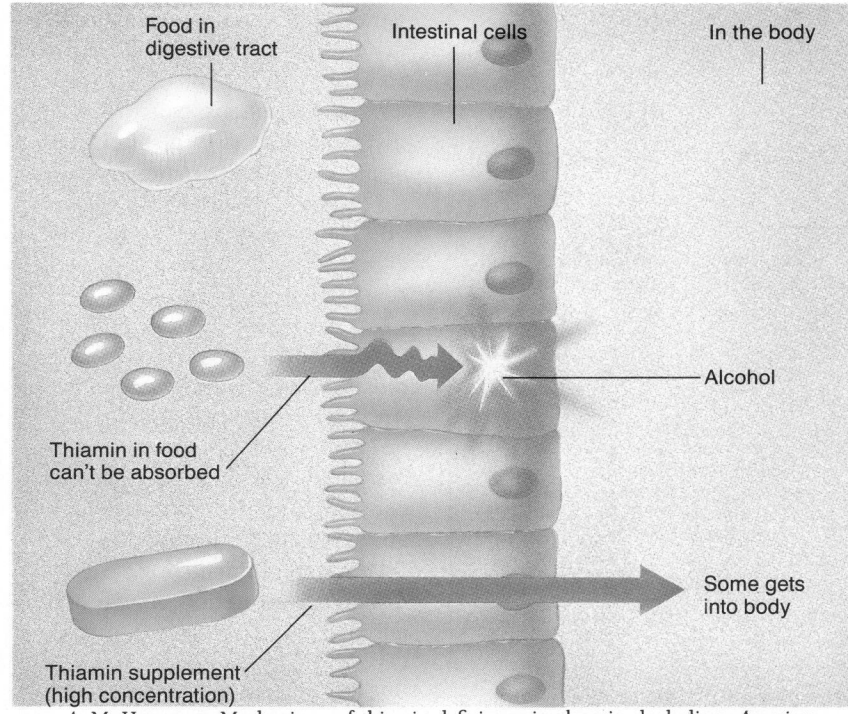

Food in digestive tract

Intestinal cells

In the body

Thiamin in food can't be absorbed

Alcohol

Some gets into body

Thiamin supplement (high concentration)

SOURCE: A. M. Hoyumpa, Mechanisms of thiamin deficiency in chronic alcoholism, *American Journal of Clinical Nutrition* 33 (1980): 2750–2761.

Nutrient deficiencies are thus a virtually inevitable consequence of alcohol abuse, not only because alcohol displaces food but also because alcohol directly interferes with the body's use of nutrients, making them ineffective even if they are present. Over a lifetime, excessive drinking, whether or not accompanied by attention to nutrition, brings about deficits of all the nutrients mentioned in this discussion and many more besides.

▦ Alcohol and Drugs

The liver's reaction to alcohol affects its handling of drugs as well as nutrients. In addition to the ADH enzymes, the liver possesses an enzyme system that metabolizes *both* alcohol and drugs—any compounds that have certain chemical features in common. As mentioned earlier, at low blood alcohol concentrations, the MEOS handles about 10 to 20 percent of the alcohol consumed. However, at high blood alcohol concentrations, or if repeatedly exposed to alcohol, the MEOS is enhanced.[17]

As a person's blood alcohol concentration rises, the alcohol competes with—and wins out over—other drugs whose metabolism relies on the MEOS. If a person drinks and uses another drug at the same time, the drug will be metabolized more slowly and so will be much more potent. The MEOS is busy disposing of alcohol, so the drug cannot be handled until later; the dose may build up to where its effects are greatly amplified—sometimes to the point of killing the user.

In contrast, once a heavy drinker stops drinking and alcohol is not present to compete with other drugs, the enhanced MEOS metabolizes those drugs much faster than before. This can make it confusing and tricky to work out the correct dosages of medications. The doctor who prescribes sedatives every four hours, for example, unaware that the person has recently gone from being a heavy drinker to an abstainer, expects the MEOS to dispose of the drug at a certain predicted rate. The MEOS is adapted to metabolizing large quantities of alcohol, however. It therefore metabolizes the drug extra fast. The drug's effects wear off unexpectedly fast, leaving the client undersedated. Imagine the doctor's alarm should a patient wake up on the table during an operation! A skilled anesthesiologist always asks the patient about his drinking pattern before putting him to sleep.

▮▮▮ Miniglossary

alcohol dehydrogenase: an enzyme system that breaks down alcohol.

antidiuretic hormone (ADH): a hormone produced by the pituitary gland in response to dehydration (or a high sodium concentration in the blood); it stimulates the kidneys to reabsorb more water and so to excrete less. This ADH should not be confused with the enzyme alcohol dehydrogenase, which is sometimes also abbreviated ADH.

cirrhosis (seer-OH-sis): advanced liver disease, often associated with alcoholism in which liver cells have died and hardened and have permanently lost their function.

drink: a dose of any alcoholic beverage that delivers 1/2 ounce of pure ethanol.

fatty liver: an early stage of liver deterioration seen in several diseases, including kwashiorkor and alcoholic liver disease. Fatty liver is characterized by accumulation of fat in the liver cells.

fibrosis (fye-BROH-sis): an intermediate stage of liver deterioration seen in several diseases, including viral hepatitis and alcoholic liver disease. In fibrosis, the liver cells lose their function and assume the characteristics of connective tissue cells (fibers).

gout (GOWT): accumulation of uric acid crystals in the joints.

MEOS (microsomal ethanol oxidizing system): a system of enzymes in the liver that oxidize not only alcohol but also several classes of drugs. (The *microsomes* are tiny particles of membranes with associated enzymes that can be collected from broken-up cells; *micro* means "tiny"; *soma* means "body").

This discussion has touched on some of the ways alcohol affects health and nutrition. Despite some possible benefits of moderate alcohol consumption, the potential for harm is great, especially with excessive alcohol consumption. Consider that over 50 percent of all fatal auto accidents are alcohol related. Translated to human lives, more than 25,000 people die each year in alcohol-related traffic accidents. The best way to avoid the harmful effects of alcohol is, of course, to avoid alcohol altogether. If you do drink, do so with care—for yourself and for others—and in moderation.

Notes

1. A. B. Eisenstein, Nutritional and metabolic effects of alcohol, *Journal of the American Dietetic Association* 81 (1982): 247–251.

2. Getting pickled, *Scientific American*, April 1985, p. 76.

3. D. W. Walder and coauthors, Neuronal loss in hippocampus induced by prolonged ethanol consumption in rats, *Science* 209 (1980): 711–713.

4. Alcohol-induced brain damage and its reversibility, *Nutrition Reviews* 38 (1980): 11–12; L. A. Cala and coauthors, Alcohol-related brain damage: Serial studies after abstinence and recommencement of drink, *Australian Alcohol/Drug Review*, July 1984, pp. 127–140.

5. A. Eisenstein, Nutritional and metabolic effects of alcohol, *Journal of the American Dietetic Association* 81 (1982): 247–251.

6. J. B. McDonald, Not by alcohol alone, *Nutrition Today*, January/February 1979, pp. 14–19.

7. T. Gordon and W. B. Kannel, Drinking habits and cardiovascular disease: The Framingham Study, *American Heart Journal* 105(1983): 667–673; A. L. Klatsky, G. D. Griedman, and A. B. Siegelaub, Alcohol consumption before myocardial infarction: Results from the Kaiser-Permanente Epidemiologic Study of myocardial infarction, *Annals of Internal Medicine* 81 (1974): 294–301; K. Cullen, N. S. Stenhouse, and K. L. Wearne, Alcohol and mortality in the Busselton Study, *International Journal of Epidemiology* 11 (1982): 67–70.

8. M. J. Stampfer and coauthors, A prospective study of moderate alcohol consumption and the risk of coronary disease and stroke in women, *New England Journal of Medicine* 319 (1988): 267–273.

9. Committee on diet and health of the Food and Nutrition Board, National Academy of Sciences, *Diet and Health: Implications for Reducing Chronic Disease Risk* (Washington, D.C.: National Academy Press, 1989), pp. 443–444.

10. A. G. Shaper, G. Wannamethee, and M. Walker, Alcohol and mortality: The myth of the U-shaped curve, *Lancet* 2 (1988): 1267-1273.

11. R. Kastenbaum, Wine and the elderly person, *Journal of Nutrition for the Elderly* 4 (1985): 15–25.

12. A. Urbano-Marquez and coauthors, The effects of alcoholism on skeletal and cardiac muscle, *New England Journal of Medicine* 320 (1989): 409–415.

13. E. S. Pollack and coauthors, Prospective study of alcohol consumption and cancer, *New England Journal of Medicine* 310 (1984): 617.

14. A. Schatzkin and coauthors, Alcohol consumption and breast cancer in the epidemiologic follow-up study of the first national health and nutrition examination survey, *New England Journal of Medicine* 316 (1987): 1169–1173; a supporting review of literature provided in the same issue is S. Graham, Alcohol and breast cancer, *New England Journal of Medicine* 316 (1987): 1211–1213.

15. B. N. Ames, R. Magaw, L. S. Gold, Ranking Possible carcinogenic hazards, *Science* 236 (1987): 271–280.

16. M. J. Eckardt and coauthors, Health hazards associated with alcohol consumption, *Journal of the American Medical Association* 246 (1981): 648–666.

17. C. S. Lieber, Biochemical and molecular basis of alcohol-induced injury to liver and other tissues, *New England Journal of Medicine* 319 (1988): 1639–1650.

Lifecycle Nutrition: Mother and Infant

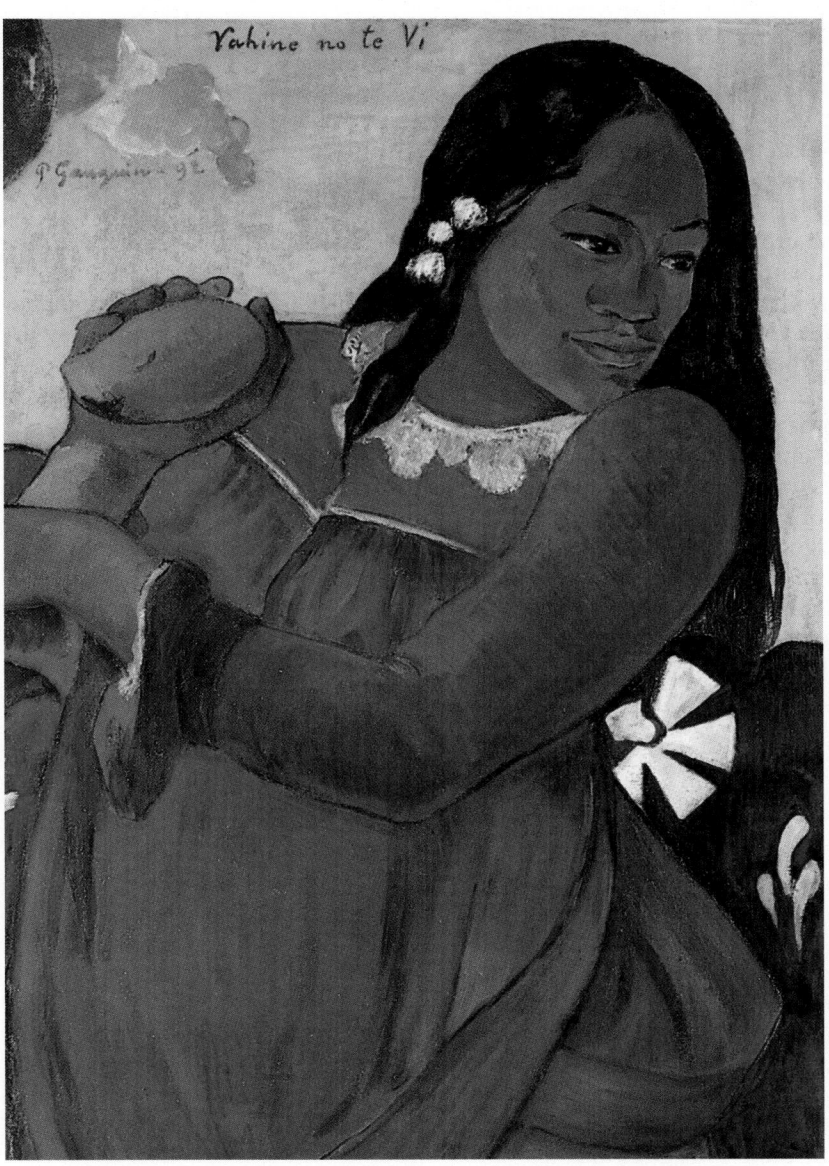

Vahine No Te Vi (Woman of the Mango) by Paul Gauguin, The Baltimore Museum of Art: The Cone Collection, formed by Dr. Claribel Cone and Miss Etta Cone of Baltimore, Maryland. BMA 1950-213

CONTENTS

low birthweight (LBW): a birthweight
of 5 1/2 lb (2500 g) or less, used as a
predictor of increased risk of health
problems in the newborn and as a
probable indicator of poor nutrition
status of the mother during and/or
before pregnancy. Low-birthweight
infants are of two different types. Some
are **premature**; they are born early and
are the right size for their gestational
age. Others have suffered growth failure
in the uterus; they may or may not be
born early, but they are **small for
gestational age (small for date)**.

uterus (YOO-ter-us): the womb, the
muscular organ within which the infant
develops before birth.

placenta (pla-SEN-tuh): the organ that
develops inside the uterus in early
pregnancy in which the mother's and
fetus's circulatory systems intertwine
and in which exchange of materials
between maternal and fetal blood takes
place. The fetus receives nutrients and
oxygen across the placenta; the
mother's blood picks up carbon dioxide
and other waste materials to be
excreted via her lungs and kidneys.

amniotic (am-nee-OTT-ic) sac: the "bag
of waters" in the uterus, in which the
fetus floats.

We normally think of our nutrition as personal, affecting only our own lives. The woman who is pregnant must come to understand that her nutrition today will be critical to the health of her child for years to come. The nutrition demands of pregnancy are outstanding because the growth of a new person requires every known nutrient, and extra amounts of most of them. In terms of importance to the child's future health nourishment during infancy is equal to that of pregnancy.

Pregnancy: The Impact of Nutrition on the Future

To be sure of nourishing herself optimally for pregnancy, a woman must start beforehand. In the early weeks of pregnancy, significant developmental changes occur that depend on a woman's nutrition status at a time when she may not even be aware that she is pregnant. A woman who eats nutrient-dense foods prior to pregnancy establishes eating habits that will optimally nourish both the growing fetus and herself. If nutrient supplementation is needed, the family-planning period is a good time to start it.

Appropriate weight for height prior to pregnancy is beneficial to pregnancy outcome. Underweight women who fail to gain adequately in pregnancy are likely to bear low-birthweight babies.[1] In turn, infant birthweight is the most potent, single indicator of the infant's future health status. A **low-birthweight (LBW)** baby, defined as one who weighs less than 5 1/2 pounds (2500 grams), has a statistically greater chance than a normal-weight baby of contracting diseases and of dying early in life. Such a baby also is likely to be unable to do its job of obtaining nourishment by sucking and to win its mother's attention by energetic, vigorous cries and other healthy behavior. The low-birthweight baby can therefore become an apathetic, neglected baby, and this compounds the original malnutrition problem. Nutritional deficiency, coupled with low birthweight, is the underlying cause of more than half of all the deaths worldwide of children under five years of age. About one in every 15 infants born in the United States is a low-birthweight infant, and about one fourth of these die within the first month of life.[2]

Obese women and their babies face additional risks, as well. Obesity in the pregnant women is often associated with gestational diabetes, hypertension, and infections after the birth. The birth itself may be more likely to require drugs to induce labor or to require surgical intervention. The infant of an obese mother may be larger than normal and born late, or may be large in size even if born prematurely. In the latter case, a premature baby may not receive the special care it requires from medical staff who assume that a large baby is a mature baby.

Women who enter pregnancy 10 percent or more below or 20 percent or more above standard weight for height and age face a greater risk of impaired pregnancy outcome. Underweight women are therefore advised to try to gain weight before becoming pregnant, and overweight women are wise to lose excess weight to maximize the chances of having healthy babies as well as to maintain their own good health.

A major reason why the mother's nutrition before pregnancy is so crucial is that it determines whether her **uterus** will be able to grow a healthy **placenta** during the first month of pregnancy. If the placenta works perfectly, the fetus wants for nothing; if it doesn't, however, no alternative source of sustenance is

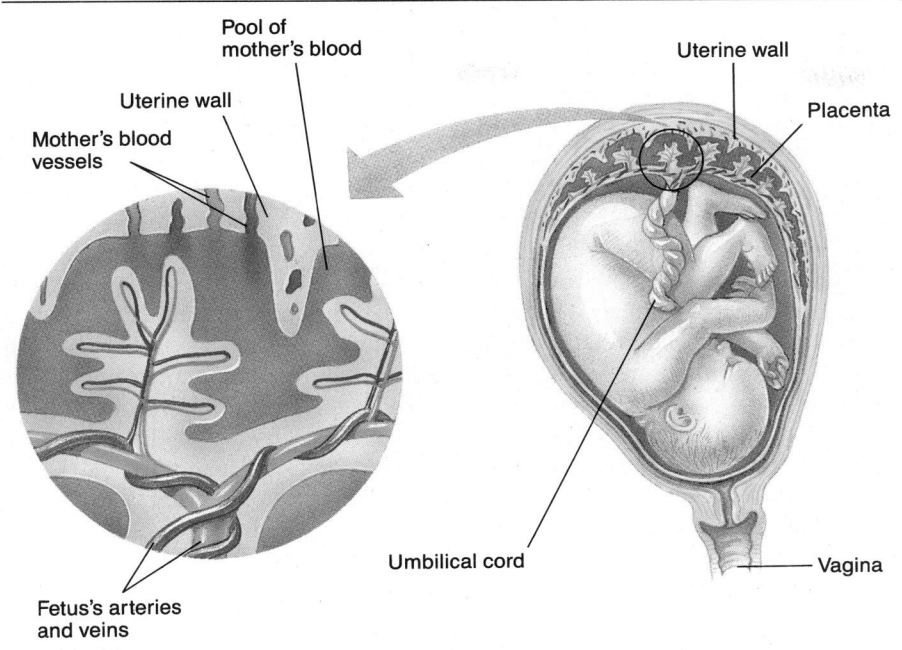

Pool of
mother's blood

Uterine wall

Mother's blood
vessels

Uterine wall

Placenta

Fetus's arteries
and veins

Umbilical cord

Vagina

■■■ Figure 12−1

The Placenta. The placenta is a sort of pillow of tissue in which maternal blood vessels lie side by side with fetal blood vessels entering it through the umbilical cord. This close association between the two circulatory systems permits the mother's bloodstream to deliver nutrients and oxygen to the fetus and to carry away fetal waste products.

available. The placenta is shown in Figure 12−1; it is a sort of cushion in which the mother's and baby's blood vessels intertwine and exchange materials—the two bloods never mix, but nutrients and oxygen enter the baby's system and wastes leave it to be excreted by the mother. The **amniotic sac** forms to house the baby, cushioning it with fluids.

Far from being passive in its transport of molecules, the placenta is a highly metabolic organ with some 60 enzymes of its own. It actively gathers up hormones, nutrients, and protein molecules such as antibodies and transfers them into the fetal bloodstream. It also produces hormones that maintain pregnancy and prepare the mother's breasts for lactation.

If the mother's nutrient stores are inadequate during development of the placenta, then the placenta will develop poorly. As a consequence, no matter how well she eats later, her unborn baby will not receive optimal nourishment. The infant is likely to be a low-birthweight baby with a risk of attendant health consequences. After getting such a poor start on life, a girl child may be ill equipped, even as an adult, to store sufficient nutrients, and so she may also be unable to grow an adequate placenta. In turn, she may bear an infant who is unable to reach full potential. Thus the poor nutrition of a woman during her early pregnancy can theoretically have an impact on the health of her *grandchild*, even after that child has become an *adult*.

Not all cases of low birthweight reflect poor nutrition. Other factors that are associated with low birthweight are heredity, disease conditions, smoking, and drug (including alcohol) use during pregnancy. Even with optimal nutrition and health during pregnancy, some women give birth to small infants for reasons unknown. Still, poor nutrition is the major factor and, ideally, an avoidable one.

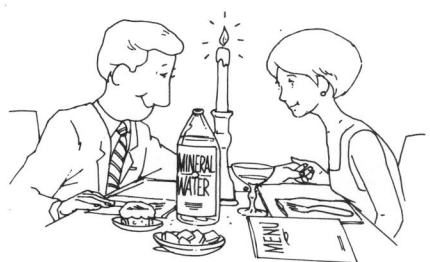

To plan a healthy pregnancy, plan to be well-nourished in advance.

implantation: the stage of development in which the fertilized egg embeds itself in the wall of the uterus and begins to develop during the first two weeks after conception.

ovum: the egg, produced by the mother, that unites with a sperm from the father to produce a new individual.

zygote (ZYE-goat): the term that describes the product of the union of ovum and sperm during the first two weeks after fertilization.

critical period: a finite period during development in which certain events may occur that will have irreversible, determining effects on later developmental stages. A critical period is usually a period of cell division in a body organ.

embryo (EM-bree-oh): the stage of human gestation from the third to eighth week after conception.

fetus (FEET-us): the stage of human gestation from eight weeks after conception until birth of an infant.

gestation: the period from conception to birth; the term of a pregnancy.

◗◗▶ *Adequate nutrition before pregnancy establishes habits that best support fetal growth. Babies who weigh less than 5 1/2 pounds at birth face greater health risks than normal weight babies.*

The Events of Pregnancy

On **implantation** of the newly fertilized **ovum** (or **zygote**) in the uterine wall, the uterus begins to grow a placenta. Placental growth depends on conditions in the uterus at the time of implantation. During the two weeks following fertilization, the zygote divides into many cells, and these cells sort themselves into three layers. Minimal growth in size takes place at this time, but it is a **critical period** developmentally. Adverse influences such as smoking, drug abuse, and malnutrition at this time lead to failure to implant or to other disturbances so severe as to cause loss of the zygote, possibly even before the woman knows she is pregnant. Both mother and child will benefit most from an optimal supply of nutrients uncontaminated by other materials.

The next six weeks of the development of the **embryo** register astonishing physical changes (Figure 12–2). At eight weeks the **fetus** has a complete central nervous system, a beating heart, a fully formed digestive system, and the beginnings of facial features.

The growth of each organ and tissue type has its own characteristic pattern and timing. Each organ is most dependent on an adequate supply of nutrients during its own intensive growth period. In the fetus, for example, the heart and brain are well developed at 14 weeks, even though the lungs are still nonfunctional ten weeks later. Therefore early malnutrition affects the heart and brain; later malnutrition affects the lungs.

◼◼◼ Figure 12-2

Stages of Embryonic and Fetal Development

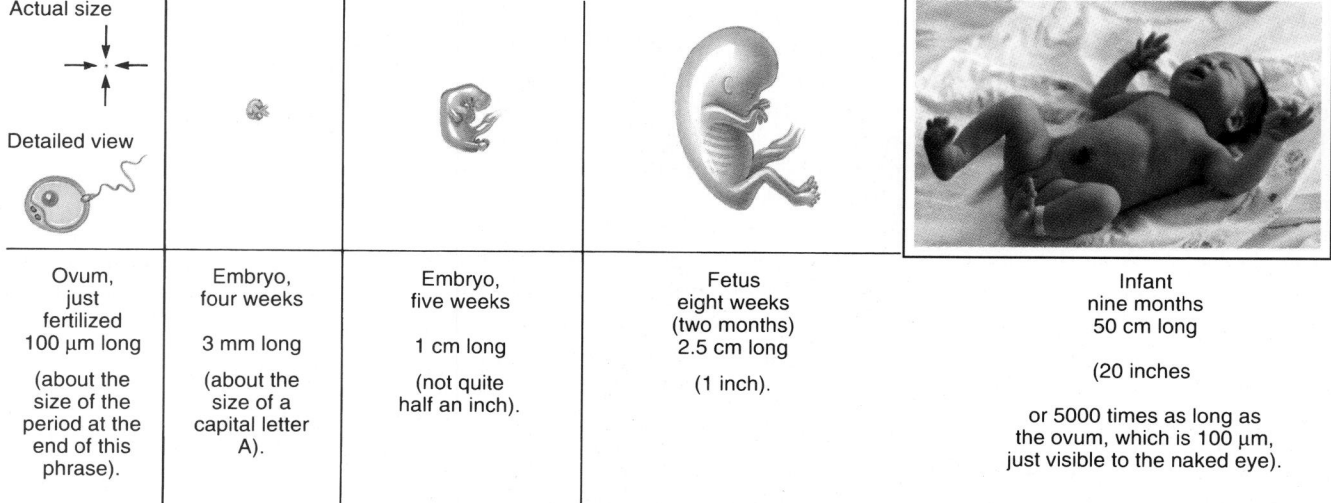

Actual size				
Detailed view				
Ovum, just fertilized 100 μm long (about the size of the period at the end of this phrase).	Embryo, four weeks 3 mm long (about the size of a capital letter A).	Embryo, five weeks 1 cm long (not quite half an inch).	Fetus eight weeks (two months) 2.5 cm long (1 inch).	Infant nine months 50 cm long (20 inches or 5000 times as long as the ovum, which is 100 μm, just visible to the naked eye).

SOURCE: Adapted from L. K. DeBruyne and S. R. Rolfes, *Life Cycle Nutrition Conception through Adolescence,* ed. E. N. Whitney (St. Paul, Minn.: West, 1989), p. 63.

■■■ Table 12–1 Effects of Nutrient Deficiencies during Pregnancy

NUTRIENT	DEFICIENCY EFFECT
Energy	Low infant birthweight
Protein	Reduced infant head circumference
Folate	Miscarriage and neural tube defect
Vitamin D	Low infant birthweight
Calcium	Decreased infant bone density
Iron	Low infant birthweight and premature birth
Iodine	Cretinism (varying degrees of mental and physical retardation in the infant)
Zinc	Congenital malformations

SOURCE: Adapted from L. K. DeBruyne and S. R. Rolfes, *Life Cycle Nutrition: Conception through Adolescence,* ed. E. N. Whitney (St. Paul, Minn.: West, 1989), p. 68.

Events during a critical period can occur at only that time and at no other. Whatever nutrients and other environmental conditions are necessary during this period must be supplied on time if the organ is to reach its full potential. If the development of an organ is limited during a critical period, recovery is impossible. Thus early malnutrition can have irreversible effects, although they may not become fully apparent until maturity. Table 12–1 provides a list of effects of nutrient deficiencies during pregnancy.

The effect of malnutrition during critical periods is seen in the shorter height of people who were undernourished in their early years and in the poor dental health of children whose mothers were malnourished during pregnancy, to give but two examples. The irreversibility of these effects is obvious when abundant, nourishing food fed after the critical time fails to remedy the growth deficit.

The last seven months of pregnancy, the fetal period, bring about a tremendous increase in the size of the fetus. Critical periods of cell division and development occur in organ after organ. The amniotic sac fills with fluid to cushion the infant. The mother's uterus and its supporting muscles increase greatly in size, her breasts may become tender and full, the nipples may darken in preparation for lactation, and her blood volume increases by half to accommodate the added load of materials it must carry. The **gestation** period, which lasts approximately 40 weeks, ends with the birth of the infant.

❚❚▶ *Nutrition before and during pregnancy affects both present and future development of the infant. Placenta development, implantation, and early critical periods depend on nutrient supply and in turn affect future growth and developmental events.*

Most severe risk factors for malnutrition in pregnancy:

■ Age 15 years or under.
■ Many pregnancies at intervals of less than a year (this depletes nutrient stores).
■ History of poor pregnancy outcome.
■ Poverty and lack of family support.
■ Low level of education.
■ Food faddism.
■ Heavy smoking.
■ Drug addiction.
■ Alcohol abuse.
■ Chronic disease requiring special diet.
■ More than 15% underweight.
■ More than 15% overweight.

These factors at the start of pregnancy indicate that poor nutrition is likely to be present and to affect the pregnancy adversely.

Nutrient Needs

Nutrient needs during periods of intensive growth are greater than at any other time and are greater for certain nutrients than for others, as shown in Figure 12–3. A study of the figure reveals some of the key needs.

One of the smallest increases recommended is for energy: pregnancy requires only 300 extra calories per day (during the second and third trimesters)

■■■ **Figure 12–3**

Comparison of Nutrient Needs of
Nonpregnant, Pregnant, and
Lactating Women.

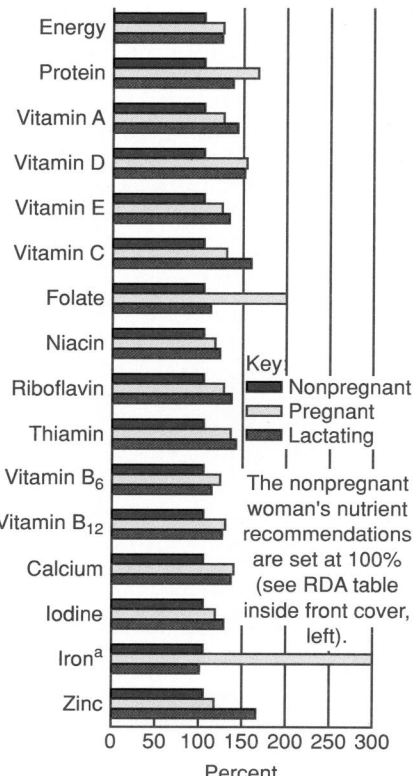

Key

■ Nonpregnant
□ Pregnant
■ Lactating

The nonpregnant
woman's nutrient
recommendations
are set at 100%
(see RDA table
inside front cover,
left).

ᵃThe increased needs of pregnancy cannot be
met by diet or by existing iron stores. Therefore,
pregnant women need to take an iron supplement.

Recommended protein intake: 60 g/day.

Recommended carbohydrate intake: about 50%
of energy intake. In a 2000 cal/day intake, this
represents 1000 cal of carbohydrate, or about
250 g.

Ordinarily a hemoglobin level below 13 g/100
ml is considered low for a woman. In
pregnancy, values of 12 g are not unusual, and
11 g is where the line defining "too low" is
often drawn. It is usually desirable to use more
sensitive measures than hemoglobin if
questions about the woman's iron status arise.

above the allowance for nonpregnant women.[3] A pregnant teenager or a physically active pregnant woman may require more. In each case, enough calories are needed to spare protein for its all-important tissue-building work.

The increase in the recommendation for protein is greater than for energy—from about 45 grams in a nonpregnant woman to about 60 grams per day for a pregnant woman. Many women in the United States exceed the recommended protein intake each day and may already take in adequate protein for pregnancy.[4] Adequate protein consumption during pregnancy is important, but excessive protein may have adverse effects, as Chapter 6 described.

Some vegetarian women limit their intakes of protein-rich foods. For them the inclusion of adequate food energy each day and several generous servings of plant-protein foods such as legumes, whole grains, nuts, and seeds are imperative. In some instances, a soy-based protein supplement can help ensure adequate protein intake. In any case, pregnant women need generous amounts of carbohydrate-rich foods to spare their protein and to provide energy.

The growing fetus and the altered hormonal activity of the pregnancy increase the metabolic demand for vitamin B_6. However, pregnant and lactating women may not eat diets that provide for their vitamin B_6 needs.[5]

The pregnant woman's Recommended Dietary Allowance (RDA) for folate is twice that of the nonpregnant woman due to the great increase in her blood volume and the rapid growth of the fetus. It is possible, but not easy, to obtain from foods alone the folate RDA for pregnancy, and folate supplements are often prescribed. However, folate supplements, especially those with iron (commonly combined in prenatal supplements) can compromise a woman's zinc status.[6] Zinc is another nutrient of concern to the pregnant woman.[7] The pregnant woman also needs greater amounts of the B vitamin that assists folate in the manufacture of new cells—vitamin B_{12}. People who eat meat, eggs, or dairy products receive all they need, even for pregnancy, but if such foods are excluded from the diet, then vitamin B_{12}-fortified soy milk or supplements are recommended.

Among the minerals, those involved in building the skeleton—calcium, phosphorus, and magnesium—are in great demand during pregnancy. Intestinal absorption of calcium doubles early in pregnancy, and the mineral is stored in the mother's bones. Later, as the fetal bones begin to calcify, there is a dramatic shift of calcium across the placenta, and the mother's bone stores are drawn upon. Women's diets are notoriously low in calcium while pregnancy and breastfeeding draw on women's skeletal reserves; thus the increases required for pregnancy may be large.

The body conserves iron even more than usual during pregnancy: menstruation ceases, and absorption of iron increases up to threefold. Still, iron stores dwindle because the developing fetus draws on its mother's iron stores to create stores of its own to carry it through the first three to six months of life. In addition, maternal blood volume increases by as much as 50 percent, and this can give the blood the appearance of anemia in blood tests. The same amount of iron is still in the blood, but it has been diluted. Few women enter pregnancy with adequate stores to meet pregnancy demands, so the committee on RDA recommends a prescribed iron supplement throughout pregnancy.

Calcification of the baby teeth begins in the fifth month of gestation. For these teeth and for the bones, fluoride may also be needed. Children whose mothers received supplemental fluoride in addition to drinking fluoridated water have more decay-free teeth at five to nine years of age than children whose mothers only used fluoridated water.[8] Keep in mind, though, that still more is not still better; the placenta freely transports even toxic levels of excess fluoride to the fetus.

Pregnancy is clearly a time of increased nutrient needs, so a woman of limited financial means may need help in obtaining food to provide those nutrients. At the Federal level she can turn to the Women's, Infants', and Children's Supplemental Feeding (WIC) program to receive nutrition counseling and coupons redeemable for nutritious foods. Federal Food Stamps can also help to stretch her grocery dollars. Her own community may provide educational services and materials, including nutrition, food budgeting, and shopping information through the local agricultural extension service.

▌▌▶ *Pregnancy induces maternal physiological adjustments that demand increases in intakes of energy and even greater increases in intakes of nutrients.*

Food Choices and Cravings

Because energy needs increase less than nutrient needs, the pregnant woman must select foods of high nutrient density. Appropriate choices include nonfat milk, lean meats, legumes, eggs, liver, dark green vegetables, and whole-grain breads and cereals. Vitamin C-rich foods at every meal will ensure maximum iron absorption from other foods. A suggested food pattern is shown in Table 12–2.

Does pregnancy give a woman the right to nudge her mate out of bed at 2 AM to fetch pickles and ice cream? Perhaps not for nutrition's sake, but he may choose to humor her anyway. Food cravings and aversions during pregnancy, although common, do not seem to reflect real physiological needs.[9] In other words, a woman who craves pickles is not likely in need of salt. Food aversions and cravings that arise during pregnancy are usually due to changes in taste and smell sensitivities, and they quickly disappear after the baby's birth.

Sometimes cravings may reflect a diet that is nutrient-poor. A pregnant woman who is deficient in certain nutrients may crave and eat clay, ice, cornstarch, and other nonnutritious substances. This is pica (first mentioned in Chapter 8) and may be a symptom of a need for iron or zinc. Still, such cravings are not adaptive; the substances she craves do not deliver the nutrients she needs.

▌▌▌ **Table 12–2 Four Food-Group Plan for Pregnant and Lactating Women**[a]

	NUMBER OF SERVINGS	
FOOD GROUP	ADULT	PREGNANT OR LACTATING WOMEN
Meat and meat alternates	2	3
Milk and milk products	2	4
Vegetables and fruits	4	4
Breads and cereals	4	4

[a]See Figure 2–4 on page 36 of Chapter 2 for details on serving sizes and food sources.

Apgar score: a system of scoring an infant's physical condition right after birth, based on heart rate, respiration rate, muscle tone, response to stimuli, and color.

■■■ **Table 12–3 Components of Ideal Weight Gain During Pregnancy**

DEVELOPMENT	WEIGHT GAIN (POUNDS)
Infant at birth	7 1/2
Placenta	1
Increase in mother's blood volume to supply placenta	4
Increase in size of mother's uterus and muscles to support it	2 1/2
Increase in size of mother's breasts	3
Fluid to surround infant in amniotic sac	2
Mother's fat stores	2 to 8
Total	22 to 28

■■ ▶ *Careful food choices can ensure optimal nutrition during pregnancy. Food cravings usually do not reflect physiological needs.*

Weight Gain

The pregnant woman must gain a certain amount of weight during pregnancy as a defense against bearing a low-birthweight baby.[10] Ideally she will have begun her pregnancy at the appropriate weight for her height, but even more important is that she will gain from 22 to 28 pounds, most of it in the second half of pregnancy (Table 12–3). The ideal pattern is thought to be about 2 to 4 pounds during the first three months and a pound per week thereafter. Women who are 10 percent or more above the standard weight for height at the start of pregnancy should gain but should gain less— 16 to 24 pounds. (Dieting during pregnancy is not recommended.[11]) Weight-gain standards must be adjusted if the woman is still growing herself, if she is obese or underweight, or if she is carrying twins or triplets. Women have been known to gain up to 60 pounds in pregnancy without ill effects. (A *sudden*, large weight gain, however, is a danger signal that may indicate the onset of pregnancy-induced hypertension; see section entitled "Troubleshooting" below.)

The weight the pregnant woman puts on is nearly all lean tissue: placenta, uterus, blood, milk-producing glands, and, of course, the baby itself. The fat she gains is needed later for lactation. Some of the weight gained during pregnancy is lost at delivery; most of the remainder is generally lost within a few weeks or months as blood volume returns to normal and accumulated fluids are lost. After the birth, fat stores are mobilized for lactation.

Exercise is important to the pregnant woman, not only to help her carry the extra weight of pregnancy without strain, but also to ease the process of her upcoming childbirth. In the old days pregnant women were admonished to "stay off their feet," and to "take it easy." However, research indicates that taking it too easy may be as detrimental to a pregnant woman and her fetus as overexertion. A balanced, 45-minute exercise session three days per week has been associated in one study with heavier birthweight babies, fewer surgical births, higher **Apgar scores**, and shorter hospital stays after birth.[12] Pregnant women should consult with their health care providers before taking on any exercise program and should follow the rules listed in the margin.

Rules for exercise during pregnancy:

■ Stop exercising if you feel overheated.
■ Drink plenty of fluids before you exercise.
■ Avoid exercising in hot, humid weather; do not sit in saunas, steam rooms, or hot tubs.
■ Protect the abdomen from injury, especially in games like baseball or basketball, in which accidents are likely.
■ Discontinue any exercise that causes discomfort.
■ Do not exercise while lying on your back after about the fourth month.
■ Do not allow your heart rate to exceed 140 beats per minute.

◖◗▷ *Weight gain is essential to a healthy pregnancy. The pregnant woman should gain 22 to 28 pounds during pregnancy by eating a balanced diet of nutrient-dense foods.*

Practices to Avoid

A general guideline can be offered to the pregnant woman: eat a normal, healthy diet, and practice moderation. Some substances can be harmful, though, and their potential impact is too great to ignore.

One such substance to limit is caffeine. Caffeine is a drug that crosses the placenta, and the fetus has only a limited ability to metabolize it. Intakes of up to four cups of coffee or tea a day are generally thought to be safe.[13] However, one recent study links the use of 2 cups' worth of caffeine or more per day to an increased risk of spontaneous abortion.[14]

A clearly harmful practice is smoking. Smoking restricts the blood supply to the growing fetus and so limits the delivery of oxygen and nutrients and the removal of wastes. It stunts growth, thus increasing the risk of retarded development. Nicotine and cyanide from cigarette smoke also pose a danger to the fetus as well as other components of smoke. One study found the incidence of cancer and leukemia in children of women who smoked while pregnant to be twice as high as normal.[15] The surgeon general has warned that smoking can be lethal to an otherwise normal fetus or newborn. Even inhaling smoky air from others' smoking may be a hazard for pregnant women and children.

Other drugs taken during pregnancy can cause serious birth defects. The use of unprescribed drugs, even over-the-counter drugs or vitamin supplements, is inadvisable.

Dieting, even for short periods, is also hazardous during pregnancy. Low-carbohydrate diets or fasts that cause ketosis deprive the growing brain of needed glucose and may impair its development. Such diets are also likely to be deficient in other nutrients vital to fetal growth. Energy restriction during pregnancy is dangerous, regardless of the woman's prepregnancy weight.

Research shows that mothers who use drugs such as marijuana and cocaine during pregnancy inflict serious health consequences, including nervous system disorders, on their future infants.[16] Alcohol consumption is common in our society, yet its effects can be so devastating to the developing fetus that the next whole section is devoted to the consequences of drinking during pregnancy.

◖◗▷ *Moderation in the use of caffeine and abstinence from smoking and other drugs, and avoiding dieting are recommended during pregnancy.*

▮▮▮ Drinking During Pregnancy

Drinking excess alcohol during pregnancy threatens the fetus with the irreversible brain damage and mental and physical retardation known as **fetal alcohol syndrome,** or **FAS**. The fetal brain is extremely vulnerable to a glucose or oxygen deficit, and alcohol causes both. In addition, alcohol itself crosses the placenta freely and is directly toxic to the fetal brain. FAS is not curable, only preventable. The only way to prevent it is to refrain from drinking too much alcohol during pregnancy. For women who want to drink during their pregnancies, then, the important question is how much alcohol is too much.

fetal alcohol syndrome (FAS): the cluster of symptoms seen in an infant or child whose mother consumed excess alcohol during her pregnancy; includes mental and physical retardation with facial and other body deformities.

Caffeine amounts in beverages and medications are provided in this chapter's Controversy.

How Much Alcohol Is Too Much?

Clearly, 3 ounces of alcohol (about 6 drinks) a day is too much early in pregnancy, even if the woman stops drinking immediately after she learns that she is pregnant.[17] Birth defects have been observed in the children of some women who drank 2 ounces (4 drinks) of alcohol daily during pregnancy. Low birthweight has been observed in infants born to some women who drank 1 ounce (2 drinks) per day during pregnancy. At that level of alcohol intake, a sizable and significant increase occurs in the rate of spontaneous abortions, perhaps by poisoning of the fetus or perhaps by causing the placenta to detach.[18] FAS is also known to occur with as few as 2 drinks a day. One study presents evidence of an association between 2 drinks a *week* and miscarriages.[19]

In all studies of alcohol levels and damage to the fetus, it is important to take into account that drinking patterns, in addition to total alcohol intake, may play a role. For example, a woman who drinks an average of 1 ounce of alcohol a day may not drink at all during the week but then might have 14 drinks each weekend. Thus the fetus might be exposed, albeit intermittently, to high alcohol levels.[20] For all intake levels and patterns, the most severe impact is likely to occur in the first month, before the woman may be aware that she is pregnant.

Alcohol's Effects

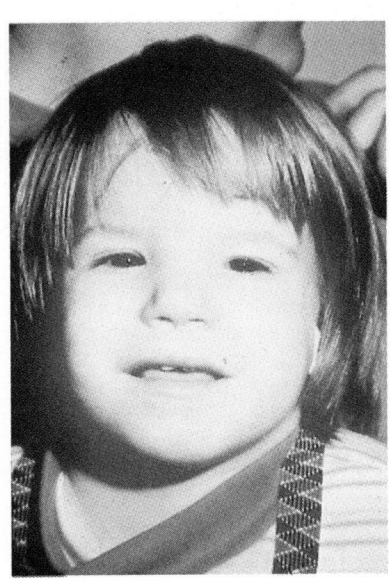

These facial traits reflect fetal alcohol syndrome, caused by maternal drinking in early pregnancy. Irreversible abnormalities of the brain and internal organs accompany these surface features.

Research using animals shows that one-fifth of the level of alcohol needed to produce major, outwardly visible defects will surely produce learning impairment in the offspring. No sign of this impairment will be apparent, but the damage will be there on the inside. An individual exposed to alcohol before birth may respond differently to it in adulthood than if no exposure had occurred—and also to certain drugs. Even before fertilization, alcohol may damage the ovum and so lead to abnormalities in offspring. In males the same is true—drinking before impregnation damages sperm and can also produce an infant of low birthweight.[21]

Although the syndrome was named for damage evident at birth, it has been shown that children born with it remain damaged—they may live, but they never fully recover.[22] About 1 to 3 in every 1000 children are victims of this preventable damage, making FAS the leading known cause of mental retardation in the world.[23] Moreover, for every baby born with these symptoms, another may go undiagnosed until problems develop later in the preschool years.[24] In addition, many others are born with **subclinical FAS.** The mothers of these children drank but not enough to cause visible, obvious effects. Even a child without external damage may have a lower IQ than peers.[25]

Thus, apparently even moderate drinking can affect a fetus negatively. Oxygen is indispensable, on a minute-to-minute basis, to the development of the fetus's central nervous system, and a sudden dose of alcohol can halt the delivery of oxygen through the umbilical cord. During the first month of pregnancy, even a few minutes of such exposure can have a major effect on the fetal brain, which at that time is growing at the rate of 100,000 new brain cells a minute. Alcohol also interferes with placental transport of nutrients to the fetus.[26]

Every container of beer, wine, or liquor for sale in the United States is now required to warn pregnant women of FAS. Before this, many women who would have ceased drinking during pregnancy had they known the danger unwittingly damaged their infants. Lawsuits against alcoholic beverage companies for failure to warn are pending in the courts.

Experts' Advice

The editors of the *Journal of the American Medical Association* have taken the position that women should stop drinking as soon as they *plan* to become pregnant. The editors of *Nutrition Today* magazine have stated the following:

- The pregnant woman who drinks is more likely to give birth to a baby with FAS defects.
- The woman who is pregnant should not drink.
- The woman who is addicted to alcohol should be advised to avoid pregnancy at all costs.

They also take the position that should a woman *addicted* to alcohol become pregnant, she should be urged to have a preventive abortion.[27] It is important to know, though, that if a woman has drunk heavily during the first two-thirds of her pregnancy, she can still prevent some organ damage by stopping heavy drinking during the third trimester.[28]

Not everyone agrees that women need to abstain totally from using alcohol during pregnancy. The American Council on Science and Health (ACSH) took the position, for a while, that women who drink only a little during pregnancy should not be harassed with overly conservative advice. Recently, however, the ACSH has modified this opinion. It now says the following:

Undoubtedly, there is a level of alcohol intake, as yet undetermined, that is not hazardous during pregnancy. Probably an occasional glass of beer or wine is tolerable in pregnancy, just as in the case of driving an automobile, provided that one drink does not lead to another. Total prohibition of drinking is an unacceptable rule for many people. Nevertheless, we believe that many pregnant women will prefer to give up drinking 'for the duration.'[29]

Researchers looking for a "safe" limit concur with the abstinence policy.[30] The authors of this book do, too. It is a personal choice, but if we had it to make, we would opt for the healthy baby. We would give up even the pleasure of wine with meals for the duration of pregnancy and drink a glass of champagne if at all, only to celebrate after the baby's birth.

▌▶ *Abstinence from or strict restriction of ingesting alcohol is critical to prevent irreversible damage to the fetus.*

▌▌▌ Troubleshooting

To avoid the most common problems encountered during pregnancy, some additional measures are helpful. Pregnancy precipitates the onset of **gestational diabetes** in some women; it is recommended that all pregnant women be screened for diabetes at about the sixth month. Thereafter, at every checkup, routine testing of urine for ketone bodies is in order. Without proper management, diabetes can lead to fetal or infant sickness and death. Properly managed, it will cause no harm at all.

A certain degree of **edema** is to be expected in late pregnancy, but in some women it is often part of a larger problem known as **pregnancy-induced**

> **subclinical FAS**: a subtle version of FAS, with hidden defects including learning disabilities, behavioral abnormalities, and motor impairments.
>
> **gestational diabetes**: abnormal glucose tolerance appearing during pregnancy, with subsequent return to normal after the end of pregnancy.
>
> **edema**: accumulation of fluid in the tissues. Also defined in Chapter 6.

pregnancy-induced hypertension (PIH): a cluster of symptoms seen in pregnancy, including edema, hypertension, and kidney complications. PIH was formerly known as *toxemia*. Other terms associated with PIH are *eclampsia* (symptoms include convulsions and coma, associated with high blood pressure; edema; and protein in the urine) and its predecessor, *preeclampsia*, characterized by edema, increasing hypertension, and protein in the urine.

The normal edema of pregnancy responds to gravity; fluid from blood pools in the ankles. The edema of toxemia causes swelling elsewhere.

hypertension (**PIH**, formerly known as *toxemia*). Pre-existing hypertension and PIH are the most common medical complications of pregnancy. They can cause maternal death, infant death, retarded growth, lung problems, and other birth defects. It is important to keep track of maternal blood pressure throughout pregnancy and if PIH is indicated, to initiate treatment promptly.* Treatment is medical, and salt restriction is not usually part of the treatment. A normal salt intake is necessary for health.

The nausea of "morning" (actually, anytime) sickness seems unavoidable because it arises from the hormonal changes of early pregnancy. It can often be alleviated by sipping water and nibbling soda crackers or other bland, carbohydrate-rich food before getting out of bed. Carbonated beverages also may help. Should morning sickness interfere with normal eating for more than a week or two, the woman should seek medical treatment to prevent nutrient deficiencies.

Later, as the hormones of pregnancy alter her muscle tone and the thriving infant crowds her intestinal organs, an expectant mother may complain of heartburn or constipation. To remedy nighttime heartburn, try raising the head of the bed with two or three pillows. A high-fiber diet and a plentiful water intake helps relieve constipation. Exercise may also help, and it should be treated as a daily necessity. The woman should use laxatives or heartburn medication only if prescribed by her physician.

Pregnancy is a time of adjustment to major changes—physical, social, emotional, and financial. The couple who are expecting a baby will have to change their lifestyles as they take on the responsibility of caring for a child. Ideally the mother will be encouraged to develop this sense of responsibility by caring for herself during pregnancy. The expectant couple needs support in thinking of themselves as important people with a new and challenging task that they can and will perform well.

▮▮▶ *Common medical problems associated with pregnancy are gestational diabetes and pregnancy-induced hypertension (PIH). These should be managed to minimize associated risks.*

▮▮▮ Breastfeeding: Concerns for the Mother

Toward the end of her pregnancy, a woman who plans to breastfeed her baby should begin to prepare. No elaborate or expensive preparations are needed, but the expectant mother might want to read at least one of the many handbooks available on breastfeeding.† Among the preparations is to learn what dietary changes are needed. Adequate nutrition is essential to successful lactation; without it, lactation may falter.

---

*Blood pressure of 140/90 millimeters of mercury during the second half of pregnancy in a woman who has not previously exhibited hypertension indicates PIH. So does a rise in systolic blood pressure of 30 millimeters or in diastolic blood pressure of 15 millimeters on at least two occasions more than six hours apart. R. J. Worley, Pathophysiology of pregnancy-induced hypertension, *Clinical Obstetrics and Gynecology* 27 (1984): 821–835.

†An international organization that helps women with breastfeeding concerns is LaLeche League. (See Appendix E for the address.) Among the League's publications are the *LaLeche League News* (a newsletter) and *The Womanly Art of Breastfeeding* (a manual), and they recommend the manual by P. B. Brewster, *You Can Breastfeed Your Baby. . .Even in Special Situations* (Emmaus, Pa.: Rodale Press, 1979).

A nursing mother produces about 30 ounces of milk a day (more in early lactation, less when the baby begins eating other foods). At 20 calories an ounce, this milk costs 600 calories per day. In addition, producing the milk takes more energy, so that the total energy output is about 750 calories a day above normal.

The food energy consumed by the nursing mother should carry with it abundant nutrients—especially those needed to make milk, such as calcium, protein, magnesium, zinc, and plenty of fluid. Figure 12–3 showed the differences between a lactating woman's nutrient needs and those of a nonpregnant woman, and Table 12–2 suggested a food pattern that meets them.

Breast-milk volume depends not on how much fluid the mother drinks but on how much milk the baby demands.[31] The nursing mother is nevertheless advised to drink at least 2 quarts of liquids each day to protect herself from dehydration. To help themselves remember to drink, many women drink a glass of milk, juice, or water each time the baby nurses as well as at mealtimes.

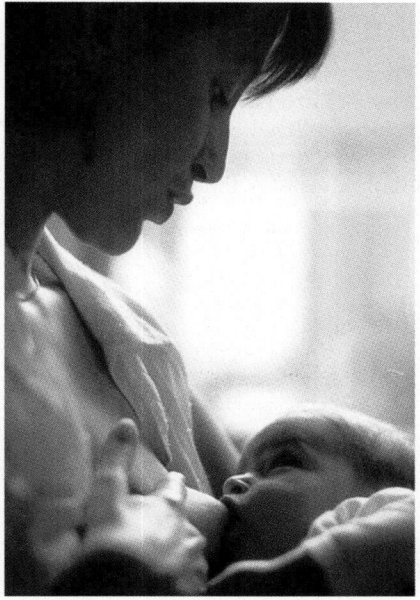

Breastfeeding goes most smoothly for the woman who prepares.

People often ask about the old adage "beer makes good milk." Beer does seem to stimulate prolactin, a hormone important to lactation. However, the alcohol in beer enters breast milk and can easily overwhelm an infant's immature alcohol-degrading system. A woman's hormones need no external assistance to perform perfectly, and even beer should be strictly limited to an occasional one serving. The only drugs permissible are those prescribed to the breastfeeding mother by a physician. Even excess caffeine can make a baby jittery and wakeful; other drugs do much worse.

Another question often raised is whether a mother's milk may lack a nutrient if she fails to get enough in her diet. The answer differs from one nutrient to the next, but in general, the effect of nutritional deprivation of the mother is to reduce the *quantity,* not the *quality,* of her milk. For protein, carbohydrate, and most minerals, the milk of a healthy mother has a fairly constant composition. Any excess, water-soluble vitamins the mother may take in are excreted in the urine; they are not allowed in the milk. The levels of fat-soluble vitamins in human milk can be altered, however, by the mother's excessive or deficient intakes. For example, large doses of vitamin A correspondingly raise the concentration of this vitamin in breast milk. Vitamin supplementation of *under-nourished* women appears to raise the vitamin concentrations in their milk and may be beneficial.[32]

If a mother does not breastfeed, she may find it hard to lose the fat she gained during pregnancy.[33] This does not mean that a breastfeeding woman can eat unlimited calories of food and still effortlessly return to prepregnancy weight. Breastfeeding costs energy, true; but a carefully chosen program of diet and exercise are still the cornerstones of weight loss. A gradual loss (1 pound per week) is safe and has no effect on milk output. However, too large an energy deficit, especially soon after birth, will inhibit lactation. A new mother's exercise program is contingent on her physician's approval.

Infants may be sensitive to foods in the mother's diet, and they may become uncomfortable when she eats those foods. However, while a few babies may be sensitive to cow's milk or onions, it is not a reason for all nursing mothers to avoid those foods. Similarly, some foods with strong flavors, such as garlic, may affect some babies' liking for the milk. A mother who is nursing her baby is advised to eat whatever nutritious foods she chooses; then, if she suspects a particular food of causing the infant discomfort, she can try eliminating that food from her diet for a few days and see if the problem goes away.

Weight Gain of Human Infants in Their First Five Years of Life. The colored vertical bars show how the yearly increase in weight gain diminishes over the years.

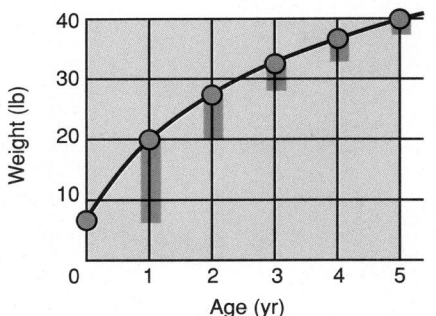

Baby's metabolism:

   Heart rate: 120 to 140 beats per minute.
   Respiration rate: 20 beats per minute.

Adult's metabolism:

   Heart rate: 70 to 80 beats per minute.
   Respiration rate: 12 to 14 beats per minute.

At six months, the infant's energy needs are reduced by slower growth but increased by increased activity.

■■▶ *The lactating woman needs extra fluid and the energy and nutrients needed to make 30 ounces of milk a day. Malnutrition most often diminishes the quantity of the milk produced, while quality remains unaffected. Weight loss is facilitated by lactation.*

■■■ Feeding the Infant

For a while the infant drinks only breast milk or formula, but later it becomes able to handle other foods. Early nutrition affects later development, and early feedings set patterns for eating habits that influence nutrition throughout life.

   While trends change and experts argue the fine points, nourishing a baby is relatively simple, overall. Common sense in the selection of infant foods and a nurturing, relaxed environment go far to promote the infant's well-being.

Nutrient Needs

A baby grows faster during the first year of life than ever again, as Figure 12−4 shows. Pediatricians carefully monitor the growth of infants and children, since growth is an important reflection of nutrition status. The birthweight doubles around four months of age and triples by the age of one year. (If an adult were to do this, the person's weight would increase from 150 to 450 pounds in a single year.) By the end of the first year, the growth rate slows considerably, so that between the first and second birthdays, the weight gained amounts to less than 10 pounds.

   The rapid growth and metabolism of the infant demands an ample supply of all the nutrients. However, the energy nutrients and those vitamins and minerals critical to the growth process, such as vitamin A, vitamin D, calcium, and iron, have special importance during infancy.

   Babies, because they are small, need smaller, total amounts of these nutrients than adults do; but as a percentage of body weight, babies need over twice as much of most nutrients. Figure 12−5 compares a three-month-old baby's needs (by weight) with those of an adult man. As you can see, some of the differences are extraordinary. Sometime around six months of age, energy needs increase less rapidly as the growth rate begins to slow down, but some of the energy saved by slower growth is spent in increased activity. When their growth slows, infants spontaneously reduce their energy intakes.[34] This means that parents should expect their babies to adjust their food intakes downwards when appropriate, and they should not force or coax them to eat more.

   The most important nutrient of all, for infants as for everyone, is the one easiest to forget: water. The younger a child the greater the percentage of the body weight is water, and the more rapid the turnover. Proportionately more of the infant's body water than the adult's is between the cells and in the vascular space, and this water is easy to lose. Conditions that cause fluid loss, such as vomiting, diarrhea, or sweating, can rapidly propel an infant into life-threatening dehydration. In early infancy, breast milk or infant formula normally provides enough water for a healthy infant to replace water losses from the skin, lungs, feces, and urine.[35] If an infant is exposed to hot weather, has diarrhea, or vomits repeatedly, supplemental water is needed to prevent dehydration. Infants cannot tell you what they are crying for; remember that they may need plain water, and let them drink it until they quench their thirst.

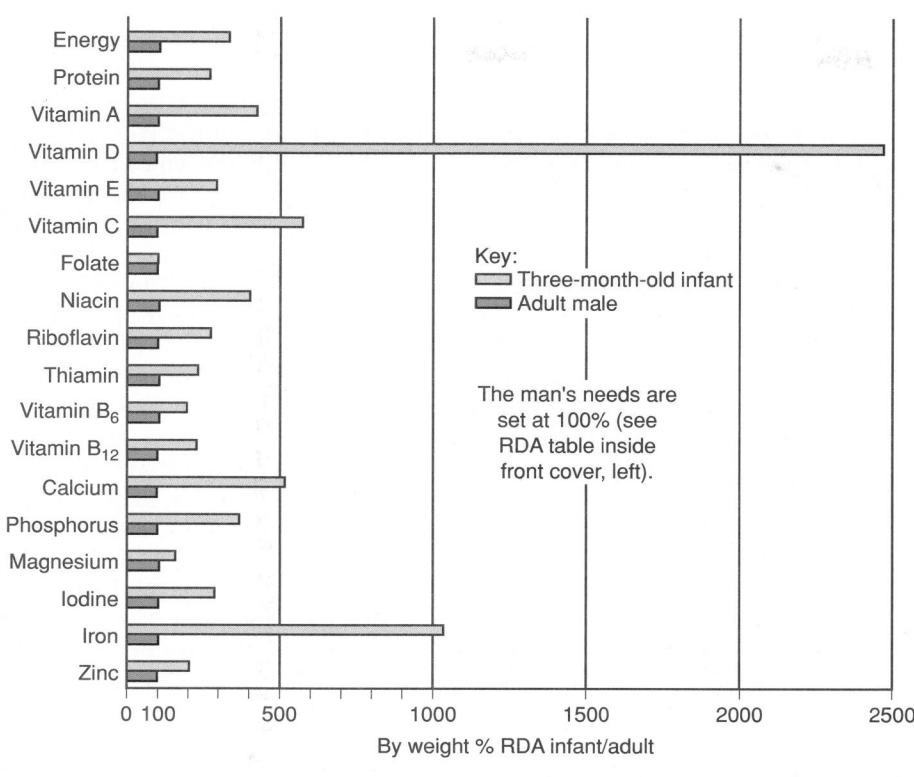

Nutrient Recommendations for a Three-Month-Old Infant and an Adult Male, per Unit of Body Weight

The type of milk the infant receives and the age at which solid foods are introduced are major areas of concern in infant nutrition research. The remainder of this discussion is devoted to feeding the infant and identifying the nutrients most often deficient in infant diets.

Under most circumstances a woman can freely choose to feed breast milk or formula, knowing that either way, the infant's nutrient needs will be met. However, if the family has a low income or if other factors act to the baby's disadvantage, then the *other* advantages of breast milk tip the balance in favor of breastfeeding.

◗◗▶ *Infants' rapid growth and development depend heavily on adequate nutrient supplies. Adequate water is also crucial.*

Breastfeeding

Before choosing a mode of feeding, a woman should be aware of some things about breastfeeding. Over ten years ago, the Committee on Nutrition of the American Academy of Pediatrics (AAP) and the Nutrition Committee of the Canadian Pediatric Society issued this statement: "Breastfeeding is strongly recommended for full-term infants, except in the few instances where specific contraindications exist."[36] This view still holds true today.

With the possible exceptions of vitamin D and fluoride, breast milk provides all the nutrients needed by the healthy infant for the first four to six months

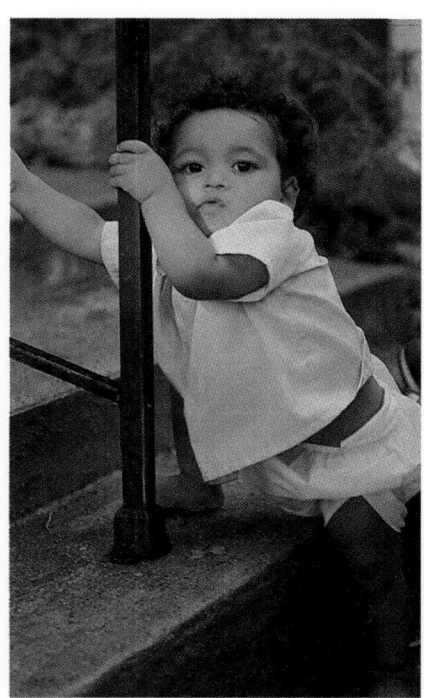

After age six months, energy saved by slowing of growth is spent on increasing activity.

alpha-lactalbumin (lact-AL-byoo-min): the chief protein in human breast milk, as opposed to casein (CAY-seen), the chief protein in cow's milk.

lactoferrin (lak-toe-FERR-in): a factor in breast milk that binds iron and keeps it from supporting the growth of the infant's intestinal bacteria.

colostrum (co-LAHS-trum): a milklike secretion from the breast, rich in protective factors, present during the first day or so after delivery, before milk appears.

bifidus (BIFF-id-us, by-FEED-us) factors: factors in colostrum and breast milk that favor the growth, in the infant's intestinal tract, of the "friendly" bacteria Lactobacillus (lack-toh-ba-SILL-us) bifidus, so that other, less desirable intestinal inhabitants will not flourish.

of life. But the attributes of breast milk go beyond its nutrient ingredients, as the later section on immunological protection describes.

Breast milk is tailor-made to meet the nutrient needs of the human infant. Its carbohydrate is lactose, and its fat provides a generous proportion of the essential omega-6 fatty acid linoleic acid. In addition, a mother who consumes food rich in omega-3 fatty acids will pass these beneficial nutrients on to her child through her milk. Breast milk contains fat-digesting enzymes that help ensure efficient fat absorption by the infant. Breast milk even changes in composition to meet the developmental needs of a preterm infant in ways that full-term mother's milk can't match. For the premature infant, then, the milk of its own mother provides more protein and less volume—just the right mix to support the rapid growth required to help a premature infant survive its first critical weeks.

The protein in breast milk is largely **alpha-lactalbumin**, a protein the human infant can easily digest. Another protein of breast milk, **lactoferrin**, indirectly benefits the baby's iron nutrition and at the same time acts as an antibacterial agent. Lactoferrin is an iron-gathering compound that keeps intestinal bacteria from getting enough iron to grow out of control, helps absorb iron into the infant's bloodstream, and also works directly to kill some bacteria.

The vitamin content of breast milk is ample. Even vitamin C, for which cow's milk is a poor source, is supplied generously by breast milk from a well-nourished mother. The concentration of vitamin D in breast milk is low,[37] but this is not a threat to infants who are taken out into the sunshine regularly.

As for minerals, the 2-to-1 calcium-to-phosphorus ratio of breast milk is ideal for the absorption of calcium, and both of these minerals, along with magnesium, are present in amounts appropriate for the rate of growth expected in a human infant. Breast milk is also low in sodium. The iron in breast milk is highly absorbable, and its zinc, too, is absorbed better than from cow's milk, thanks to the presence of a zinc-binding protein. Given the nutrient composition of breast milk, supplements are not necessary, with the possible exceptions of vitamin D, fluoride, and iron (for details, see the Consumer Caution).

CONSUMER CAUTION▮▮▮ Supplements for the Infant

A mother who is breastfeeding her healthy, full-term, newborn infant need not offer supplements of most nutrients. Breast milk and the infant's own internal stores will ensure that most nutrient needs are met for the first four to six months of life. The only exceptions to this statement are vitamin D, fluoride, and, possibly, iron.

Most experts agree that breast milk does not provide enough vitamin D for the infant who has little exposure to sunlight. A light-skinned baby wearing light-weight clothing in bright sunlight might make enough vitamin D in a few minutes to meet daily needs. A dark-skinned baby wrapped up for cold weather in a smoggy city might not make enough even if outside for several hours. Because so many variables exist regarding vitamin D and sunlight

continued on next page

exposure, the AAP recommends vitamin D supplementation beginning at birth for breastfed babies.

If the baby's only source of fluoride is breast milk, then the pediatrician is likely to prescribe fluoride supplements too. Fluoride does not appear to be secreted into breast milk even if the mother's fluoride supply is ample.[38] Infants who consume formula that is mixed with fluoridated water do not need additional fluoride. For those who consume formula made with non-fluoridated water, fluoride supplementation may be desirable until they begin drinking fluoridated water on a regular basis. In areas of nonfluoridated water, continued fluoride supplementation is recommended through young life.

As for iron, it may be desirable to begin iron supplements for the breastfed infant at about four months. Iron before this time is unnecessary because babies are born with enough iron in their livers to last through the first four months of life. When a baby can eat iron-fortified infant cereal, iron supplementation is no longer necessary.

For the formula-fed infant, the makeup of the formula determines what further supplementation may be necessary. The AAP and most pediatricians recommend iron-fortified formula.

Breast milk offers the infant unsurpassed protection against infection. This barrier of protection includes antiviral and antibacterial agents and other infection inhibitors.

During the first two or three days of lactation, the breasts produce **colostrum**, a premilk substance containing antibodies and white cells from the mother's blood. Colostrum is relatively sterile as it leaves the breast, and the baby cannot contract a bacterial infection from it even if the mother has one. Because it contains immunity factors, colostrum helps protect the newborn infant from those infections against which the mother has developed immunity—precisely those in the environment likely to infect the infant. Maternal antibodies from colostrum inactivate harmful bacteria within the infant's digestive tract. Later, breast milk also delivers antibodies, although not as many as colostrum.

Certain factors in colostrum and breast milk, known as **bifidus factors**, favor the growth of the "friendly" bacteria *Lactobacillus bifidus* in the infant's digestive tract, so that other, harmful bacteria cannot grow there. Another factor present in colostrum and breast milk stimulates the development of the infant's digestive tract. Worn-out cells in the infant's digestive tract are promptly replaced, facilitating the tract's functioning.

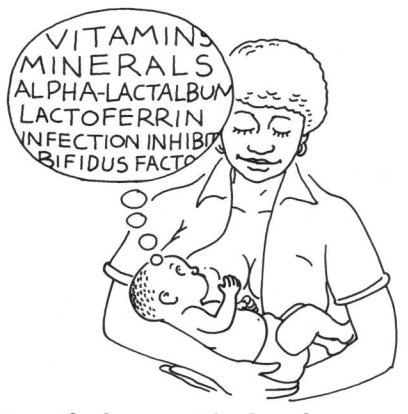

Breastfeeding provides benefits.

Other factors in breast milk include several enzymes, several hormones, and lipids, all of which protect the infant against infection. Prolonged breastfeeding (six months or more) has been shown to reduce the incidence of allergic disease in babies with a family history of allergies.[39] Much remains to be learned about the composition and characteristics of human milk, but clearly it is a very special substance.

▌▌▶ *Breast milk is normally the ideal food for infants. It contains not only the needed nutrients in the right proportions but also protective factors. It is especially valuable for premature infants.*

When Not to Breastfeed

If a woman has an ordinary cold, she can go on nursing without worry. If susceptible, the infant will catch it from her anyway, and thanks to immunological protection, a breastfed baby may be less susceptible than a formula-fed baby would be. If a woman has a communicable disease such as AIDS, tuberculosis, or hepatitis that could threaten the infant's health, then mother and baby have to be separated.‡ Breastfeeding is possible in some diseases by pumping the mother's breasts several times a day, a time-consuming process.

Similarly, if a nursing mother must take medication that is secreted in breast milk and that is known to affect the infant, then breastfeeding is contraindicated. Drug addicts, including alcohol abusers, are capable of taking such high doses that their infants can become addicts by way of breast milk; in these cases, too, breastfeeding is contraindicated. Many prescription drugs do not, but some do, reach nursing infants in sufficient quantities to affect them adversely. As a precaution, a nursing mother should consult with the prescribing physician prior to ingesting any drug.

A woman sometimes hesitates to breastfeed because she has heard that environmental contaminants may enter breast milk and harm her infant. The decision whether to breastfeed on this basis might best be made after consultation with a physician or dietitian familiar with the local circumstances.

For more about contaminants and nutrition, turn to Chapter 14.

■■▶ *Most ordinary infections such as colds have no effect on breastfeeding. Should illness require drug therapy, a physician should advise the woman about the safety of the drug in breast milk. Breastfeeding may be inadvisable if milk is contaminated with drugs or environmental pollutants.*

Formula Feeding and Weaning to Milk

The substitution of formula feeding for breastfeeding involves copying nature as closely as possible. Human and cow's milks differ; cow's milk is significantly higher in protein, calcium, and phosphorus, for example, to support the calf's faster growth rate. But a formula can be prepared from cow's milk that does not differ significantly from human milk in these respects; the formula makers first dilute the milk and then add carbohydrate and nutrients to make it nutritionally comparable to human milk.

Formula feeding offers a major advantage to the mother whose attempts at breastfeeding have met with frustration. Nourishment for the infant in formula is adequate, and a mother can choose this course with confidence. Other advantages are that parents can see that the baby is getting enough milk during feedings. Also, other family members can enjoy participating in feeding sessions, offering them a chance to develop the special closeness that feeding fosters, and freeing the mother to give time to her other children or to herself. As more mothers resume employment earlier after giving birth, more may choose formula for their infants, but they have another option. Breast milk can be pumped into bottles and given to the baby in day care. At home, they may breastfeed as usual.

Many mothers use both methods—they breastfeed at first but wean to formula within the first six months. Other milk is not appropriate for infants up to age six months or even to one year. Only formula contains enough iron (to

‡Evidence exists that AIDS may be passed from an infected mother to her infant during pregnancy, at birth, or through breastfeeding.

■■ Table 12–4 AAP Standard Compared with Human Milk and
Infant Formula

CONTENT	MATURE HUMAN MILK	AAP STANDARD	INFANT FORMULA[a]
Energy (cal/100 ml)	67–75	60–80	67
Protein (% of cal)	5.2	7–18	9
Fat (% of cal)	35–58	30–55	47–50
Carbohydrate (% of cal)	35–44	35–50	41–43

[a]Five formulas were used to generate these data: Similac (Ross), Similac 60/40 (Ross), Enfamil
(Mead Johnson), SMA (Wyeth), and Nan (Nestlé).

SOURCE: Adapted from K. Brostrom, Human milk and infant formulas: Nutritional and
immunological characteristics, In *Textbook of Pediatric Nutrition,* ed. R. M. Suskind (New York:
Raven Press, 1981).

name but one of many factors) to support normal development in the baby's
first months of life.

National and international standards have been set for the nutrient contents
of infant formulas. The Infant Formula Act of 1980 requires that formulas meet
nutrient standards based on the AAP recommendations, and in 1982 the FDA
adopted quality control procedures to be sure that they do. Formulas that meet
the standards are nutritionally similar; small differences in nutrient content are
not usually important.

Table 12–4 shows the AAP standard for the bulk ingredients of infant
formulas and permits comparison with human milk and typical formulas. As
you can see, the AAP standard recommends higher protein than is in human
milk; this is because the cow's milk protein does not present as perfect a
balance of amino acids for the human infant. You can also see that the formulas
meet the AAP standard for the nutrients listed.

For infants with special problems, formulas can be adapted to make them
closer in composition to human milk (adjusted protein ratio, lower linoleic
acid, lower sodium and other minerals). For premature babies, special premature formulas are available. Special formulas based on soy protein are available
for infants of vegetarians or for those allergic to milk protein; formulas with the
lactose replaced can be used for infants with lactose intolerance. For infants
with other special needs, many other variations are available.

As long as formula is the baby's major food, ordinary milk is an inappropriate replacement—primarily because cow's milk provides insufficient vitamin C and iron. Once the baby is obtaining at least a third of the total daily
food energy from a balanced mixture of cereals, vegetables, fruits, and other
foods (usually after six months of age), then whole cow's milk in any form,
fortified with vitamins A and D, is acceptable as an accompanying beverage.

The AAP recommends the introduction of cow's milk at six months, but
many pediatricians advise continued use of infant formula throughout the first
year because of the iron it provides. Don't offer plain, unmodified cow's milk
before six months; the infant's digestive tract may be sensitive to the protein
content and, if so, may bleed. The infant's immature kidneys are also stressed
by the composition of unmodified cow's milk. Infants under a year old should
not drink low-fat or nonfat milk routinely; they need the fat and vitamins A
and D of fortified whole milk. Canned milk once caused lead poisoning in

Formula preparation:

■ Liquid concentrate (inexpensive, relatively
easy)—mix with equal part water.
■ Powdered formula (cheapest, lightest for
travel)—read label directions.
■ Ready-to-feed (easiest, most expensive)—
pour directly into clean bottles.
■ Whole milk—do not use before six months.

▮▮▮ Milk Terms

casein or sodium caseinate: the principal protein of cow's milk. Other milk proteins, found in a higher percentage in human milk, include **lactalbumin**, found in the milk's **whey**.

condensed milk: evaporated milk to which a large amount of sugar (sucrose) is added during processing—intended for making desserts, not for feeding babies. Accidental use of condensed milk in preparation of infant formula can cause dehydration.

evaporated milk: milk concentrated to half volume by evaporation. Adding water reconstitutes the milk; the taste, however, is altered by the processing.

evaporated milk formula: formula made at home from evaporated milk, sugar, and water—seldom used today.

fortified (with respect to milk): milk to which vitamins A and D have been added.

homogenized milk: milk treated to mix the fat evenly with the watery part (fat ordinarily floats to the top as cream). Heated milk is forced under high pressure through small openings to emulsify the fat.

lactalbumin: see *casein*.

pasteurized milk: milk that is heat treated to eliminate disease-causing microbes and to reduce its total bacterial count to an acceptable level.

powdered milk: dehydrated milk solids. Some powdered milks rehydrate easily (instant milk); others require extensive blending. Both whole and nonfat milks can be powdered.

whey: the liquid that remains after milk has coagulated (see also *casein*).

whole milk: full-fat cow's milk. The standard of identity for whole milk in most states requires not less than 3.25% milk fat and not less than 8.25% nonfat milk solids.

---

babies because the cans were sealed with lead solder. Today, canned milk is virtually lead-free thanks to new canning materials.[40]

▮▮ ▶ *Infant formulas are designed to resemble breast milk and must meet an AAP standard for nutrient composition. Special formulas are available for premature babies, allergic babies, and others. Formula should be replaced with milk only after the baby is eating a balanced assortment of foods, at the earliest six months; a year is preferred.*

First Foods

Young babies depend solely on powerful sucking to obtain food and can swallow only liquids that are well back in the throat. Later (at two months or so) the baby's tongue can move against the palate to swallow semisolid food. Still later, the first teeth erupt, but it is not until sometime during the second year that a baby can begin to handle chewy food. The stomach and intestines are immature at first; they can digest milk sugar (lactose) but not starch. At about four months, most babies can begin to digest starchy foods.

The baby's kidneys are unable to concentrate waste efficiently, so a baby must excrete relatively more water than an adult to carry off a comparable amount of waste. This means that the risk of dehydration is even greater once solid foods are introduced.

Iron deficiency is prevalent in children between the ages of six months and three years due to their rapid growth rate and the significant place that milk has in their diets. This can lead to iron-deficiency anemia, popularly called **milk anemia**.

Investigators who performed research comparing preschool children with and without iron deficiency found that those who were deficient were "less likely to pay attention to relevant cues in problem-solving situations."[41] By the end of the first year, half or more of all infants are receiving less than the RDA for iron, and one-fourth are receiving less than two-thirds of the RDA. Six-month-old infants who are weaned to cow's milk have lower blood-iron measures than those who remain on formula.[42] Iron ranks highest on the list of nutrients most needing attention in infant nutrition. A baby's stored iron supply from before birth runs out after the birthweight doubles, so formula with iron, iron-fortified cereals, and, later, meat or meat alternates are recommended at or before that time.

The timing for adding solid foods to a baby's diet depends on several factors. Formula or breast milk is sufficient until age four to six months, but babies not fed solid foods when they are ready for them within the first year suffer delayed growth. Any of the following indicates readiness:

■ When the infant has doubled its birthweight.
■ When the infant can consume 8 ounces of formula and is hungry again in less than four hours.
■ When the infant is consuming 32 ounces (about 1 liter) of formula a day and wanting more.
■ When the infant is six months old.

All babies develop according to their own schedules, and some are ready before others. Table 12–5 presents a suggested sequence but should be used as a flexible guide, taking individuality into account.

The addition of foods should be governed by three considerations: the baby's nutrient needs, the baby's physical readiness to handle different forms of foods,

> **milk anemia:** iron-deficiency anemia caused by drinking so much milk that iron-rich foods are displaced from the diet.

■■■ **Table 12–5 First Foods for the Infant**

AGE (MONTHS)	ADDITION
4–6	Iron-fortified rice cereal, followed by other cereals (for iron; baby can swallow and can digest starch now)[a]
5–7	Strained vegetables and/or fruits and their juices,[b] one by one (perhaps vegetables before fruits, so the baby will learn to like their less sweet flavors)
6–8	Protein foods (cheese, yogurt, tofu, cooked beans, meat, fish, chicken, egg yolk)
9	Finely chopped meat (baby can chew now), toast, teething crackers (for emerging teeth)
10–12	Whole egg (allergies are less likely now), whole milk

[a]Later you can change cereals, but don't forget to keep on using the iron-fortified varieties.
[b]All baby juices are fortified with vitamin C. Orange juice causes allergies in some babies; apple juice is often recommended.
SOURCE: Adapted from the 1979 *Recommendations for Infant Feeding Practices of the California Department of Health Services,* as presented in Current infant feeding practices, *Nutrition and the M. D.,* January 1980.

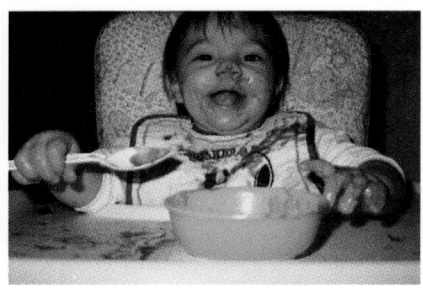

Ideally, the one-year-old eats much of what everyone else eats.

and the need to detect and control allergic reactions. With respect to nutrient needs, iron has already been mentioned as primary; next is vitamin C.

Physical readiness to handle foods that supply these nutrients develops in many small steps. For example, the ability to swallow solid food develops at around four to six months, and experience with solid food at that time helps to develop swallowing ability by desensitizing the gag reflex. Later still, a baby can sit up, can handle finger foods, and is teething. Then hard crackers and other hard finger foods may be introduced under the watchful eye of an adult: they promote the development of manual dexterity and control of the jaw muscles, but the infant can also choke on them.

Some parents want to feed solids at an earlier age, on the theory that "stuffing the baby" at bedtime promotes sleeping through the night. There is no proof for this theory. Babies start to sleep through the night whenever they are ready, regardless of when solid foods are introduced; by three months, most are sleeping through the night whether or not they are receiving any solid foods.

New foods should be introduced one at a time, so that allergies can be detected. For example, when cereals are introduced, first try rice cereal for several days; it causes allergy least often. Try wheat cereal last; it is a common offender, along with egg whites, soy products, and citrus fruits. If a cereal causes an allergic reaction (irritability due to skin rash, digestive upset, or respiratory discomfort), discontinue its use before going on to the next food. About nine times out of ten the allergy won't be evident immediately but will manifest itself in vague symptoms occurring up to five days after the offending food is eaten. Wait a month or two to try the food again; many sensitivities disappear with maturity. If there is a family history of allergies, extra caution in introducing new foods is prudent. If parents detect allergies in an infant's early life, they can spare the whole family much grief. (Chapter 13 offers more information on allergies.)

As for the choice of foods, baby foods commercially prepared in the United States and Canada are generally safe, nutritious, and of high quality. In response to consumer demand, baby food companies have removed much of the added salt and sugar their products contained in the past, and baby foods also contain few or no additives. They generally have high nutrient density, except for mixed dinners and heavily sweetened desserts. Parents should not feed directly from the jar but should remove the portion to be fed to a dish for feeding so as not to contaminate the unused food that will be stored in the jar.

It has been suggested that the early introduction of sweet fruits to babies' diets might favor their developing a preference for sweets and lessen their liking for vegetables introduced later. To prevent this the order can be reversed: vegetables first, fruits later. As for sweets of any other kind (including baby food "desserts"), they have no place in a baby's life. The added food energy they contribute can promote obesity, and they convey few nutrients to support growth.

An alternative to commercial baby food for the parent who wants the baby to have family foods is to "blenderize" a small portion of the table food at each meal. This necessitates cooking without salt or sugar, though, as the baby food manufacturers do. The adults can season their own food after taking out the baby's portion.

Canned vegetables are not appropriate for babies; not only is the sodium content too high, but some nutrient value is lost in the canning process. Also, awareness of food poisoning and precautions against it are imperative; honey

■■■ Table 12–6 Meal Plan for a One-Year-Old

Breakfast	**Snack**
1 c milk	1/2 c milk
3 tbsp cereal	Teething crackers
2 to 3 tbsp fruit	1 tbsp peanut butter
Teething crackers	
Lunch	**Supper**
1 c milk	1 c milk
2 to 3 tbsp vegetables	1 egg
2 tbsp chopped meat or well-cooked, mashed legumes	2 tbsp cereal or potato
	2 to 3 tbsp vegetables
	2 to 3 tbsp fruit

should never be fed to infants because of the risk of botulism. (For more on these topics, see Chapter 14.) Babies and even young children have difficulty swallowing popcorn, nuts, hot dogs, raw carrots, and hard candy. An infant can easily choke on foods like these; they are not worth the risk.

Ideally the one-year-old is sitting at the table, eating many of the same foods everyone else eats, and drinking liquids from a cup—not a bottle. Infants and children thrive best on water, milk, or juice, so avoid feeding them nonnutritious soft drinks, sports drinks, sugary juice drinks, or punches. A meal plan that meets the requirements for the one-year-old is shown in Table 12–6.

Ⅱ▶ *Solid food additions to a baby's diet should begin at about six months and should be governed by the baby's nutrient needs and readiness to eat. By one year the baby should be receiving foods from all food groups.*

Looking Ahead

The first year of a baby's life is the time to lay the foundation for future health. From the nutrition standpoint, the relevant problems most common in later years are obesity and dental disease. Prevention of obesity can also help prevent the development of the obesity-related diseases—atherosclerosis, diabetes, and cancer.

Obesity in all but the youngest babies predicts obesity in later life. Probably the most important single measure to prevent it is to encourage eating habits that will support continued normal weight as the child grows. Primarily this means introducing a variety of nutritious foods in an inviting way, not forcing the baby to finish the bottle or to empty the baby food jar, avoiding concentrated sweets and empty-calorie foods, and encouraging vigorous physical activity.

To discourage development of the behaviors and attitudes that worsen obesity, parents should not teach babies to seek food as a reward, to expect food as comfort for unhappiness, or to associate food deprivation with punishment. If they cry for thirst, give them water, not milk or juice. If they cry for companionship, pick them up, don't feed them.

Beyond these recommendations, some thought has been given to the idea of a "prudent diet" for infants, like that recommended for adults to reduce heart disease risk: restrict fat, increase the ratio of polyunsaturated to saturated fat,

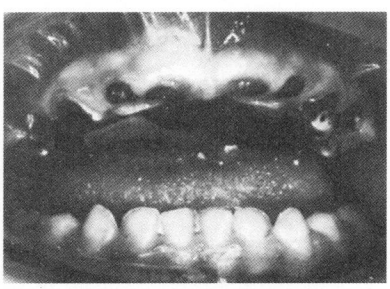

Nursing bottle syndrome, an extreme example. This child was frequently put to bed sucking on a baby bottle filled with apple juice, so that the teeth were bathed in carbohydrate for long periods of time—a perfect medium for bacterial growth. The upper teeth have decayed all the way to the gum line.

For a perspective on the notion that sugar affects behavior in children, turn to Controversy 4.

and reduce cholesterol intake. The AAP recommends against a fat-modified diet during infancy, stating that the evidence in its favor so far is scanty and does not warrant dietary manipulation to lower blood cholesterol. Dietary fat is necessary for proper development of the central nervous system. Furthermore, growth failure has been observed in children on fat-restricted diets, even when energy from other sources was constant.

Babies need the food energy and fat of whole milk until two years of age. The only exception might be the obese older baby, a case that would require physician consultation. Tampering with the amount of protein in a baby's diet could be especially risky. Protein is the single most important nutrient for growth.

Normal dental development is promoted by the same strategies outlined above: supplying nutritious foods, avoiding sweets, and discouraging the association of food with reward or comfort. In addition, the practice of giving a baby a bottle as a pacifier is strongly discouraged by dentists on the grounds that sucking for long periods of time pushes the normal jawline out of shape and causes a bucktoothed profile: protruding upper and receding lower teeth. Furthermore, prolonged sucking on a bottle of milk or juice bathes the upper teeth in a carbohydrate-rich fluid that favors the growth of decay-producing bacteria. Babies permitted to do this are sometimes seen with their upper teeth decayed all the way to the gum line.

▌▌▶ *The early feeding of the infant lays the foundation for lifelong eating habits. It is desirable to foster preferences that will, throughout life, support normal weight and development and help avert common lifestyle diseases.*

 Food Feature

Mealtimes with Infants

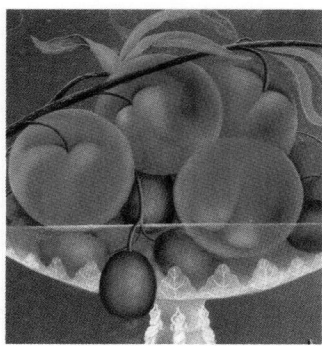

The wise parent of a one-year-old offers nutrition and love together. Both promote growth. It is literally true that "feeding with love" produces better growth in both weight and height of children than feeding the same food in an emotionally negative climate.[43] It also promotes better brain development. The formation of nerve-to-nerve connections in the brain depends both on nutrients and on environmental stimulation.[44]

The person feeding a one-year-old has to be aware that this is a period in the child's life when exploring and experimenting are normal and desirable behaviors. The child is developing a sense of autonomy that, if allowed to flower, will provide the foundation for later assertiveness in choosing when and how much to eat and when to stop eating as well as general confidence and effectiveness as an individual. The child's self-direction, if consistently overriden, can later turn into shame and self-doubt. In light of the developmental and nutrient needs of one-year-olds and in the face of their often contrary and willful behavior, a few feeding guidelines may be helpful. Following are several problem situations with suggestions for handling them:

▌ *He stands and plays at the table instead of eating.* Don't let him. This is unacceptable behavior and should be firmly discouraged. Put him down, and let him wait until later to eat again. Be consistent and firm, not punitive. If he is really hungry, he will soon learn to sit still while eating. A baby's appetite is less keen at a year than at eight months, and his energy needs are relatively lower. A one-year-old will get enough to eat if you let his hunger be his guide.

■ *She wants to poke her fingers into her food.* Let her. She has much to learn from feeling the texture of her food. When she knows all about it, she'll naturally graduate to the use of a spoon.

■ *He wants to manage the spoon himself, but can't handle it.* Let him try. As he masters it, withdraw gradually until he is feeding himself competently. This is the age at which a baby can learn to feed himself and is most strongly motivated to do so. He will spill, of course, but he'll grow out of it soon enough.

■ *She refuses food that her mother knows is good for her.* This way of demonstrating autonomy, one of the few available to the one-year-old, is most satisfying. Don't force. It is in the one- to two-year-old stage that most of the feeding problems develop that can last throughout life. As long as she is getting enough milk and is offered a variety of nutritious foods to choose from, she will gradually acquire a taste for different foods—provided that she feels she is making the choice. This year is the most important year of a child's life in establishing future food preferences. If a baby refuses milk, provide an alternative source of the bone- and muscle-building nutrients it supplies. Milk-based puddings, custards, and cheese are often successful substitutes. For the baby who is allergic to milk, soy milk and other formulas are available.

■ *He prefers sweets—candy and sugary confections—to foods containing more nutrients.* Human beings of all races and cultures have a natural inborn preference for sweet-tasting foods. Limit them strictly. If they are kept in the house, keep them out of sight. There is no room in a baby's daily 1000 calories for the calories from sweets, except occasionally. The meal plan shown in Table 12–6 provides more than 500 calories from milk; one or two servings of each of the other types of food provide the other 500. If a candy bar were substituted for any of these foods, the baby would lose out on valuable nutrients; if it were added daily, the baby would become obese.

These recommendations reflect a spirit of tolerance that serves the best interest of the child emotionally as well as physically. The wise parent of a one-year-old offers nutrition and love together.

Notes

1. M. Mitchell and E. Lerner, Weight gain and pregnancy outcome in underweight and normal weight women, *Journal of the American Dietetic Association* 89 (1989): 634–638, 641.

2. National Institute of Child Health and Human Development, *Facts about Premature Birth*, publication no. 461-338-814/25324 (Washington, D.C.: Government Printing Office, 1985).

3. Food and Nutrition Board, *Recommended Dietary Allowances*, 10th ed. (Washington, D.C.: National Academy of Sciences, 1989), p. 34.

4. B. H. Dennis and coauthors, Nutrient intakes among selected North American populations in the Lipid Research Clinics prevalence study: Composition of energy intake, *American Journal of Clinical Nutrition* 41 (1985): 312–329.

5. R. D. Reynolds, M. Polansky, and P. B. Moser, Analyzed vitamin B_6 intakes of pregnant and postpartum lactating and nonlactating women, *Journal of the American Dietetic Association* 84 (1984): 1339–1344.

6. K. Simmer and coauthors, Are iron-folacin supplements harmful? *American Journal of Clinical Nutrition* 45 (1987): 122–125.

7. K. M. Hambidge and coauthors, Zinc nutritional status during pregnancy: A longitudinal study, *American Journal of Clinical Nutrition* 37 (1983): 429–442.

8. F. B. Glenn, W. D. Glenn, and R. C. Duncan, Fluoride tablet supplementation during pregnancy for caries immunity: A study of the offspring produced, *American Journal of Obstetrics and Gynecology* 143 (1982): 560–564.

9. B. Worthington-Roberts and coauthors, Dietary cravings and aversions in the postpartum period, *Journal of the American Dietetic Association*: 89 (1989): 647–651.

10. Mitchell and Lerner, 1989.

11. R. L. Naeye, Weight gain and the outcome of pregnancy, *American Journal of Obstetrics and Gynecology* 135 (1979): 3–9; J. E. Brown and coauthors, Prenatal weight gains related to the birth of healthy-sized infants to low-income women, *Journal of the American Dietetic Association* 86 (1986): 1679–1683.

12. D. Hall and D. Kaufmann, Effects of aerobic and strength conditioning on pregnancy outcomes, *American Journal of Obstetrics and Gynecology* 157 (1987): 1199–1203.

13. National Institute of Nutrition in Canada, Caffeine: A perspective on current concerns, *Nutrition Today* July/August 1987, pp. 36–38.

14. W. Srisuphon and B. M. Bracken, Caffeine consumption during pregnancy and association with late spontaneous abortion, *American Journal of Obstetrics and Gynecology* 154 (1986): 14–20.

15. M. Stjernfeldt and coauthors, Maternal smoking during pregnancy and risk of childhood cancer, *Lancet* 1 (1986): 1350–1352.

16. B. Zuckerman and coauthors, Effects of maternal marijuana and cocaine use on fetal growth, *New England Journal of Medicine* 320 (1989): 762–768.

17. Alcohol and pregnancy, *Nutrition and the MD*, August 1984.

18. J. Kline and coauthors, Drinking during pregnancy and spontaneous abortion, *Lancet*, 26 July 1980, pp. 176–180; M. C. Marbury and coauthors, The association of alcohol consumption with outcome of pregnancy, *American Journal of Public Health* 73 (1983): 1165.

19. Kline and coauthors, 1980.

20. C. Raymond, Birth defects linked with specific level of maternal alcohol use, but abstinence still the best policy, *Journal of the American Medical Association* 258 (1987): 177–178.

21. M. H. Kaufman, Ethanol-induced chromosomal abnormalities at conception, *Nature* 302 (1983): 258–260; R. E. Little and C. F. Sing, Father's drinking and infant birthweight, *Teratology* 36 (1987): 59–65.

22. A. P. Streissguth, S. K. Clarren, and K. L. Jones, Natural history of the fetal alcohol syndrome: A 10-year follow-up of eleven patients, *Lancet*, 13 July 1985, pp. 85–91.

23. K. R. Warren and R. J. Bast, Alcohol-related birth defects: an update, *Public Health Reports* 103 (1988): 638–642.

24. J. M. Graham and coauthors, Independent dysmorphology evaluations at birth and 4 years of age for children exposed to varying amounts of alcohol in utero, *Pediatrics* 81 (1988): 772–778.

25. B. Bower, Drinking while pregnant risks child's IQ, *Science News* 135 (1989): 68.

26. S. Fisher and P. Karl, Maternal ethanol use and selective fetal malnutrition, *Alcoholism* (New York: Plenum Press, 1988), pp. 277–289.

27. *Nutrition Today* letter, 8 April 1981.

28. H. L. Rosett, L. Weiner, and K. C. Edelin, Treatment experience with pregnant problem drinkers, *Journal of the American Medical Association* 249 (1983): 2029–2033.

29. *Alcohol Use During Pregnancy*, December 1981 (a booklet available from the American Council on Science and Health, 47 Maple St., Summit, NJ 07901).

30. C. Ernhart and coauthors, Alcohol teratogenicity in the human: A detailed assessment of specificity, critical period, and threshold, *American Journal of Obstetrics and Gynecology* 156 (1987): 33–39.

31. Maternal nutrition during lactation, *Nutrition and the MD*, February 1987.

32. Maternal nutrition, 1987.

33. M. Brewer, M. Bates, and L. Vannoy, Postpartum changes in maternal weight and body fat depots in lactating vs nonlactating women, *American Journal of Clinical Nutrition* 49 (1989): 259–265.

34. R. G. Whitehead and coauthors, A critical analysis of measured food energy intakes during infancy and early childhood in comparison with current international recommendations, *Journal of Human Nutrition* 35 (1981): 339–348.

35. American Academy of Pediatrics, Committee on Nutrition, *Pediatric Nutrition Handbook*, 2d ed. (Elk Grove Village, Ill.: American Academy of Pediatrics, 1985), p. 31.

36. American Academy of Pediatrics, Committee on Nutrition, and Nutrition Committee of the Canadian Pediatric Society, Breastfeeding: A commentary in celebration of the International Year of the Child, 1979, *Pediatrics* 62 (1978): 591–601.

37. American Academy of Pediatrics, Committee on Nutrition, 1985, pp. 37–48.

38. J. Ekstrand, No evidence of transfer of fluoride from plasma to breast milk, *British Medical Journal* 283 (1981): 761–764.

39. C. Briggs, Recent developments in infant feeding and nutrition, in *Nutrition Update,* vol. 1, eds. J. Weininger and G. M. Briggs (New York: Wiley, 1983), pp. 227–261.

40. R. Miller, The metal in our mettle, *FDA Consumer* December 1988-January 1989, pp. 24–27.

41. E. Pollitt and coauthors, Iron deficiency and behavioral development in infants and preschool children, *American Journal of Clinical Nutrition* 43 (1986): 555–565.

42. Ross Laboratories, Perspectives on nutrition in latter infancy, *Public Health Currents* 28 (1988): 17–20.

43. E. M. Widdowson, Mental contentment and physical growth, *Lancet* 1 (1951): 1316–1318.

44. J. Cravioto, Nutrition, stimulation, mental development and learning, *Nutrition Today*, September/October 1981, pp. 4–8, 10–15.

Medicines, Other Drugs, and Nutrition

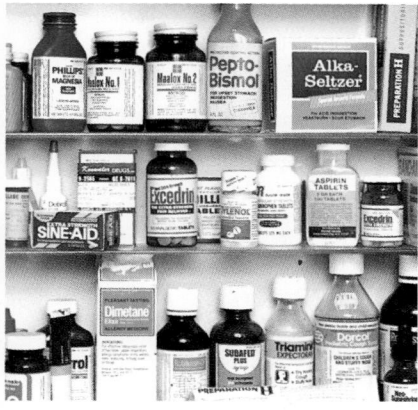

The ways in which alcohol affects health and nutrition status were described in the last Controversy. Other drugs also interact with body systems and can affect nutrient needs. This Controversy describes the effects of the major drugs other than alcohol—medicines, illicit drugs, and the two commonly used drugs, caffeine and nicotine.

■■■ Medicines

People sometimes think that medicines are unlike other drugs, that they do only good, no harm. The Food and Drug Administration (FDA) monitors the safety and effectiveness of medicines. But just as alcohol and other drugs can interact in potentially dangerous ways, so too can drugs interact with each

other. For example, one drug can inhibit or negate the action of another drug. And just as alcohol and nutrition interact, so do drugs and nutrition:

■ Foods can slow down the absorption of drugs from the digestive tract.
■ Drugs can make nutrients unavailable for absorption.
■ Drugs can alter food intake by modifying taste or the appetite.
■ Nutrients can interfere with the action or excretion of drugs.
■ Drugs can interfere with the action or excretion of nutrients.

These effects occur not only with **prescription drugs** but also with **over-the-counter (OTC) drugs** such as aspirins and laxatives. This discussion focuses on a few of the more commonly used medicines; Table C12–1 (next page) gives some examples of possible drug-nutrient interactions for a variety of commonly used OTC and prescription drugs.

OTC drugs are readily available and widely used in the United States

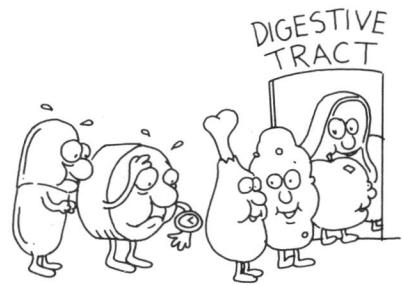

Foods can slow down the absorption of drugs in the digestive tract.

and harm people's nutrition status, especially when they are misused. For example, people who use laxatives daily for weeks or months may find that their intestines can no longer function without them. Laxative dependence can lead to malnutrition, since laxatives can cause nutrients to travel so rapidly through the intestines that many vitamins do not have time to be absorbed. The laxative mineral oil can rob a person of fat-soluble vitamins because they dissolve in the indigestible oil and are excreted. Vitamin D deficiencies can occur this way; calcium, too, may be excreted with the oil, accelerating adult bone loss.

Advertisers promote antacids as a panacea for those who overindulge themselves in rich food and drink, but people should think twice before taking them. Recurrent stomach pain should be checked by a physician—it could indicate a serious condition such as an ulcer. Also, the presence of aluminum hydroxide in an antacid can promote the excretion of both phosphorus and calcium. Therefore chronic use of some antacids can eventually impair bone health. In one case an elderly woman had to be admitted to the hospital because over the last few months the pain in her legs had gotten so bad she could barely stand up or walk unassisted. During this same period of time she had more than doubled her consumption of antacids. Once she stopped taking the antacids, the pain in her legs subsided.

Many people take large doses of aspirin each day to relieve the pain

■■■ **Table C12−1 Examples of Drug−Nutrient Interactions for Selected, Commonly Used Drugs**

DRUG	POSSIBLE EFFECT ON NUTRITION STATUS				
	REDUCES ABSORPTION	RAISES BLOOD CONCENTRATIONS	LOWERS BLOOD CONCENTRATIONS	INCREASES EXCRETION	OTHER
Antacids (aluminum containing)	Iron			Phosphorus Calcium	Thiamin[a]
Antibiotics	Fats Amino acids Carbohydrates Folate Vitamin B_{12} Fat-soluble vitamins Calcium Iron Potassium Magnesium Zinc			Potassium Niacin Riboflavin Folate Vitamin C	Vitamin K[b]
Aspirin			Folate	Vitamin C Thiamin Vitamin K	Iron[c]
Caffeine				Calcium Magnesium	Cholesterol[d]
Diuretics		Zinc Calcium	Potassium Chloride Magnesium Phosphorus Folate Vitamin B_{12}	Calcium Sodium Thiamin Potassium Chloride Magnesium	Zinc[e]
Laxatives	Fat Glucose Vitamin D Calcium Potassium Fat-soluble vitamins Carotene				
Oral Contraceptives	Folate	Vitamin A Copper Iron	Vitamin B_6 Riboflavin Folate Vitamin B_{12} Vitamin C		Riboflavin[f] Vitamin B_6[f] Calcium[g]

[a] Antacids may accelerate the destruction of thiamin.
[b] Some antibiotics may interfere with intestinal synthesis of vitamin K.
[c] Aspirin use may cause blood loss, thus compromising iron status.
[d] Large doses of caffeine may raise blood cholesterol concentrations.
[e] Some diuretics may interfere with zinc storage in the liver.
[f] Some oral contraceptives may augment the requirements for riboflavin and vitamin B_6.
[g] Some oral contraceptives may improve the absorption of calcium.

SOURCE: Adapted from: R. E. Hodges, *Nutrition in Medical Practice* (Philadelphia: Saunders, 1980), pp. 323−331; R. C. Theuer and J. J. Vitale, Drug and nutrient interactions, in *Nutritional Support of Medical Practice,* eds. H. A. Schneider; C. F. Anderson; and D. B. Coursin (Hagerstown, Md.: Harper and Row, 1977), pp. 297−305; D. A. Roe, *Drug Induced Nutritional Deficiencies* (Westport, Conn.: AVI, 1985).

of arthritis, backaches, and headaches. Taking large quantities of aspirin, say 10 to 12 tablets per day (not an unusual amount for people with chronic pain) increases blood loss from the stomach by as much as ten times or so, enough to cause iron-deficiency anemia in some people.[1] People who take aspirin regularly should make sure they eat iron-rich foods regularly as well.

Prescription drugs are true miracles of our time when they are used correctly. For example, a person with diabetes depends on drugs to raise insulin levels—literally a life-saving treatment. They can also wreak havoc with nutrition; the dangers of overuse or misuse are great.

This discussion focuses on the nutrition effects of just one prescription medication, **oral contraceptives**, to illustrate that interactions between just one drug and nutrients can be complex. Millions of women use oral contraceptives, daily doses of hormones that prevent pregnancy by creating a hormonal climate similar to that of pregnancy itself. In its 30-year history, the pill has become the most studied drug in the United States.[2] The identification of a number of risk factors has prompted changes in the dosages and formulations of the pill to produce an effective contraceptive with a wide margin of safety.

Oral contraceptives clearly do alter the concentrations of nutrients in the blood. One of their most significant health effects is to alter blood lipids, raising the risk of car-diovascular disease.[3] For young, healthy women who do not smoke, no association between oral contraceptives and heart disease appears to exist.[4] Later in life, however, most oral contraceptives raise total cholesterol and triglyceride concentrations and lower HDL, amplifying the risk of heart disease. The risk is greatest for women over 35 years of age who smoke and for all women over 45 years.[5] All women should stop smoking, and after 45 years of age should find alternative contraceptive methods.

Each nutrient responds differently to oral contraceptive use. Oral contraceptives depress blood concentrations of vitamin B_6, folate, vitamin C, and zinc, while they raise blood concentrations of vitamin A, vitamin K, iron, and copper. At first glance this might seem to indicate that women using them are at risk for deficiency of the first four nutrients named but have somehow increased their body stores of the last four. The research in the area has yielded conflicting results, however, so any such assumptions would be premature. Research suggests that the changed blood concentrations of some nutrients may reflect a redistribution of the nutrients within the body and not a changed total-body content of the nutrients.

Take vitamin A, for example. The higher-than-usual vitamin A blood concentrations in oral contraceptive users appears to be due to extra vitamin A's being released from storage in the liver. Knowing this, researchers became concerned that this might deplete vitamin A in the liver and lead to deficiency.[6] They found otherwise. Oral contraceptives do not appear to cause liver depletion of vitamin A or a deficiency of any sort.

Oral contraceptive users also have higher blood concentrations of iron. Unlike vitamin A, this is probably due to enhanced conservation of iron by the body. Oral contraceptive use brings about both less blood loss in menstruation and greater absorption of iron in the intestine. However, iron in the blood of oral contraceptive users stays well within the normal range.

The vitamin B_6 status of oral contraceptive users has been extensively studied. Research shows that some oral contraceptive users have low blood concentrations of vitamin B_6. Since vitamin B_6 assists in the body's handling of the amino acid tryptophan, this pathway is impaired. Because other vitamin B_6-dependent functions remain normal, confusion persists about whether oral contraceptive users require more vitamin B_6 than nonusers. Excess vitamin B_6 can be toxic (Chapter 7), so oral contraceptive users are generally advised to rely on vitamin B_6-rich foods to replenish their supply and to avoid supplements.

For some women, however, depressed blood concentrations of vitamin B_6 may warrant special attention. Research shows that pregnant and lactating women may actually develop vitamin B_6 deficiencies after long-term use of oral contraceptives. One study showed that pregnant women who had used oral contraceptives for 30 months or more had significantly reduced blood concentrations of vitamin B_6 at delivery and five months later, and the vitamin's concentration in their milk and in their newborn infants' blood showed similar patterns.[7] It seems important, therefore, to monitor the vitamin B_6 status of long-term oral contraceptive users who become pregnant. A mother's deficiency in pregnancy could affect the future infant.

If a woman on the pill thinks she may have a nutrient deficiency, she should refrain from taking individual supplements and seek testing and a diagnosis from a health care professional to rule out other causes of her symptoms. For most women a nutritious diet is all that is needed. However, if a woman feels compelled to take a supplement, a multivitamin-mineral supplement that does not exceed the RDA is probably harmless, as long as it is in addition to (not a replacement for) a well-balanced diet. Controversy 7 showed how to select one.

▮▮▮ Illicit Drugs

People know that illicit drugs are harmful, but in spite of the risks, many choose to abuse them anyway. Like over-the-counter and prescription drugs, illegal drugs modify body functions. They are unlike medicines, however, in that no watchdog agency such as the FDA monitors them for safety, effectiveness, or even for purity. The risks of using illicit drugs are many and diverse—ranging from health risks to imprisonment to early death.

Marijuana and cocaine are the most notorious illicit drugs.

Smoking a marijuana cigarette has several characteristic effects on the body, altering, among other things, the sense of taste. Among the apparent taste changes induced by marijuana is an enhanced enjoyment of eating, especially of sweets, commonly known as "the munchies." Why or how this effect occurs is not known. Some investigators speculate that the hunger induced by marijuana is actually a social effect caused by the suggestibility of the group in which it is smoked. Prolonged use of the drug does not seem to bring about a weight gain.

Despite increased food intakes, marijuana abusers often consume fewer nutrients than do nonabusers. This is probably because the extra foods they choose are usually high-calorie, low-nutrient snack foods.

Marijuana users may think that because they usually smoke fewer marijuana cigarettes in a day than tobacco cigarettes, they will incur fewer harmful, long-term effects on their lungs. This is a myth. Research shows that one marijuana cigarette is as bad for the body as four or five tobacco cigarettes. People may smoke fewer marijuana cigarettes than tobacco cigarettes, but they inhale more smoke and hold it in their lungs longer. As a result, regular marijuana users may face the same risk of lung cancer as people who smoke a pack of cigarettes a day.[8]

Cocaine elicits effects such as intense euphoria, restlessness, heightened self-confidence, irritability, insomnia, and loss of appetite. Weight loss is a common side effect, and cocaine abusers often develop eating disorders.[9] Repeated use can cause rapid heart rate, irregular heart beats, heart attacks, and even death. Cocaine use continues to escalate as cheaper and more dangerous forms of the drug become available. Cocaine in its smokable form, crack, is more addicting than any other drug.[10] The addictive power of the drug is overwhelming and frightening. One former crack addict tells the story of holding a gun to his brother's head to steal money for his next crack purchase.

Unlike marijuana use, cocaine use brings nutritional consequences. Notably, the craving for the drug replaces hunger; the stronger the craving for cocaine, the less a drug abuser wants food. Rats given unlimited cocaine will choose the drug over food until they die of starvation.[11]

The effects of other addictive drugs vary in degree but are similar in kind to those of cocaine. Drug abusers face multiple nutrition problems:

▮ They spend money for drugs that could be spent on food.
▮ They lose interest in food during "high" times.
▮ Some drugs induce at least a temporary depression of appetite.
▮ Their lifestyle often lacks the regularity and routine that promote good eating habits.
▮ They may contract hepatitis, a liver disease common in drug abusers, which causes taste changes and loss of appetite. They risk contracting AIDS.
▮ Their nutrition status may be altered by treatments and medicines.

■ They often become ill with infectious diseases, which increase their need for nutrients.

During withdrawal from drugs, an important aspect of treatment is the identification and correction of nutrition problems.

■■■ Caffeine

The well-known "wake-up" effect of caffeine is the primary reason that people in every society use it in some form. Compared with the drugs discussed so far, though, caffeine's interactions with foods and nutrients are subtle. And yet in one important way caffeine's relationship to nutrition is more distinct—people usually ingest caffeine by way of foods and beverages, and they may even be unaware that they are consuming it at all. For this reason, and because caffeine's effects on health and nutrition continue to be controversial, it warrants discussion.

Caffeine is a true stimulant drug. Like all stimulants, it increases the respiration rate, heart rate, blood pressure, and secretion of stress and other hormones. It stimulates the digestive tract, promoting efficient elimination, and promotes water loss from the body as well.

Caffeine is the most popular and widely consumed drug in the United States.[12] One in three people in the United States consumes about 200 milligrams of caffeine per day (the amount in 2 small cups of coffee), but many others consume much more—amounts that may be harmful to some people.[13] Like alcohol's effects, the effects of caffeine vary according to how much people consume, how much they weigh, and how much tolerance they have developed to the drug. Because they are small and, at first, not adapted to its use, children are especially vulnerable to caffeine's effects.

Despite caffeine's tremendous popularity, many people today are cutting their use of it because they fear it will harm them. Research in the last decade has yielded sporadic reports linking caffeine to health problems such as hypertension, fibrocystic breast disease, birth defects, clinical anxiety, and cancer, to name a few.[14] However, much other research refutes these findings. For example, the weight of evidence now seems to suggest no link between caffeine and cancer or birth defects.[15]

Recent studies reveal still more links between caffeine and health. A study of women attempting to become pregnant reported conception difficulties in women who consumed more than 1 cup of coffee per day.[16] However, these findings were later refuted in a study of thousands of women that showed no link between fertility and caffeine consumption.[17] It did, however, find that increased caffeine intake accompanies advanced age, higher body weight, and more cigarette and alcohol use.

In contrast to the finding that heavier women use more caffeine, results of another study suggest possible benefits of moderate caffeine ingestion for weight control.[18] As little as 100 milligrams of caffeine noticeably raised the metabolic rates of both lean and previously obese people for several hours after caffeine consumption.

Chapter 10 stated that athletes sometimes use caffeine to facilitate the release of free fatty acids into the blood. Research now in progress is asking whether the blood lipid alterations caused by caffeine may be related to raised blood cholesterol and thus to the risk of heart disease.

Caffeine seems relatively harmless when used in moderation (the equivalent of fewer than, say, 2 to 4 average-sized cups of coffee a day). In amounts greater than this it can cause the symptoms associated with anxiety—sweating, tenseness, and inability to concentrate—and is suspected of raising heart disease and heart attack risks and of causing the possibly painful but benign fibrocystic breast disease.

If you like consuming caffeine-containing foods or beverages, the most reasonable approach may be to limit your intake to the equivalent of about 2 small cups of coffee per day. For most people this is enough to produce the desired effects of reduced drowsiness and keener awareness of tasks at hand without paying too high a price. Pregnant women, especially, should exercise moderation in using caffeine, and parents should monitor and control their children's intakes. Table C12−2 lists the caffeine contents of beverages and foods, and Table C12−3 displays the caffeine amounts in selected over-the-counter drugs.

◼◼◼ Table C12-2 Caffeine Content of Beverages and Foods

DRINKS AND FOODS	AVERAGE (MG)	RANGE (MG)
Coffee (5-oz cup)		
Brewed, drip method	130	110–150
Brewed, percolator	94	64–124
Instant	74	40–108
Decaffeinated, brewed or instant	3	1–5
Tea (5-oz cup)		
Brewed, major U.S. brands	40	20–90
Brewed, imported brands	60	25–110
Instant	30	25–50
Iced (12-oz glass)	70	67–76
Soft drinks (12-oz can)		
Dr. Pepper		40
Colas and cherry colas:		
Regular		30–46
Diet		2–58
Caffeine free		0–trace
Jolt		72
Mountain Dew, Mello Yello		52
Big Red		38
Fresca, Hires Root Beer, 7–Up, Sprite,		0
Squirt, Sunkist Orange		0
Cocoa beverage (5-oz cup)	4	2–20
Chocolate milk beverage (8 oz)	5	2–7
Milk chocolate candy (1 oz)	6	1–15
Dark chocolate, semisweet (1 oz)	20	5–35
Baker's chocolate (1 oz)	26	26
Chocolate-flavored syrup (1 oz)	4	4

SOURCE: Data from C. Lecos, The latest caffeine scoreboard, *FDA Consumer*, March 1984, p. 14; Measuring your life with coffee spoons. *Tufts University Diet and Nutrition Letter*, April 1984, pp. 3–6; Institute of Food Technologists, Expert Panel on Food Safety and Nutrition, *Evaluation of Caffeine Safety*, a publication (1986) available from the Institute of Food Technologists, 221 N. LaSalle St., Chicago, IL 60601.

◼◼◼ Nicotine

Cigarette and other smoking is a pervasive health problem causing thousands of people to suffer from cancer and diseases of the cardiovascular, digestive, and respiratory systems. These effects are beyond the scope of nutrition, but smoking does influence hunger, body weight, and nutrient status. Links between smoking's nutrition effects and lung cancer are also known.

Smoking a cigarette eases feelings of hunger. A smoker who receives a hunger signal can quiet it with a cigarette instead of food. Such behavior ignores body signals and postpones energy and nutrient intake. Thus smokers tend to weigh less than nonsmokers and to gain weight upon cessation of smoking.[19] Weight gain is often a concern for people contemplating giving up cigarettes. The decision to quit weighs unhealthy smoking against unattractive (and potentially unhealthy) weight gain. The message to smokers wanting to quit is to adjust diet and exercise habits to maintain weight during and after cessation.

Nutrient intakes of smokers and nonsmokers differ. Smokers have lower intakes of dietary fiber, vitamins, and minerals, even when their energy intakes are quite similar to those of nonsmokers.[20] The association between smoking and low vitamin intake may be noteworthy, considering the altered metabolism of vitamin C in smokers and the protective effect of vitamin A against lung cancer.

Research shows that the vitamin C requirement of smokers exceeds that of nonsmokers.[21] Smokers break down vitamin C faster, thus requiring more vitamin C to achieve steady body pools comparable to those of nonsmokers. It is estimated that the vitamin C requirement of smokers may be twice as high as that of nonsmokers. The evidence for this is so strong that it is reflected in the vitamin C RDA—at least 100 milligrams per day for smokers compared to 60 for nonsmokers.[22]

Beta-carotene, a precursor to vitamin A found in vegetables, has anticancer activity.[23] Specifically, the risk of lung cancer is greatest for smokers who have the lowest intake of carotene. Of course, conclusions from such evidence should not be

■■■ Table C12-3 Caffeine Content of Selected OTC Drugs

DRUGS[a]	AVERAGE (MG)	RANGE (MG)
Cold remedies (standard dose)		
Dristan	0	
Coryban-D, Triaminicin	30	
Diuretics (standard dose)		
Aqua-ban, Permathene H₂Off	200	
Pre-Mens Forte	100	
Pain relievers (standard dose)		
Excedrin	130	
Midol, Anacin	65	
Aspirin, plain (any brand)	0	
Stimulants		
Caffedrin, NoDoz, Vivarin	200	
Weight-control aids (daily dose)		
Prolamine	280	
Dexatrim, Dietac	200	

[a]Because products change, contact the manufacturer for an update on products you use regularly.
SOURCES: Same as for Table C12–2.

misinterpreted. People cannot be led to believe that as long as they eat their carrots they can safely smoke their cigarettes. Smokers are ten times more likely to get lung cancer than nonsmokers.[24] People who do smoke, however, as well as those who do not, can lower their cancer risks by eating fruits and vegetables rich in carotene.

Users of smokeless tobacco products also affect their nutrition status. Many chewing tobaccos contain a licorice compound that, while not a nutrient, can be toxic in excess. Moreover, tobacco products have been shown to carry the risk of worsened hypertension due to sodium or other unknown factors in the tobacco. Additionally, the risk of cancer of the mouth and throat skyrockets with chewing tobacco use, and chewers who believe this a safer practice than smoking are mistaken.

All drugs—medicines, illicit drugs, and even the common drugs caffeine and nicotine—can interact with foods and nutrients to affect health and nutrition status. Of course, not all the interactions discussed here occur every time a person takes a drug; but some people are more vulnerable to drug–nutrient interactions than others. The potential for undesirable drug–nutrient interactions is greatest for those who:

■ Take medication or any drug for a long period of time.
■ Take two or more drugs at the same time.
■ Are not well nourished to begin with or are not eating adequate diets.

In conclusion, when you need to take a medicine, do so wisely. Ask your health care provider for specific instructions about the doses and when to take them—with meals or on an empty stomach. If you notice new symptoms or if the drug does not seem to be working well, consult your health care provider.

No matter how hard people try to protect themselves from the ill effects of illicit drugs, they cannot. The risks such drugs pose cannot be calculated. The only instructions people need about illicit drugs is to avoid them altogether for the reasons mentioned earlier and for countless others as well. As for smoking and chewing tobacco, the same advice applies—don't take these habits up, and if you already have them, take steps to quit. For drugs of lesser consequences to health, such as caffeine, use moderation.

Try to live life in a way that requires less chemical assistance. If sleepy, try a 15-minute nap or meditation instead of a 15-minute coffee break. The coffee will stimulate your nerves for an hour, but the alternatives will refresh your attitude for the rest of the day. If you suffer constipation, try getting enough exercise, fiber, and water for a few days. Chances are that a laxative will be unnecessary. The attitude being demonstrated here is one of taking control of your body, allowing your reliable, self-healing nature to make fine adjustments in functioning without overriding them with chemicals. Bodies have few requests: adequate nutrition, rest, exercise, and hygiene. Give yours what it needs, and let it function naturally, without interference from drugs on a day-to-day basis.

Notes

1. Why food and medicine don't always make a good mix, *Tufts*

■■■ Miniglossary

oral contraceptives: pill containing synthetic hormones that disrupt the female menstrual cycle and prevent ovulation; used to prevent conception, often called birth control pills.

over-the-counter (OTC) drug: a drug legally available without a prescription.

prescription drug: a drug available only with a physician's order.

University Diet and Nutrition Letter, July 1989, pp. 3–6.

2. B. D. Shepard, Oral contraceptives—An overview, *Journal of the Florida Medical Association* 73 (1986): 763–767.

3. E. L. Marut, Oral contraceptives—Who, which, when, and why? *Postgraduate Medicine* 82 (1987): 66–70.

4. J. K. Williams, Oral contraceptives—The long-term perspective, *Journal of the Florida Medical Association* 73 (1986): 769–771.

5. Marut, 1987.

6. K. Amatayakul and coauthors, Oral contraceptives: Effect of long-term use on liver vitamin A storage assessed by the relative dose response test, *American Journal of Clinical Nutrition* 49 (1989): 845–848.

7. L. T. Miller, Do oral contraceptive agents affect nutrient requirements—vitamin B_6? *Journal of Nutrition* 116 (1986): 1344–1345.

8. T. C. Wu and coauthors, Pulmonary hazards of smoking marijuana as compared with tobacco, *New England Journal of Medicine* 318 (1988): 347–351.

9. J. M. Jonas and M. S. Gold, Cocaine abuse and eating disorders, *Lancet* 1 (1986): 390–391.

10. J. V. Lamar, Crack, *Time* 2 June 1986, pp. 16–18.

11. M. A. Bozarth and R. A. Wise, Toxicity associated with long-term intravenous heroin and cocaine self-administration in the rat, *Journal of the American Medical Association* 254 (1985): 81–83.

12. T. K. Leonard, R. R. Watson, and M. E. Mohs, The effects of caffeine on various body systems: A review, *Journal of the American Dietetic Association* 87 (1987): 1048–1053.

13. R. Watson, Caffeine: Is it dangerous to health? *American Journal of Health Promotion* Spring 1988, pp. 13–22.

14. R. Watson, Caffeine: Is it dangerous to health? *American Journal of Health Promotion*, Spring 1988, pp. 13–22.

15. *Tufts University Diet and Nutrition Letter,* February 1990, pp. 3–6.

16. A. Wilcox, C. Weinberg, and D. Baird, Caffeinated beverages and decreased fertility, *Lancet*, 24/31 December 1988, pp. 1453–1455.

17. M. R. Joesoef and coauthors, Are caffeinated beverages risk factors for delayed conception? *Lancet* 335 (1990): 136–137.

18. A. G. Dulloo and coauthors, Normal caffeine consumption: Influence on thermogenesis and daily energy expenditure in lean and postobese human volunteers, *American Journal of Clinical Nutrition* 49 (1989): 44–50.

19. M. E. Mohs, R. R. Watson, and T. Leonard-Green, Nutritional effects of marijuana, heroin, cocaine, and nicotine, *Journal of the American Dietetic Association* 90 (1990): 1261–1267.

20. A. M. Fehily, K. M. Phillips, and J. W. G. Yarnell, Diet, smoking, social class, and body mass index in the Caerphilly Heart Disease Study, *American Journal of Clinical Nutrition* 40 (1984): 827–833.

21. G. Schectman, J. C. Byrd, and H. W. Gruchow, The influence of smoking on vitamin C status in adults, *American Journal of Public Health* 79 (1989): 158–162.

22. Food and Nutrition Board, Committee on Dietary Allowances, *Recommended Dietary Allowances*, 10th ed. (Washington, D.C.: National Academy of sciences, 1989), pp. 115–124.

23. Dietary carotene and the risk of lung cancer, *Nutrition Reviews* 40 (1982): 265–268; R. Shekelle and coauthors, Dietary vitamin and risk of cancer in the Western Electric Study, *Lancet* 28 November 1981, pp. 1185–1189; D. Mackerras and coauthors, Carotene intake and the risk of laryngeal cancer in coastal Texas, *American Journal of Epidemiology* 128 (1988): 980–988.

24. B. Liebman, Carrots against cancer? *Nutrition Action Health Letter* December 1988, pp. 1, 5–7.

Child, Teen, and Older Adult

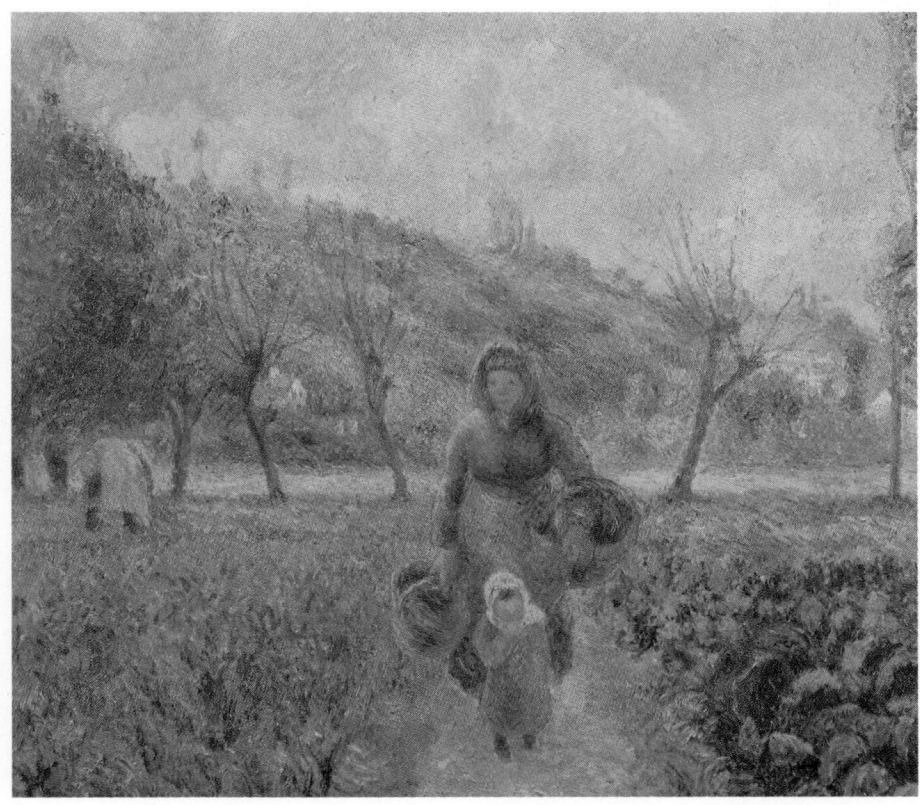

CONTENTS

In the Garden by Camille Pissarro, Narodni Gallery, Prague. Giraudon/Art Resource, N.Y.

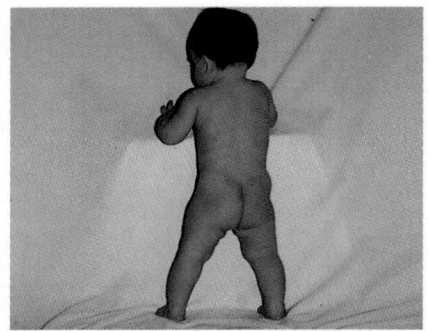

The body shape of a one-year-old (above) changes dramatically by age two (below). The two-year-old has lost much of the baby fat; the muscles (especially in the back, buttocks, and legs) have firmed and strengthened; and the leg bones have lengthened.

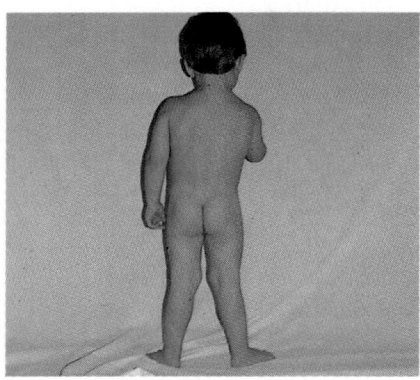

Cues to eating were discussed in Chapter 9.

Parents look forward to being proud of strong, healthy, competent, and happy sons and daughters. To grow to function well in the adult world, children need a solid background of sound eating habits that will help to determine their future health. These habits begin at babyhood with the introduction of solid foods, as shown in the last chapter. But at that point nutrition has just begun; the plot thickens. Nutrient needs change steadily throughout life, depending on the rate of growth, gender, and many other factors. Nutrient needs also vary from individual to individual, but generalizations are possible and useful.

Early and Middle Childhood

After the age of one year, a child's growth rate slows, but the body continues to change dramatically. At age one, infants have just learned to stand and toddle; by two years they can take long strides with solid confidence and are learning to run, jump, and climb. These new accomplishments are possible thanks to the accumulation of a larger mass and greater density of bone and muscle tissue. Thereafter the same trend—a lengthening of the long bones and an increase in musculature—continues, unevenly and more slowly, until adolescence.

Growth and Nutrient Needs of Young Children

An infant's appetite decreases markedly near the first birthday, in line with the great reduction in growth rate. Thereafter the appetite fluctuates; at times children seem to be insatiable, and at other times they seem to live on air and water. Parents need not worry about this—a child will need and demand more food during periods of rapid growth than during slow periods. The perfection of appetite regulation in children of normal weight guarantees that their food energy intakes will be right for each stage of growth.[1] One caution: some children may eat in response to external cues, disregarding appetite regulation signals, setting the stage for obesity.

A one-year-old child needs perhaps 1000 calories a day; a three-year-old needs only 300 to 500 calories more. At age ten a child needs only about 2000 calories a day. Thus even though total energy needs have doubled by age ten, the child's energy need per pound of body weight has steadily declined. Active children of any age need more energy because they spend more, and an inactive child can become obese even when consuming a diet that is below average in calories.

Growth increases the demand for all the nutrients (see the Recommended Dietary Allowance [RDA] tables in the inside front cover or the Recommended Nutrient Intakes [RNI] tables for Canadians in Appendix B). Before their adolescent growth spurt, children accumulate stores of nutrients that they will need in the years ahead. Then, when they take off on that growth spurt, there comes a time during which their nutrient intakes cannot meet the demands of rapid growth, and they draw on the nutrients they stored earlier. This is especially true of calcium; the denser the bones are in childhood, the better prepared they will be to support teen growth and still withstand the inevitable bone losses of later life. The RDA and Canadian RNI tables reflect the gradually increasing nutrient needs of the growing years to provide all these nutrients.

■■■ Table 13–1 Children's Daily Food Patterns for Good Nutrition

FOOD GROUP	SERVINGS PER DAY	AVERAGE SIZE OF SERVING		
		1 TO 3 YEARS	4 TO 6 YEARS	7 TO 12 YEARS
Milk and milk products[a]	4	½–¾ c	¾ c	¾–1 c
Meat and meat alternates[b]	2 or more	1–2 oz	1–2 oz	2–3 oz
Fruits and vegetables[c]	4 or more	2–4 tbsp or ½ c juice	¼–½ c or ½ c juice	½–¾ c or ½ c juice
Bread and cereals (whole grain or enriched)[d]	4 or more	½ slice	1 slice	1 to 2 slices

[a]½ c milk = ½ c cottage cheese, pudding, yogurt; ¾ oz cheese; 2 tbsp dried milk.
[b]1 oz meat, fish, poultry = 1 egg, 1 frankfurter, 2 tbsp peanut butter, ½ c legumes.
[c]Vitamin C source (citrus fruits, berries, tomatoes, broccoli, cabbage, cantaloupe) daily; Vitamin A source (spinach, carrots, squash, tomato, cantaloupe) 3 to 4 times weekly.
[d]1 slice bread = ¾ c dry cereal; ½ c cooked cereal; ½ c potato, rice, or noodles.

SOURCE: Adapted from P. M. Queen and R. R. Henry, Growth and nutrient requirements of children, in *Pediatric Nutrition,* eds. R. J. Grand, Jr., L. Sutphen, and W. H. Dietz, Jr. (Boston: Butterworths, 1987), p. 347.

The Four Food Group Plan is tried and true, and its recommendations for children are reflected in Table 13–1.

Careful food selection is essential to ensure that a child receives the right amounts of nutrients. When a child skips breakfast or is allowed to choose sugary foods in place of nourishing ones, it is virtually certain that the child will fail to get enough of several nutrients. The nutrients missed from a skipped breakfast won't be "made up" at lunch and dinner but will be completely left out that day. A child can't be trusted to choose nutritious foods on the basis of taste alone; the preference for sweets is inborn, as Figure 13–1 shows.

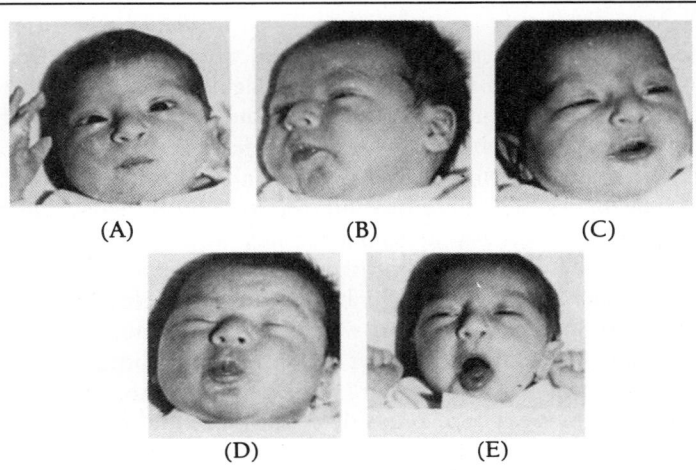

(A)   (B)   (C)

(D)   (E)

■■■ Figure 13–1

The Innate Preference for Sweet Taste. This newborn baby is (A) resting and (B) tasting distilled water, (C) sugar, (D) something sour, and (E) something bitter.

SOURCE: Taste-induced facial expressions of neonate infants from the studies of J. E. Steiner, in *Taste and Development: The Genesis of Sweet Preference,* ed. J. M. Weiffenbach, HHS publication no. NIH 77-1068 (Bethesda, Md.: U.S. Department of Health and Human Services, 1977), pp. 173–189, with permission of the author.

Active, normal-weight children may enjoy occasional treats of high-calorie but nutritious foods—ice cream or pudding from the milk group, whole-grain or enriched cakes and cookies from the bread group—in addition to a balanced diet. These foods are made from milk and grain, they carry valuable nutrients, and they encourage a child to learn, appropriately, that eating is fun. However, should a child eat large quantities of less nourishing treats such as candy or cola, the only possible outcomes are nutrient deficiencies, obesity, or both. Parents of school children should be aware that wandering school children may spend pocket money on candy at a nearby store and fill up on sweets.

While it is important to teach children to avoid obesity, it is also important to use moderation. Children are impressionable and can easily get the idea that their worthiness or lovability is somehow tied to body weight. Some parents fail to realize that society's ideal of slimness can be perilously close to starvation, and that a child encouraged to "diet" cannot obtain the nutrients required for normal growth and development. Even healthy children without diagnosable eating disorders have been observed to dwarf their own growth through "dieting."[2] Weight loss in truly overweight children can be accomplished safely without compromising growth, but should be overseen by a registered dietitian.

It is, however, appropriate to teach children to relax while eating, to pause and enjoy their table companions, and to stop eating when they are full. Parents can assist further by serving small portions of food that can be followed by additional servings, if needed, and by providing healthy snacks such as milk, peanuts, and fruit rather than colas and chips. The next section presents other tips for feeding children.

▌▌▷ *Children's nutrient needs reflect their stage of growth. Parental guidance and encouragement are critical to establishing food patterns that provide adequate nourishment for growth.*

Mealtimes

The childhood years are a parent's last chance to influence food choices. By fostering the development of healthy eating habits, parents help to ensure positive development, not just during growth but for all the years after. Food choices can help prevent obesity and the degenerative diseases of later life.

Children naturally like nutritious foods in all the food groups, with one exception—vegetables, which young children frequently refuse. Here the presentation may be the key. Try to remember how you felt when first offered a cup of vegetable soup, a serving of runny spinach, or a pile of peas and carrots. If the soup burned your tongue, it may have been years before you were willing to try it again. As for the spinach, it was suspiciously murky looking. (Who could tell what might be lurking in that ugly, dark-green liquid?) The peas and carrots troubled your sense of order. Before you could eat them, you felt compelled to sort the peas onto one side of the plate and the carrots onto the other. Then you had to separate, into a reject pile, all those that got mashed in the process or contaminated with gravy from the potatoes. Only then might you be willing to eat the intact, clean peas and carrots one by one—perhaps with your fingers, since the peas, especially, kept rolling off the fork.

Children prefer vegetables that are slightly undercooked and crunchy, bright in color, served separately, and easy to eat. Cooked foods should be served warm, not hot, because a child's mouth is much more sensitive than an adult's. The flavor should be mild (a child has more taste buds), and smooth foods such as mashed potatoes or pea soup should have no lumps in them (a child wonders, with some disgust, what the lumps might be). Children prefer foods that are familiar to them, and fear of unfamiliar foods is practically universal among children. Try introducing small amounts of new foods at the beginning of the meal, when the child is hungry.

When feeding children, parents must always be alert to the dangers of choking. A child may make no clamor or sound when choking, so an adult should always observe children who are eating. Encouraging the child to sit when eating is also a good practice; choking is more likely when a child is running or reclining. Round foods such as grapes, nuts, hard candies, and hot-dog pieces can easily become lodged in the small opening of a child's windpipe. Other potentially dangerous foods include tough meat, popcorn, and snack chips.

Wise parents allow children to help make the family's choices, including the right to say their favorite word: *NO!* (Don't allow them to dominate the family though.) Children can help plan and prepare the family's meals; in that way they are likely to eat the foods they helped choose or prepare.

Little children like to eat at little tables and to be served little portions of food. If a child is offered large portions, chances are excellent that the child will fill up on favorite foods while ignoring less preferred items. In fact, toddlers may go on food jags during which they will eat nothing but one or two favored foods. The best response to food jags lasting a week or so is no response—attention is a valuable reward to the two-year-old. After two weeks of indulging the jag, try serving tiny portions of many foods, including the favored items. Distract the child with friends at meals, and make other foods as attractive as possible.

Remember, too, that parents have likes and dislikes to which they feel entitled; a child who genuinely and consistently rejects a food should be offered the same privilege. The "clean-your-plate" dictum should be stamped out for all time. Children who are forced to override their own satiety signals are essentially in training to develop obesity. Encourage children to stop eating when they are full and to listen to their bodies. Also, do not make an issue of food acceptance. When children are pushed to try new foods, even by way of rewards, they are less likely to try those foods again than children who are left to decide for themselves. The parent is responsible for *what* the child is offered to eat, but the child is responsible for *how much* and even *whether* to eat.[3]

Parents may find that their children often snack so much that they are not very hungry at mealtimes. This need not be a problem as long as children know *how* to snack. Snacks that are as nutritious as the foods served at mealtime become like small meals as far as nutrition is concerned. Even mealtime foods make good snacks when served throughout the day. Easy, readily available snacks are attractive to tired children after a day of school. Keep them simple. Milk, cheese, fruit, yogurt, peanut butter sandwiches, and cereal are all beloved snacks that help meet nutrient needs.

A bright, unhurried atmosphere free of conflict is conducive to good appetite. Parents who serve meals in a relaxed and casual manner, without anxiety, provide the climate in which a child can learn to enjoy eating. Parents who beg, cajole, and demand that their child eat deny the child an opportunity to develop self-control. A power struggle is sure to result. For example, if a child sits down to the table and is confronted with a barrage of accusations—"Susie, your hands are filthy . . . your report card . . . and clean your plate! Your mother cooked that food!"—mealtimes may be unbearable. Her stomach may recoil because her body as well as her mind react to stress of this kind.

Many parents may overlook perhaps the single, most important influence on their child's food habits—themselves. Parents who don't serve and eat carrots shouldn't be surprised when their child refuses to eat carrots. A child learns much through imitation. Parents set an irresistible example by enjoying nutritious foods.

While serving and enjoying food, caretakers can promote not only physical but also emotional growth at every stage of a child's life. It is important for parents to help Joey or Susie to remember that they are good kids. What they *do* may sometimes be unacceptable; but what they *are* on the inside are normal, healthy, growing, fine human beings.

▌▌▶ *Healthy eating habits learned in childhood can help forestall many lifestyle diseases of adulthood. Parents train children in attitudes about food by their actions and by example.*

The Effects of Nutrient Deficiencies on Behavior

A child who suffers from nutrient deficiencies also exhibits physical and behavioral symptoms—the child is sick and out of sorts. The connections between diet and behavior are of keen interest to caretakers who not only feed children but also must live with them.

Other than iron's role in carrying the blood's oxygen, one of iron's main functions is transporting that oxygen within cells, where it works as part of large molecules to release energy. A lack of iron not only causes an energy crisis but also directly affects behavior, mood, attention span, and learning ability. Iron also plays key roles in many molecules of the brain and nervous system. Deficiencies of iron produced experimentally in animals have caused abnormal metabolism of neurotransmitters, notably those that regulate the ability to pay attention, and paying attention is crucial to learning.[4]

Iron deficiency is the most common nutrient deficiency in children and adolescents.[5] Iron deficiency manifests itself in a lowering of the child's ability to pay attention and to learn.[6] Anemic children perform less well on tests and have more conduct disturbances than their classmates.[7] One might label such children "hyperactive," "depressed," or "unlikable," when in fact these traits might arise from any of a number of marginal nutrient deficiencies. In the case of iron deficiency, most studies show improvement of these symptoms with iron supplements.[8]

Malnutrition is often a complex condition involving multiple nutrients and other factors. One such factor is lead poisoning; it can cause iron-deficiency anemia, and iron deficiency impairs the body's defenses against absorption of lead. A child with iron-deficiency anemia is three times as likely to have elevated blood-lead concentrations as a child with normal iron status.[9]

▌▌▶ *Iron deficiency is the most widespread nutrition problem of children and expresses itself in abnormalities of both physical health and behavior.*

The Problem of Lead

In their early years, normal-appearing babies can be silently building up toxic concentrations of lead in their bodies through normal baby activities. Babies like to explore, and they put everything into their mouths, including things that may harm them, such as chips of old paint, pieces of metal, and other unlikely substances. Not until much later, after lead toxicity has set in, do caretakers notice unusual symptoms.

Joey was such a child. This normal-appearing baby grew up in an inner city, where dust from heavily traveled streets settled on his playthings, sprinkling lead from gasoline into his environment. He loved to taste everything—table legs, toys, the spindles of flaky paint railings were all within his reach. Furthermore, his mother had often mixed his morning formula with the first water from the tap, water that had spent the night absorbing lead from the old building's lead pipes.

Joey grew into a cautious, quiet preschooler who clung to stair railings with both hands as he slowly climbed up or down. Joey was late in walking, small for his age, seldom played as vigorously as other children, and was prone to small health disturbances—diarrhea, irritability, and lethargy. While his health quietly deteriorated, his parents shrugged off subtle symptoms as just normal variations in children. They explained away his small size, his clinging to stair railings, his hearing difficulties, and his slowness in learning. Finally, an astute pediatrician concluded that lead toxicity was inflicting its toll on young Joey, and treatment was begun. Except for persistent, minor learning disabilities, Joey is now growing and functioning normally.

For kids like Joey, the truth can easily come too late, since even one year of lead exposure can permanently impair the brain, nervous system, and psychological functioning.[10] Furthermore, recent experiments have shown that the effects occur with lower doses than has been thought in the past.[11] The Public Health Service has singled out lead poisoning as the worst environmental threat to children.[12]

Lead is an indestructible metal, unchangeable by body chemistry. Similar chemically to nutrient minerals like iron, calcium, and zinc, lead displaces these minerals from the body, but then lead is unable to perform their biological functions. Consequently lead interferes with many of the body's systems, particularly the vulnerable tissues of the nervous system, kidney, and bone marrow.[13]

The body absorbs lead greedily during times of rapid growth and hoards it possessively thereafter.[14] During pregnancy, lead invades the developing fetus by crossing the placenta, and once in, lead inflicts severe damage on the fetal nervous system. Infants and young children absorb five to ten times as much lead as do adults. One out of every six children between the ages of six months and five years and one out of every nine fetuses are exposed to threatening levels of lead.[15]

As toddlers, children expand their ranges for exploring, and they still taste and chew everything. Thus the toddler years see a marked rise in blood concentrations of lead.[16] While the neuromuscular system is maturing, high blood concentrations of lead interfere with balance, motor development, and the relay of nerve messages to and from the brain. Children with the highest blood-lead concentrations at ages two and three years suffer the greatest developmental delays at age four.[17] Researchers who wish to study the develop-

allergy: an immune reaction to a foreign substance (such as some components of food). Also called *hypersensitivity* by researchers.

antigen: a substance foreign to the body that elicits the formation of antibodies or an inflammation reaction from immune system cells. Food antigens are usually glycoproteins (large proteins with glucose molecules attached).

antibody: a large protein that is produced in response to an antigen and that inactivates the antigen.

histamine: a substance produced by cells of the immune system as part of a local immune reaction to an antigen; participates in causing inflammation.

food intolerance: an adverse effect from a food or food additive not involving immune response, such as Chinese restaurant syndrome (see Chapter 7).

anaphylactic (an-AFF-ill-LAC-tic) **shock**: a whole-body allergic reaction to an offending substance. Symptoms: abdominal pain, nausea, vomiting, diarrhea, inflamed nasal membranes, chest pain, hives, swelling, low blood pressure.

food aversion: an intense dislike of a food, possibly biological in nature, resulting from an illness or other negative association with that food.

ment of young children must now consider the possibility that lead intoxication may affect their results.[18]

Reductions in the use of leaded gasolines and other products mandated by federal law in recent years have helped to limit the amounts of lead in the environment—and in children's blood. The decline in blood lead concentrations in children during the late 1970s paralleled exactly the decline in the nation's use of leaded gasoline, leaded house paint, and lead-soldered food cans.[19] Even so, many children's blood lead concentrations are still unacceptably high because some lead is still discharged into their environment.* Chapter 15 discusses environmental contaminants such as lead and proposes what must still be done to reduce their impact on human health.

As mentioned earlier, lead competes in the body with iron, calcium, and zinc, and deficiencies of these minerals are common in young children. Just as iron deficiency enhances uptake of lead, an inadequate calcium intake also enhances lead absorption and retention.[20] Prevention of lead toxicity rests primarily on reduced exposure, but parents can protect their children, at least to some degree, by making sure that they receive adequate intakes of calcium and other minerals.[21]

Nutrient deficiencies and even lead toxicity are easy to treat once diagnosed; the trick is in identifying these conditions early, before real damage sets in. Parents and medical practitioners often overlook malnutrition or lead toxicity as causes of odd or unpleasant behavior. Of course, such behavior can be caused by many other problems, but consider the behavior of a well-nourished child: alert, energetic, responsive to external stimuli; in other words, healthy. Sometimes abnormal behavior is the only observable sign of poor nutrition.

▌▶ *Lead poisoning is the worst environmental threat to children. It can inflict severe, irreparable damage on developing systems. Lead levels have declined in recent years but not enough to safeguard children's health.*

Food Allergies

Food **allergy** is frequently blamed for physical and behavioral abnormalities in children. A true food allergy occurs when a whole food protein or other large molecule enters the body tissues. (Recall that most large molecules of food are normally dismantled in the digestive tract to smaller ones before absorption.) The body's immune system reacts to a food protein or other large molecules as it does to an **antigen**—by producing **antibodies**, **histamine**, or other defensive agents. A problem not involving the immune system that results from exposure to food substances is known as a **food intolerance**.

Allergies may have one or two components. They always involve antibodies; they may or may not involve symptoms. A person may produce antibodies *without* having any symptoms or may produce antibodies *and* have symptoms. Symptoms without antibody production are *not* due to allergy. This means that allergies cannot be diagnosed from symptoms alone; they have to be diagnosed by testing for antibodies.

Depending on the location of the allergic reaction in the body, a symptomatic allergy will exhibit different symptoms. In the digestive tract it may cause

Acceptable was defined in 1988 by Centers for Disease Control as 30 micrograms per deciliter of blood.

nausea or vomiting; in the skin it may cause rashes; and in the nasal passages and lungs it can cause inflammation or asthma. A severe, generalized reaction is **anaphylactic shock**.

Allergic reactions to food can occur with different timings; the appearance of symptoms may come within minutes or after several (up to 24) hours. Identifying a food that causes an immediate allergic reaction is easy because symptoms correlate closely with the time of eating the food. If the reaction is delayed, though, identifying the offending food is more difficult because the symptoms may not appear until a day or more has passed; and by that time many other foods will have been eaten too.

The foods that most often cause allergic reactions are listed in Table 13–2. According to one investigator, 91 percent of adverse reactions are caused by only four major foods—nuts (43 percent), eggs (21 percent), milk (18 percent), and soy (9 percent).[22] Many people are allergic to just one food, but some are allergic to many.

A number of tests and food challenges are required to identify a true food allergy. However, the tests are time consuming and expensive, and so people, and even physicians, sometimes try to guess the cause of an adverse reaction to foods and use the term *food allergy* loosely. A parent whose child has any kind of discomfort after eating—stomachache, headache, pain, rapid pulse rate, nausea, wheezing, hives, bronchial irritation, cough, or any other—may decide that an allergy is responsible, when in fact the cause is something else entirely. These reactions should be called *hypersensitivity reactions* or *adverse reactions*, not *allergies*. Only careful, skilled testing by a physician can distinguish the many possibilities, and such testing is seldom done.

Because reliable food allergy tests are inconvenient and expensive, people are tempted to believe quacks bearing sophisticated-sounding, but quick and easy laboratory work. For example, "cytotoxic testing" involves mixing blood with foods to see what blood cells "react" to. As you might guess, this test is invalid for detecting allergy because isolated blood cells are cut off from the body's immune system, which produces the allergic response. Other terms relating to allergy quackery are *brain allergy*, *metabolic rejectivity syndrome*, and the term *ecology* when applied to body functions.

A **food aversion**, an intense dislike of a food, may be a biological response to a food that once caused trouble. Children's food aversions may be the result of nature's efforts to protect them from allergic or other adverse reactions. Parents are advised to watch for signs of food dislikes and to take them seriously. Such a dislike may turn out to be a whim or fancy, but it should be respected. Although many cases of suspected allergies turn out to be something else, real allergies do exist, as do other valid reasons to avoid certain foods. Don't prejudge, in any case. Test. Then if a food is excluded from the diet, find other foods to provide the omitted nutrients to ensure the child's continued good nutrition.

Allergies are often blamed when behavior problems arise. While a child who is sick from any cause is likely to be cranky, evidence does not support the hypothesis that allergy can cause misbehavior without other symptoms. However, hyperactivity often expresses itself accurately as misbehavior.

▶ *Food allergies cause illness, but diagnosis is difficult. To determine whether allergy exists, tests are imperative. Food aversions can be related to food allergies or to adverse reactions to foods.*

■■■ **Table 13–2 Foods That Most Often Cause Allergies**

Nuts	Peanuts
Eggs	Chicken
Milk	Fish
Soybeans	Shellfish
Wheat	Mollusks

SOURCE: Information from F. M. Atkins, The basis of immediate hypersensitivity reactions to foods, *Nutrition Reviews* 41 (1983): 229–234.

hyperactivity in children: a syndrome characterized by inattention, impulsivity, and high levels of motor activity. Usually occurs before age seven, lasts six months or more, and does not entail mental illness or mental retardation. Also called *attention deficit disorder* or *hyperkinesis* and may be associated with minimal brain damage.

learning disability: an altered ability to learn basic cognitive skills such as reading, writing, and mathematics.

tension-fatigue syndrome: transient hyperactivity produced in a child by the combination of lack of sleep and overstimulation with anxiety.

dental caries: decay of the teeth (*caries* means "rottenness").

Hyperactivity and Diet

In searching for explanations for a child's misbehavior, many people have looked to the kitchen. One such attempt is to blame food for **hyperactivity**. Hyperactivity, one kind of **learning disability**, occurs in 5 to 10 percent of young, school-aged children, that is, in 2 or 3 in every classroom of 30 children.[23] It can lead to academic failure and major behavioral problems. Parents and teachers need to deal effectively with it wherever it appears to avert the grief that can otherwise result.

Physicians often diagnose hyperactivity by conducting a trial with stimulant drugs. Stimulants normally speed up people's activity, but they have a paradoxical effect in children with hyperactivity—the drugs calm them. (Perhaps they stimulate centers in the brain that control behavior.) If a child responds to stimulant drugs by calming down, that indicates that the drugs may be correcting a biochemical imbalance in the nervous system and can be used to help control the behavior. *In children who are responsive,* prescription medication should at least be considered as the treatment of choice.

Many parents, resistant to the idea of drugs for children, hope that altering children's diets might affect their behavior. While optimal nutrition is critical to mental and physical health, appealing-sounding but unfounded dietary "treatments" may only serve to delay effective medical help for a child who sorely needs it.

The dietary approach to hyperactivity, when it occasionally seems to work, probably does so by way of psychology. A child who "learns" that hyperactive behavior is caused by food and that now the family is going to eat differently may believe the problem is thus eliminated. This can bring about a cure by way of the placebo effect mentioned in Chapter 7. The child's needs for love and attention may now be filled with family activities centering around preparing and eating meals, eliminating the child's need to act up for attention. It is not the nature of the diet that works but the changed lifestyle that the diet demands.

Food allergies have been blamed for hyperactivity. Research to date does not support the idea that allergy and behavior are linked, but studies continue.[24] There is nothing to suggest that food allergies or intolerances cause hyperactivity in children.

One proven link between food and behavior is the effect of caffeine on the nervous system. Excess caffeine can overstimulate children. A 12-ounce cola beverage may contain as much as 50 milligrams caffeine; two or more such beverages are equivalent in the body of a 60-pound child to the caffeine in 8 cups of coffee for a 175-pound man. Chocolate bars also contribute caffeine. Children can be troubled by sleeplessness, restlessness, irregular heartbeats, and general misery due to excess caffeine consumption. A survey of over 1000 children between the ages of 1 and 17 years found that 77 percent consumed caffeine.[25] (Controversy 12 presented a table of caffeine amounts in certain products.) Children cannot be expected to resist tempting colas and candy bars—it is the task of concerned adults to limit their access to such foods. Eventually children develop self-control, but it will be patterned on limits they encountered while young.

Without any magical answers, parents still have to deal with excitable, rambunctious, and unruly children. Common sense says that all children at times get wild and "hyper." There are many normal, everyday causes of such behavior:

■ Desire for attention.
■ Lack of sleep.
■ Overstimulation.
■ Too much television.
■ Lack of exercise.

Together these produce the **tension-fatigue syndrome**, which can be relieved by giving more consistent care to the child's welfare. It helps especially to insist on regular hours of sleep, regular mealtimes, and regular outdoor exercise.

❚❚▶ *Hyperactivity is not caused by poor nutrition but may reflect genetics, poor management of the child, or other causes. A wise parent will limit children's caffeine intakes and meet their needs for structure to prevent tension-fatigue syndrome.*

The Effects of Television

In addition to its contribution to tension-fatigue syndrome, television has other adverse effects on children. On the average, children in the United States spend as much time watching television as they do attending school. Watching television affects children's nutritional health adversely in several ways. First, television viewing requires no energy beyond the resting metabolic rate. Second, it contributes to physical inactivity and replaces time spent in more vigorous activities. Third, watching television correlates with between-meal snacking and with buying and eating the calorically dense foods most heavily advertised on children's programs. The more television children view, the more likely they are to become obese. In fact, the prevalence of obesity increases by 2 percent for each hour of television viewed.[26] Also, children who watch more than two hours a day of television may have higher serum cholesterol levels than do more active children.

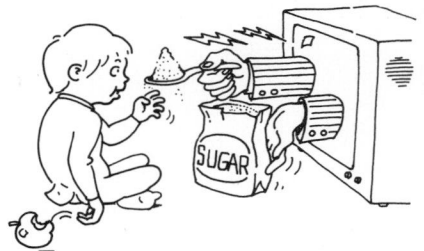

Children love sweets, and they trust the ads they see on television.

Children who watch hours of television a day are also prone to frequent snacking on high-sugar foods, a major factor in **dental caries** development. Sticky, sugary snack foods stay on the teeth and provide an ideal environment for the growth of mouth bacteria that cause caries. What child can resist the delicious-looking, fun foods, full of sugar, that dance across their television screens? Television commercials aimed at children are intended only to promote purchase and consumption of sugary foods—they have no stake in promoting dental health. Parents must combat this influence by teaching children to do the following:

■ Restrict sweets to mealtimes, when they are less likely to cause caries.
■ Brush and floss daily, and brush or rinse after eating snacks.
■ Choose foods that are swallowed quickly, not those that stick to teeth.
■ Eat a variety of crisp or fibrous foods to stimulate the rinsing action of the salivary glands.

The foods listed in Table 13–3 promote dental health and are excellent choices for nutrients too.

❚❚▶ *Television advertising of sugary foods promotes sugar consumption and tooth decay and can contribute to obesity through lack of exercise and overconsumption of snacks.*

■■■ Table 13–3 Dietary Recommendations for Controlling
Dental Caries

FOOD GROUP	FREQUENT USE RECOMMENDED	INFREQUENT USE SUGGESTED[a]
Dairy	Milk, cheese, plain yogurt	Chocolate milk, ice cream, ice milk, milk shakes, fruited yogurt
Meat/meat alternates	Lean meat, fish, poultry; eggs; legumes	Peanut butter with added sugar, lunch meats with added sugar, meats with sugared glazes
Fruits	Fresh or packed in water	Dried, packed in syrup or juice, jams, jellies, preserves, fruit juices or drinks
Vegetables	Salad greens, cauliflower, cucumbers, radishes, carrots, celery	Candied sweet potatoes, glazed carrots
Bread/cereal	Popcorn, soda crackers, toast, hard rolls, pretzels, corn chips, pizza	Cookies, sweet rolls, pies, cakes, potato chips, ready-to-eat sweetened cereals as between-meal snacks
Other	Sugarless gum, coffee or tea without sugar	Sugared soft drinks, candy, fudge, caramels, honey, sugars, syrups

[a]It is particularly important to practice good oral hygiene after eating those foods.

SOURCE: For all but potato chips, S. R. Rolfes and E. N. Whitney, *Say Cheese and Smile: The Nutrition and Oral Health Picture,* a monograph (1988) available from Stickley Publishing Co., 210 Washington Sq., Philadelphia, PA 19106; for potato chips, W. Bowen and coauthors, A method to assess cariogenic potential of foodstuffs, *Journal of the American Dietetic Association* 100 (1980): 677–681.

The Importance of Breakfast

Children who eat no breakfast perform poorly in tasks of concentration, their attention spans are shorter, and they even show lower IQs on testing than their well-fed peers.[27] Common sense tells us that it is unreasonable to expect anyone to learn and to perform work when no fuel has been provided. By the late morning, discomfort from hunger may become distracting even if a child has eaten breakfast.

The disadvantage faced by children who attempt morning schoolwork on an empty stomach appears to be at least partly due to hypoglycemia. The average child up to the age of ten or so needs to eat every four to six hours to maintain a blood glucose concentration high enough to support the activity of the brain and nervous system. A child's brain is as big as an adult's, and the brain is the body's chief glucose consumer. A child's liver is considerably smaller, and the liver is the organ responsible for storing glucose (as glycogen) and for releasing it into the blood as needed. The liver can't store more than about four hours' worth of glycogen; hence the need to eat fairly often. Teachers aware of the late-morning slump in their classrooms wisely request that a midmorning snack be provided; it improves classroom performance all the way to lunch time. But for the child who hasn't had breakfast, the morning may be lost altogether.

❚❚▷ *Breakfast is critical to children's school performance.*

Nutrition at School

While parents are doing what they can to establish favorable eating behaviors for children, other factors begin to enter the picture. During preschool or grade school, the child encounters foods prepared and served by outsiders. The U.S. government funds several programs to provide nutritious, high-quality meals to children at school. (School lunches in Canada are administered locally and therefore vary from area to area.) School lunches are designed to meet certain requirements. They must include specified servings of milk, protein-rich foods (meat, poultry, fish, cheese, eggs, legumes, or peanut butter), vegetables, fruits, and breads or other grain foods. The design is intended to provide at least a third of the RDA for each of the nutrients. Table 13–4 shows school lunch patterns for different ages. Many schools also serve breakfast for early-arriving children.

Parents rely on school lunches to meet a significant part of their children's nutrient needs on school days. Indeed, students who participate in the school lunch program have higher intakes of energy and nutrients than students who do not. Children don't always like what they are served, and school lunch programs attempt to feed them both what they want and what will nourish them. In response to children's differing needs and tastes, the program operates best as follows:

❚ To offer a variety of selections and to allow children to choose what they are served.

❚ To vary portion sizes so that little children may take little servings, thus reducing waste.

■■■ Table 13–4 School Lunch Patterns for Different Ages

FOOD GROUP	PRESCHOOL (AGE)		GRADE SCHOOL THROUGH HIGH SCHOOL (GRADE)		
	1 TO 2	3 TO 4	K TO 3	4 TO 6	7 TO 12
Meat or Meat Alternate 1 serving:					
Lean meat, poultry, or fish	1 oz	1½ oz	1½ oz	2 oz	3 oz
Cheese	1 oz	1½ oz	1½ oz	2 oz	3 oz
Large egg(s)	1	1½	1½	2	3
Cooked dry beans or peas	½ c	¾ c	¾ c	1 c	1½ c
Peanut butter	2 tbsp	3 tbsp	3 tbsp	4 tbsp	6 tbsp
Vegetable and/or Fruit 2 or more servings, both to total	½ c	½ c	½ c	¾ c	¾ c
Bread or Bread Alternate Servings[a]	5 per week	8 per week	8 per week	8 per week	10 per week
Milk 1 serving of fluid milk	¾ c	¾ c	1 c	1 c	1 c

[a]A serving is 1 slice of whole-grain or enriched bread; a whole-grain or enriched biscuit, roll, muffin, and so on; or ½ c cooked pasta or other cereal grain such as bulgur or grits.

SOURCE: School lunch patterns: Ready, set, go! *School Food Service Journal,* August 1980, p. 31.

■ To involve students (in secondary schools) in the planning of menus.
■ To schedule lunches so that children can eat when they are hungry and can have enough time to eat well.

In keeping with the National Research Council (NRC) recommendations to reduce dietary fat, some schools offer low-fat (chocolate or white) or nonfat milk as alternatives to whole milk. Many schools mimic fast-food cuisines, with salad bars, potato bars, and taco bars. This gives kids an opportunity to practice selecting from nutritious foods to create the meals *they* want to eat.

Some children purchase snacks from vending machines. The American Dental Association (ADA) would like to eliminate the sale of confections as snacks in schools but so far has met with little success. Most progress has been made by way of individual, voluntary initiatives. Experiments have shown that children will choose nutritious snacks over sugary confections if the two are offered side by side. When apples are made available in vending machines, children choose chocolate bars less often. When milk is made available, soft drink use drops considerably. Coincident with the school lunch program is a program of nutrition education and training (NET program) in all public schools. This program is minimally funded, but program administrators are ingenious and creative in accomplishing its highest priority objectives. Children need not only to be fed well but to learn enough about nutrition to become able to make healthy food choices when the choices become theirs to make.

❚❚▶ *School lunches are designed to meet the needs of growing children. Schools also have the responsibility of offering nutrition education.*

❚❚❚ The Teen Years

Teenagers are not fed; they eat. Few become interested in nutrition, except as crash diets to lose weight or as supplement fads to enhance physique. Still, nutrition affects their health for good or for ill, and teenagers need to develop food habits to support health through adulthood.

Growth and Nutrient Needs of Teenagers

With the onset of adolescence, children embark upon an intensive growth spurt. The growth spurt begins at the age of 10 or 11 years in girls and reaches its peak at about 12 years. A boy's growth spurt begins at 12 or 13 years and peaks at about 14 years, ending at about 19 years. All the nutrients needed to support growth are needed in large quantities, and the need for iron is especially great to support menstruation in girls and to develop lean body mass in boys. As they grow to adults, girls develop a somewhat higher percentage of body fat than do boys. In fact, nutrient needs in adolescence are greater than at any other stage of life, except in women during pregnancy and lactation. This intensive growth period brings hormonal changes that profoundly affect every organ of the body (including the brain).

Teenagers' rates and patterns of growth vary tremendously. Growth charts used for children mean less during adolescence. Two boys of the same age may vary in height by a foot, but if both have been growing steadily, each is fulfilling his genetic destiny according to an inborn schedule of events. Worried parents should watch only for reasonably smooth progress. To apply external standards that a child cannot "live up to" is to invite a diminished self-image, since these are years of development of one's identity that will last a lifetime. The only way to be sure a teenager is growing normally is to compare his or her height and weight with previous measures taken at intervals. If reasonably smooth progress is being made, be assured and reassure the teenager that all is well.

There is also tremendous variation in the energy needs of adolescents. An active, rapidly growing boy of 15 may need 4000 calories or more a day just to maintain his weight. An inactive girl of the same age, however, whose growth is nearly at a standstill may need fewer than 2000 calories if she is to avoid becoming obese. Teen athletes are especially in need of energy and nutrients, and the nutrition advice to athletes in Chapter 10 is especially important for them.

Teenagers are notorious for eating large quantities of foods, and many are well nourished. However, some have nutritional problems. One study of adolescent nutrient intake found that boys met the RDA for all nutrients except iron. The girls in this study failed to meet the RDA for iron, calcium, and vitamin A.[28] Other studies have reported dietary inadequacies of vitamin B_6, zinc, folate, iodine, vitamin D, and magnesium prevalent among adolescent girls.[29] The more food a teenager eats, the greater the likelihood that the teen will be well nourished, especially if foods chosen are of high nutrient density.

The insidious problem of obesity may first become apparent in adolescence, mostly in girls, especially black girls, and may last a lifetime.

⫿▶ *The nutrient needs of teens can be enormous, especially for energy to support growth. Surveys show that few teens meet their RDA for nutrients.*

> **gatekeeper:** with respect to nutrition, a key person who controls other people's access to foods and thereby has a profound impact on their nutrition; examples are the spouse who buys and cooks the food, the parent who feeds the children, and the caretaker in a day-care center.

Eating Patterns and Food Choices

Teenagers come and go as they choose and eat what they want when they have time. With a multitude of after-school, social, and job activities, they almost inevitably fall into irregular eating habits. The adult becomes a **gatekeeper**, controlling the availability but not the consumption of food in the teenager's environment. Teens typically turn a deaf ear to adults' attempts at coercion or persuasion to eat particular foods. The wise gatekeeper will provide access to nutritious foods that are low in sugar and fat and will welcome their teenaged sons and daughters and their friends into the kitchen with the invitation, "Help yourselves! There's plenty of food in the refrigerator" (meats for sandwiches, raw vegetables, milk, fruit juices) "and more on the table" (fruits, nuts, popcorn, cereals).

On the average, about a fourth of a teenager's total daily energy intake comes from snacks. This is one way that teens with irregular schedules can receive substantial amounts of protein, thiamin, riboflavin, vitamin B_6, magnesium, and zinc. Their calcium intakes may fall short unless they snack on dairy products, and they often fail to obtain enough iron and vitamin A. For iron, a teen might snack on hard-boiled eggs, bran muffins, or peanut butter and crackers. For vitamin A, why not carrot sticks, or cheese, tomato juice, cantaloupe, or some dried apricots?

Inevitably teenagers do a lot of eating away from home. A fast-food lunch of a hamburger, a chocolate shake, and french fries supplies nutrients in the amounts shown in Table 13–5 at a calorie cost of 820. For the most part these

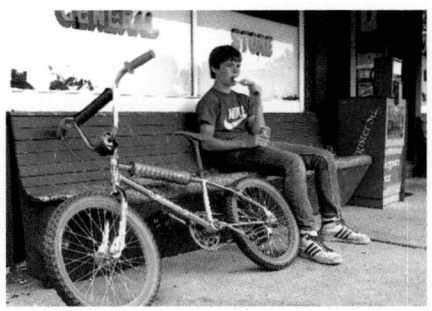

Teenagers often grab snacks on the run.

■■■ Table 13–5 Selected
Nutrients in a Hamburger,
Chocolate Shake, and Fries
(Percentage of RDA)

NUTRIENT	MALE[a]	FEMALE[a]
Energy	27	37
Protein	41	55
Calcium	32	32
Iron	30	24
Zinc	23	28
Vitamin A	8	10
Thiamin	34	47
Riboflavin	53	73
Niacin	32	43
Folate	23	26
Vitamin C	16	16

[a]RDA for an 18-year-old, moderately active,
person of average height and weight.

The nutritive value of selected fast foods is
presented in Appendix A.

are substantial percentages of recommended intakes at an energy cost some teenagers can afford. Depending on how they adjust their breakfast and dinner choices, lean, active teenagers may meet their nutrient needs more than adequately with this sort of lunch. They need only select fruits and vegetables (for vitamins A and C), good fiber sources, and more good iron and zinc sources at their other meals. For those who tend to gain weight, such a meal is ill advised.

Calcium is sometimes a problem nutrient for teenagers. The requirement for calcium reaches its peak during these years. Unfortunately many teens reject milk as a "child's drink" and opt instead for soft drinks with their lunches, dinners, and snacks. As might be expected, the more soft drinks teenagers drink, the less likely they are to meet their RDA for calcium.[30]

Teenagers are intensely involved in day-to-day life with their peers and in preparation for their future lives as adults. Adults need to remember that teenagers have the right to make their own decisions—even if they are in opposition to the adults' own views. The gatekeeper can set up the environment so that nutritious foods are available and can stand by with reliable nutrition information and advice, but the rest is up to the teens themselves. Ultimately they make the choices.

❚❚▶ *With planning, the gatekeeper can encourage teens to meet nutrient requirements by providing nutritious snacks.*

Acne

No one knows why some people get **acne** while others do not, but heredity plays a role—acne runs in families. The hormones of adolescence also play a role by stimulating the glands in the skin. The skin's natural oil is made in deep glands and is supposed to flow out through tiny ducts to the skin's surface. In acne, the ducts become clogged, and oily secretions cannot escape; they build up under the surface of the skin.

One medical treatment for acne is to apply a vitamin A relative—retinoic acid—directly to the skin. This loosens the plugs that form in the ducts, allowing the oil to flow normally. But care is necessary because the acid may burn the skin and cause pimples to form, making the acne look worse at first. Another prescription treatment—antibiotic ointment—works well in many has caused and doesn't burn the skin. The oral prescription medicine Accutane is synthesized from vitamin A but is much more powerful than the vitamin itself, and it is effective against the deep lesions of cystic acne. Accutane is highly toxic and has caused serious birth defects in the infants of women who have taken it during their pregnancies. Women with acne who wish to use Accutane are well advised to use an effective form of contraception before beginning treatment and for a time after treatment has ceased.

While it is true that medicines made from vitamin A are successful in treating acne, vitamin A itself has no effect, and supplements of the vitamin can be toxic. Quacks remain undaunted by these facts, though, and market vitamin A supplements to people hoping to cure acne. Enough vitamin A is essential for healthy skin; too much can damage the body.

Among foods charged with aggravating acne are chocolate, cola beverages, fatty or greasy foods, milk, nuts, sugar, and foods or salt containing iodine. None of these foods has been shown to worsen acne, and two have been shown not to worsen it—chocolate and sugar. Stress, though, clearly worsens acne.

Vacations from school often bring acne relief. Sun and swimming also help, perhaps because they are relaxing and also because the sun's rays kill bacteria and water cleanses the skin.

One remedy always works: time. While waiting, attend to basic needs. Petal-smooth, healthy skin reflects a tended, cared-for body whose owner provides it with nutrients and fluids to sustain it, exercise to stimulate it, and rest to restore its cells.

❚❚▷ *While foods are not proven to aggravate acne, stress can worsen it. Supplements are useless against acne, but sunlight and proved medications can help.*

acne: a chronic inflammation of the skin's follicles and oil-producing glands, which leads to an accumulation of oils inside the ducts that surround hairs, usually associated with the maturation of young adults.

premenstrual syndrome (PMS): a cluster of symptoms, including both physical and emotional pain, that some women experience prior to and during menstruation.

Nutrition and the Menstrual Cycle

One of the many changes girls face as they become women is the onset of menstruation. The hormones that regulate the menstrual cycle are powerful, and they affect more than just the uterus and the ovaries. They alter the metabolic rate, glucose tolerance, appetite, food intake, mood, and behavior. Most women live easily with the cyclic rhythm of the menstrual cycle, but some are afflicted with physical and emotional pain prior to menstruation, a condition given the name **premenstrual syndrome**, or **PMS**.

All menstruating women can benefit from some recent findings on nutrition and the menstrual cycle. Many women just plain get hungry during the week or two before menstruation. Reliable research shows that two things happen during that time:

◻ Basal metabolic rate speeds up.[31]
◻ Appetite and calorie intake pick up.[32]

About 20 percent of the women in two studies indicated, when asked, that their appetites increased before menstruation.[33] But, in fact, most or all women may actually eat more during this time without being aware that they do. They report that they crave sweets, and when their food intakes are actually measured, they are seen to be eating an average of 500 calories a day more during the ten days prior to menstruation than during the ten days after—principally from carbohydrate.[34]

At least one application of these findings seems obvious at first glance. Many women attempt to restrict their calories, sometimes severely, in the effort to control their weight. During the two weeks following menstruation, they may find this relatively easy to do, but during the two weeks before the next menstruation, they may find it hard because they are fighting a natural, hormone-governed increase in metabolic rate, appetite, and possibly even a built-in craving for carbohydrate.

For women who suffer from physical pain before and during the menstrual period, it is important to know that it can have a wide variety of causes, some of which should clearly *not* be labeled PMS. Inflammation or infection of the lining of the uterus, a potentially dangerous condition, can cause symptoms like those ascribed to PMS; but a diagnosis and treatment are imperative. Muscular abnormalities of the uterus and its opening (the cervix) can cause cramping during menstruation; again, treatment depends on diagnosis. Once these causes are ruled out, cases remain that are, at least for the present, grouped together as PMS.

prostaglandins: hormonelike
compounds (eicosanoids) related to
and derived from polyunsaturated fatty
acids (*prostagland* because the first
such compound discovered was from
the prostate gland).

A woman suffering from PMS may complain of any or all of the following symptoms: cramps and aches in the abdomen, back pain, headaches, acne, swelling of face and limbs associated with water retention, food cravings (especially for sweets), abnormal thirst, pain and lumps in the breasts, diarrhea, and mood changes, including both nervousness and depression. Some researchers are attempting to define clusters of these symptoms in hopes of assigning each cluster to a different cause.

Among the candidates for causes of PMS are abnormal secretion of **prostaglandins** and altered secretion of the two major regulatory hormones associated with the menstrual cycle, estrogens and progesterone. Other possibilities include an abnormality of the muscle tissue, emotional illness, or lack of exercise. Many sedentary women find that taking up regular exercise greatly reduces menstrual discomfort, and for some a brisk walk can relieve the symptoms completely.

Medical therapies can be useful in some cases of PMS.[35] For example, the aspirin-derivative drug ibuprofen works by reducing prostaglandin action and is alone effective against the symptoms of PMS in many cases.† Prescriptions of hormones seem to help in some cases. Muscle relaxants relieve cramps. Physicians sometimes prescribe tranquilizers such as Valium (diazepam) to relax muscles. These seem to work, but they may do so by putting the woman out of touch with the problem rather than solving it; they also can cause a dangerous dependency.

Do emotional problems contribute to PMS? Researchers believe that at least some PMS may be psychological in origin, but it is hard to tell. After all, people are suggestible, and PMS is something of a fad. When women are expecting their periods, they may have learned to expect PMS. As for nutrition-related causes, this chapter devotes a box ("Nutrition and Premenstrual Syndrome") to them because they often lead people to consider taking supplements.

†Ibuprofen is sold under the names Advil, Motrin, Nuprin, and Rufen.

CONSUMER CAUTION ▌▌▌ **Nutrition and Premenstrual Syndrome**

Among possible nutrition-related causes of PMS, one is sodium and water retention caused by the hormones that dominate the premenstrual weeks. Some doctors prescribe diuretics to get rid of the excess sodium and water, and some researchers have reported that diuretics relieve all PMS symptoms except painful breasts; others, though, have tried to confirm this finding and have failed. The placebo effect is extraordinarily powerful in PMS, so much so that even an agent that appears to relieve PMS symptoms for several months may not in the long run prove to be a cure.[36] Diuretic therapy has been criticized on the basis that it may cause losses of needed minerals such as potassium or magnesium, possibly making PMS symptoms worse. Also, if women *do* retain sodium and water just before menstruation, it may be a normal and desirable state.

Another nutrient that may have some connection with PMS is magnesium. When magnesium status was studied in "normal" and PMS subjects, the

continued on next page

levels of this mineral in the red blood cells were found to be lower in the PMS group.[37] The naive reader might jump to the conclusion that people with PMS need more magnesium, but this may not be the case at all. The subjects' diets weren't studied, so it is impossible to tell whether they had a dietary deficiency, were absorbing less, or were excreting more magnesium. In fact, it is possible that the women's total-body contents of magnesium hadn't changed but that there had been a shift of magnesium from the red blood cells into some other body compartment. Red blood cells, like all cells, "decide" what their contents should be; that is, they actively take in or reject available substances in response to signals from elsewhere—hormones, for example. The PMS group might have too much or too little of some other substance, and this difference might cause their red blood cells to take up less magnesium. Clearly, on the basis of the one finding, it is impossible to say whether people with PMS need more magnesium or less or more or less of something else.

In these studies the researchers measured inside-the-body indicators of nutrition status in PMS sufferers versus those in other women. Other research has involved simply trying different agents and asking the women by questionnaire how they felt in response. One nutrient researched in this fashion has been vitamin B_6.

The logic of ascribing PMS to a vitamin B_6 deficiency is that women with PMS may have abnormal levels of hormones that regulate the menstrual cycle—hormones that require vitamin B_6 for their action. One of the symptoms of PMS is depression, a disorder of mood that many people, both male and female, experience under a wide variety of conditions and in many different physical and mental disorders. Vitamin B_6 deficiency has been implicated as one of many possible causes of depression too. [38]

Trials of vitamin B_6 in PMS have produced mixed results at best. Typical is one study in which the researchers attempted to use vitamin B_6 to relieve premenstrual depression and found a dramatic positive response in only 1 of 13 women and a slight positive response in 4—balanced by a positive response in 5 women on placebo medication, no response in 2, and a strong *negative* response in 1![39]

We might conclude from this that vitamin B_6 is not effective in PMS, but it is also possible to conclude that it may occasionally be just what is needed—witness the one woman who did respond positively. Confirming this, another pair of researchers tested a particular woman who claimed to be responsive to vitamin B_6. They gave her the vitamin (50 milligrams/day) and a placebo in alternate months for six months without telling her and also without knowing, themselves, which was which until the end of the study (a double-blind experiment). She experienced relief from her symptoms consistently with the vitamin and not with the placebo, showing clearly that in her case PMS was related to vitamin B_6.[40] It is possible that "the cause" of PMS is not the same in all women. For some women a relative or absolute vitamin B_6 deficiency may aggravate or even cause PMS, whereas for others it might have no relation to the syndrome. Note that the effective dose mentioned above was 50 milligrams a day. No need exists for megadoses of

continued on next page

vitamin B$_6$, and the hazards associated with such doses are well documented (p. 213).

Vitamin E deficiency is another candidate for contributor to PMS, and one creditable attempt has demonstrated that vitamin E has some effectiveness in relieving one symptom often experienced in PMS—sore breasts. One research study, a double-blind, placebo-controlled study of 75 women, suggested that vitamin E (300 IU) brought relief, while the placebo did not.[41] However, some women *without* PMS also have sore breasts that can sometimes be relieved by vitamin E.[42] Possibly the correct logic is that vitamin E deficiency can cause sore breasts and the menstrual cycle can make them worse but not that vitamin E deficiency causes PMS.

One recent study pointed to tea consumption as strongly related to PMS.[43] Women who drank the most tea seemed to have the worst symptoms. Which component of tea, the caffeine, the pigments, or other substances, might be responsible for the finding has yet to be studied.

Before we can really know what to recommend to women who suffer with PMS, several kinds of studies are needed. One type of study will have to answer the question, "How do the diets of women with PMS differ from those of women unaffected by PMS?" One report suggests that women with PMS eat more refined sugar and salt and less of several nutrients than other women—in other words, that they tend to choose foods of lower nutrient density and have lower intakes of B vitamins, iron, and zinc as a consequence.[44] However, the study may be biased because its chief author is employed by a company that sells nutrient supplements. An opposing study found no evidence that PMS was caused by nutrient deficiencies.[45] Without several more such studies carefully performed by a variety of independent investigators, we cannot really know what the typical nutrition status of PMS women is. It seems far too early for any woman who thinks she suffers from PMS to leap to the conclusion that she needs a particular supplement. She had better see a competent health care provider and find out what the real possibilities are.

One thing seems clear: the woman with PMS should look to her total lifestyle, diet being only part of it. She may not have complete control over her condition, but many aspects of her lifestyle *are* under her control. If she has any nutrient deficiencies, then she isn't doing all she can to help herself be well. She should also be sure to get adequate sleep. Physical activity helps too; she should exercise regularly. She should be sensible about her intakes of sugar, caffeine, salt, alcohol, and any other abusable substances. She should watch out for snake-oil salespeople selling PMS "cures"—there are a lot of them out there.

Only one other nutrition problem teens face will be discussed here: teen pregnancy. But another set of problems affecting nutrition may crop up during the teen years, for they are a critical time in the development of problem behaviors such as drug use. Three of every five high school seniors report that they have at least tried an illicit drug, most commonly marijuana.[46] Controversy 11 discussed the nutrition effects of alcohol, and Controversy 12 described those related to other drug use, including that of tobacco.

▌▌▶ *The menstrual cycle affects women's metabolism and appetites in a cyclic fashion. Some women have the uncomfortable symptoms associated with the cycle—so-called premenstrual syndrome (PMS), which is probably a diverse set of conditions with no single cause. A sound diet without extremes is part of the recommended lifestyle to minimize PMS.*

Teenage Pregnancy

Teenaged pregnancy presents a special case of nutrient needs. Each year one out of every ten teenaged girls becomes pregnant; of these one million, about half give birth. Even when not pregnant, a teenaged girl is hard put to meet her own nutrient needs, but when pregnant, a teenaged girl is likely to be deficient in many vitamins and minerals, including vitamins A and C, niacin, iron, and chromium. Figure 13–2 compares nutrient requirements of a pregnant 15-year-old with those of a nonpregnant teen. Nourishing a growing fetus adds to her burden. Her own high nutrient requirements can compete with those of her fetus, especially if she is going through her most rapid growth phase. To support the needs of both mother and fetus, young teenagers (13 to 16 years old) are encouraged to gain approximately 35 pounds during pregnancy. Young teenagers who gain less, even if they gain the 24 to 27 pounds recommended

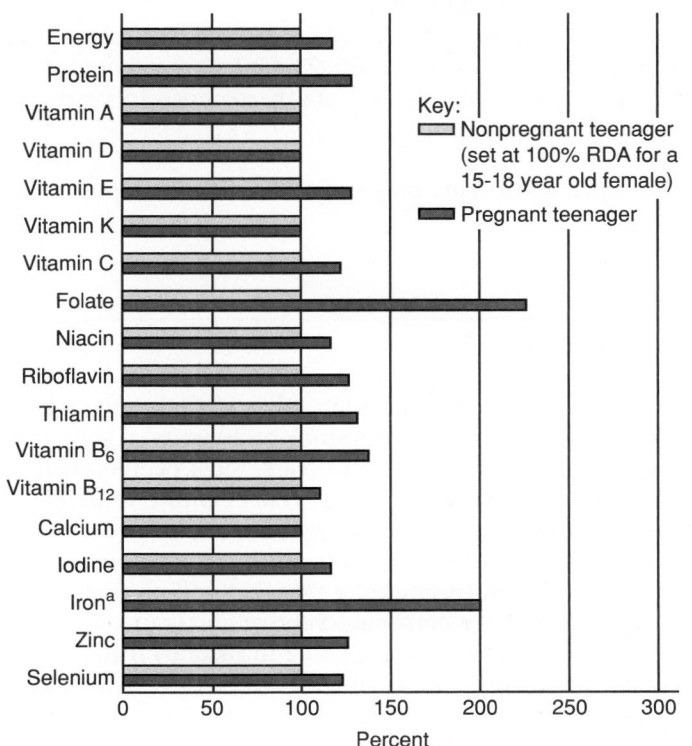

▌▌▌ Figure 13–2

Comparison of the Nutrient Needs of a Nonpregnant Teenager with Those of a Pregnant Teenager. These values derive from adding the increment of recommended nutrients for the pregnant adult woman to the RDA for females 15 to 18 years of age.

[a]The pregnant teenager may need to take an iron supplement.

■■■ Table 13–6 Four Food Group Plan for Pregnant and Lactating Teenagers[a]

	NUMBER OF SERVINGS	
	---	---
FOOD GROUP	TEENAGERS	PREGNANT OR LACTATING TEENAGERS
Meat and meat alternates	2	3
Milk and milk products	4	5
Vegetables and fruits	4	4
Breads and cereals	4	4

[a]See Figure 2–4 in Chapter 2 for a more detailed summary of serving sizes and food sources.

for older pregnant women, have smaller newborns. As discussed in Chapter 12, small newborns have a high risk of disease and death.

Little information is available on the specific nutrient needs of pregnant adolescents. Estimates of their nutrient needs are usually made by adding the increments of recommended nutrients for the pregnant adult woman to the RDA for nonpregnant girls 15 to 18 years of age. A pregnant teenager's needs for many nutrients double, although her energy allowance increases by only a few percent. If a young woman starts pregnancy already malnourished or lacks education, resources, and support, she may encounter serious medical problems. Table 13–6 provides a daily food guide for pregnant and lactating teenagers based on the Four Food Group Plan.

Complications are common in pregnant teenagers. The greatest risk of a teenage pregnancy is death of the infant. The infant mortality rate for mothers under the age of 20 years is high, with mothers under 15 years of age having the highest rate of all age groups.

❚❚▶ *Of all the population groups, pregnant teenaged girls have the highest nutrient needs.*

■■■ Our Aging Population

This looks like a section about older people, but it is relevant even if the reader is only 20 years old. How you live and think at 20 years of age can profoundly affect the quality of your life at 60 or 80 years. Most people, without realizing it, hold a stereotype, largely negative, of what it is like to be old—and then, later, they become that way. An old saying has it that "as the twig is bent, so grows the tree"—only, unlike a tree, you can bend your own twig.

Before you will adopt nutrition behaviors that will enhance your health in old age, you must accept on a personal level that you yourself are aging. People who fear age try to deny that it is happening to them by distancing themselves from the older generations. But, of course, everyone ages, so people who are prejudiced against older people are therefore prejudiced against *everyone*, including their own future selves. (Another form of prejudice is to view all old people as good, generous, and kind, when in fact thieves and crooks age too.)

To see what negative and positive views you hold about aging, try answering the following questions:

■ In what ways do you expect your appearance to change as you grow older?
■ What physical activities do you see yourself engaging in at age 70?
■ What will be your financial status? Will you be independent or dependent?
■ What will your sex life be like? Will others see you as sexy?
■ How many friends will you have? What will you do together?
■ Will you be happy? Cheerful? Curious? Depressed? Uninterested in life or new things?

Your answers reveal not only what you think of other people now but also what will probably become of you. You may wish to review some of the reasons for your answers and, if they are not supported by science, to change your beliefs.

Older people are an incredibly diverse group, and for the most part they are self-sufficient, socially sophisticated, mentally lucid, fully participating members of society who report themselves to be happy and healthy.[47] Most live in their own or relatives' homes, and only 5 percent live in nursing homes. Three-fifths of the elderly are women. Most have planned ahead financially, and about half need no financial assistance from the government. Planning ahead is important, since the average income of older men in the United States is about $10,000 per year, and for women it is only half that amount. Of aged black women, nearly half have yearly incomes of under $1000.[48]

The majority of the U.S. population is now middle-aged. As that group ages, the ratio of old people to young is growing larger, as Figure 13–3 shows. The fastest growing age group is people over 85 years.

In 1983 in the United States, the **life expectancy** for women was 78 years and for men was 71 years, up from about 45 years in 1900. Advances in medical science—antibiotics and other treatments—are largely responsible for almost doubling the life expectancy in this century. Still, a biological schedule is built into the human organism (we call it aging) that cuts off life at a genetically fixed point in time. The **life span** (the maximum length of life possible for a species) of human beings— 115 years—has not changed over the years and is probably the upper limit of human **longevity**. The controversy at the end of this chapter addresses research about how nutrition affects length of life.

■■■ Nutrition in the Later Years

Knowledge of nutrition through aging is limited. There are no RDA for older age groups—everyone over 50 years of age is grouped together, even though needs change as aging progresses. The problems include a lack of data on the effects of aging on nutrition.[49] The changes many times depend on individual genetics and medical history. For example, one individual may need more iron because that person's stomach acid secretion has declined (stomach acid helps in iron absorption), while another person may excrete more folate (and thus need to obtain more) due to past liver disease. Despite its shortcomings, the RDA are still reasonable standards against which to gauge nutrient intakes. The following sections pay attention to a few nutrients of concern.

life expectancy: the average number of years lived by people in a given society.

life span: the maximum number of years of life attainable by a member of a species.

longevity: long duration of life.

■■■ Figure 13–3

The Aging of the Population. In 1900, 4 percent of the U.S. population were over 65 years of age; today 12.7 percent are over 65 years; by 2040, 21.7 percent will have reached age 65; and a century from now, 25 percent will be 65 years and older.

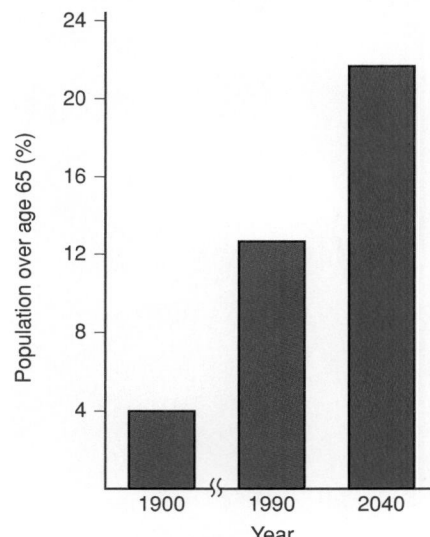

SOURCE: Data from K. Flieger, Why do we age? *FDA Consumer,* October 1988, pp. 20–25.

Water recommendation for adults: 1 to 1 1/2 oz/kg actual body weight.

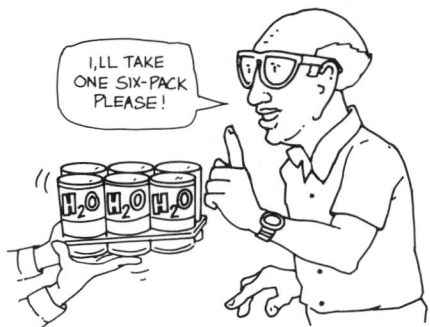

Adults of all ages need six to eight glasses of water each day.

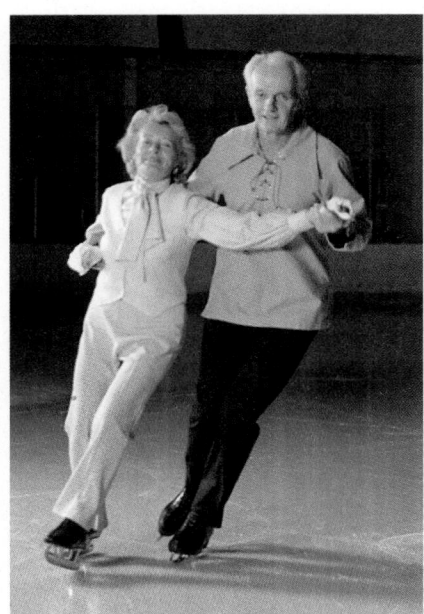

Energy like this requires continued physical activities and all the nutrients to support it.

Nutrient Needs

Dehydration is a major risk for older adults, who may not notice or pay attention to their thirst. With age, the thirst mechanism may become imprecise, and older people may go for long periods without drinking fluids. This causes some problems and worsens others—constipation, other intestinal problems, even muscle weakness and mental confusion can result. Regardless of age, adults need to drink six to eight glasses of water each day.

A person we know uses this trick to ensure getting enough water: he keeps six inexpensive 8-ounce cups in the cupboard. Through the day he uses each one to drink water only once and then collects them in the drainer. In the evening he checks the cupboard and drinks from any remaining cups. For him, drinking has become a habit, and seldom are there cups left in the cupboard.

Energy needs decrease with advancing age. For one thing, the number of active cells in each organ decreases, reducing the body's overall metabolic rate (although this is not inevitable). For another, older people usually reduce their physical activity (although they need not do so). After about the age of 50 years, the RDA for energy assumes about a 5 percent per decade reduction in energy output. The variation is great, so the ranges are wide (see inside front cover). On such a limited energy allowance, there is little leeway for low-nutrient–density foods, and older people must limit sugars, fats, oils, and, of course, alcohol.

Physical activities of all kinds help to maintain high energy and general good health. Older people especially should be sure to meet the exercise recommendations of Chapter 10 — 20 minutes of aerobic exercise three or four days a week. Many older persons believe that strenuous exercise is out of reach for them, but studies have shown that they can do more than they think they can. Even frail, institutionalized people in their *nineties* have been able to gain muscle bulk and strength and to put some pep in their walking steps after just eight weeks of weight training.[50] Any exercise—even a ten-minute walk a day—is better than nothing. Training not only improves muscles but also increases the blood flow to the brain; additionally, a person spending energy in physical activity can afford to eat more food, and with it comes more nutrients.

Among carbohydrates, fiber takes on extra importance for its role against constipation—a common complaint among older adults and especially among nursing home residents. Neither independent-living older adults or nursing home residents generally meet current recommendations of from 20 to 35 grams of fiber daily.[51] When low fiber intakes are combined with low fluid intakes, inadequate exercise, and constipating medications, constipation becomes almost inevitable.

Fats should be limited in the diet of older adults for many reasons. Foods low in fat are often rich in needed vitamins and minerals and may also help retard the development of cancer, atherosclerosis, obesity, and many other diseases.

Among the vitamins, vitamin A stands alone in that absorption appears to increase with aging.[52] For this reason researchers have proposed lowering of the RDA for vitamin A in aged populations. Some resist such a change, though, citing research that finds the vitamin A compound beta carotene to be active in cancer prevention.

Older adults face a greater risk of vitamin D deficiency than younger people do. Many older adults drink little or no vitamin D-fortified milk, and many go day after day with no exposure to sunlight, especially if they reside in nursing homes.[53] Additionally, as people age, vitamin D synthesis declines, setting the stage for deficiency. These age-related changes have inspired the suggestion that the RDA for vitamin D be raised for the elderly, but a more effective approach would be to ensure that elderly people drink more vitamin D-fortified milk and get outside more often or even just sit by a sunny window some of the time.

Adequate vitamin intakes can be ensured by including foods from all food groups. Studies have shown that the elderly most often omit foods of the vegetable group either to save money or because preferences have changed.[54] About 18 percent of older people are reported to eat no vegetables at all. Fruit is also lacking in many diets, and people who omit foods of both groups are almost sure to become nutrient deficient. Some older adults do not eat whole-grain breads and cereals, a significant source of many B vitamins. Controversy 13 discusses the importance of some B vitamins to the aging brain.

Among the minerals, iron deserves mention. Iron-deficiency anemia is not as common in older adults as it is in younger people, but it still occurs in some, especially in those with low food energy intakes. Aside from diet, other factors in many older people's lives increase the likelihood of iron deficiency:

- Chronic blood loss from ulcers, hemorrhoids, or other disease conditions.
- Poor iron absorption due to reduced stomach acid secretion.
- Antacid use, which interferes with iron absorption.
- Use of medicines that cause blood loss, including anticoagulants, aspirin, and arthritis medicines.

Older people take more medicines than others, and nutrition effects are common.

Zinc deficiencies are common in older people; as many as 95 percent of older adults may not get the zinc they need, and many miss the mark by more than half. Some research suggests that older adults absorb zinc less efficiently than younger people do.[55] The bright side of the zinc story is that some healthy older adults may need less than they did when they were younger.

Abundant dietary calcium throughout life is important to protect against osteoporosis, which can set in during later life. Controversy 8 took up the question of what intake of calcium is appropriate for older adults. While researchers attempt to reach agreement about the calcium requirements of older adults, especially those of women, one aspect of calcium nutriture is not controversial—calcium intakes of many people, especially women, in the United States are well below the RDA. If fresh milk causes stomach discomfort, as some older people report, then other calcium-rich foods should take its place.

▌▌▶ *Aging brings changed vitamin and mineral needs; some are increased, some decreased.*

Cataracts and Arthritis

An age-related change occurs in the lens of the eye: **cataracts**, a thickening of the lenses that impair vision and ultimately leads to blindness. Cataracts occur even in well-nourished individuals due to injury, viral infections, toxic substances, and genetic disorders, but most cataracts are vaguely called senile cataracts, meaning "caused by aging." Scientists have searched for possible roles

cataracts (CAT-uh-racts): thickenings of the lens of the eye that can lead to blindness. Cataracts can be caused by injury, viral infection, toxic substances, genetic disorders—and possibly by some nutrient deficiencies or imbalances.

Figure 8–7 of Chapter 8 showed some calcium-rich foods.

arthritis: a usually painful inflammation of a joint caused by many conditions, including infections, metabolic disturbances, or injury; joint structure is usually altered, with loss of function.

Not effective against arthritis:

- Alfalfa tea.
- *Aloe vera* liquid.
- Any of the amino acids.
- Burdock root.
- Calcium.
- Celery juice.
- Copper or copper complexes.
- Dimethyl sulfoxide (DMSO).
- Fasting.
- Fresh fruit.
- Honey.
- Inositol.
- Kelp.
- Lecithin.
- Para-aminobenzoic acid (PABA).
- Raw liver.
- Selenium.
- Superoxide dismutase (SOD).
- Vitamin D, E, C, or any B vitamin supplements.
- Watercress.
- Yeast.
- Zinc.
- 100 other substances.

of nutrient deficiencies, excesses, and imbalances in cataract causation. They have observed several possible (and, it should be emphasized, highly tentative) links: to protein, fat, or sugar (fructose derived from sucrose) excess; to excess food energy intake (in people with diabetes); to deficiencies of the vitamins riboflavin or vitamin E; and to deficiencies of the minerals selenium or zinc. Micronutrient-dense diets may, from one preliminary study, help protect against cataracts: of 112 people in this study, those who ate less than 1½ servings of fruit or 2 of vegetables were 3½ times more like to have cataracts then comparable other people.[56] A link between lactose intolerance and cataracts is worth exploring, and researchers are trying to determine whether the presence of the milk sugar itself, or the dehydration caused by diarrhea in lactose-intolerant people, is the associated factor.[57]

One certain cause of cataracts is radiation from sunlight and tanning booths. To avoid this source of preventable damage, wear sunglasses that filter out the sun's ultraviolet radiation and avoid tanning parlors, or at least protect your eyes if you must use them. Aside from protection from the sun and an adequate, balanced diet, no measure to avoid cataracts has yet proved effective.

Another major disease that disables the elderly is **arthritis**, a painful swelling of the joints that troubles many people as they grow older. During movement, the normal ends of bones are protected from wear by cartilage and by small sacs of fluid that act as a lubricant; but with age, bones sometimes disintegrate, and the joints become malformed and painful to move. The cause of arthritis is unknown, but it afflicts millions around the world and is a major problem of the elderly.

Arthritis has for centuries been ascribed to poor diet, and many quack remedies for it have been promoted, including many bizarre diets and supplements advertised as arthritis cures. Two or three new popular books on diet for arthritis come out every year, urging people to eat no meat, or to drink no milk, or to eat all their food raw, or to take supplements of "antioxidants," or to avoid all additives, or—who knows what will be next? Actually no known diet prevents, relieves, or cures arthritis, but as long as people keep buying the books that make these claims, the law of supply and demand dictates that such books will keep coming out.[58]

One possible true link between arthritis and diet is through the immune system. It could be that in some cases of arthritis, the immune system has become defective and attacks the tissues of the bone coverings as it normally would an invader. The integrity of the immune system depends on adequate nutrition, and a poor diet probably worsens the condition. It is also possible that foods might stimulate the immune system to attack.[59] Other nutrients linked to arthritis are the now-famous omega-3 fatty acids in fish oil. Chapter 11 described possible connections of omega-3 acids with heart health; research shows, too, that the same diet recommended there—one low in saturated fat from red meats and dairy products and adequate in omega-3 fatty acids—can reduce the suffering of people with arthritis.[60] The seemingly all-purpose low-fat diet that includes foods rich in omega-3 fatty acids may prevent the inflammation in the joints that makes arthritis so painful. Researchers hypothesize that omega-3 acids probably alter the action of prostaglandins, chemicals involved in the inflammatory response of body tissues, but more research is needed to test this idea fully.

Weight loss is important for overweight persons with arthritis because the joints affected are often weight-bearing joints that are stressed and irritated by having to carry excess poundage. Weight-loss diets alone often relieve the worst of the pain in arthritis clients, even that of arthritis in the hands (not weight bearing). Perhaps the drastic reduction in fat intake that accompanies the adoption of a calorie-restricted diet is beneficial for arthritis relief, with or without omega-3 fatty acids added. Important to note: jogging and other weight-bearing exercise is not related to the development of arthritis—even in marathon runners, although exercise can irritate an existing condition.[61] Drugs are commonly used to relieve arthritis. Some drugs may affect nutrient availability and require attention to nutrition status when used over a prolonged time.

These brief discussions of cataracts and arthritis could be multiplied many-fold, both to provide further details and to add other diseases, but they have sufficed to show that nutrition probably can provide at least some protection against certain diseases commonly associated with aging. Nutrition through the prime years may play a greater role than has been realized in preventing many changes once thought to be inevitable consequences of growing older.

This chapter's Controversy explores other relationships between nutrition and aging.

■■▶ *Several nutrients are being investigated for their relationships to cataracts. Omega-3 fatty acids and weight control may both play roles in helping to prevent arthritis.*

Sources of Assistance

Some older people may need assistance in obtaining proper, nourishing meals because of financial or other difficulties. Three major federal programs can help older persons with money problems, at least a little. Under Social Security, employees and employers pay into a fund from which the employee collects benefits at retirement. The Food Stamp program enables people who qualify to obtain stamps with which to buy food. The Supplemental Security Income program is aimed at directly improving the financial plight of the very poor by increasing a person's or a family's income to the defined poverty level. This sometimes helps older people retain their independence.

Another program to benefit the elderly is the Older Americans Act of 1965. Title IIIC (formerly Title VII) of this act is the "Nutrition Program for the Elderly." The major goals of this program are to provide:

■ Low-cost nutritious meals.
■ Opportunity for social interaction.
■ Homemaker education and shopping assistance.
■ Counseling and referral to other social services.
■ Transportation services.

The program is intended to improve older people's nutrition status and to enable them to avoid medical problems, to continue living in communities of their own choice, and to stay out of institutions.

Sites chosen for congregate meals under this program must be accessible to most of the target population. Volunteers may also deliver meals to those who are homebound either permanently or temporarily; these efforts are known as Meals on Wheels. The program ensures nutrition, but its recipients miss out on the social benefit of the congregate meal sites; every effort is made to persuade them to come to the shared meals if they can. Despite these programs, many eligible people are still missing meals and are malnourished simply because

Source of support for the elderly:

■ Social Security.
■ Food Stamps.
■ Supplemental Security Income.
■ Title IIIC of the Older Americans Act
■ Meals on Wheels.

they don't know of the programs available. Identification of such people should become a higher priority.

Food banks have been established in several areas to help older people stretch their food dollars. A food bank project buys industry's "irregulars"—good products that have been mislabeled, underweighted, redesigned, or mis-packaged and would ordinarily therefore be thrown away. Whenever government money dwindles, the nutrition status of low-income people of all ages depends more and more on private efforts such as food banking.

Although studies focus on foods and nutrients, another facet of eating is as important—the psychological well-being of the individual. Dr Jack Weinberg, professor of psychiatry of the University of Illinois, wrote perceptively:

> It is not *what* the older person eats but *with whom* that will be the deciding factor in proper care for him. The oft-repeated complaint of the older patient that he has little incentive to prepare food for only himself is not merely a statement of fact but also a rebuke to the questioner for failing to perceive his isolation and aloneness and to realize that food . . . for one's self lacks the condiment of another's presence which can transform the simplest fare to the ceremonial act with all its shared meaning.[62]

Nutrition knowledge meets health in the real world of cooking, cleaning, and shopping, but many older people, even able-bodied ones with financial resources, find themselves unable to perform these tasks; the following story illustrates this point. A man who had never prepared food for himself became a widower and suddenly became responsible for planning and preparing his own meals. During the year following his wife's death, he subsisted on a diet of black coffee, hamburgers, martinis, and steaks. He developed symptoms, and his health care providers treated him for many ailments. Finally, he was seen by a registered dietitian who made the correct diagnosis: scurvy from vitamin C deficiency. Even an occasional baked potato with his steak would have improved his vitamin C status, but without knowledge he was at a loss to select it, and baking it was beyond his skill. Furthermore, his loneliness robbed him of self-concern. With no one to share his meals, self-care became unimportant, and food lost its appeal.

For anyone living alone and for those of advanced age especially, it is important to work through the problems food preparation presents. This chapter's Food Feature may give you some ideas.

◖◗▶ *Financial planning is needed to ensure support in later years. Assistance programs are available for older people. Many programs directly improve nutrition status; some are aimed at helping to relieve financial problems. Wise adults will plan ahead to maximize their enjoyment of the later years.*

This Food Feature appears in a section on nutrition for older people, but it could be for anyone. Singles of all ages face problems concerning food purchasing, storing, and preparing. Large packages of meat and vegetables are often suitable for a family of four or more, and even a head of lettuce can spoil before one person can use it all. Many singles live in small dwellings, some without kitchens and freezers—for them, purchasing and storage problems are compounded. Following is a collection of ideas gathered from single people who have devised answers to these problems.

Buy only what you will use: the small-sized containers of food may be expensive, but it is also expensive to let the unused portion of a large-sized container spoil before using. Buy only three pieces of each kind of fresh fruit: a ripe one, a medium-ripe one, and a green one. Eat the first right away and the second soon, and let the last one ripen to eat days later. Don't be timid about asking the grocer to break open a family-sized package of wrapped meat or fresh vegetables.

Think up a variety of ways to use a vegetable when you must buy it in large quantity. For example, you can divide a head of cauliflower into thirds. Cook one third and eat it as a hot vegetable. Put another third into a salad dressing marinade for use as an appetizer, and save the rest to use raw in salad. Make mixtures using what you have on hand. A thick stew prepared from any leftover vegetables and bits of meat, with some added onion, pepper, celery, and potatoes, makes a complete and balanced meal—except for milk. If you like creamed gravy, you can add nonfat dry milk to your stew.

Buy fresh milk in the sizes best suited for you. If your grocer doesn't carry pints or quarts of milk, try a nearby convenience store.

Design a space for rows of glass jars containing shelf staple items that you can't buy in single-serving quantities—rice, tapioca, lentils and other dry beans, flour, cornmeal, dry nonfat milk, and cereal, to name only a few possibilities. Place each jar, tightly sealed, in the freezer for a few days to kill any eggs or organisms before storing it on the shelf. Then the jars will keep bugs out of the foods indefinitely. The jars make an attractive display and will remind you of possibilities for variety in your menus. Cut the directions-for-use label from the package of each item and store it in the jar.

Cook for several meals at a time. For example, boil three potatoes with skins. Eat one hot, mashed with chives. When the others have cooled, use one to make a potato-cheese casserole ready to be put into the oven for the next evening's meal. Slice the third one into a covered bowl, and pour some pickle juice over it. The pickled potato will keep several days in the refrigerator and can be used in a salad.

Experiment with stir-fried foods. Use a frying pan if you don't have a wok. A variety of vegetables and meats can be enjoyed this way; inexpensive vegetables such as cabbage and celery are delicious when crisp cooked in a little oil with soy sauce or lemon added. Cooked, leftover vegetables can be dropped in at the last minute. Frozen mixtures of Chinese or Polynesian vegetables are available in the larger grocery stores. Bonus: only one pan to wash. If you can afford a microwave oven, buy one; it will eliminate the need for most pots and pans, and allow you to freeze meals in microwavable containers so that you can reheat them at your convenience. Many frozen, single-serving meals come in microwave containers that you can reuse—place extra servings of home-cooked food in them and freeze.

Single Survival

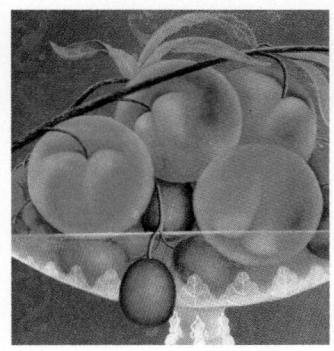

Remember, light destroys riboflavin, so use opaque jars for enriched pasta and dry milk.

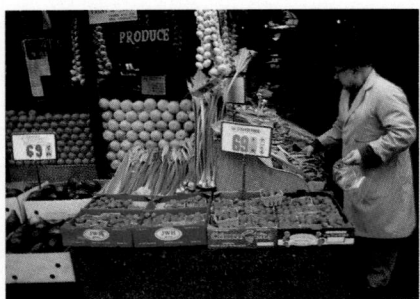

Take time to nourish your body well.

Depending on your freezer space, make double or even six times as much as you need of a dish that takes time to prepare: a casserole, vegetable pie, or meat loaf. Freeze individual portions in containers that can be microwaved or oven heated for serving later as just described. Be sure to date these so you will use the oldest first.

Buy a loaf of bread and immediately store half, well wrapped, in the freezer (not the refrigerator, which will make it stale). Buy frozen vegetables in large bags rather than in small cartons. You can take out the exact amount you need and close the bag tightly with a rubber band or spring clothes pin. Season the bag of vegetables by adding some fresh herbs. Buy bunches of parsley, dill, and oregano or basil; keep just a few sprigs out for use during the next few days; and chop up the rest to add to the frozen vegetable bags for low-cost elegance. Wrap individual portions of meat you wish to bake or broil before freezing so that you can defrost just the amount you need for a meal. Put the portions in a brown bag marked "hamburger" or "chicken thighs." The bag is easy to locate in the freezer, and you'll know when your supply is running low.

For nutrition's sake, it is important to attend to loneliness at mealtimes; the person who is living alone must learn to connect food with socializing. Cook for yourself with the idea that you are also preparing for guests you might want to invite. Or invite guests and make enough food so that you will have some left for a later meal. With leftovers on hand you can invite a single friend on the spur of the moment to "come over and share my frozen dinners with me tonight."

When you are alone at mealtime, make it a special occasion. One way to do this is to let cooking become a pleasant ritual of luxury. Try something like this: set the table with tablecloth, napkin, a full complement of utensils, and a flower if you can. Set a pot of stew with vegetables and fresh herbs on low heat to cook, and make a salad. Go settle in a stuffed chair and enjoy a book, some soothing music, and a crackling cold glass of lemoned sparkling water until the rich aroma of stew calls you to dinner. After serving your plate, light a candle, dim the lights, savor the food, and relish some of the best company you will ever have—your own.

Notes

1. L. L. Birch and M. Deysher, Caloric compensation and sensory specific satiety: Evidence for self-regulation of food intake by young children, *Appetite* 7 (1986): 323–331.

2. F. Lifshitz and N. Moses, Nutritional dwarfing: Growth, dieting, and fear of obesity, *Journal of the American College of Nutrition* 7 (1988): 367–376.

3. E. M. Satter, *Child of Mine: Feeding with Love and Good Sense* (Palo Alto, Calif.: Bull Publishing, 1986).

4. *Iron Nutrition Revisited—Infancy, Childhood, Adolescence*, 82nd Ross Conference on Pediatric Research (Columbus, Oh.: Ross Laboratories, 1981), p. 1.

5. D. M. Tucker and H. H. Sandstead, Body iron stores and cortical arousal, in *Iron Deficiency: Brain Biochemistry and Behavior*, eds. E. Pollitt and R. L. Leibel (New York: Raven Press, 1982), pp. 161–182.

6. S. Soewondo, M. Husaini, and E. Pollitt, Effects of iron deficiency on attention and learning processes in preschool children: Bandung, Indonesia, *American Journal of Clinical Nutrition* 50 (1989): 667–674.

7. R. L. Leibel, Behavioral and biochemical correlates of iron deficiency: A review, *Journal of the American Dietetic Association* 71 (1977): 399–404.

8. One of many studies that show the effect is S. Seshadi and T. Gopaldas, Impact of iron supplementation on cognitive functions in preschool and school-aged children: The Indian experience, *American Journal of Clinical Nutrition* 50 (1989): 675–686.

9. M. Clark, J. Royal, and R. Seeler, Interaction of iron deficiency and lead and the hematologic findings in children with lead poisoning, *Pediatrics* 81 (1988): 247–254; W. S. Watson

and coauthors, Food iron and lead absorption in humans, *American Journal of Clinical Nutrition* 44 (1986): 248–256.

10. Getting the lead out, *Science News* 132 (1987): 269.

11. D. Faust and J. Brown, Moderately elevated blood lead levels: Effect on neuropsychological functioning in children, *Pediatrics* 80 (1987): 623–629.

12. U.S. Department of Health and Human Services, Public Health Service, *Promoting Health, Preventing Disease: Objectives for the Nation* (Washington, D.C.: Government Printing Office, 1980), p. 34.

13. Y. H. Neggers and K. R. Stitt, Effects of high lead intake in children, *Journal of the American Dietetic Association* 86 (1986): 938–940.

14. Neggers and Stitt, 1986.

15. R. W. Miller, The metal in our mettle, *FDA Consumer,* December 1988–January 1989, pp. 24–27.

16. J. Raloff, Lead effects show in child's balance, *Science News* 135 (1989): 54.

17. A. J. McMichael and coauthors, Port Pirie Cohort study: Environmental exposure to lead and children's abilities at the age of four years, *New England Journal of Medicine* 319 (1988): 468–475.

18. Environmental exposure to lead and cognitive deficits in children, *New England Journal of Medicine* 320 (1989): 595–596.

19. E. Yetley, Nutritional applications of the Health and Nutrition Examination Surveys (HANES), *Annual Review of Nutrition* 7 (1987): 441–463; Miller, 1989.

20. K. Mahaffey and coauthors, Blood lead levels and dietary calcium intake in 1- to 11-year-old children: The Second National Health and Nutrition Examination Survey, 1976–1980, *Pediatrics* 78 (1986): 257–262.

21. K. R. Mahaffey, P. S. Gartside, and C. J. Glueck, Inverse associations of dietary calcium and blood lead in 3513 one to eleven year old black and white children: The NHANES II study, *American Journal of Clinical Nutrition* 41 (1985): 836.

22. C. D. May, Food allergy: Perspective, principles, practical management, *Nutrition Today,* November–December 1980, pp. 28–31.

23. *Diagnostic and Statistical Manual (DSM III),* 3rd ed. (Washington, D.C.: American Psychiatric Association, 1980), p. 41.

24. F. M. Atkins, Food allergy and behavior: Definitions, mechanisms, and a review of the evidence, *Nutrition Reviews Supplement,* May 1986, pp. 104–112.

25. M. L. Arbeit and coauthors, Caffeine intakes of children from a biracial population: The Bogalusa Heart Study, *Journal of the American Dietetic Association* 88 (1988): 466–471.

26. W. H. Dietz, Jr. and S. L. Gortmaker, Do we fatten our children at the television set? Obesity and television viewing in children and adolescents, *Pediatrics* 75 (1985): 807–812.

27. E. Pollitt, R. Leibel, and D. Greenfield, Brief fasting, stress and cognition in children, *American Journal of Clinical Nutrition* 34 (1981): 1526–1533.

28. J. Skinner and coauthors, Appalachian adolescents' eating patterns and nutrient intakes, *Journal of the American Dietetic Association* 85 (1985): 1093–1099.

29. J. Driskell, A. Clark, and S. Moak, Longitudinal assessment of vitamin B_6 status in southern adolescent girls, *Journal of the American Dietetic Association* 87 (1987): 307–310; P. Thompson and coauthors, Zinc status and sexual development in adolescent girls, *Journal of the American Dietetic Association* 86 (1986): 892–897; H. McCoy and coauthors, Nutrient intakes of female adolescents from eight southern states, *Journal of the American Dietetic Association* 84 (1984): 1453–1460; A. Clark, S. Mossholder, and R. Gates, Folacin status in adolescent females, *American Journal of Clinical Nutrition* 46 (1987): 302–306.

30. P. M. Guenther, Beverages in the diets of American teenagers, *Journal of the American Dietetic Association* 86 (1986): 493–499.

31. S. J. Solomon, M. S. Kurzer, and D. H. Calloway, Menstrual cycle and basal metabolic rate in women, *American Journal of Clinical Nutrition* 36 (1982): 611–616.

32. S. P. Dalvit, The effect of the menstrual cycle on patterns of food intake, *American Journal of Clinical Nutrition* 34 (1981): 1811–1815.

33. J. H. Morton and coauthors, A clinical study of premenstrual tension, *American Journal of Obstetrics and Gynecology* 65 (1953): 1182–1191; and H. Sutherland and I. Stewart, A critical analysis of the premenstrual syndrome, *Lancet* 1 (1965): 1180–1183, as cited by D. Y. Jones and S. K. Kumanyika, Premenstrual syndrome: A review of possible dietary influences, *Journal of the Canadian Dietetic Association* 44 (1983): 194–203.

34. S. P. Dalvit-McPhillips, The effect of the human menstrual cycle on nutrient intake, *Physiology and Behavior* 31 (1983): 209–212.

35. Emotional problems, Chapter 4 in F. S. Sizer and E. N. Whitney, *Life Choices: Health Concepts and Strategies* (St. Paul, Minn.: West, 1988), pp. 88–89.

36. "There is a very striking placebo effect in this disorder. Symptoms often disappear during a woman's first month on sugar pills," but gradually return over the next four to five months. R. L. Reid, as quoted by E. R. Gonzalez, Premenstrual syndrome, an ancient woe deserving of modern scrutiny (Medical News), *Journal of the American Medical Association* 245 (1981): 1393–1396.

37. G. E. Abraham and M. M. Lubran, Serum and red cell magnesium levels in patients with premenstrual tension, *American Journal of Clinical Nutrition* 34 (1981): 2364–2366.

38. C. S. Russ and coauthors, Vitamin B_6 status of depressed and obsessive-compulsive patients, *Nutrition Reports International* 27 (1983): 867–873.

39. J. Stokes and J. Mendels, Pyridoxine and premenstrual tension (letter to the editor), *Lancet* 1 (1972): 1177–1178.

40. J. A. Mattes and D. Martin, Pyridoxine in premenstrual tension, *Human Nutrition: Applied Nutrition* 36A (1982): 131–133.

41. R. S. London and coauthors, The effect of alpha-tocopherol on premenstrual symptomatology, a double-blind study, *Journal of the American College of Nutrition* 2 (1983): 115–122.

42. E. R. Gonzalez, Vitamin E relieves most cystic breast disease; may alter lipids, hormones (Medical News), *Journal of the American Medical Association* 244 (1980): 1077–1078.

43. A. Rossignol and coauthors, Tea and premenstrual syndrome in the People's Republic of China, *American Journal of Public Health* 79 (1989): 67–69.

44. G. S. Goei, J. L. Ralston, and G. E. Abraham, Dietary patterns of patients with premenstrual tension, *Journal of Applied Nutrition* 34 (1982): 4–11.

45. M. Mira, P. Stewart, and S. Abraham, Vitamin and trace element status in premenstrual syndrome, *American Journal of Clinical Nutrition* 47 (1988): 636–641.

46. Data presented in this discussion are from the national surveys of roughly 17,000 high school seniors entitled Monitoring the Future: A Continuing Study of the Lifestyles and Values of Youth, funded by the National Institute on Drug Abuse, conducted every spring since 1975, as cited in L. Johnston, P. O'Malley, and J. Bachman, Psychotherapeutic, licit, and illicit use of drugs among adolescents, *Journal of Adolescent Health Care* 8 (1987): 36–51.

47. S. M. Golant, *A Place to Grow Old: The Meaning of Environment in Old Age* (New York: Columbia University Press, 1984), pp. 137, 316.

48. Senate Special Committee on Aging, American Association of Retired Persons, National Center for Health Statistics, Bureau of Labor Statistics, and the Population Reference Bureau as cited in Numbers show aging of America, *Tallahassee Democrat,* 17 February 1985.

49. H. Smicklas-Wright, Aging, in *Present Knowledge in Nutrition,* ed. M. L. Brown (Washington, D.C.: International Life Sciences Institute—Nutrition Foundation, 1990), pp. 333–340.

50. M. A. Fiatrone and coauthors, High-intensity strength training in nonagenarians, *Journal of the American Medical Association* 263 (1990): 3029–3034.

51. Position of the American Dietetic Association: Health implications of dietary fiber, *Journal of the American Dietetic Association* 88 (1988): 216.

52. P. J. Garry and coauthors, Vitamin A intake and plasma retinol levels in healthy elderly men and women, *American Journal of Clinical Nutrition* 46 (1987): 989–994.

53. Vitamin D status of the elderly: Contributions of sunlight exposure and diet, *Nutrition Reviews* 43 (1985): 78–80.

54. V. Holt, J. Nordstrom, and M. B. Kohrs, Food preferences of older adults (abstract), *Journal of the American Dietetic Association* 87 (1987): 1597.

55. J. R. Turnlund and coauthors, Stable isotope studies of zinc absorption and retention in young and elderly men (abstract), *Journal of the American Dietetic Association* 86 (1986): 1762.

56. P. F. Jacques and coauthors, conference report, October 1989, *American Journal of Clinical Nutrition* (supplement), in preparation.

57. The nutritional origin of cataracts, *Nutrition Reviews* 42 (1984): 377–379; F. Rosales and coauthors, Lactose digestion and milk consumption pattern in Guatemalan cataract patients (abstract), *American Journal of Clinical Nutrition* 43 (1986): 700.

58. The items shown in the margin were listed by K. A. Meister, Can diet cure arthritis? *ACSH News and Views,* September–October 1980, p. 10; and in Morsels and tidbits, *Nutrition and the MD,* January 1982.

59. L. G. Darlington, N. W. Ramsey, and J. R. Mansfield, Placebo-controlled, blind study of dietary manipulation therapy in rheumatoid arthritis, *Lancet* 1 (1986): 236–238.

60. J. M. Kremer and coauthors, Fish-oil fatty acid supplementation in active rheumatoid arthritis: A double-blind, controlled crossover study, *Annals of Internal Medicine* 106 (1987): 497–503.

61. N. E. Lane, D. A. Block, and H. H. Jones, Long distance running, bone density, and osteoarthritis, *Journal of the American Medical Association* 255 (1986): 1147–1151.

62. J. Weinberg, Psychologic implications of the nutritional needs of the elderly, *Journal of the American Dietetic Association* 60 (1972): 293–296.

◼◼◼ C O N T R O V E R S Y   13 ◼◼◼

Can Nutrition Influence Aging?

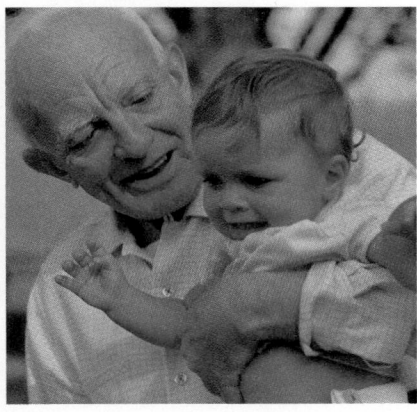

People have tried everything to delay or to reverse aging. Charlatans who sell hoaxes to the elderly nibble away their retirement funds in exchange for vitamins, "nutrients," or. "essences" falsely promoted as aging "remedies." With advancing age, people experience more aches and pains; if doctors cannot provide a cure, they may fall into the hands of quacks who promise unlimited help. To a person who experiences symptoms, money may seem less important than even the slightest chance of a miracle, and even brilliant, sophisticated people let themselves be bamboozled.

The legitimate study of aging is a young science, not nearly ready to offer potions, regimens, or gadgets to bestow longevity or restored health on anyone.[1] Instead, researchers are asking basic questions about how and why human beings age, such questions as:

◼ What factors determine the life span of human beings, and which others influence the life expectancy of an individual? Can we extend either through lifestyle choices?
◼ What roles does nutrition play in aging of the mind, and what roles can it play in retarding such aging?

This Controversy takes up the first of these questions first and presents results of research in the area of life extension. The last section considers the aging of the brain and what roles nutrition may play in the process.

◼◼◼ The Aging Process

Aging is a normal, inevitable process that affects cells, tissues, organs, and the whole person. Cells of each type of tissue age at different rates, and thus organs also age somewhat independently of one another. Most types of cells constantly renew themselves throughout a person's life; cells are born, and they reproduce, age, and finally die, each according to its own internal clock. Cell turnover is affected by many factors, including nutrition, and the whole process tends to slow down as the person ages. Notable as an exception to this pattern are the cells of the central nervous system, including many brain cells, which do not renew themselves but live out the person's entire life span.

These cells are sensitive to conditions within the body and are affected by whatever affects the rest of the body throughout life.

Many people mistakenly assume that the aging process expresses itself similarly in everyone—that all old people are physiologically much the same. Nothing could be further from the truth. As people get older, each one becomes less and less like anyone else. The older that people are, the more time has elapsed for such factors as diet, genetics, exercise, illnesses, and everyday stress to influence the physical and psychological progress of aging. Each of these factors can interact with one or more of the others, and each can affect the aging process positively or negatively.

Chapter 1 presented the concept that as people age, the effects of a lifetime of nutrition choices compound for the better or for the worse. While each day's intakes of nutrients may have only a minute effect on body organs and their functions, over years and decades their repeated effects accumulate to have major impacts. One writer has put it this way: "By age 65, the average American will have consumed 100,000 pounds of food, give or take a few tons. . . . Neglect will almost certainly be reflected in the state of his or her health by age 65, if not long before."[2] This being the case, it is of great importance for everyone to pay close attention now to nutrition and other lifestyle changes. Table C13–1 sums up the changes with age that a person with advanced know-how might avoid and some that are inevitable.

■■■ Table C13–1 Changes with Age: Inevitable vs Preventable

CHANGES WITH AGE	YOU PROBABLY CANNOT CHANGE THESE	YOU PROBABLY CAN SLOW OR PREVENT THESE CHANGES BY EXERCISING, EATING AN ADEQUATE DIET, REDUCING STRESS AND PLANNING AHEAD
Appearance		
Graying of hair	✓	
Balding	✓	
Drying and wrinkling of skin	✓	
Nervous System		
Impairment of near vision	✓	
Some loss of hearing	✓	
Reduced taste and smell sensitivity	✓	
Reduced touch sensitivity	✓	
Slowed reactions (reflexes)	✓	
Slowed mental function	✓	
Mental confusion		✓
Diminished visual memory	✓	
Heart, Circulatory System, and Lungs		
Increased blood pressure		✓
Increased resting heart rate		✓
Decreased breathing capacity and oxygen uptake		✓
Body Composition/Metabolism		
Increased body fatness		✓
Raised blood cholesterol		✓
Slowed energy metabolism		✓
Other Physical Characteristics		
Decreased maximum work rate		✓
Menopause (women)	✓	
Loss of fertility (men)	✓	
Loss of sexual functioning		✓
Joints: loss of elasticity	✓	
Joints: loss of flexibility		✓
Oral health: loss of teeth, gum disease		✓
Bone loss		✓
Digestive problems, constipation		✓

SOURCE: Adapted from F. S. Sizer and E. N. Whitney, *Life Choices: Health Concepts and Strategies* (St. Paul: West, 1988), p. 398.

■■■ Can Nutrition Affect Longevity?

Much of what has been learned regarding nutrition's role in longevity may be true only with regard to the experimental animals that were affected and may be of only academic interest to people. However, at least some evidence of nutrition's effect on longevity in human beings is worthy of notice.

The first evidence that diet might increase longevity in rats surfaced more than half a century ago.[3] Researchers fed young rats on diets adequate in all the nutrients essential for growth but short in calories. The rats stopped growing on this

When researchers added calories, growth resumed. Control rats were allowed to eat and grow normally. The rats from the experimental groups outlived the control rats. Furthermore, the experimental rats developed the diseases of old age later in life than did the controls. However, the degree of food restriction in the study was severe enough to cost many animal lives early on and to produce in the survivors permanent malformations and stunting, lasting into later life on normal feed. This drastic side effect of early starvation obviously limits this study's usefulness to human beings.

A later group of researchers decided to explore further the effects of food restriction on disease onset.[4] One group of rats received a diet containing half the calories of normal chow, the other group received a diet providing two-thirds the normal calories. Again, the life-extension effect was evident. Compared with control rats, nearly twice as many rats in both restricted groups lived to 800 days. Disease incidence was lower in the calorie-restricted groups too. The restricted animals contracted the same diseases as the others but did so at later times of life.

In the studies just described, food restriction began as soon as the animals were weaned. Researchers have also investigated the effects on rat longevity of food restriction initiated later in life. Rats fed normally through growth, then later placed on energy-restricted diets survived as long as had the rats that had been restricted during growth.[5] In this study food restriction in later

life extended longevity without incurring the physical malformations caused by early restriction. Other studies have repeated these results— even short-term food restriction of adult rats has been shown to extend the animals' lives.[6] In view of knowledge about the importance of nutrition during critical growth periods, it is not surprising that animals who are allowed to grow normally survive periods of food restriction better than those starved during growth.

To apply the results of animal studies to human beings is often unrealistic and, in this case, even dangerous. While these studies show an effect, they are not intended as an example for people. Restricting the diets of infants or young children impairs growth and development, and no one would take this risk on the theoretical chance of prolonging life. But what about animal studies suggesting that moderate energy restriction later in life increases life expectancy? Does research on people show a similar effect?

The relationships between diet, body weight, and longevity are less clear-cut for human beings than for experimental animals, but they do exist. Researchers in California studied nearly 7000 adults and noticed that some were young for their ages, others old for their ages.[7] To find out what made the difference, the researchers focused on factors relating to health habits that affect **physiological age**. Of the factors studied, four were related to nutrition: alcohol consumption, breakfast habits, snacking habits, and weight control. (The others were sleep, smok-

ing, and exercise habits.) In this study, overweight, especially high degrees of overweight, correlated with poor health. Irregular eating habits also seemed detrimental to health. The effects of all these factors were cumulative, that is, those who followed all of the practices were in better health, even if older in calendar years, than people who failed·to do so. In fact, the physical health of those who reported all positive health practices was comparable to that of people *30 years younger* who followed few of them. These findings demonstrate that although you cannot alter the year of your birth, you can alter the *probable* length of your life.

Insurance companies have also compiled many years of data on mortality with relation to people's weights and heights. Generally their findings indicate that the more overweight an individual is, the greater the risk of mortality.[8] The same is true for severely underweight individuals. If overweight individuals have an increased mortality risk, why, then, do many live long, healthy lives? The answer is unknown, but the question shows that body weight alone is not responsible for the increased mortality of obese people. Unlike controlled studies of animals, however, these associations can be affected by many other factors—genetics, disease state, and medical care, just to name a few. Nevertheless, data confirm that people who live to advanced ages are leaner than those who die younger.[9]

Does it follow, then, that people who restrict their energy intakes live the longest? Evidence supporting a correlation between food energy restriction and longevity in human beings is limited but not totally absent. For example, people living on the island of Okinawa take in much less energy each day than do people living on mainland Japan. (The foods consumed, mainly fish and vegetables, are highly nutritious.) The Okinawan people suffer from cerebral disease, heart disease, and cancer much less frequently than do people of mainland Japan.[10] Okinawa also has up to 40 times the number of mainland people reaching their 100th birthday. Other factors such as stress, exercise, climate, or genetics may turn out to be factors, but a low-energy, nutrient-dense diet appears to have some association with enhanced longevity of the people of Okinawa.

One other piece of evidence contributes to the energy-longevity picture. Long ago, when restrictions on scientific research involving human beings were less rigorous, researchers at a religious institution for the elderly fed some of the residents an alternating diet—2300 calories every odd-numbered day and 1000 calories each even-numbered day.[11] A control group received the 2300-calorie diet every day. Those on the alternating diet had a lower incidence of illness (as indicated by admissions to the infirmary) and half as many deaths as the control group during the study period.

Although evidence from animal studies and observations about human beings seems to support a link between low-calorie diets and increased longevity, much more re-

search is needed to establish a cause-and-effect relationship. For one thing, we would need to understand the metabolic means by which energy restriction and body weight contribute to longevity. This would mean ruling out such factors as genetics, fitness, and stress. But evidence about these factors is not dismissed lightly.

■■■ Evidence on Genetics, Fitness, and Stress

Researchers have a difficult time separating the effects of genetics from those of fitness or stress. This section shows that each affects longevity.

GENETICS. Heredity is a major factor that determines a person's chances of contracting diseases that shorten life. A person's family history of certain diseases is a powerful indicator of that person's probability of contracting those diseases. Still, environmental factors are often pivotal in determining whether a tendency to develop a disease will be expressed. Environment, in this sense, is everything other than genetics—including air, food, and water. The relationship between genetics and environmental factors is often synergistic; for instance, the effect of cigarette smoking in augmenting the risk of coronary heart disease is especially strong in people who are genetically predisposed to develop the disease.[12]

Families with adopted children are of interest to researchers who

wish to study the effects of similar environmental conditions on genetically different people. A study of causes of deaths in adoptees and their biological parents illustrates this point.[13] The results were startling. Death of a biological parent before the age of 50 years from natural causes doubled the mortality rate for adoptees. Death of an adoptive parent from natural causes before the age of 50 years had no effect on the mortality rate for adoptees. Adoptees whose biological parents died from vascular causes were five times as likely to die of vascular diseases as adoptees whose adoptive parents died that way. Thus susceptibility to certain diseases seems largely affected by heredity.

This picture changes, however, in the case of cancer. Deaths of adoptive parents from cancer before the age of 50 years increased the adoptees' mortality from cancer fivefold, whereas deaths of biological parents from cancer had no effect on adoptees' death rates from cancer. Cancer is well known as a disease with its roots in the environment.

The authors offer some important cautions in generalizing the results of their study. The population studied was homogeneous—all white and of similar cultural background. Also, adopted individuals are usually not able to change their environments to counteract genetic tendencies toward diseases, since they are usually unaware of such biological tendencies. In contrast, biological children are aware and can take preventive measures against diseases they might inherit. This difference may heighten the contrast in studies of adoptive versus biological children and overstate the impact of genetics on disease.

FITNESS. Physical activity and fitness are among the factors related to disease and longevity that researchers classify as environmental. Research continues to confirm what athletes, trainers, and most people who exercise already know: the mental and physical benefits of regular physical activity are many and remarkable. Chapter 10 presented a long list of such benefits as increased lean body mass, reduced body fatness, reduced blood pressure, a reduced risk of cardiovascular disease—and even a longer life.

The mechanism by which exercise may extend life is still to be determined, but an extensive study of more than 16,000 Harvard alumni indicates that regular exercise can prolong life.[14] The men were between 35 and 74 years of age and were studied for 12 to 16 years. The group whose members expended 2000 or more calories in exercise per week (equal to walking or running about 20 miles per week) had a death rate 25 to 33 percent lower than the less active group's rate. Furthermore, lack of exercise seemed to influence risk of death even more than did heredity. Even if the subjects' parents had died before the age of 65 years, active subjects' risks of death were lower than those of inactive subjects with the same parental history. Also, the

mortality rates of physically active men were lower with or without regard to smoking, hypertension, or extremes in body weight.

Physical activity, then, slows cardiovascular aging and positively affects risk factors for heart disease. The ever more numerous benefits derived from regular physical activity emphasize the importance of making it a priority in everyone's life.

STRESS. Stress is also considered to be a factor in longevity. The body has remarkable ability to maintain a steady internal condition by adapting to stressors that would otherwise cause life-threatening changes. Controversy 3 outlined the fight-or-flight reaction that occurs in the body at stressful times. If stress is prolonged or severe and especially if physical action is not a permitted response to the stressor, then it can drain the body of its reserves and leave it weakened, aged, and vulnerable to illness.

Older individuals have less ability to adapt to both external and internal disturbances. Animals show a reduced tolerance to cold (a source of physical stress) as they age, and epidemiological studies of human beings show that the death rate from heat stroke rises abruptly after the age of 60 years.[15] As for internal stressors, with advancing age, glucose tolerance declines. A marked increase in blood sugar concentration occurs after a glucose challenge.[16] Fasting blood glucose concentrations, on the other hand, rise only slightly with age.[17]

The stress response begins in the brain, and it is here that researchers have elucidated some specific effects of stress hormones on brain tissues. When researchers examine the brain's sites of regulation of stress hormone release, they find that repeated exposure of those sites to the stress hormones reduces their ability to respond to stress.[18] This diminished response is reflected in three measurable characteristics.[19] First, higher concentrations of the stress hormones are needed to elicit a response from the brain; second, the adaptation response is slower; and third, recovery is delayed, that is, once the stress response is turned on, it takes longer to turn it off. The researchers also point out that the metabolic changes induced by stress hormones, such as increases in blood glucose concentrations and heart rate, while essential for dealing with stress, are harmful if prolonged.

As aging progresses, inevitable changes in structure and function of each of the body's organs contribute to the decline in function of the body as a whole. When disease strikes and further impairs function, the reduced ability to adapt makes the aging individual more vulnerable to death than the younger, more adaptive person.

In none of the studies do individual nutrients affect longevity. No supplement, nutrient, food, or any other product has been shown to extend life or to have antiaging effects, regardless of the many claims by quacks that they do. Furthermore, many "life-extending"

■■■ Table C13-2 Examples Of Unproved Anti-Aging Products and Regimens

PRODUCT OR REGIMEN	"ACTIVE" INGREDIENT OR SUPPOSED BASIS	COMMENTS
Gerovital H-3 (GH-3)	The anesthetic procaine hydrochloride (Novocaine) and various pseudonutrients	Originally available only in Romania. Now sold through clinics in many countries and by mail.
Barleygreen	Barley juice	
Megadophilus	A culture of the bacterium *Lactobacillus acidophilus*	
Live Cell Therapy	Cell suspensions from fetal animals injected into patients	Extremely expensive. No research available to support claims of efficacy.
Superoxide dismutase (SOD)	Destroys free radicals	A totally useless product. SOD supplements are digested by the body and never reach body cells intact.
Butylated hydroxyanisole (BHA) and butylated hydroxytoluene (BHT)	Destroy free radicals	Although safe in the amounts used in processed foods, these antioxidant food additives may be toxic in the larger doses recommended by food faddists.
MaxiLife supplements containing vitamins E and B_6, methionine, and selenium	Destroy free radicals	Unnecessary supplements. B_6 is toxic in large doses.
The amino acids arginine and ornithine	Supposedly improve the immune function	
Dimethylaminoethanol (DMAE) with para-aminobenzoic acid (PABA)	Supposed brain stimulant	
The amino acid L-cysteine	Supposedly protects against environmental agents that damage DNA	

SOURCE: J. A. Lowell, *Quackery and the Elderly,* a booklet available from The American Council on Science and Health, 1995 Broadway, 16th Floor, New York, NY 10023-5860. Reprinted with permission.

regimens can be dangerous. Many popular books on the topic cite scientific-sounding references but misinterpret scientific writings and twist the facts to support their claims. Table C13-2 lists some nutrients and other chemicals *not* effective in prolonging life. Neither do they improve mental functioning or cure mental illnesses of old age, as many quacks claim.

These studies have provided valuable insight into the roles of genetics and environment in disease and longevity. As researchers learn more about the genes and environmental factors that influence disease susceptibility, so do they learn more about how to help people from susceptible families avoid diseases. A person cannot change an inherited genetic map but can control nutri-

tion, exercise, and other lifestyle habits to enhance the quality of life and to make more likely the attainment of maximal life expectancy.

Strongly related to the quality of life in later years is mental acuity. Evidence about the brain's aging and lifestyle factors is presented next.

■■■ The Aging Brain

The brain, like all of the body's organs, is influenced by both genetic and environmental factors that can enhance or impair its capacities. One of the challenges researchers face when studying the aging process in human beings is to distinguish among disease processes, normal age-related physiological changes, and changes that are the result of cumulative, extrinsic factors such as diet.

The brain ages in some characteristic ways. The number of neurons decreases as people age, and so does blood flow to the brain. When the number of nerve cells in one part of the cerebral cortex diminishes, hearing and speech are affected. Losses of neurons in other parts of the cortex can impair memory and cognitive function. When the number of neurons in the hindbrain diminishes, balance and posture are affected. Losses of neurons in other parts of the brain affect still other functions.

Clinicians now recognize that much of the cognitive loss and forgetfulness generally attributed to aging is due in part to extrinsic, and therefore controllable, factors. In some instances cognitive loss is attributable to a specific disorder. Moderate, long-term nutrient deficiencies may contribute to the loss of memory and cognition that some older adults may experience. However, in some cases deterioration of the brain is genetically determined and will not yield to external approaches.

■■■ Alzheimer's Disease and Aluminum

Lately much attention has focused on the *abnormal* deterioration of the brain called senile dementia of the **Alzheimer's** type (SDAT). SDAT may be the most common acquired progressive brain syndrome, afflicting 5 percent of the population by the age of 65 years and 20 percent of those over 80 years.[20] Although diagnosis of SDAT is difficult, its symptoms make its presence known: gradual losses of memory and reasoning, of ability to communicate, of physical capabilities, and, eventually, loss of life. To date, causes are unknown and no cure exits. Treatment involves providing relief and support to both the clients and their families.

Nutrition may be relevant to some SDAT characteristics. For example, normally, as blood flow to the brain diminishes with age, the brain compensates by absorbing more glucose and oxygen. In SDAT, no such compensation occurs, and glucose and oxygen concentrations decline. Whether the brain's diminished capacity to get glucose and oxygen causes or results from SDAT remains unclear.

Most people have heard of an association between aluminum and the development of SDAT, although a causative role of aluminum, if any, has yet to be defined. Brain concentrations of aluminum in SDAT people exceed normal brain concentrations by some 10 to 30 times, but blood and hair concentrations remain normal, indicating that the accumulation is caused by something in the brain itself, and not by an overload of aluminum in the body. This may be a result, rather than a cause, of SDAT. However, an epidemiological survey found that the risk of SDAT was 1 1/2 times greater in areas where water aluminum concentrations were high compared with areas where concentrations were low, indicating that environmental aluminum might play some yet unknown role.[21] Current research is investigating the relationship between dietary aluminum and SDAT in individuals; aluminum cookware can increase the aluminum content of foods slightly, but the idea that this can significantly affect the progress of SDAT is doubtful.

■■■ Nutrient Deficiencies and Brain Function

SDAT is an identifiable disease, the course of which is probably unaffected by even superb nutrition, similar to the genetic diseases multiple sclerosis or cystic fibrosis. Many promising trials involving drugs that enhance memory and cognition may lead to future treatments.[22] But general poor nutrition does affect the brain in other ways. We know that the enzymes involved in neurotransmitter synthesis require vitamins and minerals to function properly.[23] Research on animals and human beings clearly shows that severe dietary deficiencies of thiamin, niacin, vitamin B_6, vitamin B_{12}, folate, and vitamin C impair mental ability, including memory.[24] Trace elements such as iodine, iron, copper and zinc also support normal brain function.[25] One nutrient, choline, has been linked to SDAT through altered choline handling by the brain, but to date, supplements of choline or lecithin (which contains choline) have had no effect on the disease. The most recent trials that combine highly concentrated lecithin with other drugs have appeared to show improvements in limited areas of cognitive deficiencies without improving others.[26]

Researchers have begun exploring the possibility that the memory impairments observed in people and animals with severe nutrient deficiencies could develop in older adults who have experienced moderate (subclinical) deficiencies for long times. A lifetime of multiple nutrient deficiencies could conceivably contribute to mental impairment in later life by way of brain cell degeneration.

One group of researchers studied the relationship between nutrition status and cognitive functioning in older, healthy adults and found that subjects with low blood concentrations of vitamin C or vitamin B_{12} scored worse in short-term memory and problem solving than better nourished participants. Those with low blood concentrations of riboflavin or folate also scored worse on the problem-solving test.[27]

It is important to note that even the lowest scores in this study were still within the normal range for men and women of the same age.

Also the relationship between poor cognition and poor nutrition might be compared with the question of whether the chicken or the egg came first. Poor cognition is itself a risk factor for poor nutrition because people with impaired thinking ability might be less adept at meal preparation. However, the participants in this study had no history of dementia or impaired mental status, and so the researchers concluded that poor nutrition status might contribute to poor cognitive functioning in healthy, elderly people.

Memory impairment due to vitamin B_{12} deficiency can precede the blood symptoms of deficiency by years.[28] Evidence that vitamin B_{12} deficiency accounts for some cognitive deficits in older people comes from a study that revealed abnormal short-term memory in more than two-thirds of clients with pernicious anemia.[29] Treatment with vitamin B_{12} restored memory within one month in three-fourths of the clients. The researchers recommend that a diagnosis of senile dementia should not be made, even in the absence of anemia, until vitamin B_{12} status is determined biochemically.

Among people with alcoholism, dementia is common. As Controversy 11 described, alcohol displaces food from the diet and alters normal nutrient metabolism, causing multiple nutrient deficiencies and, among them, thiamin deficiency. Thiamin deficiency without alcoholism brings on dementia, and it is thought that abnormal thiamin metabolism may contribute to the mental symptoms that can accompany alcoholism.[30] When people addicted to alcohol become abstinent and resume eating, dementia often subsides. That which remains is the result of damage to brain tissue by the toxin alcohol.

It could be that older people are more sensitive to dietary thiamin restriction than are younger people.[31] When thiamin was restricted in the diets of ten women between the ages of 52 and 72 years, they experienced irritability, fatigue, and headaches after only 12 days. Women between the ages of 18 and 21 years eating the same diet experienced no symptoms at all.

When rats are fed experimental diets low in copper and vitamin B_6, they incur brain changes that resemble the degenerative changes that occur in the brains of human beings as they age.[32] The rats' diets were extremely deficient in vitamin B_6, an unlikely situation for human beings, but vitamin B_6 intakes of many older adults vary, and many people are ingesting amounts well below recommendations.[33]

Iron deficiency is known to affect mental functioning. Research on children shows a relationship between iron deficiency and cognitive function.[34] Researchers examining iron status and cognition in college students found a relationship between body iron stores and cognition.[35] The exact relationship is unclear, but iron status appeared to influence tasks dominated by the left side of the brain differently from tasks dominated by the right side. For example, higher iron status was

■■■ Table C13–3 Strategies for Growing Old Gracefully

1. Maintain appropriate body weight.
2. Reduce your stress.
3. For women, see your physician about estrogen replacement against osteoporosis.
4. Do not smoke; if you do smoke, quit.
5. Expect to enjoy sex, and learn new ways of enhancing it.
6. Maintain physical fitness, and change activities to suit changing abilities and tastes.
7. Use alcohol only moderately, if at all; use drugs only as prescribed.
8. Take care to prevent accidents.
9. Expect good vision and hearing throughout life; obtain glasses and hearing aids if necessary.
10. Be alert to confusion as a disease symptom, and seek diagnosis.
11. Control depression through activities and friendships.
12. Drink eight glasses of water every day.
13. Practice your mental skills. Keep on solving math problems, reading, following directions, writing, imagining, and creating.
14. Make financial plans early to ensure your security.
15. Accept change. Work at recovering from losses; make new friends.
16. Cultivate spiritual health. Consult your values, and make meaning in your life.

associated with better word fluency performance (a left brain-dominated task) but with poorer performance of right brain-dominated tasks. Animal research supports a relationship between iron deficiency and cognition.[36] The offspring of rats fed an iron-deficient diet were less responsive to adverse stimuli than were the offspring of iron-sufficient mice. In view of the wide-spread occurrence of iron deficiency, the role of lifelong deficiencies on mental function in the aged deserves further research.

A study in England showed that people with senile dementia had much lower blood concentrations of zinc than those without dementia.[37] Among older women in the United States, as many as 25 percent take in less than half of their recommended allowance.[38]

Aside from clinical dementia, many older people become easily confused, or senile. But senility is often caused by correctable factors—and many are preventable. One, of course, is poor nutrition, as the preceding sections made clear. Others include:

■ Abuse of drugs, especially alcohol. (Their effects can sometimes resemble those of strokes and seizures.)
■ Accidents. (Falls can cause concussions or bleeding, and confusion follows.)

■ Poor vision and hearing. (Misunderstanding is easy when sensory input is faulty.)
■ Disease states. (Diseases present different symptoms in older people than in younger ones. Tuberculosis, diabetes, meningitis, encephalitis, and even heart attack can all begin with confusion.)
■ Stroke. (This is a major cause of senility.)
■ Depression. (A distracted grieving person can seem senile.)
■ Dehydration. (The thirst signal may become faint, and one of its major symptoms is confusion.)
■ Disuse. (People lose what they do not use, but practicing mental skills reinstates them.[39])

Beware of charlatans selling nutrients, especially large doses of nutrients, as "megavitamin therapy" to correct mental illness. When any "therapy" includes nutrient megadoses, this should sound an alarm in your mind to warn you of the possibility that you are dealing with quackery.[40]

There are many things people can do, besides obtaining adequate nutrition, to support a high quality of life into old age. Table C13–3 shows some of them.

■■■ Miniglossary

Alzheimer's disease: a relentless, irreversible brain disease that attacks some people as they age; the final stage is complete helplessness and death.

physiological age: age as estimated from the body's health and probable life expectancy; as opposed to **chronological age**, age measured in years from the date of birth.

Notes

1. E. L. Schneider and J. D. Reed, Life extension, *New England Journal of Medicine* 312 (1985): 1159–1168.

2. L. Hofmann, ed., *The Great American Nutrition Hassle* (Palo Alto, Calif.: Mayfield Publishing, 1978), p. 89.

3. C. M. McCay, M. F. Crowell, and L. A. Maynard, The effect of retarded growth upon the length of life span and upon the ultimate body size, *Journal of Nutrition* 10 (1935): 63–79.

4. B. N. Berg and H. S. Simms, Nutrition and longevity in the rat: II. Longevity and onset of disease with different levels of food intake, *Journal of Nutrition* 71 (1960): 255–263.

5. G. A. Nolen, Effect of various restricted dietary regimens on growth, health, and longevity of albino rats, *Journal of Nutrition* 102 (1972): 1477–1494.

6. M. H. Ross, Length of life and caloric intake, *American Journal of Clinical Nutrition* 25 (1972): 834–838.

7. N. B. Belloc and L. Breslow, Relationship of physical health status and health practices, *Preventive Medicine* 1 (1972): 409–421.

8. T. Harris and coauthors, Body mass index and mortality among nonsmoking older persons, *Journal of the American Medical Association* 259 (1988): 1520–1524.

9. E. D. Schlenker, Obesity and the life span, in *Nutrition, Physiology, and Obesity,* ed. R. Schemmel (Boca Raton, Fla.: CRC Press, 1980), pp. 151–166; Y. Kagawa, Impact of westernization on the nutrition of Japanese: Changes in physique, cancer, longevity and centenarians, *Preventive Medicine* 7 (1978): 205–217.

10. Kagawa, 1978.

11. E. A. Vallejo, Restricted diet on alternate days in the nutrition of the aged, *Revista Clinica Espanola* 63 (1956): 25–27.

12. K. T. Khaw and E. Barrett-Connor, Family history of heart attack: A modifiable risk factor, *Circulation* 74 (1986): 239–244.

13. T. I. A. Sorensen and coauthors, Genetic and environmental influences on premature death in adult adoptees, *New England Journal of Medicine* 318 (1988): 727–732.

14. R. S. Paffenbarger and coauthors, Physical activity, all-cause mortality, and longevity of college alumni, *New England Journal of Medicine* 314 (1986): 605–611.

15. A. J.Harper, Nutrition, aging, and longevity, *American Journal of Clinical Nutrition* 36 (1982): 737–749. D. M. Driscoll, The relationship between weather and mortality in the major metropolitan areas in the United States, 1962–1965, *International Journal of Biometeorology* 15 (1971): 23–39; as cited by D. M. Watkin, The physiology of aging, *American Journal of Clinical Nutrition* 36 (1982): 750–758.

16. J. W. Rowe, Physiologic interface of aging and nutrition, in *Nutrition and Aging,* eds. M. L. Hutchinson and H. N. Munro (Orlando, Fla.: Academic Press, 1986), pp. 11–21.

17. Rowe, 1986.

18. P. W. Landfield, R. K. Baskin, and T. A. Pitler, Brain aging correlates: Retardation by hormonal-pharmacological treatments, *Science* 214 (1981): 581–584.

19. R. M. Sapolsky, L. C. Krey, and B. S. McEwen, The adrenocortical stress-response in the aged male rat: Impairment of recovery from stress, *Experimental Gerontology* 18 (1983): 55–64, as cited by M. L. Zoler, Hormones and aging: Turning off "the aging switch," *Geriatrics* 38 (1983): 107–112.

20. Much of the discussion on Alzheimer's disease is based on M. S. Claggett, Nutritional factors relevant to Alzheimer's disease, *Journal of the American Dietetic Association* 89 (1989): 392–396.

21. C. N. Martyn and coauthors, Geographical relation between Alzheimer's disease and aluminum drinking water, *Lancet* 1 (1989): 59–62.

22. U. Schindler, Pre-clinical evaluation of cognition enhancing drugs, *Progess in Neuro-Psychopharmocology and Biological Psychiatry* 13 (1989): S99–S115.

23. W. M. Lovenberg, Biochemical regulation of brain function, *Nutrition Reviews* (supplement), May 1986, pp. 6–11.

24. K. Yoshimura and coauthors, Animal experiments on thiamine avitaminosis and cerebral function, *Journal of Nutritional Science and Vitaminology* 22 (1976): 429–437, as cited by A. Cherkin, Effects of nutritional factors on memory function, in *Nutritional Intervention in the Aging Process,* eds. H. J. Armbrecht, J. M. Prendergast, and R. M. Coe (New York: Springer-Verlag, 1984), pp. 229–249; M. K. Horwitt, Niacin, in *Modern Nutrition in Health and Disease,* 6th ed., eds. R. S. Goodhart and M. S. Shils

(Philadelphia: Lea and Febiger, 1980), pp. 204–208; C. S. Russ and coauthors, Vitamin B$_6$ status of depressed and obsessive-compulsive patients, *Nutrition Reports International* 27 (1983): 867–873; J. S. Goodwin, J. M. Goodwin, and P. J. Garry, Association between nutritional status and cognitive functioning in a healthy elderly population, *Journal of the American Medical Association* 249 (1983): 2917–2921.

25. H. Sandstead, A brief history of the influence of trace elements on brain function, *American Journal of Clinical Nutrition* 43 (1986): 293–298.

26. S. Gauthier and coauthors, Progress report on the Canadian Multicentre Trial of tetrahydroaminoacridine with lecithin in Alzheimer's disease, *Canadian Journal of Neurological Sciences* 16 (1989): S543–S546.

27. Goodwin, Goodwin, and Garry, 1983.

28. Cherkin, 1984.

29. R. W. Strachan and J. G. Henderson, Psychiatric syndromes due to avitaminosis B$_{12}$ with normal blood and marrow, *Journal of Medicine* 34 (1965): 303–317, as cited by Cherkin, 1984.

30. M. Victor, Alcohol and nutritional diseases of the nervous system, *Journal of the American Medical Association* 167 (1958): 65–71.

31. H. G. Oldham, Thiamin requirements of women, *Annals of the New York Academy of Sciences* 378 (1982): 542–549, as cited by R. H. Haas, Thiamin and the brain, in *Annual Review of Nutrition*, eds. R. E. Olson, E. Beutler, and H. P. Broquist (Palo Alto, Calif.: Annual Reviews, 1988), pp. 483–515.

32. E. J. Root and J. B. Longenecker, Brain cell alterations suggesting premature aging induced by dietary deficiency of vitamin B$_6$ and/or copper, *American Journal of Clinical Nutrition* 37 (1983): 540–552.

33. P. J. Garry and coauthors, Nutritional status in a healthy elderly population: Dietary and supplemental intakes, *American Journal of Clinical Nutrition* 36 (1982): 319–331.

34. E. Pollitt and coauthors, Iron deficiency and behavioral development in infants and preschool children, *American Journal of Clinical Nutrition* 43 (1986): 555–565.

35. D. M. Tucker and coauthors, Iron status and brain function: Serum ferritin levels associated with asymmetries of cortical electrophysiology and cognitive performance, *American Journal of Clinical Nutrition* 39 (1984): 105–113.

36. J. Weinberg, Behavioral and physiological effects of early iron deficiency in the rat, in *Iron Deficiency: Brain Biochemistry and Behavior,* eds. E. Pollitt and R. L. Leibel (New York: Raven Press, 1982), pp. 93–123.

37. R. Hullin, Zinc deficiency: Can it cause dementia? *Therapaecia,* September 1983, pp. 26, 27, 30.

38. Garry and coauthors, 1982.

39. Mental skills of the elderly; lost and found, *Science News* 129 (1986): 244.

40. S. Barrett, Claims and cautions: Megavitamin therapy, *Priorities,* Spring 1989, pp. 27–29.

Food Technology and Food Safety

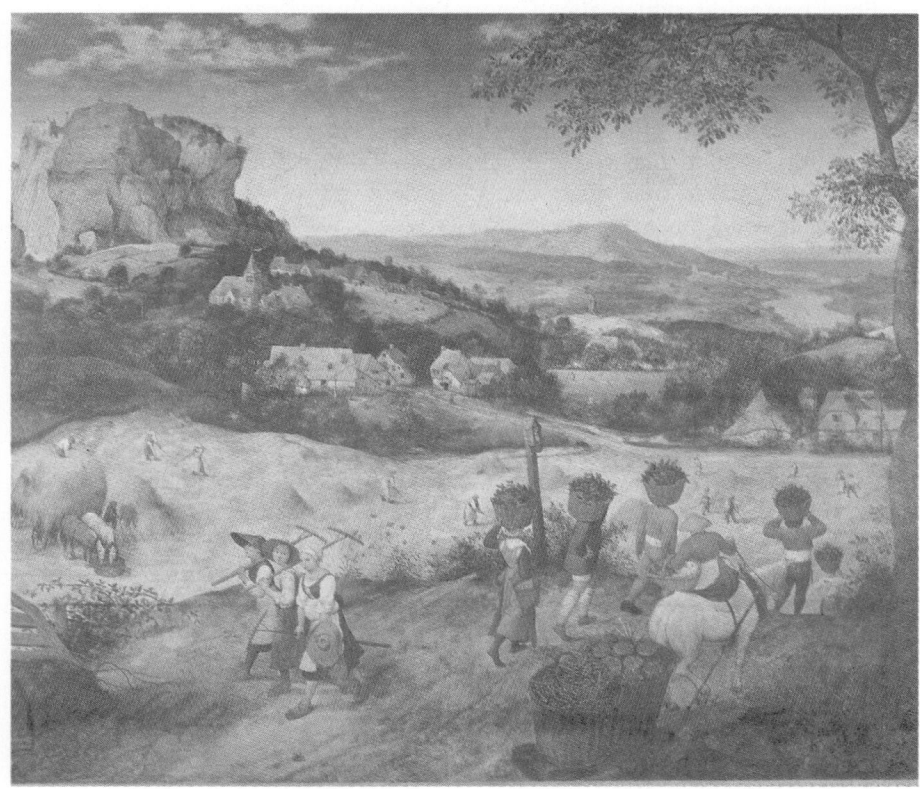

CONTENTS

La Fenaison by Pieter Brueghel, the Elder, Narodni Gallery, Praque. Giraudon/Art Resource, N.Y.

food poisoning: illness transmitted to human beings through food, caused by a poisonous substance (*food intoxication*) or an infectious agent (*foodborne infection*).

botulism: an often-fatal food poisoning caused by botulin toxin, a toxin produced by bacteria that grow without oxygen in nonacidic canned foods.

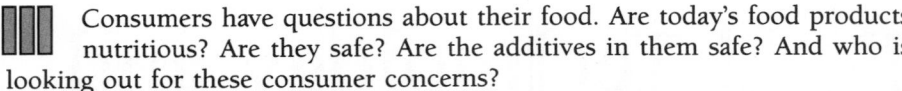 Consumers have questions about their food. Are today's food products nutritious? Are they safe? Are the additives in them safe? And who is looking out for these consumer concerns?

The Food and Drug Administration (FDA) is the agency charged with much of the responsibility of monitoring the food supply. The FDA lists food hazards in order of their impact on human health. What is it about our food supply that actually causes or has the potential to cause the greatest harm to people? FDA ranks risks in order from highest to lowest:

1. Food poisoning, which affects more people every year.
2. Nutrient content, which requires close attention as more and more artificially constituted foods appear on the market.
3. Environmental contaminants (other than pesticides) such as household and industrial chemicals, which are increasing yearly in number and concentration and whose consequences are difficult to foresee and to forestall. The next chapter on global nutrition addresses this concern.
4. Naturally occurring toxicants in foods, which occur randomly and constitute a hazard whenever people turn to consuming single foods either by choice (fad diets) or by necessity (poverty). This topic is addressed in Controversy 14.
5. Pesticide residues, also a topic of the next chapter.
6. Intentional food additives, listed last because so much is known about them and because they are well regulated.

In this free market, where food companies compete for sales, consumers receive benefits—the safest, most pleasing, and most abundant food supply in the world. With these benefits comes the consumers' responsibility of looking out for their own best interests. This chapter provides the information you need to make your food-purchasing decisions with confidence. It begins with the most pressing concern on FDA's list—food poisoning. Nutrient density of processed foods is the second of FDA's priorities and is covered second here. The last item on FDA's list is food additives, a concern for many people who hear about them in the news; the section on additives later in the chapter clears up some common misconceptions. Finally, the Food Feature describes how to store and cook food in ways that preserve its freshness and nutrients.

▐▐▐ Preventing Food Poisoning

Episodes of **food poisoning** cause illness in at least one-third of the U.S. population each year, and their number is increasing yearly. It may be that just about everyone experiences illness from this source within a year's time but may mistakenly pass the incidents off as the "flu."[1]

The term *food poisoning* refers either to foodborne infection—illness caused by infectious microorganisms, such as *Salmonella* varieties, that infect people, or to food intoxication—illness from toxins produced by microorganisms in food such as *Streptococcus* and others. In most illnesses the acute symptoms are mild, with abdominal cramps, headache, vomiting, and diarrhea, the same symptoms that accompany a number of other minor conditions. For people who are otherwise ill or malnourished or for the very old or young, even these relatively mild disturbances can be fatal. If you experience the acute symptoms listed above as the major or only symptoms of your next bout of "flu," chances are excellent that what you really have is food poisoning. (Some viruses do

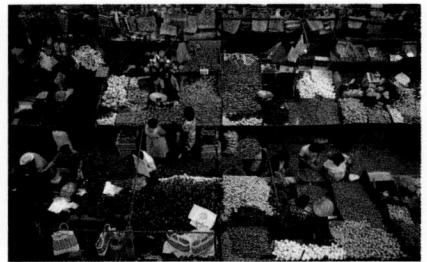

With the privileges of abundance comes the responsibility to choose wisely.

cause intestinal distress, and those that do are usually transmitted via food; the rules for food-poisoning prevention hold for preventing these viruses.) The symptoms of one intoxication stand alone as severe and commonly fatal— those of **botulism,** caused by the toxin of a microbe that grows inside some kinds of canned or vacuum-packed foods. Botulism danger signs constitute a true medical emergency. Even with medical assistance, survivors suffer the effects for months, years, or a lifetime. An amount of botulin toxin as tiny as a single crystal of salt can kill several people within an hour.

It is estimated that between 21 million and 81 million and possibly more cases of diarrhea treated in the United States each year are from food poisoning. Infection from one major food supplier can cause many thousands of cases of illness. For example, when a major dairy developed a flaw in its pasteurization system, over 16,000 confirmed and as many as 200,000 suspected cases of food poisoning resulted. In another episode 100 people died of infection.[2] Consumers have little protection against such large-scale calamities; they must trust government inspectors to enforce strict standards to prevent all but truly unavoidable accidents. Luckily large-scale incidents, while dramatic, make up only a fraction of the total food-poisoning cases each year. Most arise from one person's error in a small setting and affect just a few victims. Some people have come to accept a yearly bout or two of intestinal illness as inevitable, but in truth, most of these illnesses can be prevented. To protect themselves, consumers need to learn how to select, prepare, and store food safely.

Commercially prepared food is usually safe. Batch numbering makes it possible to recall contaminated foods through public announcements via newspapers, television, and radio, and FDA monitors large suppliers. Home-canned food can be prepared safely as long as proper canning techniques are followed to the letter. Local U.S. Department of Agriculture (USDA) extension agents can provide these instructions. Raw food, especially meats and poultry, from the grocery store contains microbes, as all things do. Food picks up microbes during processing or in transit, and as the microbes multiply, the foods can become unsafe. Whether or not microbes from these sources multiply and cause illness can be largely a matter of what you do or fail to do in the grocery store and in your own kitchen.

In the store, carefully inspect the seals and wrappers of packages; reject leaking or bulging cans. Many jars have safety "buttons," areas of the lid designed to pop up once opened; make sure that they and other jars are firmly sealed. Frozen foods should be solidly frozen and stored below the frost line in the freezer case. Notice how the majority of the packages on the shelf appear. If the one you have chosen looks ragged or soiled or if it has holes or tears in it, do not buy the product—turn it in to the store manager. A broken seal, a badly dented can, or a mangled package cannot ensure protection from microorganisms, insects, spoilage, or even vandals.

Food Safety in the Kitchen

Food can provide ideal conditions for bacteria to thrive. Bacteria require:

■ Warmth (40 to 140° F).
■ Moisture.
■ Nutrients.

To defeat them, people who prepare food can do these three things: keep hot food hot, keep cold food cold, and keep the kitchen clean. Keeping hot food

Most cases of food poisoning clear up spontaneously. See a doctor if symptoms seem severe or if the victim is young or weak. If you suspect botulism, seek help at once. Symptoms of botulism:
■ Double vision.
■ Weakening muscles.
■ Difficulty swallowing.
■ Difficulty breathing.

Remember the rule of 2, 40–140: hold food no longer than two hours at temperatures between 40 and 140° F.

hot includes allowing sufficient cooking time for food to reach internal temperatures sufficient to kill microbes during cooking (these temperatures are listed on meat thermometers) and holding it at a high enough temperature to prevent bacterial growth until served. Temperatures between 140 and 165° F are usually safe for up to two hours. After that the food should be chilled. Another two-hour rule: keep food at room temperature (between 40 and 140° F) no longer than two hours.

Keeping cold food cold starts when you leave the grocery store; if you are running errands, shop last, so that the groceries will not stay in the car too long. (If ice cream begins to melt, it has been too long.) Pack foods into the refrigerator or freezer immediately upon arrival at home.

Keeping a clean kitchen includes using freshly washed hands and utensils and laundered towels. If you are ill, it includes staying away from food to prevent its contamination.

Microbes love to nestle down in small, damp spaces such as those between the fibers of wooden cutting boards or in the inner cells of sponges. To eliminate the microbes you have three choices, each with benefits and drawbacks. One is to poison the microbes where they reside, by washing items with toxic chemicals such as bleach (one capful per gallon of water). The benefit here is that chlorine can kill even the hardiest organism. The obvious drawback is that chlorine that washes down household drains into the water supply forms chemicals that can harm waterways and fish.

A second option is to treat sponges and boards with heat. Soapy water heated to 140 degrees Fahrenheit kills most harmful organisms and washes most others away. This takes effort, though, for you have to use truly scalding water.

The third option is to use nonporous boards for cutting and launderable dishcloths for wiping (change the dishcloths often). For a small initial investment you reap truly safe utensils with which to prepare your food.

❚❚▶ *To prevent food poisoning, hold foods at their proper temperatures, keep them in sanitary conditions, and remember that food poisoning is always a possibility.*

Troublesome Foods

Meat requires special handling. It may contain all sorts of bacteria, and it provides a moist, nutritious environment—just right for microbial growth. If you take burgers out to the grill on a plate, wash that plate in hot, soapy water before using it to hold the cooked burgers. Otherwise the bacteria inevitably left on the plate from the raw meat can contaminate and grow in the cooked food that people plan to eat.

Especially susceptible to bacterial contamination is ground meat. It is handled more than other kinds of meat and has much more surface exposed to the air for bacteria to land on. It is best to cook hamburgers to at least medium well done. For a meatloaf, use a thermometer to test the internal temperature.

It goes without saying that any food with an off appearance or odor should not be used or even tasted. However, you cannot rely on your senses of smell or sight alone to warn you of hazards because most contamination is not detectable by odor, taste, or appearance. To protect yourself, you must remember that food poisoning is always a possibility; so comply with food safety rules before eating. For example, if you are at a buffet and some meatballs in a warming tray are warm but not hot when you choose them, remember the rule of 2, 40–140. Food at 140° F feels hot, not just warm. The likelihood of illness is strong in this situation, and the pleasure of eating meatballs isn't worth the

■■■ TABLE 14–1 How to Prevent Food Poisoning

To keep hot foods hot

When cooking meats or poultry, use a meat thermometer to test the internal temperature. Insert the thermometer between the thigh and the body of the turkey or in the thickest part of other meats, making sure the tip of the thermometer is not in contact with bone. Cook to the temperature indicated for that particular meat; cook hamburgers to at least medium well done.

Cook stuffing separately or stuff poultry just prior to cooking.

Do not cook large cuts of meats or turkeys in a microwave oven because large, solid meats may not cook evenly, and cool spots can harbor microbes.

Cook eggs before eating them (simmered for seven minutes, poached for five, or fried for three minutes on each side).

When serving foods, maintain temperatures above 140° F.

Heat leftovers thoroughly to at least 140° F.

To keep cold foods cold

When running errands, stop at the grocery store last. When you get home, refrigerate the perishables immediately.

Buy only those foods stored below the frost line in store freezers.

Keep cold foods at 40° F or less.

Refrigerate leftovers promptly; use shallow containers to help foods cool faster.

Thaw meats or poultry in the refrigerator, not at room temperature. If you must hasten thawing, use cool running water or a microwave oven.

Tote lunches in a thermal lunch bag. Freeze plastic bottles or pouches of beverages and let them keep the lunch cool as they thaw out through the morning.

To keep a clean kitchen

Use warm, soapy water to wash hands, utensils, dishes, cutting boards, and countertops.

Avoid cross contamination by washing all surfaces that have been in contact with raw meats, poultry, or eggs before reusing.

Mix foods with utensils, not hands; keep hands and utensils away from mouth, nose, and hair.

Avoid coughing or sneezing over food. A person with a skin infection or infectious disease should not prepare food.

Wash or replace sponges and towels regularly.

Clean up food spills and crumb-filled crevices.

In general

Throw out foods with off odors.

Do not even taste food that is suspect.

Do not buy or use items that appear to have been opened.

Follow label instructions for storing and preparing packaged and frozen foods.

risk, even if you must go hungry for awhile. Study Table 14–1; if you learn and follow the rules given there, you can apply them to avoid illnesses.

Picnics are fun and can be safe too. Choose foods that last without refrigeration, such as fresh fruits and vegetables, breads and crackers, and canned spreads and cheeses that you can open and use on the spot. Aged cheeses, such as cheddar and Swiss, do well for an hour or two, but for longer periods, carry them in an ice chest. The advice not to add mayonnaise to picnic foods such as meat or pasta salads has been reversed by some who cite a study that found that mayonnaise was resistant to spoilage because of its acid content. Still, whether or not they contain mayonnaise, mixed salads of chopped ingredients spoil easily because they have extensive surface area for bacteria to invade and because they have been in contact with cutting boards, hands, and kitchen utensils that easily transmit bacteria to food. Chill them well before, during, and after the picnic. Keep mayonnaise itself cold. To be safe, follow the two, 40°-140° temperature safety rules.

Another danger concerns honey. Honey has been found to contain dormant bacterial spores that can awaken in the human body to produce the deadly botulin toxin mentioned earlier. Adults are big and strong enough to withstand the doses usually encountered, but infants under one year of age should never be fed honey.[3] (It can also be contaminated with environmental pollutants

sushi: vinegar-flavored rice and seafood, typically wrapped in seaweed and stuffed with colorful vegetables. Some sushi is stuffed with raw fish; other varieties contain only cooked ingredients.

picked up by the bees.) Honey has been implicated in several cases of sudden infant death.[4]

For adults and children alike, eating raw or lightly steamed seafood is a risky proposition even if it is eaten in **sushi** prepared by a master Japanese chef. The microorganisms that lurk there are undetectable, even to an expert.

People who like sushi know that not all varieties are made from raw fish. Many types are made with cooked crabmeat and vegetables, avocado, or other delicacies and are perfectly safe to enjoy. Also, rumor has it that freezing fish will make it safe to eat raw, but this is only partly true. Freezing fish will kill mature parasitic worms, but only cooking can kill all worm eggs and other microorganisms that can cause illness.

As population density increases along the shores of seafood-harvesting waters, pollution of those waters inevitably invades the seafood living there. Watchdog agencies monitor commercial fishing waters and try to keep harvesters out of the worst areas, and they eventually do catch cheaters. But meanwhile, unwholesome food can reach the market.[5] In one season alone, black-market dealers may sell millions of dollars worth of clams and oysters taken illegally from closed harvesting areas.[6]

The foodborne infections that lurk in normal-appearing seafood can be even worse than those of spoilage—hepatitis; worms, flukes, and other parasites; severe viral intestinal disorders; and other diseases. Hepatitis is a prolonged illness of months' or years' duration and also causes severe damage to the liver and other serious symptoms. Hepatitis also greatly increases the risk of developing liver cancer, and is transmissible to others through sexual activity. Many types of worms depend on the blood of their host for food and reproduction; they attack digestive membranes, sometimes causing life-threatening perforations. Flukes attack the liver, damaging it. People who love raw seafood and have eaten it for years may try to brush off these threats because they have never experienced serious illness. Now, though, experts say that the risks of consuming raw or lightly cooked seafood have become unacceptably high.

CONSUMER CAUTION ▌▌▌ Food Safety While Traveling

If you travel to places where cleanliness standards are lacking, chances are about even that you will suffer from digestive infections that can ruin your trip—traveler's diarrhea. You can take steps to protect your health against disease-causing organisms not found at home. To avoid illness:

■ Wash your hands often with soap and water, especially before handling food or eating.

■ Eat only cooked food and canned foods. Eat raw fruits or vegetables only if you have washed them in boiled water and peeled them yourself. Skip salads.

■ Be aware that water, and ice made from it, may be unsafe, too. Drink only boiled, canned, or bottled beverages, and drink them without ice, even if they are not chilled to your liking.

■ Avoid using the local water supply, even if you are just brushing your teeth, unless you boil or disinfect it first.

continued on next page

■ Take along disinfecting tablets or an element that boils water in a cup.
■ Before you leave on the trip, check with your physician for recommendations on which medicines to take with you in case your efforts to avoid illness fail.

Do not take the medicines in hopes of warding off illness unless your physician directs you to do so. Chances are excellent, if you follow the rules above, that you will remain well.

▌▌▶ *Disease and illness can be transmitted to people through foods that harbor microbes or their toxins. Almost all cases of food poisoning can be averted by following the rules of safe food preparation, storage, and cleanliness. Organisms in seafood may cause serious illness unless the seafood is thoroughly cooked.*

▌▌▌ Food Processing and Nutrient Density

The first question about foods that most people want answered is how processing affects nutritional quality. The FDA ranks this concern second in importance only to food poisoning because of its far-reaching impact on health. A great percentage of the total food consumed, whether eaten in restaurants or at home, has been prepared in some way by industry. People often ask what processing does to foods and which kinds of foods are most and least nutritious.

In general, food processing involves a tradeoff: it makes food safer and gives it a longer usable lifetime than fresh food, but at the cost of some vitamin and mineral losses. A process such as **pasteurization,** the heating of milk to make it safe from disease-causing organisms, is clearly worth the cost of small nutrient losses. Other processed foods may even gain a nutritional edge over their unprocessed counterparts, such as when fat is removed by processing from milk or other foods. This section explains each of the processing techniques, **canning, freezing, drying,** and **extrusion,** and the effects they have on nutrients.

Canning

Which nutrients are affected by canning, and how are they affected? Canning is one of the better methods for preserving food against the microbes (bacteria, fungi, and yeasts) that might otherwise spoil it, but canned foods, unfortunately, do have fewer nutrients. Like other heat treatments, the canning process is based on time and temperature. Each small increase in temperature has a major killing effect on microbes with only a minor effect on nutrients. By contrast, long treatment times are costly in terms of nutrient losses. Therefore industry chooses treatments that employ the **high-temperature–short-time (HTST) principle** for canning.

To determine how much of a food's nutritional value is lost in canning, food scientists have performed many experiments. They have paid particular attention to three vulnerable water-soluble vitamins—thiamin, riboflavin, and vitamin C.

Acid stabilizes thiamin, but heat rapidly destroys it; therefore the foods that lose the most thiamin during canning are the low-acid foods such as lima

pasteurization: the treatment of milk with heat sufficient to kill certain pathogens (disease-causing microbes) commonly transmitted through milk, not a sterilization process. Pasteurized milk retains bacteria that causes milk spoilage. Raw milk, even if labeled "certified," transmits many foodborne diseases to people each year and should be avoided.

canning: preservation by killing all microorganisms present in food and sealing out air. The food, its container, and its lid are heated until sterile; as the food cools, the lid makes an airtight seal, preventing contamination.

freezing: preservation by lowering food temperature to the point at which life processes cease. Microorganisms are not destroyed but are held dormant as long as the food is frozen.

drying: preservation by removing sufficient water from food to inhibit microbial growth.

extrusion: a heat process by which the form of food is changed, such as changing corn to corn chips; not a preservation measure.

high-temperature–short-time (HTST) principle: every 10° C (18° F) rise in processing temperature gives approximately a tenfold increase in microbial destruction, while it only doubles nutrient losses.

To see the effect of canning on thiamin in foods, look at Appendix A, items 563 and 564 (3 oz of raw clams versus 3 oz of canned clams). Or check the thiamin in items 890 and 891 (½ cup frozen green peas versus ½ cup canned green peas). While you are looking, what other effects of canning on thiamin do you see?

beans, corn, and meat. Up to half, or even more, of the thiamin in these foods can be lost during canning. Unlike thiamin, riboflavin is stable to heat but sensitive to light; so glass-packed, not canned, foods are most likely to lose riboflavin. Vitamin C's special enemy is an enzyme (ascorbic acid oxidase) present in fruits and vegetables as well as in microorganisms. By destroying this enzyme, HTST processes such as canning actually aid in preserving vitamin C, while the short time of treatment means less of the vitamin is destroyed. As for the fat-soluble vitamins, they are relatively stable and are not affected much by canning.

Minerals are unaffected by heat processing because they cannot be destroyed, as vitamins can be. However, both minerals and the vitamins can be lost when they leak into water that the consumer may throw away. Losses are closely related to the extent to which a food's tissues have been broken, cut, or chopped and to the length of time the food is in the water.

Some minerals are added when foods are canned. Important in this regard is sodium chloride. In general, the more highly a food is processed, the more sodium chloride and the less potassium it is likely to contain, as Chapter 8 demonstrated. Many food companies have begun making low-salt varieties, although these usually cost more than the higher salt versions.

▌▌▷ *Food contents of some water-soluble vitamins are slightly reduced by canning, but many more diffuse into the canning liquid. Fat-soluble vitamins and minerals are not affected by canning, but minerals also leach into canning liquid.*

Freezing

An alternative to canning, as a means of preserving food, is freezing. People often ask how frozen foods compare with canned. In general, frozen foods' nutrient contents are similar to those of fresh foods; losses are minimal. The freezing process itself does not destroy any nutrients, but some losses may occur during the steps taken in preparation for freezing, such as the quick dunking into boiling water (blanching), washing, trimming, or grinding. Vitamin C losses are especially likely because they occur whenever tissues are broken and exposed to air (oxygen destroys vitamin C). Uncut fruits, especially if they are acidic, do not lose their vitamin C; strawberries, for example, may be kept frozen for over a year without losing any vitamin C.

Fresh foods are often shipped long distances, and to make the trip without bruising or spoiling, they are often harvested unripe. Frozen foods are shipped frozen, so that produce is allowed to ripen in the field and to develop nutrients to their fullest potential. If foods are frozen and stored under proper conditions, they will often contain more nutrients when served at the table than fresh fruits and vegetables that have stayed in the produce department of the grocery store even for a day.

Frozen foods have to be kept frozen to retain their nutrients. To be solidly frozen, a food has to be colder than 32° F or 0° C. Conversion of vitamin C to its inactive forms occurs rapidly at warmer temperatures. Food may seem frozen at 2° C, but much of it is actually unfrozen, and enzyme-mediated changes occur more rapidly than if it were solidly frozen. Under these conditions the vitamin C in a frozen food can be completely lost in as short a time as two months.

In general, for frozen foods, the lower the temperature the longer the storage life and the greater the nutrient retention. If you want to maximize the nutritive value of the foods you store at home, invest in a freezer thermometer, monitor the temperature of your frozen-food storage place, and keep it below freezing.

◨▷ *Foods frozen promptly and kept frozen lose few nutrients.*

Drying

Consumers wonder how dried or dehydrated foods compare with canned and frozen foods. Dried or dehydrated foods have their own special characteristics. Drying offers several advantages. It eliminates microbial spoilage (because microbes need water to grow), and it greatly reduces the weight and volume of foods (because foods are mostly water). Furthermore, commercial drying does not cause major nutrient losses. However, foods dried in heated ovens at home may sustain dramatic nutrient losses. Vacuum puff drying and freeze drying, which take place in cold temperatures, conserve nutrients especially well.

Sulfite additives are added during the drying of fruits such as peaches, grapes (raisins), and plums (prunes) to prevent browning. (Some people suffer allergic reactions when they consume sulfites, as discussed later.) Sulfur dioxide helps to preserve vitamin C as well, but it is highly destructive of thiamin. The overall effect of its addition is probably beneficial because most dehydrated products with added sulfur dioxide are not major sources of thiamin anyway.

Extrusion

Some food products, particularly snack foods, have undergone a process known as extrusion. In this process the food is heated, ground, and pushed through various kinds of screens to yield different shapes, usually bite-sized or smaller, such as pieces of breakfast cereal or the "bits" you sprinkle on salad— so-called food novelties. Considerable nutrient losses occur during extrusion processes, and nutrients are usually added to compensate. But foods this far removed from the original fresh state are still lacking significant nutrients (notably vitamin E), and consumers should not rely on them as staple foods. Enjoy them, but only as occasional snacks and as additions to enhance the appearance, taste, and variety of meals.

◨▷ *Commercially dried foods retain most of their nutrients. When sulfur dioxide is added, thiamin may be destroyed. Extrusion involves heat and destroys nutrients.*

Choosing Wisely

In general, the more heavily processed foods are, the less nutritious they become. Does that mean, then, that everyone should avoid all processed food? The answer is not simple: in each case it depends on the food and on the process. Consider the case of orange juice and vitamin C. Orange juice is available in several forms, each processed a different way. Fresh juice is simply squeezed from the orange—a process that extracts the fluid juice from the fibrous structures that contain it. The fresh-squeezed juice, per 100 calories, contains 111 milligrams of vitamin C. If this juice were condensed by heat, frozen, and then reconstituted, as is the juice in the freezer case of the grocery store, 100 calories of the reconstituted juice would contain just 88 milligrams

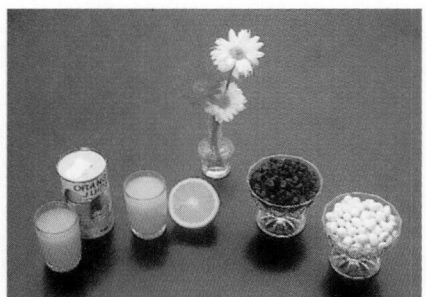

Canned juice is almost as nutritious as fresh, but yogurt-covered raisins are *not* as nutritious as plain raisins.

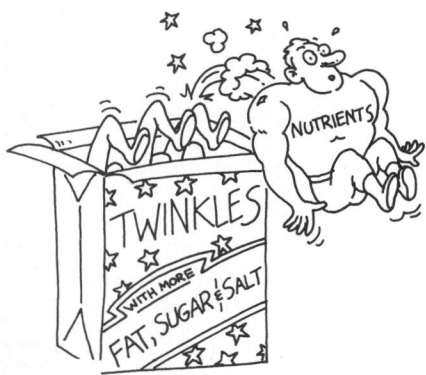

Many heavily processed foods have lost nutrients and have gained fat, sugar, and salt.

of vitamin C—vitamin C is destroyed in the condensing process. Canning is even harder on the vitamin C content of orange juice— 100 calories of canned juice has 82 milligrams of vitamin C.

These figures may seem to indicate that fresh juice is the superior food, and so it is, but consider this: the U.S. Recommended Dietary Allowance (U.S. RDA) for vitamin C is 60 milligrams, an amount covered single-handedly by one serving of any of the above choices. In this case, at least for vitamin C, the losses due to processing are not a problem, and there is an enormous convenience and distribution advantage to the processing. Fresh orange juice spoils. Shipping it cold to distant points uncondensed is much more expensive than shipping frozen juice (which takes up less space) or canned juice (which requires no refrigeration). The fresh product cannot be stored indefinitely without compromising nutrient quality. Without canned or frozen juice, people who have no access to the fresh juice would be deprived of this excellent food.

Some processing stories are not so rosy. In Chapter 8, for instance, you saw how processed foods are often loaded with sodium as their potassium is leached away. A related mischief of processing is the addition of sugar and fat—palatable, high-calorie additives that reduce nutrient density. An example is nuts and raisins covered with "natural yogurt." This may sound like one healthy food being added to another, but a look at the ingredient panel warns that generous amounts of fat and sugar accompany the yogurt. About 75 percent of the weight of the product is fat and sugar, about 8 percent is yogurt. To pick just one nutrient for an example, here is what happens to the iron density of the raisins: 100 calories of raisins = 0.71 milligrams iron; 100 calories of "yogurt" raisins = 0.26 milligrams of iron. These foods taste so good that wishful thinking can easily take hold, but the reality is that fat- and sugar-coated food is candy. The word *yogurt* on the label means only that one of the ingredients of the candy coating is some small amount of yogurt. Names, even whole-food names, written on labels do not prove that the foods so named confer any nutritional benefit on the consumer unless the foods themselves are nutritious.

Incidentally, do not conclude from this example that raisins are a good source of iron. Compared with other food sources of iron on a per-calorie basis, raisins fall short. If you relied on raisins to supply 100 percent of the U.S. RDA for iron, you would have to eat 2600 calories of them in one day. In contrast, 114 calories of spinach meets the U.S. RDA for iron. Figures 8–10 and 8–11 in Chapter 8 showed some iron-rich foods.

A generalization for optimal food choices might be to choose whole foods to the greatest extent possible. Being realistic, few people have the time to bake all their own bread from scratch, to shop every few days for fresh meats, or to wash, peel, chop, and cook fresh fruits and vegetables at every meal. This is where food processing comes in. Commercially prepared whole-grain breads, frozen cuts of meats, bags of frozen vegetables, and canned or frozen fruit juices do little disservice to nutrition and enable the consumer to eat a wide variety of foods. The nutrient contents of processed foods exist on a continuum:

Whole-grain bread > refined white bread > sugared doughnuts.
Milk > fruit-flavored yogurt > canned chocolate pudding.
Corn on the cob > canned creamed corn > caramel popcorn.
Oranges > orange juice > orange-flavored drink.
Baked ham > deviled ham > fried bacon.

Another continuum parallels it—the nutrition status of the consumer. The closer to the farm the foods you eat, the better nourished you are, but that doesn't mean you have to live in the fields.

These pointers have answered the specific questions people most often ask about processed foods. What about fresh foods, then? Another generalization may be useful: as fresh food quality (appearance, taste, and texture) deteriorates, its nutrient content often deteriorates to match. For example, when a food smells bad, the odor reveals that oxidative or enzymatic changes have occurred—the same kinds of reactions as those that have adverse effects on nutrients. Thus some unprocessed foods sold as "natural" foods may be a poor choice in spite of the claims made for them. If they have lost their freshness, they may well have lost their vitamins, too, because "no processing" means no measures have been taken to prevent oxidative and enzymatic changes. Thus your common sense, which tells you that a food "doesn't look quite right," can often be trusted to give you valid information.

In modern commercial processing, losses of vitamins seldom exceed 25 percent. In contrast, losses in food preparation at home can be close to 100 percent, and it is not unusual to see losses in the 60 to 75 percent range. These facts put the matter of food processing into perspective and reveal that while the kinds of foods you buy certainly make a difference, what you do with them in your kitchen can make an even greater difference. This chapter's Food Feature shows ways you can make sure that your food delivers nutrients to its fullest potential.

||▶ *Many processed foods are wise choices because they are nutritious, convenient, and available. In some foods, fat and sugar have been processed in, nutrients processed out, and these should be used sparingly.*

▮▮▮ Food Additives

Most people want to know about **additives.** What are they, why are they there, and are they dangerous in any way? Are the foods labeled "no additives" better for health than others? Those questions are valid, and FDA lists food additives among its concerns, as shown on the list that was given at the start of this chapter.

The safety of food additives is not first, or even third, on the FDA's list of priority concerns; it is sixth and last. This doesn't mean that additives are of no concern—they are, to many people. It does mean, though, that the other five hazards present greater causes for concern.

Some definitions will assist understanding of these crucial concerns. Substances put into foods on purpose are **intentional food additives,** while **incidental food additives** are those that may get in unintentionally during processing. This discussion begins with the intentional additives, and after taking them up class by class, it goes on to the incidental additives.

Intentional food additives are substances put into foods to give them some desirable characteristic: color, flavor, texture, stability, or resistance to spoilage. Some are nutrients added to foods to increase their nutritional value, such as vitamin C added to fruit drinks or potassium iodide added to salt. Additives, classed by their functions, are listed as glossary terms on this page, and each is treated in a section of its own to follow.

additives: substances not normally consumed as foods by themselves but added to foods either intentionally or unintentionally.

intentional food additives: additives intentionally added to food, such as nutrients or colors. See the Miniglossary on page 494.

incidental food additives: substances that can get into food not through intentional introduction but as a result of contact with the food during growing, processing, packaging, storing, or some other stage before the food is consumed. The terms *accidental* or *indirect additives* mean the same thing.

safety: the practical certainty that injury will not result from the use of a substance.

GRAS (generally recognized as safe) list: a list of food additives, established by the FDA, that had long been in use and were believed safe. The list is subject to revision as new facts become known.

Regulations Governing Additives

The agency charged with the responsibility for deciding what additives shall be in foods is the FDA. The FDA's authority over additives hinges primarily on their **safety.** A manufacturer has to go through a special procedure that can take many years to get permission to use a new additive in food products. The manufacturer must test it to satisfy the FDA of the following:

■ It is effective (it does what it is supposed to do).
■ It can be detected and measured in the final food product.

Then the manufacturer has to feed the additive in large doses to animals under strictly controlled conditions and prove that:

■ It is safe (it causes no cancer, birth defects, or other injury).

Finally, the manufacturer must submit all test results to the FDA.

The FDA then calls a public hearing and announces the topic, date, and location in its official publication, *FDA Consumer.* Consumers are invited to participate at these hearings, where experts present testimony for and against granting permission to use the additive. Thus the consumer's rights and responsibilities are written into the provisions for deeming additives safe.

If the FDA approves the additive's use, that does not mean the manufacturer can add it in any amount to any food. On the contrary: the FDA writes a regulation stating in what amounts and in what foods the additive may be used. No additives are permanently approved; all are periodically reviewed.

Many substances were exempted from complying with this procedure at the time it was first instituted because they had been used a long time and their use entailed no known hazards. Some 700 substances in all were put on the **generally recognized as safe (GRAS) list**. However, any time substantial scientific evidence or public outcry has questioned the safety of any of the substances on the GRAS list, it has been reevaluated. All substances about which any legitimate question was raised have been removed or reclassified. A set of 2100 flavoring agents has similarly been reviewed, as well as some 200 coloring agents. Meanwhile the entire GRAS list is subjected to an ongoing review.

To remain on the GRAS list, an additive must not have been found to be a carcinogen in any test on animals or human beings. The Delaney clause (the part of the law that states this criterion) is uncompromising in addressing carcinogens in food and drugs; in fact, it has been under fire in recent years for being too strict and inflexible.

The Delaney clause states that "no additive shall be deemed to be safe if it is found to induce cancer when ingested by man or animal." That sounds simple and clear enough, yet you may be aware of additives in products on the market that fail to meet that criteria. Saccharin paved the way for exceptions to the rule. In the 1970s, when FDA tried to ban saccharin because tests had revealed that it caused cancer in animals, Congress made a special exception that allowed saccharin to remain on the market as long as products containing it carried a warning. This was their best effort in trying to balance the Delaney clause with current food safety and cancer knowledge. A little historical background may provide some insight.

The Delaney clause was adopted over 30 years ago, at a time when scientists knew only that radiation, tobacco smoke, a chemical used to make dyes, and soot caused cancer. Since then researchers have identified more than three dozen human carcinogens and several hundred animal carcinogens. In addition, technology has advanced so that substances once detectable only in parts per thousand can now be measured in parts per billion or even per trillion. (One part per trillion is equivalent to about one grain of sugar in an Olympic-sized swimming pool or one hair on ten million heads, assuming none are bald.) An FDA official states, "Given the extraordinarily low levels at which analytical chemists could measure chemical contaminants in food or anything else, all substances, no matter how pure, could be shown to be contaminated with one carcinogen or another."[7] In other words, we cannot provide absolute protection from all carcinogens in foods, as Congressman Delaney once thought we could. For practical purposes, FDA deems additives "safe" if they present no more than a one-in-a-million risk of human cancer.

An important distinction that governs determinations of additives' safety is the distinction between **toxicity** as a property of substances and **hazard** associated with substances. "Toxicity—the capacity of a chemical substance to harm living organisms—is a general property of matter; hazard is the capacity of a chemical to produce injury under conditions of its use. All substances are potentially toxic but are hazardous only if consumed in sufficiently large quantities."[8] An additive is not considered to be a hazard if some immense amount that people never consume is toxic. The additive is a hazard only if it is toxic under the conditions of its actual use. A food additive is supposed to have a wide **margin of safety**.

Most additives that involve risk are allowed in foods only at levels 100 times below those at which the risk is still known to be zero; their margin of safety is 1/100. Experiments to determine the extent of risk involve feeding test animals the substance at different concentrations throughout their lifetimes. The additive is then permitted in foods at 1/100 the level that can be fed under these conditions without causing any harmful effect whatever. In many foods, naturally occurring substances appear at levels that bring their margins of safety closer to 1/10. Even nutrients, as you have seen, involve risks at high dosage levels. The margin of safety for vitamins A and D is 1/25 to 1/40; it may be less than 1/10 in infants. For some trace elements it is about 1/5. People consume common table salt daily in amounts only three to five times less than those that cause serious toxicity.

The margin-of-safety concept also applies to nutrients when they are used as additives. Iodine has been added to salt to prevent iodine deficiency, but it has had to be added with care because it is a deadly poison in excess. Similarly, iron has been added to refined bread and other grains (enrichment) and has doubtless helped prevent many cases of iron-deficiency anemia in women and children who are prone to that disease. But the addition of too much iron could put men (who usually have enough iron in their bodies) at risk for iron overload. The upper limit has to be remembered.

All the additives just named are in foods for a reason. They offer benefits that outweigh the risks they present or that make the risks worth taking. In the case of color additives that only enhance the appearance of foods but do not improve their health value or safety, no amount of risk may be deemed worth taking. Only 33 of an original 200 color additives are still approved by the FDA for use in foods, and screening of these continues.

toxicity: the ability of a substance to harm living organisms. All substances are toxic if high enough concentrations are used.

hazard: state of danger; used to refer to any circumstance in which harm is possible under normal conditions of use.

margin of safety: as used when speaking of food additives, a zone between the concentration normally used and that at which a hazard exists. For common table salt, for example, the margin of safety is 1/5 (five times the concentration normally used would be hazardous).

A carcinogen is a cancer-causing agent.

■■■ **Miniglossary of Intentional Food Additives by Function**

antimicrobial agents: preservatives that keep microorganisms from growing.

antioxidants: chemicals that prevent rancidity of fats and other damage to food caused by oxygen. (See also definition in Chapter 5.)

artificial colors: certified food colors, added to enhance appearance. (*Certified* means approved by the FDA.)

artificial flavors, flavor enhancers: chemicals that mimic natural flavors and those that enhance flavor.

nutrient additives: vitamins and minerals added to improve nutritive value.

radiation: ionizing rays that disrupt chemical structures within cells.

It is also the manufacturers' responsibility to use only the amounts of additives necessary to get the needed effects, not more. Additives must also *not* be used:

■ To disguise faulty or inferior products.
■ To deceive the consumer.
■ Where they significantly destroy nutrients.
■ Where their effects can be achieved by economical, sound manufacturing processes.

The regulations in force governing the management of intentional additives are well conceived and have been effective, on the whole. Cutbacks in funding in the mid-1980s limit the capabilities of watchdog agencies such as the FDA, however, and some mistakes and cases of false reporting are bound to slip by.

■■▶ *FDA regulates the use of intentional additives; additives must be safe, effective, and measurable in the final product. Additives on the GRAS list are assumed to be safe because they have long been used. No additive may be used that has been found to cause cancer in animals or people, and those used must have wide margins of safety.*

A Closer Look at Selected Food Additives

The following sections focus on a few individual food additives—notably, those that have received the most negative publicity because people ask questions about them most often. The order is alphabetical; it does not imply an order of importance. The Miniglossary above defines the six categories of additives that follow; the margin definitions describe examples within each category.

ANTIMICROBIAL AGENTS. Foods can go bad in two ways: one dangerous, one not. The dangerous way is by becoming hazardous to health; the other way is by losing their flavor and attractiveness. An example of the former: bacteria, yeasts, and molds and other fungi growing in foods can cause food poisoning. Preservatives known as **antimicrobial agents** protect foods from these microbes.

The best known, most widely used antimicrobial agents are the two common substances salt and sugar. Salt has been used since before recorded history to preserve meat and fish; sugar serves the same purpose in canned and frozen fruits as well as jams and jellies. (Any jam or jelly that toots its "no preservatives" horn is exaggerating. There is no need to add extra preservatives, so most makers do not.) Both salt and sugar work by withdrawing water from the food; microbes cannot grow without water. Today, other additives such as potassium sorbate and sodium propionate are also used to extend the shelf life of baked goods, cheese, beverages, mayonnaise, margarine, and many other products.

Another group of antimicrobial agents, the **nitrites,** is added to foods for three main purposes: to preserve their color (especially the pink color of hotdogs and other cured meats); to enhance their flavor by inhibiting rancidity (especially in cured meats); and to protect against bacterial growth. In particular, in amounts much smaller than needed to confer color, nitrites prevent the growth of the botulinum bacteria that produce the deadly toxin described earlier in the chapter.

Nitrites clearly perform important jobs, but they have been the object of controversy because they can be converted in the human body to nitrosamines, which cause cancer in animals. Some cured meats are available without nitrites. However, reducing nitrites consumed in meats would hardly make a difference in a person's overall exposure to nitrosamine-related compounds. For example, an average cigarette smoker inhales 100 times the nitrosamines that the average bacon eater ingests; a beer drinker ingests up to roughly five times the amount of the bacon eater. Cosmetics deliver via absorption through skin about twice the amount delivered from bacon, and even the air inside automobiles delivers a measurable amount.[9]

ANTIOXIDANTS. The other way in which food can go bad is by undergoing changes in color and flavor caused by exposure to oxygen in the air (oxidation). Often these changes involve no hazard to health, but they damage the food's appearance, taste, and nutritional quality. Familiar examples of these changes are the way sliced apples or potatoes turn brown or oil goes rancid. Preservatives known as **antioxidants** protect food from this kind of spoilage.

A total of 27 antioxidants are approved for use in foods. Vitamin C (ascorbate) and vitamin E (tocopherol) are among them. Vitamin E is added to bacon to prevent nitrosamine formation while assisting nitrite's antioxidant activity. When the vitamin E additive is present in bacon along with the regular amount of nitrite preservative, nitrosamine formation is inhibited by more than half.

Another group of preservatives is the **sulfites.** They are cheaper than the vitamins and are used to prevent oxidation in many processed foods, in alcoholic beverages (especially wine), and in drugs. They used to be popular with restaurant owners for use on salad bars because they keep raw fruits and vegetables looking fresh, but this use has been banned. The ban came after some people experienced allergic reactions to the sulfites—reactions that were sometimes dangerous, and for a few, deadly.[10] The FDA has taken a number of steps to protect people who are allergic to sulfites. It prohibits sulfite use on food intended to be consumed raw; it requires that foods declare sulfite additives on their labels' ingredient lists and that drug labels warn that sulfites are present. For most people the sulfites do not pose a hazard in the amounts used in products,[11] but there is one more consideration: sulfiting agents destroy an appreciable amount of the vitamin thiamin in foods. A person choosing a food that contains sulfites should not count on that food to provide a share of the daily need for thiamin.

The ban on sulfites has stimulated research to look for alternatives. For example, some producers use honey to clarify browned apple juice. Agriculturists have also created a hybrid apple that doesn't brown.[12] One manufacturer

nitrites: salts added to food to prevent botulism. Compounds called **nitrosamines** (nigh-TROHS-uh-meens) are derivatives of nitrites that may be formed in the stomach when nitrites combine with amines, and nitrosamines are carcinogenic.

sulfites: salts containing sulfur, added to fresh and frozen fruits and vegetables to prevent spoilage.

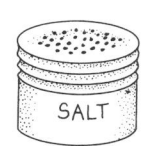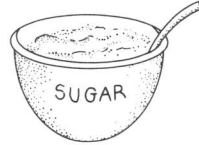

Two long-used preservatives.

has combined four GRAS additives* to create a product that can substitute for sulfites.[13]

Two other antioxidants in wide use are the well-known BHA and BHT, which prevent rancidity in baked goods and snack foods. BHT provides a refreshing change from the tales of woe and cancer scares associated with many of the other additives. Among the many tests that were performed on BHT were several showing that animals fed large amounts of this substance developed less cancer when exposed to carcinogens and lived longer than controls. BHT apparently protects against cancer through its antioxidant effect, similar to that of vitamin E. To obtain this effect from BHT, though, a large amount of the substance must be present in the diet—larger by far than the amount in the U.S. diet. (A caution: at levels of intake even higher than this, the substance has experimentally *produced* cancer.) Vitamin E and vitamin C remain the most important dietary antioxidants to strengthen defenses against cancer.[14]

Upon learning of the studies that show BHA and BHT to inhibit cancer in rats, some people came to a wrong conclusion—that what works for rats must work for people too. Manufacturers have begun marketing capsules of the preservatives as anticancer pills and recommending taking amounts far beyond the FDA's limit of safety. In fact, the daily dose recommended by the makers of these pills is almost a lethal dose and is high enough to cause possibly serious reactions in those with allergy to BHT. Ironically health food stores sell capsules of BHT and BHA alongside the packages of "no additives" foods.

This discussion provides the opportunity to mention an important point about additives. No two additives are alike, and therefore generalizations about them are meaningless. Whenever questions about the safety of "additives" are being discussed, you might as well leave the room, because no valid statement can be made that applies to the 3000-odd different substances commonly added to foods. Questions about which additives are safe, under what conditions of use, have to be asked and answered on an item-by-item basis.

⬛⬛▷ *Preservatives are added to food to prevent microbial spoilage; the most widely used of these are sugar and salt. Antioxidants, including vitamin E, prevent rancidity of fats and have been found to prevent cancer in certain laboratory tests.*

ARTIFICIAL COLORS. As just mentioned, only about 30 **artificial colors** are still on the GRAS list, a highly select group that has survived considerable screening. They are among the most intensively investigated of all additives. In fact, they are much better known than the *natural* pigments of plants, and the limits on the safety of their use can be stated with greater certainty.[15]

Still, the food colors have been more heavily criticized than almost any other group of additives. This is because they are dispensable. Simply stated, they only make foods pretty, whereas other additives, such as preservatives, make foods safe. Hence with food colors we can afford to require that their use entail no risk, whereas with other additives we may have to compromise between the risks of using them and the risks of *not* using them.

An infamous food-coloring agent of an earlier time was red dye number 2, which came under suspicion as a carcinogen in 1970 on the basis of two studies conducted in Russia. It was never shown to cause cancer, but it proved impossible to demonstrate that it did *not* cause cancer either, and so it was

*Monsanto Company has developed a sulfite alternative called Snow Fresh from citric acid, ascorbic acid, sodium acid pyrophosphate, and calcium chloride.

banned in the United States in 1976. On the same evidence, Canada concluded that it was not likely to cause cancer and continued to permit its use. (Red candies in this country do not contain red dye number 2.)

More recently, the food color tartrazine (yellow number 5) has received publicity because it causes an allergic reaction in susceptible people. Symptoms include hives, itching, and nasal congestion, sometimes severe enough to require medical treatment. People who are allergic to aspirin are especially likely to be affected, but tartrazine sensitivity also occurs in people without aspirin allergy. It is not a common problem; only one or two in 10,000 individuals may have the reaction, but still, that is over 20,000 individuals in the nation as a whole, and these people rightly demand to know where the dye is in foods so that they can avoid it. It is not enough to avoid yellow-colored foods because tartrazine is used to confer turquoise, green, and maroon colors in foods and drugs as well.[16]

Tartrazine was for a while blamed for causing many (some people said most) cases of hyperactivity in children, and a special diet (the Feingold diet), composed entirely of additive-free foods, was recommended for these children. By 1980 it was clear that the majority of cases of hyperactivity are not caused by tartrazine or other additives, but legislation is now in force requiring that tartrazine must be listed on all labels of foods that contain it so that consumers can avoid it if they wish.

ARTIFICIAL FLAVORS AND FLAVOR ENHANCERS. While only 33 colors are currently permitted in foods, there are close to 2000 **artificial flavors** and **flavor enhancers**, making them the largest single group of food additives. One of the best known members of this group is monosodium glutamate, or MSG (tradename, Accent)—the monosodium salt of the amino acid glutamic acid. MSG is used widely in restaurants, especially Asian restaurants, as a flavor enhancer. In addition to enhancing their flavors, research indicates that MSG may itself possess a basic taste independent of the well-known sweet, salty, bitter, and sour.[17] MSG has received publicity because it may produce an adverse reaction in some individuals—the so-called Chinese restaurant syndrome—involving burning sensations, chest and facial flushing or pain, and throbbing headaches. MSG has been investigated extensively enough to be deemed safe for adults to use (except people who react adversely to it, of course), but it is kept out of foods for infants because very large doses have been shown to destroy brain cells in developing mice. Infants have not yet developed the capacity to fully exclude such substances from their brains and so are more sensitive to them.

No one really knows how common Chinese restaurant syndrome is or why it might occur. It may have some relationship to vitamin B_6 deficiency, but that does not account for all cases. Researchers are looking for a link between the development of the syndrome and elevated blood levels of the MSG component glutamate. So far the results are mixed.

Some of the research indicates that MSG is not the only cause of the syndrome and that if people do not know they are eating MSG, they may not have the symptoms.[18] This seems to indicate a strong placebo effect at work. In addition, it has been difficult to correlate blood glutamate levels with symptoms. Recently it has been discovered that when MSG is administered along with some carbohydrate, as in a juice or other sweetened drink, the expected rise in blood glutamate does not occur.[19] When MSG is given with just water

Foods containing tartrazine:

- Orange drinks (Tang, Daybreak, Awake).
- Gatorade (lime flavored).
- Gelatin desserts (Jell-O, Royal).
- Golden Blend Italian dressing (Kraft).
- Some cake mixes and icings (Duncan Hines, Pillsbury, Cake Mate).
- Imitation banana or pineapple extract (McCormick).
- Seasoning salt (French's).
- Macaroni and cheese dinner (Kraft).
- 'Cheez' curls and balls (Planter's).
- Fruit chews (Skittles).
- Butterscotch squares and candy corn (Brach's).

Chapter 13 addresses the idea that hyperactivity might be "cured" by diet.

The placebo effect is defined in Chapter 1.

irradiated foods: foods that have been treated with radiation.

unique radiolytic (RAY-dee-oh-LIT-ic) products (URPs): products formed during the irradiation of food.

ultrahigh temperature(UHT): short-time exposure of a food to temperatures above those normally used to sterilize it.

or broth, the blood glutamate zooms up.[20] This effect might explain some of the confusing results of early studies. For example, when researchers delivered the MSG in water or broth, they reported elevated blood glutamate levels, but still had mixed results as to symptoms; those researchers who used sweet beverages reported no effects and little rise in blood glutamate levels.

There is still much to learn about Chinese restaurant syndrome because it is still not known for certain whether only a few sensitive people are affected, whether the syndrome occurs universally with a high enough dose, or even whether elevated blood glutamate is the cause. However, it can do no harm to apply what is known to restaurant eating. For example, even if a restaurant chef has not added extra MSG, many industrial soup mixes and flavorings already contain it. Thus soups may contain substantial MSG even when the restaurant claims "no MSG added." To make use of what has been discovered so far, a person who wishes to avoid Chinese restaurant syndrome might want to skip the soup or to order the kind with noodles (carbohydrate). As for the rest of the meal, eat plenty of rice with each bite, as the Chinese themselves do, to provide carbohydrate.

▋▶ *Among colorings and flavorings added to foods, the yellow color tartrazine and the flavoring MSG are suspected of causing reactions in people with sensitivities to them.*

NUTRIENT ADDITIVES. Another class of additives is nutrients added to improve or to maintain the nutritional value of foods. Included among **nutrient additives** are the nutrients added to refined grains to enrich them; the iodine added to salt; vitamins A and D added to dairy products; and the nutrients added to fortified breakfast cereals. When nutrients are added to a nutrient-poor food, it may appear from its label to be nutrient rich. It is, but only in those nutrients chosen for addition, and the absorption of these nutrients may be poor (see the Food Feature of Chapter 1). Nutrients are sometimes also added for other purposes. Vitamins C and E are examples already mentioned.

▋▶ *Nutrients are added to foods to enrich or to fortify them but still do not necessarily make them nutrient rich, except in the vitamins and minerals that have been added.*

RADIATION. Ionizing **radiation** kills living cells and thus sterilizes foods that are treated with it.† Radiation kills microorganisms and insect pests, inhibits the growth of sprouts on potatoes and onions, and delays ripening in some fruits.[21] In a sense radiation is an additive if it is applied to foods, as additives are, to improve their quality. However, unlike additives, it does not itself remain in the food, nor does the food become radioactive. FDA classifies radiation with additives because it slightly alters the chemistry of food treated with it.

People fail to understand that **irradiated foods** do not themselves produce rays. They have learned to think of radiation as causing cancer, birth defects, and mutations; they think they should avoid all forms of radiation for their

†Ionizing rays include X rays, gamma rays, and beta rays (electrons). Radiation sources include x-ray machines and electron accelerators, or the source may be a radioactive isotope such as cobalt 60 or cesium 137.

health's sake. When they hear talk of irradiated food, they naturally have doubts, if not strong emotions, about it ("Don't nuke my food!"). Irradiating foods does not damage foods, though. It sterilizes them while altering their flavors and textures little, if at all.

Radiation works by breaking up molecules. Some broken pieces called **unique radiolytic products (URP)** are being studied for safety. The higher the dose of radiation, the more of these substances are formed. Most are not unlike the substances found in food anyway, and realistically URPs probably present no hazard.[22] However, studies on their safety continue.

The FDA has approved irradiation treatment, at low concentrations, to perform those functions mentioned earlier, to replace post-harvest pesticide fumigation of certain foods, and to kill *Trichinella,* the dangerous parasitic worms that are sometimes found in pork. It has also approved high-dose treatment of dried spices, other seasonings, and teas to sterilize them. Milk products change flavor when irradiated and so are not candidates for the treatment. (Incidentally, those boxes of milk kept at room temperature on the shelves of the grocery store are not irradiated but have been treated with a process called **ultrahigh temperature** (UHT); the milk is exposed to temperatures above those of the normal milk treatment for a short time, just long enough to sterilize it.)

Irradiation cuts down on food wastage and can replace some costly pesticides, thus reducing those residues in food. Unfortunately, poor countries that have many hungry people and little food for them lack irradiation technology, and much of their food rots or is eaten by insects. Where technology is available, its use must be carefully scrutinized. Reports of accidental exposure of workers to radiation and liberation of radioactive waste from irradiation plants into public sewage and water systems are causes for concern.[23] There is no possibility of a meltdown or other nuclear disaster because food irradiation plants are not nuclear reactors, but strict controls on irradiation facilities and the wastes they generate are needed to prevent hazards to workers and to the environment.

In the United States the FDA has published regulations governing the use of irradiation.[24] Among requirements for dose levels and specific allowed uses is a requirement that each food treated with radiation bear a label indicating that the food was "treated with radiation" or "treated by irradiation."[25] This requirement informs consumers of this method of preservation but also could mislead them. Consumers could misinterpret the *absence* of the irradiation label to mean that the food was produced without treatment of any kind. This, of course, is not true; it is just that statements about the other treatments that perform similar functions, such as post-harvest fumigation with pesticides, are not required on labels. Some people urge that all treatment methods be declared so that consumers can make fully informed choices.[26]

Related to irradiation by virtue of its creative use of radiation on food is the microwave oven. Like irradiation, microwaves sterilize foods. Unlike irradiation, though, microwaves cook the food as they pass through it, and they do not create URPs in food.

◗◗▶ *Radiation is used to sterilize food after harvest, to kill* Trichinella *worms in pork, to slow ripening, and to prevent sprouting. URPs are chemicals produced by the splitting of large molecules in foods by radiation; most have been tested and found safe in the quantities in which they occur in food.*

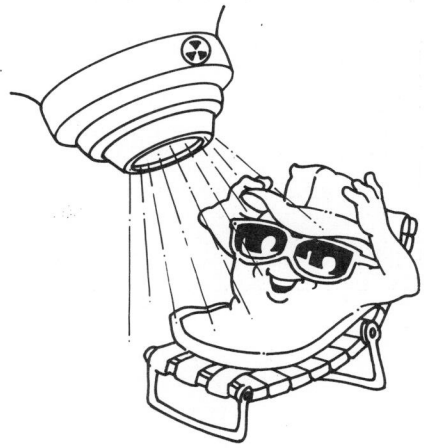

Irradiation can make some foods safer to eat by destroying organisms that cause illness.

The irradiation symbol.

Incidental Food Additives

Incidental or indirect additives are all substances that find their way into food as the result of some phase of production, processing, storage, or packaging. For example, among incidental additives are tiny bits of plastic, glass, paper, tin, and other substances from packages, as well as chemicals from processing, such as the solvent used to decaffeinate some types of coffee.

Incidental additives sometimes find their way into foods, but adverse effects are rare. These additives are well regulated, just as intentional additives are. All food packagers are required to perform specific tests to discover whether materials from packages are migrating into foods; if they are, their safety must be confirmed by strict procedures similar to those governing intentional additives.

In contrast to additives, some substances that find their way into foods are extremely hazardous to consumers. These are contaminants from industry and other sources. Chapter 15 shows where these materials come from and how they get into foods.

 Incidental additives are substances that get into food during processing. They are well regulated, and most present no hazard.

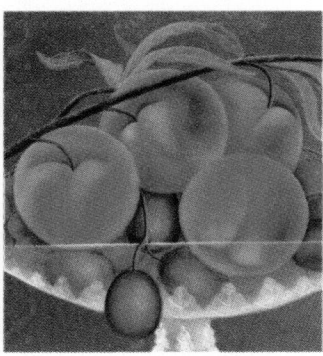

▮▮▮ Food Feature

Storing and Cooking Food Wisely

Once you have selected the most nutritious foods at the market and brought them home, you have the task of storing and preparing them so that they deliver the nutrients to you when you eat them. This requires some understanding of ways to conserve the vitamin value of foods in the kitchen. Vitamins are organic compounds synthesized and broken down by enzymes found in the foods that contain them. The enzymes in fruits and vegetables, like all enzymes, have a temperature optimum. They work best at the temperatures at which the plants grow, normally about 70° F (25° C), which is also the room temperature in most homes. After a fruit has been picked, the enzymes that synthesize vitamins (which have depended on a continued influx of energy from sunlight) largely stop working; those enzymes that degrade vitamins, a process that releases energy, continue to do so. Chilling the fruit slows down this degradation. To protect the vitamin content, fruits and vegetables should be vine ripened (if possible), chilled immediately after picking, and kept cold until used.

Riboflavin is light sensitive; it can be destroyed by the ultraviolet rays of the sun or by fluorescent light. For this reason milk is not sold (and should not be stored) in transparent glass containers. Cardboard or plastic containers screen out light, protecting the riboflavin.

Some vitamins are acids or antioxidants and so are most stable in an acid solution, away from air. Citrus fruits, tomatoes, and many juices are acid. As long as the skin is uncut or the can is unopened, their vitamins are protected from air. If you store a cut vegetable or fruit or an opened container of juice, cover it with an airtight wrapper and store it in the refrigerator.

You have seen labels on frozen foods that tell you "Do not refreeze." As food freezes, the cellular water expands into long, spiky ice crystals that puncture cell membranes and disrupt tissue structures, changing the texture of the food. People sometimes wonder if there is any danger in eating a twice-frozen food. Provided that they haven't let it spoil while it was thawed, the only problem is that the food may be less appealing. Be sure that the refrigerator keeps food at 40° F or below and the freezer at 0° F or below (use a freezer thermometer).

The water-soluble vitamins readily dissolve into the water in which cut vegetables are washed or boiled. If the water is discarded, as much as half of the vitamin content of the food is poured down the drain with it. To minimize this kind of loss, steam vegetables over water rather than in it, or microwave them. Wash the food vigorously and briefly, don't soak it, and cut it after cooking.

The nutrient contents of canned foods are usually shown as "solids and liquids." If you throw away the liquid from a canned food, you are throwing away all the nutrients that have leaked into that liquid, up to half the amount in the original product. A bit of southern folk wisdom is to serve the cooking liquid with the vegetable rather than throwing it away; this liquid is known as the "pot liquor." The user of canned vegetables who can think of a way to use the "liquor"—for example, by saving it to make soups, cook rice, or moisten casseroles—is displaying similar wisdom.

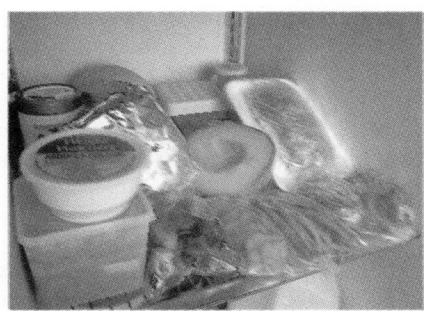
To preserve nutrients, wrap food tightly and refrigerate it.

Microwave ovens are excellent for conserving nutrients. They cook fast without requiring the addition of fats or excess liquid. They do have drawbacks, though. For one thing, large, thick, dense foods, such as meatloaf or meat roast may not cook evenly and thoroughly enough to ensure that all microorganisms have been destroyed. Such foods are best cooked by another method or divided into small, thin portions to be microwaved individually. Another potential hazard from microwave cooking is that food can heat to temperatures above those encountered in food cooked by other methods and thus may burn an unsuspecting diner. Avoid this by allowing steam to escape from covered containers and by allowing for a few minutes of sitting time following cooking.

During other types of cooking, minimize the destruction of vitamins by avoiding high temperatures and long cooking times. Iron destroys vitamin C by catalyzing its oxidation, but perhaps the benefit of increasing the iron content of foods by cooking in iron utensils outweighs this disadvantage. Each of these tactics is small by itself, but saving a small percentage of the vitamins in foods daily can mean saving significant amounts in a year's time.

Meanwhile, however, a law of diminishing returns operates. Most vitamin losses under reasonable conditions are not catastrophic. (For example, frozen orange juice that has been reconstituted and refrigerated typically retains 80 percent of its original vitamin C activity after eight days of storage.) You need not fret over small vitamin losses that occur in your kitchen; you may waste energy or time that is valuable to you in other ways. Be assured that if you start with fresh, whole foods containing ample amounts of vitamins and are reasonably careful in their preparation, you will receive a bounty of the nutrients that they contain.

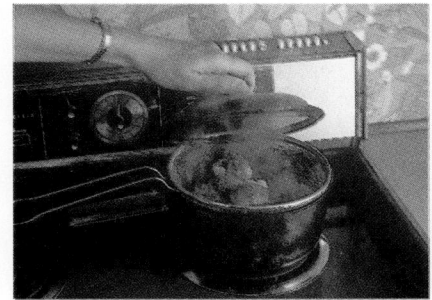
Steam vegetables.

Notes

1. Sanford A. Miller, director of FDA's Center for Food Safety and Applied Nutrition, in C. Lecos, Worrying about the *right* issues in food safety, *FDA Consumer,* November 1986, pp. 24–27.

2. Lecos, 1986.

3. Corn syrup can also be contaminated with *C. botulinum* spores. D. A. Kautter and coauthors, *Clostridium botulinum* spores in infant foods—a survey, *Journal of Food Protection* 45 (1982): 1028–1029.

4. I. B. Vyhmeister, What about honey? *Life and Health,* August 1980, pp. 5–7; R. W. Miller, Honey: Making sure it's pure, *FDA Consumer,* September 1979, pp. 12–13.

5. D. L. Morse and coauthors, Widespread outbreaks of clam- and oyster-associated gastroenteritis: Role of Norwalk virus, *New England Journal of Medicine* 314 (1986): 678–681; H. L. Dupont, Consumption of raw shellfish—is the risk now unacceptable? (editorial), *New England Journal of Medicine* 314 (1986): 707–708; Sushi lovers: Beware of parasites, *Science News,* 2 March 1985, p. 141.

6. V. Modeland, Fishing for facts on fish safety, *FDA Consumer,* February 1989, pp. 16–24.

7. Dr W. Gary Flamm of FDA's Center for Food Safety and Applied Nutrition, as cited by K. Flieger, The Delaney dilemma, *FDA Consumer,* September 1988, pp. 18–19.

8. F. M. Strong, Toxicants occurring naturally in foods, in *Nutrition Review's Present Knowledge in Nutrition,* 4th ed. (Washington, D. C.: Nutrition Foundation, 1976), pp. 516–527.

9. J. Hotchkiss and R. Cassens, Nitrate, nitrite, and nitroso compounds in foods (a scientific status summary by the Institute of Food Technologists' Expert Panel on Food Safety and Nutrition), April 1987, available from Institute of Food Science, Department of Food Science, Cornell University, Ithaca, NY 14853.

10. C. W. Lecos, Sulfites: FDA limits uses, broadens labeling, *FDA Consumer,* October 1986, pp. 10–13.

11. S. L. Taylor and R. K. Bush, Sulfites as food ingredients, *Contemporary Nutrition,* a publication (1986) available from the Nutrition Department, General Mills, Inc., PO Box 1172, Minneapolis, MN 55440.

12. One honey of an alternative to sulfites, *Science News* 134 (1988): 218.

13. New "food freshener," *Nutrition Forum* 5 (1988): 49.

14. W. F. Wilkens and J. I. Gray, Reduce N-nitrosamines formation in bacon, *Food Engineering* 58 (1986): 68–69; E. N. Frankel, Lipid oxidation: Mechanisms, products and biological significance, *Journal of the American Oil Chemists' Society* 61 (1984): 1908–1917.

15. T. M. Parkinson and J. P. Brown, Metabolic fate of food colorants, *Annual Reviews of Nutrition* 1 (1981): 175–205.

16. Tartrazine, *Nutrition and the MD,* January 1983.

17. Institute of Food Technologists' Expert Panel on Food Safety and Nutrition, (a scientific status summary) Monosodium Glutamate (MSG), May 1987, available from Institute of Food Technologists, 221 N. La Salle St, Chicago, IL 60601.

18. M. Gore, The Chinese Restaurant Syndrome, in *Adverse Effects of Foods,* eds. E. F. P. Jelliffe and D. B. Jelliffe (New York: Plenum Press, 1982), pp. 211–223.

19. L. D. Stegink and coauthors, Effect of sucrose ingestion on plasma glutamate concentrations in humans administered monosodium L-glutamate, *American Journal of Clinical Nutrition* 43 (1986): 510–515.

20. L. D. Stegink, L. J. Filer, and G. L. Baker, Plasma glutamate concentrations in adult subjects ingesting monosodium L-glutamate in consomme, *American Journal of Clinical Nutrition* 42 (1985): 220–225.

21. Irradiated foods, a report (December 1988) by the American Council on Science and Health, available from the ACSH at 1995 Broadway, New York, NY 10023–5860; D. Blumenthal, Food irradiation toxic to bacteria, safe for humans, *FDA Consumer*, November 1990, pp. 11–15.

22. A. Rogan and G. Glaros, Food irradiation: The process and implications for dietitians, *Journal of the American Dietetic Association* 88 (1988): 833–838.

23. E. Blume and M. F. Jacobson, Food irradiation: Is the time ripe? *Nutrition Action,* November 1986, pp. 1–7.

24. *Federal Register,* 27 March 1981, as cited in Food irradiation: Ready for a comeback, *Food Engineering,* April 1982, pp. 71–80.

25. C. W. Lecos, The growing use of irradiation to preserve food, *FDA Consumer,* July-August 1986, pp. 12–15.

26. Food irradiation under attack, *Nutrition Forum,* October 1986, p. 79.

▊▊▊ C O N T R O V E R S Y   1 4 ▊▊▊▊▊▊▊▊▊▊▊▊▊▊▊▊▊▊▊▊▊ ▊▊▊▊

Nonnutrients in Foods

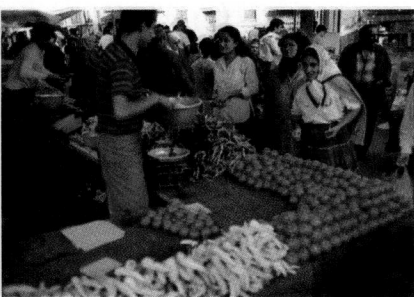

[20,000 years ago] The camp was quiet, settling down for the night. By the dim glow of hot coals, Iza checked the contents of several small pouches spread out in orderly rows on her cloak. . . . Earlier, she had inspected the vegetation growing around the cave, wanting to know the availability of plants to replenish and enlarge her pharmacopoeia. She always carried certain things with her in the otter-skin bag, but to her, the small pouches of dried leaves, flowers, roots, seeds, and barks in her medicine bag were only first aid. In the new cave she would have room for greater quantity and variety.
—J. M. Auel, The Clan of the
Cave Bear

From earliest times human beings have valued plants and animals not only for the nourishment they convey but for other properties. Substances from both flora and fauna have offered ways to stop bleeding, to relieve pain, to quell coughing, to calm inflammation, to fight infection, to soften dry skin, and to ease the way to sleep, as well as many other remedies. And in the last hundred years, many of the active ingredients from plant and animal tissues have been isolated and identified and are now sold by pharmacists in purified form, in standard formulations, and in measured doses. Many of today's drugs are produced synthetically, but they still copy drugs that occur naturally in **herbs** and other plant and animal tissues.[1]

Nutrients are thus not the only chemicals in foods, although they are by far the best-known ones. Foods, after all, come from the tissues of living things. Living tissues contain thousands of different chemicals, only some 40-odd of which happen to serve as nutrients for the human body. Among the familiar nonnutrients are fibers (in plants), a constituent vital to human nutrition, although not nourishing in the sense of directly promoting growth or repair of body tissues. The fibers of legumes and oats may lower blood cholesterol, as first reported in Chapter 4. Foods also contain pigments, such as chlorophyll, hemoglobin, myoglobin, and others, which give them their green, red, and other hues. They also may contain poisons, including the toxins of poisonous mushrooms, naturally occurring pesticides, agricultural pesticide residues (see Chapter 15), and many others. Then there are the subjects of the present discussion.

The subjects of this discussion are those nonnutrient components of foods other than fiber that are reputed to have beneficial health effects. Among these are some microbes; flavor compounds, such as the heat chemical in hot peppers; and other molecules that have a variety of physiological effects. Technically, because "a molecule with a physiological effect" is the definition of a drug, these latter compounds should all be called drugs—although in many cases their identity is not yet known, and they make their presence apparent only as "something in the food."

Nonnutrient food constituents that have beneficial health effects have led people to believe, wrongly, that certain *foods* have special power to promote health. They do not, but because they contain physiologically active substances, they may be more likely to support health than nutrient supplements are. By eating a variety of foods, a person receives a variety of both nutrients and nonnutrients.

Seriously ill people in hospitals drink all-synthetic liquid diets described as "nutritionally complete," meaning that they contain all of the essential nutrients in the amounts needed to support life. On such diets people maintain physical well-being for up to six months.[2] Yet real food apparently supports health better. Foods convey more value than just that carried by the nutrients in them, although it is not clear just how they do so.[3] Certainly one possibility is that a variety of nonnutrients confer extra benefits.

◼◼◼ Warnings

Let us begin with a few warnings. *Warning #1*: when people consume plant or animal tissues to obtain a specific physiological effect, they don't always get the substance they think they are getting. Neither can they always know its concentration in a food when it is present. Foods vary from batch to batch, from strain to strain, from one part of a plant or animal to another, from season to season, from one geographical region to another, and from one preparation method to the next. When foods are transformed into powders and potions, their ingredients change, and so do their effects. Unlike the chemical composition of standardized drugs, that of foods taken from plants and animals is unreliable and unpredictable. The potential dangers are amplified when a food is mislabeled or misidentified. A root sold as the rare and expensive ginseng root may actually be that of a different plant, indistinguishable to an untrained eye.

As an example of the mistaking of one herb for another, a man confused **foxglove** (from which the potent heart medication digoxin is extracted) with **comfrey** (a plant popular for making tea). He brewed a tea from the foxglove and drank a little more than a quart of it over several days. As a result, he suffered digoxin poisoning.[4] Comfrey itself becomes toxic when used regularly (see later), but foxglove is even more so. Such stories involving the use of herbal preparations are common.

Warning #2: people differ in their reactions to biologically active compounds. Children are particularly susceptible to the effects of biologically active compounds, and special care must be taken when feeding foods that contain them to children. Adults, too, can suffer from the careless use of natural sources of drugs, especially if they have current disease or inherited disease susceptibility.

Warning #3: some foods for which special health-promoting claims are made do *not* contain chemical components that benefit the human body—or at least not in quantities or potencies worth anyone's special attention.

Warning #4: when people consume plant or animal tissues to obtain a specific physiological effect, they may get an unexpected, even harmful, effect. Whenever a food is prized for one compound it contains, the likelihood exists that it contains others for which it might be condemned. Many commonly used plants and plant products contain naturally occurring toxic substances. Mushrooms are a familiar example; but a number of other common foods have been observed to cause toxic effects. Consider this list:

◼ Cabbage, mustard, and other plants contain goitrogens; if these plants are consumed as a steady diet, they can enlarge the thyroid gland.

◼ Spinach and rhubarb contain oxalates, tolerable as usually consumed; but one normal serving of rhubarb contains one fifth the toxic dose for humans.

◼ Potatoes contain solanine, a powerful inhibitor of nerve impulses; ordinary consumption of potatoes delivers one tenth the dose of solanine that would be toxic. When potatoes are exposed to light, they develop more solanine; it is the green layer that develops just beneath the skin. Throw such potatoes away; don't eat them.

Some 700 other plants have caused serious illnesses or deaths in the Western hemisphere.[5] Some fish are also naturally toxic, presenting a range of hazards, from mild illness to instant death. A well-known environmental scientist has said, "One can predict that if the standards used to test manmade chemicals were applied to 'natural' foods, fully half of the human food supply would have to be banned."[6]

These warnings translate into a pair of questions any health-minded person would be wise to ask in relation to any food for which health effects are claimed. Examine the available scientific evidence, and ask:

1. Does it really do what is claimed? (Is there scientifically valid evidence that conclusively demonstrates that the claimed benefits are real?)

2. Does it do any harm? (Be sure that harmful effects have been looked for.)

When the answer to the first question is affirmative, other questions arise. At what concentration does the substance provide the beneficial effect? Is the concentration of the substance in the food, when the food is consumed in ordinary amounts, great enough to produce the desired effect? Even if it is, the chemical interactions that accompany digestion of the food and the body's handling of the components might interfere with the physiological action, thus altering the effect. This leads us to *Warning #5*: before nonnutrients can be assumed safe to take for their drug effects, their absorption and metabolism must be understood.

Keep in mind, too, that in many instances the reported benefits of a food came from serendipitous observations and personal accounts or even wishful thinking. Unfortunately the periodic publication of bits of new information about the true, beneficial effects of food components on health sets people up to believe larger claims made by misguided or unscrupulous individuals. The object, here, is to sort valid, useful information from the unfounded claims. Within this perspective, then, this Controversy looks at some foods that contain nonnutrients with supposedly beneficial effects and asks what significance, if any, the available information has for consumers.

■■■ Alfalfa

The **alfalfa** plant is a good example of a food for which claims have been overly enthusiastic. Like any plant, alfalfa contains hundreds of chemicals, including proteins, fats, organic acids, vitamins, minerals, fibers, pigments, and others. Alfalfa is a forage plant, and it supports the healthy growth of cattle both when they graze on it in summer and when they eat the dried hay in winter. Promoters of alfalfa claim that if it is good for cattle, it must be good for people, too— but that people should eat its nutrients directly, not "via the steer." Such a viewpoint may appeal to people consuming a vegetarian diet, but to equate the nutritional benefits of an alfalfa salad with those of beef from a cow that grazed on alfalfa is to overlook many biochemical transformations. However, the alfalfa promoters do argue a valid point that the earth benefits when people eat plants instead of animal-derived products. Plants require less land to produce a given amount of protein and food energy than animals do.

Claims that alfalfa cures arthritis, reduces blood cholesterol, treats diabetes, stimulates the appetite, and acts as a general tonic are overstated. For example, in a test tube, alfalfa saponins bind with cholesterol; in a rat, the effect is evident, but insignificant.[7] To claim beneficial effects in human beings at this time is to exaggerate the research findings.

Like the positive physiological effects of alfalfa, the negative effects are minimal, if any, and so alfalfa is safe to consume. Indeed, consumers should feel free to eat alfalfa sprouts, and mung bean sprouts, and wheat berry sprouts, and radish seed sprouts, and a variety of other sprouts—in moderation, of course. Sprouted seeds are reasonably nutritious and lend variety to the diet. Like most seeds and sprouts, alfalfa sprouts contain a variety of vitamins and minerals and provide relatively few calories. They are also, like all plant-derived foods, rich in fibers. However, even with these nutrition benefits, alfalfa has no special health-promoting powers greater than other plants.

Although the alfalfa *plant* is neither particularly effective in promoting health nor particularly hazardous when consumed in moderation, alfalfa *tablets*, which are made from the crushed, dehydrated plant, are a different story. They deliver much more alfalfa, enough to be hazardous, particularly for people with systemic lupus erythematosus (SLE), a rare disease involving inflammation of the joints. A study of two people whose SLE had been in remission showed that the disease was reactivated after they had been taking doses of 8 to 15 tablets daily for a long time. Researchers found that the alfalfa tablets contained a substance that was shown to reactivate SLE in susceptible animals.[8] For most healthy people, though, taking the tablets a few at a time does little harm except to the pocketbook.

The unexpected harmful effect of alfalfa tablets illustrates the warnings issued at the start. First (recall Warning #1), the effects of a plant may differ from the effects of that same plant after it has been processed. The chemical compositions and concentrations of oils, extracts, and powders are not necessarily the same as those of their sources. Also (Warning #2), what is good, bad, or neutral for one person may not be for another. Each individual has a unique genetic endowment and health status that influence the body's reactions to various

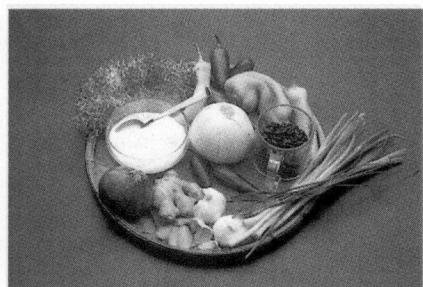

Some foods offer more than just nutrients.

compounds. Still another lesson is a variation of "if it's not broken, don't fix it." For people to consume products on a whim or on the advice of a friend, store clerk, or advertisement is to play Russian roulette. The chances of receiving beneficial, neutral, or harmful reactions from a product are, for the most part, unknown (Warnings #3 and #4).

▆▆▆ Ginseng

The root of the wild, slow-growing **ginseng** plant (actually several species of plants) is so valued for its supposed antifatigue and aphrodisiac properties that it has been gathered almost to extinction. In the United States, ginseng has been declared an endangered species. Ginseng has been intensively studied, and over a thousand books and papers have been written about it, but much of the writing has been in the tradition of folklore and Oriental mysticism. Scientific work is incomplete.

The answers to two important questions about ginseng are apparent, though. To the question of

whether it offers any beneficial health effects, the answer is yes; and to the question of whether it does any harm, the answer is also yes.

Like alfalfa, ginseng plants contain saponins—a family of chemicals that affect specific body functions, that is, they act as drugs. This makes ginseng, just like the multitude of other plants from which drugs are derived, both potentially valuable and potentially dangerous, since drugs can be misused or abused. Chinese folklore credits ginseng for providing health, strength, and happiness to people who are exhausted by stress, injury, or fatigue.

Like those in alfalfa, ginseng's saponins are largely responsible for its pharmacological activities. Saponin extracts of ginseng, depending on the particular batch from which they are made, have been reported to be effective in relieving inflammation in rats. In the test tube, their inhibitory effect on the reaction of human white blood cells to a stressor proves more potent than that of hydrocortisone (a common anti-inflammatory drug).[9] Chewing the ginseng root is reported to be effective in raising HDL cholesterol levels and reducing cardiovascular disease risk ratings (as estimated from HDL) from high to zero.[10]

These reported effects of ginseng must be considered with caution. They are unpredictable—probably because ginseng potencies and chemical composition vary according to the strain, the part of the plant used, the season, and the mode of preparation. Thus ginseng has also been observed to raise

blood pressure and to cause insomnia, nervousness, confusion, and depression—a cluster of symptoms observed often enough to be worth naming: the **ginseng abuse syndrome**.[11] Many of these harmful effects appear to be due to a physiological action like that of the stress hormones or the female hormone estrogen. Excessive use of ginseng is associated with physiological changes in the vaginal mucosa in women, and one case is reported in which a daily ginseng tablet was associated with vaginal bleeding in an elderly woman.[12]

Ginseng is not commonly eaten as a food. Its druglike components can be extracted by chewing the root or by chemical processing. Ginseng teas and sodas are also available. When consumed for specific physiological actions, ginseng is a drug—a drug that may not work as desired because its side effects can occur at about the same dose levels as its desired effects. The cost of purifying the chemicals from ginseng is high, and they are not in wide use pharmaceutically.

The cases of alfalfa and ginseng illustrate two different sets of answers to the questions asked at the start (Does the food do what is claimed? Does it do any harm?). In the case of alfalfa, the answers to both questions are no; in the case of ginseng, the answers to both are a qualified yes, although much of the evidence has been obtained from studies on animals, not human beings.

▮▮▮ Wine

One of the most potent and dangerous drugs used by human beings arises when carbohydrates in plants are fermented by microorganisms, namely, alcohol. Its effects are too numerous and its impacts too great for the scope of this discussion. Controversy 11 provided greater insights into the effects of alcohol on the brain and on nutrition status. Setting alcohol aside, though, and granting that its moderate use may not be harmful, we might ask whether fermented beverages have special health effects. Wine, in particular, is certainly credited with many such effects—naturally, many of them claimed by wine makers and merchants but some that have been scientifically validated. Test tube experiments suggest that grape juice has an antiviral effect that carries over (to a lesser extent) when the grape juice is made into wine.[13] The substance responsible for inactivating viruses is found in the skin of grapes, which explains why red wines are more antiviral than white. (White wines are fermented from the juice only, while red wines are made from the entire grape.) Strawberries and several other fruits also provide an antiviral effect.

Alcoholic beverages also affect the appetite. Usually they take the edge off people's hunger by providing a few calories and a measure of relaxation. Sometimes, because they can be high in calories, they contribute to obesity. In people who are tense and unable to eat, though, small doses of wine taken 20 minutes before meals help because they stimulate the appetite. Acid compounds in the wine that are known as **congeners** are credited with this effect. For undernourished people and for people with severely depressed appetites, wine may facilitate eating even when psychotherapy fails to do so. At the same time, because it relaxes people, wine may help obese people lose weight. Its success in that connection is thought to stem from its ability to relieve emotional stress, which is a common reason for overeating. Certain of the congeners in wine may contribute to the tranquilizing effect, and some are said to be nearly 100 times more effective than alcohol.[14] French wine also contains a compound known to lower liver lipids and cholesterol in rats.[15]

It goes without saying that people need not drink wine to obtain many of these effects. The chemicals responsible for them are present in the original juice from which the wine was fermented, and they are still present when the alcohol is again removed from the wine. If people who drink wine give it up, they can still enjoy its benefits by learning to drink moderate amounts of fruit juices or dealcoholized wine in its place—or, of course, by eating grapes. The point of discussing wine rather than grape juice or grapes is to give another example of how science can help to sift reality out of folklore. The folklore surrounds the wine, but science finds the truth in the grapes.

How, then, would wine be evaluated in response to the two questions asked at the start? Does it really do what is claimed? Yes—although grape juice, grapes, or other fruits do many of the same things as well or better. Does it do any harm? Since the harmful effects of overconsumption of alcohol are well known, this question might have to be answered by saying yes, possibly so; and grape juice, grapes, or other fruits would not. In short, use wine in moderation, if at all, but do eat a variety of fruits—boring advice, perhaps, but safe and beneficial to health.

▮▮▮ Garlic

People who are seeking an edge over heart disease might hear that garlic has a nonnutrient effect on heart health. Garlic has been considered a "magic" food for centuries— the first Olympic athletes believed it conferred stamina, and they chewed it before competitive events. For those ancients who perceived themselves to be pestered by vampires, garlic was a well-known repellent. These claims remain untested, but the effect of garlic on blood lipids is supported by some research. The essential oil of garlic (equivalent to about 1 ounce, or one bulb, of raw garlic a day) appears not only to lower the blood lipids associated with heart disease but also to oppose clot formation.[16] The effect is seen in both healthy people and in people with coronary heart disease and is maintained for two months after garlic treatments are discontinued.

When people learned of the effects of garlic on blood lipids, many wanted to employ it for its heart health benefits. However, large quantities of garlic may bring more than the desired results (Warning #3). The effects may include nausea, vomiting, diarrhea, and excessive intestinal gas; and garlicky body odor is noticeable in people who regularly consume large quantities. In addition, the immediate breath odor is unmistakable and considered unpleasant. (To improve garlic breath, brush the teeth and tongue after eating, and chew some fresh parsley. The chlorophyll in the parsley *may* help eliminate the garlic odor compounds, although this effect is more hearsay than science.[17]) Capsules of odorless garlic extract available at health-food stores are untested, and they are likely to lack the very chemicals that are candidates for imparting health benefits.

Garlic is commonly used to enhance the flavor of foods. When used in small quantities on an occasional basis, garlic confers minimal, if any, health benefits. However, when used in larger quantities on a regular basis, its components reach concentrations that do have both beneficial drug effects and unpleasant side effects. Thus, like ginseng, garlic does not work well as a drug, and for purposes of minimizing its potential for harm, moderate use is recommended—use at a level such that its benefits, other than its pleasing taste, may be insignificant as well.

▣▣▣ Hot Peppers

Some groups of people have low incidences of the fatal blood clotting associated with heart and artery disease. A food associated with this effect is hot peppers, as indicated by reports from Thailand, Mexico, and Hungary, where these peppers are dietary staples. For example, Thai people eat hot peppers many times a day. Each time they eat them, a temporary anticlotting action takes place in their blood.[18] This effect is attributed to the pungent chemical **capsaicin** in the hot peppers. Conceivably this anticlotting action, repeated several times daily, is sufficient to reduce the risk of fatal blood clotting.

Hot peppers have another interesting effect: immediately after a person eats a meal spiced with them, the person's metabolic rate rises by up to 65 percent, whereas the meal alone raises it by only 40 percent. If you like hot food, you may have noticed this effect as increased body heat and sweating after eating hot pepper-spiced food. The excess heat persists for three hours or more.[19] This makes a difference of only a few calories in the day's energy total (we calculate that a 25 percent rise in energy spent on metabolism might amount to a pound of fat every three months); but for the person concerned with weight control, the difference is in the right direction.

In some people, and especially in those with ulcers, food spiced with hot peppers can cause gastric distress, although such food does not appear to actually injure the tissues of the digestive tract.[20] Again, caution is necessary when using the components in foods to achieve an effect. Advantages and disadvantages must be weighed carefully. Asking Question 1 of hot peppers, then, we might respond that there appear to be small but real benefits. To Question 2: moderation is recommended.

Hot peppers and garlic are only two of the foods related to reducing the risk of heart disease. Unprocessed or lightly processed fruits, vegetables, legumes, and grains all play roles, thanks to the actions of their fibers—and possibly other constituents. These and other foods also play roles in defenses against cancer, as the following sections suggest.

▣▣▣ Cabbages and Their Relatives

In the last 20 years it has become apparent that many cancers originate from lifestyle factors that are within people's power to control—food choices among them. Among dietary factors related to cancer are the diet's fat content; deficiencies of nutrients such as vitamin C, folate, vitamin A and its precursor carotene;[21] food additives (to a limited extent); food contaminants; and nonnutrients in foods. Chapter 11 mentioned each of these, but it is useful to look in depth at several candidates among the nonnutrients that may help prevent cancer: among them, the **indoles**[22] and **dithiolthiones**[23] among the cruciferous vegetables, and enzyme inhibitors in seeds and grains.

A table of the cruciferous vegetables appeared in Chapter 11. They include broccoli, cauliflower, brussels sprouts, and other vegetables with cross-shaped flowers. Research indicates that people who consume large amounts of these vegetables have lower cancer rates than those who do not.[24] This finding has led to studies of the vegetables themselves and to the further finding that the indoles and dithiolthiones they contain induce the activity of certain enzymes in the liver. These enzymes, among other things, inactivate certain carcinogens (cancer-causing chemicals).[25] Often such effects are seen only in compounds purified and concentrated from plants, but the dithiolthiones in cabbage have this effect in mice even when the cabbage is fed in amounts comparable to servings people could normally eat.[26] It seems, therefore, that consuming these vegetables could tend to tip the balance toward a slightly lower likelihood of contracting cancer, but direct confirmation or rejection by way of experiments on human beings is not possible for ethical reasons.

Other vegetables contain constituents that may activate the enzyme system that degrades carcinogens.[27] These constituents are so widespread among plants that the single most valuable application of the information obtained to date is *not* to eat cabbage in particular but to eat a wide variety of vegetables in generous quantities. Balancing this advice, notice that the next section advocates the use of grains and seeds and the next one milk and milk products—so that in the end, the tried-and-true recommendation to eat a balanced diet also seems to apply to the person wishing to avoid cancer.

▌▌▌ Seeds and Grains

Another class of foods that may contain cancer-fighting substances is the **seed foods,** including grains, nuts, and legumes. Many of them contain **protease inhibitors**— substances that prevent digestive enzymes from doing their work.[28] These inhibitors prevent digestion of the seeds themselves, or at least enough of them to ensure passage intact through the digestive tract, so that they can return to the soil and sprout. However, the inhibitors also prevent digestion of other proteins. The inhibitor in raw soybeans is so powerful that it can prevent digestion of other foods eaten with the soybeans—the basis for the imperative that soybeans must be cooked before eating. Some investigators believe that these inhibitors may convey an anticancer advantage,[29] although whether they could convey this advantage as eaten is an unanswered question. Among the plants under study are soybeans, lima beans, other beans, and potatoes (in which the eyes are similar to seeds), all of which contain factors that may inhibit the process by which carcinogens are formed.[30] Answers to the interesting question of whether these foods play a role in cancer prevention are still to come, but some practical implications are apparent.

Seed foods add variety to the diet and can be eaten in moderation. Overconsumption is probably possible and would have adverse effects.

▌▌▌ Yogurt

Years ago, when some long-lived people of another culture were asked their longevity secret, they gave the credit to their daily meals of yogurt—hence the start of yogurt mania in developed countries. Since then researchers have studied both yogurt and yogurt-eating people to try to detect whether yogurt has health-promoting qualities.

Yogurt is made from milk that has been fermented by the **Lactobacillus** bacteria group. Yogurt is nutritionally equivalent to the same quantity of milk, except that some of the lactose has been fermented to lactic acid. It is rich in calcium, protein, and the other nutrients normally found in milk. Its high calcium content may help protect against cancer, since diets high in calcium seem to protect against cancer generally, especially that of the colon (large intestine).[31] *Fermented* milk products (yogurt, buttermilk, kefir, and others) contain, in addition to nutrients, the bacteria from which they were made, and these bacteria, or products of their metabolism, seem to have additional, special effects of their own. Specific strains of the yogurt-making bacteria produce enzymes that act against a number of transplanted and chemically induced cancers in animals, although exactly how they work is not yet known.[32]

Groups of people who include yogurt as a staple food suffer less colon cancer than people who do not. This is so even if their diets are high enough in fat to be expected to promote a high cancer rate. The bacteria of yogurt are known to survive the digestion process and take up residence in the large intestine, so it seems logical to look to bacterial action in the colon for an explanation of yogurt's apparent anticancer effect. Researchers studying the colon contents of yogurt-eating people have found that they contain fewer enzyme-produced carcinogens than the colons of other people. It seems that *Lactobacillus* bacteria growing in the intestine inhibit those intestinal enzymes that convert at least some food chemicals into carcinogens in the colon.[33] In a study of mice, intestinal tumors stopped growing when the mice ate yogurt, presenting another possibility—that the by-products of bacterial growth inhibit tumor growth after it has begun.[34]

This is not to say that these researchers have proven that yogurt can prevent intestinal cancer. Their findings must be followed by more research, particularly research that uses the commercially available yogurt ordinarily consumed by people, to determine whether the products on the grocery store shelves have any anticancer effect. Assuming, though, that the *Lactobacillus* bacteria do inhibit carcinogen production in the colon, how can consumers apply this information?

The bacterial strain present in yogurt takes up only temporary residence in the digestive tract. It must be included in the diet regularly (daily or several times weekly) to achieve any possible benefits. Also, the yogurt must contain live cultures.[35] Some manufacturers provide this information on the label. Canned yogurt products do not contain live cultures.

Two other products also deliver *Lactobacillus:* **acidophilus milk** and tablets. *Lactobacillus acidophilus* bacteria are grown in a medium, then harvested and added to milk. The bacteria are not grown in the milk, where they would ferment the lactose, since if they did, they would produce a sour by-product—lactic acid. The lactose content of acidophilus milk is therefore the same as that of milk, but it provides the beneficial bacteria, together with a medium suitable for their growth within the digestive tract. Acidophilus tablets taken without a milk product do not supply the needed medium in which the bacteria can multiply and so do not establish a large *Lactobacillus* colony in the intestine.

Other research has led to other claims for yogurt. For example, yogurt cultures fed to rats produce and secrete an antibiotic effective against *other* bacteria that might cause harm—such as the ones that cause food poisoning.[36] Although supported by some research, these claims were derived from research in animals. Like all such claims, they need further investigation before they can be applied to human health.

Milk group foods may confer advantages against heart disease, too. Milk contains both saturated fat and cholesterol, which might be expected to raise blood cholesterol, and yet both milk and yogurt (even whole milk and yogurt in some experiments) have been shown to *lower* blood cholesterol.[37] Nonfat milk would be preferable, of course, for the person seeking to escape the cancer-promoting effects of fat. Among compounds present in milk that may account for the cholesterol-lowering effect are lactose[38] and two acids that, when purified and fed in higher doses, lower blood cholesterol.[39] Cheese also buffers salivary pH, inhibiting the caries-producing action of mouth bacteria. This makes it a good choice for a snack for people who can't brush their teeth right after eating—if they can afford the calories.[40]

It is a disservice to one's nutrition to overemphasize yogurt and milk at the expense of other, equally valuable foods from other food groups. But for calcium nutrition's sake, people are advised to include a minimum of two or more servings of yogurt or milk a day among the foods they choose. The possible nonnutrient benefits these foods convey make both of them excellent choices.

Other Foods

This discussion has included several foods with reputations for service to human nutrition beyond the call of duty; it has left out others that have popular reputations the reader might wonder about. What about brewer's yeast, honey, wheat germ, chocolate, and other foods considered by some to be especially health promoting? Perhaps a word about each might not be amiss. In the old days **brewer's yeast** was a by-product of beer making; dead, bitter-tasting yeasts would settle to the bottom of the vats. Today cultures of nonbitter yeasts are grown by a somewhat different method for use as food supplements and are still called brewer's yeast, or nutritional yeast. Brewer's yeast is a source of B vitamins, iron, and protein (1 tablespoon has 3 grams of usable protein or about 5 percent of the recommended amount for adults) and can be used to improve the quality of a vegetarian diet. Cereal grains combined with brewer's yeast are especially nutritious. Many vegetarian recipes for breads, cereals, soups, and rice dishes therefore recommend the addition of 1 to 2 tablespoons of yeast to their other ingredients. Brewer's yeast is highly nutritious, but for now it seems to be true that it exerts health benefits only by donating the traditional nutrients. For example, people who lack the mineral chromium in their diets may suffer from high blood pressure or from a diabetes-like condition caused by resistance to the hormone insulin (insulin needs chromium to do its work). These conditions may be corrected by adding brewer's yeast or any other high-chromium food to the diet.

As for honey, it confers no proven benefits, although some people like to believe that eating locally harvested honey can reduce hay fever by introducing small amounts of the local pollens into the system, much as allergy shots do. It seems equally possible, though, that exposure to local pollens could aggravate hay fever, and bee pollen is known to do so. Pollens also pick up high concentrations of environmental contaminants. Spores of the organism that causes botulism, a deadly form of food poisoning, can get into honey, and parents are warned not to feed it to infants. Given the high-sugar, low-nutrient content of honey and the risk of botulism, honey remains in its proper place as an occasional treat and only for older children and adults.

Wheat germ is high in B vitamins, vitamin E, magnesium, iron, and zinc and has a justified place in the diet of those who enjoy it, but it has no demonstrated nonnutrient benefits. Wheat germ oil is nutritionally inferior to wheat germ itself, it is much more expensive than other oils, and it has no apparent advantage over any other equally unsaturated oil.

And chocolate? Rumor has it that it relieves depression, but there is no proof that it does so physiologically. It does contain phenylethylamine, which is a biologically active amine, and could conceivably have an effect on mood. However, a search through the literature cited in support of the rumor reveals no connections established by actual research—doubtless a disappoint-

ment to chocoholics everywhere.[41] Perhaps chocolate's caffeine content, together with the sugar that is always added to it, accounts for its perceived effects on mood. (Controversy 6 discussed the effects of carbohydrate on mood.)

Many other foods contain substances that have nonnutrient effects. A fun example is the old Jewish remedy for a cold, chicken soup, which helps to speed the flow of mucus, ridding the body of infection.[42] Cinnamon, cloves, cranberries, and other plants contain benzoic acid and its esters, which act as preservatives, preventing microbial action in foods. The herb thyme contains one or more compounds that kill certain bacteria in food, as do cloves and clove oil. The herb ginger may prove to contain an effective motion-sickness drug.[43] However, as mentioned earlier, herbs can be misused and can cause harm. Like many other foods and like drugs, herbs require the user to have adequate knowledge to use them properly. Unfortunately, because of the rampant quackery associated with herbs, that knowledge is not easy for users to sort out from the accompanying misinformation. This Controversy's reference, *The Honest Herbal*, is refreshingly different from most.*

*V. E. Tyler, *The New Honest Herbal: A Sensible Guide to Herbs and Related Remedies* (Philadelphia: Stickley, 1987). Varro E. Tyler, Ph.D. (pharmacognosy), formerly on the faculties of the Universities of Nebraska and Washington, is Dean of the Schools of Pharmacy, Nursing, and Health Services at Purdue University.

■■■ Miniglossary

acidophilus milk: milk to which a culture of *Lactobacillus acidophilus* has been added (but not allowed to grow).

alfalfa: a perennial herb, used as cattle fodder and as food for people (as seeds or sprouts); claims of extraordinary health benefits from alfalfa are unfounded.

brewer's yeast: a preparation of yeast cells, often praised for its high nutrient content. It is especially rich in B vitamins, as are many other foods. Also called nutritional yeast, it is not useful for making bread rise.

capsaicin (cap-SAY-ih-sin): the chemical in peppers responsible for their "hot" taste.

comfrey: an herb, used mostly for making tea.

congeners (CON-jen-ers): chemical substances other than alcohol that account for the physiological effects, such as taste and aftereffects, that are unique to different alcoholic beverages.

dithiolthiones: a class of chemical compounds, significant in this discussion because those occurring in the cruciferous vegetables are believed to exhibit some anticancer action. Also defined in Chapter 11.

foxglove: a plant (digitalis) containing a chemical (digoxin) of value as a drug for heart clients.

ginseng (JIN-seng): a plant containing chemicals that have physiological effects on human beings.

ginseng abuse syndrome: a cluster of syndromes associated with the overuse of ginseng, including high blood pressure, insomnia, nervousness, confusion, and depression.

herbs: nonwoody plants or plant parts valued for their flavor, aroma, or medicinal qualities.

indoles: a class of chemical compounds, significant in this discussion because those occurring in the cruciferous vegetables are believed to exhibit some anticancer action. Also defined in Chapter 11.

Lactobacillus: a genus of bacteria that includes several species that grow in milk and in the human intestine. *Lactobacillus acidophilus* is one of these species, sometimes added to milk to help ferment the sugar lactose in the intestine to make the milk usable by people who cannot digest that sugar.

protease inhibitors: chemicals that inhibit the action of enzymes that break down proteins. The inhibitors referred to here are those found in some seed foods; they make seed foods somewhat indigestible, a benefit to the seed but a hindrance to the eater's nutrition.

seed foods: foods made from seeds—grains, nuts, beans, peas, and the like.

Health-food stores sell a variety of herbal preparations to "remedy" a multitude of problems. One example is the use of comfrey capsules and tablets, prepared from the leaves or the roots of the comfrey plant, to aid digestion. A woman took two such tablets with each meal for four months. She became ill with liver disease due to the toxic accumulation of a substance found in comfrey.[44]† Comfrey tea is carcinogenic in rats, and its use is discouraged because of its reported toxicity in human beings.[45]

The spices and herbs mentioned here are only a few among the many plants that people use in hopes of reaping health benefits. Table C14–1 presents some other plants that have been said to benefit health, and readers are referred to its source for further information.

■■■ Conclusions

That many foods contain compounds that have real physiological effects in people is interesting. A rational response to this reality is to keep an open mind, at first, about all such claims, that is, neither discredit nor hail a newly discovered food effect until it has been scientifically studied. Wait until the evidence is in. Although claims of special effects of foods are usually surrounded by a chaff of speculation, they may contain kernels of truth, and it is becoming increasingly interesting to watch the research sift them out. Maintain a

---

†The toxic substances found in comfrey are pyrrolizidine alkaloids. Tyler, 1987, p. 77.

■■■ **Table C14–1 A Sampling of Plants for Which Claims of Nonnutrient Benefits Are Made**

Selected are some of the more familiar plants of the more than 100 reviewed by Tyler (see source). The judgments are Tyler's, and they are based on an honest scientific scrutiny of thousands of papers, books, and articles, many of which, however, are more in the realm of folklore than of science. The judgments are based on uses of the plants as described in the book (indiscriminate use of a plant called "safe," here, would not necessarily be safe). Much remains to be learned about these plants and the constituents responsible for their effects.

COMMON NAME	CLAIM MADE	EFFECTIVE? (FROM AVAILABLE EVIDENCE)	SAFE? (FROM AVAILABLE EVIDENCE)
Alfalfa (leaves, tops)	Cures arthritis,	No	Yes
	lowers blood cholesterol	No	Yes
Aloe (fresh juice)	Heals wounds and burns when applied to skin	Yes	Yes
Apricot pits (Laetrile)	Cures cancer	No	No
Caffeine-containing plant parts	Acts as a stimulant	Yes	Yes/no
Chamomile (flowers)	Relieves intestinal gas,	Yes	Yes[a]
	soothes inflammation,	Yes	Yes[a]
	prevents or relieves spasms,	Yes	Yes[a]
	acts against infection	Yes	Yes[a]
Comfrey (roots, leaves)	Aids healing	Yes	No
Fennel (fruits, seeds)	Stimulates the stomach,	Yes	Yes
	relieves intestinal gas	Yes	Yes
Feverfew (leaves)	Prevents migraine headaches	Yes[b]	Yes[b]
Garlic and other onionlike bulbs	Reduces high blood pressure	Yes	Yes
Gentian (roots)	Stimulates the appetite,	Yes	Yes
	aids digestion	Yes	Yes
Hawthorn (fruits, leaves, flowers)	Dilates blood vessels, lowers blood pressure	Yes	Yes
Hibiscus (flowers)	Acts as a laxative and diuretic	Yes (?)	Yes
Honey	Cures arthritis,	No	Yes
	acts as a sedative	No	Yes
Horehound (leaves, tops)	Acts as an expectorant (causes productive coughing)	Yes	Yes
Papaya (dried leaves)	Aids digestion,	No	Yes
	expels intestinal worms	No	Yes
Peppermint (leaves)	Stimulates the stomach,	Yes	Yes
	relieves intestinal gas	Yes	Yes
Sassafras (root bark)	Acts as a stimulant,	No	No
	prevents or relieves spasms,	No	No
	produces sweating,	No	No
	relieves rheumatism,	No	No
	acts as a general tonic	No	No
Savory (above ground plant)	Relieves intestinal gas,	Yes	Yes
	stimulates appetite,	Yes	Yes
	opposes diarrhea,	Yes	Yes
	acts as an aphrodisiac,	No	Yes
	reduces sex drive	No	Yes
Valerian (roots)	Tranquilizes and calms	Yes	Yes

[a]Except for allergic reactions.

[b]J. J. Murphy, S. Heptinstall, and J. R. A. Mitchell, Randomized double-blind placebo-controlled trial of feverfew in migraine prevention, *Lancet*, 23 July 1988, p. 189, as cited in *Journal of the American Dietetic Association* 88 (1988): 1621.

SOURCE: Adapted from V. E. Tyler, *The New Honest Herbal: A Sensible Guide to Herbs and Related Remedies* (Philadelphia: Stickley, 1987), with permission.

healthy skepticism, and evaluate the sources from which they come. Scientists have much to learn about foods and their effects, and true scientists will be the first to tell you so.

Meanwhile, to apply the information now available: strive for variety in the foods you choose to eat. Even if scientific research supports the claims associated with the foods discussed here, it is unwise to eat the same foods day after day. To opt for the benefits of only a few to the exclusion of many others is to put all your health eggs in one basket and perhaps to deny yourself many benefits not yet discovered. By eating a variety of foods you can diversify your investment, obtain maximum benefits, and at the same time dilute the undesirable substances in all the foods consumed. Notice that the foods that seem to have won most endorsement in this discussion are members of every major food group except meat (we have nothing against meat; it just did not turn up among the foods for which the health claims are most often made). They include vegetables, fruits, nuts, seeds, grains, and milk products, as well as herbs. So make selections from all of these categories, just as you would for nutrient adequacy.

Also, stay with whole foods, as close to the unrefined, farm-grown products as possible, because they are the ones most likely to contain both needed trace nutrients and beneficial nonnutrients. This or that fraction extracted from a food may not be an improvement upon the food itself. Chances are the beneficial effect of a food depends on a synergy among its nutrients, its structure, and its active nonnutrient components.

Notes

1. This discussion is adapted from E. N. Whitney, S. R. Rolfes, and F. S. Sizer, *Nonnutrients in Foods,* a monograph (1987) available from the Stickley Publishing Co., 210 Washington Sq., Philadelphia, PA 19106.

2. R. L. Koretz and J. H. Meyer, Elemental diets—facts and fantasies, *Gastroenterology* 78 (1980): 393–410.

3. F. D. Moore, Current thoughts on malabsorption: Parenteral, enteral, and oral feeding (commentary), *Journal of the American Dietetic Association* 86 (1986): 1169–1170.

4. R. J. I. Bain, Accidental digitalis poisoning due to drinking herbal tea (letter to the editor), *British Medical Journal* 290 (1985): 1624.

5. A. Brynjolfsson, Food irradiation and nutrition, *Professional Nutritionist,* Fall 1979, pp. 7–10.

6. R. Dubos, The intellectual basis of nutrition science and practice. Paper presented at the NIH Conference on the Biomedical and Behavioral Basis of Clinical Nutrition, 19 June 1978, in Bethesda, Md., and reprinted in *Nutrition Today,* July/August 1979, pp. 31–34.

7. J. A. Story and coauthors, Interactions of alfalfa plant and sprout saponins with cholesterol in vitro and in cholesterol-fed rats, *American Journal of Clinical Nutrition* 39 (1984): 917–929.

8. The substance the alfalfa tablets contained was an amino acid not normally found in proteins, L-canavanine. One person's SLE was reactivated after taking 15 tablets daily for nine months; the other person's, after taking eight tablets daily for two and a half years. J. L. Roberts and J. A. Hayashi, Exacerbation of SLE associated with alfalfa ingestion (letter to the editor), *New England Journal of Medicine* 308 (1983): 1361.

9. S. K. F. Chong and coauthors, Effect of ginseng saponins and hydrocortisone on phytohaemagglutinin transformation of lymphocytes, *Lancet,* 18 September 1982, pp. 662–663.

10. F. H. Schultz, Jr., R. Lowe, and R. A. Woodley, A possible effect of ginseng on serum HDL cholesterol (abstract no. 1522), *Federation Proceedings* 39, 1 March 1980.

11. M. A. Dubick, Historical perspectives on the use of herbal preparations to promote health, *Journal of Nutrition* 116 (1986): 1348–1354.

12. V. E. Tyler, *The New Honest Herbal: A Sensible Guide to the Use of Herbs and Related Remedies* (Philadelphia: Stickley, 1982), p. 108; E. M. Greenspan, Ginseng and vaginal bleeding (letter to the editor), *Journal of the American Medical Association* 249 (1983): 2018.

13. J. Konowalchuk and J. I. Speirs, Virus inactivation by grapes and wines, *Applied and Environmental Microbiology,* December 1976, pp. 757–763; A vintage medicine, *New York Times,* 12 June 1977, p. E7.

14. D. J. Forkner, Should wine be on your menu? *Professional Nutritionist,* Spring 1982, pp. 1–3.

15. P. N. Chaudhari and V. G. Hatwalne, Effect of epicatechin on liver lipids of rats fed with choline defi-

cient diet, *Indian Journal of Nutrition and Dietetics* 14 (1977): 136–139.

16. A. Bordia, Effect of garlic on blood lipids in patients with coronary heart disease, *American Journal of Clinical Nutrition* 34 (1981): 2100–2103; A. Bordia, Effect of garlic on human platelet aggregation in vitro, *Atherosclerosis* 30 (1978): 355–360; A. A. Qureshi and coauthors, Suppression of avian hepatic lipid metabolism by solvent extracts of garlic: Impact on serum lipids, *Journal of Nutrition* 113 (1983): 1746–1755; B. S. Kendler, Garlic (*Allium sativum*) and onion (*Allium cepa*): A review of their relationship to cardiovascular disease, *Preventive Medicine* 16 (1987): 670–685.

17. Garlic, *Journal of Nutrition Education* 15 (1983): 124.

18. S. Visudhiphan and coauthors, The relationship between high fibrinolytic activity and daily capsicum ingestion in Thais, *American Journal of Clinical Nutrition* 35 (1982): 1452–1458.

19. C. J. K. Henry and B. Emery, Effect of spiced food on metabolic rate, *Human Nutrition: Clinical Nutrition* 40C (1986): 165–168.

20. D. Graham, J. Smith, and A. Opekun, Spicy food and the stomach: Evaluation by videoendoscopy, *Journal of the American Medical Association* 260 (1988): 3473–3475.

21. G. A. Colditz and coauthors, Increased green and yellow vegetable intake and lowered cancer deaths in an elderly population, *American Journal of Clinical Nutrition* 41 (1985): 32–36.

22. L. W. Wattenberg, Inhibition of neoplasia by minor dietary constit-

uents, *Cancer Research* 43 (1983): 24485–24535.

23. S. S. Ansher, P. Dolan, and E. Bueding, Biochemical effects of dithiolthiones, *Food and Chemical Toxicology* 24 (1986): 405–415.

24. B. S. Reddy and coauthors, Nutrition and its relationship to cancer, *Advances in Cancer Research* 32 (1980): 238–345.

25. The enzymes are the microsomal mixed-function oxidases and, in particular, aryl hydrocarbon hydroxylase. L. W. Wattenberg and coauthors, Dietary constituents altering the responses to chemical carcinogens, *Federation Proceedings* 35 (1976): 1327–1331; L. W. Wattenberg and W. D. Loub, Inhibition of polycyclic aromatic hydrocarbon-induced neoplasia by naturally occurring indoles, *Cancer Research* 38 (1978): 1410–1413.

26. S. J. Stohs and coauthors, Effects of oltipraz, BHA, ADT and cabbage on glutathione metabolism, DNA damage and lipid peroxidation in old mice, *Mechanisms of Aging and Development* 37 (1986): 137–145.

27. Among the other inducers of the mixed-function oxidase system, found in plants, are flavones, aromatic isothiocyanates, coumarin, and selenium salts. Wattenberg and Loub, 1978.

28. W. Troll, K. Frenkel, and R. Wiesner, Protease inhibitors: Their role as modifiers of carcinogenic processes, in *Nutritional and Toxicological Significance of Enzyme Inhibitors in Foods,* ed. M. Friedman (New York: Plenum Press, 1986), pp. 153–165.

29. B. Merz, Adding seeds to the diet may keep cancer at bay, *Journal of the American Medical Association* 249 (1983): 2746.

30. J. Lauerman, A nutritional block against cancer? *Harvard Magazine,* May/June 1987, pp. 41–42; An alternative theory that plant-derived estrogen antagonists may be responsible for part of the effect on breast cancer is explained in S. Barnes and coauthors, Soybeans inhibit mammary tumors in models of breast cancer, in *Mutagens and Carcinogens in the Diet: Proceedings of a Satellite Symposium of the Fifth International Conference on Environmental Mutagens,* held in Madison, Wisconsin, July 5–7, 1989 ed. M. W. Pariza (New York: Wiley-Liss, 1990), pp. 239–253.

31. M. Lipkin and H. Newmark, Effect of added dietary calcium on colonic epithelial-cell proliferation in subjects at high risk for familial colonic cancer, *New England Journal of Medicine* 313 (1985): 1381–1384.

32. B. A. Friend and K. M. Shahani, Antitumor properties of lactobacilli and dairy products fermented by lactobacilli, *Journal of Food Protection* 47 (1984): 717–723.

33. B. R. Goldin and S. L. Gorbach, The effect of milk and *Lactobacillus* feeding on human intestinal bacterial enzyme activity, *American Journal of Clinical Nutrition* 39 (1984): 756–761.

34. G. V. Reddy and coauthors, Antitumor activity of yogurt compounds, *Journal of Food Protection* 46 (1983): 8–11.

35. Goldin and Gorbach, 1984.

36. A. D. Hitchins and coauthors, Amelioration of the adverse effect of a gastrointestinal challenge with *Salmonella enteritidis* on weanling rats by a yogurt diet, *American Journal of Clinical Nutrition* 41 (1985): 92–100.

37. In an experiment using rats, both whole and nonfat milk lowered serum cholesterol significantly. D. Kritchevsky and coauthors, Influence of wholeor skim milk on cholesterol metabolism in rats, *American Journal of Clinical Nutrition* 32 (1979): 597–600. In adolescent boys, nonfat milk, but not whole milk, lowered serum cholesterol. J. E. Rossouw and coauthors, The effect of skim milk, yogurt, and full cream milk on human serum lipids, *American Journal of Clinical Nutrition* 34 (1981): 351–356.

38. B. D. Agarwal and coauthors, Effect of lactose on serum lipids in cases of coronary artery disease, *Journal of the Indian Medical Association* 75 (1980): 153–156.

39. These acids are hydroxymethylglutaric acid and orotic acid. L. Aftergood and R. B. Alfin-Slater, Adverse effects of some food lipids, in *Adverse Effects of Foods,* eds. E. F. P. Jelliffe and D. B. Jelliffe, (New York: Plenum Press, 1982), p. 498.

40. N. Jenkins, Diet and dental caries, *Food and Nutrition News,* November/December 1984, p. 1.

41. R. Tomelleri and K. K. Grunewald, Menstrual cycle and food cravings in young college women, *Journal of the American Dietetic Association* 87 (1987): 311–315; W. J. Hurst; R. A. Martin; and B. L. Zoumas, Biogenic amines in chocolate—a review, *Nutrition Reports International* 26 (1982): 1081–1086; J. H. Burn and M. J. Rand, The action of sympathomimetic amines in animals treated with reserpine, *Journal of Physiology* 144 (1958): 314–336; B. Blackwell, Hypertensive crisis due to monoamine oxidase inhibitors, *Lancet* 2 (1963): 849–851; M. D. McDougal and G. B. West, The inhibition of the peristaltic reflex by sympathomimetic amines, *British Journal of Pharmacology* 9 (1954): 131–137.

42. Tidbits and morsels, *Nutrition and the MD,* January 1979.

43. Ginger aid, *Health,* August 1982, p. 14.

44. P. M. Ridker and coauthors, Hepatic venocclusive disease associated with the consumption of pyrrolizidine-containing dietary supplements, *Gastroenterology* 88 (1985): 1050–1054, as cited in R. J. Huxtable, J. Luthy, and U. Zweifel, Toxicity of comfrey-pepsin preparations, *New England Journal of Medicine* 315 (1986): 1095.

45. Questions and answers, *Nutrition and the MD,* December 1982.

Hunger and Hope: Nutrition and the Environment, 1990s

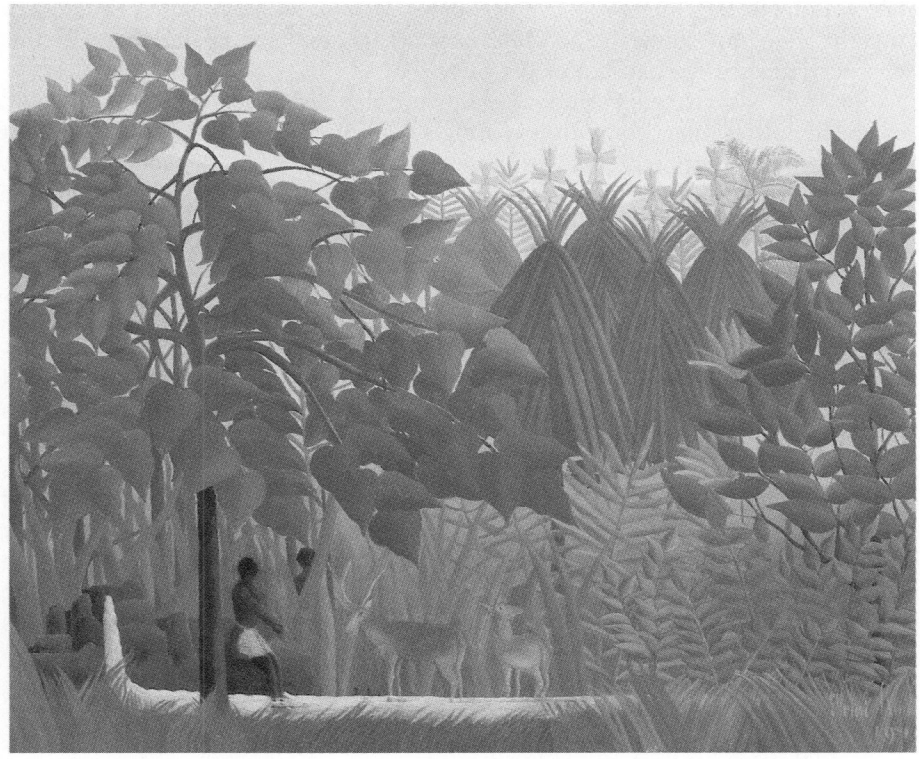

CONTENTS

Henri Rousseau, French, 1844–1910, *The Waterfall* (La Cascade), oil on canvas, 1910, 116.2 × 150.2 cm, Helen Birch Bartlett Memorial Collection. Photograph © 1990, The Art Institute of Chicago. All Rights Reserved.

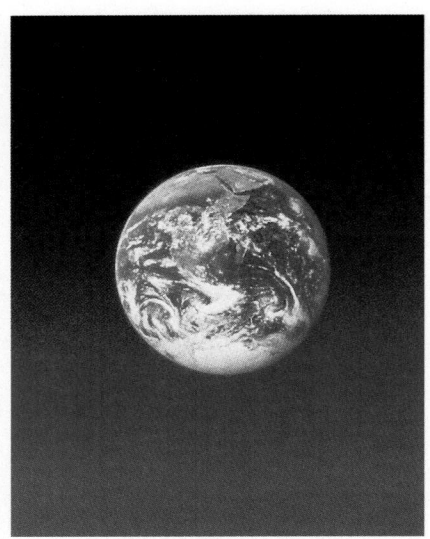

Planet earth—our home.

■■■ What if a global disaster were scheduled for today but didn't come off? What if everybody worked so hard to prevent it that it didn't happen? The premise of this chapter is that the rescue scenario can take place.

This is not an attempt to make light of a very serious subject—for the subject of this chapter is a life-and-death matter for everyone. Rather it is an attempt to introduce the kind of thinking being espoused by today's experts on the future—the people studying the population explosion, world hunger, global warming, and the other growing problems of the earth today that affect tomorrow's food and water supplies. It is positive thinking. The idea is that *if* we are willing to face the problems we have created, think together, and work together, we can solve them. Time is short, though (as is the space in this chapter), and so we had better get busy.

It is not easy to grasp and face the problems described in this chapter, especially all at once. As with any tough reading assignment, this one might best be tackled in increments with breaks between (perhaps at each key point). It resembles any other tough learning task in another way too, though: the reward is proportional to your mastery of the task. In this case the reward is the personal power that comes with understanding the problems well enough to take action to help solve them.

The 1980s, at the end of which this chapter was being written, were an eventful and scary decade in world history. Major news included AIDS (it was named in 1981); the most severe droughts and floods ever seen on several continents (Asia, 1984; Africa, 1984–1985; United States, 1988); a massive, deadly pesticide leak from a factory (Bhopal, India, 1984); the biggest nuclear accident ever (Chernobyl, USSR, 1986); the biggest oil spill ever (Alaska's Prince William Sound, 1989); and the confirmation that global warming was indeed taking place (1989). Also new were signs of new hope for world peace (Gorbachev became leader in the USSR in 1985), freedom (the iron curtain began to crumble late in 1989), and cooperation among nations in solving the world's problems (by 1990 many nations agreed to a reduction in their outputs of chemicals that destroy the earth's protective ozone layer). Earth Day, in 1990, involved all people everywhere in honoring the planet and in promoting human survival and health.

Among the most important perspectives on world nutrition and the environment are views that have appeared in publications by the Worldwatch Institute of Washington, D.C. and in a special issue of *Scientific American* entitled *Managing Planet Earth.** Both sources convey the strong conviction that poverty, hunger, and worldwide environmental degradation are very closely linked and can and must be solved in concert, and both employ terms to help conceptualize the solution—terms such as "sustainable development," "environmental feedback into pricing," and "low-input agriculture."

Watch for these concepts as you read. Watch especially for mention of **renewable resources, appropriate technology,** and **sustainable methods,** since these seem to be keys to the solutions for today's global problems. Notice, too, that both the poor (largely agricultural) and the well-to-do (largely industrial) nations make major contributions to these problems and share the responsibility for solving them.

*Worldwatch Institute is a nonprofit research organization created to analyze and focus attention on global problems; it is funded by private foundations and United Nations organizations. Its *State of the World* report, which comes out annually, is used as a text in more and more college courses and is helping to make tomorrow's leaders aware of the areas on which they need to focus their attention. The *Scientific American* issue was published in September 1989.

The experts seem to agree that we need to learn some radically new ways of thinking if humankind is to succeed at the unique experiment in earth life that it is presently conducting. And not only is new thinking needed but also new feeling: our attitudes and motivation need to be transformed. As one set of writers put it, it is not enough to know we need to change our behaviors in some ways; we must actually buckle down and do so; and this "will require that we plow through some new emotional territory."[1]

Part One of this chapter presents the pieces of the puzzle; Part Two of the chapter shows how they are all connected. Part Three then presents proposed solutions, and the chapter concludes with personal agendas for action.

▐▐▐ ▶ Part One: Puzzle Pieces

The world's supply of stored grain has diminished. Soil depletion worldwide is reaching crisis proportions; so are water shortages. Both droughts and floods are becoming more common. Pesticide and industrial contamination of the environment is widespread and increasing. Forests are dwindling everywhere, and species losses are occurring at an unprecedented rate. The climate is heating up, and a hole in the outer atmosphere's protective ozone layer has formed and is growing larger fast. The world's population is growing by larger increments every year, poverty and hunger are growing worse, and the poor nations' debts to the wealthy nations are huge and growing larger. These are the pieces of the puzzle that all fit together into a massive problem for humanity on earth that demands immediate action. This section discusses each in turn.

Declining Grain Stores

The world's food supply is often measured in grain output, since grain is the world's single largest crop. Between 1950 and 1984, the world's grain supply increased faster than the population did, encouraging world leaders to believe that continued expansion would be possible. Then in 1984, the picture suddenly changed. Grain output per person leveled off, and in 1987 it began to fall sharply. Whereas at the start of 1987 stored grain surpluses were sufficient to feed the world's people for 101 days, at the end of 1988 they were sufficient for only 54 days.[2] Droughts accounted for much of the decline in reserves; they and other environmental factors such as air pollution, soil loss, and climate change were suspected causes of the slowdown in food output.[3]

In the past, any nation that has run short of grain has had two options—to buy, borrow, or beg other countries' stored surpluses or to take measures to increase its own grain outputs. Now the stored surpluses are dwindling, and outputs cannot be increased much more. Nearly all of the world's suitable land is already under cultivation. Farming *unsuitable* land (such as the land on steep, erodible mountainsides or in rainforests) results in losses of soil and water to an extent that cannot be sustained for more than a few years. Furthermore, expanding human populations and industrial development are claiming for homes, highways, and industrial parks the very same land, labor, and water that might be recruited for farming.

▐▐ ▶ *Remedies for grain shortages that have worked in the past are now failing because they are based on the fallacy that the world's resources are infinite. The*

renewable resources: resources that constantly renew themselves, such as forests (if allowed to do so), sunlight, and rain. In contrast, *nonrenewable resources* are those of which a limited supply exists, such as oil and ground water.

appropriate technology: technology suited to local need, not excessive in its use of resources or in its use of machines to replace human labor. As an example, it is not necessary to use a bulldozer to bury a quart of garbage in your back yard. An ordinary shovel will do.

sustainable methods (for example, of agriculture or industry): methods that employ renewable resources at a rate that can be sustained indefinitely without depleting them. Examples: use of solar energy is a sustainable method of fueling energy-requiring processes; recycling is a sustainable method of using any resource.

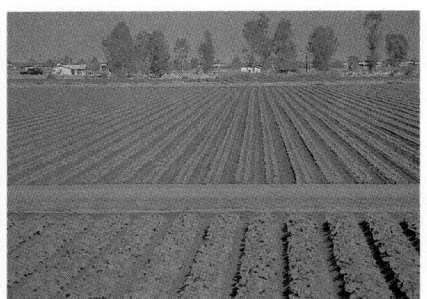

Vast areas are under the plow, and if they must be irrigated they are becoming salty and unusable.

truth is that soil, water, and land are all being depleted. These resources are limited, and we stand within sight of their exhaustion.

Soil Loss

To grow food requires soil—soil that can hold water long enough for plants to drink it up, soil with nutrients in it. However, soil is being lost all over the globe at a tremendous rate; its loss has been called the most serious environmental calamity the earth's living things are facing. Soil is being picked up by winds and blown away; washed down slopes into rivers and down rivers into the ocean; dried out; polluted; paved over; leached of nutrients to the point of uselessness; and rendered too salty by irrigation for use. New soil is created continuously by the action of wind and water on rocks, but losses are greatly outpacing gains and are increasing every year—essentially, soil is not a renewable resource. Soil loss due to human misuse of the land today is taking place so fast that a quarter of the world's farmable land is fated to become permanent wasteland. With less soil, plants become stressed and vulnerable to disease and insect pests, so that they require more care.

In the past the chief means employed by agriculture to bolster failing cropland where soil loss has occurred has been to plow, irrigate, fertilize, and apply pesticides more intensively. (This is known as **high-input agriculture.**) Unfortunately, though, plowing exposes bare soil unprotected by roots to erosion from wind and water. Also, irrigation damages the soil, and all four practices pollute surface and ground water.

Irrigation damages the soil by causing salt to accumulate on the land (**salinization**). All water, even fresh water, contains some salts, and water evaporates, while salts do not. Currently, about 20 percent of all the irrigated land in the United States is becoming salinized to the point of no return, and possibly about a quarter of the world's irrigated land is being similarly affected.[4]

Irrigation also pollutes the water, taking a heavy environmental toll on neighboring lands. The water that does not evaporate from an agricultural field runs off—together with the fertilizers and pesticides it picked up from the soil and plants. Drainage water laced with toxic chemicals drains into wetlands that are crucial habitats for fish and wildlife. Accumulating evidence of reproductive failure and grotesque deformities of wildlife indicates that this problem is widespread in many Western states, which use irrigation heavily. Agricultural pollution is also destroying major lakes that provide people's drinking water in Florida and elsewhere in the southeast.

High-input agriculture is, for this and many other reasons, not sustainable over the long term. A preferable way to replenish soil and restore its fertility—and this is the sustainable way that we must look to in the future—is to build and improve the soil by returning plant material and manure to it. It will also help to rotate crops and return vulnerable areas to forest and grassland for periods long enough to permit renewal rather than letting the soil become worn out and wash or blow away. (See the later section on sustainable development.)

▐▐ ▷ *The earth's soil is being depleted faster than it is being formed. High-input agriculture causes soil losses by way of erosion and damages soil by way of irrigation, which makes it so salty that plants cannot grow on it.*

Water Shortages and Contamination

Of all the bounties of the world, water is the most abundant, pure, and life-giving—or was, that is, until recently. Now the quantity of water available to meet human needs worldwide is running short, and the quality is also deteriorating.

Rain is the ultimate source of all the world's water, and after falling on the earth, much of it returns to the sky as vapor or runs off in rivers to the oceans. The water that remains on the land long enough to be used is what we depend on for our lives, and there is enough to support the lives of about 20 billion people—about four times the world's 1990 population of five-plus billion. However, the supply is uneven; in many places there is not enough water to grow the food needed to sustain human life.[5] Agriculture uses about three-fourths of all the water people withdraw from the earth. Vast areas of the world are irrigated to grow crops—a total land area nearly as large as all of India.

Irrigated areas are increasing, but recently at the rate of only about 1 percent per year, only a little more than half as fast as the world's population. The heyday of new irrigation projects, seen earlier in this century, is over, because the rivers and ground waters usable for irrigation have already been tapped by increasing populations. Now water tables are falling, and pumping costs are rising. Little significant expansion of irrigation is thought to be possible henceforth; the only reasonably priced hope for providing water to larger land areas in the future is to reduce the wastage of the water already being used, so that it will spread further.

Where there are water shortages, people turn to three ways of gaining the additional amounts needed. They dam rivers, they "mine" water from underground **aquifers** where it has been trapped since prehistoric times, or they conserve—ceasing to waste water on nonessential uses. As mentioned, most of the world's usable rivers have already been dammed. As for the mining of aquifers, theoretically they are a renewable resource if no more water is drawn out than is replaced by rain. However, in many places water is being removed so fast that rain cannot maintain the water levels. In many parts of the world, including much of the United States, the land is drying out and collapsing below sea level due to overpumping of underground water in this fashion. Along coastlines, as underground fresh water levels drop, salt water from the ocean moves in to fill the space and so invades aquifers, ruins people's wells, and makes it impossible to grow crops.

The way in which irrigation pollutes surface water has already been described. It also depletes the ground water supply because once the ground water is spread on the land, it is lost by evaporation. Ironically this adds to the *drying out* of the irrigated land—**desertification**—by lowering the water table. Irrigated land thus grows more dry from below the surface and more salty on top (by salinization, already described) and finally reaches a point where it cannot support the growth of any sort of vegetation—even weeds die out. The vast desert of North Africa was once a wheat-producing area that fed the Roman Empire until, due to irrigation, water became too scarce and the soil too salty to grow wheat.

Water pollution is also increasing worldwide, creating a further shortage of *usable* water—both the water in surface waterways and the water of aquifers (ground water). One major pollutant of waterways is eroding soil—beneficial on land but harmful to waterways. It fills them with silt and clouds them so that their normal vegetation cannot grow—vegetation that feeds aquatic

high-input agriculture: agriculture that uses intensive applications of irrigation, pesticides, fertilizers, and fossil fuel.

salinization (of soil): the progressive accumulation of salt in soil.

aquifer: an underground, water-bearing stratum of rock, sand, or other sediment, the source of so-called *ground water.*

desertification: the conversion of fertile land to desert.

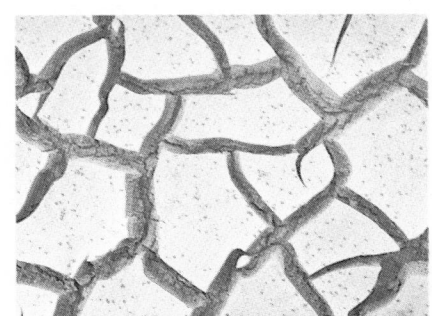

As ground water is used up, deserts spread.

eutrophication (you-tro-fi-CAY-shun): the process by which excess nutrients such as nitrogen and phosphorus support the overgrowth of algae in a water body and lead to the "death" of the water body—its inability to support normal aquatic life.

runoff: the water that drains into waterways from pavement, agricultural fields, and other areas rather than sinking into the ground.

food chain: the order of predation in nature in which each organism eats others. Microorganisms and plants are at the base of the food chain; herbivorous animals near the base; small carnivores next; and large carnivores such as eagles, large fish, large cats, and human beings at the top.

organisms and fish. Another pollutant, often accompanying soil, is fertilizers from agriculture, which are full of compounds that can serve as nutrients to plants. These support the overgrowth of algae, which form thick sheets on the water's surface. As some algae are crowded out of the sunlight they need, they die and become food for bacteria. The bacteria that decompose them use up the water's oxygen in doing so, making the water unlivable for fish and other organisms. By this process of overgrowth, or **eutrophication,** lakes fill with organic matter and die.

Whereas in farming regions agricultural water affects an area's waterways, in urban areas city or industrial water affects them. Cities generate sewage by the thousands of tons, and even if they extract the solids from it in treatment plants, the effluent they release is full of dissolved pollutants. Sewage effluent also often carries toxic compounds from industrial plants that have discarded their wastes into drains. Urban areas pollute the waterways in another way too: whenever it rains, sheets of water wash the accumulated oil, grease, and other toxic compounds (**runoff**) from streets, parking lots, and highways into nearby water bodies. Unlike sewage, which can be treated at collection points, runoff enters waterways all along their boundaries.

Pollutants affect lakes, rivers, bays, and deltas not only now but later by way of contaminating their bottom mud. The amount of contamination along a river and in its bay varies directly, both with the number of people there and with those people's monetary wealth—the number because people create sewage and agricultural pollution; and the wealth because wealth is often gained through industry, and industry brings pollution. If a project involves dredging up polluted bottom mud (for example, to create more land to grow crops), the dredging process often kills aquatic life in the water body, and the mud itself often proves too toxic for agricultural use or even as earth on which to build homes.[6] The suspended silt can cover nesting sites, clog gills of fish, block sunlight needed by aquatic plants, and more; it is a highly destructive substance even when not toxic.

Water pollution aggravates food shortages. More than half of the world's population lives on seacoasts, around the mouths of rivers, and near bays, and most of the fish on which vast populations depend are caught in and near these very same areas. Coastal waters are the world's most biologically productive areas, since most marine organisms conduct crucial parts of their life cycles there—reproduction, incubation of eggs, foraging for feed. In many parts of the world, both where agricultural populations are growing and where industrialization is now taking place, degradation of water resources is considered the most threatening of all environmental problems to human life and to all life.[7]

Some water pollution is reversible, albeit at great cost. A surface water body such as a river or lake can be restored to usable purity over years with massive effort. However, ground water (aquifer) pollution is, for all practical purposes, not reversible. Once salt water has invaded a coastal aquifer, that aquifer will never again be fresh. Once oil has leaked from an underground tank to contaminate an aquifer, the water can never again be used as drinking water. Surface and ground water are not completely separate either; pollution of surface water today may work its way into ground water tomorrow.

Although this chapter's main mission is to show the connections between all the puzzle pieces, consumers are rightly concerned about possible pollution of their own water supplies. Some consumers buy bottled water, hoping for purity, but they may not be getting what they bargained for. No place in the

United States has totally pure water, and even the deepest cold springs now contain pollutants.[8] While bottled water must comply with purity standards set for municipal tap water, it need be tested only once each year, and no additional standards of purity are mandatory.[9] Some bottled water *is* municipal water that has been filtered to remove specific contaminants (while others remain in the water). Sometimes bacteria and other contaminants are allowed to enter the water during bottling, setting the stage for illness in those who would drink it. In addition, most bottled water does not contain fluoride, and if it is distilled, beneficial constituents such as calcium and other minerals are removed.

The purest drinking water is unpolluted rain water without excess acid, collected directly or withdrawn pure from the earth. Since water is vital to all life, this is one of the most compelling reasons why we need clean air and an unpolluted environment.

▌▶ *Surface water supplies are a renewable resource; ground water aquifers are not. Ground water is being depleted, mostly by agriculture (irrigation), and surface waters are being polluted by agriculture, industry, and growing human populations. Conservation and protection of water supplies is a vital need.*

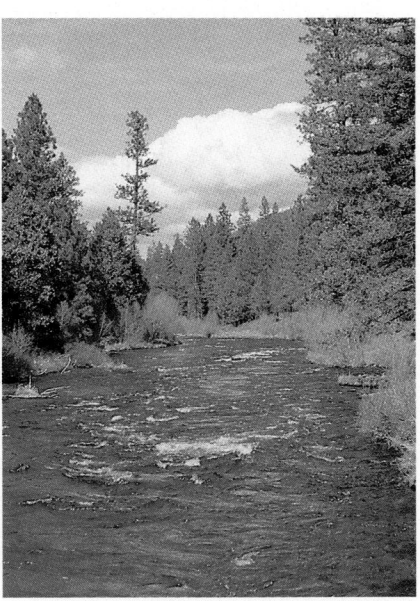

Pure rivers represent irreplaceable water resources.

Pesticide Use in Agriculture

One of the most notable features of high-input agriculture is pesticide use. Pesticides are intended to help produce and protect an adequate supply of food for a reasonable price. They are relatively new in the world; and their widespread use is very new. In U.S. agriculture, their use is regulated, and their presence in food is monitored in such a way that the food supply itself presents few hazards to consumers. But the damage pesticides do to the environment is considerable and increasing. Furthermore, there is some question about whether the widespread use of pesticides has really improved the overall yield of food. In 1945, when pesticide use was minimal, about one-fifth of the nation's food supply was lost to pests; today we still lose about one-fifth of our crops to pests.[10] Also the high prices of pesticides cut into farmers' profits.

Pesticides doubtless do help preserve some crops from some pests, but at a considerable cost in other respects. Many are broad-spectrum poisons that damage all living cells, not just those of pests. Their use, therefore, is hazardous, and poisoning episodes involving farm workers are not uncommon. During the production and transport of poisons, leaks and spills are especially likely; the episode at Bhopal, India, cited earlier with other disasters of the decade, killed 3000 people immediately, many more later, and maimed more still. Table 15–1 shows how pesticides work biologically.

Also, pesticides kill pests' natural predators, as well as the pests themselves, since predators are one step higher on the **food chain** than the pests they prey on. For example, many insect pests eat leaves and are eaten in turn by birds. An insect may eat many times its weight in leaves each day and so accumulate a large dose of poison, but a bird eats so many insects that it accumulates even more. The still higher animals that prey on the bird ingest more poison still, and it is they—the animals highest on the food chain—that are most likely to be poisoned. Since human beings eat high on the food chain (for example, they eat large fish that eat small fish that eat plants), they are vulnerable too (Figure 15–1).

■■■ Table 15–1 Biological Effects of Pesticides

TYPE OF USE	COMMON NAMES (EXAMPLES)	BIOLOGICAL EFFECTS
Insecticides	Parathion, Malathion	Toxic to nerves; acute poisoning causes respiratory failure.
	Aldicarb, Zectran	Toxic to nerves.
	DDT, Dieldrin,	Accumulate in fatty tissues, inhibit electrolyte transport, impair
	Heptachlor, Chlordane,	reproduction in birds.
	Mirex	
	Ethylene dibromide (EDB)	A carcinogen.
Herbicides	2,4,5-T	Toxic generally and to nerves.
	Paraquat	Toxic generally; causes edema in the lungs.
	Prophan	Allergenic.
	Simazine	Carcinogenic.
Fungicides	Captan	Causes birth defects.
	Pentachlorophenol (PCP)	Toxic generally.
Rodenticides	Warfarin	An anticoagulant.
	Red squill	Causes heart failure.
	Compounds 1080, 1081	Inhibit cellular respiration.
	ANTU	Causes edema in the lungs.

SOURCE: Adapted from M. G. Mustafa, Agricultural chemicals, in *Adverse Effects of Foods,* eds. E. F. P. Jelliffe and D. B. Jelliffe (New York: Plenum Press, 1982), Table 1, pp. 112–113.

The use of DDT provides a well-known example of failure of a pesticide to do its job safely. Intended only to poison pests, DDT accumulated to such levels in higher animals that it threatened their survival, including that of the American national symbol, the bald eagle. DDT also accumulated in human tissues, and its use on agricultural crops in the United States was finally banned. (Other countries still use DDT, however, and in fact they import it from the United States.)

Pesticides also induce resistance in pests. A pesticide may kill *almost* 100 percent of the insects that are attacking a crop, but thanks to the inevitable genetic variability of large populations, a very few insects are likely to be able to survive exposure. The resistant insects can then multiply free of competition and soon will produce large numbers of offspring that inherit their resistance to the pesticide and can attack the crop with enhanced vigor. This requires application of a new and more powerful pesticide, and so the cycle continues.

Pesticides also pollute the environment. They are carried by wind and washed by rain into many areas for which they are not intended and can end up killing wildlife and polluting people's drinking water. Farmers in many states are now becoming aware that pesticides do more harm than good and are demanding support for development of alternatives to their use. In Iowa, for example, the result has been a tax on pesticides that finances programs designed to reduce the use of farm chemicals.[11]

This chapter comes back later to the problems of pesticides and the environment, but for the consumer, their presence in food is of most immediate concern: "Are the foods I buy safe to eat?" The answer to this question seems to be yes, almost without exceptions, because this nation's food safety regulations and procedures are stringent and effective. This chapter's Consumer Caution addresses the problem of how to protect yourself from pesticides.

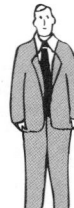

Level 4
a 150 lb person

Level 3
100 lb of larger fish

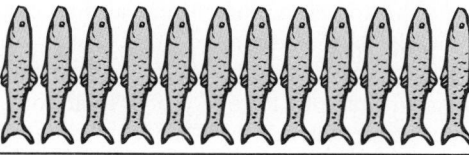

Level 2
a few tons of small
plant-eating fish

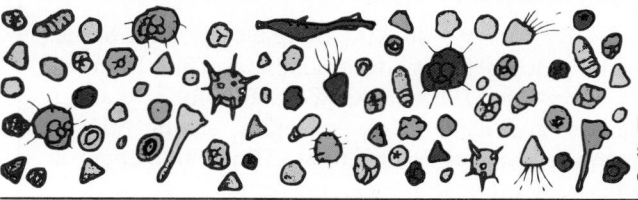

Level 1
several tons of producer
organisms

███ **Figure 15–1**

Accumulation of Toxins in the Food Chain. A person whose principal animal protein source is fish may consume about 100 pounds of fish in a year. These fish will, in turn, have consumed a few tons of plant-eating fish in the course of their lifetimes. The plant eaters, in their lifetimes, will have consumed several tons of photosynthetic producer organisms. If the producer organisms have become contaminated with toxic chemicals, these chemicals become more concentrated in the bodies of the fish that consume them. If none of the chemicals are lost along the way, *one person* ultimately eats the same amount of contaminant as was present in the original *several tons* of producer organisms.

| CONSUMER CAUTION‖‖ | **Protection from Pesticides** |

You read of pesticide scares all the time, and always they seem to be affecting just the foods you were about to buy: apples, grapes, or oranges. Should you be alarmed? How alarmed should you be? What should you do to protect yourself from pesticide residues in foods?

The first thing to do is to know enough to appreciate the excellent protection provided for you by government agencies. The Environmental Protection Agency (EPA) and the Food and Drug Administration (FDA) have joint responsibility for registering pesticides and regulating their use. To register a pesticide, the maker submits data to EPA on the results of studies on its biological effects, persistence in crops on which the pesticide may be used, and environmental fate. EPA then evaluates the risks and benefits of the pesticide's use (How dangerous is it? How much residue is left in the crop? How much harm does it do to the environment? How necessary is it? What are the alternatives to its use?), registers the pesticide (if approved), and establishes a **tolerance** level for its presence in foods. In 1987 there were 320

continued on next page

tolerance: the maximum amount of a residue permitted in a food when a pesticide is used according to label directions, provided that the level does not present an unacceptable health risk.

certification: inspection by a private laboratory of shipments of a product for selected chemicals, followed by the laboratory's guarantee that the product is free of violative levels of those chemicals.

pesticide chemicals with established food and/or feed tolerances in the United States.

FDA then monitors foods and feeds for the presence of pesticides. Based on 25 years' worth of data, FDA seldom finds residues above tolerance levels, so it appears that pesticides are generally used according to label directions. Where violations are found, they are usually due to misuse, to unusual weather conditions, or to unapproved use of the pesticide—for example, use on a product for which no tolerance has been set (any amount is then illegal). For example, FDA still finds DDT in foods occasionally, a finding that triggers prosecution of the user.

The way that FDA monitors foods is to collect samples of both domestic and imported foods and to analyze them using methods that can detect residues well below tolerances. If FDA finds violative levels, it can seize the products or stop the manufacturer from selling them. FDA may also invoke a **certification** requirement: this forces manufacturers, at their own expense, to have their foods periodically inspected and certified safe by an independent testing agency. FDA also cooperates with states to scan for pesticides and industrial chemicals. As an example, for one year's "food-contam" effort, 15,000 samples in five states were analyzed.† (A "feedcon" program operates similarly.)

FDA then conducts selective surveys—looking more closely for a particular pesticide in a particular group of foods—for example, bananas from five countries. (The selective surveys for 1987 included a search for aldicarb in potatoes, captan in cherries, and diaminozide in apples, among others.) Actions taken in 1987 required several certifications. Thus one shipper in Australia had to certify his apples, one in Canada his peppers, one in Costa Rica his chayotes, eight in the Dominican Republic their eggplant, 11 in Spain their lemons; and there were other similar actions. All grapes from Mexico had to be certified in 1987; so did all mangoes from anywhere. (This shows, incidentally, how many foods come from abroad—apples, peppers, chayotes, bitter melons, eggplant, long beans, okra, snow peas, squash, broccoli, coriander, cucumbers, grapes, okra, peppers, strawberries, currants, lemons, and mangoes—but it also shows that FDA monitors them as carefully as it monitors the domestic food supply.)

A summary of FDA's findings indicates that no residues were found in over 50 percent of all samples, domestic and imported, analyzed in 1987. Of the violations found, nearly all (87 percent) of the violations involved use of pesticides for which no tolerance had been established (these are illegal at any level). Fewer than 1 percent had residues that exceeded tolerances. The list of "pesticides that could have been detected or were found in 1987" included 253 chemical names from acephate to zytron. "These data illustrate that pesticide chemicals are rarely used in a manner that results in residue levels that exceed tolerances."[12] Figure 15–2 illustrates the proportions of contaminated foods among foods selected for inspection.

†To better monitor imported foods, FDA purchased in 1986 the Battelle World Agrochemical Data Bank, a computerized data base containing information on foreign pesticide use, so as to better target particular pesticides likely to have been used on particular crops.

continued on next page

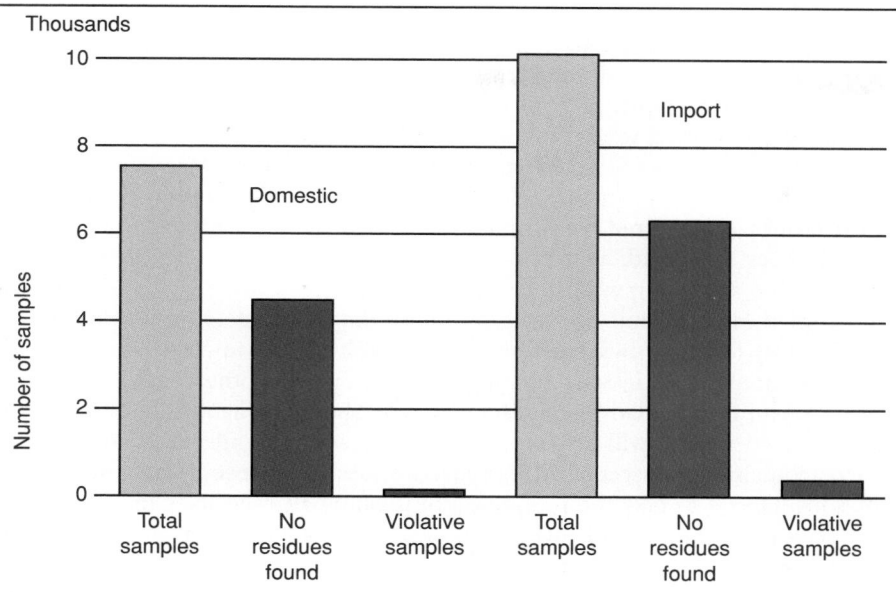

■■■ **Figure 15–2**

Results of Surveys of Selected Foods, FDA, 1988.
Of over 6000 domestic samples fewer than 1% had pesticide residues that exceeded tolerances. Of about 8000 imported foods, the same result: fewer than 1% had violative residues.
Source: From *Residues in Foods— 1988* (Washington, D.C.: Food and Drug Administration, 1989), Figure 5.

While monitoring foods on the market for pesticides on the one hand, FDA also monitors people's actual intakes on the other. It runs the Total Diet Study (the "Market Basket Survey") to estimate the dietary intakes of pesticide residues by eight age/sex groups from infants to senior citizens. (It also monitors their intakes of essential minerals, industrial chemicals, heavy metals, and radioactive materials.) The surveyors buy over 200 foods four times a year in U.S. grocery stores, each time in several cities, prepare them table ready, and then analyze them. Because food preparation often reduces levels of contaminants in foods, FDA must use procedures that measure levels at least five times lower than permitted limits. In all, the survey reports on over 10,000 samples a year, and recently more than half have been imported foods. Most heavily sampled are fresh vegetables, then fruits, then dairy foods.

The Total Diet Study provides a direct estimate of people's dietary intakes of pesticides. In one recent year 200 were sought, and 55 were found. For almost all pesticides, the dietary intake was found to be less than 1 percent of the amount considered acceptable. (The amount considered acceptable is "the daily intake of a chemical which, if ingested over a lifetime, appears to be without appreciable risk"; it is established by the United Nations Food and Agriculture Organization and the World Health Organization.) All in all, these findings corroborate "the continuing safety of the U.S. food supply relative to pesticide residues."[13]

Despite these reassuring reports, consumers worry that the monitoring of foods may not be adequate, for several reasons. For one, new pesticides keep appearing before the EPA can act to evaluate and register them. For another, as described, other countries use pesticides that are illegal for use here— some even exported from here to those countries—and imported foods are

continued on next page

not always tested for the presence of those pesticides. Also, the maximum amount of a pesticide allowed in a food assumes that a person will only consume moderate quantities of that food, whereas in reality people sometimes overeat certain foods.

Besides, diagnosing toxic effects of pesticides is difficult. Many cause delayed reactions, especially those that poison the nerves. Toxins may collect in fatty tissues, sequestered away from the rest of the body—harmless until that fat becomes mobilized, as may occur in animals when food is scarce or in people who are losing weight.

All of these problems are real and imply that consumers have some responsibility for their own health and safety with respect to pesticides. Consumers should read reliable literature, discuss it with others, advise their government representatives on how pesticides should be handled, and apply pressure wherever it will help change procedures. Meanwhile, to avoid using foods containing unacceptably high levels of pesticides, people have several options. One is to take the precaution of washing all vegetables in running water, scrubbing them with a vegetable brush, or soaking uncut vegetables in a weak vinegar and water solution to remove pesticides. Irradiated fruits and vegetables are also a reasonable choice because they are spared post-harvest pesticide sprayings.

Another is, whenever possible, to buy fresh foods grown locally, especially when you can confirm that they have been grown using responsible methods. Don't look for "perfect" fruits and vegetables; pesticide-free produce may have a few blemishes, but blemishes are not a hazard. Importantly, it is sensible to buy a variety of foods and not to rely too heavily on any one. The food supply is protected well enough so that with these precautions consumers can feel secure that the foods they eat are safe. If you have questions, call the EPA's pesticide hotline‡—but probably the most important thing consumers can do to protect their *food* supply is to be active in defending the *environment* (see this chapter's Food Feature).

While our domestic food supply seems to be relatively safe, the widespread use of pesticides in U.S. agriculture contributes to major environmental problems such as the pollution of our air, water, and soil. As you will see, an agenda item for the future is to reduce pesticide use in U.S. agriculture as well as worldwide and to develop more environmentally benign means of controlling pests.

‡The National Pesticide Hotline, funded by EPA, is 1–800–858–PEST. Call any time day or night, 365 days a year.

◖◗▷ *Pesticide use on agricultural crops is widespread. Domestic and imported foods are carefully monitored and generally well within safe limits, but environmental damage and the risks of accidents involving pesticides are of concern.*

Other Contaminants

Related to the problem of pesticides in foods and of equal concern to consumers is the problem of other contaminants, especially those released by industry. The number of contaminants and the amount of information available about them is far beyond this book's scope. Instead of dealing superficially with many of them, let us illustrate principles that apply to all contaminants by giving details about just a few. A list of some of the chemical contaminants of greatest concern in foods is presented in Table 15–2. Table 15–3 gives more details on four of them.

Table 15–3 shows how pervasively a contaminant can affect the body. Look at the case of lead for a particularly telling example. Then note that thousands of U.S. children aged six months to five years have symptoms caused by lead toxicity: 1 out of every 50 in rural areas and more than 1 out of every 10 in inner cities.[14] Chapter 13 told the story of Joey, one such child afflicted with lead poisoning. Similar stories could be told about many other contaminants, since contamination of the environment is becoming more widespread.

The single major reason for this is that the earth's people are multiplying. As they do so, they demand more and more food and more and more of the products of industry. Food means agriculture with its associated pesticides and fertilizers; industry means other contaminants. These two huge, human activities dominate the earth; almost every human community centers on one or the other or both. And people themselves are a third source of pollution in the form of human sewage and throwaways such as garbage and plastics. All these problems grow in proportion to our population's growth, another puzzle piece to be discussed later.

▌▌▶ *Contaminants are potentially dangerous compounds that can accidentally find their way into food; lead is an example. Contaminants also affect the environment. They come from both agricultural and industrial enterprises, as well as from centers of human habitation, and so are most abundant where people are numerous. They are becoming more widespread as the human population grows.*

Deforestation

Another problem that is growing worse as the human population increases is the loss of trees all over the world. Trees are vital to many natural balances and cycles. They help replenish the soil, and they play a major role in replenishing fresh water. By preserving soil, they help the earth hold moisture; but more than that, they return vast amounts of underground water to the atmosphere by a process known as **transpiration.** Transpired water is pure and forms clouds that will fall again as rain (fresh water) rather than running down rivers to join the ocean and become unusable salt water.

Trees have covered much of the earth since prehistoric times. They provide a deep layer of vegetation that engages in many processes that support and renew the environment and sustain the lives of other plants and animals. Consider the trees in a rainforest, for example. They may be more than 100 feet tall and 20 feet across at the base. They support a mass of vegetation and animal life. They create shade and hold moisture. By transpiration, they help create rain clouds, and these rain clouds burst frequently, releasing drenching torrents. They absorb carbon dioxide and generate oxygen by photosynthesis, permitting all living things in the forest to breathe. By capturing moisture, they help to regulate the earth's temperature. They drop tons of leaf litter, bark, branches, and animal droppings to the ground beneath them, where molds, fungi, and bacteria break down this litter as fast as it falls, keeping the system

transpiration: the process by which trees and other plants shift water from below the ground to the air.

▌▌▌ Table 15–2 Chemical Contaminants of Concern in Foods, U.S., 1870–1980

Heavy Metals
Lead
Mercury
Cadmium
Selenium
Arsenic
Halogenated Compounds
Chlorine
Iodine
Vinyl chloride
Ethylene dichloride
Trichloroethylene (TCE)
Polychlorinated biphenyls (PCBs)
Polybrominated biphenyls (PBBs)
Others
Asbestos
Dioxins
Acrylonitrile
Lysinoalanine
Diethylstilbestrol (DES)
Heat-induced mutagens
Antibiotics (in animal feed)

SOURCE: E. M. Foster, How safe are our foods? *Nutrition Reviews* (supplement), January 1982, pp. 28–34.

■■■ Table 15–3 Examples of Contaminants in Foods

NAME AND DESCRIPTION	SOURCES	TOXIC EFFECTS	TYPICAL ROUTE TO FOOD CHAIN
Cadmium (heavy metal)	Used in industrial processes including electroplating, plastics, batteries, alloys, pigments, smelters, and burning fuels. Present in cigarette smoke.	No immediately detectable symptoms; slowly and irreversibly damages kidneys and liver.	Enters air in smokestack emissions, settles on ground, absorbed into food plants, consumed by farm animals, and eaten in meat and vegetables by people. Sewage sludge and fertilizers leave large amounts in the soils; runoff contaminates shellfish.
Lead (heavy metal)	Added to gasoline, added to paints, used in batteries, used to seal cans of food, used in pesticides. Also pollutes air and water, originating from industrial plants.	Displaces calcium, iron, zinc, and other minerals from their sites of action in the nervous system, bone marrow, kidneys, and liver, causing failure to function. Severe effects in fetuses, infants, and children who easily absorb and retain lead. Causes breakage of red blood cells (anemia) and interferes with the immune response.	Food can seals, air pollution, water pollution, gasoline, water pipes. Lead in foods comes largely from air pollution from gasoline, which makes its way through rainfall and soil into plants and animals used as food.
Mercury (heavy metal)	Widely dispersed in gases from earth's crust; local high concentrations from industry, electrical equipment, paints, and agriculture.	Methylmercury poisons the nervous system, especially in fetuses.	Inorganic mercury released into waterways by industry and acid rain is converted to methylmercury by bacteria and ingested by food species of fish (tuna, swordfish, and others).
Polychlorinated biphenyls (PCBs) (organic compounds)	No natural source; produced for use in electrical equipment (transformers, capacitors).	Long-lasting skin eruptions, eye irritations, growth retardation in children of exposed mothers, anorexia, fatigue, many others.	Discarded electrical equipment; accidental industrial leakage, or reuse of PCB containers for food.

in balance. (Only an inch of soil lies below the litter, and below that is impermeable clay; that is why tropical forest lands are so unsuitable for clearing and agricultural use.) The rainforest meets two basic human needs by generating oxygen and rain.

Rainforests are important in other senses too, though. They have covered the earth for millions of years, and they hold a treasure trove of biological diversity. Millions and millions of species of animals and plants not yet known to science thrive in their honeycombs of multitudinous spaces. Within one acre of a rainforest may dwell 800,000 pounds of living things.[15]

The loss of rainforests worldwide in these last years of the twentieth century is one of the most devastating effects of the developing world's galloping increase in population and the developed world's accelerating demands for resources. According to a letter from Conservation International in December 1988, some 27 million acres of tropical forests and other woodlands are being cleared *each year* to make way for large-scale, misguided "development" projects and for desperately poor people seeking land on which to live. Once

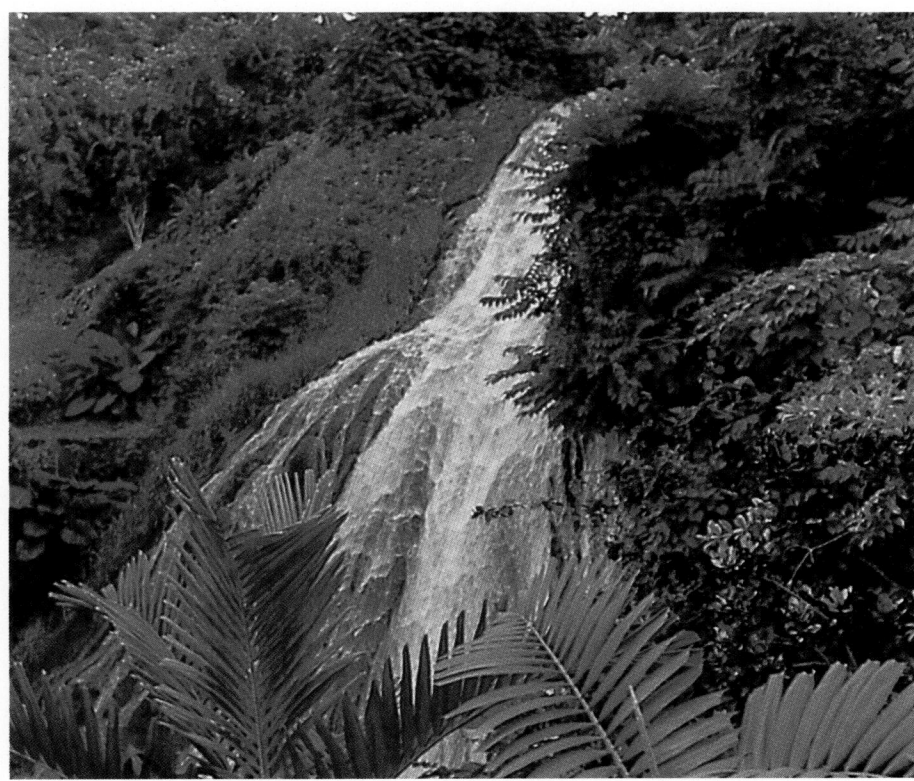

The rain forest meets two basic needs of life by generating oxygen and rain.

the trees are cut, the land's richness degenerates quickly beyond supporting even basic food crops. Floods become more common because rain runs off rather than sinking in and being again transpired by trees to the air. Droughts become more common because the region becomes hotter and dryer. Soil loss and degradation forces the people to move on, cutting deeper and deeper into the forest, continuing to live in poverty and desperation.

The tropics occupy only 6 percent of the earth's surface today, yet they are home to more than 60 percent of the species living on this planet. That diversity reflects a vast storehouse of genetic blueprints specifying plants and animals with the potential to adapt to widely varying conditions. It is a kind of bank of information that can permit different species to take over and carry on even if climatic changes or diseases render the world's currently dominant species unable to survive. It also has direct economic value for human beings; about 25 percent of the medicines now produced commercially in the United States have been developed from plants found in the world's rainforests. To lose those that remain before they are ever even identified and studied would be to lose forever a potentially vast storehouse of the future's medical and scientific knowledge and possible future foods.

Still, as of this writing, the destruction of rainforests is accelerating. In China alone, a forested area the size of Italy has become a *desert* in the last 30 years due to firewood cutting, timbering, and clearing for agricultural use. Floods and droughts are both common in this area now. In Southeast Asia and sub-Saharan Africa, two-thirds of the wildlife habitat has recently disappeared. The loss of tropical rainforests is now bringing about the greatest destruction of life forms that has ever occurred on earth. The shaving off of the earth's protective layer of vegetation not only deprives local people of needed firewood and causes mudslides that bury whole villages but also contributes to global environmental problems—our atmosphere itself is deteriorating.

▐▌▶ *Deforestation is accelerating worldwide, leading to the loss of irreplaceable wild species, of soil, and of rain. Forest losses lead ultimately to desertification, render land unfit for any use, and contribute to harmful atmospheric changes.*

Global Climate Change

Human beings, and indeed all animals, require oxygen to obtain the energy they need to support their lives. While using oxygen, they exhale carbon dioxide. People's fuel-burning processes such as cooking, heating homes, and running cars or factories do the same thing; they consume oxygen and release carbon dioxide. As plants balance these processes, they use the sun's energy directly during the day; they *consume* carbon dioxide and *return* oxygen to the air.[§]

Green plants use the carbon dioxide they consume in two ways. One way is to store it in sugar and starch molecules (for example, in their seeds) that they themselves can later metabolize as fuel when they need to (for example, when seeds need to grow in the dark, underground). They return all of this carbon dioxide to the atmosphere. The other way they use carbon dioxide is as the building material for their own structural elements—the fibers of roots, stems, and leaves. This carbon dioxide they keep for as long as they are alive, and some is held even longer in wood and undecomposed litter.

It is that second way of using carbon dioxide that makes trees—and especially rainforest trees—particularly significant because they are so big and (in forests) so numerous. For as long as they stand, they withhold a giant bank of carbon dioxide from the atmosphere. When they are felled, however, no matter whether they are burned or left to rot, they release that carbon dioxide back into the atmosphere. The destruction of rainforests actually threatens the earth's atmosphere in three ways: it adds directly to the air's carbon dioxide content, it takes away the trees that are the means for carbon dioxide removal, and it permits dedication of the land to carbon dioxide-*producing* activity such as human habitation or industry.

Now that we human beings have become so numerous on earth, we—and especially our fuel-burning activities—are among the earth's major carbon dioxide producers. When human beings burn **fossil fuels** such as gasoline, oil, or coal, they are releasing carbon dioxide from plants that trapped it from the air long ago. The more of us there are and the more intense our use of fossil fuels, the more plants (especially forests) we need to balance our activities.

Carbon dioxide in the outer atmosphere blocks the escape of heat and helps to keep the earth warm. The amount of carbon dioxide in the atmosphere has remained about the same for billions of years and has made possible life on earth as we know it. Beginning some 30 years ago, however, the concentration

[§]Green plants, too, require energy to support their lives, and during the night they obtain it the same way as animals do—by consuming oxygen and releasing carbon dioxide. However, during the day, thanks to their capacity for photosynthesis, green plants can use the sun's energy directly to build their own supporting materials and energy stores. This is a privilege that animals do not enjoy.

of carbon dioxide in the earth's air has increased by 25 percent, mostly as the result of increased burning of oil and coal. The added gas is holding more heat around the earth than before, and so the earth is warming up—the so-called **greenhouse effect.**[16] Other gases associated with human activity are contributing to the greenhouse effect in similar ways.

The greenhouse effect is expected to have major impacts on life on earth; some are already occurring. Rainfall appears to be declining across the corn and wheat belts in the United States, Europe, Russia, and Asia, resulting in more frequent droughts than in the past, with loss of crops and range lands. Water tables, already falling due to human demands for water mentioned earlier, are further depleted by evaporation caused by global warming. Inland, rivers are shrinking, creating hardship for areas that depend on their water. Along the coastlines, salt water is invading, depriving both vegetation and people of needed fresh water. The oceans are expanding as they warm up, and the polar ice caps are melting, so the sea level is rising. Governments are faced with the choice of seeing coastal cities and shores go under water or of building dikes and levees to try to hold the water back. Forests and agricultural crops, stressed by rising temperatures, are yielding to diseases and insect pests. Whole species of animals and plants, including food crops, are threatened with extinction as the earth's climate changes by only a few degrees.

Carbon dioxide is thought to cause about half of the heating caused by the greenhouse effect. Agricultural practices, including deforestation, account for much of it. The burning of felled rainforest trees alone accounts for up to 20 percent of greenhouse gas emissions worldwide.

According to a letter from M. Oppenheimer, president of the Environmental Defense Fund, in December 1988, thinning of the **ozone** layer in the outer atmosphere causes another quarter of the global warming. The outer atmosphere's ozone layer protects life on earth. The ozone layer has for billions of years screened out 99 percent of the ultraviolet rays of the sun, allowing just enough through to support plant growth. Today's living things probably did not begin to evolve until after the earth's protective ozone layer was formed.

Ozone has for millennia been formed and destroyed constantly at equal rates—formed by sunlight's action on the earth's outermost gases and destroyed by chemicals floating up from underneath. Now air pollution from human activities all over the earth is eating away at the ozone layer faster than it can be reformed. As a result, ultraviolet radiation of higher and higher intensities is reaching the earth's surface each year. This radiation causes cancers and mutations in animals and people and damages plants and crops.

Chief among the pollutants that destroy ozone are compounds known as **chlorofluorocarbons** (the trade name of one product made from them is *Freon*). These chemicals are used as coolants in refrigerators, freezers, and air conditioners; to create plastic foams (including some styrofoams); and to expel liquids (such as deodorants) under pressure from aerosol cans. As of this writing, industrial use of them is still rising. Since it takes these molecules up to 40 years to reach the outer ozone layers, the destruction of atmospheric ozone will continue for a long time even if their production ceases altogether.[17] At the current rate of increase, according to several independent predictions, the ozone layer will be seriously depleted within 100 years. Skin cancer rates are already on the increase, but individual cases of cancer do not constitute the biggest threat. Ultraviolet rays in excess of the norm disrupt the genetic

fossil fuels: fuels that originated as living plants and have been preserved below the ground for ages—natural gas, oil, and coal are examples.

greenhouse effect: the effect by which heat is prevented from rising—accomplished by the glass roof of a greenhouse and by the so-called greenhouse gases carbon dioxide, methane, and others in the earth's atmosphere.

ozone: a gas produced by (among other things) the action of sunlight on oxygen in the outer atmosphere. Ozone is an unwanted air pollutant near the earth's surface but a needed protective shield in the outer atmosphere.

chlorofluorocarbons: chemicals used as coolants, propellants, and for other purposes in industry; of interest here because they destroy ozone.

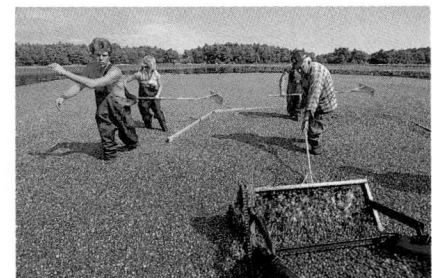

Kept unpolluted and free of climatic stress, the earth brings forth crops abundantly.

---

acid rain: rain containing acid due to the combination of normal rain water with air pollutants.

demographic transition: the change in population dynamics that takes place when a nation reaches a certain level of economic development; death and birth rates both fall, and the population may then hold steady or even decline as long as prosperity persists.

---

material in all living tissues, damaging all future generations of forests, agricultural crops, grasslands, gardens, and animal life on land and in the seas as well.

As mentioned, air pollution cannot help but affect the water and soil as well. One problem arising from air pollution is **acid rain.** Each time it rains, the air is scrubbed of its pollutants; they fall to the earth. Many of them, when combined with water, form acids, which affect living things profoundly.

Air pollution and acid rain reduce the effectiveness of the remaining forests in their air-cleansing work of photosynthesis. Beneath polluted air, trees, crops, and other vegetation grow slowly and are vulnerable to disease. All of these effects are now noticeably slowing production of the world's food. This is reflected in the dwindling grain supply mentioned at the start and also in damage to both hard and soft wood forests all over the world.

▐▐▶ *Global climate change is apparent as global warming, outer-atmosphere ozone depletion, and acid rain. Among major contributors are industrial and individual fossil fuel use, deforestation, and industrial use of chlorofluorocarbons.*

The Population Problem

All of the foregoing problems are aggravated by this one—the world's growing population. Each year, these days, there are 100 million more people alive on the earth than there were the year before. A hundred million people—that's ten cities the size of New York in one year. It is one *billion* people per decade— 100 cities the size of New York *added* to those we already have. How to feed them? How to dispose of their wastes? How to handle the pollution from their cars?

People sometimes fail to understand that this problem, already familiar for decades to every educated person today, is growing *worse,* but it is. Don't ever misunderstand when the demographers tell you that the rate of population growth has declined. Nothing is declining. Yes, the *rate* was 2 percent in the 1960s, and it is 1.7 percent today, but the absolute *number* of people added each year is *greater* than the year before. Don't get jaded, hearing the word *crisis,* either. You may become bored with the word, but it was a crisis yesterday, and it is a greater one today. The margin table illustrates that each billion has been added in a shorter time than the last.[18] If we continue at this rate, then by the year 2585, the average population density over the entire surface of the earth, *including the oceans,* will be equal to the average density, today, of Manhattan at noon.[19] That is impossible, of course; the earth already cannot support us in our present numbers, but the bomb is still ticking, and the time has grown shorter until it goes off.[20]

Those who are increasing most rapidly are the poor—people without land, possessions, or jobs.[21] The industrialized countries have only a little over one billion people, birthrates are low, and population growth is slowing. It has virtually ended in Europe. But the developing countries have about four billion people, and many families there produce five, six, seven or more children. Twenty years later, each of their children does the same thing.

Whereas the wealthy create major environmental problems by being polluters, the poor do so by simply being so numerous. Unfortunately their very poverty is one factor that makes them multiply, since with no social security, medicare, or social assistance, one's children are one's only source of support in later years. To stop the population explosion, one indispensable agenda item is to improve the lot of the poor because that can help stabilize their numbers.

■ 1 billion in 1835 — 1,000,000s of years.
■ 2 billion in 1930 — 95 years.
■ 3 billion in 1960 — 30 years.
■ 4 billion in 1975 — 15 years.
■ 5 billion in 1985 — 10 years.
■ 6 billion by ?

For reasons not fully understood, every nation that reaches a certain level of economic development goes through a **demographic transition**: death and birth rates both fall to new levels. A nation's population may actually fall while its prosperity holds steady after it has gone through this transition.[22] Poverty, then, is a key puzzle piece.

❚❚ ▷ *The world's population is huge and growing faster all the time. Of five+ billion in 1990, four billion were poor and multiplying the fastest. Economic development can help arrest this process by bringing growing populations to a demographic transition.*

The Poverty/Hunger Problem

To point to poverty as a cause of the population increase is to simplify the problem; more accurately, it is the poverty *cluster*—a constellation of lacks: of income, of land, of property, of resources, of literacy, of physical strength, of health, of power, and even of food. To visualize this cluster clearly, translate the generalities into the case of one person who is *average* for the poorest one-fifth of the world's population—the poorest one billion people. This person makes less than $500 a *year,* sleeps on the ground, has no access to formal education, and owns no assets. The person has nowhere to turn for health care, no organization through which to fight an exploitative economic system, no information to help open the way out of poverty, and no access to ideas that will lead to betterment. The person cannot read; illiteracy is an almost invariable accompaniment to the most extreme poverty. The person is physically weak due to malnutrition and disease; and the weakness makes sickness chronic and further debilitating. The person has no way to influence the government that extorts taxes, cannot get a loan to start climbing out of poverty, and has no appeal when fired from work or told that he owes more money than he owns. Take this description of one poor person, multiply it by a billion, and you have a picture of the plight one-fifth of the world's population finds itself in today. The death and disease rate in most countries of the world is high and rising. More than a billion people lack clean drinking water, and over two billion have no sanitation facilities—prime causes of infectious disease.[23] Living conditions are unimaginably atrocious among the poor. In some parts of China, parents are reported to be killing one out of every three girl babies because they feel they cannot afford to support them.[24]

Look a little more closely at the land part of this cluster. The poorest people have the poorest land. The harder they work the land, the more denuded of soil, water, and trees it becomes, aggravating their poverty.

With uncanny regularity, the world's most impoverished regions also suffer the worst ecological damage; maps of the two are almost interchangeable. . . . The poor live in shanty towns that sprawl through insect-infested floodplains, up perilous slopes, and around hazardous industrial plants. [They] live in degraded semiarid and arid regions or in . . . crowded hill country . . . vanishing forests . . . wasted lands . . . exhausted soils . . . gully-riven highlands . . . parched plains . . . overcrowded slopes . . . inhospitable drylands . . . infertile scrub. . . . [They are] thus as disenfranchised environmentally as they are politically.[25]

Deprived of what they need on their own land to eke out a living, the poor then turn to the "common lands," nonagricultural lands where they can gather

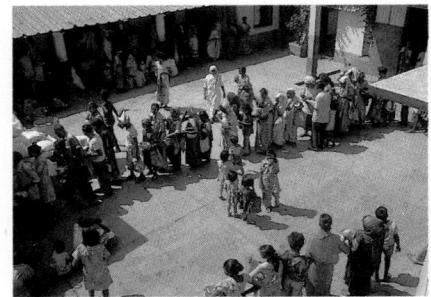

Without land, people must beg for food.

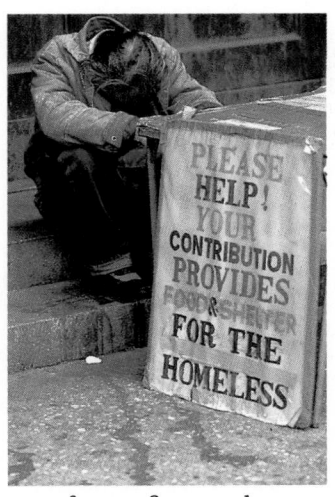

One out of every five people owns no land and no assets.

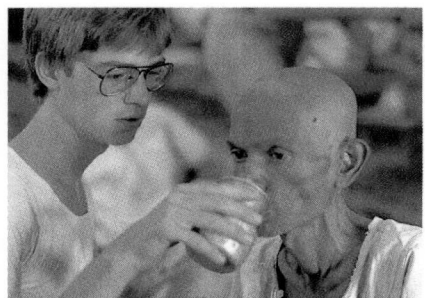

Malnutrition is rampant everywhere.

Marasmus and kwashiorkor are defined in Chapter 6.

"Third World" is a convenient term for the developing countries. The "First World" refers to the nations with developed market economies—Western Europe, North America, Japan, Australia, and New Zealand. The "Second World," a term seldom used, refers to developed nations with centrally planned economies (much of Eastern Europe and the USSR). "Fourth World" is sometimes used to refer to the very poorest of the developing countries.

berries, fruits, nuts, fish, and game and wood with which to cook them. The more deprived they are the more they deplete these resources too—the environment that surrounds them and all of us. The result over vast areas is deforestation and desertification, leading, in turn, to regional heat waves, droughts, floods, and storms. These disasters then lead to shorter food supplies and higher prices.

Consider, now, the hunger part of the poverty cluster. Everyone knows the feeling of hunger as the urge to eat that signals the time for the next meal. But many know hunger as a constant companion because that meal does not follow. Then hunger is ceaseless discomfort, weakness, and pain.

Chronic hunger afflicts millions of people. Many are children, some ten million of whom weigh less than 60 percent of the standard weight for their age. Some 50,000 children and adults die each day as the result of malnutrition; many more die of diseases precipitated and aggravated by malnutrition and poverty: measles, tuberculosis, malaria, and diarrhea; these, in turn, aggravate malnutrition. It is estimated that one child dies of these causes every two seconds.[26] Besides children, groups especially vulnerable to malnutrition and its effects are pregnant women, the ill, and the elderly.

The most widespread form of malnutrition in the developing world today is protein-energy malnutrition, or PEM (see p. 171). PEM takes two forms. Children who are thin for their height may be suffering from **acute PEM,** or recent severe food restriction, whereas children who are short for their age have experienced **chronic PEM,** or long-term food restriction. Stunted growth due to PEM, rather than symptoms of vitamin and mineral deficiency diseases, may be the most common sign of malnutrition in developing countries. Breast-feeding permits infants in many developing countries to achieve weight and height gains equal to children in developed countries until about six months of age, but then the majority of these children fall behind in weight and height. Failure of children to grow is a warning that one of the extreme forms of PEM, marasmus or kwashiorkor, may soon follow.

The descriptions here are largely of Third World poverty and hunger, but poverty and hunger as severe as in the Third World exist in developed countries too, including the United States. Of the 11 million people around the mouth of the Mississippi River, for example, 40 percent had incomes below the federal poverty line as of 1990, which was $15,000 a year for a family of four.[27] Many other examples, both rural and urban, exist. That poverty and hunger go hand in hand in the United States is apparent from the findings of the 1985 Physician's Task Force on Hunger in America, which found that "at least 20 million citizens suffer from hunger at least some days each month."[28] Despite economic gains over the last few years, millions of Americans still experience this dehumanizing and debilitating specter of hunger—especially homeless people and families, low-income women and their children, the elderly, the mentally ill, drug and alcohol abusers and their families, former blue-collar families forced out of manufacturing (oil, natural gas, steel, mining), and former farm families who have lost their farms. Children are now the poorest age group in the nation; one out of five children is in a family below the poverty line.

Each nation's political system aggravates the problem of the poor, since tax and other laws favor the few over the many. Aid arriving in a country where poverty is widespread seldom reaches the poorest people. National budgets favor industrial over rural development and military over social expenditures. Roads, electricity, and piped drinking water are built for the well-to-do, not for the poor. Assistance workers consult with and advise the well-to-do, not the poor. Credit, education, health care—seldom do these filter down to the people whose needs are most acute. Without a change in the policies that perpetuate poverty, global environmental degradation can only worsen. It already is threatening the stability of the planetary ecosystem.

International trade agreements also aggravate the problem of poverty, as the next section shows. And because those agreements are made to benefit the wealthy producers and consumers of nations like the United States, the problem of the poor seems to be one of our own making.

▌▐ ▶ *Poverty and hunger afflict billions and contribute to worsening environmental degradation. Many nations' political systems are ineffective in remedying poverty and hunger.*

acute PEM: acute protein-energy malnutrition, caused by recent severe food restriction, characterized by thinness for height.

chronic PEM: chronic protein-energy malnutrition, caused by long-term food deprivation, characterized in children by short height for age. For *PEM*, see p. 171.

The Problems of Third World Debt and First World Investments

The two problems just discussed are linked—the population problem (people are multiplying) and the poverty/hunger problem (they are multiplying because they are poor and hungry). Other problems tie in with these, and they have to do with economics.

One is the problem of third world debt. The poorest nations owe "us" (the rich nations) money, so much money that they cannot make headway in solving their poverty problem because they are constantly struggling instead to pay the interest on their debts to us. "The poor world's debt to the rich is so colossal as to sound surreal." The Philippines, for example, owes 87 percent of its gross national product to lender countries, largely the United States, while Zambia owes 334 percent of its gross national product (GNP). Putting it graphically, Zambia could pay off its national debt beginning in 1991 if everyone in the country were to give every penny they earned to the foreign lender nations and did not eat again for 3 ½ years.[29]

The international debt situation has been worsening. In the mid-1980s the debtor nations were making some headway against it, but in 1984 the flow reversed, and now it has become a torrent. By 1988 the poor nations were paying the rich nations $50 billion a year.[30] This has led to widespread destruction, within their own countries, of the only resources they have access to—those of the land itself. "Forests have been recklessly logged, mineral deposits carelessly mined, fragile lands put to the plow, and fisheries overexploited, all to pay foreign financiers."[31] In an attempt to struggle out of their many problems such as high debt and burgeoning populations, the developing economies are destroying the last of the resources on which they and all of us depend. By underpaying them for the resources they are sacrificing, we in the wealthy nations are making the Third World debt problem worse. Then, to make it still worse, when we produce products that compete with theirs, we tax their products to make them less desirable to consumers. Then they lose even the inadequate sales that might help them out of their indebtedness.

Another problem, ironically, is that of First World investments in Third World economies. Through the World Bank, the International Monetary Fund, and other gigantic economic institutions, we invest in "helping" the Third World countries to "develop"—but often along lines that are inappropriate and unsustainable. Notorious examples are that we help them to clear rainforests to grow beef or to dam rivers to provide power for energy-intensive industrial projects without taking into account the grave losses of forests and rivers that these projects entail. While economic benefits accrue to the investors and perhaps to some of the recipients, the social and environmental costs of such projects often spell oppression for numerous poor and hungry people.

Foreign aid is also flawed in that it often provides less money than what is demanded back in interest charges; it seldom flows to the neediest countries; and it is often skewed in favor of supporting countries that buy from us rather than those that are seeking self-sufficiency. Processes such as lending, investing, and aiding other countries in these ways are, at best, well intentioned but misguided and, at worst, greedy and destructive. The world is so tightly knit that environmental damage anywhere is felt everywhere else, so such apparently self-serving moves in fact are simply short sighted.

▯▯▷ *The debts Third World countries owe to world banks aggravate their internal poverty-hunger problems and cause them to overexploit their nonrenewable resources. Citizens of developed nations contribute to the problem by investing in ill-conceived "development" schemes and by providing foreign aid that costs more than it helps.*

The Problems of Agribusiness

Despite the world's rapidly growing numbers of poor, unemployed, and hungry people, there is still a grain surplus. It is dwindling, to be sure, but as of this writing there is enough food available, in theory, to feed all the hungry and still have some left over. That the production of food is so successful is largely a credit to the agriculture of the United States and a few other nations such as Canada and Australia. These countries have abundant fertile lands and tremendously successful systems of producing food on those lands. You might think, then, that the solution to the world hunger problem would be to enlarge and extend what we already do so well—produce more food by these highly productive agricultural methods. As stated earlier, though, these agricultural methods are in some ways contributing to rather than helping solve the world hunger problem and the environmental degradation that threatens life on earth. Because this puzzle piece is one that is right here at home, literally on our own soil, it deserves close scrutiny.

This puzzle piece completes the puzzle. U.S. agriculture is an example; it has become big business—**agribusiness.** It is highly productive because it is high-input agriculture at its most extreme, using intensive inputs of costly fertilizers, pesticides, irrigation, and machinery driven by more calories of fuel energy than they produce in food energy. Agribusiness is also highly successful because it is politically powerful and receives many favorable tax breaks, subsidies, and trade advantages in competition against the products of Third World markets. As a result, it contributes to all of the following problems:

- ▪ Soil and water pollution, by way of overuse of fertilizers and pesticides.
- ▪ Desertification, soil loss, and water shortages, by way of overirrigation.
- ▪ Deforestation, by claiming still-forested lands for new agriculture.
- ▪ Air pollution, by extensive use of fossil fuels.
- ▪ Global warming, by way of desertification, deforestation, and fossil fuel use.
- ▪ Loss of farmable land, because owners of small farms, failing to compete with agribusiness, yield to pressure and sell their land for development.

■ Poverty in the United States, by way of putting farm families out of work.
■ Third World debt and poverty, by subsidizing domestic goods and creating trade barriers against foreign goods.
■ Vulnerability of crops to global warming and new pests or diseases by way of reliance on **monocultures.**

Agribusiness is such big business that it overflows national boundaries. Food-producing corporations in the United States buy up prime farmland in other countries; hire cheap labor there; overuse pesticides, fertilizers, irrigation, and powerful fuel-guzzling machinery; and then sell their products here, leaving the land exhausted and polluted and the people as poor as or poorer than before. Other **multinational corporations** do the same thing—oil companies, tobacco companies, cotton growers, sugar growers, soft drink companies, fast food makers, pesticide makers, drug companies, and others. Export-oriented enterprises in Third World countries use land, capital, technology, and labor that are needed to help local families produce their own food. Africa has the highest incidence of PEM of any continent, yet *exports* barley, beans, peanuts, fresh vegetables, beef, coffee, and cocoa. Mexico suffers from one of the world's highest infant death rates caused by malnutrition, yet sells the United States over half its supply of many vegetables. Central America exports, for the profit of a few, half of the food its lands produce while half of its people eat less than half of the protein they need.

Besides diverting acreage from domestic people's traditional dietary staples, multinational corporations contribute to hunger by way of their marketing techniques. Their advertisements lead many consumers with limited incomes to associate products like cola beverages, cigarettes, infant formula, and snack foods with prosperity and health. These promotions are inappropriate for poor people; their nutrition status suffers when their tight budgets are drained by purchases of such goods.

‖▷ *Agribusiness produces abundant crops for dollar profits, but at high, hidden costs in pollution, soil loss, ground water depletion, desertification, deforestation, fuel, land loss, displacement of farm families and small landowners, poverty, hunger, and others.*

agribusiness: agriculture as practiced by large corporations; high-input agriculture with large investments of capital, fuel, fertilizer, pesticides, and irrigation, supported by subsidies, tax breaks, and trade advantages against Third World imports.

monocultures: vast acreages planted to single, genetically uniform crops that can suddenly be wiped out by environmental change (*mono* means "one").

multinational corporations: corporations that do their business in many nations.

▋▋▋ Part Two: The Puzzle Pieces Assembled

It must now be clear why this chapter started with the statement that the puzzle pieces just presented all have to do with world hunger and malnutrition. Each contributes to the others, and all are rapidly growing worse. An observer notes that "the exponential growth of population and its attendant assault on the environment is so recent that it is difficult for people to appreciate how much damage is being done."[32] It is vital that we try, though, because the processes have tremendous momentum. To stop them we must act in advance of the endpoints and without waiting to understand their dynamics as well as we might like to. An example: no one knows exactly how fast the ozone hole is developing, or exactly what the consequences will be, or exactly what measures may be most effective in halting the process. Yet we must act now, anyway, basing our actions on the best guesses we can make and being willing to alter our actions based on new data as they become available.

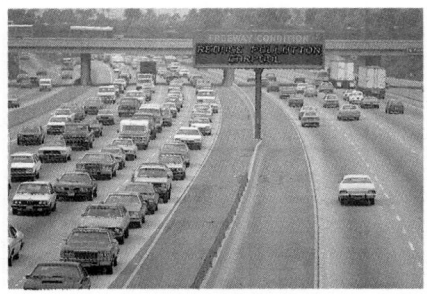

People-generated pollution today comes largely from our cars . . .

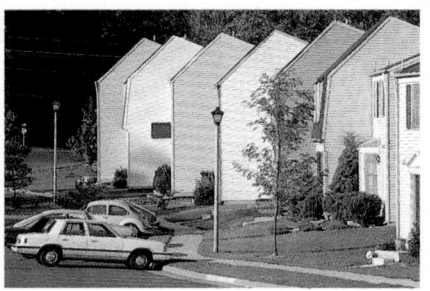

. . . and from our houses.

Solutions are forthcoming only if we all do our share—individuals and nations, the poor and the rich alike. This does not mean building polluting industries in other countries to keep from polluting our own air and water. Rather it means curbing our greed—the demands we place on Third World economies and underpay them for. Each individual person can help by regulating behavior in countless small ways (see the Food Feature that concludes this book). At the same time, nations must make and enforce rational laws regulating trade, agriculture, finance, and environmental management. The wealthy nations must help the poor nations to better their people's lots so that they can get their numbers under control. The well-to-do nations must also cease to generate the consumer demands that are driving the destruction of the world's environment.

This chapter has focused much on how the multiplying poor are contributors to the crisis. An example is due of how consumer demand is contributing. Global deforestation provides such an example. Even though we consumers may not personally be clearing rainforest land, our demands for products are driving the process. We panel and furnish our homes and offices with teak and mahogany from giant trees harvested from deep within virgin rainforest lands. We fuel our cars, homes, malls, and factories with fossil fuels that intensify acid rain and global warming, destroying forests. We dress in rayon blouses manufactured from the last of the old-growth forests of the Pacific Northwest. We also recklessly cut the remaining forests from our own environments, enthusiastically endorsing the expansion of our suburbs, cities, amusement parks, and industrial parks.

We eat more than 330 million pounds of beef from Central American countries alone. To pursue this example for a moment, that beef is grown on cleared rainforest land and represents 90 percent of that region's beef exports.[33] International banks have provided billions of dollars to convert rainforests to grasslands. U.S. investors, in turn, provide most of the banks' money either directly, by investing in the banks, or indirectly, by buying Japanese goods. The Japanese investors have then invested those surplus dollars to exploit lands and resources in other countries—cutting forests, for example.

For another example of consumers' responsibility for environmental problems, consider air pollution. Natural processes such as forest fires, volcanoes, and the natural rotting of organic matter have always released temporary bursts of contamination into the air, but people-generated pollution is continuous, concentrated, and in many cases growing more intense from year to year.

Two of the four major sources today are fuel burned to run *cars* and other forms of transportation and fuel burned to heat and cool *homes* and run home appliances. These reflect personal individual choices—our own lifestyle choices. The days when we could blame major industrial polluters for most of our problems are over—they still do their share, but *small consumers are now the major contributors to the pollution of our environment*. When asked at a major conference on the rainforest what we as individuals could do to help reverse the growing deforestation tragedy, several world experts said, "Convince U.S. consumers to change their own lifestyles."[34]

An irony of consumerism is that it makes things both worse and better at the same time. Follow this line of thought for a moment, beginning with a poor family who has nothing. Suppose that the family gains the means to support itself reliably. Then it is able to buy a home and perhaps a car. Then, with education, the family may become able to free itself from the psychological need to produce large numbers of children (earlier its only form of security) and even to see the advantages of raising, say, only two children. This is, of course, how economic benefits better the situation, since the world needs stability of population size.

But now the family is a consumer family. As its wealth increases, it becomes able to buy a dishwasher, a washing machine, an air conditioner, a furnace. It becomes able to travel long distances on airplanes, to shop in air-conditioned malls, to play with boats or horses. It is now a major polluter family. "Everywhere there is this symmetry between numbers of people on the one hand and harmful practices on the other."[35] As people become better off, they may multiply less rapidly, but they generate much more pollution.

That is the dilemma posed by the problem of development of Third World countries: if they do not develop economically, their numbers will increase astronomically; if they do develop, they may become major polluters, contributing even more to destabilization of the planetary ecosystem. Already, at a population size of five + billion, human beings each year consume the equivalent of two tons of coal per person, use 40 percent of the energy that land plants make by photosynthesis, and withdraw from the rain-evaporation cycle a volume of water equivalent to that of Lake Huron.[36] What will we do if there are twice as many of us? What will we do if more of us industrialize? The United States, with only some 6 percent of the world's population, already uses 60 percent of the resources people use.

The need is clear: development must proceed fast—fast enough to bring the developing world to the demographic transition as quickly as possible. While development proceeds, a high priority is to help people get enough to eat—but not a Western-type, high-meat food pattern and not by way of high-input agriculture that will aggravate environmental degradation. Instead, the development must involve appropriate technology. It must be *sustainable*. The solution to the world's population/environment problem can be phrased as follows. Three tasks must be accomplished simultaneously:

1. To disseminate the knowledge and the means necessary to control human population growth.
2. To facilitate vigorous economic development and equitable distribution of its benefits to meet the basic needs of the whole human population in this and subsequent generations.
3. To structure this development so as to keep its enormous potential for environmental transformation within safe limits.[37]

❚❚▶ *Population growth, environmental degradation, and poverty are all worsening each other. To reverse the growing crisis demands action from all: individuals and their governments, poor and rich. Consumer uses of nonrenewable resources must slow; sustainable development must proceed fast to halt population growth.*

❚❚❚ Part Three: Proposed Solutions

How can we accomplish the three tasks just named? The actions taken will be most effective if they are governed by the concepts mentioned at the start of this chapter—sustainable development, environmental feedback into pricing, and low-input agriculture—headed by population control.

Population Control

Most experts agree that population control is more urgent today than ever before. The Worldwatch Institute's position, under the heading of "Biting the Bullet," is as follows:

Avoiding a life-threatening food situation during the nineties may depend on quickly slowing world population growth to bring it in line with food output. The only reasonable goal will be to try and cut it in half by the end of the century. . . . For the United States, the obvious first step is to restore its funding of the United Nations Population Fund and International Planned Parenthood. . . . It may now be appropriate for the United Nations' secretary general, the president of the World Bank, and national political leaders to urge couples everywhere to stop at two surviving children. Difficult and harsh though this may seem, bringing population and food into balance by lowering birthrates is surely preferable to doing so inadvertently by allowing death rates to rise.[38]

To this end, the provision of birth control is most important. Birth control and access to contraceptives have been major contributors to declining fertility in all countries.[39]

Birth rates in the less developed countries will decline only as the countries develop. Their development is hindered by large and growing populations, however, and so the scale of development will have to be enormous in order for the benefits to reach everyone. The strain on the environment will therefore be unprecedented. Brazil says it cannot develop without cutting down Amazon forests, and it resents foreign demands for this restraint. Population growth in some areas is now so great that the limits of materials and the environment have already been reached; this strain has slowed the economic development that would check births. In the face of such a danger, the urgency of birth-control programs cannot be stressed enough.[40]

Development must hasten, then, but it must be sustainable development.

▌▌▶ *Most future watchers view population control as imperative to the world's future environmental stabilization. Together with rapid economic development, it may prevent the looming crisis.*

Sustainable Development

For the poor, sustainable development means one thing, for the wealthy, another. For the poor it means adopting policies that put them first. For the well-to-do it means voluntarily adopting or politically requiring alterations of lifestyle that will reduce fossil fuel use and other environmentally destructive activities.

Consider the poor first. A Worldwatch Institute writer quotes Gandhi's guideline for evaluating policies to help the poor: "Whenever you are in doubt . . . apply the following test. Recall the face of the poorest and the weakest man whom you may have seen, and ask yourself, if the step you contemplate is going to be of any use to him. Will he gain anything by it? Will it restore him to a control over his own life and destiny?"[41]

The poor must be involved in deciding how their lots can be bettered. Whatever the details, the end result must be to reverse the cluster of lacks of income, land, property, resources, literacy, physical strength, health, and power that aggravate their poverty. They must become able to take action for themselves. To provide just one provocative observation, where people are wretchedly poor and have no rights to grow and harvest trees on the land there are vast common areas nearby that are deforested. If they could *own* that land, they would not mistreat it so.[42] In support of this view, in one village the villagers have registered under a new law that gives them ownership of some land—and that land has become lush green and full of grass. "Even during the severe drought of 1987, when cattle died by the thousands in neighboring areas, [that village's people] filled 80 bullock carts with grass."[43]

Other efforts to improve the poverty picture include provision, with involvement of local populations, of low-cost, clean drinking water and basic health care; of birth control education and supplies; and of enforced equity under the law for the very poor. International debt reduction and relief from trade restrictions is also indispensable to helping those in developing countries obtain relief from crushing burdens. To help bring Third World populations under control, the developed countries will have to welcome and pay for their products.[44]

Meanwhile it is urgent among the well-to-do to slow down our burning of fossil fuels and to stabilize the atmosphere. Fossil fuel use is closely tied to the global poverty rate. The more heavily we use fossil fuels, the more the poor in other countries become poorer, the more severe becomes deforestation and desertification, and the narrower becomes the planet's remaining survival margin. The wealthy and the poor are tightly bonded together through the land, water, and air: on an endangered planet, the poverty of the poor is a luxury the wealthy can no longer afford. The actions consumers can take are summarized in the Food Feature, Strategies for Consumers. Only by taking these actions immediately can we buy ourselves time in which to develop alternative sources of energy and get our numbers under control.

Nations as well as individuals can take, and are taking, initiatives to curb environmental degradation too. China is now planting vast areas in reforestation projects, the world's largest such effort. Reforestation reduces the amount of land presently being farmed but with a difference from development: the plants and trees are preserved. Thailand, as hard as it is on the country economically to give up the income, has ceased exporting all timber from its rainforests. The same principle applies—the loss in present dollars may be severe, but the consequence of loss of the forest in the long run would be far more so.

▐▌▶ *To develop sustainably, the poor nations must get their numbers under control and adopt policies to alleviate poverty and hunger. The rich nations must cease demanding nonrenewable resources and desist from policies that keep the Third World nations poor.*

Environmental Feedback into Pricing

To slow down our burning of fossil fuels and our pollution of the environment, it will help to price things right. The prices of things are information signals. They tell us whether things are scarce or abundant, valuable or worthless, costly or free to produce. Famous works of art are scarce and highly valued, so they have high prices. Fancy cars are expensive because much skilled labor goes into their production. The air is free because it is abundant, and obtaining it is effortless.

■■ **Figure 15–3**

Sustainable Development versus Exploitation of Nonrenewable Resources

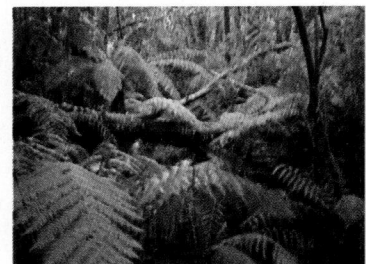

Sustainable development. The forest can produce fruits and other products year after year.

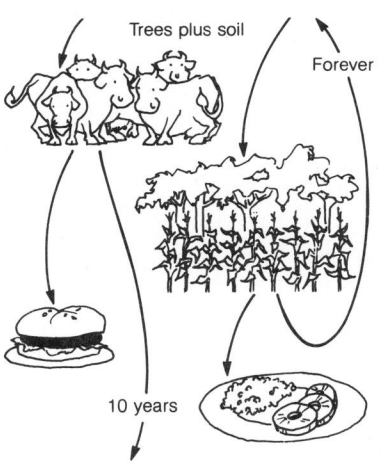

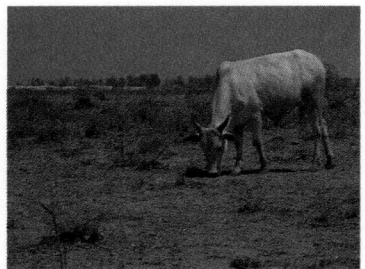

Traditional development. People drain the earth's resources, and the earth ceases to support them.

People use free things freely and high-priced things more conservatively. Thus high prices serve as signals to conserve: Consumers say, "Let's reuse this; let's not buy that at all, let's find an alternative."

Prices are imperfect signals, however, because they do not always reflect the true value of things. The air is a prime example; nothing could be more valuable, yet it is "free," at least, in terms of dollars. Many other environmental "givens" have also been free up to now, but some economists are questioning whether they should be. They are suggesting that prices should reflect environmental as well as labor and material costs. If a valuable resource such as ground water has too low a price, people use it inefficiently. When the government helps keep water's price low by using tax money (**subsidies**) to supply it to farmers or ranchers for irrigation, then it is overused. Government subsidies encourage the abuse of land, too, to grow products at artificially low prices. Examples are sugar, tobacco, and grain that is fed to beef, which are supported by government subsidies for overirrigation, overfertilization, and overuse of pesticides.[45] (You do pay much more for these than you realize, actually, but with your tax dollars, not your food dollars, and with your losses of environmental quality.)

Policies that encourage such environmental abuses may no longer be tolerable in today's world. "Good policies will make expensive to citizens that which is expensive to the nation."[46] According to this thinking, the true cost of a resource such as water should be borne by the users and passed on to consumers. Take, for example, the case of a grower of sugar cane (or rice, or a citrus crop, or cattle) who irrigates his fields with water paid for by everyone's taxes and then drains the polluted water into waterways whose degradation "no one" pays for (the environment pays). Suppose, now, that the price of the product reflected the *true* cost of the irrigation water plus the cost of preventing the pollution of the receiving water bodies. Then the product would be much higher in price, consumer demand for it would fall, and the producer would have to shift into producing other products to uphold his profits.[47]

A second example is that of the rainforest. Its true value is hard to measure but must be very high, since it makes contributions to the world's oxygen-carbon dioxide balance, temperature, water balance, purity of rivers and ocean, and species richness, to name just a few things. A land speculator who buys an acre of rainforest at $30 an acre is not paying for its true value; the price is a signaling failure. When the landowner clears the land of its trees because they are "worthless" to him and then puts beef cattle to graze on the land and markets the beef, he profits on paper because the beef brings a dollar price, but the environmental loss is severe. When an acre of forest is cleared, its soil's fertility is used up within about eight years. The land is then useless for any purpose whatever; however, the speculator walks away with a profit.

Eight years is a short time for a million-year-old acre of forest to die. Within that time span the acre will produce only 50 pounds of cattle per year—400 pounds total. Only 200 pounds of that is usable meat, enough to yield 800 4-ounce hamburgers. The tradeoff: 55 square feet of forest, representing half a ton of forest life, lost permanently for each hamburger (Figure 15-3).[48] If the consumers at innumerable fast food establishments had to pay for the real value of the rainforest acreage destroyed to produce that beef, they might not buy so many hamburgers.

This pricing concept can even be applied to population control, since each child born represents a drain on the earth's nonrenewable resources. Suppose that the true cost of bearing extra children was borne by those responsible for people's producing those children—not by society in general and not by the environment. If the policy makers, nations, and families who encouraged over-multiplication were to pay its true costs, they would be motivated to take measures to curb population growth.[49]

When a nation begins to conceptualize the links between economy and environment in this way, another insight follows. Environmental changes are themselves a form of feedback to the economic system. The same is true on a worldwide scale: the hole in the ozone layer is a form of feedback from the earth's environment to the world's economy.[50] It therefore deserves to be reflected in the prices of things so that the demands for those things will be in proportion to their true costs. Concretely: the costs of air-conditioner coolants, Styrofoam cups, and aerosol sprays should be much higher than they are—high enough to help put the ozone layer back. This price would be so high as to put these products out of reach of consumers; then they would disappear from the market, and the market would respond by developing alternative, sustainable means of achieving comfort and convenience.

❚❚▶ *Prices of consumer goods do not reflect their environmental costs. The result is that everyone pays them, not in dollars but in losses of forests, clean air, climate stability, and other environmental values. Environmentally destructive products need to cost more.*

Low-Input Agriculture

Agribusiness may be the kind of agricultural system that produces the most food on the smallest land area, but it is environmentally destructive. When its environmental costs are calculated in, agribusiness turns out to be too costly, economically, to be sustainable. If food bills reflected the true costs of producing food using so much irrigation, pesticides, fertilizers, and fossil fuel, food prices would be much higher than they are. It has been suggested that food prices also should pay for "the costs of unemployment when farms fail . . . national security to protect our supply of imported petroleum [for tractor fuel] . . . medical care for the thousands of workers injured each year by pesticides . . . ground water contamination,"[51] and many other costs.

In contrast, **low-input agriculture** is seen as "an idea whose time has come,"[52] and it is being pioneered by six states. It is seen as "a food production system that can indefinitely sustain a healthy food supply, restore our soil and water resources, and revitalize individual farms and rural communities, all with little reliance on fossil fuels."[53] The National Academy of Sciences formally recognized the need to develop this kind of agriculture in a report, *Alternative Agriculture,* released late in 1989.[54]

Low-input agriculture would produce food that might *appear* to cost more, but the *environmental* cost of the food would be far lower than it is now. It works, and apparently people are ready to pay for it. As of this writing, 30,000 of the nation's farms are successfully using sustainable techniques such as recycling animal manure into fertilizer; alternating nutrient-devouring crops with nutrient-restoring crops; conserving soil by means of cover crops, crop rotation, and contour plowing; and controlling pests biologically rather than with herbicides and pesticides (**integrated pest management**). Not all crops can grow reliably without pesticides, but many can; evidence suggests that if

subsidies: moneys paid by governments to support enterprises so that producers can sell their products at prices lower than their true costs.

low-input agriculture: an agricultural system that uses more labor and fewer capital inputs and operates on a smaller scale than agribusiness and is therefore more sustainable.

integrated pest management: control of pests using many techniques simultaneously—chemicals (to a limited extent); mechanical manipulation of the soil; frequent mechanical removal of pests; and biological strategies such as releasing predators that prey on crop pests or releasing sterilized males to compete with fertile male pests.

> **agroforestry:** a sustainable means of farming within a forest by rotating crops from site to site and refraining from cutting down any, or many, trees.

price supports were eliminated, farmers would use pesticides perhaps a third more sparingly and to better effect.[55] Optimism runs high that new agricultural techniques such as these can produce food fast enough to keep pace with the world's population growth. (Many of those techniques are not really new, incidentally, and would be familiar to our great grandparents. They were superseded by high-tech methods and are now coming back into favor.)

People can even produce food in the rainforest sustainably rather than by cutting the forest down. The technique, practiced for millennia by the forests' original people, is known as **agroforestry.** The original natives in a rainforest area, living on small, cleared patches beneath the undisturbed forest canopy, were able to grow 5000 pounds of shelled corn *and* 4000 pounds of root and vegetable crops each year on each acre of plots for five to seven years. Then they would allow the plots to return to forest and clear others. They rotated their crops of citrus, rubber, cacao, avocado, and papaya in a way that could be continued indefinitely. To solve their people's hunger problems, governments of rainforest countries can do no better than to encourage sustainable agricultural methods such as these. Food production systems practiced by traditional rainforest Indians are, without exception, more productive than the pasturelands that often replace them.[56] People can also grow commercial, exportable crops beneath the forest canopy—crops such as rubber, nuts, fruits, oils, and many others.[57] The rubber tappers in the Amazon River basin are conserving the rainforest while making a living from growing rubber.[58] If such a forest's goods are sold, they are worth much more over time than the trees are worth in a one-time sale, since the forest products can be produced indefinitely.[59] Consumers can help by learning which imported products to support with their demands (no to teak, mahogany, and beef; yes to rubber, cashew nuts, and bananas).

In some areas of the world the application of intensive inputs may still be appropriate, but in much of the Third World it is probably not. Peasant agriculture is a repository for crop and wild-plant resources. Rural development projects can improve traditional farming systems but should emphasize food self-sufficiency, preservation of adjacent natural ecosystems, and conservation of local resources and cultural diversity.[60]

▐▌▶ *Low-input agriculture is not as productive per unit of land as high-input agriculture, but it is sustainable. It is seen by many as the preferable alternative for the future.*

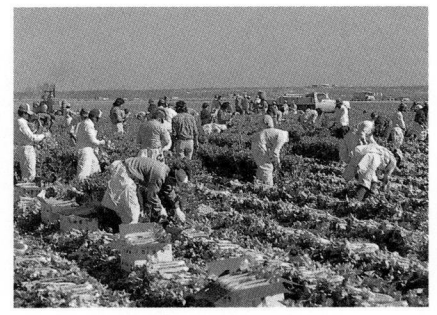

Labor intensive agriculture, low in technical inputs is often the most appropriate form of agriculture in developing countries.

International Cooperation

The nations of the world are coming to realize that they must cooperate in managing the population-environmental crisis they are facing. Fortunately this is now possible in ways it has never been before thanks to two current trends: the explosion of scientific knowledge about environmental problems and the world's increasing use of fast communications to make that knowledge available to all governments simultaneously. Knowledge and awareness shared among people and governments can bring about rapid decision making and action.

Worldwatch suggests obvious but ingenious allocations of efforts among nations. Those that have the greatest power to affect a given problem should focus on that problem. For example, of the people added to the world's population each year, China and India account for about a third of the total. Those two countries should therefore emphasize population control the most heavily and be supported in doing so by the others. Similarly, of all the world's fossil fuel use, half occurs in only three nations—the United States, the Soviet Union, and China. These countries should aim major efforts at that problem. Similarly, three nations contain more than half of the world's remaining tropical rainforests—Brazil, Indonesia, and Zaire—so efforts at conservation should focus on them. Substantial progress can be made if the right efforts are made by the right groups.[61]

The rapid pace of change has already been mentioned, as has the irony that in many instances hard decisions are having to be made before scientific knowledge is sufficient to be sure that they are right. To help rank those decisions, it makes most sense to take actions that will yield tie-in benefits even if the projected changes do not materialize exactly as expected.[62] For example, to counter global warming, all nations should adopt energy conservation measures and shift from fossil fuels to renewable energy sources as quickly as possible. Even if global warming does not occur as predicted, these measures will help prevent pollution and other environmental problems.

Nations must adapt policies to motivate changes in the behavior of millions and millions of individuals. This is hard to do, since the science is uncertain and the action generates pain, but it is urgent nonetheless. "Something enormous may be happening to our world. Our species may be pushing up against some immovable limits on the combustion of fossil fuels and damage to ecosystems."[63] A third revolution in human history is needed. The first was the agricultural revolution ten thousand years ago, and the second was the industrial revolution just 200 years ago. The third "will have to be a fully conscious operation, guided by the best foresight that science can provide—foresight pushed to its limit. If we actually do it, the undertaking will be absolutely unique in humanity's stay on the earth."[64]

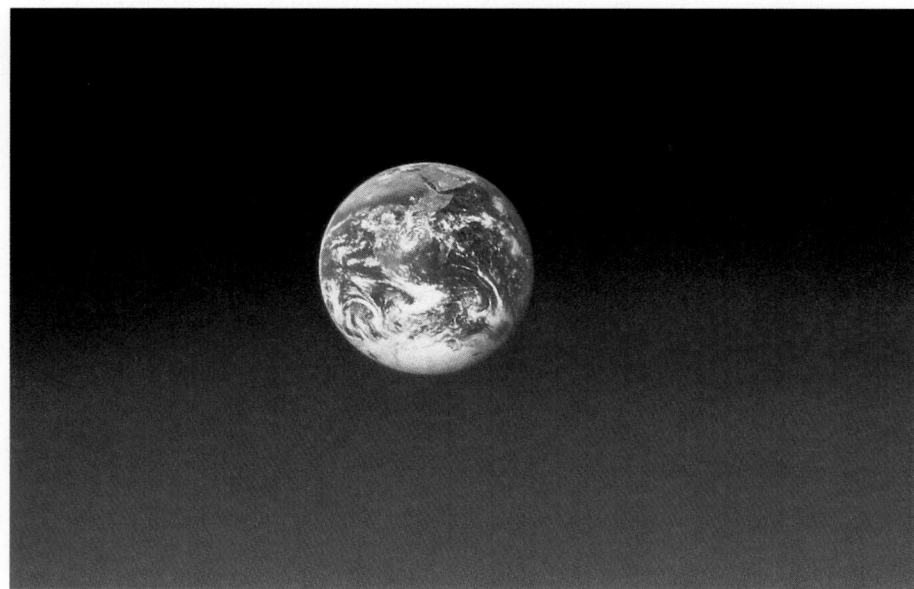

Good planets are hard to find.

The attitude we need to cultivate is new to us but is really very old. It is similar to that of long ago, when "sustainability was the original economy of our species" and "the people were spiritually connected to the animals and plants on which they subsisted; they were part . . . of nature, not set apart as masters."[65] Humankind, especially in much of the developed world, has lost this consciousness. Even those who call themselves environmentalists give little more than lip service to its tenets; the United States espouses strict environmental statutes, but its citizens engage in "the world's most wasteful and most polluting style of life."[66] Our *actions* must now square with our environmental consciousness. The three beliefs that must guide our *actions* henceforth are:

1. We are part of nature and we must not destroy it.
2. We must pay for what we take from nature and for what we do to it.
3. We are all one family, and we must all work to improve our common lot.[67]

◖◗▶ *Global cooperation in resolving the population and environmental crisis is needed and is feasible. Nations must adopt policies to motivate millions of individuals to change their lifestyles—to bear fewer children, to use fewer resources, and to pollute less.*

All of this book's previous chapters have ended with Food Features that applied the chapter contents to personal lifestyles. This chapter does so too, but the applications merit more than the usual emphasis. The Food Feature therefore occupies the slot that would normally be occupied by a Controversy, and concludes the book.

Notes

1. J. H. Gibbons, P. D. Blair, and H. L Gwin, Strategies for energy use, *Scientific American Special Issue: Managing Planet Earth,* September 1989, pp. 136–143.

2. L. R. Brown, The changing world food prospect: The nineties and beyond, *Worldwatch Paper* 85 (1988), p. 5.

3. L. R. Brown, Feeding six billion, *World Watch,* September-October 1989, pp. 32–40.

4. J. W. M. la Riviere, Threats to the world's water, *Scientific American Special Issue: Managing Planet Earth,* September 1989, pp. 80–94; S. Postel, *Worldwatch Paper 93, Water for Agriculture: Facing the Limits,* December 1989, p. 16.

5. La Riviere, 1989.

6. La Riviere, 1989.

7. La Riviere, 1989.

8. E. P. Jorgensen, ed., *The Poisoned Well: New Strategies for Groundwater Protection* (Washington, D.C.: Island Press, 1989), p. xix and Chapter 3.

9. S. Woodruff, Drinking water: Present problems, future directions, *Nutrition Clinics,* March-April 1990.

10. A. Levin, Pesticides: How dangerous are they? *Building Economic Alternatives* (a quarterly publication of Co-op America, 2100 M Street NW, Suite 310, Washington, DC 20063), Summer 1989, p. 16.

11. *Organic Agriculture: What the States are Doing* (Washington, D.C.: Center for Science in the Public Interest, 1989).

12. *Residues in Foods—1987* (Washington, D.C.: Food and Drug Administration, 1988). Reprint of an article published in *Journal of the Association of Official Analytical Chemists* 71, November/December 1988, p. 11.

13. *Residues in Foods—1988* (Washington, D.C.: Food and Drug Administration, 1989).

14. Update: Childhood lead poisoning, *Journal of the American Dietetic Association* 80 (1982): 592, 594.

15. C. Uhl and G. Parker, Viewpoint: Our steak in the jungle, *BioScience,* November 1986, p. 642.

16. S. Begley, M. Miller, and M. Hager, The endless summer? *Newsweek,* 11 July 1988, pp. 18–20.

17. R. Crum, More on less ozone, *Harvard Magazine,* May/June 1987, pp. 4, 6.

18. B. Bull, Voodoo demography: What population problem? *The Amicus Journal,* Fall 1984, pp. 36–40.

19. I. Asimov, Is anyone listening? *Animal Kingdom,* September/October 1989, pp. 8, 52–53.

20. C. Haub, Trial by numbers, *Sierra,* November/December 1988, pp. 40–42. The United Nations projected in May of 1989 that because of failed family-planning efforts, the world's pop-

ulation would not level off as earlier expected at 10 billion, but would go to 14 billion before it stopped increasing; Brown 1989.

21. N. Keyfitz, The growing human population, *Scientific American Special Issue: Managing Planet Earth,* September 1989, pp. 119–126.

22. Keyfitz, 1989.

23. Bull, 1984.

24. Robert McNamara, as cited by Bull, 1984.

25. A. B. Durning, Poverty and the environment: Reversing the downward spiral, *Worldwatch Paper 92* (Washington, D.C.: Worldwatch Institute, 1989), p. 45.

26. D. R. Gwatkin, How many die? A set of demographic estimates of the annual number of infant and child deaths in the world, *American Journal of Public Health* 70 (1980): 1286–1289.

27. Delta commission report shows Third World poverty in America (AP), *Tallahassee Democrat,* 28 August 1989.

28. Harvard University School of Public Health, *Physician Task Force on Hunger in America* (Cambridge, Mass.: Harvard University School of Public Health, 1986).

29. Durning, 1989, p. 35.

30. Durning, 1989, p. 35.

31. Durning, 1989, pp. 35–36.

32. Keyfitz, 1989.

33. J. D. Nations and D. I. Komer, Rainforests and the hamburger society, *Environment,* April 1983, pp. 12–20.

34. Tropical rainforests: Strategies for wise management, a conference, 27–31 January 1988, Florida International University, Miami, FL.

35. Keyfitz, 1989.

36. W. C. Clark, Managing planet earth, *Scientific American Special Issue: Managing Planet Earth,* September 1989, pp. 47–54.

37. Clark, 1989.

38. Brown, 1989.

39. Keyfitz, 1989.

40. Keyfitz, 1989.

41. Gandhi quote from Robert Chambers, private communication, as cited by Durning, 1989, p. 54.

42. T. Shah, Gains from social forestry: Lessons from Wet Bengal, IDS Discussion Paper 243, Brighton, April 1988, as cited by Durning, 1989, p. 58.

43. A. Agarwal and S. Narain, The greening of India, *Illustrated Weekly of India,* 4 June 1989, as cited by Durning, 1989, p. 58.

44. Keyfitz, 1989; MacNeil, 1989.

45. Clark, 1989.

46. Keyfitz, 1989.

47. P. R. Crosson and N. J. Rosenberg, Strategies for agriculture, *Scientific American Special Issue: Managing Planet Earth,* September 1989, pp. 128–135.

48. Uhl and Parker, 1986.

49. Keyfitz, 1989.

50. J. MacNeill, Strategies for sustainable economic development, *Scientific American Special Issue: Managing Planet Earth,* September 1989, pp. 155–165.

51. C. Mitlo-Shartel and the Land Stewardship Project, Regenerating America's Agriculture, *Building Economic Alternatives* (a quarterly publication of Co-op America, 2100 M Street NW, Suite 310, Washington, DC 20063), Summer 1989, pp. 9-12.

52. *Organic Agriculture: What the States Are Doing,* 1989. The quote is from the assistant secretary of agriculture, Orville G. Bentley, in a USDA press release, February 1988.

53. Mitlo-Shartel and the Land Stewardship Project, 1989.

54. National Research Council recommends changes in U.S. agriculture, *Forum* (a newsletter of the American Institute of Biological Sciences), September/October 1989, p. 3.

55. K. Mattes, Kicking the pesticide habit, *The Amicus Journal* Fall 1989, pp. 10–17.

56. Nations and Komer, 1983.

57. First "extractive reserve" is to be created in Brazilian rainforest, *EDF Letter,* June 1988, p. 3.

58. B. M. Rich, Development alternatives for third world conservation, *EDF Letter,* Date? 1988, p. 4.

59. A hectare of forest produces $400 in fruit and $22 in rubber annually, year after year. One-time harvesting of the trees earns $1000. C. M. Peters, A. H. Gentry, and R. O. Mendelsohn, Valuation of an Amazonian rainforest, *Nature* 339 (1989): 655–656.

60. M. A. Altieri, L. C. Merrick, and M K. Anderson, Peasant agriculture and the conservation of crop and wild plant resources, *Conservation Biology* 1, May 1987, pp. 49–58; K. A. Dahlberg, Redefining development priorities: Genetic diversity and agroecodevelopment, *Conservation Biology* 1, December 1987, pp. 311–322.

61. *State of the World 1987: A Worldwatch Institute Report on Progress toward a Sustainable Society* (New York, Norton, 1987).

62. S. H. Schneider, The changing climate, *Scientific American Special Issue: Managing Planet Earth,* September 1989, pp. 70–79.

63. W. D. Ruckelshaus, Toward a sustainable world, *Scientific American Special Issue: Managing Planet Earth,* September 1989, pp. 166–174.

64. Ruckelshaus, 1989.

65. Ruckelshaus, 1989.

66. Ruckelshaus, 1989.

67. Ruckelshaus, 1989.

███ C O N T R O V E R S Y   15

Strategies for Consumers

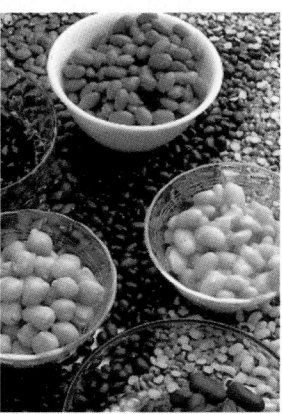

Up to now, this book's Controversies have been controversial. This one is not; its subject is more like that of a Food Feature, for it deals with food purchases and preparation. It deserves more attention than it might receive as the concluding section of a chapter, though, for it asks an important question: how you, as a consumer, can most responsibly manage your food and related lifestyle elements as a citizen of Planet Earth.

Most of the following suggestions are taken from a resource developed by the Center for Science in the Public Interest, which set itself the task of identifying ways for individuals to simplify their lives for the benefit of all.[1] A sampling of the ideas they have generated is presented in Table C15−1. Interestingly the suggestions closely resemble those already made throughout the book to bring about the greatest possible improvement in your own

nutrition. It seems that the same solutions will promote sustainable food production for the well-being of the earth and its people.

You may already be implementing many of these suggestions. Consider taking just one more this month and maybe adding another each month this year. It takes some effort to get started on each of them, but over a year's time each can become a habit whose cumulative effects become impressive over time.

The first item on the list, "Select nutrient-dense foods most often," captures in a sentence possibly the most important personal nutrition advice in this book. For the earth, too, it is vitally important. The concept of nutrient density was introduced in Chapter 2, and discussions of foods thereafter have made clear

that most often, foods low on the food chain—plant foods, especially vegetables—are richest in nutrients. If people use more vegetables to attain nutrient adequacy each day, they eat less meat, and, as this chapter has made clear, vegetables demand far fewer of the earth's limited resources, measured in calories, land, and environmental costs, than do meats. In contrast, fats and sugars *lower* the nutrient density of foods and are also costly to the earth to produce.

The second item on the list is "Select unprocessed foods, grown locally." You cannot only do this yourself but can ask local restaurants, schools, and hospitals to do it too. Its benefits are equally applicable to self and world. Unprocessed, in this sense, means "with the nutri-

███ Table C15−1 Foodways to Simplify Life

1. Select nutrient-dense foods most often.
2. Select unprocessed foods, grown locally.
3. Buy staple foods in bulk containers.
4. Buy fresh foods in season.
5. Learn to preserve foods.
6. Conserve food, and conserve its nutritional value. Buy all foods in recyclable containers.
7. Eat lower on the food chain—more plant foods, less meat.
8. If you eat beef, look for forage-fed or grass-fed beef.
9. If you eat beef, choose domestic, not foreign-grown beef. Don't feed beef to pets.
10. Reduce your intakes of refined sugar and other nonnutritive products.
11. Grow your own fruits and vegetables whenever possible. Use organic fertilizer and biological pesticides.
12. Eat wild foods.
13. Organize a food co-op.
14. Bake bread, home prepare other foods.
15. Drink homemade beverages.

SOURCES: Ideas from Center for Science in the Public Interest, Simple Lifestyle Team, *99 Ways to a Simple Lifestyle* (Garden City, N.Y.: Anchor Books, 1977), and D. Katz and M. T. Goodwin, *Food: Where Nutrition, Politics, and Culture Meet* (Washington, D.C.: Center for Science in the Public Interest, 1976), p. 155.

ents left in, sugar and fat left out." You already know why you should select unprocessed, or whole, foods for personal nutrition. To appreciate why they are also good for the earth and why the local varieties are preferred, consider how apples grown far away might become a processed food, say cinnamon apple chips, in your grocery store. To make the chips the whole apples are transported on fuel-burning, air-polluting trucks from the orchard to the factory, where power-driven, water-polluting machines strip the apples of some of their parts (and some of their nutrients); other machines alter their shape and consistency; and others add sugar, salt, and fat (each additive produced at its own factory). Then the mixture is cooked and dried in electrical equipment, and still more machines portion out the finished cinnamon apple chips into plastic or cardboard containers or perhaps containers sealed with cellophane, all produced with many other fuel-gobbling machines at many other factories and trucked in at the cost of still more fuel. Then they are shipped: the containers are boxed together and hauled by still other fuel-burning trucks to the distribution center from which they will be delivered to the air-conditioned or heated grocery store and stacked in brightly lighted cases for the consumer to purchase. Now compare: a consumer stops at a roadside stand to buy apples within viewing distance of the orchard. Not only is the apple-eater's personal nutrition best served, but the cost of apple nutrition per calorie of the earth's resources is immeasurably lower. Even if the apples are brought in from the next county and sold in the grocery store, they are far preferable in energy cost and pollution burden to the cinnamon apple chips.

Often "unprocessed foods, grown locally" cost *less* than packaged foods from the grocery store thanks to the ease with which they were collected and delivered. But if they cost *more,* consider buying them anyway. Some of the environmental costs of producing them are reflected in the price. More direct costs may be involved in raising food on a small, local farm than in raising it on a corporation's giant tract of land. By paying the higher price for the food, you are expressing the willingness to carry your share of the price for treating the environment with respect.

Energy considerations also apply to item 3 — "Buy staple foods in bulk or recyclable containers." Bulk containers involve much less energy at the manufacturing end, and when you get home you can distribute the foods into small jars or canisters that you can use over and over again. Recyclable containers require replacement infrequently. Carry your purchases home in reusable bags too—then you don't have to accept either paper or plastic at the grocery store.

While you are at it, recycle everything else you can as well. Disposal of your trash costs land area and soil and water pollution (if it is buried), air pollution (if it is burned), energy, and nonrenewable resources (to replace all the items that will be needed again). Recycle your glass, newspapers, plastics, aluminum, and other cans. Compost your garbage. Carry your toxic trash (paint cans, for example) to your community's toxic collection center. Don't even buy aerosol cans or styrofoam. Take it as a personal challenge; see if you can get your personal, nonrecyclable trash down to less than one small bag a week.

As for item 4, "Buy fresh foods in season," such a choice saves all the costs, not only of packing but also of refrigeration during transport and storage.

While you are at it, conserve energy in other ways too. You can learn to conserve energy in many ways without even sacrificing your luxuries; West Germany uses only half the energy per person that we use while maintaining a standard of living similar to ours.[2] Consider traveling less. Much of the damage to earth's ecosystems is related to the unprecedented mobility of modern city dwellers.[3] (Exceptions: do consider an exchange program that lets you see alternative lifestyles to your own. And do visit a tropical rainforest; your tourist dollars spent there will help to preserve it.) Consider walking, biking, or using mass transit more and using your car less. The planet presently bears the burden of some 500 million registered automobiles, and they use about one third of the world's production of oil. At current rates of increase there will be four times as many cars by the year 2025 — too many for the earth to support.[4] (A fringe benefit to reduced car use will be your own improved fitness.) Regulate your thermostat, water heater, stove, windows, and lighting fixtures with energy awareness. (It takes five acres of trees to balance the carbon dioxide produced by a typical U.S. four-person home. Right now more energy passes through the windows of buildings in the United States than flows through the Alaska pipeline.[5] High-efficiency fluorescent light bulbs are now available that can be screwed into regular incandescent light sockets; if the whole United States were to conserve energy by means of applications such as these it could pay off its national debt by the year 2000.[6]) Remember that anything that saves on your fuel bill also saves in environmental tolls, since even "clean heat" (electricity) is produced at the cost of environmental pollution. (Coal, oil, or gas is burned to make electricity—it may seem clean in your kitchen, but it is not clean at the power plant end of your electric line.) Many resources are available to advise you on specific steps you can take along these lines; some are mentioned at the end of this feature.

"Learn to preserve food" is item 5. When local produce is in season, it is least expensive. If you buy more than you need and quickcook and freeze some, you can then eat that food later for a price no higher, except for what it has cost you to store it. Home canning is more expensive than industrial canning but still permits you to keep this summer's produce for the winter.

Item 6 on the list is "Conserve food, and conserve its nutritional value." Once you have purchased the food, whatever the cost to the earth in producing it, be sure to obtain the full nutrient contribution it can make to your health. Prepare no more than you will serve; serve no more than you will eat. And cook it with care: the plant captured sunlight and used fertilizer to synthesize and store its nutrients. The animal consumed plants to do the same thing. The Food Feature of Chapter 7 showed ways of conserving those nutrients to make a difference to people's nutritional health. Here, too, what is good for you is good for the earth.

While you are at it, conserve water too, and promote water conservation. Question whether it still makes sense to irrigate vast areas to grow grain for cattle. Question whether it makes sense to water lawns with drinking water when recycled water would do and when alternative landscaping styles are available and beautiful. Lawns cost considerable fuel too, and fertilizers used on them enter runoff and pollute waterways.

Items 7 through 10 say to eat less meat, particularly less beef, and less sugar (and to this we would add less fat). These are the converse of item 1, since implicit in them is the admonition to eat more vegetables, legumes, and whole foods of all sorts and to appreciate the natural flavors of foods without sugar and fat. Meats, fats, and sugars cost as much energy to produce as any processed food and often more. The

land on which sugar cane and oil seeds grow yields products devoid of nutrients and rich in energy, excesses of which are linked to obesity and associated ills. That same land could be used instead to produce vitamin-rich plant foods or forests or both and to support human health and the natural environment upon which all life depends.

To reduce the demands you make on world resources, depend less on animal-based protein and use more plant-based proteins. Even one meal a week per person can make a difference. Meat can remain a part of the diet, since ruminants—cattle, sheep, and goats—can use forage crops and crop residues produced on land not suitable to other crops. In so doing these animals convert plants indigestible by humans into high-quality animal protein, and the wastes they excrete return as natural fertilizer to the soil. Today, however, many meat animals eat feed grown on rich cropland that could instead grow plant foods for human use. The animals eat these grain and protein feeds in feedlots, where they grow fat much faster than if they had grazed on pastureland, and excrete wastes that cause a major water-pollution problem. If we simply cut back on our beef consumption and substitute less land-costly plant protein sources, we can perhaps help rescue some of the last of the rainforests and can certainly help make large amounts of land available for human food production. We can also reduce water and fertilizer requirements in this way. Irrigation for beef alone requires four to 45 times more water than for other field crops.[7]

Item 11 suggests that you grow your own fruits and vegetables whenever possible. If you can do so, it can promote your health in a nonenergy-consuming way—you expend your own energy outdoors in a healthful environment instead of in an air-conditioned spa or a heated ice-skating rink. Then you eat the food you've produced—requiring less food to be produced for you by others. Even if you don't have a garden, you can grow a few patio vegetables, even in a window-box. Or consider a community plot where you and your friends and other community members can share the land and the work. Activities like these can help you discover your direct connection with, and dependence on, the earth's simple gifts.

Item 12 says "Eat wild foods." For many people this is not a possibility, but for some it is. The same principles apply: it is the simplest and most cost-free way of obtaining nourishment, and it connects you with the earth. Many people are not aware of foods that grow in wild places near their homes, or even as weeds in nearby public parks. Local botanical societies can inform you about these plants and also about the importance of harvesting conservatively and replacing the seeds so that they will be there again next year.

Item 13 recommends that you "Organize a food co-op," that is, a grocery store that you and your neighbors or friends run for your-selves. The theory is that cooperatives generate self-reliance and expand the human potential of their participants. Their members, who pay minimal dues, can save money on food and other basic items and more money by volunteering their labor.

Most supermarkets make it their first objective to make money. Highly processed impulse items increase their profit margin: supermarkets make more money from sugared cereals, sodas, candy, and other end-of-aisle displays than from nutritious foods. In contrast, cooperative stores are more responsive to their customers—they are owned by the consumers, so there is no conflict of interest. They can offer bulk quantities of unprocessed foods for very little above wholesale prices and resist low-quality foods in jazzy packages. If they produce profits, they return them to their members or reinvest them in a way the members approve. Many communities already have food cooperatives operating; for those that do not, resources are available to show how to start them.*

Items 14 and 15 recommend that you prepare your own bread, other food products, and beverages. Not everyone thinks they have the time or the will to bake bread, but there is much to be said for considering it. Home-baked bread can be more delicious than any bread bought

*Examples: G. Stern, *How to Start Your Own Food Co-op: A Guide to Wholesale Buying* (New York: Walker and Company, 1974); T. Vellela, *Food Coops for Small Groups* (New York: Workman Publishing Company, 1975).

from the store. The time and energy spent baking it are time and energy not spent doing something else (driving a car, consuming luxury goods and services). The choice requires only that you be willing to exchange some other activity for it. People who learn to enjoy producing their own food obtain a satisfaction from it that may make it less necessary for them to consume items that are more costly in terms of land, resources, and other people's energy.

Above all, even though you may live in the city, cultivate country mentality. Cities rely on outlying water reservoirs and farms to supply their water and food. People in cities do not help maintain the water supply—they use it to dispose of their sewage and industrial wastes. They do not maintain the earth to produce food—they have paved it. Today those who live in cities are depending on the rest of the world to provide their water and food, and they are making it increasingly difficult for the "rest of the world" to do so. Be aware of that.

Importantly, instill earth consciousness in your children too. After all, we do not inherit the land, we only borrow it from our children. Besides, care of the earth and its living things matters for its own sake as well as for people's sake. The earth is truly our mother; its preservation and that of other species is a moral and ethical responsibility that concerns us in a deep, spiritual way.[8] Our native American predecessors, the Indians, have always known:

This we know. The Earth does not belong to man; man belongs to the Earth. This we know. All things are connected like the blood which unites one family. All things are connected. Whatever befalls the Earth befalls the sons of the Earth. Man did not weave the web of life, he is merely a strand in it. Whatever he does to the web, he does to himself.

—Chief Seattle, 1854

Even if we worship in towering cathedrals deep within mighty cities, we must remain aware of and act responsibly toward the trees, the rivers, the birds, and the fish, since they are as much a part of the web as we are.

No doubt everyone can make some of the choices suggested here; a lucky few can make them all. Personal lifestyles do matter, since a society is nothing more than the sum of its individuals. As we go, so goes our world. And if we can't take care of our earth, who on earth can?

■■■ Suggested References

One book of excellent suggestions for meeting personal responsibilities to the world is produced under the auspices of the American Friends Service Committee: J. Bodner, ed., *Taking Charge of Our Lives: Living Responsibly in a Troubled World* (San Francisco: Harper and Row, 1984). Another is produced by the Center for Science in the Public Interest, Simple Lifestyle Team, *99 Ways to a Simple Lifestyle* (Garden City, N.Y.: Anchor Books, 1977).

Another reference is the video tape, Koyaanisqatsi (available from Pacific Arts Video Records, Carmel, CA 93923), a thought-provoking series of scenes set to music showing the massiveness of our consumer demands and their impacts on the environment. Koyaanisqatsi is a Hopi Indian word meaning "life out of balance," or "a state of life that calls for another way of living."

John Robbins, scion of the Baskin-Robbins ice cream chain, has written a thought-provoking book, *Diet for a New America: How Your Food Choices Affect Your Health, Happiness, and the Future of life on Earth* (Walpole, NH: Still point Publishing, 1987).

Notes

1. Also C. Mitlo-Shartel and the Land Stewardship Project, 1989 Regenerating America's Agriculture, *Building Economic Alternatives* (a quarterly publication of Co-op America, 2100 M Street NW, Suite 310, Washington, DC 20063), Summer 1989, pp. 9–12.

2. T. Wicker, We have battered, abused planet, *Tallahassee Democrat,* 29 November 1988.

3. N. Keyfitz, The growing human population, *Scientific American Special Issue: Managing Planet Earth,* September 1989, pp. 119–126.

4. W. D. Ruckelshaus, Toward a sustainable world, *Scientific American Special Issue: Managing Planet Earth,* September 1989, pp. 166–174.

5. Ruckelshaus, 1989.

6. Saving energy to save ourselves: Amory Lovins (interview), *Calypso Log,* October 1989, pp. 8–10,22.

7. C. G. Knight and R. P. Wilcox, *Triumph or Triage? The World Food Problem in Geographical Perspective,* Resource paper no. 75–3 (Washington, D.C.: Association of American Geographers, 1976), p. 53.

8. E. O. Wilson, *Biophilia: The Human Bond with Other Species* (Cambridge, Mass.: Harvard University Press, 1984), pp. 119–140.

Appendixes

A

B

C

D

E

F

Table of Food Composition

This table of food composition is not the standard table found in most nutrition textbooks. The list of foods chosen is an expanded version of that presented in the 1986 edition of the USDA *Home and Garden Bulletin Number 72, Nutritive Value of Foods*. The *Bulletin*, however, does not contain the values for dietary fiber, vitamin B₆, folate, magnesium, or zinc. Also, many additional foods have been added (such as frozen yogurt, canola oil, and imitation seafood items) to reflect current food patterns. The latest data for beef is also included. It is from the USDA data tapes and reflects the leaner cuts of beef now sold.

To achieve a complete and reliable listing of nutrients for all the foods, many sources of information had to be researched. Government sources of information are the primary base for all of the data: USDA *Handbooks 8–1* through *8–18; Handbook 8–21;* prepublication material on cereals, grains, and pasta; current supplemental data on vegetables and other foods; and provisional USDA information on nutrient values—both published and unpublished. Many conversations with professional staff members at the USDA Human Information Service in Hyattsville, Maryland also contributed to the refinement and completion of the data.

Even with all the government sources available, there are still many missing nutrient values; and, as the various government data are updated, conflicting values are often reported from the USDA. To fill in the missing values and resolve discrepancies, other sources of reliable information were used: journal articles, food composition tables from Canada and England, information from other nutrient data banks and publications, unpublished scientific data, and manufacturers' data.

Estimates of nutrient amounts for foods include all possible adjustments. When multiple values are reported for a nutrient, the numbers are averaged and weighted with consideration of the original number of samples in the separate sources. Whenever water percentages are available, estimates of nutrient amounts are adjusted for water content. When no water is given, water percentage is assumed to be that shown in the table. Whenever a reported weight appears inconsistent (cooked eggplant and collards, for example), many kitchen tests are made, and the average weight of the typical product is given as tested.

When estimates of nutrient amounts in cooked foods are derived from reported amounts in raw foods, published retention factors are applied. Some reported data for combination foods are modified in this table to include newer data available for major ingredients. For example, since the "pies" were analyzed and reported, newer data on fruits has been published. Older reported data on certain bakery items are updated for the new enrichment levels for certain nutrients.

Considerable effort has been made to report the most accurate data available and to eliminate missing values. There will always be future changes, and the authors welcome any suggestions or comments from readers.

■ It is important to know

that there can be many different values reported for the same nutrient. Many factors influence the amounts of nutrients in foods: the mineral content of the soil, the method of processing, genetics, the diet of the animal or the fertilizer of the plant, the season of the year, methods of analysis, the differences in moisture contents of the samples analyzed, the length and method of storage, and methods of cooking the food.

Even reliable sources report conflicting data. Although each nutrient from USDA government data is presented as a single number in some USDA publications, each number is actually an average of a range of data. In the more detailed reports (Handbook 8 series), the number of samples is identified, and the standard deviation is also noted. USDA data will report different values for foods as well, because old information is being updated in the more recent publications. Therefore, nutrient data should be used only as a guide, a close approximation of nutrient content.

Dietary fiber deserves a special word. It is important to remember that changes will be made to dietary fiber data, as research continues and analytical techniques are modified. Estimates of dietary fiber are included for all the foods in this table. The sources of this information are primarily extensive published and unpublished information from the USDA human Nutrition Information Service in Hyattsville, Maryland; *Composition of Foods by Southgate* (England); and many journal articles.

Dietary fiber is composed of cellulose, hemicellulose, lignin, pectin, gums, and mucilages. Very little data is available for gum and mucilage, but there is considerable data for the other components.

Many different analytical techniques are used to measure various components of fiber, and these methods are undergoing their own review of accuracy in the scientific community. In this table, either an estimate of the total dietary fiber (a specific analytical technique) or a combination of measures for the insoluble components and pectin, when available, are used.

Vitamin A is reported in retinol equivalents. The amount of this vitamin can vary with the season of the year. Reported values in both dairy products and plants are higher in summer and early fall than in winter. The values reported here represent year-round averages. In the organ meats of all animal products (liver especially), there are large amounts of vitamin A, and these amounts vary widely with the background of the animal. The vitamin is present in very small amounts in regular meat and is often reported as a trace.

Newer reported vitamin A values for some plant foods have increased significantly due to additional information and sometimes to newer plant genetics. New vitamin A values for canned pumpkin, for example, are 3.5 times greater than the previously reported values. This information was used to modify the vitamin A value of pumpkin pie, which had not yet been updated.

The energy and nutrients in recipes and combination foods vary widely, depending on the ingredients. The various fatty acids and cholesterol are influenced by the type of fat used (the specific type of oil, vegetable shortening, butter, margarine, etc.).

Total fat, as well as the breakdown of total fat to saturated, monounsaturated, and polyunsaturated fat, is listed in the table. The fatty acids seldom add up exactly to the total. This is due to rounding and to the existence of small amounts of other fatty acid components that are not included in the three basic categories.

Niacin values are for preformed niacin and do not include additional niacin that may form in the body from the conversion of tryptophan.

The items in this table have been organized into several categories, which are listed at the head of each right-hand page. As the key shows, each group has a number and that number is indicated in the first column. For ease in paging through this table, the category listed on the page you are on is highlighted in color. Thus if 7-GRAIN is colored and you are looking for dairy foods, turn back a few pages; if you are looking for sweets, turn forward.

A

Note: This table has been prepared for West Publishing Company and is copyrighted by ESHA Research in Salem, Oregon—the developer and publisher of "The Food Processor®" computerized nutrition systems. The major sources for the data from the U.S. Department of Agriculture are supplemented by over 450 additional sources of information. Because the list of references is so extensive, it is not provided here, but it is available from the publisher.

Table A–1   Food Composition

Grp	Computer Code No.	Food Description	Measure	Wt (g)	H₂O (%)	Ener (cal)	Prot (g)	Carb (g)	Dietary Fiber (g)	Fat (g)	Fat Breakdown (g) Sat	Mono	Poly
BEVERAGES													
		Alcoholic:											
		Beer:											
1	1	Regular (12 fl oz)	1½ c	356	92	146	1	13	1	0	0	0	0
1	2	Light (12 fl oz)	1½ c	354	95	100^1	1	5	1	0	0	0	0
		Gin, rum, vodka, whiskey:											
1	3	80 proof	1½ fl oz	42	67	97	0	<.1	0	0	0	0	0
1	4	86 proof	1½ fl oz	42	64	105	0	<.1	0	0	0	0	0
1	5	90 proof	1½ fl oz	42	62	110	0	<.1	0	0	0	0	0
		Liqueur:											
1	1359	Coffee Liqueur, 53 proof	1½ fl oz	52	31	174	0	24	0	<1	.1	t	.1
1	1360	Coffee & cream liqueur, 34 proof	1½ fl oz	47	47	154	1	10	0	7	4.5	2.1	.3
1	1361	Creme de menthe, 72 proof	1½ fl oz	50	28	186	0	21	0	<1	t	t	.1
		Wine:											
1	6	Dessert (4 fl oz)	½ c	118	72	181^2	<1	14^2	0	0	0	0	0
1	7	Red	3½ fl oz	103	88	74	<1	2	0	0	0	0	0
1	8	Rosé	3½ fl oz	103	89	73	<1	2	0	0	0	0	0
1	9	White medium	3½ fl oz	103	90	70	<1	1	0	0	0	0	0
		Carbonated^3:											
1	10	Club soda (12 fl oz)	1½ c	355	100	0	0	0	0	0	0	0	0
1	11	Cola beverage (12 fl oz)	1½ c	370	89	151	0	39	0	0	0	0	0
1	12	Diet cola (12 fl oz)	1½ c	355	100	2	0	<1	0	0	0	0	0
1	13	Diet soda pop–average (12 fl oz)	1½ c	355	100	2	0	<1	0	0	0	0	0
1	14	Ginger ale (12 fl oz)	1½ c	366	91	124	0	32	0	0	0	0	0
1	15	Grape soda (12 fl oz)	1½ c	372	89	161	0	42	0	0	0	0	0
1	16	Lemon-lime (12 fl oz)	1½ c	368	90	149	0	38	0	0	0	0	0
1	17	Orange (12 fl oz)	1½ c	372	88	177	0	46	0	0	0	0	0
1	18	Pepper-type soda (12 fl oz)	1½ c	368	89	151	0	38	0	0	0	0	0
1	19	Root beer (12 fl oz)	1½ c	370	89	152	<1	39	0	0	0	0	0
		Coffee^3:											
1	20	Brewed	1 c	240	99	2^4	<1	1	<1	0	0	0	0
1	21	Prepared from instant	1 c	240	99	2^4	<1	1	0	0	0	0	0
		Fruit drinks, noncarbonated^5:											
1	22	Fruit punch drink, canned	1 c	253	88	118	<1	30	0	<1	t	t	t
1	1358	Gatorade	1 c	230	99	39	0	11	0	0	0	0	0
1	23	Grape drink, canned	1 c	250	88	112	0	35	<1	<1	t	t	t
1	1304	Koolade, sweetened with sugar	1 c	240	100	100	0	25	0	0	0	0	0
1	1356	Koolade, sweetened with nutrasweet	1 c	240	100	4	0	0	0	0	0	0	0
		Lemonade, frozen:											
1	26	Concentrate (6-oz can)	¾ c	219	52	397	1	103	1	<1	.1	t	.1
1	27	Lemonade prepared from frozen concentrate	1 c	248	89	100	<1	26	<1	<1	t	t	t
		Limeade, frozen:											
1	28	Concentrate (6-oz can)	¾ c	218	50	408	<1	108	1	<1	t	t	.1
1	29	Limeade prepared from frozen concentrate	1 c	247	89	102	<1	27	<1	<1	t	t	t
1	24	Pineapple grapefruit, canned	1 c	250	88	117	1	29	0	<1	t	t	.1
1	25	Pineapple orange, canned	1 c	250	87	125	3	29	0	<1	t	t	.1
		Fruit and vegetable juices: see Fruit and Vegetable sections											

$^{(1)}$Calories can vary from 78 to 131 for 12 fl oz.
$^{(2)}$Values are for sweet dessert wine. Dry dessert wines contain 149 cal and 5 g of carbohydrate.
$^{(3)}$Mineral content varies depending on water source.
$^{(4)}$Calorie values from USDA vary from 1 to 4 calories per cup.
$^{(5)}$Usually less than 10% fruit juice.

(Computer code number is for West Diet Analysis program)

A

GRP KEY: 1 = BEV   2 = DAIRY   3 = EGGS   4 = FAT/OIL   5 = FRUIT   6 = BAKERY   7 = GRAIN   8 = FISH   9 = BEEF   10 = POULTRY
11 = SAUSAGE   12 = MIXED/FAST   13 = NUTS/SEEDS   14 = SWEETS   15 = VEG/LEG   16 = MISC   22 = SOUP/SAUCE

Chol (mg)	Calc (mg)	Iron (mg)	Magn (mg)	Phos (mg)	Pota (mg)	Sodi (mg)	Zinc (mg)	VT-A (RE)	Thia (mg)	Ribo (mg)	Niac (mg)	V-B6 (mg)	Fola (µg)	VT-C (mg)
0	18	.11	23	44	89	19	.07	0	.02	.09	1.61	.18	21	0
0	18	.14	18	43	64	10	.11	0	.03	.11	1.39	.12	15	0
0	0	.02	0	2	1	<1	.02	0	<.01	<.01	<.01	t	0	0
0	0	.02	0	2	1	<1	.02	0	<.01	<.01	<.01	0	0	0
0	0	.02	0	2	1	<1	.02	0	<.01	<.01	<.01	0	0	0
0	1	.03	1	3	15	4	.01	0	<.01	.01	.08	—	0	0
—	7	.06	1	23	15	43	.08	—	0	.03	.04	—	0	0
0	0	.04	0	0	0	3	—	0	0	0	<.01	0	0	—
0	9	.24	11	11	109	11	.08	0	.02	.02	.25	0	<1	0
0	8	.44	13	14	115	6	.10	0	<.01	.03	.08	.04	2	0
0	9	.39	10	15	102	5	.06	0	<.01	.02	.08	.03	1	0
0	9	.33	11	14	82	5	.07	0	<.01	<.01	.07	.01	<1	0
0	17	.15	4	0	6	75	.36	0	0	0	0	0	0	0
0	9	.13	3	46	4	15	.05	0	0	0	0	0	0	0
0	12	.11	4	30	0	21[6]	.28	0	.02	.08	0	0	0	0
0	14	.14	3	38	7	21[6]	.10	0	0	0	0	0	0	0
0	12	.66	3	1	5	25	.18	0	0	0	0	0	0	0
0	12	.31	4	0	3	57	.26	0	0	0	0	0	0	0
0	9	.25	2	1	4	41	.18	0	0	0	.06	0	0	0
0	19	.23	4	4	9	46	.38	0	0	0	0	0	0	0
0	12	.14	1	41	2	38	.15	0	0	0	0	0	0	0
0	19	.19	4	2	3	49	.26	0	0	0	0	0	0	0
0	4	.12	14	3	130	5	.08	0	0	.02	.53	0	<1	0
0	8	.12	9	8	87	8	.07	0	0	<.01	.69	0	0	0
0	19	.52	5	3	64	56	.31	4	.06	.06	.05	0	3	75
0	23	—	—	0	23	123	—	0	—	—	—	—	—	—
0	3	.41	5	3	13	16	.28	<1	.08	.02	.07	.02	1	85
0	0	0	0	0	0	0	0	0	0	0	0	0	0	6
0	0	0	0	0	0	0	0	0	0	0	0	0	0	6
0	15	1.58	11	19	148	8	.17	21	.06	.21	.16	.06	22	39[7]
0	4	.41	3	5	38	8	.05	5	.02	.05	.04	.02	6	10[7]
0	11	.22	60	13	129	<1	.11	<1	.02	.02	.22	.11	25	26
0	3	.06	15	3	33	<1	.03	<1	<.01	<.01	.05	.03	6	7
0	18	.77	15	14	154	34	.15	9	.08	.04	.67	.10	26	115
0	13	.67	14	10	116	9	.14	133	.08	.05	.52	.12	27	56

[6] Value for product sweetened with aspartame only; sodium is 32 mg if a blend of aspartame and sodium saccharin is used; 75 mg if just sodium saccharin is used.
[7] Vitamin C can range from 5 to 72 mg in a small can of frozen concentrate, and from 1 to 18 mg in l c of prepared lemonade.

(For purposes of calculations, use "0" for t, <1, <.1, <.01, etc.)

A

Table A–1   Food Composition

Grp	Computer Code No.	Food Description	Measure	Wt (g)	H$_2$O (%)	Ener (cal)	Prot (g)	Carb (g)	Dietary Fiber (g)	Fat (g)	Fat Breakdown (g) Sat	Mono	Poly
		BEVERAGES—Con.											
1	1357	Perrier® bottled water, 6.5 fl oz bottle	1 ea	192	100	0	0	0	0	0	0	0	0
		Tea[8]:											
1	30	Brewed	1 c	240	100	2	<.01	1	0	0	0	0	0
1	31	From instant, unsweetened	1 c	237	100	2	0	<1	0	0	0	0	0
1	32	From instant, sweetened	1 c	262	91	86	0	22	0	0	0	0	0
		DAIRY											
		Butter: see Fats and Oils, #158, 159, 160											
		Cheese, natural:											
2	33	Blue	1 oz	28	42	100	6	1	0	8	5.3	2.2	.2
2	34	Brick	1 oz	28	41	105	6	1	0	8	5.3	2.4	.2
2	35	Brie	1 oz	28	48	95	6	<1	0	8	5.0	2.3	.3
2	36	Camembert	1 oz	28	52	85	6	<1	0	7	4.3	2.0	.2
		Cheddar:											
2	37	Cut pieces	1 oz	28	37	114	7	<1	0	9	6.0	2.7	.3
2	38	1" cube	1 ea	17	37	69	4	<1	0	6	3.6	1.6	.2
2	39	Shredded	1 c	113	37	455	28	1	0	37	24	11	1
		Cottage:											
2	40	Creamed, large curd	1 c	225	79	235	28	6	0	10	6.4	3.0	.3
2	41	Creamed, small curd	1 c	210	79	215	26	6	0	9	6.0	2.7	.3
2	42	With fruit	1 c	226	72	279	22	30	0	8	4.9	2.2	.3
2	43	Low fat 2%	1 c	226	79	205	31	8	0	4	2.8	1.2	.1
2	44	Low fat 1%	1 c	226	82	164	28	6	0	2	1.5	.7	.1
2	45	Dry curd	1 c	145	80	123	25	3	0	1	.4	.2	<.1
2	46	Cream	1 oz	28	54	99	2	1	0	10	6.2	2.8	.4
2	47	Edam	1 oz	28	42	101	7	<1	0	8	5.0	2.3	.2
2	48	Feta	1 oz	28	55	75	5	1	0	6	4.2	1.3	.2
2	49	Gouda	1 oz	28	42	101	7	1	0	8	5.0	2.2	.2
2	50	Gruyère	1 oz	28	33	117	8	<1	0	9	5.4	2.9	.5
2	51	Gorgonzola	1 oz	28	39	111	7	0	0	9	5.5	2.4	.5
2	52	Liederkranz	1 oz	28	53	87	5	0	0	8	5.3	2.2	.2
2	53	Monterey jack	1 oz	28	41	106	7	<1	0	9	5.4	2.4	.2
		Mozzarella, made with:											
2	54	Whole milk	1 oz	28	54	80	5	1	0	6	3.7	1.9	.2
2	55	Part skim milk, low moisture	1 oz	28	49	80	8	1	0	5	3.1	1.4	.1
2	56	Muenster	1 oz	28	42	104	6	<1	0	8	5.4	2.5	.2
		Parmesan, grated:											
2	57	Cup, not pressed down	1 c	100	18	455	42	4	0	30	19	8.7	.7
2	58	Tablespoon	1 tbsp	5	18	23	2	<1	0	2	1	.4	<.1
2	59	Ounce	1 oz	28	18	129	12	1	0	9	5.4	2.5	.2
2	60	Provolone	1 oz	28	41	100	7	1	0	8	4.8	2.1	.2
		Ricotta, made with:											
2	61	Whole milk	1 c	246	72	428	28	7	0	32	20	8.9	1
2	62	Part skim milk	1 c	246	74	340	28	13	0	19	12	5.7	.6
2	63	Romano	1 oz	28	31	110	9	1	0	8	4.9	2.2	.2
2	64	Swiss	1 oz	28	37	107	8	1	0	8	5.0	2.1	.3
		Pasteurized processed cheese products:											
2	65	American	1 oz	28	39	106	6	<1	0	9	5.6	2.5	.3
2	66	Swiss	1 oz	28	42	95	7	1	0	7	4.6	2.0	.2
2	67	American cheese food	1 oz	28	44	93	6	2	0	7	4.4	2.0	.2
2	68	American cheese spread	1 oz	28	48	82	5	2	0	6	3.8	1.8	.2

[8]Mineral content varies depending on water source.

(Computer code number is for West Diet Analysis program)

GRP KEY: 1=BEV 2=DAIRY 3=EGGS 4=FAT/OIL 5=FRUIT 6=BAKERY 7=GRAIN 8=FISH 9=BEEF 10=POULTRY
11=SAUSAGE 12=MIXED/FAST 13=NUTS/SEEDS 14=SWEETS 15=VEG/LEG 16=MISC 22=SOUP/SAUCE

Chol (mg)	Calc (mg)	Iron (mg)	Magn (mg)	Phos (mg)	Pota (mg)	Sodi (mg)	Zinc (mg)	VT-A (RE)	Thia (mg)	Ribo (mg)	Niac (mg)	V-B6 (mg)	Fola (µg)	VT-C (mg)
0	26	0	1	0	0	3	0	0	0	0	0	0	0	0
0	0	.05	7	1	89	7	.05	0	0	.03	.1	0	12	0
0	5	.05	5	3	47	8	.07	0	0	<.01	<.01	<.09	1	0
0	1	.04	3	3	49	1	.06	0	0	.04	.09	0	5	0
21	150	.09	7	110	73	396	.75	65	.01	.11	.29	.05	10	0
27	191	.13	7	128	38	159	.73	86	<.01	.1	.03	.02	6	0
28	52	.14	6	53	43	178	.7	57	.02	.15	.11	.07	18	0
20	110	.09	6	98	53	236	.68	71	.01	.14	.18	.06	18	0
30	204	.20	8	146	28	176	.92	86	.01	.11	.02	.02	5	0
18	124	.12	5	88	17	107	.54	52	<.01	.07	.01	.01	3	0
119	815	.77	31	579	111	701	3.51	342	.03	.42	.09	.08	21	0
34	135	.26	11	297	190	911	.8	108	.05	.37	.30	.14	27	<1
31	126	.30	11	277	177	850	.8	101	.04	.34	.27	.14	26	<1
25	108	.25	9	236	151	915	.66	81	.04	.29	.23	.12	22	<1
19	155	.36	14	340	217	918	.95	45	.05	.42	.33	.17	30	0
10	138	.32	12	302	193	918	.86	25	.05	.37	.29	.15	28	t
10	46	.33	6	151	47	19	.68	12	.04	.21	.23	.12	21	0
31	23	.34	2	30	34	84	.33	124	<.01	.06	.03	.01	4	0
25	207	.13	8	152	53	274	1.06	72	.01	.11	.02	.02	5	0
25	140	.18	5	96	18	316	.81	36	.04	.23	.29	.02	3	0
32	198	.07	8	155	34	232	1.1	49	<.01	.10	.02	.02	6	0
31	287	.06	4	172	23	95	1	98	.02	.08	.03	.02	3	0
25	149	.12	8	121	26	513	.57	103	.01	.09	.2	.04	9	0
21	110	.12	7	100	68	390	.7	91	.01	.18	.1	.04	34	0
26	212	.2	8	126	23	152	.85	81	<.01	.11	.02	.02	3	0
22	147	.05	5	105	19	106	.7	68	<.01	.07	.02	.02	2	0
15	207	.08	8	149	27	150	.83	54	<.01	.1	.03	.02	3	0
27	203	.13	8	133	38	178	.84	90	<.01	.09	.03	.02	3	0
79	1376	.95	51	807	107	1862	3.19	173	.04	.39	.32	.11	8	0
4	69	.05	3	40	5	93	.16	9	<.01	.02	.02	<.01	<1	0
22	390	.27	14	229	30	528	1	49	.01	.11	.09	.03	2	0
20	214	.15	8	141	39	248	.89	75	<.01	.09	.04	.02	3	0
124	509	.94	28	389	257	207	2.85	330	.03	.48	.26	.11	14	0
76	669	1.09	4	449	307	307	3.29	278	.05	.46	.19	.05	14	0
29	302	.23	12	215	26	340	1	40	.01	.11	.02	.03	2	0
26	272	.05	10	171	31	74	1.1	72	<.01	.1	.03	.02	2	0
27	174	.11	6	211	46	406	.93	82	.01	.1	.02	.02	2	0
24	219	.17	8	216	61	388	1.02	65	<.01	.08	.01	.01	2	0
18	163	.24	9	130	79	337	.85	62	.01	.13	.04	.02	2	0
16	159	.09	8	201	69	381	.78	54	.01	.12	.04	.03	2	0

A

(For purposes of calculations, use "0" for t, <1, <.1, <.01, etc.)

Table A–1   Food Composition

Grp	Computer Code No.	Food Description	Measure	Wt (g)	H$_2$O (%)	Ener (cal)	Prot (g)	Carb (g)	Dietary Fiber (g)	Fat (g)	Fat Breakdown (g) Sat	Mono	Poly
DAIRY—Con.													
		Cream, sweet:											
		Half and half (cream and milk):											
2	69	Cup	1 c	242	81	315	7	10	0	28	17	8	1
2	70	Tablespoon	1 tbsp	15	81	20	<1	1	0	2	1.1	.5	.1
		Light, coffee or table:											
2	71	Cup	1 c	240	74	469	6	9	0	46	29	13	1.7
2	72	Tablespoon	1 tbsp	15	74	30	<1	1	0	3	1.8	.8	.1
		‑ Light whipping cream, liquid:											
2	73	Cup	1 c	239	64	699	5	7	0	74	46	22	2.1
2	74	Tablespoon	1 tbsp	15	64	44	<1	<1	0	5	2.9	1.4	.1
		Heavy whipping cream, liquid[9]:											
2	75	Cup	1 c	238	58	821	5	7	0	88	55	25	3.3
2	76	Tablespoon	1 tbsp	15	58	51	<1	<1	0	6	3.5	1.6	.2
		Whipped cream, pressurized[9]:											
2	77	Cup	1 c	60	61	154	2	7	0	13	8.3	3.9	.5
2	78	Tablespoon	1 tbsp	4	61	10	<1	<1	0	1	.5	.2	<.1
		Cream, sour, cultured:											
2	79	Cup	1 c	230	71	493	7	10	0	48	30	14	1.8
2	80	Tablespoon	1 tbsp	14	71	30	<1	1	0	3	1.8	.9	.1
		Cream products—imitation and part dairy:											
		Coffee whitener:											
2	81	Frozen or liquid	1 tbsp	15	77	20	<1	2	0	2	1.4	t	t
2	82	Powdered	1 tsp	2	2	11	<1	1	0	1	.6	t	t
		Dessert topping, frozen:											
2	83	Cup	1 c	75	50	239	1	17	0	19	16	1.2	.4
2	84	Tablespoon	1 tbsp	5	50	15	<1	1	0	1	1.0	.1	t
		Dessert topping from mix:											
2	85	Cup	1 c	80	67	151	3	13	0	10	8.6	.7	.2
2	86	Tablespoon	1 tbsp	5	67	9	<1	1	0	1	.5	<.1	t
		Dessert topping, pressurized:											
2	87	Cup	1 c	70	60	185	1	11	0	16	13	1.4	.2
2	88	Tablespoon	1 tbsp	4	60	11	<1	1	0	1	.8	.1	t
		Sour cream imitation:											
2	91	Cup	1 c	230	71	479	6	15	0	45	41	1.4	.1
2	92	Tablespoon	1 tbsp	14	71	29	<1	1	0	3	2.5	.1	t
		Sour dressing, part dairy:											
2	89	Cup	1 c	235	75	416	8	11	0	39	31	4.6	1.1
2	90	Tablespoon	1 tbsp	15	75	25	<1	1	0	2	2.0	.3	.1
		Milk, fluid:											
2	93	Whole milk	1 c	244	88	150	8	11	0	8	5.1	2.4	.3
2	94	2% low-fat milk	1 c	244	89	121	8	12	0	5	2.9	1.4	.2
2	95	2% milk solids added[10]	1 c	245	89	125	9	12	0	5	2.9	1.4	.2
2	96	1% low-fat milk	1 c	244	90	102	8	12	0	3	1.6	.8	.1
2	97	1% milk solids added[10]	1 c	245	90	105	9	12	0	2	1.5	.7	.1
2	98	Skim milk	1 c	245	91	86	8	12	0	<1	.3	.1	t
2	99	Skim milk solids added[10]	1 c	245	90	91	9	12	0	1	.4	.2	t
2	100	Buttermilk	1 c	245	90	99	8	12	0	2	1.3	.6	.1

[9]For whipped cream, (non-pressurized), double the liquid cream volume of codes 75,76 or 73,74. One tablespoon liquid cream becomes 2 Tablespoons when "whipped".

[10]Milk solids added, label claims less than 10 g protein per cup.

(Computer code number is for West Diet Analysis program)

GRP KEY: 1 = BEV   2 = DAIRY   3 = EGGS   4 = FAT/OIL   5 = FRUIT   6 = BAKERY   7 = GRAIN   8 = FISH   9 = BEEF   10 = POULTRY
11 = SAUSAGE   12 = MIXED/FAST   13 = NUTS/SEEDS   14 = SWEETS   15 = VEG/LEG   16 = MISC   22 = SOUP/SAUCE

Chol (mg)	Calc (mg)	Iron (mg)	Magn (mg)	Phos (mg)	Pota (mg)	Sodi (mg)	Zinc (mg)	VT-A (RE)	Thia (mg)	Ribo (mg)	Niac (mg)	V-B6 (mg)	Fola (µg)	VT-C (mg)
89	254	.17	25	230	314	98	1.23	259	.09	.36	.19	.09	6	2
6	16	.01	2	14	20	6	.08	16	.01	.02	.01	<.01	<1	<1
159	231	.1	21	192	292	95	.65	437	.08	.36	.14	.08	6	2
10	14	.01	1	12	18	6	.04	27	<.01	.02	.01	<.01	<1	<1
265	166	.07	17	146	231	82	.60	705	.06	.30	.1	.07	9	1
17	10	<.01	1	9	15	5	.04	44	<.01	.02	.01	<.01	1	<1
326	154	.07	17	149	179	89	.55	1002	.05	.26	.09	.06	10	1
20	10	<.01	1	9	11	6	.03	63	<.01	.02	.01	<.01	1	<1
46	61	.03	6	54	88	78	.22	124	.02	.04	.04	.03	1	0
3	4	<.01	<1	3	5	5	.01	8	<.01	<.01	<.01	<.01	<1	0
102	268	.14	26	195	331	123	.69	448	.08	.34	.15	.04	25	2
6	16	.01	2	12	20	7	.04	27	<.01	.02	.01	<.01	2	<1
0	1	<.01	<1	10	29	12	<.01	1[10]	0	0	0	0	0	0
0	<1	.02	<1	8	16	4	.01	<1[10]	0	<.01	0	0	0	0
0	5	.09	1	6	14	19	.03	65[11]	0	0	0	0	0	0
0	<1	.01	<1	<1	1	1	<.01	4[11]	0	0	0	0	0	0
8	72	.03	8	69	121	53	.22	39[11]	.02	.09	.05	.02	3	1
<1	5	<.01	<1	4	8	3	.14	3[11]	<.01	<.01	<.01	<.01	<1	<1
0	4	.01	1	13	13	43	.01	33[11]	0	0	0	0	0	0
0	<1	<.01	<1	1	1	3	<.01	2[11]	0	0	0	0	0	0
0	6	.01	—	102	369	235	0	0	0	0	0	0	0	0
0	<1	<.01	—	6	23	14	0	0	0	0	0	0	0	0
213	266	.07	23	205	381	113	.87	5[11]	.09	.38	.17	.04	28	2
1	17	<.01	2	13	24	7	.05	<1[11]	.01	.02	.01	<.01	2	<1
33	291	.12	33	228	370	120	.94	76	.09	.4	.2	.1	12	2
22	297	.12	33	232	377	122	.96	140	.1	.4	.21	.1	12	2
18	314	.12	35	245	397	128	.98	140	.1	.42	.22	.11	12	2
10	300	.12	34	235	381	123	.96	145	.1	.41	.21	.11	12	2
10	314	.12	35	245	397	128	.98	145	.1	.42	.22	.11	12	2
4	302	.1	28	247	406	126	.92	149	.09	.34	.22	.1	14	2
5	316	.12	37	255	419	130	1	149	.1	.43	.22	.11	12	2
9	285	.12	26	219	371	257	1.03	20	.08	.38	.14	.08	12	2

[11]Vitamin A value is from beta-carotene used for coloring.

A

(For purposes of calculations, use "0" for t, <1, <.1, <.01, etc.)

Table A–1   Food Composition

Grp	Computer Code No.	Food Description	Measure	Wt (g)	H$_2$O (%)	Ener (cal)	Prot (g)	Carb (g)	Dietary Fiber (g)	Fat (g)	Fat Breakdown (g)		
											Sat	Mono	Poly
DAIRY—Con.													
		Milk, canned:											
2	101	Sweetened condensed	1 c	306	27	982	24	166	0	27	17	7.4	1
2	102	Evaporated, whole	1 c	252	74	340	17	25	0	20	12	5.9	.6
2	103	Evaporated, skim	1 c	255	79	200	19	29	0	1	.3	.2	t
		Milk, dried:											
2	104	Buttermilk	1 c	120	3	464	41	59	0	7	4.3	2.0	.3
		Instant, nonfat:											
2	105	Envelope[12]	1 ea	91	4	326	32	48	0	1	.4	.2	t
2	106	Cup	1 c	68	4	244	24	36	0	1	.3	.1	t
2	107	Goat milk	1 c	244	87	168	9	11	0	10	6.5	2.7	.4
2	108	Kefir[13]	1 c	233	82	122	9	9	0	5	2.9	1.2	.1
		Milk beverages and powdered mixes:											
		Chocolate:											
2	109	Whole	1 c	250	82	210	8	26	4	8	5.3	2.5	.3
2	110	2% fat	1 c	250	84	180	8	26	4	5	3.1	1.5	.2
2	111	1% fat	1 c	250	84	160	8	26	4	3	1.5	.8	.1
		Chocolate-flavored beverages:											
2	112	Powder containing nonfat dry milk:	1 oz	28	1	100	4	23	<1	1	.7	.4	t
2	113	Drink prepared with water	¾ c	206	86	100	4	23	<1	1	.7	.4	t
2	114	Powder without nonfat dry milk:	¾ oz	22	<1	75	1	20	<1	1	.4	.2	t
2	115	Drink prepared with whole milk:	1 c	266	81	226	9	31	<1	9	5.5	2.6	.3
2	116	Eggnog, commercial	1 c	254	74	342	10	34	0	19	11	5.7	.9
		Instant Breakfast:											
2	1027	Envelope, dry powder only	1 ea	37	3	130	7	23	0	0	0	0	0
2	1028	Prepared with whole milk	1 c	281	87	280	15	34	0	8	5.1	2.4	.3
2	1029	Prepared with 2% milk	1 c	281	88	251	15	35	0	5	2.9	1.4	.2
2	1283	Prepared with 1% milk	1 c	281	89	232	15	35	0	3	1.5	.7	.1
2	1284	Prepared with skim milk	1 c	282	89	216	15	35	0	<1	.3	.1	t
		Malted milk, chocolate flavor:											
2	117	Powder[14], 3 heaping tsp:	¾ oz	21	1	79	1	18	<1	1	.5	.2	.1
2	118	Drink prepared with whole milk	1 c	265	81	229	9	30	<1	9	5.2	2.6	.4
		Malted milk, natural flavor:											
2	119	Powder[14], 3 heaping tsp:	¾ oz	21	2	87	2	16	<1	2	.9	.4	.3
2	120	Drink prepared with whole milk	1 c	265	81	237	10	27	<1	10	6.0	2.8	.6
		Milk shakes:											
2	121	Chocolate (10 fl oz)	1¼ c	283	72	360	10	58	<1	11	6.6	3.0	.4
2	122	Vanilla (10 fl oz)	1¼ c	283	75	314	10	51	<1	8	5.3	2.4	.3
		Milk desserts:											
2	134	Custard, baked	1 c	265	77	305	14	29	0	15	6.8	5.4	.7
		Ice cream, regular vanilla (about 11% fat):											
		Hardened:											
2	123	½ gallon	½ gal	1064	61	2153	38	254	0	115	71	33	4
2	124	Cup	1 c	133	61	269	5	32	0	14	8.3	4.1	.5
2	125	Fluid ounces	3 oz	50	61	101	2	12	0	5	3.3	1.6	.2
2	126	Soft serve	1 c	173	60	377	7	38	0	22	14	6.7	1.0
		Ice cream, rich vanilla (about 16% fat):											
		Hardened:											
2	127	½ gallon	½ gal	1188	59	2805	33	256	0	190	118	55	7
2	128	Cup	1 c	148	59	349	4	32	0	24	15	6.8	.9

[12]Yields 1 qt fluid milk when reconstituted according to package directions.
[13]Most values provided by product labeling.
[14]The latest USDA data from *Handbook 8–14* on beverages updates previous USDA data.

(Computer code number is for West Diet Analysis program)

GRP KEY: 1 = BEV 2 = DAIRY 3 = EGGS 4 = FAT/OIL 5 = FRUIT 6 = BAKERY 7 = GRAIN 8 = FISH 9 = BEEF 10 = POULTRY
11 = SAUSAGE 12 = MIXED/FAST 13 = NUTS/SEEDS 14 = SWEETS 15 = VEG/LEG 16 = MISC 22 = SOUP/SAUCE

Chol (mg)	Calc (mg)	Iron (mg)	Magn (mg)	Phos (mg)	Pota (mg)	Sodi (mg)	Zinc (mg)	VT-A (RE)	Thia (mg)	Ribo (mg)	Niac (mg)	V-B6 (mg)	Fola (µg)	VT-C (mg)
104	868	.58	78	775	1136	389	2.88	248	.28	1.27	.64	.16	34	8
74	657	.48	60	510	764	267	1.94	136	.12	.8	.49	.13	18	5
10	738	.7	68	497	845	293	2.18	300	.11	.8	.4	.14	22	3
83	1421	.36	131	1119	1910	621	4.82	65	.47	1.9	1.05	.41	57	7
16	1120	.28	107	896	1552	500	4.01	646[15]	.38	1.59	.81	.31	45	5
12	837	.21	80	670	1160	373	3.06	483[15]	.28	1.19	.61	.24	34	4
28	326	.12	34	270	499	122	.73	137	.12	.34	.68	.11	2	3
10	350	.5	28	319	205	50	.9	155	.45	.44	.3	.09	20	6
31	280	.6	33	251	417	149	1.02	73	.09	.41	.31	.1	12	2
17	284	.6	33	254	422	151	.91	143	.09	.41	.32	.1	12	2
7	287	.6	33	256	425	152	1.02	148	.1	.42	.32	.1	12	2
1	89	.29	23	88	223	139	1.26	1	.03	.17	.18	.04	3	1
1	89	.29	23	88	223	139	1.26	1	.03	.17	.18	.04	3	1
0	8	.68	21	28	128	45	.33	1	.01	.03	.11	<.01	4	<1
33	300	.8	54	256	498	165	1.26	76	.1	.43	.32	.1	12	3
149	330	.51	47	278	420	138	1.17	203	.09	.48	.27	.13	2	4
0	10	7.9	80	15	0	166	3.00	175	.30	.07	5.00	.40	100	27
33	301	8.0	113	243	370	286	3.95	251	.39	.46	5.20	.50	112	29
18	307	8.0	113	247	377	289	3.96	315	.40	.47	5.21	.51	112	29
10	310	8.0	124	250	381	289	3.96	315	.40	.48	5.21	.51	112	29
4	312	8.0	108	262	406	292	3.96	327	.39	.41	5.22	.50	113	29
1	13	.48	15	37	130	53	.17	4	.04	.04	.42	.03	4	<1
34	304	.6	47	265	499	172	1.09	80	13	.44	.63	.14	16	3
4	63	.16	20	75	159	103	.21	19	.11	.19	1.1	.09	10	1
37	354	.27	52	303	529	223	1.14	94	.2	.59	1.31	.19	22	3
37	319	.88	47	288	567	273	1.15	64	.16	.69	.46	.14	10	1
32	344	.26	35	289	492	232	1.01	90	.13	.52	.52	.15	9	2
213	297	1.1	37	310	387	209	1.53	146	.11	.5	.3	.13	24	1
478	1405	.96	149	1075	2053	926	11.3	1064	.42	2.63	1.08	.49	22	6
59	176	.12	18	134	257	116	1.41	133	.05	.33	.13	.06	3	1
23	66	.05	7	50	97	44	.53	50	.02	.12	.05	.02	1	<1
153	236	.43	25	199	338	153	1.99	199	.08	.45	.18	.1	9	1
701	1212	.83	131	927	1770	867	9.74	1758	.36	2.27	.93	.43	23	5
88	151	.1	16	115	221	108	1.21	219	.04	.28	.12	.05	2	1

(15)With added vitamin A.

A

(For purposes of calculations, use "0" for t, <1, <.1, <.01, etc.)

Table A–1   Food Composition

Grp	Computer Code No.	Food Description	Measure	Wt (g)	H$_2$O (%)	Ener (cal)	Prot (g)	Carb (g)	Dietary Fiber (g)	Fat (g)	Fat Breakdown (g) Sat	Mono	Poly
DAIRY—Con.													
		Milk Desserts—Con.											
		Ice milk, vanilla (about 4% fat):											
		Hardened:											
2	129	½ gallon	½ gal	1048	69	1467	41	232	0	45	28	13	1.7
2	130	Cup	1 c	131	69	184	5	29	0	6	3.5	1.6	.2
2	131	Soft serve (about 3% fat)	1 c	175	70	223	8	38	0	5	2.9	1.3	.2
		Pudding, canned, 5 oz can = .55 cup:											
2	135	Chocolate	1 ea	142	68	205	3	30	<1	11	9.5	.5	.1
2	136	Tapioca	1 ea	142	74	160	3	28	0	5	4.8	t	t
2	137	Vanilla	1 ea	142	69	220	2	33	0	10	9.5	.3	.1
		Puddings, prepared from dry mix with whole milk:											
2	138	Chocolate, instant	1 c	260	71	310	8	54	<1	8	4.6	2.2	.4
2	139	Chocolate, regular, cooked	½ c	130	73	150	4	25	<1	4	2.4	1.1	.1
2	140	Rice, cooked	½ c	132	73	155	4	27	<1	4	2.3	1.1	.1
2	141	Tapioca, cooked	½ c	130	75	145	4	25	0	4	2.3	1.1	.1
2	142	Vanilla, instant	½ c	130	73	150	4	27	0	4	2.2	1.1	.2
2	143	Vanilla, regular, cooked	½ c	130	74	145	4	25	0	4	2.3	1	.1
		Sherbet (2% fat):											
2	132	½ gallon	½ gal	1542	66	2158	17	469	0	31	19	8.8	1.1
2	133	Cup	1 c	193	66	270	2	59	0	4	2.4	1.1	.1
2	144	Soy milk	1 c	240	93	79	7	4	0	5	.5	.8	2.0
2	1584	Yogurt, frozen, low fat[16]	½ c	87	70	110	4	17	0	2	1.1	.5	<1
		Yogurt, low fat:											
2	145	Fruit added[17]	1 c	227	74	231	10	43	<1	2	1.6	.7	.1
2	146	Plain	1 c	227	85	144	12	16	0	3	2.3	1.0	.1
2	147	Vanilla or coffee flavor	1 c	227	79	193	11	31	0	3	1.8	.8	.1
2	148	Yogurt, made with nonfat milk	1 c	227	85	127	13	17	0	<1	.3	.1	t
2	149	Yogurt, made with whole milk	1 c	227	88	138	8	11	0	7	4.8	2.0	.2
EGGS[18]													
		Raw, large:											
3	150	Whole, without shell	1 ea	50	75	75	6	1	0	5	1.6	1.6	.7
3	151	White	1 ea	33.4	88	17	4	<1	0	0	0	0	0
3	152	Yolk	1 ea	16.6	49	59	3	<1	0	5	1.6	1.9	.7
		Cooked:											
3	153	Fried in margarine	1 ea	46	69	91	6	1	0	7	1.9	2.7	1.3
3	154	Hard-cooked, shell removed	1 ea	50	75	79	6	1	0	5	1.6	2.0	.7
3	155	Hard-cooked, chopped	1 c	136	75	211	17	2	0	14	4.5	5.5	2.0
3	156	Poached, no added salt	1 ea	50	75	75	6	1	0	5	1.5	1.9	.7
3	157	Scrambled with milk and margarine	1 ea	61	73	100	7	1	0	7	2.2	2.9	1.3
FATS and OILS													
		Butter:											
4	158	Stick	½ c	113	16	813	1	<1	0	92	57	27	3.4
4	159	Tablespoon	1 tbsp	14	16	100	<1	<1	0	12	7.2	3.3	.4
4	160	Pat (about 1 tsp)[19]	1 ea	5	16	34	<1	<1	0	4	2.5	1.2	.2

[16] Data is a composite of USDA information and several manufacturers.

[17] Carbohydrate and calories vary widely—consult label if more precise values are needed.

[18] This data is newest revised information from the USDA with 24% less cholesterol.

[19] Pat is 1″ square, ⅓″ thick; about 1 tsp; 90 per lb.

(Computer code number is for West Diet Analysis program)

GRP KEY: 1 = BEV   2 = DAIRY   3 = EGGS   4 = FAT/OIL   5 = FRUIT   6 = BAKERY   7 = GRAIN   8 = FISH   9 = BEEF   10 = POULTRY
11 = SAUSAGE   12 = MIXED/FAST   13 = NUTS/SEEDS   14 = SWEETS   15 = VEG/LEG   16 = MISC   22 = SOUP/SAUCE

Chol (mg)	Calc (mg)	Iron (mg)	Magn (mg)	Phos (mg)	Pota (mg)	Sodi (mg)	Zinc (mg)	VT-A (RE)	Thia (mg)	Ribo (mg)	Niac (mg)	V-B6 (mg)	Fola (µg)	VT-C (mg)
146	1404	1.47	147	1035	2117	838	4.40	419	.61	2.78	.94	.68	21	6
18	176	.18	19	129	265	105	.55	52	.08	.35	.12	.09	3	1
13	274	.28	29	202	412	163	.86	44	.12	.54	.18	.13	5	1
1	74	1.2	24	117	254	285	.70	31	.04	.17	.6	.03	3	<1
1	119	.3	24	113	212	252	.70	<1	.03	.14	.4	.03	3	<1
1	79	.2	24	94	155	305	.70	<1	.03	.12	.6	.03	3	<1
28	260	.6	48	658	352	880	1.18	66	.08	.36	.22	.13	10	2
15	146	.2	24	120	190	167	.59	34	.05	.2	.13	.06	4	1
15	133	.5	16	110	165	140	.60	33	.10	.18	.6	.05	6	1
15	131	.1	16	103	167	152	.50	34	.04	.18	.1	.05	6	1
15	129	.1	16	273	164	375	.50	33	.04	.17	.1	.05	6	1
15	132	.1	16	102	166	178	.50	34	.04	.18	.1	.05	6	1
113	827	2.47	124	594	1588	709	10.6	308	.26	.71	1.05	.2	108	31
14	103	.31	15	74	198	88	1.33	39	.03	.09	.13	.03	14	4
0	10	1.38	45	117	338	30	.54	8	.39	.17	.35	.10	4	0
7	120	.05	5	980	148	45	.56	17	.03	.14	.07	.03	7	<1
10	345	.16	31	325	442	125	1.68	25	.08	.4	.22	.09	21	2
14	415	.18	40	326	531	159	2.02	36	.10	.49	.26	.11	25	2
11	388	.16	36	306	497	150	1.88	30	.10	.46	.24	.10	23	2
4	452	.2	43	354	579	173	2.20	5	.11	.53	.28	.12	28	2
30	275	.11	27	216	352	104	1.34	68	.07	.32	.17	.07	16	1
213	25	.72	5	89	60	61	.55	97	.03	.25	.04	.07	25	0
0	2	.01	4	4	48	55	<.1	0	<.01	.15	.03	<.01	1	0
213	23	.7	1	81	16	7	.54	97	.03	.11	.01	.07	24	0
211	25	.72	5	89	61	162	.55	114	.03	.24	.04	.07	18	0
215	25	.72	5	86	63	62	.55	84	.03	.26	.03	.06	22	0
574	68	1.95	14	233	171	169	1.5	227	.09	.70	.09	.16	61	0
212	25	.72	5	89	60	61	.55	95	.03	.22	.03	.06	18	0
215	44	.72	7	104	84	171	.6	119	.03	.26	.05	.07	18	0
247	27	.18	2	26	29	933[20]	.06	852[21]	.01	.04	.05	<.01	3	0
31	3	.02	<1	3	4	116[20]	.01	106[21]	<.01	<.01	.01	t	<1	0
11	1	.01	<1	1	1	41[20]	<.01	38[21]	t	<.01	<.01	t	<1	0

[20] For salted butter; unsalted butter contains 12 mg sodium per stick or ½ c, 1.5 mg/tbsp, or .5 mg/pat.
[21] Values for vitamin A are a year-round average.

(For purposes of calculations, use "0" for t, <1, <.1, <.01, etc.)

A

Table A–1   Food Composition

Grp	Computer Code No.	Food Description	Measure	Wt (g)	H₂O (%)	Ener (cal)	Prot (g)	Carb (g)	Dietary Fiber (g)	Fat (g)	Fat Breakdown (g)		
											Sat	Mono	Poly
FATS and OILS—Con.													
		Fats, cooking:											
4	1363	Bacon fat	1 tbsp	14	<1	126	0	0	0	14	5.0	6.7	1.7
4	1362	Beef fat/tallow	1 c	205	0	1837	0	0	0	205	102	85.6	8.2
4	1364	Chicken fat	1 c	205	<1	1846	0	0	0	205	61.2	92.0	43.0
		Vegetable shortening:											
4	161	Cup	1 c	205	0	1812	0	0	0	205	51	91	54
4	162	Tablespoon	1 tbsp	13	0	15	0	0	0	13	3.3	5.8	3.4
		Lard:											
4	163	Cup	1 c	205	0	1849	0	0	0	205	80	93	23
4	164	Tablespoon	1 tbsp	13	0	115	0	0	0	13	5.1	5.9	1.5
		Margarine:											
		Imitation (about 40% fat), soft:											
4	165	8-oz container	8 oz	227	58	785	1	1	0	88	18	36	31
4	166	Tablespoon	1 tbsp	14	58	50	<.1	<.1	0	6	1.1	2.2	2.0
		Regular, hard (about 80% fat):											
4	167	Cup	½ c	113	16	812	1	1	0	91	18	41	29
4	168	Tablespoon	1 tbsp	14	16	100	<1	<1	0	11	2.3	5.1	3.6
4	169	Pat[19]	1 ea	5	16	36	<.1	<.1	0	4	.8	1.8	1.3
		Regular, soft (about 80% fat):											
4	170	8-oz container	8 oz	227	16	1626	2	1	0	183	31	65	79
4	171	Tablespoon	1 tbsp	14	16	100	1	<.1	0	11	2.0	4.0	4.9
		Spread (about 60% fat), hard:											
4	172	Cup	½ c	113	37	610	1	0	0	69	16	29	20
4	173	Tablespoon	1 tbsp	14	37	75	<.1	0	0	9	2.0	3.6	2.5
4	174	Pat[19]	1 ea	5	37	25	<.1	0	0	3	.7	1.3	.9
		Spread (about 60% fat), soft:											
4	175	8 oz container	8 oz	227	37	1225	1	0	0	138	29	72	31
4	176	Tablespoon	1 tbsp	14	37	75	<.1	0	0	9	1.8	4.4	1.9
		Oils:											
		Canola:											
4	1585	Cup	1 c	218	0	1927	0	0	0	218	13.1	128	65
4	1586	Tablespoon	1 tbsp	14	0	125	0	0	0	14	.8	8.2	4.1
		Corn:											
4	177	Cup	1 c	218	0	1927	0	0	0	218	28	53	128
4	178	Tablespoon	1 tbsp	14	0	125	0	0	0	14	1.8	3.4	8.2
		Olive:											
4	179	Cup	1 c	216	0	1909	0	0	0	216	29	159	18
4	180	Tablespoon	1 tbsp	14	0	125	0	0	0	14	1.9	10	1.2
		Peanut:											
4	181	Cup	1 c	216	0	1909	0	0	0	216	36	100	69
4	182	Tablespoon	1 tbsp	14	0	125	0	0	0	14	2.4	6.5	4.5
		Safflower:											
4	183	Cup	1 c	218	0	1927	0	0	0	218	20	26	162
4	184	Tablespoon	1 tbsp	14	0	125	0	0	0	14	1.3	1.7	10
		Soybean:											
4	185	Cup	1 c	218	0	1927	0	0	0	218	33	94	82
4	186	Tablespoon	1 tbsp	14	0	125	0	0	0	14	2	6	5
		Soybean/cottonseed:											
4	187	Cup	1 c	218	0	1927	0	0	0	218	39	64	105
4	188	Tablespoon	1 tbsp	14	0	125	0	0	0	14	2.5	4	7

[19] Pat is 1″ square, ⅓″ thick; about 1 tsp; 90 per lb.

(Computer code number is for West Diet Analysis program)

GRP KEY: 1 = BEV   2 = DAIRY   3 = EGGS   4 = FAT/OIL   5 = FRUIT   6 = BAKERY   7 = GRAIN   8 = FISH   9 = BEEF   10 = POULTRY
11 = SAUSAGE   12 = MIXED/FAST   13 = NUTS/SEEDS   14 = SWEETS   15 = VEG/LEG   16 = MISC   22 = SOUP/SAUCE

A

Chol (mg)	Calc (mg)	Iron (mg)	Magn (mg)	Phos (mg)	Pota (mg)	Sodi (mg)	Zinc (mg)	VT-A (RE)	Thia (mg)	Ribo (mg)	Niac (mg)	V-B6 (mg)	Fola (μg)	VT-C (mg)
84	–	–	–	–	–	140	–	<1	–	–	–	0	–	–
223	2	.41	–	27	0	0	–	<1	<.01	<.01	<.01	<.01	<1	0
174	–	–	–	–	–	–	–	350	–	–	–	0	0	0
0	0	0	0	0	0	0	.10	0	0	0	0	0	0	0
0	0	0	0	0	0	0	0	0	0	0	0	0	0	0
195	<1	0	<1	6	<1	<1	.23	0	0	0	0	0	0	0
12	<1	0	<1	<1	<1	<1	.01	0	0	0	0	0	0	0
0	40	0	3	31	57	2178[22]	.23	2254[23]	.01	.05	.03	.01	2	<1
0	3	0	<1	2	4	136[22]	.03	141[23]	<.01	<.01	<.01	<.01	<1	<1
0	34	.07	3	26	48	1066[22]	.23	1122[23]	.01	.04	.03	.01	1	<1
0	4	.01	<1	3	6	133[22]	.03	139[23]	<.01	<.01	<.01	<.01	<1	<1
0	2	.01	<1	1	2	47[22]	.01	50[23]	t	<.01	<.01	t	<1	<1
0	60	0	5	46	86	2448[22]	.46	2254[23]	.02	.07	.05	.02	2	<1
0	4	0	<1	3	5	153[22]	.03	140[23]	<.01	<.01	<.01	<.01	<1	<1
0	24	0	2	18	34	1123[22]	.17	1122[23]	<.01	.03	.02	.01	1	<1
0	3	0	<1	2	4	139[22]	.02	139[23]	<.01	<.01	<.01	<.01	<1	<1
0	1	0	<1	1	2	50[22]	.01	50[23]	t	<.01	<.01	t	<1	<1
0	47	0	4	37	68	2256[22]	.35	2254[23]	.16	.06	.04	.01	2	<1
0	3	0	<1	2	4	139[22]	.02	139[23]	.01	<.01	<.01	<.01	<1	<1
0	0	0	0	0	0	0	–	0	0	0	0	0	0	0
0	0	0	0	0	0	0	–	0	0	0	0	0	0	0
0	0	.01	0	2	0	0	.02	0	0	0	0	0	<1	0
0	0	0	0	0	0	0	.03	0	0	0	0	0	0	0
0	<1	.83	<1	3	0	0	.13	0	0	0	0	0	<1	0
0	<1	.05	<1	<1	0	0	.01	0	0	0	0	0	0	0
0	t	.06	<1	0	0	0	.02	t	0	0	0	0	<1	0
0	t	<.01	<1	0	0	0	<.01	t	0	0	0	0	0	0
0	0	0	–	0	0	0	.41	0	0	0	0	0	0	0
0	0	0	–	0	0	0	.03	0	0	0	0	0	0	0
0	<1	.05	<1	1	0	0	.4	0	0	0	0	0	<1	0
0	t	0	<1	t	0	0	.03	0	0	0	0	0	t	0
0	0	0	–	0	0	0	.4	0	0	0	0	0	<1	0
0	0	0	–	0	0	0	.03	0	0	0	0	0	0	0

[22] For salted margarine.
[23] Based on average vitamin A content of fortified margarine. Federal specifications require a minimum of 15,000 IU/lb.

(For purposes of calculations, use "0" for t, <1, <.1, <.01, etc.)

Table A–1   Food Composition

Grp	Computer Code No.	Food Description	Measure	Wt (g)	H₂O (%)	Ener (cal)	Prot (g)	Carb (g)	Dietary Fiber (g)	Fat (g)	Fat Breakdown (g) Sat	Mono	Poly
FATS and OILS—Con.													
		Oils—Con.											
		Sunflower:											
4	189	Cup	1 c	218	0	1927	0	0	0	218	23	43	143
4	190	Tablespoon	1 tbsp	14	0	125	0	0	0	14	1.4	2.7	9.2
		Salad dressings/ sandwich spreads:											
4	191	Blue cheese salad dressing	1 tbsp	15	32	75	1	1	<1	8	1.5	1.9	4.3
		French salad dressing:											
4	192	Regular	1 tbsp	16	35	85	<.1	1	<1	9	1.4	4	3.5
4	193	Low calorie	1 tbsp	16	75	24	<.1	2	<1	2	.2	.3	1
		Italian salad dressing:											
4	194	Regular	1 tbsp	14	34	80	<1	1	<1	9	1.3	3.7	3.2
4	195	Low calorie	1 tbsp	15	86	5	<.1	1	<1	1.5	.2	.3	.9
		Mayonnaise:											
4	196	Regular	1 tbsp	14	15	100	<1	<1	0	11	1.7	3.2	5.8
4	197	Imitation, low calorie	1 tbsp	15	63	35	0	2	0	3	.5	.7	1.6
4	198	Ranch style salad dressing	½ c	119	35	435	4	6	0	45	6.7	19	17
		Mayo type salad dressing:											
4	199	Regular	1 tbsp	15	40	58	<1	4	0	5	.7	1.4	2.7
4	1030	Low calorie	1 tbsp	15	63	35	<1	2	0	3	.5	.8	1.4
4	200	Tartar sauce	1 tbsp	14	34	74	<1	1	<1	8	1.2	2.6	3.9
		Thousand Island salad dressing:											
4	201	Regular	1 tbsp	16	46	60	<1	2	<1	6	1.0	1.3	3.2
4	202	Low calorie	1 tbsp	15	69	25	<1	2	<1	2	.2	.4	.9
		Salad dressings, prepared from home recipe:											
4	203	Cooked type[24]	1 tbsp	16	69	25	1	2	0	2	.5	.6	.3
4	204	Vinegar and oil	1 tbsp	16	47	70	0	0	0	8	1.5	2.4	3.9
FRUITS and FRUIT JUICES													
		Apples:											
		Fresh, raw, with peel:											
5	205	2¾″ diam (about 3 per lb with cores)	1 ea	138	84	80	<1	21	3	<1	.1	t	.1
5	206	3¼″ diam (about 2 per lb with cores)	1 ea	212	84	125	<1	32	5	1	.1	t	.2
5	207	Raw, peeled slices	1 c	110	84	65	<1	16	3	<1	.1	t	.1
5	208	Dried, sulfured	10 ea	64	32	155	1	42	8	<1	t	t	.1
5	209	Apple juice, bottled or canned	1 c	248	88	116	<1	29	<1	<1	.1	t	.1
		Applesauce:											
5	210	Sweetened	1 c	255	80	195	<1	51	4	<1	<.1	t	.1
5	211	Unsweetened	1 c	244	88	106	<1	28	4	<1	<.1	t	<.1
		Apricots:											
5	212	Raw, without pits (about 12 per lb with pits)	3 ea	106	86	51	1	12	2	<1	t	.2	.1
		Canned (fruit and liquid):											
5	213	Heavy syrup	1 c	258	78	214	1	55	4	<1	t	.1	t
5	214	Halves	3 ea	85	78	70	<1	18	1	<.1	t	t	t
5	215	Juice pack	1 c	248	87	119	2	31	4	<.1	t	t	t
5	216	Halves	3 ea	84	87	40	1	10	1	<.1	t	t	t
		Dried:											
5	217	Dried halves	10 ea	35	31	83	1	22	3	<1	t	.1	t
5	218	Cooked, unsweetened, with liquid	1 c	250	75	210	3	55	7	<1	t	.2	.1
5	219	Apricot nectar, canned	1 c	251	85	141	1	36	2	<1	t	.1	t

[24]Fatty acid values apply to product made with regular margarine.

(Computer code number is for West Diet Analysis program)

GRP KEY: 1 = BEV   2 = DAIRY   3 = EGGS   4 = FAT/OIL   5 = FRUIT   6 = BAKERY   7 = GRAIN   8 = FISH   9 = BEEF   10 = POULTRY
11 = SAUSAGE   12 = MIXED/FAST   13 = NUTS/SEEDS   14 = SWEETS   15 = VEG/LEG   16 = MISC   22 = SOUP/SAUCE

Chol (mg)	Calc (mg)	Iron (mg)	Magn (mg)	Phos (mg)	Pota (mg)	Sodi (mg)	Zinc (mg)	VT-A (RE)	Thia (mg)	Ribo (mg)	Niac (mg)	V-B6 (mg)	Fola (µg)	VT-C (mg)
0	0	0	0	0	0	0	—	0	0	0	0	0	0	0
0	0	0	0	0	0	0	—	0	0	0	0	0	0	0
3	12	.03	11	11	6	164	.04	10	<.01	.02	.01	<.01	4	t
0	2	.06	<1	1	2	188	.01	t	t	t	t	<.01	0	t
0	6	.07	—	5	3	306	.03	t	t	t	t	0	t	t
0	1	.03	<1	1	5	162	.02	3	t	t	t	.03	0	t
0	1	.03	<1	1	4	136	0	t	t	t	t	0	t	t
8	2	.07	<1	4	5	80	.02	12	<.01	<.01	<.01	<.01	<1	0
4	0	0	—	0	2	75	—	0	0	0	0	0	t	0
47	119	.31	12	100	158	522	.43	86	.04	.17	.08	.05	6	1
4	2	.03	<1	4	1	105	0	13	<.01	<.01	t	<.01	t	0
4	3	.03	—	4	1	75	.02	10	.03	t	t	—	t	—
4	3	.1	<1	4	11	182	.02	9	<.01	<.01	<.01	<.01	<1	t
4	2	.09	<1	3	18	110	.03	15	<.01	<.01	.03	<.01	6	t
2	2	.09	<1	3	17	153	0	14	<.01	<.01	.03	<.01	<1	t
9	13	.08	—	14	19	117	0	20	.01	.02	.04	0	<1	t
0	0	0	—	0	1	0	—	0	0	0	0	0	—	0
0	10	.25	6	10	159	1	.05	7	.02	.02	.11	.07	4	8
0	15	.38	9	23	244	1	.08	11	.04	.03	.16	.1	6	12
0	4	.1	3	8	124	1	.04	5	.02	.01	.1	.05	<1	4
0	9	.9	10	24	288	56[25]	.13	0	0	.1	.59	.08	1	3
0	17	.92	8	17	295	7	.07	<1	.05	.04	.25	.07	1	2[26]
0	10	1	7	18	156	8	.1	3	.03	.07	.50	.07	2	4[26]
0	7	.29	7	18	183	5	.06	7	.03	.06	.46	.06	2	3[26]
0	15	.58	8	21	313	1	.28	166	.03	.04	.64	.06	9	11
0	23	.77	18	33	361	10	.27	317	.05	.06	.97	.14	4	8
0	7	.26	6	10	119	3	.09	105	.02	.02	.32	.05	1	3
0	30	.74	24	50	409	9	.27	419	.05	.05	.85	.18	5	12
0	10	.25	8	17	139	3	.1	142	.02	.02	.29	.06	2	4
0	16	1.65	16	41	482	4	.26	253	<.01	.05	1.05	.06	4	1
0	40	4.2	42	103	1222	8	.66	591	.02	.08	2.36	.28	0	4
0	18	.96	13	23	286	8	.23	330	.02	.04	.65	.16	3	2[27]

[25] Sodium bisulfite used to preserve color; unsulfured product would contain lower levels of sodium.
[26] Value based on products without added vitamin C. Bottled apple juice with added vitamin C usually contains 41.6 mg/100 g, or 103 mg per cup. Check label for specific vitamin C values.
[27] Without added vitamin C. Products with added vitamin C contain 136 mg per cup. Check label.

(For purposes of calculations, use "0" for t, <1, <.1, <.01, etc.)

Table A–1   Food Composition

	Computer Code			Wt (g)	H₂O (%)	Ener (cal)	Prot (g)	Carb (g)	Dietary Fiber (g)	Fat (g)	Fat Breakdown (g)		
Grp	No.	Food Description	Measure								Sat	Mono	Poly
FRUITS and JUICES—Con.													
		Avocados, raw, edible part only:											
5	220	California (½ lb with refuse)	1 ea	173	73	305	4	12	17	30	4.5	19	3.5
5	221	Florida (1 lb with refuse)	1 ea	304	80	340	5	27	29	27	5	15	5
5	222	Mashed, fresh, average	1 c	230	74	370	5	17	22	35	6	22	5
		Bananas, raw, without peel:											
5	223	Whole, 8¾" long (weighs 175 g w/peel)	1 ea	114	74	105	1	27	2	1	.2	<.1	.1
5	224	Slices	1 c	150	74	138	2	35	3	1	.3	.1	.1
5	1285	Bananas, dehydrated slices	1 c	100	3	346	4	88	8	2	.7	.2	.3
5	225	Blackberries, raw	1 c	144	86	74	1	18	10	1	.3	.1	.1
		Blueberries:											
5	226	Fresh	1 c	145	85	82	1	21	4	1	<.1	.2	.3
		Frozen, sweetened:											
5	227	10-oz container	10 oz	284	77	230	1	62	7	<1	.1	.1	.2
5	228	Cup	1 c	230	77	185	1	51	5	<1	.1	.1	.2
		Cherries:											
5	229	Sour, red pitted, canned water pack	1 c	244	90	90	2	22	3	<1	.1	.1	.1
5	230	Sweet, raw, without pits	10 ea	68	81	49	1	11	1	1	.1	.2	.2
5	231	Cranberry juice cocktail[28]	1 c	253	85	145	<1[29]	36	1	<1	t	t	.1
5	232	Cranberry-apple juice	1 c	253	86	169	<1	43	1	1[30]	.2	.1	.4
5	233	Cranberry sauce, canned, strained	1 c	277	61	419	1	108	6	<1	<.1	.1	.2
		Dates:											
5	234	Whole, without pits	10 ea	83	22	228	2	61	7	<1	.2	.1	t
5	235	Chopped	1 c	178	22	489	4	131	15	1	.3	.2	.1
5	236	Figs, dried	10 ea	187	28	477	6	122	21	2	.4	.5	1.1
		Fruit cocktail, canned, fruit and liquid:											
5	237	Heavy syrup pack	1 c	255	80	185	1	48	3	<1	<.1	<.1	.1
5	238	Juice pack	1 c	248	87	115	1	29	3	<1	t	t	t
		Grapefruit:											
		Raw 3¾" diam-weight with rind is 241g for one-half											
5	239	Pink/red, half fruit, edible part	1 half	123	91	37	1	9	2	<1	t	t	<.1
5	240	White, half fruit, edible part	1 half	118	90	39	1	10	2	<1	t	t	<.1
5	241	Canned sections with liquid	1 c	254	84	152	1	39	3	<1	<.1	<.1	.1
		Grapefruit juice:											
5	242	Fresh, raw	1 c	247	90	96	1	23	1	<1	<.1	<.1	.1
		Canned:											
5	243	Unsweetened	1 c	247	90	93	1	22	1	<1	<.1	<.1	.1
5	244	Sweetened	1 c	250	87	115	1	28	1	<1	<.1	<.1	.1
		Frozen concentrate, unsweetened:											
5	245	Undiluted, 6-fl-oz can	¾ c	207	62	300	4	72	3	1	.2	.2	.3
5	246	Diluted with 3 cans water	1 c	247	89	102	1	24	1	<1	<.1	<.1	.1
		Grapes, raw, European type (adherent skin):											
5	247	Thompson seedless	10 ea	50	81	35	<1	9	1	<1	.1	t	.1
5	248	Tokay/Emperor, seeded types	10 ea	57	81	40	<1	10	1	<1	.1	t	.1
		Grape juice:											
5	249	Bottled or canned	1 c	253	84	155	1	38	1	<1	.1	t	.1
		Frozen concentrate, sweetened:											
5	250	Undiluted, 6-fl-oz can	¾ c	216	54	385	1	96	4	1	.2	<.1	.2
5	251	Diluted with 3 cans water	1 c	250	87	128	<1	32	1	<1	.1	t	.1

[28] Data here are from the newest USDA *Handbook 8–14* on beverages. These data are somewhat different from that presented in *Handbook 8–9* on fruits and fruit juices.
[29] The newest USDA *Handbook 8–14* data on beverages indicates "0" for protein.
[30] The newest USDA *Handbook 8–14* data on beverages indicates "0" for fat.

(Computer code number is for West Diet Analysis program)

GRP KEY: 1 = BEV 2 = DAIRY 3 = EGGS 4 = FAT/OIL 5 = FRUIT 6 = BAKERY 7 = GRAIN 8 = FISH 9 = BEEF 10 = POULTRY
11 = SAUSAGE 12 = MIXED/FAST 13 = NUTS/SEEDS 14 = SWEETS 15 = VEG/LEG 16 = MISC 22 = SOUP/SAUCE

A

Chol (mg)	Calc (mg)	Iron (mg)	Magn (mg)	Phos (mg)	Pota (mg)	Sodi (mg)	Zinc (mg)	VT-A (RE)	Thia (mg)	Ribo (mg)	Niac (mg)	V-B6 (mg)	Fola (µg)	VT-C (mg)
0	19	2.04	70	73	1097	21	.73	106	.19	.21	3.32	.48	113	14
0	33	1.6	104	119	1484	14	1.28	186	.33	.37	5.84	.85	162	24
0	25	2.3	90	95	1378	24	.97	141	.25	.28	4.42	.64	142	18
0	7	.35	32	22	451	1	.19	9	.05	.11	.62	.66	24	10
0	9	.46	43	29	593	1	.25	12	.07	.15	.81	.87	31	14
0	22	1.15	108	74	1491	3	.61	31	.18	.24	2.80	.54	40	7
0	46	.8	29	30	282	0	.39	24	.04	.06	.58	.08	49	30
0	9	.24	7	15	129	9	.16	15	.07	.07	.7	.05	9	20
0	16	1.11	7	20	169	4	.14	12	.06	.15	.72	.17	19	3
0	13	.9	6	16	138	3	.14	10	.05	.12	.58	.14	16	2
0	27	3.34	15	25	240	17	.17	184	.04	.1	.43	.11	20	5
0	10	.3	8	13	152	0	.04	15	.03	.04	.3	.02	3	5
0	8	.38	5	5	45	5	.18	1	.02	.02	.09	.05	<1	90[31]
0	18	.15	5	7	68	5	.1	<1	.01	.05	.15	.06	<1	81[31]
0	11	.61	8	17	72	80	.09	6	.04	.06	.28	.05	3	6
0	27	1	29	33	541	2	.24	4	.08	.08	1.83	.16	14	0
0	58	2.14	63	70	1161	5	.52	9	.16	.18	3.92	.34	29	0
0	269	4.18	111	128	1331	21	.94	25	.13	.17	1.3	.42	16	1
0	16	.73	14	28	224	15	.21	52	.05	.05	.95	.11	1	5
0	20	.53	17	34	235	10	.21	76	.03	.04	0	.13	2	7
0	13	.15	10	11	158	0	.09	32[32]	.04	.03	.24	.05	15	47
0	14	.07	11	9	175	0	.08	1	.04	.02	.32	.05	12	39
0	36	1.02	25	25	328	4	.21	0	.1	.05	.62	.05	22	54
0	22	.49	30	37	400	2	.13	2[33]	.1	.05	.49	.11	52	94
0	17	.49	24	27	378	2	.22	2	.1	.05	.57	.05	26	72
0	20	.9	24	28	405	5	.15	2	.1	.06	.8	.05	26	67
0	56	1.02	78	101	1002	6	.38	6	.3	.16	1.6	.32	26	248
0	20	.34	26	34	337	2	.12	2	.1	.05	.54	.11	52	83
0	5	.13	3	7	92	1	.03	4	.05	.03	.15	.06	4	5
0	6	.15	4	8	105	1	.03	4	.05	.03	.17	.06	4	6
0	22	.61	24	27	334	8	.13	2	.07	.09	.66	.16	7	<1
0	28	.78	32	32	160	15	.28	6	.11	.2	.93	.32	9	179[34]
0	10	.26	11	11	53	5	.10	2	.04	.07	.31	.11	4	60[34]

[31] Nutrient added.
[32] Vitamin A in Texas red grapefruit would be 74 RE.
[33] This is Vitamin A for white grapefruit juice; pink or red grapefruit juice = 109 RE per cup.
[34] With added Vitamin C (ascorbic acid).

(For purposes of calculations, use "0" for t, <1, <.1, <.01, etc.)

Table A–1   Food Composition

Grp	Computer Code No.	Food Description	Measure	Wt (g)	H₂O (%)	Ener (cal)	Prot (g)	Carb (g)	Fiber (g)	(g)	Fat Breakdown (g) Sat	Mono	Poly
		FRUITS and FRUIT JUICES—Con.											
5	252	Kiwi fruit, raw, peeled (88g with peel)	1 ea	76	83	46	1	11	3	<1	t	.2	.2
5	253	Lemons, raw, without peel and seeds (about 4 per lb whole)	1 ea	58	89	17	1	5	1	<1	t	t	.1
		Lemon juice:											
		Fresh:											
5	254	Cup	1 c	244	91	60	1	21	1	t	t	t	t
5	255	Tablespoon	1 tbsp	15	91	4	<.1	1	<1	t	t	t	t
		Canned or bottled, unsweetened:											
5	256	Cup	1 c	244	92	52	1	16	1	<1	.1	<.1	.2
5	257	Tablespoon	1 tbsp	15	92	3	<1	1	<1	<.1	t	t	t
		Frozen, single strength, unsweetened:											
5	258	Cup	1 c	244	92	54	1	16	1	<1	.1	<.1	.2
5	259	Tablespoon	1 tbsp	15	92	3	<1	1	<1	<.1	t	t	t
		Lime juice:											
		Fresh:											
5	260	Cup	1 c	246	90	65	1	22	1	<1	<.1	<.1	.1
5	261	Tablespoon	1 tbsp	15	90	4	<1	1	<1	<.1	t	t	t
5	262	Canned or bottled, unsweetened	1 c	246	92	50	1	16	1	1	.1	.1	.2
5	263	Mangos, raw, edible part (weighs 300 g with skin and seeds)	1 ea	207	82	135	1	35	7	1	.1	.2	.1
		Melons, raw, without rind and cavity contents:											
5	264	Cantaloupe, 5″ diam (2⅓ lb whole with refuse), orange flesh	½ ea	267	90	94	2	22	3	1	.1	.1	.2
5	265	Honeydew, 6½″ diam (5¼ lb whole with refuse), slice = 1/10 melon	1 slice	129	90	45	1	12	1	<1	t	t	<.1
5	266	Nectarines, raw, without pits, 2½″ diam	1 ea	136	86	67	1	16	3	1	.1	.2	.3
		Oranges, raw:											
5	267	Whole without peel and seeds, 2⅝″ dm. (weighs 180 g with peel and seeds)	1 ea	131	87	60	1	15	3	<1	t	<.1	<.1
5	268	Sections, without membranes	1 c	180	87	85	2	21	4	<1	<.1	<.1	<.1
		Orange juice:											
5	269	Fresh, all varieties	1 c	248	88	111	2	26	1	<1	.1	.1	.1
5	270	Canned, unsweetened	1 c	249	89	105	1	25	<1	<1	<.1	.1	.1
5	271	Chilled	1 c	249	88	110	2	25	<1	1	.1	.1	.2
		Frozen concentrate:											
5	272	Undiluted (6-oz can)	¾ c	213	58	339	5	81	2	<1	.1	.1	.1
5	273	Diluted with 3 parts water by volume	1 c	249	88	110	2	27	<1	<1	t	<.1	<.1
5	1345	Orange juice, from dry crystals	1 c	248	89	114	2	27	0	<1	.1	.1	.1
5	274	Orange and grapefruit juice, canned	1 c	247	89	105	1	25	<1	<1	<.1	<.1	.1
		Papayas, raw:											
5	275	½″ slices	1 c	140	89	60	1	14	2	<1	.1	.1	<.1
5	276	Whole fruit, 3½″ diam by 5⅛″, without seeds and skin (1 lb with refuse)	1 ea	304	89	117	2	30	5	<1	.1	.1	.1
5	1031	Papaya nectar, canned	1 c	250	85	142	<1	36	2	<1	.1	.1	.1
		Peaches:											
5	277	Raw, whole, 2½″ diam, peeled, pitted (about 4 per lb whole)	1 ea	87	88	37	1	10	2	<1	t	<.1	<.1

(Computer code number is for West Diet Analysis program)

GRP KEY: 1 = BEV   2 = DAIRY   3 = EGGS   4 = FAT/OIL   5 = FRUIT   6 = BAKERY   7 = GRAIN   8 = FISH   9 = BEEF   10 = POULTRY
11 = SAUSAGE   12 = MIXED/FAST   13 = NUTS/SEEDS   14 = SWEETS   15 = VEG/LEG   16 = MISC   22 = SOUP/SAUCE

A

Chol (mg)	Calc (mg)	Iron (mg)	Magn (mg)	Phos (mg)	Pota (mg)	Sodi (mg)	Zinc (mg)	VT-A (RE)	Thia (mg)	Ribo (mg)	Niac (mg)	V-B6 (mg)	Fola (µg)	VT-C (mg)
0	20	.3	23	30	252	4	.08[35]	13	.02	.04	.4	.05[35]	17[35]	75
0	15	.35	2	9	80	1	.06	2	.02	.01	.06	.05	7	31
0	18	.08	16	14	303	2	.12	5	.07	.02	.24	.12	32	112
0	1	<.01	1	1	19	<1	.01	<1	<.01	<.01	.02	.01	2	7
0	26	.31	22	21	248	50[36]	.15	4	.10	.02	.48	.11	25	61
0	2	.02	1	1	15	3[36]	.01	<1	.01	<.01	.03	.01	2	4
0	19	.30	20	20	218	4	.12	4	.14	.03	.33	.15	23	77
0	1	.02	1	1	14	<1	.01	<1	.01	<.01	.02	.01	1	5
0	22	.08	14	18	268	2	.15	3	.05	.03	.25	.11	21	72
0	1	<.01	1	1	17	<1	.01	<1	<.01	<.01	.02	.08	1	5
0	30	.6	16	25	185	39[36]	.15	4	.08	.01	.4	.07	20	16
0	21	2.6	18	22	323	4	.07	806	.12	.12	1.21	.28	39	57
0	29	.56	19	45	825	24	.43	861	.1	.06	1.53	.31	80	113
0	8	.09	9	13	350	13	.11	5	.1	.02	.77	.08	39	32
0	6	.21	11	22	288	0	.12	100	.02	.06	1.35	.03	5	7
0	52	.14	13	18	237	<1	.09	27	.11	.05	.37	.08	40	70
0	72	.19	18	25	326	<1	.4	37	.16	.07	.51	.11	83	96
0	27	.50	27	42	496	2	.12	50	.22	.07	.99	.1	109	124
0	20	1.1	27	35	436	5	.17	44	.15	.04	.4	.1	15	86
0	25	.42	28	27	473	2	.11	19[37]	.28	.05	.7	.13	45[37]	82[37]
0	68	.75	73	121	1436	6	.38	59	.6	.14	1.53	.33	331	294
0	22	.27	24	40	474	2	.13	19	.2	.04	.5	.11	109	97
0	40	.02	5	31	50	1	—	.50	.20	.07	1.00	0	0	80
0	20	1.1	24	35	390	7	.18	29	.14	.07	.83	.06	20	72
0	33	.3	14	12	247	9	.10	282	.04	.05	.47	.03	26	92
0	72	.3	31	16	780	8	.22	612	.08	.10	1.03	.06	48	188
0	24	.86	8	1	78	14	.38	28	.02	.01	.38	.02	5	8
0	4	.1	6	10	171	0	.12	47	.02	.04	.86	.02	3	6

[35] Data are estimated from other fruit data.
[36] Sodium benzoate and sodium bisulfite added as preservatives.
[37] Values for juice from California oranges indicate the following values for 1 c: 36 RE of vitamin A, 72µg of folacin, and 106 mg of vitamin C.

(For purposes of calculations, use "0" for t, <1, <.1, <.01, etc.)

Table A–1   Food Composition

	Computer Code								Dietary		Fat Breakdown (g)		
Grp	No.	Food Description	Measure	Wt (g)	H₂O (%)	Ener (cal)	Prot (g)	Carb (g)	Fiber (g)	Fat (g)	Sat	Mono	Poly

Grp	No.	Food Description	Measure	Wt (g)	H_2O (%)	Ener (cal)	Prot (g)	Carb (g)	Dietary Fiber (g)	Fat (g)	Sat	Mono	Poly
		FRUITS and FRUIT JUICES—Con.											
		Peaches—Con.											
5	278	Raw, sliced	1 c	170	88	73	1	19	3	<1	t	.1	.1
		Canned, fruit and liquid:											
		Heavy syrup pack:											
5	279	Cup	1 c	256	79	190	1	51	3	<1	<.1	.1	.1
5	280	Half	1 ea	81	79	60	<1	16	1	<1	t	<.1	<.1
		Juice pack:											
5	281	Cup	1 c	248	88	109	2	29	3	<1	t	<.1	<.1
5	282	Half	1 ea	77	88	34	<1	9	1	<1	t	t	t
		Dried:											
5	283	Uncooked	10 ea	130	32	311	5	80	11	1	.1	.4	.5
5	284	Cooked, fruit and liquid	1 c	258	78	200	3	51	4	1	.1	.2	.3
		Frozen, sliced, sweetened:											
5	285	10-oz package	1 ea	284	75	267	2	68	6	<1	<.1	.1	.2
5	286	Cup, thawed measure	1 c	250	75	235	2	60	4	<1	<.1	.1	.2
5	1032	Peach nectar, canned	1 c	249	86	134	1	35	1	<1	t	<.1	<.1
		Pears:											
		Fresh, with skin, cored:											
5	287	Bartlett, 2½″ diam (about 2½ per lb)	1 ea	166	84	98	1	25	5[38]	1	<.1	.1	.2
5	288	Bosc, 2½″ diam (about 3 per lb)	1 ea	141	84	85	1	21	4[38]	1	<.1	.1	.1
5	289	D'Anjou, 3″ diam (about 2 per lb)	1 ea	200	84	120	1	30	6[38]	1	<.1	.2	.2
		Canned, fruit and liquid:											
		Heavy syrup pack:											
5	290	Cup	1 c	255	80	188	1	49	4[38]	<1	t	.1	.1
5	291	Half	1 ea	79	80	59	<1	15	1[38]	<1	t	t	t
		Juice pack:											
5	292	Cup	1 c	248	86	123	1	32	4[38]	<1	t	<.1	<.1
5	293	Half	1 ea	77	86	38	<1	10	1[38]	<1	t	t	t
5	294	Dried halves	10 ea	175	27	459	3	122	19	1	.1	.2	.3
5	1033	Pear nectar, canned	1 c	250	84	149	<1	39	2	<1	t	t	t
		Pineapple:											
5	295	Fresh chunks, diced	1 c	155	86	76	1	19	2	1	<.1	<.1	.2
		Canned, fruit and liquid:											
		Heavy syrup pack:											
5	296	Crushed, chunks, tidbits	1 c	255	79	199	1	52	2	<1	t	<.1	.1
5	297	Slices	1 ea	58	79	45	<1	12	1	<.1	t	t	<.1
		Juice Pack:											
5	298	Crushed, chunks, tidbits	1 c	250	84	150	1	39	2	<1	t	<.1	.1
5	299	Slices	1 ea	58	84	35	<1	9	1	<.1	t	t	t
5	300	Pineapple juice, canned, unsweetened	1 c	250	86	140	1	34	1	<1	t	t	.1
		Plantains, without peel:											
5	301	Raw slices (one whole plantain weighs 179 g without peel)	1 c	148	65	181	2	47	7[39]	1	.2	.1	.1
5	302	Cooked, boiled, sliced	1 c	154	67	179	1	48	7	<1	.1	<.1	.1
		Plums, canned:											
		Fresh:											
5	303	Medium 2⅛″ diam	1 ea	66	85	36	1	9	1	<1	<.1	.3	.1
5	304	Small, 1½″ diam	1 ea	28	85	15	<1	4	1	<1	t	.1	<.1

[38]Dietary fiber data vary 2.4 to 3.4 g/100 g for fresh pears; 1.6 to 2.6 g/100 g for canned pears.
[39]Dietary fiber value partially derived from data for bananas.

(Computer code number is for West Diet Analysis program)

GRP KEY: 1 = BEV   2 = DAIRY   3 = EGGS   4 = FAT/OIL   5 = FRUIT   6 = BAKERY   7 = GRAIN   8 = FISH   9 = BEEF   10 = POULTRY
11 = SAUSAGE   12 = MIXED/FAST   13 = NUTS/SEEDS   14 = SWEETS   15 = VEG/LEG   16 = MISC   22 = SOUP/SAUCE

A

Chol (mg)	Calc (mg)	Iron (mg)	Magn (mg)	Phos (mg)	Pota (mg)	Sodi (mg)	Zinc (mg)	VT-A (RE)	Thia (mg)	Ribo (mg)	Niac (mg)	V-B6 (mg)	Fola (µg)	VT-C (mg)
0	9	.19	11	20	335	1	.18	91	.03	.07	1.68	.03	6	11
0	8	.69	13	29	235	16	.22	85	.03	.06	1.57	.05	8	7
0	3	.22	4	9	75	5	.07	27	.01	.02	.5	.01	3	2
0	15	.72	18	43	317	11	.26	94	.02	.04	1.44	.05	8	9
0	5	.21	6	13	98	3	.09	29	.01	.01	.45	.02	3	3
0	37	5.28	54	155	1295	9	.74	281	<.01	.28	5.69	.09	6	6
0	23	3.37	35	99	825	6	.46	51	.01	.05	3.92	.1	<1	10
0	9	1.05	14	31	369	17	.14	81	.04	.10	1.9	.05	9	268[40]
0	8	.93	12	28	325	16	.13	71	.03	.09	1.63	.04	8	236[40]
0	13	.47	11	16	101	10	.20	64	.01	.04	.72	.03	2	13
0	19	.42	9	18	208	1	.20	3	.03	.07	.17	.03	12	7
0	16	.40	8	16	176	<1	.17	3	.03	.06	.1	.03	10	6
0	22	.50	11	22	250	<1	.24	4	.04	.08	.2	.04	14	8
0	13	.56	11	18	166	13	.21	1	.03	.06	.62	.04	3	3
0	4	.17	3	5	51	4	.06	<1	.01	.02	.19	.01	1	1
0	22	.71	17	29	238	10	.22	1	.03	.03	.5	.04	5	4
0	7	.22	5	9	74	3	.07	<1	.01	.01	.15	.01	2	1
0	59	3.68	58	103	932	10	.68	1	.01	.25	2.4	.01	21	12
0	11	.65	6	7	33	8	.16	<1	<.01	.03	.32	.03	2	3
0	11	.57	21	11	175	2	.12	4	.14	.06	.65	.14	16	24
0	36	.97	40	18	265	3	.31	4	.23	.06	.73	.19	12	19
0	8	.22	9	4	60	1	.70	1	.05	.02	.17	.04	3	4
0	35	.70	35	15	305	3	.25	10	.24	.05	.71	.19	12	24
0	8	.16	8	4	71	1	.06	2	.06	.02	.17	.04	3	6
0	43	.65	34	20	335	3	.28	1	.14	.06	.64	.24	58	27[41]
0	4	.89	55	50	739	6	.27	167[42]	.08	.08	1.02	.44	33	27
0	3	.89	49	43	716	8	.21	140	.07	.08	1.16	.37	40	17
0	3	.07	4	7	114	<1	.07	21	.03	.06	.33	.05	3	6
0	1	.03	2	3	48	<1	.03	9	.01	.03	.14	.02	1	3

[40] With added vitamin C (ascorbic acid).
[41] If vitamin C is added, it contains 96 mg per cup.
[42] Vitamin A values range from 1.5 RE for white-fleshed varieties to 178 RE for yellow-fleshed varieties.

(For purposes of calculations, use "0" for t, <1, <.1, <.01, etc.)

Table A–1   Food Composition

	Computer Code									Dietary		Fat Breakdown (g)		
Grp	No.	Food Description	Measure	Wt (g)	H₂O (%)	Ener (cal)	Prot (g)	Carb (g)	Fiber (g)	Fat (g)	Sat	Mono	Poly

				Wt (g)	H$_2$O (%)	Ener (cal)	Prot (g)	Carb (g)	Dietary Fiber (g)	Fat (g)	Sat	Mono	Poly
FRUITS—Con.													
		Plums—Con.											
		Canned, purple, with liquid:											
		Heavy Syrup pack:											
5	305	Cup	1 c	258	76	230	1	60	4	<1	t	.2	.1
5	306	Plums	3 ea	110	76	98	<1	25	2	<1	t	.1	t
		Juice pack:											
5	307	Cup	1 c	252	84	146	1	38	4	<.1	t	<.1	t
5	308	Plums	3 ea	95	84	55	<1	14	2	<.1	t	t	t
		Prunes, dried, pitted:											
5	309	Uncooked (10 prunes weigh 97 g with pits, 84 g without pits.)	10 ea	84	32	201	2	53	8[43]	<1	<.1	.3	.1
5	310	Cooked, unsweetened, fruit and liquid (250 g with pits)	1 c	212	70	227	2	60	9	<1	<.1	.3	.1
5	311	Prune juice, bottled or canned	1 c	256	81	181	2	45	3	<.1	t	<.1	t
		Raisins, seedless:											
5	312	Cup, not pressed down	1 c	145	15	435	5	115	9	1	.2	<.1	.2
5	313	One packet, ½ oz	½ oz	14	15	41	<1	11	1	<.1	t	t	t
		Raspberries:											
5	314	Fresh	1 c	123	87	60	1	14	8	1	t	.1	.4
		Frozen, sweetened:											
5	315	10-oz container	10 oz	284	73	293	2	74	15	<1	t	<.1	.3
5	316	Cup, thawed measure	1 c	250	73	255	2	65	12	<1	t	<.1	.2
5	317	Rhubarb, cooked, added sugar	1 c	240	68	279	1	75	5	<1	t	t	.1
		Strawberries:											
5	318	Fresh, whole, capped	1 c	149	92	45	1	11	4	1	<.1	.1	.3
		Frozen, sliced, sweetened:											
5	319	10-oz container	10 oz	284	73	273	2	74	6	<1	t	.1	.2
5	320	Cup, thawed measure	1 c	255	73	245	1	66	8	<1	t	.1	.2
		Tangerines, without peel and seeds:											
5	321	Fresh (2⅜″ whole) 116g with refuse	1 ea	84	88	37	1	9	2	<1	t	<.1	<.1
5	322	Canned, light syrup, fruit and liquid	1 c	252	83	154	1	41	4	<1	<.1	<.1	.1
5	323	Tangerine juice, canned, sweetened	1 c	249	87	125	1	30	1	<1	<.1	<.1	.1
		Watermelon, raw, without rind and seeds:											
5	324	Piece, 1″ thick by 10″ diam (weighs 2 lb with refuse or 926g)	1 pce	482	92	152	3	35	2	2	.3	.2	1
5	325	Diced	1 c	160	92	50	1	12	1	1	.1	.1	.4
BAKED GOODS:													
BREADS, CAKES, COOKIES, CRACKERS, PIES, PANCAKES, TORTILLAS													
6	326	Bagels, plain, enriched, 3½″ diam	1 ea	68	32	180	7	35	1	1	.2	.3	.4
		Biscuits:											
6	327	From home recipe	1 ea	28	28	100	2	13	1	5	1.2	2	1.3
6	328	From mix	1 ea	28	29	94	2	14	1	3	.8	1.4	.9
6	329	From refrigerated dough	1 ea	20	30	65	1	10	<1	2	.6	.9	.6
6	330	Bread crumbs, dry grated (see 364, 365 for soft crumbs)	1 c	100	7	390	13	73	4	5	1.5	1.6	1
		Breads:											
6	331	Boston brown bread, canned, 3¼″ slice	1 pce	45	45	95	2	21	2	1	.26	.13	.14
		Cracked wheat bread (¼ cracked-wheat flour, ¾ enr wheat flour):											
6	332	1-lb loaf	1 ea	454	35	1190	42	227	23	16	3.1	4.3	5.7
6	333	Slice (18 per loaf)	1 pce	25	35	65	2	13	1	1	.2	.2	.3
6	334	Slice, toasted	1 pce	21	26	65	2	13	1	1	.2	.2	.3

[43]Dietary fiber data can vary between 8 and 13 g for 10 prunes.

(Computer code number is for West Diet Analysis program)

GRP KEY: 1 = BEV   2 = DAIRY   3 = EGGS   4 = FAT/OIL   5 = FRUIT   6 = BAKERY   7 = GRAIN   8 = FISH   9 = BEEF   10 = POULTRY
11 = SAUSAGE   12 = MIXED/FAST   13 = NUTS/SEEDS   14 = SWEETS   15 = VEG/LEG   16 = MISC   22 = SOUP/SAUCE

Chol (mg)	Calc (mg)	Iron (mg)	Magn (mg)	Phos (mg)	Pota (mg)	Sodi (mg)	Zinc (mg)	VT-A (RE)	Thia (mg)	Ribo (mg)	Niac (mg)	V-B6 (mg)	Fola (μg)	VT-C (mg)
0	23	2.17	13	34	235	49	.18	67	.04	.1	.75	.07	7	1
0	10	.92	6	14	100	21	.08	29	.02	.04	.32	.03	3	<1
0	25	.86	20	38	388	3	.28	254	.06	.15	1.19	.1	8	7
0	10	.32	8	15	147	1	.11	96	.02	.06	.45	.04	3	3
0	43	2.08	38	66	626	3	.45	167	.07	.14	1.65	.22	3	3
0	49	2.35	43	74	708	4	.51	65	.05	.21	1.53	.46	<1	6
0	31	3.02	36	64	707	10	.54	1	.04	.18	2.01	.56	1	11
0	71	3.02	48	140	1089	17	.46	1	.23	.13	1.19	.36	5	5
0	7	.29	5	14	105	2	.05	<1	.02	.01	.12	.04	1	<1
0	27	.7	22	15	187	0	.57	16	.04	.11	1.11	.07	32	31
0	43	1.85	37	48	324	3	.51	17	.05	.13	.65	.1	74	47
0	38	1.62	32	43	285	3	.45	15	.05	.11	1.5	.09	65	41
0	348	.5	30	19	230	2	.19	17	.04	.06	.48	.05	13	8
0	21	.57	16	28	247	2	.19	4	.03	.1	.34	.09	28	85
0	31	1.7	20	37	278	9	.17	7	.05	.14	1.1	.09	47	118
0	28	1.5	18	33	250	8	.15	6	.04	.13	1.02	.08	42	106
0	12	.08	10	8	132	1	.38	77	.09	.02	.13	.06	17	26
0	18	.93	19	25	197	15	.60	212	.13	.11	1.1	.11	34	50
0	45	.5	20	35	443	2	.08	105	.15	.05	.25	.08	8	55
0	38	.82	52	41	560	10	.34	176	.39	.1	.96	.69	10	47
0	13	.27	17	14	186	3	.11	59	.13	.03	.32	.23	3	15
0	20	2.1	15	61	65	300	.61	0	.26	.20	2.4	.03	16	0
t	48	.7	6	36	32	195	.15	3	.08	.08	.8	.01	2	t
t	59	.58	7	129	57	265	.18	4	.12	.11	.85	.01	2	t
1	4	.47	4	78	18	249	.09	0	.08	.05	.67	.01	1	0
5	122	4.1	31	141	152	736	.50	0	.35	.35	4.8	.02	28	0
3	41	.90	40	72	131	113	.35	0	.06	.04	.7	.06	8	0
0	295	12.1	218	581	608	1966	6.36	0	1.73	1.73	15.3	.42	218	t
0	16	.67	12	32	34	106	.35	0	.1	.1	.84	.02	12	t
0	16	.67	12	32	34	106	.35	0	.07	.1	.84	.02	9	t

(For purposes of calculations, use "0" for t, <1, <.1, <.01, etc.)

Table A–1   Food Composition

	Computer Code								Dietary		Fat Breakdown (g)		
Grp	No.	Food Description	Measure	Wt (g)	H₂O (%)	Ener (cal)	Prot (g)	Carb (g)	Fiber (g)	Fat (g)	Sat	Mono	Poly
		BAKED GOODS—Con.											
		Breads—Con.											
		French/Vienna bread, enriched:											
6	335	1-lb loaf	1 ea	454	34	1270	43	230	8	18	4	6	6
6	336	French, slice, 5 × 2½ × 1"	1 pce	35	34	100	3	18	1	1	.3	.4	.5
6	337	Vienna, slice 4¾ × 4 × ½"	1 pce	25	34	70	2	13	1	1	.2	.3	.3
		French toast: see Mixed Dishes, and Fast Foods, code # 691											
		Italian bread, enriched:											
6	338	1-lb loaf	1 ea	454	32	1255	41	256	5	4	.6	.3	1.6
6	339	Slice, 4½ × 3¼ × ¾"	1 pce	30	32	83	3	17	<1	<1	<.1	t	.1
		Mixed grain bread, enriched:											
6	340	1-lb loaf	1 ea	454	37	1165	45	212	18	17	3	4	7
6	341	Slice (18 per loaf)	1 pce	25	37	65	2	12	2	1	.2	.2	.4
6	342	Slice, toasted	1 pce	23	27	65	2	12	2	1	.2	.2	.4
		Oatmeal bread, enriched:											
6	343	1-lb loaf	1 ea	454	37	1145	38	212	16	20	4	7	8
6	344	Slice (18 per loaf)	1 pce	25	37	65	2	12	1	1	.2	.4	.5
6	345	Slice, toasted	1 pce	23	30	65	2	12	1	1	.2	.4	.5
6	346	Pita pocket bread, enr, 6½" round	1 ea	60	31	165	6	33	1	1	.1	.1	.4
		Pumpernickel bread (⅔ rye flour, ⅓ enr. wheat flour):											
6	347	1-lb loaf	1 ea	454	37	1160	42	218	19	16	3	4	6
6	348	Slice, 5 × 4 × ⅜"	1 pce	32	37	80	3	15	2	1	.2	.3	.5
6	349	Slice, toasted	1 pce	29	28	80	3	15	1	1	.2	.3	.5
		Raisin bread, enriched:											
6	350	1-lb loaf	1 ea	454	33	1260	37	239	12	18	4	7	7
6	351	Slice (18 per loaf)	1 pce	25	33	68	2	13	1	1	.2	.4	.4
6	352	Slice, toasted	1 pce	21	24	68	2	13	1	1	.2	.4	.4
		Rye bread, light (⅓ rye flour, ⅔ enr. wheat flour):											
6	353	1-lb loaf	1 ea	454	37	1190	38	218	30	17	3.3	5.2	5.5
6	354	Slice, 4¾ × 3¾ × ⁷⁄₁₆"	1 pce	25	37	65	2	12	2	1	.2	.3	.3
6	355	Slice, toasted	1 pce	22	28	65	2	12	2	1	.2	.3	.3
		Wheat bread (blend of enr. wheat flour and whole-wheat flour):[44]											
6	356	1-lb loaf	1 ea	454	37	1160	43	213	25	19	3.9	7.3	4.5
6	357	Slice (18 per loaf)	1 pce	25	37	65	2	12	1	1	.2	.4	.3
6	358	Slice, toasted	1 pce	23	28	65	2	12	1	1	.2	.4	.3
		White bread, enriched:											
6	359	1-lb loaf	1 ea	454	37	1210	38	222	12	18	5.6	6.5	4.2
6	360	Slice (18 per loaf)	1 pce	25	37	65	2	12	<1	1	.3	.4	.2
6	361	Slice, toasted	1 pce	22	28	65	2	12	<1	1	.3	.4	.2
6	362	Slice (22 per loaf)	1 pce	20	37	55	2	10	<1	1	.2	.3	.2
6	363	Slice, toasted	1 pce	17	28	55	2	10	<1	1	.2	.3	.2
		White bread cubes, crumbs:											
6	364	Cubes, soft	1 c	30	37	80	2	15	1	1	.4	.4	.3
6	365	Crumbs, soft	1 c	45	37	120	4	22	1	2	.6	.6	.4
		Whole-wheat bread:											
6	366	1-lb loaf	1 ea	454	38	1110	44	206	51	20	6	7	5
6	367	Slice (16 per loaf)	1 pce	28	38	70	3	13	2	1	.4	.4	.3
6	368	Slice, toasted	1 pce	25	29	70	3	13	2	1	.4	.4	.3

[44]A blend of white and whole-wheat flour—no official ratio specified.

(Computer code number is for West Diet Analysis program)

GRP KEY: 1 = BEV   2 = DAIRY   3 = EGGS   4 = FAT/OIL   5 = FRUIT   6 = BAKERY   7 = GRAIN   8 = FISH   9 = BEEF   10 = POULTRY
11 = SAUSAGE   12 = MIXED/FAST   13 = NUTS/SEEDS   14 = SWEETS   15 = VEG/LEG   16 = MISC   22 = SOUP/SAUCE

Chol (mg)	Calc (mg)	Iron (mg)	Magn (mg)	Phos (mg)	Pota (mg)	Sodi (mg)	Zinc (mg)	VT-A (RE)	Thia (mg)	Ribo (mg)	Niac (mg)	V-B6 (mg)	Fola (µg)	VT-C (mg)
0	499	14	91	386	409	2633	2.9	0	2.09	1.59	18.2	.24	168	t
0	39	1.08	7	30	32	203	.22	0	.16	.12	1.4	.02	13	t
0	28	.77	5	21	23	145	.16	0	.12	.09	1	.01	9	t
0	77	12.7	106	350	336	2656	3.1	0	1.86	1.06	15.1	.24	160	0
0	5	.8	7	23	22	176	.21	0	.12	.07	1	.02	11	0
0	472	14.8	222	962	990	1870	5.45	t	1.77	1.73	18.9	.47	295	0
0	27	.8	12	55	56	106	.3	t	.1	.1	1.1	.03	16	t
0	27	.8	12	55	56	106	.3	t	.08	.1	1.1	.02	12	t
0	267	12	154	563	707	2231	4.45	0	2.09	1.2	15.4	.07	15	0
0	15	.7	9	31	39	124	.25	0	.12	.07	.85	<.01	1	0
0	15	.7	9	31	39	124	.25	0	.09	.07	.85	<.01	1	0
0	49	1.45	16	60	71	339	.50	0	.27	.13	2.32	.01	12	0
0	322	12.4	309	990	1966	2461	5.18	0	1.54	2.36	15	.72	222	0
0	23	.88	22	71	141	177	.4	0	.11	.17	1.06	.05	16	0
0	23	.88	22	71	141	177	.4	0	.09	.17	1.06	.05	12	0
0	463	14.1	114	395	1058	1657	2.81	1	1.5	2.81	18.6	.15	159	t
0	25	.78	6	22	59	92	.16	t	.08	.16	1.02	.01	9	t
0	25	.80	6	22	59	92	.16	t	.06	.16	1.02	.01	8	t
0	363	12.3	109	658	926	3164	5.77	0	1.86	1.45	15	.43	177	0
0	20	.68	8	36	51	175	.38	0	.1	.08	.83	.02	10	0
0	20	.68	6	36	51	175	.38	0	.08	.08	.83	.02	8	0
0	572	15.8	209	835	627	2447	4.77	t	2.09	1.45	20.5	.50	204	t
0	32	.87	12	47	35	135	.26	t	.12	.08	1.13	.03	11	t
0	32	.87	12	47	35	135	.26	t	.10	.08	1.20	.02	8	t
0	572	12.9	95	490	508	2334	2.81	t	2.13	1.41	17.0	.15	159	t
0	32	.71	5	27	28	129	.16	t	.12	.08	.94	.01	9	t
0	32	.71	5	27	28	129	.16	t	.09	.08	.94	.01	9	t
0	25	.57	4	22	22	103	.12	t	.09	.06	.75	.01	7	t
0	25	.6	4	21	22	103	.12	t	.07	.06	.75	.01	7	t
0	38	.85	6	32	34	154	.19	t	.14	.09	1.13	.01	11	t
0	57	1.28	9	49	50	231	.28	t	.21	.14	1.69	.02	16	t
0	327	15.5	422	1180	799	2887	7.63	t	1.59	.95	17.4	.85	250	t
0	20	.97	26	74	50	180	.50	t	.10	.06	1.09	.05	16	t
0	20	.97	26	74	50	180	.50	t	.08	.06	1.08	.05	12	t

(For purposes of calculations, use "0" for t, <1, <.1, <.01, etc.)

A

Table A–1   Food Composition

Grp	Computer Code No.	Food Description	Measure	Wt (g)	H$_2$O (%)	Ener (cal)	Prot (g)	Carb (g)	Dietary Fiber (g)	Fat (g)	Fat Breakdown (g) Sat	Mono	Poly
		BAKED GOODS—Con.											
		Bread stuffing, prepared from mix:											
6	369	Dry type	1 c	140	33	500	9	50	4	31	6	13	10
6	370	Moist type, with egg	1 c	203	61	420	9	40	4	26	5	11	8
		Cakes, prepared from mixes:[45]											
		Angel food cake:											
6	371	Whole cake, 9 ¾″ diam tube	1 ea	635	38	1510	38	342	3	2	.4	.2	1
6	372	Piece, 1/12 of cake	1 pce	53	38	125	3	29	<1	<1	t	t	.1
6	373	Boston cream pie, 1/8 of cake	1 pce	120	35	260	3	44	1	8	2.8	3.1	1.5
		Coffee cake:											
6	374	Whole cake, 7¾ × 5⅛ × 1¼″	1 ea	430	30	1385	27	225	3	41	12	17	10
6	375	Piece, 1/6 of cake	1 pce	72	30	230	5	38	2	7	2.0	2.8	1.6
		Devil's food with chocolate frosting:											
6	376	Whole cake, 2 layer, 8 or 9″ diam	1 ea	1107	24	3755	49	645	5	136	56	51	20
6	377	Piece, 1/16 of cake	1 pce	69	24	235	3	40	1	8	3.5	3.2	1.2
6	378	Cupcake, 2½″ diam	1 ea	42	24	143	2	25	<1	5	2.1	2.0	.7
		Gingerbread:											
6	379	Whole cake, 8″ square	1 ea	570	37	1575	18	291	3	39	10	16	11
6	380	Piece, 1/9 of cake	1 pce	63	37	174	2	32	2	4	1.1	1.8	1.2
		Yellow, with chocolate frosting, 2 layer:											
6	381	Whole cake, 8 or 9″ diam	1 ea	1108	26	3735	45	638	5	125	48	49	22
6	382	Piece, 1/16 of cake	1 pce	69	26	235	3	40	<1	8	3	3.1	1.4
		Cakes from home recipes with enriched flour:											
		Carrot cake, cream cheese frosting:[46]											
6	383	Whole, 9 × 13″ cake	1 ea	1792	23	6496	63	832	20	328	69	135	114
6	384	Piece, 1/16 of 9 × 13″ cake 2¼ × 3¼″	1 pce	112	23	406	4	52	1	21	4.3	8.5	7.1
		Fruitcake, dark, 7½″ diam tube, 2¼″ high:[46]											
6	385	Whole cake	1 ea	1361	18	5185	74	783	38	228	48	113	52
6	386	Piece, 1/32 of cake, ⅔″ arc	1 pce	43	18	165	2	25	2	7	1.5	3.6	1.6
		Sheet cake, plain, no frosting:[47]											
6	387	Whole cake, 9″ square	1 ea	777	25	2830	35	434	3	108	30	45	26
6	388	Piece, 1/9 of cake	1 pce	86	25	315	4	48	<1	12	3.3	5	2.8
		Sheet cake, plain, uncooked white frosting:[48]											
6	389	Whole cake, 9″ square	1 ea	1096	21	4020	37	694	3	129	42	50	26
6	390	Piece, 1/9 of cake	1 pce	121	21	445	4	77	<1	14	5	6	3
		Pound cake:[48]											
6	391	Loaf, 8½ × 3½ × 3¼″	1 ea	514	22	2025	33	265	4	94	21	41	27
6	392	Piece, 1/17 of loaf, ½″ slice	1 pce	30	22	120	2	15	<1	5	1.2	2.4	1.6
		Cakes, commercial:											
		Pound cake:											
6	393	Loaf, 8½ × 3½ × 3″	1 ea	500	24	1935	26	257	4	94	52	30	4
6	394	Slice, 1/17 of loaf, ½″ slice	1 pce	29	24	110	2	15	<1	5	3.0	1.7	.2
		Snack cakes:											
6	395	Chocolate w/creme filling, 2 small cakes per package	1 ea	28	20	105	1	17	<1	4	1.7	1.5	.6
6	396	Sponge cake w/creme filling, 2 small cakes per package	1 ea	42	19	155	1	27	<1	5	2.3	2.1	.5

[45]Excepting angel food cake, cakes were made from mixes containing vegetable shortening, and frostings were made with margarine. All mixes use enriched flour.
[46]Made with vegetable oil.
[47]Cake made with vegetable shortening.
[48]Made with margarine.

(Computer code number is for West Diet Analysis program)

A

GRP KEY: 1 = BEV 2 = DAIRY 3 = EGGS 4 = FAT/OIL 5 = FRUIT 6 = BAKERY 7 = GRAIN 8 = FISH 9 = BEEF 10 = POULTRY
11 = SAUSAGE 12 = MIXED/FAST 13 = NUTS/SEEDS 14 = SWEETS 15 = VEG/LEG 16 = MISC 22 = SOUP/SAUCE

Chol (mg)	Calc (mg)	Iron (mg)	Magn (mg)	Phos (mg)	Pota (mg)	Sodi (mg)	Zinc (mg)	VT-A (RE)	Thia (mg)	Ribo (mg)	Niac (mg)	V-B6 (mg)	Fola (µg)	VT-C (mg)
0	92	2.2	30	136	126	1254	.55	273	.17	.20	2.50	.02	14	0
67	81	2.03	45	134	118	1023	.78	256	.10	.18	1.62	.04	20	t
0	527	2.73	51	1086	845	3226	.82	0	.32	1.27	1.6	.08	51	0
0	44	.23	4	91	71	269	.07	0	.03	.11	.13	.01	4	0
20	26	.6	11	70	40	225	.23	70	.01	.18	.7	.05	7	0
279	262	7.30	27	748	469	1853	3.70	194	.82	.90	7.70	.12	30	1
47	44	1.22	5	125	78	310	.62	32	.14	.15	1.29	.02	5	t
598	653	22.1	200	1162	1439	2900	7.95	498	1.11	1.66	10	.32	82	1
37	41	1.40	12	72	90	181	.53	31	.07	.1	.6	.02	1	t
23	25	.85	7	44	55	110	.40	19	.04	.06	.37	.01	3	t
6	513	10.8	41	570	1562	1733	5.52	0	.86	1.03	7.4	.07	36	1
1	57	1.20	5	63	173	192	.61	0	.10	.11	.82	.01	4	t
576	1008	15.5	72	2017	1208	2515	3.31	465	1.22	1.66	11.1	.45	80	1
36	63	.97	5	126	75	157	.21	29	.08	.10	.69	.03	5	t
912	440	20	185	1040	1856	2336	7.2	10,600	1.92	1.97	15.0	1.12	192	23
57	27	1.2	12	65	116	146	.45	663	.11	.14	1.0	.06	12	1
640	1293	37.6	340	1592	6138	2123	6.8	422	2.41	2.55	17	1.72	54	504
20	41	1.2	11	50	194	67	.22	13	.08	.08	.5	.05	2	16
552	497	11.7	108	793	614	2331	2.75	373	1.24	1.40	10.1	.26	54	2
61	55	1.3	12	88	68	258	.31	41	.14	.15	1.1	.03	15	t
636	548	11	108	822	669	2488	2.90	647	1.21	1.42	9.9	.27	110	2
70	61	1.2	12	91	74	275	.32	71	.13	.16	1.1	.03	12	t
555	339	9.3	48	473	483	1645	2.69	1033	.93	1.08	7.8	.39	55	1
32	20	.5	3	28	28	98	.16	60	.05	.06	.5	.02	3	t
1100	146	9.3	48	517	443	1857	1.95	715	.96	1.12	8.1	.38	55	1
64	8	.5	3	30	26	108	.11	41	.06	.06	.5	.02	3	t
15	21	1.0	3	26	34	105	.17	4	.06	.09	.7	.01	3	0
7	14	.6	3	44	37	155	.21	9	.07	.06	.6	.02	4	0

(For purposes of calculations, use "0" for t, <1, <.1, <.01, etc.)

Table A–1 Food Composition

Grp	Computer Code No.	Food Description	Measure	Wt (g)	H₂O (%)	Ener (cal)	Prot (g)	Carb (g)	Dietary Fiber (g)	Fat (g)	Fat Breakdown (g) Sat	Mono	Poly
		BAKED GOODS—Con.											
		Cakes—Con.											
		White cake with white frosting, 2-layer:											
6	397	Whole cake, 8 or 9″ diam	1 ea	1140	24	4170	43	670	5	148	33	62	42
6	398	Piece, ¹⁄₁₆ of cake	1 pce	71	24	260	3	42	<1	9	2.1	3.8	2.6
		Yellow cake with chocolate frosting, 2-layer:											
6	399	Whole cake, 8 or 9″ diam	1 ea	1108	23	3895	40	620	5	175	92	59	10
6	400	Piece, ¹⁄₁₆ of cake	1 pce	69	23	245	3	39	<1	11	5.7	3.7	.6
		Cheesecake:											
6	401	Whole cake, 9″ diam	1 ea	1110	46	3350	60	317	5	213	120	66	15
6	402	Piece, ¹⁄₁₂ of cake	1 pce	92	46	278	5	26	1	18	9.9	5.4	1.2
6	1035	Cheese puffs/Cheetos®	1 oz	28.4	1	158	2	14	<1	10	4.8	3.4	.6
		Cookies made with enriched flour:											
		Brownies with nuts:											
6	403	Commercial with frosting, 1½ × 1¾ × ⅞	1 ea	25	13	100	1	16	<1	4	1.6	2	.8
6	404	Home recipe, 1¾ × 1¾ × ⅞″[49]	1 ea	20	10	95	1	11	<1	6	1.4	2.8	1.2
		Chocolate chip cookies:											
6	405	Commercial, 2¼″ diam	4 ea	42	4	180	2	28	<1	9	2.9	3.1	2.6
6	406	Home recipe, 2¼″ diam[50]	4 ea	40	3	185	2	26	1	11	3.9	4.3	2
6	407	From refrigerated dough, 2¼″ diam	4 ea	48	5	225	2	32	1	11	4	4.4	2
6	408	Fig bars	4 ea	56	12	210	2	42	3	4	1	1.5	1
6	409	Oatmeal raisin cookies, 2⅝″ diam	4 ea	52	4	245	3	36	1	10	2.5	4.5	2.8
6	410	Peanut butter cookies, home recipe, 2⅝″ diam[50]	4 ea	48	3	245	4	28	1	14	4	5.8	2.8
6	411	Sandwich-type cookies, all	4 ea	40	2	195	2	29	<1	8	2	3.6	2.2
		Shortbread cookies:											
6	412	Commercial, small	4 ea	32	6	155	2	20	1	8	2.9	3	1.1
6	413	From home recipe, large[51]	2 ea	28	3	145	2	17	1	8	1.3	2.7	3.4
6	414	Sugar cookies from refrigerated dough, 2½″ diam	4 ea	48	4	235	2	31	<1	12	2.3	5	3.6
6	415	Vanilla wafers	10 ea	40	4	185	2	29	<1	7	1.8	3	1.8
6	416	Corn chips	1 oz	28	1	155	2	16	1	9	1.8	3.4	3.7
		Crackers:[52]											
6	1034	Armenian cracker bread	4 pce	28.4	4	117	5	19	4	2	.4	.7	1.1
6	417	Cheese crackers	10 ea	10	4	50	1	5	<1	3	.9	1.2	.3
6	418	Cheese crackers with peanut butter	4 ea	30	3	150	4	19	<1	8	1.6	3.2	1.2
6	419	Graham crackers	2 ea	14	4	60	1	11	<1	1	.4	.6	.4
6	420	Melba toast, plain	1 pce	5	4	20	1	4	<1	<1	.1	.1	.1
6	421	Rye wafers, whole grain	2 ea	14	5	55	1	10	2	1	.3	.4	.3
6	422	Saltine® crackers[53]	4 ea	12	4	50	1	9	<1	1	.5	.4	.2
6	423	Snack-type crackers, round	3 ea	9	3	45	1	6	<1	3	.6	1.2	.3
6	424	Wheat crackers, thin	4 ea	8	3	35	1	5	1	1	.4	.5	.4
6	425	Whole wheat wafers	2 ea	8	4	35	1	5	1	2	.5	.6	.4
6	426	Croissants, 4½ × 4 × 1¾″	1 ea	57	22	235	5	27	1	12	3.5	6.7	1.4
		Danish pastry:											
6	427	Packaged ring, plain, 12 oz	1 ea	340	27	1305	21	152	3	71	22	29	16
6	428	Round piece, plain, 4¼″ diam 1″ high	1 ea	57	27	220	4	26	1	12	3.6	4.8	2.6

[49] Made with vegetable oil.
[50] Made with vegetable shortening.
[51] Made with margarine.
[52] Crackers made with enriched white (wheat) flour except for rye wafers and whole-wheat wafers.
[53] Made with lard.

(Computer code number is for West Diet Analysis program)

GRP KEY: 1 = BEV 2 = DAIRY 3 = EGGS 4 = FAT/OIL 5 = FRUIT 6 = BAKERY 7 = GRAIN 8 = FISH 9 = BEEF 10 = POULTRY
11 = SAUSAGE 12 = MIXED/FAST 13 = NUTS/SEEDS 14 = SWEETS 15 = VEG/LEG 16 = MISC 22 = SOUP/SAUCE

A

Chol (mg)	Calc (mg)	Iron (mg)	Magn (mg)	Phos (mg)	Pota (mg)	Sodi (mg)	Zinc (mg)	VT-A (RE)	Thia (mg)	Ribo (mg)	Niac (mg)	V-B6 (mg)	Fola (µg)	VT-C (mg)
46	536	15.5	60	1585	832	2827	1.77	194	3.19	2.05	27.6	.16	64	0
3	33	1	4	99	52	176	.11	12	.2	.13	1.7	.01	4	0
609	366	19.9	72	1884	1972	3080	3.3	488	.78	2.22	10	.45	80	0
38	23	1.24	5	117	123	192	.21	30	.05	.14	.62	.03	5	0
2053	622	5.33	111	977	1088	2464	4.66	833	.33	1.44	5.11	.71	200	56
170	52	.44	9	81	90	204	.39	69	.03	.12	.42	.06	17	5
5	18	.20	7	29	23	344	—	26	.01	.03	.20	—	—	0
14	13	.61	14	26	50	59	.36	18	.08	.07	.33	.04	5	t
18	9	.40	11	26	35	51	.31	6	.05	.05	.3	.04	4	t
5	16	.8	10	41	56	140	.3	15	.1	.23	.9	.02	4	t
18	13	1	14	34	82	82	.22	5	.06	.06	.58	.03	4	0
22	13	1.04	10	34	62	173	.24	8	.06	.10	.89	.01	4	0
27	40	1.36	15	34	162	180	.36	6	.08	.07	.73	.07	4	t
2	18	1.1	26	58	90	148	.53	12	.09	.08	1	.03	6	0
22	21	1.1	19	60	110	142	.36	5	.07	.07	1.9	.04	12	0
0	12	1.4	15	40	66	189	.21	0	.09	.07	.8	.01	1	0
27	13	.8	4	39	38	123	.15	8	.10	.09	.9	.01	3	0
0	6	.55	4	31	18	125	.13	89	.08	.06	.71	.01	2	t
29	50	.9	8	91	33	261	.24	11	.09	.06	1.1	.02	4	0
25	16	.8	6	36	50	150	.12	14	.07	.1	1	.01	4	0
0	35	.5	21	52	52	233	.44	11	.04	.05	.4	.04[54]	3[55]	1
0	21	.45	41	1	77	—	.90	1	.06	.04	1.05	.03	12	2
6	11	.35	3	17	17	112	.07	5	.05	.04	.4	.01	—	0
4	26	1.2	2	94	64	338	.06	3	.16	.12	2.4	.03	—	0
0	6	.37	6	20	36	86	.11	0	.02	.03	.6	.01	2	0
0	6	.1	1	10	11	44	—	0	.01	.01	.1	.01	.7	0
0	7	.5	16	44	65	115	1.60	0	.06	.03	.5	.03	10	0
4	3	.5	3	12	17	165	.09	0	.06	.05	.6	<.01	2	0
0	9	.3	2	18	12	90	.05	t	.03	.03	.3	<.01	1	0
.6	3	.25	6[56]	15	17	69	.24[56]	t	.04	.03	.4	.01	3[55]	0
0	3	.24	8[56]	22	31	59	.23	0	.02	.03	.4	.01	3[55]	0
13	20	2.1	9	64	68	452	.32	13	.17	.13	1.3	.03	18	0
292	360	6.5	68	347	316	1302	2.86	99	.95	1.02	8.5	.12	84	t
49	60	1.1	11	58	53	218	.48	17	.16	.17	1.4	.02	14	t

[54]B_6 values vary from 0 to .04 g between various brands—check label.
[55]Folacin values estimated and derived from values for cornmeal and corn tortillas.
[56]Values derived from whole-wheat recipes and retention values.

(For purposes of calculations, use "0" for t, <1, <.1, <.01, etc.)

Table A–1   Food Composition

	Computer Code								Dietary		Fat Breakdown (g)		
Grp	No.	Food Description	Measure	Wt (g)	H₂O (%)	Ener (cal)	Prot (g)	Carb (g)	Fiber (g)	Fat (g)	Sat	Mono	Poly

Grp	No.	Food Description	Measure	Wt (g)	H$_2$O (%)	Ener (cal)	Prot (g)	Carb (g)	Fiber (g)	Fat (g)	Sat	Mono	Poly
		BAKED GOODS—Con.											
		Danish Pastry—Con.											
6	429	Ounce, plain	1 oz	28	28	110	2	13	<1	6	1.8	2.4	1.3
6	430	Round piece with fruit	1 pce	65	30	235	4	28	1	13	3.9	5.2	2.9
		Desserts, 3 × 3 inch piece:											
6	1348	Apple crisp	1 pce	78	58	146	1	25	1	5	1.0	2.3	1.7
6	1353	Apple cobbler	1 pce	104	56	201	2	35	2	6	1.4	2.7	1.9
6	1349	Cherry crisp	1 pce	138	73	157	2	27	2	5	1.0	2.3	1.7
6	1352	Cherry cobbler	1 pce	129	65	199	2	34	1	6	1.4	2.7	1.9
6	1350	Peach crisp	1 pce	139	72	166	2	30	2	5	1.0	2.3	1.7
6	1351	Peach cobbler	1 pce	130	64	130	2	37	2	6	1.4	2.7	1.9
		Doughnuts:											
6	431	Cake type, plain, 3¼″ diam	1 ea	50	21	210	2	25	1	12	3.4	5.8	2
6	432	Yeast-leavened, glazed, 3¾″ diam	1 ea	60	27	235	4	26	1	13	5.2	5.5	.9
		English muffins:											
6	433	Plain, enriched	1 ea	57	42	140	5	26	2	1	.3	.2	.3
6	434	Toasted	1 ea	50	29	140	5	26	2	1	.3	.2	.3
		Muffins, 2½″ diam, 1½″ high:											
		From home recipe:											
6	435	Blueberry[57]	1 ea	45	37	135	3	20	2	5	1.5	2.1	1.2
6	436	Bran, wheat[58]	1 ea	45	35	125	3	19	3	6	1.4	1.6	2.3
6	437	Cornmeal	1 ea	45	33	145	3	21	2	5	1.5	2.2	1.4
		From commercial mix:											
6	438	Blueberry	1 ea	45	33	140	3	22	2	5	1.4	2	1.2
6	439	Bran	1 ea	45	28	140	3	24	3	4	1.3	1.6	1
6	440	Cornmeal	1 ea	45	30	145	3	22	2	6	1.7	2.3	1.4
		Pancakes, 4″ diam:											
6	441	Buckwheat, from mix with egg and milk	1 ea	27	58	55	2	6	1	2	.9	.9	.5
6	442	Plain, from home recipe	1 ea	27	50	60	2	9	1	2	.5	.8	.5
6	443	Plain, from mix; egg, milk, oil added	1 ea	27	54	60	2	8	1	2	.5	.9	.5
		Piecrust, with enriched flour, vegetable shortening, baked:											
6	444	Home recipe, 9″ shell	1 ea	180	15	900	11	79	4	60	15	26	16
		From mix:											
6	445	Piecrust for 2-crust pie	1 ea	320	19	1485	21	141	6	93	23	41	25
6	446	1 pie shell	1 ea	180	19	835	12	79	4	52	13	23	14
		Pies, 9″ diam; pie crust made with vegetable shortening, enriched flour:											
		Apple pie:[59]											
6	447	Whole pie	1 ea	945	48	2420	22	360	19	105	25	46	29
6	448	Piece, ⅙ of pie	1 pce	158	48	405	4	60	3	18	4.1	7.6	4.9
		Banana cream pie:[60]											
6	449	Whole pie	1 ea	1190	66	1915	38	282	10	77	27	29	15
6	450	⅙ of pie	1 pce	198	66	319	6	47	2	13	4.5	4.9	2.5
		Blueberry pie:[59]											
6	451	Whole pie	1 ea	945	51	2285	23	330	22	102	24	45	28
6	452	Piece, ⅙ of pie	1 pce	158	51	380	4	55	4	17	4.0	7.5	4.7

[57]Made with vegetable shortening.
[58]Made with vegetable oil.
[59]Recipes updated for latest USDA values for fruits/nuts/fruit juice.
[60]Recipe based on pie crust, cooked vanilla pudding, 2 bananas.

(Computer code number is for West Diet Analysis program)

GRP KEY: 1 = BEV   2 = DAIRY   3 = EGGS   4 = FAT/OIL   5 = FRUIT   6 = BAKERY   7 = GRAIN   8 = FISH   9 = BEEF   10 = POULTRY
11 = SAUSAGE   12 = MIXED/FAST   13 = NUTS/SEEDS   14 = SWEETS   15 = VEG/LEG   16 = MISC   22 = SOUP/SAUCE

A

Chol (mg)	Calc (mg)	Iron (mg)	Magn (mg)	Phos (mg)	Pota (mg)	Sodi (mg)	Zinc (mg)	VT-A (RE)	Thia (mg)	Ribo (mg)	Niac (mg)	V-B6 (mg)	Fola (µg)	VT-C (mg)
24	30	.55	6	29	27	109	.24	9	.08	.09	.7	.01	7	t
56	17	1.3	13	80	57	233	.55	11	.16	.14	1.4	.02	16	t
0	20	.77	12	15	112	66	.09	65	.05	.04	.41	.03	3	4
1	32	.76	7	42	86	305	.17	76	.08	.07	.70	.04	3	<1
0	29	2.16	16	22	163	73	.14	144	.06	.08	.56	.05	10	3
1	39	1.78	10	46	113	311	.21	135	.09	.10	.81	.05	9	2
0	24	.997	18	30	197	71	.19	104	.05	.05	1.01	.03	5	5
1	35	.90	11	52	139	309	.24	105	.08	.08	1.15	.03	5	3
20	23	.8	12	111	58	192	.25	5	.12	.12	1.1	.02	4	t
21	17	1.4	13	55	64	222	.30	<1	.28	.12	1.8	.28	13	0
0	96	1.7	11	67	331	378	.41	0	.26	.18	2.14	.02	18	0
0	96	1.7	11	67	331	378	.41	0	.23	.18	2.14	.02	15	0
19	54	.9	11	46	47	198	.29	9	.10	.11	.9	<.01	12	1
24	60	1.4	34	125	99	189	.37	30	.11	.13	1.3	.01	9	3
23	66	.9	11	59	57	169	.31	15	.11	.11	.9	.04	5	t
45	15	.9	7	90	54	225	.21	11	.11	.13	1.17	<.01	14	<1
28	27	1.7	28	182	50	385	.95	14	.08	.12	1.9	.12	19	0
42	30	1.3	11	128	31	291	.34	16	.09	.09	.8	.04	5	t
20	59	.4	18	91	66	125	.5	17	.04	.05	.2	.06	6	t
16	27	.5	7	38	33	115	.23	10	.06	.07	.5	.02	4	t
16	36	.7	7	71	43	160	.23	7	.09	.12	.8	.01	3	t
0	25	4.5	31	90	90	1100	1.50	0	.54	.40	5.0	.17	32	0
0	131	9.3	44	272	179	2600	1.19	0	1.07	.79	9.89	.27	57	0
0	74	5.23	25	153	101	1462	.79	0	.60	.44	5.57	.15	32	0
0	170	10	69	300	600	2844	1.6	28	1.04	.76	9.5	.5	48	2
0	28	1.67	12	50	100	476	.27	5	.18	.13	1.6	.08	8	<1
90	880	6.54	186	809	2000	2532	4.17	222	.94	1.75	7.40	1.77	116	26
15	147	1.09	31	135	333	422	.69	37	.16	.29	1.23	.30	19	4
0	155	12.3	60	274	756	2533	1.68	85	1.04	.85	10.4	.43	84	36
0	26	2.1	10	46	126	423	.28	14	.17	.14	1.73	.07	14	6

(For purposes of calculations, use "0" for t, <1, <.1, <.01, etc.)

Table A–1   Food Composition

Grp	Computer Code No.	Food Description	Measure	Wt (g)	H$_2$O (%)	Ener (cal)	Prot (g)	Carb (g)	Dietary Fiber (g)	Fat (g)	Fat Breakdown (g)		
											Sat	Mono	Poly
BAKED GOODS—Con.													
		Pies—Con.											
		Cherry pie:[59]											
6	453	Whole pie	1 ea	945	47	2465	26	363	15	107	25	47	30
6	454	Piece, ⅙ of pie	1 pce	158	47	410	4	61	2	18	4.2	7.8	4.9
		Chocolate cream pie:[61]											
6	455	Whole pie	1 ea	1051	63	1863	45	255	4	76	27	30	15
6	456	Piece, ⅙ of pie	1 pce	175	63	311	7	42	1	13	4.5	5.0	2.5
		Custard pie:											
6	457	Whole pie	1 ea	910	58	1760	46	204	4	84	28	35	17
6	458	Piece, ⅙ of pie	1 pce	152	58	293	8	34	1	13	.9	5.8	2.8
		Lemon meringue pie:[59]											
6	459	Whole Pie	1 ea	840	47	2140	31	317	5	84	21	37	22
6	460	Piece, ⅙ of pie	1 pce	140	47	355	5	53	1	14	3.5	6.2	3.7
		Peach pie:[59]											
6	461	Whole pie	1 ea	945	48	2410	24	361	17	105	25	46	29
6	462	Piece, ⅙ of pie	1 pce	158	48	405	4	61	3	17	4.1	7.7	4.8
		Pecan pie:[59]											
6	463	Whole pie	1 ea	825	20	3500	38	551	10	142	24	75	34
6	464	Piece, ⅙ of pie	1 pce	138	20	583	6	92	5	24	3.9	13	5.7
		Pumpkin pie:[59]											
6	465	Whole Pie	1 ea	910	59	2200	54	308	15	94	34	37	17
6	466	Piece, ⅙ of pie	1 pce	152	59	367	9	51	5	16	5.7	6.1	2.8
		Pies, fried, commercial:											
6	467	Apple	1 ea	85	43	255	2	32	2	14	5.8	6.6	.6
6	468	Cherry	1 ea	85	43	250	2	32	1	14	5.8	6.7	.6
		Pretzels, made with enriched flour:											
6	469	Thin sticks, 2¼" long	10 ea	3	2	10	<1	2	<1	<1	t	<.1	<.1
6	470	Dutch twists, 2¾ × 2⅝"	1 ea	16	2	65	2	13	<1	1	.1	.2	.2
6	471	Thin twists, 3¼ × 2¼ × ¼"	10 ea	60	3	240	6	48	2	2	.4	.8	.6
		Rolls and buns, enriched:											
		Commercial:											
6	472	Cloverleaf rolls, 2½" diam, 2" high	1 ea	28	32	85	2	14	1	2	.5	.8	.6
6	473	Hotdog buns	1 ea	40	34	115	3	20	1	2	.5	.8	.6
6	474	Hamburger buns	1 ea	45	34	129	4	23	1	2	.6	.9	.7
6	475	Hard rolls, white, 3¾" diam, 2" high	1 ea	50	25	155	5	30	1	2	.4	.5	.6
6	476	Submarine rolls or hoagies, 11½ × 3 × 2½	1 ea	135	31	400	11	72	2	8	1.8	3	2.2
		From home recipe:											
6	477	Dinner rolls 2½" diam, 2" high	1 ea	35	26	120	3	20	1	3	.8	1.2	.9
6	478	Toaster pastries, fortified	1 ea	54	13	210	2	38	1	6	1.7	3.6	.4
		Tortilla chips:											
6	1271	Plain	1 oz	28	4	139	2	17	1	8	1.1	3.1	3.1
6	1036	Nacho flavor	1 oz	28	1	139	2	18	1	7	1.4	2.5	2.8
6	1037	Taco flavor	1 oz	28	1	140	3	18	1	7	1.4	2.5	2.7
		Tortillas:											
6	479	Corn, enriched, 6" diam	1 ea	30	45	65	2	13	2	1	.1	.3	.6
6	480	Flour, 8" diam	1 ea	35	27	105	3	19	1	3	.4	1.2	1.0
6	1301	Flour tortilla, 10.5" diam.	1 ea	57	27	168	4	31	2	4	.6	1.9	1.6
6	481	Taco shells	1 ea	14	4	59	1	9	1	2	.2	.6	1.2

[59] Recipes updated for latest USDA values for fruits/nuts/fruit juice.
[61] Based on value for pie crust, cooked chocolate pudding with meringue.

(Computer code number is for West Diet Analysis program)

GRP KEY: 1 = BEV   2 = DAIRY   3 = EGGS   4 = FAT/OIL   5 = FRUIT   6 = BAKERY   7 = GRAIN   8 = FISH   9 = BEEF   10 = POULTRY
11 = SAUSAGE   12 = MIXED/FAST   13 = NUTS/SEEDS   14 = SWEETS   15 = VEG/LEG   16 = MISC   22 = SOUP/SAUCE

Chol (mg)	Calc (mg)	Iron (mg)	Magn (mg)	Phos (mg)	Pota (mg)	Sodi (mg)	Zinc (mg)	VT-A (RE)	Thia (mg)	Ribo (mg)	Niac (mg)	V-B6 (mg)	Fola (µg)	VT-C (mg)
0	220	19	91	350	920	2873	1.87	416	1.13	.85	9.50	.50	93	5
0	37	3.17	15	58	153	480	.31	70	.19	.14	1.58	.08	16	1
90	958	6.46	176	881	1332	2565	4.46	204	.91	1.80	6.38	.54	66	3
15	160	1.08	29	147	222	427	.74	34	.15	.30	1.06	.09	11	<1
705	742	8.64	110	880	1040	2000	4.75	573	.82	1.60	5.50	.51	91	1
118	124	1.44	18	147	173	333	.79	96	.14	.27	.92	.08	15	4
822	150	8.4	54	412	420	2369	3.06	395	.59	.84	.50	.30	78	25
137	25	1.4	9	69	70	395	.51	66	.10	.14	.83	.05	13	4
0	160	11.3	98	332	1408	2533	2.11	690	1.04	.93	13.9	.39	72	28
0	27	1.90	16	55	235	423	.35	115	.18	.16	2.30	.07	12	5
822	210	12.0	192	777	781	1823	8.8	248	1.63	.99	6.6	.51	110	0
137	35	1.85	32	130	130	304	1.47	41	.22	.17	1.1	.08	18	0
655	1273	15.8	240	1269	2400	2029	5.96	11170[62]	.82	1.76	7.3	.64	120	6
109	212	2.63	40	211	400	338	.99	1861[62]	.14	.29	1.22	.11	20	1
14	12	.94	6	34	42	326	.14	3	.09	.06	1.0	.03	4	1
13	11	.70	7	41	61	371	.15	19	.06	.06	.60	.04	8	1
0	1	.06	1	3	3	48	.03	0	.01	.01	.13	<.01	<1	0
0	4	.32	4	15	16	258	.17	0	.05	.04	.70	<.01	3	0
0	16	1.2	15	55	61	966	.42	0	.19	.15	2.6	.01	10	0
t	33	.81	6	44	36	155	.22	t	.14	.09	1.10	.01	11	<1
0	54	1.19	8	44	56	241	.36	t	.20	.13	1.58	.01	15	<1
0	61	1.34	9	50	63	271	.41	t	.22	.15	1.78	.02	17	<1
0	24	1.40	14	46	49	313	.44	0	.20	.12	1.70	.02	17	0
0	100	3.80	31	115	128	683	1.17	0	.54	.33	4.50	.09	49	0
12	16	1.10	10	36	41	98	.32	8	.12	.12	1.20	.01	12	0
0	104	2.16	10	104	91	248	.31	150[63]	.17	.18	2.27	.2	43	4
0	82	1.00	22	74	30	140	.42	1	.01	.02	.20	.08	<1	<1
0	17	.40	13	98	109	107	.42	13	.04	.03	.40	.10	—	0
0	45	.70	27	91	72	191	.42	15	.08	.09	.80	.10	—	0
0	42	.60	19	55	43	1	.36	8	.05	.03	.40	.09	6	0
0	21	.55	12	59	35	134	.27	0	.13	.08	1.20	.01	16	0
0	34	.88	19	94	56	215	.43	0	.21	.13	1.93	.02	25	0
0	26	.26	9	33	25	62	.22	1	<.01	.01	.25	.02	2	0

[62]Latest USDA values of Vitamin A for canned pumpkin are almost 3.5 times greater than previously published values. Canned pumpkin is usually a blend of pumpkin and winter squash.
[63]Vitamin A values from label declaration varies from 100 to 150 RE for major brands.

(For purposes of calculations, use "0" for t, <1, <.1, <.01, etc.)

Table A–1   Food Composition

Grp	Computer Code No.	Food Description	Measure	Wt (g)	H$_2$O (%)	Ener (cal)	Prot (g)	Carb (g)	Dietary Fiber (g)	Fat (g)	Sat	Mono	Poly
											Fat Breakdown (g)		
		BAKED GOODS—Con.											
		Waffles, 7″ diam:											
6	482	From home recipe	1 ea	75	37	245	7	26	1	13	4	4.9	2.6
6	483	From mix, egg/milk added	1 ea	75	42	205	7	27	1	8	2.7	2.9	1.5
		GRAIN PRODUCTS: CEREAL, FLOUR, GRAIN, PASTA and NOODLES, POPCORN											
		Barley, pearled:											
7	484	Dry, uncooked	1 c	200	11	700	16	158	31	2	.4	.3	1.1
7	485	Cooked	1 c	157	69	193	4	44	4	1	.1	.1	.3
		Breakfast cereals, hot, cooked:											
		Corn grits (hominy) enriched cooked:											
7	486	Regular and quick, prepared	1 c	242	85	146	4	31	5	<1	t	.1	.3
7	487	Instant, prepared from packet, white	1 pkt	137	85	80	2	18	3	<1	t	.1	.1
		Cream of Wheat®, cooked:											
7	488	Regular, quick, instant	1 c	244	86	140	4	29	3	1	.1	.1	.2
7	489	Mix and eat, plain, packet	1 ea	142	82	100	3	21	2	<1	<.1	<.1	.1
7	490	Malt-O-Meal® cereal, cooked	1 c	240	88	122	4	26	3	<1	<.1	<.1	.1
		Oatmeal or rolled oats, cooked:											
7	491	Regular, quick, instant, nonfortified	1 c	234	85	145	6	25	4	2	.4	.8	1
		Instant, fortified:											
7	492	Plain, from packet	¾ c	177	86	104	4	18	3	2	.3	.6	.7
7	493	Flavored, from packet	¾ c	164	76	160	5	31	3	2	.3	.7	.8
7	494	Whole wheat cereal, cooked	1 c	242	84	150	5	33	4	1	.1	.1	.3
		Breakfast cereals, ready to eat:											
7	495	All-Bran®	⅓ c	28	3	70	4	22	9	<1	.1	.1	.3
7	1306	Alpha Bits®	1 c	28	1	111	2	25	1	1	.1	.2	.3
7	1307	Apple Jacks®	1 c	28	2	110	2	26	<1	<1	<.1	<.1	<.1
7	1308	Bran Buds®	1 c	84	3	217	12	64	23	2	.4	.3	1.1
7	1305	Bran Chex®	1 c	49	2	156	5	39	9	1	.2	.2	.8
7	1309	Buc Wheats®	¾ c	28	3	110	2	24	2	1	.1	.1	.5
7	1310	C.W. Post® plain	1 c	97	2	432	9	69	2	15	11.3	1.7	1.4
7	1311	C.W. Post® with raisins	1 c	103	4	446	9	74	2	15	11.0	1.7	1.4
7	496	Cap'n Crunch®	1 c	37	2	156	2	30	1	3	2.2	.4	.5
7	1312	Cap'n Crunchberries®	1 c	35	3	146	2	29	<1	3	1.9	.4	.5
7	1313	Cap'n Crunch®, peanut butter	1 c	35	2	154	3	27	<1	5	1.9	1.4	1.0
7	497	Cheerios®	1 c	23	5	89	3	16	2	1	.3	.5	.6
7	1314	Cocoa Krispies®	1 c	36	3	139	2	32	<1	<1	.2	.2	.2
7	1316	Cocoa Pebbles®	⅔ c	21	2	87	1	18	<1	1	<.1	<.1	<.1
7	1315	Corn Bran®	1 c	36	3	124	3	30	7	1	.2	.3	.7
7	1317	Corn Chex®	1 c	28	2	111	2	25	<1	<1	.1	.3	.6
7	498	Corn Flakes, Kellogg's®	1¼ c	28	3	110	2	24	1	<1	t	t	.1
7	499	Corn Flakes, Post Toasties®	1¼ c	28	3	110	2	24	1	<1	t	t	.1
7	1318	Cracklin' Oat Bran®	1 c	60	4	229	6	41	9	9	2.1	2.3	3.5
7	1038	Crispy Wheat 'N Raisins®	1 c	43	7	150	3	35	2	1	.1	.1	.4
7	1319	Fortified oat flakes	1 c	48	3	177	9	35	1	1	.1	.3	.3
7	500	40% Bran Flakes, Kellogg's®	1 c	39	3	125	5	35	5	1	.14	.14	.4
7	501	40% Bran Flakes, Post®	1 c	47	3	152	5	37	6	1	.2	.2	.3
7	502	Froot Loops®	1 c	28	2	111	2	25	<1	1	.2	.1	.1

(Computer code number is for West Diet Analysis program)

GRP KEY: 1 = BEV   2 = DAIRY   3 = EGGS   4 = FAT/OIL   5 = FRUIT   6 = BAKERY   7 = GRAIN   8 = FISH   9 = BEEF   10 = POULTRY
11 = SAUSAGE   12 = MIXED/FAST   13 = NUTS/SEEDS   14 = SWEETS   15 = VEG/LEG   16 = MISC   22 = SOUP/SAUCE

A

Chol (mg)	Calc (mg)	Iron (mg)	Magn (mg)	Phos (mg)	Pota (mg)	Sodi (mg)	Zinc (mg)	VT-A (RE)	Thia (mg)	Ribo (mg)	Niac (mg)	V-B6 (mg)	Fola (µg)	VT-C (mg)
102	154	1.50	17	135	129	445	.65	39	.18	.24	1.50	.03	13	t
59	179	1.20	14	257	146	515	.52	49	.14	.23	.90	.03	4	t
0	32	4.2	51	378	320	6	4.47	0	.24	.1	7.9	.45	40	0
0	17	2.1	35	85	146	5	1.29	0	.13	.1	3.2	.18	25	0
0	1	1.55[64]	11	29	54	0[65]	.18	15[66]	.24[64]	.15[64]	1.96[64]	.06	2	0
0	7	1[64]	5	16	29	343	.08	0	.18[64]	.08[64]	1.3[64]	.03	1	0
0	54[64]	10.9[64]	12	43[67]	46	5[67,68]	.35	0	.24[64]	.07[64]	1.5[64]	.02	9	0
0	20[64]	8.10[64]	7	20[64]	38	241	.20	376[64]	.43[64]	.28[64]	5.0[64]	.01	5	0
0	5	9.6[64]	14	24[64]	31	2[68]	.17	0	.48[64]	.24[64]	5.8[64]	.02	5	0
0	19	1.59	56	178	131	2[68]	1.15	5	.26	.05	.3	.05	9	0
0	163[64]	6.32[64]	51	133	99	285[64]	1	453[64]	.53[64]	.29[64]	5.49[64]	.74	150	0
0	168[64]	6.7[64]	51	148	137	254[64]	1	460[64]	.53[64]	.38[64]	5.9[64]	.77	150	<1
0	17	1.5	53	168	171	3	1.16	0	.17	.12	2.13	.07	25	0
0	23	4.5[64]	106	264	320	260	3.7	375[64]	.37[64]	.43[64]	5.0[64]	.5	100	15[64]
0	8	1.80	17	51	100	219	1.50	375	.40	.40	5.0	.50	100	—
0	3	4.50	6	30	23	125	3.70	375	.40	.40	5.0	.50	100	15
0	56	13.4	267	729	930	516	11.1	1112	1.10	1.30	14.8	1.50	297	45
0	29	7.80	126	327	394	455	2.14	11	.60	.26	8.6	.90	173	26
0	60	8.10	24	60	—	235	.30	682	.68	.77	9.0	.90	—	27
0	47	15.4	67	224	198	167	1.64	1284	1.30	1.50	17.1	1.70	342	—
0	51	16.4	74	232	260	160	1.64	1364	1.30	1.50	18.1	1.90	364	—
0	6	9.83[64]	15	47	48	278	4.01	5[64]	.66[64]	.71[64]	8.64[64]	1	238	0
0	11	9.04	14	47	49	243	3.56	0	.59	.67	8.14	.93	128	—
0	7	9.10	19	49	57	268	3.79	0	.60	.70	8.97	1.04	244	—
0	38	3.6[64]	31	109	82	246	.63	304[64]	.32[64]	.32[64]	4.0[64]	.4	5	12[64]
0	6	2.30	12	47	53	275	1.90	477	.50	.50	6.3	.60	127	19
0	4	1.30	9	16	35	102	1.10	282	.30	.30	3.7	.40	75	—
0	41	12.2	18	52	70	310	4.00	—	.38	.70	10.9	.86	232	—
0	3	1.80	4	11	23	271	.10	14	.40	.07	5.0	.50	100	15
0	1	1.8[64]	3	18	26	351	.06	375[64]	.37[64]	.43[64]	5.0[64]	.51	100	15[64]
0	1	.7[64]	3	12	33	297	.06	375[64]	.37[64]	.43[64]	5.0[64]	.51	100	0
0	40	3.80	116	241	355	402	3.20	794	.80	.90	10.6	1.10	212	32
0	71	6.80	35	117	174	204	.51	569	.60	.60	7.6	.80	40	—
0	68	13.7	58	176	343	429	1.50	636	.60	.70	.39	.90	169	—
0	19	11.2[64]	71	192	248	363	5.15	522[64]	.51[64]	.59[64]	6.86[64]	.7	138	0
0	21	7.47[64]	102	296	251	431	2.5	629[64]	.62[64]	.72[64]	8.3[64]	.85	166	0
0	3	4.5[64]	9	28	30	125	3.7	225[64]	.4[64]	.4[64]	5.0[64]	.5	100	15[64]

[64] Nutrient added (values sometimes based on label declaration).
[65] Cooked without salt. If salt is added according to label recommendation, sodium content is 540 mg.
[66] Value for yellow corn grits; cooked white corn grits contain 0 RE of Vitamin A.
[67] Values for regular and instant cereal. For quick cereal, phosphorus is 102 mg, and sodium is 142 mg.
[68] Cooked without salt. If added according to label recommendations, sodium content is 390 mg for Cream of Wheat; 324 mg for Malt-O-Meal; 374 mg for oatmeal.

(For purposes of calculations, use "0" for t, <1, <.1, <.01, etc.)

Table A–1   Food Composition

Grp	Computer Code No.	Food Description	Measure	Wt (g)	H₂O (%)	Ener (cal)	Prot (g)	Carb (g)	Dietary Fiber (g)	Fat (g)	Fat Breakdown (g) Sat	Mono	Poly
		GRAIN PRODUCTS—Con.											
		Cereals—Con.											
7	1320	Frosted Mini-Wheats®	4 ea	31	5	111	3	26	2	<1	.1	<.1	.2
7	1321	Frosted Rice Krispies®	1 c	28	3	109	1	26	1	<1	<.1	<.1	<.1
7	1323	Fruit & Fiber® w/apples	½ c	28	2	90	3	22	4	1	.2	.2	.6
7	1324	Fruit & Fiber® w/dates	½ c	28	2	90	3	21	4	1	.2	.2	.6
7	1325	Fruitful Bran® cereal	¾ c	34	3	110	3	27	5	0	0	0	0
7	1322	Fruity Pebbles® cereal	⅞ c	28	3	113	1	24	<1	2	.3	.2	.4
7	503	Golden Grahams®	1 c	39	2	156	2	33	2	2	1.0	.1	.2
7	504	Granola, homemade	1 c	122	3	595	15	67	13	33	5.8	9.4	17
7	505	Grape Nuts®	½ c	57	3	210	6	46	5	<1	t	t	.2
7	1326	Grape Nuts® flakes	⅞ c	28	3	102	3	23	2	<1	<.1	<.1	.1
7	1327	Honey & Nut Corn flakes	¾ c	28	4	113	2	23	<1	2	.2	.5	.7
7	506	Honey Nut Cheerios®	1 c	33	3	127	4	27	1	1	.2	.4	.5
7	1328	Honey Bran	1 c	35	3	119	3	29	4	1	.1	.1	.4
7	1329	Honeycomb®	1 c	22	1	86	1	20	<1	<1	.1	.1	.2
7	1330	King Vitamin® cereal	1 c	21	2	85	1	18	<1	1	.7	.2	.2
7	1039	Kix®	1 c	19	3	73	2	16	<1	<1	.1	.1	.2
7	1331	Life®	1 c	44	5	162	8	32	1	1	.1	.2	.4
7	507	Lucky Charms®	1 c	32	3	125	3	26	1	1	.2	.4	.5
7	508	Nature Valley® Granola	1 c	113	4	503	12	76	12	20	13	2.8	2.8
7	1332	Nutri-Grain™—Barley	1 c	41	3	153	5	34	2	<1	<.1	<.1	.1
7	1333	Nutri-Grain™—Corn	1 c	42	3	160	3	36	3	1	.1	.3	.6
7	1334	Nutri-Grain™—Rye	1 c	40	3	144	4	34	3	<1	.1	.1	.1
7	1335	Nutri-Grain™—Wheat	1 c	44	3	158	4	37	3	<1	.1	.1	.3
7	1336	100% Bran	1 c	66	3	178	8	48	20	3	.6	.6	1.9
7	509	100% Natural® cereal, plain	¼ c	28	2	135	3	18	3	6	4.1	1.2	.5
7	1337	100% Natural® with apples	1 c	104	2	478	11	70	5	20	15.5	1.8	1.3
7	1338	100% Natural® with raisins & dates	1 c	100	4	496	11	72	4	20	13.7	3.7	1.7
7	510	Product 19®	1 c	33	3	126	3	27	<1	<1	t	t	.1
7	1339	Quisp®	1 c	30	2	124	2	25	<1	2	1.5	.3	.3
7	511	Raisin Bran, Kellogg's®	1 c	49	8	158	5	37	6	1	.2	.1	.4
7	512	Raisin Bran, Post®	1 c	56	9	170	5	42	6	1	.2	.2	.4
7	1040	Raisins, Rice & Rye™	1 c	46	9	155	3	39	<1	<1	<.1	<.1	<.1
7	1041	Rice Chex®	¾ c	19	3	75	1	17	1	1	.2	.2	.3
7	513	Rice Krispies, Kellogg's®	1 c	29	2	112	2	25	<1	<1	t	t	.1
7	514	Rice, puffed	1 c	14	3	55	1	13	<1	<1	t	t	<.1
7	515	Shredded Wheat®	¾ c	32	5	115	3	25	4	1	.1	.1	.3
7	516	Special K®	1½ c	32	2	125	6	24	<1	<1	t	t	t
7	1340	Sugar Corn Pops®	1 c	28	3	108	1	26	<1	<1	t	<.1	.1
7	518	Sugar Frosted Flakes®	1 c	35	3	133	2	32	1	<1	t	t	t
7	517	Super Sugar Crisp®	1 c	33	2	123	2	30	<1	<1	t	t	.1
7	519	Sugar Smacks®	¾ c	28	3	106	2	25	<1	<1	.1	.1	.2
7	1341	Tasteeos®	1 c	24	2	94	3	19	1	1	.2	.2	.3
7	1342	Team®	1 c	42	4	164	3	36	<1	1	.2	.2	.3
7	520	Total®, wheat, with added calcium	1 c	33	4	122	3	26	2	1	.1	.1	.4
7	521	Trix®	1 c	28	2	109	1	25	<1	1	.2	.1	.1
7	1042	Wheat & Raisin Chex®	1 c	54	7	185	5	43	4	<1	.1	.1	.2
7	1344	Wheat Chex®	1 c	46	3	169	5	38	3	1	.2	.2	.6
7	1043	Wheat, puffed	1 c	12	3	44	2	10	2	<1	t	t	.1
7	522	Wheaties®	1 c	29	5	101	3	23	3	1	.1	.1	.2

(Computer code number is for West Diet Analysis program)

GRP KEY: 1 = BEV   2 = DAIRY   3 = EGGS   4 = FAT/OIL   5 = FRUIT   6 = BAKERY   7 = GRAIN   8 = FISH   9 = BEEF   10 = POULTRY
11 = SAUSAGE   12 = MIXED/FAST   13 = NUTS/SEEDS   14 = SWEETS   15 = VEG/LEG   16 = MISC   22 = SOUP/SAUCE

A

Chol (mg)	Calc (mg)	Iron (mg)	Magn (mg)	Phos (mg)	Pota (mg)	Sodi (mg)	Zinc (mg)	VT-A (RE)	Thia (mg)	Ribo (mg)	Niac (mg)	V-B6 (mg)	Fola (µg)	VT-C (mg)
0	10	2.00	26	81	106	9	1.60	410	.40	.50	5.5	.60	109	16
0	1	1.80	5	27	21	240	.31	375	.40	.40	5.0	.50	100	15
0	10	4.50	60	150	168	195	1.50	375	.38	.43	5.0	.50	100	0
0	10	4.50	60	100	168	170	1.50	378	.38	.43	5.0	.50	100	0
0	10	8.10	60	150	150	240	3.75	378	.38	.43	5.0	.50	100	0
0	4	1.80	6	16	22	157	2	375	.40	.40	5.0	.50	100	0
0	24	6.2[64]	16	56	82	476	.34	521[64]	.5[64]	.6[64]	6.9[64]	.7	136	21[64]
0	76	4.84	141	494	612	12	4.47	4	.73	.31	2.14	.43	99	1
0	20	16	52	153	183	341	2	753[64]	.7[64]	.9[64]	10.0[64]	1	200	0
0	11	4.50	31	84	99	218	.57	375	.40	.40	5.0	.50	100	—
0	3	1.80	6	13	36	225	.11	375	.40	.40	5.0	.50	100	15
0	23	5.2[64]	39	122	115	299	.87	437[64]	.4[64]	.5[64]	5.8[64]	.6	4	17[64]
0	16	5.60	46	132	151	202	.90	463	.50	.50	6.2	.60	23	19
0	4	1.40	8	22	70	166	1.20	291	.30	.30	3.9	.40	78	—
0	—	12.7	7	—	26	161	.16	717	.09	1.06	12.9	1.18	286	33
0	23	5.40	8	26	29	226	.17	250	.27	.27	3.33	.33	2	10
0	154	11.6	55	238	197	229	1.55	0	.95	1.00	11.6	.05	37	—
0	36	5.1[64]	27	88	66	227	.56	424[64]	.4[64]	.5[64]	5.6[64]	.6	—	17[64]
0	71	3.78	116	354	389	232	2.19	8	.39	.19	.83	.32	85	0
0	11	1.45	32	126	108	277	5.40	540	.50	.60	7.2	.70	145	22
0	1	.89	27	120	98	276	5.50	556	.50	.60	7.4	.75	148	22
0	8	1.13	31	104	72	272	5.30	530	.50	.60	7.0	.70	141	21
0	12	1.24	34	164	120	299	5.80	583	.60	.70	7.7	.80	155	23
0	46	8.12	312	801	824	457	5.74	0	1.60	1.80	20.9	2.10	200	63
0	49	.83	34	104	138	12	.63	2	.09	.15	.6	.64	8	0
0	157	2.89	71	350	513	52	2.00	8	.33	.58	1.88	.11	17	—
0	160	3.12	124	347	538	47	2.11	8	.30	.64	2.08	.17	45	—
0	4	21[64]	12	47	51	378	.5	1769[64]	1.7[64]	2[64]	23.3[64]	2.3	466	70[64]
0	9	6.31	12	25	45	241	.18	—	.54	.76	5.80	.91	8	—
0	25	24[64]	73	200	307	293	5.0	500[64]	.51[64]	.57[64]	6.67[64]	.67	133	0
0	27	9.01[64]	96	237	349	370	3.01	750[64]	.74[64]	.85[64]	10[64]	1.02	200	0
0	10	5.60	20	50	144	350	4.70	467	.50	.60	6.30	.60	125	0
0	3	1.20	5	19	22	158	.26	1	.27	.20	3.34	.33	67	10
0	4	1.8[64]	10	34	30	340	.48	388[64]	.4[64]	.4[64]	5.0[64]	.5	100	15[64]
0	1	.15[64]	4	14	16	<1	.14	0	.02[64]	.01[64]	.42[64]	.01	3	0
0	12	1.35	42	112	115	3	1.05	0	.08	.09	1.67	.08	16	0
0	9	5.06[64]	18	62	55	298	4.16	429[64]	.45[64]	.45[64]	5.63[64]	.56	112	17[64]
0	2	1.80	2	8	20	90	1.50	225	.40	.40	5.00	.50	100	15
0	1	2.2[64]	3	26	22	284	.05	463[64]	.5[64]	.5[64]	6.2[64]	.6	124	19[64]
0	7	2.1[64]	20	60	123	29	1.7	437[64]	.4[64]	.5[64]	5.8[64]	.6	116	0
0	3	1.8[64]	13	31	42	75	.28	375[64]	.37[64]	.43[64]	5[64]	.5	100	15[64]
0	11	3.80	26	96	71	183	.69	318	.30	.40	4.20	.40	9	13
0	6	2.57	19	65	71	259	.58	556	.55	.63	7.40	.80	—	22
0	200	21[64]	34	137	123	330	.15	1769[64]	1.7[64]	2[64]	23.3[64]	2.3	400	70[64]
0	6	4.5[64]	6	22	27	169	.13	379[64]	.4[64]	.4[64]	4.9[64]	.5	99	15[64]
0	—	7.70	53	163	174	306	1.19	<1	.50	.60	7.10	.70	143	2
0	18	7.30	58	182	174	308	1.23	0	.60	.17	8.10	.80	162	24
0	3	.57	17	43	42	0	.30	0	.02	.03	1.30	.02	4	0
0	44	4.6[64]	32	100	108	363	.65	388[64]	.4[64]	.4[64]	5.1[64]	.5	9	15[64]

[64] Nutrient added (values sometimes based on label declaration).

(For purposes of calculations, use "0" for t, <1, <.1, <.01, etc.)

Table A–1   Food Composition

Grp	Computer Code No.	Food Description	Measure	Wt (g)	H$_2$O (%)	Ener (cal)	Prot (g)	Carb (g)	Dietary Fiber (g)	Fat (g)	Fat Breakdown (g) Sat	Mono	Poly
		GRAIN PRODUCTS—Con.											
		Buckwheat:											
		Flour:											
7	523	Dark	1 c	98	12	338	12	71	8	3	.5	.8	.9
7	524	Light	1 c	98	12	340	6	78	6	1	.2	.4	.4
7	525	Whole grain, dry	1 c	175	11	586	23	128	16	4	.8	1.4	1.5
		Bulgar:											
7	526	Dry, uncooked	1 c	140	9	479	17	106	31	2	.3	.2	.8
7	527	Cooked	1 c	182	78	151	6	34	11	<1	.1	.1	.2
		Cornmeal:											
7	528	Whole-ground, unbolted, dry	1 c	122	10	442	10	94	13	4	.6	1.2	2
7	529	Bolted, nearly whole, dry	1 c	122	10	441	10	91	12	4	.6	1.2	2
7	530	Degermed, enriched, dry	1 c	138	12	505	12	107	10	2	.3	.6	1
7	531	Degermed, enriched, cooked	1 c	240	88	120	3	26	3	<1	.1	.1	.3
		Macaroni, cooked:											
7	532	Enriched	1 c	140	66	197	7	40	2	1	.1	.1	.4
7	533	Vegetable, enriched	1 c	134	68	172	6	36	2	.1	<.1	<.1	<.1
7	534	Whole wheat	1 c	140	67	174	8	37	2	1	.1	.1	.3
7	535	Millet, cooked	½ c	120	71	143	4	28	1	1	.2	.2	.6
		Noodles:											
7	536	Egg noodles, cooked	1 c	160	69	213	8	40	4	2	.5	.7	.6
7	537	Chow mein, dry	1 c	45	.73	237	4	26	2	14	2	4	8
7	538	Spinach noodles, dry	3½ oz	100	8	372	13	75	7	2	1.0	1.1	1.1
7	1343	Oat bran, dry	¼ c	25	6	61	4	17	4	2	.3	.6	.7
		Popcorn:											
7	539	Air popped, plain	1 c	8	4	30	1	6	1	<1	t	.1	.2
7	540	Popped in veg oil/salted	1 c	11	3	55	1	6	1	3	.5	1.4	1.2
7	541	Sugar-syrup coated	1 c	35	4	135	2	30	1	1	.1	.3	.6
		Rice:											
7	542	Brown rice, cooked	1 c	195	73	217	5	45	3	2	.3	.6	.6
		White, enriched, all types:											
7	543	Regular/long grain, dry	1 c	185	12	675	13	148	2	1	.3	.4	.3
7	544	Regular/long grain, cooked	1 c	205	69	264	6	57	1	<1	.2	.2	.2
7	545	Instant, prepared without salt	1 c	165	76	162	3	35	1	<1	.1	.1	.1
		Parboiled/converted rice:											
7	546	Raw, dry	1 c	185	10	686	13	151	4	1	.3	.3	.3
7	547	Cooked	1 c	175	73	200	4	43	1	<1	.1	.2	<.1
7	548	Wild rice, cooked	1 c	164	74	166	4	35	3	<1	.1	.1	<.1
7	549	Rye flour, medium	1 c	102	10	361	10	79	15	2	.2	.2	.8
7	1044	Soy flour, low fat	1 c	88	3	370	51	34	12	6	.9	1.3	3.3
		Spaghetti, cooked:											
7	550	without salt, enriched	1 c	140	66	197	7	40	2	1	.5	.1	.4
7	551	with salt, enriched	1 c	140	66	197	7	40	2	1	.5	.1	.4
7	552	Whole wheat spaghetti, cooked	1 c	140	94	174	7	37	5	1	.1	.1	.3
7	1302	Tapioca, dry	1 c	152	11	518	.3	135	2	<.1	<.1	<.1	<.1
7	553	Wheat bran	½ c	30	10	65	5	19	8	1	.2	.2	.7
		Wheat germ:											
7	554	Raw	1 c	100	11	360	23	52	12	10	1.7	1.4	6
7	555	Toasted	1 c	113	6	432	33	56	16	12	2.1	1.7	7.5
7	556	Rolled wheat, cooked	1 c	240	80	142	4	32	5	1	.1	.1	.3
7	557	Whole-grain wheat, cooked	⅓ c	50	86	28	1	7	1	<1	<.1	<.1	.1

(Computer code number is for West Diet Analysis program)

GRP KEY: 1 = BEV   2 = DAIRY   3 = EGGS   4 = FAT/OIL   5 = FRUIT   6 = BAKERY   7 = GRAIN   8 = FISH   9 = BEEF   10 = POULTRY
11 = SAUSAGE   12 = MIXED/FAST   13 = NUTS/SEEDS   14 = SWEETS   15 = VEG/LEG   16 = MISC   22 = SOUP/SAUCE

Chol (mg)	Calc (mg)	Iron (mg)	Magn (mg)	Phos (mg)	Pota (mg)	Sodi (mg)	Zinc (mg)	VT-A (RE)	Thia (mg)	Ribo (mg)	Niac (mg)	V-B6 (mg)	Fola (µg)	VT-C (mg)
0	32	2.5	135	298	490	1	2.65	0	.58	.16	2.75	.41	125	0
0	11	1	47	86	314	1	2.56	0	.09	.05	.47	.09	100	0
0	200	6.7	335	560	740	3	4.4	0	1.05	.26	7.7	.37	53	0
0	49	3.4	230	420	574	24	2.7	0	.33	.16	7.2	.48	38	0
0	18	1.8	58	73	124	9	1.04	0	.1	.05	1.8	.15	33	0
0	7	4.2	155	294	350	43	2.22	57	.47	.25	4.4	.37	31	0
0	21	4.2	154	272	303	43	2.22	57	.37	.1	2.3	.56	29	0
0	7	5.7	55	116	224	4	1	57	1	1	7	.35	66	0
0	2	1.48	17	34	38	1	.23	14	.14	.1	1.2	.06	6	0
0	10	2	25	76	43	1	.74	0	.29	.14	2.34	.05	10	0
0	15	1	26	67	42	8	.59	7	.15	.08	1.4	.03	4	0
0	21	1.5	42	125	62	4	1.1	0	.2	.1	1	.11	7	0
0	4	1	53	120	74	2	1.1	0	.1	.1	1.6	.13	23	0
50	19	2.5	30	110	45	11	1	10	.3	.13	2.4	.06	11	0
0	14	2.1	23	72	54	197	1	4	.3	.2	3	.05	10	0
0	58	2.1	174	322	376	36	2.8	46	.37	.2	4.6	.32	48	0
0	15	1.4	59	184	142	1	.78	0	.29	.05	.23	.04	13	—
0	1	.2	23	22	20	<1	.22	1	.03	.01	.2	.02	3	0
0	3	.27	25	31	19	86	.28	2	.01	.02	.1	.02	3	0
0	2	.5	29	47	90	<1	.29	3	.13	.02	.4	.03	3	0
0	20	1	84	162	84	10	1.23	0	.19	.05	3	.28	8	0
0	52	8	46	213	213	9	2.02	0	1	1	7.76	.3	15	0
0	23	2.3	27	96	80	4	.94	0	.33	.03	3.03	.19	6	0
0	13	1.04	8	23	6.6	5[69]	.4	0	.12	.08	1.45	.017	6.6	0
0	111	7	57	252	222	9.3	1.78	0	1.1	.13	6.7	.65	32	0
0	33	2	21	74	65	5	.54	0	.44	.03	2.5	.03	7	0
0	5	1	53	135	166	5	2.2	0	.1	.14	2.1	.221	43	0
0	25	2.16	77	211	347	3	2	0	.29	.11	1.76	.273	38	0
0	165	5.27	202	522	2262	16	1.04	4	.33	.25	1.90	.46	361	0
0	10	2.00	25	76	43	1	.74	0	.29	.14	2.34	.05	10	0
0	10	2	25	76	43	140	.74	0	.29	.14	2.34	.05	10	0
0	21	1.5	42	125	62	4	1.14	0	.15	.06	1	.11	7	0
0	30	2.4	1.5	10.6	17	2	.182	0	.01	.15	0	0	6	0
0	22	3.2	183	304	355	.6	2.18	0	.16	.17	4.07	.39	24	0
0	39	6.3	239	842	892	12	12	0	1.88	.5	6	1.3	281	0
0	51	10.3	362	1295	1070	5	18.9	0	1.89	.93	6.32	1.11	398	0
0	17	1.5	58	130	165	2	1.22	0	.17	.06	2.2	.08	27	0
0	3	.3	12	26	33	<1	.24	0	.04	.01	.5	.03	4	0

[69] If prepared with salt according to label recommendation, sodium would be 608 mg.

(For purposes of calculations, use "0" for t, <1, <.1, <.01, etc.)

Table A–1   Food Composition

Grp	Computer Code No.	Food Description	Measure	Wt (g)	H₂O (%)	Ener (cal)	Prot (g)	Carb (g)	Dietary Fiber (g)	Fat (g)	Fat Breakdown (g) Sat	Mono	Poly
		Wheat flour (unbleached):											
		All-purpose white flour, enriched:											
7	558	Sifted	1 c	115	12	419	12	88	3	1	.2	.1	.5
7	559	Unsifted	1 c	125	12	455	13	95	3	1	.2	.1	.5
7	560	Cake or pastry flour, enriched, sifted	1 c	96	12	348	8	75	3	1	.1	.1	.4
7	561	Self-rising, enriched, unsifted	1 c	125	11	442	12	93	3	1	.2	.1	.5
7	562	Whole wheat, from hard wheats	1 c	120	10	407	16	87	15	2	.4	.3	1
MEATS: FISH and SHELLFISH													
8	1045	Bass, baked or broiled	3.5 oz.	100	70	125	24	0	0	4	.9	1.6	1.2
		Bluefish:											
8	1046	Baked or broiled	3.5 oz.	100	68	159	26	0	0	5	1.1	2.1	1.3
8	1047	Fried in bread crumbs	3.5 oz.	100	61	205	23	5	0	10	2.1	4.3	2.5
		Clams:											
8	563	Raw meat only	3 oz	85	82	63	11	2	<1	1	.1	.1	.2
8	564	Canned, drained	3 oz	85	64	126	22	4	t	2	.2	.2	.5
8	1290	Steamed, meat only	20 ea	90	64	133	23	5	<1	2	.2	.2	.5
		Cod:											
8	565	Baked with butter	3½ oz	100	75	132	23	0	0	3	.4	.3	.5
8	566	Batter fried	3½ oz	100	61	199	20	8	0	10	3.9	5.5	.9
8	567	Poached, no added fat	3½ oz	100	76	102	22	0	0	1	.2	.1	.3
		Crab, meat only:											
8	1048	Blue crab, cooked	1 c	135	77	138	27	0	0	2	.3	.4	.9
8	1049	Dungeness Crab, cooked	.75 c	101	74	85	18	<1	0	2	.3	.6	1.1
8	568	Canned	1 c	135	76	133	28	0	0	2	.3	.3	.6
8	1587	Crab, imitation, from surimi	3 oz	85	74	87	10	9	0	1	—	—	—
8	569	Fish sticks, breaded pollock	2 ea	57	46	155	9	14	<1	7	1.8	2.9	1.8
		Flounder/sole, baked with lemon juice:											
8	570	With butter	3 oz	85	73	120	16	<1	0	6	3.2	1.5	.5
8	571	With margarine	3 oz	85	73	120	16	<1	0	6	1.2	2.3	1.9
8	572	Without added fat	3 oz	85	78	99	21	0	0	1	.3	.3	.4
		Haddock:											
8	573	Breaded, fried[70]	3 oz	85	61	175	17	7	<1	9	2.4	3.9	2.4
8	1050	Smoked	3.5 oz	100	72	116	25	0	0	1	.2	.2	.3
8	574	Broiled with butter and lemon juice	3 oz	85	72	140	23	0	0	6	3.3	1.6	.7
8	1051	Smoked	3.5 oz	100	49	224	21	0	0	15	2.5	4.8	6.9
8	1054	Raw	3.5 oz	100	78	110	21	0	0	2	.3	.7	.8
8	575	Herring, pickled	3 oz	85	55	223	12	8	0	15	2.0	10	1.4
8	1052	Lobster meat, cooked w/ moist heat	1 c	145	77	142	30	2	0	1	.2	.2	1
8	576	Ocean perch, breaded/fried	3 oz	85	59	185	16	7	<1	11	3	5	3
8	1056	Octopus, raw	3.5 oz.	100	80	82	15	2	0	1	.2	.2	.2
		Oysters:											
8	577	Raw, Eastern	1 c	248	85	170	18	10	0	6	1.6	.6	1.8
8	578	Raw, Pacific	1 c	248	82	200	23	12	0	6	1.3	.9	2.2
		Cooked:											
8	579	Eastern, breaded, fried, medium	6 ea	88	65	173	8	10	<1	11	2.8	4.1	2.9
8	580	Western, simmered	3½ oz	100	71	135	19	7	0	2	.5	.4	.9
		Pollock, cooked:											
8	581	Baked or broiled	3 oz	85	74	96	20	0	0	1	.2	.1	.6
8	1055	Moist heat, poached	3.5 oz	100	72	128	23	0	0	1	.2	.1	.6

[70] Dipped in egg, milk and bread crumbs; fried in vegetable shortening.

(Computer code number is for West Diet Analysis program)

GRP KEY: 1 = BEV   2 = DAIRY   3 = EGGS   4 = FAT/OIL   5 = FRUIT   6 = BAKERY   7 = GRAIN   8 = FISH   9 = BEEF   10 = POULTRY
11 = SAUSAGE   12 = MIXED/FAST   13 = NUTS/SEEDS   14 = SWEETS   15 = VEG/LEG   16 = MISC   22 = SOUP/SAUCE

A

Chol (mg)	Calc (mg)	Iron (mg)	Magn (mg)	Phos (mg)	Pota (mg)	Sodi (mg)	Zinc (mg)	VT-A (RE)	Thia (mg)	Ribo (mg)	Niac (mg)	V-B6 (mg)	Fola (µg)	VT-C (mg)
0	17	5.34	25	124	123	2	.8	0	.90	.57	6.8	.05	30	0
0	19	5.8	28	135	134	3	.88	0	1.0	.62	7.4	.06	33	0
0	13	7	15	82	101	2	.6	0	.90	.41	6.5	.032	18	0
0	423	5.8	24	744	155	1587	.78	0	.80	.50	7.29	.06	53	0
0	41	4.7	166	415	486	6	3.52	0	.54	.26	7.6	.41	53	0
80	86	1.61	32	216	385	75	.70	35	.10	.03	2.40	.35	9	0
63	9	.62	42	290	477	77	1.04	127	.08	.11	7.78	.53	2	<1
60	8	.53	37	285	413	67	.90	120	.06	.08	5.50	.37	2	<1
29	39	11.9	8	144	267	47	1.16	77	.09	.18	1.5	.07	13	9
57	78	23.8	16	287	534	95	2.32	145	.01	.36	2.85	.07	4	3
60	83	25.2	17	304	565	100	2.46	154	.01	.38	3.02	.08	4	4
60	20	.49	42	140	245	224	.58	30	.09	.08	2.51	.28	10	<1
55	80	.5	36	200	370	100	.5	26	.04	.04	2.2	.24	9	<1
55	14	.49	42	138	244	78	.58	14	.09	.08	2.51	.28	11	<1
135	140	1.22	45	278	437	376	5.70	20	.14	.12	3.00	.33	20	2
64	46	.37	46	184	359	299	4.33	14	.04	.16	2.92	.33	20	2
120	137	1.13	52	351	505	450	5.42	14	.11	.11	1.85	.41	22	0
17	11	.33	—	—	77	715	—	—	—	.02	.15	—	—	—
64	11	.42	14	103	149	332	.38	18	.07	.1	1.21	.03	10	0
68	16	.28	50	187	272	145	.53	54	.07	.1	1.85	.20	10	1
55	16	.28	50	187	273	151	.53	69	.07	.1	1.85	.20	10	1
58	16	.28	50	246	292	89	.53	10	.07	.1	1.85	.20	10	1
55	34	1.15	26	183	270	123	.85	20	.06	.1	2.9	.13	14	0
77	49	1.40	54	251	415	763	.50	22	.05	.05	5.07	.40	3	<1
45	51	.91	91	242	490	100	.43	174	.06	.08	6.06	.34	6	<1
100	48	.84	83	222	450	480	.42	45	.05	.07	5.80	.33	5	<1
32	47	.84	83	222	450	54	.42	47	.06	.08	5.85	.34	12	<1
11	65	1.04	8	76	59	740	.45	219	.03	.12	2.8	.11	2	0
104	88	.57	51	268	510	551	4.23	38	<1	1	1.55	.112	16	t
46	92	1.2	26	191	241	138	.41	20	.10	.11	2	.22	6	0
48	53	5.30	—	186	—	—	1.68	<1	.03	.04	2.10	.36	—	<1
136	111	16.6	135	344	568	277	226[71]	223	.34	.41	3.3	.12	25	24
136	20	12.7	55	402	417	262	41.2[71]	223	.17	.58	5	.12	25	72
72	54	6.12	51	140	215	367	76.7[71]	86	.13	.18	1.45	.06	12	7
48	16	10.2	44	322	334	210	33[71]	81	.14	.46	3.82	.10	17	7
82	5	.24	31	250	329	98	.51	19	.06	.07	1.4	.06	4	t
70	60	.53	1	252	400	98	.54	9	.04	.18	3.14	.27	12	0

[71] Value varies widely.

(For purposes of calculations, use "0" for t, <1, <.1, <.01, etc.)

Table A–1   Food Composition

Grp	Computer Code No.	Food Description	Measure	Wt (g)	H₂O (%)	Ener (cal)	Prot (g)	Carb (g)	Dietary Fiber (g)	Fat (g)	Fat Breakdown (g) Sat	Mono	Poly
MEATS: FISH and SHELLFISH—Con.													
		Salmon:											
8	582	Canned pink, solids and liquid	3 oz	85	69	118	17	0	0	5	1.3	1.5	1.7
8	583	Broiled or baked	3 oz	85	62	183	23	0	0	9	1.6	4.5	2.1
8	584	Smoked	3 oz	85	72	99	16	0	0	4	.8	1.7	.8
8	585	Atlantic sardines, canned, drained, 2 = 24 g	3 oz	85	60	177	21	0	0	11	1.4	3.6	4.7
8	586	Scallops, breaded, cooked from frozen	6 ea	93	59	200	17	9	<1	10	2.5	4.2	2.7
8	1588	Scallops, imitation, from surimi	3 oz	85	74	84	11	9	0	<1	—	—	—
		Shrimp:											
8	587	Cooked, boiled, 18 large shrimp	3½ oz	100	77	99	21	0	0	1	.3	.2	.4
8	588	Canned, drained	⅔ c	85	73	102	20	1	0	2	.3	.3	.6
8	589	Fried, 4 large = 30g[70]	12 ea	90	53	218	19	10	<1	11	1.9	3.4	4.6
8	1057	Raw, large, about 7 g each	14 ea	100	76	106	20	1	0	2	.3	.3	.7
8	1589	Shrimp, imitation, from surimi	3 oz	85	75	86	11	8	0	1	—	—	—
8	1053	Snapper, baked or broiled	3.5 oz	100	70	128	26	0	0	2	.4	.3	.6
8	1060	Squid, fried in flour[72]	3 oz	85	65	149	15	7	<1	6	1.6	2.3	1.8
8	1590	Surimi[73]	3 oz	85	76	84	13	6	0	1	—	—	—
		Swordfish:											
8	1058	Baked or broiled	3.5 oz	100	76	121	20	0	0	4	1.1	1.6	.9
8	1059	Raw	3.5 oz	100	69	155	25	0	0	5	1.4	2.0	1.2
8	590	Trout, baked or broiled	3 oz	85	63	129	22	<1	0	4	.7	1.1	1.3
		Tuna, light, canned, drained solids:											
8	591	Oil pack	3 oz	85	60	163	25	0	0	7	1.2	1.4	3.1
8	592	Water pack	3 oz	85	71	111	25	0	0	1	.2	.1	.3
8	1061	Tuna, raw, average	3.5 oz	100	68	144	23	0	0	5	1.3	1.4	1.7
MEATS: BEEF, LAMB, PORK and others													
		BEEF, cooked:[74]											
		Braised, simmered, pot roasted:											
		Relatively fat, like choice chuck blade:											
9	593	Lean and fat, piece 2½ × 2½ × ¾″	3 oz	85	47	295	23	0	0	22	9	9	.8
9	594	Lean only	3 oz	85	55	223	26	0	0	12	5	5	.4
		Relatively lean, like choice round:											
9	595	Lean and fat, piece 4⅛ × 2¼ × ¾″	3 oz	85	52	233	24	0	0	14	5	6	.5
9	596	Lean only	3 oz	85	57	187	27	0	0	8	2.7	3.5	.3
		Ground beef, broiled, patty 3 × ⅝″:											
9	597	Extra lean, about 16% fat	3 oz	85	57	225	24	0	0	13	5.3	6.0	.5
9	598	Lean, 21% fat	3 oz	85	53	238	24	0	0	15	6	6.7	.6
		Roasts, oven cooked, no added liquid:											
		Relatively fat, prime rib:											
9	601	Lean and fat, piece 4⅛ × 2¼ × ½″	3 oz	85	46	319	19	0	0	27	11	11	1
9	602	Lean only	3 oz	85	58	204	23	0	0	12	5	5	.4
		Relatively lean, choice round:											
9	603	Lean and fat, piece 2½ × 2½ × ¾″	3 oz	85	59	204	23	0	0	12	5	5	.4
9	604	Lean only	3 oz	85	65	148	25	0	0	5	2	2	.15
		Steak, broiled, relatively lean, choice sirloin:											
9	605	Lean and fat, piece 2½ × 2½ × ¾″	3 oz	85	52	240	23	0	0	16	7	7	.6
9	606	Lean only	3 oz	85	62	171	26	0	0	7	3.0	3	.3

[70]Dipped in egg, bread crumbs, and flour; fried in vegetable shortening.
[72]Recipe is 94.6% squid, 4.9% flour, and 0.6% salt.
[73]Surimi is processed from Walleye (Alaska) pollock. Also see Imitation crab, shrimp, scallops.
[74]Outer layer of fat removed to about 1/2″ of the lean. Deposits of fat within the cut remain.

(Computer code number is for West Diet Analysis program)

GRP KEY: 1 = BEV   2 = DAIRY   3 = EGGS   4 = FAT/OIL   5 = FRUIT   6 = BAKERY   7 = GRAIN   8 = FISH   9 = BEEF   10 = POULTRY
11 = SAUSAGE   12 = MIXED/FAST   13 = NUTS/SEEDS   14 = SWEETS   15 = VEG/LEG   16 = MISC   22 = SOUP/SAUCE

A

Chol (mg)	Calc (mg)	Iron (mg)	Magn (mg)	Phos (mg)	Pota (mg)	Sodi (mg)	Zinc (mg)	VT-A (RE)	Thia (mg)	Ribo (mg)	Niac (mg)	V-B6 (mg)	Fola (µg)	VT-C (mg)
37	181[75]	.72	29	279	277	471	.78	14	.02	.16	5.6	.10	13	0
74	6	.47	26	234	319	56	.43	53	.18	.14	5.67	.19	14	0
20	9	.72	15	139	149	666	.26	22	.02	.09	4.01	.24	2	0
121	325[75]	2.5	33	417	337	429	1.11	57	.07	.19	4.5	.14	10	0
57	39	.76	55	219	310	431	.99	21	.04	.10	1.4	.18	11	0
18	7	.26	—	—	88	676	—	—	.01	.01	.26	—	—	—
195	39	3.09	34	137	182	224	1.56	18	.03	.03	2.59	.13	4	<1
147	50	2.32	35	198	179	143	1.07	15	.02	.03	2.34	.09	2	0
159	60	1.13	36	196	213	310	1.24	50	.12	.12	2.76	.09	7	1.4
152	52	2.41	37	205	185	148	1.11	3	.03	.03	2.55	.10	3	2
31	16	.51	—	—	76	599	—	—	.02	.03	.15	—	—	—
47	40	.24	37	201	522	57	.44	12	.05	.08	3.46	.27	9	<1
221	33	.86	33	213	237	260	1.5	0	.05	.39	2.21	.05	—	4
25	7	.22	—	—	95	122	—	—	.02	.02	.19	—	—	—
39	4	.81	27	263	288	90	1.15	36	.04	.10	9.68	.33	14	1
50	6	1.04	34	337	369	115	1.47	41	.04	.12	11.8	.38	16	1
62	73	2.07	33	272	539	29	1.18	19	.07	.19	2.3	.42	6	3
27	11	1.2	26	265	176	301	.77	20	.03	.09	10.1	.32	5	0
28	10	2.7	26	158	267	303	.77	20	.03	.10	13.2	.32	5	0
38	16	1.02	38	191	252	39	.60	18	.24	.25	8.65	.46	25	0
84	9	2.6	16	183	206	50	5.7	0	.06	.20	2.66	.24	8	0
90	11	3.13	20	199	223	60	8.73	0	.07	.24	2.27	.25	5	0
82	5	2.65	19	208	239	43	4.18	0	.06	.21	3.17	.28	9	0
82	4	2.94	21	231	262	43	4.66	0	.06	.22	3.47	.31	9	0
84	8	2.36	21	162	314	70	5.47	0	.06	.27	5	.27	9	0
86	10	2.08	20	155	297	76	5.27	0	.05	.2	5	.27	9	0
72	9	2	16	146	251	54	4.5	0	.06	.15	2.9	.22	6	0
69	9	2.2	21	181	319	63	5.90	0	.07	.18	3.5	.26	7	0
61	5	1.6	20	175	305	50	3.7	0	.07	.14	2.95	.3	5	0
58	4	3	23	192	335	53	4	0	.08	.15	3.2	.31	6	0
77	9	2.6	24	185	305	53	5	0	1	.22	3.3	.34	8	0
76	9	3	27	208	343	56	6	0	.1	.25	3.6	.38	9	0

[75] If bones are discarded, calcium value is greatly reduced.

(For purposes of calculations, use "0" for t, <1, <.1, <.01, etc.)

Table A–1   Food Composition

Grp	Computer Code No.	Food Description	Measure	Wt (g)	H$_2$O (%)	Ener (cal)	Prot (g)	Carb (g)	Dietary Fiber (g)	Fat (g)	Fat Breakdown (g)		
											Sat	Mono	Poly
		MEATS: BEEF, LAMB, PORK and others—Con.											
		BEEF, Cooked—Con.											
		Steak, broiled, relatively fat, choice T-bone:											
9	1063	Lean and fat	3 oz	85	50	253	21	0	0	18	7	7.5	.7
9	1064	Lean only	3 oz	85	60	182	24	0	0	9	3.5	3.5	.3
		Variety meats:											
9	1086	Brains, pan fried	3 oz	85	71	167	11	0	0	13	3.2	3.4	2.0
9	599	Heart, simmered	3 oz	85	64	149	25	<1	0	5	1.4	1.1	1.2
9	600	Liver, fried	3 oz	85	56	185	23	7	0	7	2.3	1.4	1.5
9	1062	Tongue, cooked	3 oz	85	56	241	19	<1	0	18	7.6	8.1	.7
9	607	Beef, canned, corned	3 oz	85	58	213	23	0	0	13	5	5	.5
9	608	Beef, dried, cured	1 oz	28	57	47	8	<1	0	1	.4	.5	.1
		LAMB, domestic, cooked:											
		Chop, arm, braised (5.6 oz raw with bone):											
9	609	Lean and fat	2.5 oz	70	44	244	21	0	0	17	7	7	1
9	610	Lean part of #609	1.9 oz	55	49	152	19	0	0	8	2.8	3.4	.5
		Chop, loin, broiled (4.2 oz raw with bone):											
9	611	Lean and fat	2.3 oz	64	52	201	16	0	0	15	6	6	1
9	612	Lean part of #611	1.6 oz	46	61	100	14	0	0	5	1.6	2.0	.3
9	1067	Cutlet, avg of lean cuts, cooked	3 oz	85	62	175	24	0	0	8	2.9	3.6	.5
		Leg, roasted, 3 oz piece = 4⅛ × 2¼ × ½″:											
9	613	Lean and fat	3 oz	85	57	219	22	0	0	14	5.9	5.9	1.0
9	614	Lean only	3 oz	85	64	162	24	0	0	7	2.4	2.9	.4
		Rib, roasted, 3 oz piece = 2½ × 2½ × ¾″:											
9	615	Lean and fat	3 oz	85	48	305	18	0	0	25	11	11	1.9
9	616	Lean only	3 oz	85	60	197	22	0	0	11	4	5	1
		Shoulder, roasted:											
9	1065	Lean and fat	3 oz	85	56	235	19	0	0	17	7.4	7.1	1.4
9	1066	Lean only	3 oz	85	64	163	22	0	0	8	3.1	3.2	.7
		Variety meats:											
9	1069	Brains, pan-fried	3 oz	85	61	232	14	0	0	19	4.8	3.4	1.9
9	1068	Heart, braised	3 oz	85	64	158	22	2	0	7	2.7	1.9	.66
9	1070	Sweetbreads, cooked	3 oz	85	62	196	16	0	0	13	6.3	5.1	.7
9	1071	Tongue, cooked	3 oz	85	58	234	18	0	0	17	6.7	8.5	1.1
		PORK, CURED, cooked (see also #669–672):											
9	617	Bacon, medium slices	3 pce	19	13	109	6	<1	0	9	3.3	4.5	1.1
9	1087	Breakfast strips, cooked	3 pce	34	27	156	10	<1	0	13	4.3	5.6	1.9
9	618	Canadian-style bacon	2 pce	47	62	86	11	1	0	4	1.3	1.9	.4
		Ham, roasted:											
9	619	Lean and fat, 2 pieces 4⅛ × 2¼ × ¼″	3 oz	85	58	207	18	0	0	14	5.1	7	2
9	620	Lean only	3 oz	85	66	133	21	0	0	5	1.6	2.2	.5
9	621	Ham, canned, roasted	3 oz	85	66	140	18	<1	0	7	2.4	3.5	.8
		PORK, fresh, cooked:											
		Chops, loin (cut 3 per lb with bone):											
		Braised:											
9	1291	Lean and fat	1 ea	71	44	261	19	0	0	20	7.2	9.1	2.2
9	1292	Lean only	1 ea	55	51	150	18	0	0	8	2.8	3.6	.0
		Broiled:											
9	622	Lean and fat	3.1 oz	87	50	275	24	0	0	19	7	9	2
9	623	Lean only from #622	2.5 oz	72	57	166	23	0	0	8	2.6	3.4	.9

(Computer code number is for West Diet Analysis program)

GRP KEY: 1 = BEV 2 = DAIRY 3 = EGGS 4 = FAT/OIL 5 = FRUIT 6 = BAKERY 7 = GRAIN 8 = FISH 9 = BEEF 10 = POULTRY
11 = SAUSAGE 12 = MIXED/FAST 13 = NUTS/SEEDS 14 = SWEETS 15 = VEG/LEG 16 = MISC 22 = SOUP/SAUCE

Chol (mg)	Calc (mg)	Iron (mg)	Magn (mg)	Phos (mg)	Pota (mg)	Sodi (mg)	Zinc (mg)	VT-A (RE)	Thia (mg)	Ribo (mg)	Niac (mg)	V-B6 (mg)	Fola (µg)	VT-C (mg)
71	7	2.3	21	156	302	52	3.98	<1	.09	.19	3.47	.29	6	0
68	6	2.55	25	177	346	56	4.59	<1	.09	.21	3.94	.33	7	0
1697	8	1.89	12	328	301	134	1.15	0	.11	.22	3.21	.33	5	3
164	5	6.39	21	213	198	54	2.66	0	.12	1.31	3.46	.18	2	1
410	9	5.34	20	392	310	90	4.63	9126[76]	.18	3.52	12.3	1.22	187	20
91	6	2.88	14	121	153	51	4.08	0	.03	.30	1.83	.14	4	<1
73	10	1.77	12	94	116	856	3.04	0	.02	.13	2.07	.11	8	1
12	2	1.28	9	49	126	984	1.49	0	.02	.06	1.6	1	3	4.2
84	18	1.7	18	145	216	51	4.28	2	.05	.18	4.7	.08	13	0
66	14	1.5	16	127	185	41	4.0	1	.04	.15	3.5	.07	12	0
64	13	1.15	15	125	209	49	2.22	2	.07	.16	4.5	.08	12	0
44	9	.93	13	105	175	39	1.91	1	.05	.13	3.2	.07	11	0
78	13	1.74	22	179	293	64	4.48	<1	.09	.24	5.37	.14	19	0
79	9	1.69	20	162	266	56	3.74	2	.09	.23	5.6	.13	17	0
76	7	1.81	22	175	287	58	4.2	1	.09	.25	5.4	.14	20	0
82	19	1.4	17	141	231	62	2.96	2	.07	.18	5.7	.10	13	0
74	18	1.5	20	165	268	69	3.8	<1	.08	.20	5.24	.13	19	0
78	15	1.72	19	155	220	55	3.81	<1	.08	.21	5.66	.10	17	0
73	14	1.9	22	172	236	57	4.46	<1	.08	.23	5.39	.12	21	0
2128	18	1.73	18	421	304	133	1.70	0	.14	.31	3.87	.20	6	20
212	12	4.70	21	216	160	54	3.13	0	.14	1.01	3.71	.25	2	6
347	29	1.53	20	357	221	179	1.79	0	.03	.2	1.79	.02	12	15
161	8	2.24	14	114	134	57	2.54	0	.07	.36	3.14	.14	2	6
16	2	.32	5	64	92	303	.62	0	.13	.05	1.39	.05	1	6[77]
36	5	.67	9	90	158	714	1.25	0	.25	.13	2.58	.12	1	15
27	5	.38	10	138	181	719	.79	0	.38	.09	3.22	.21	2	10[77]
53	6	.74	16	182	243	1009	1.97	0	.51	.19	3.8	.32	3	0
47	6	.8	19	193	269	1128	2.19	0	.58	.22	4.27	.4	3	0
35	6	.91	16	188	298	908	1.97	0	.82	.21	4.27	.33	4	19[77]
73	6	.82	14	141	245	46	2.15	2	.43	.21	4.24	.26	3	<1
58	5	.77	13	131	230	41	2.05	2	.38	.20	3.82	.25	3	<1
84	4	.71	22	184	312	61	1.68	3	.87	.24	4.35	.35	4	<1
71	4	.66	22	176	302	56	1.61	2	.83	.22	3.99	.34	4	<1

[76] Value varies widely.
[77] Values based on products containing added ascorbic acid or sodium ascorbate. If none added, ascorbic acid content would be negligible.

(For purposes of calculations, use "0" for t, <1, <.1, <.01, etc.)

Table A–1   Food Composition

Grp	Computer Code No.	Food Description	Measure	Wt (g)	H₂O (%)	Ener (cal)	Prot (g)	Carb (g)	Dietary Fiber (g)	Fat (g)	Fat Breakdown (g) Sat	Mono	Poly
		MEATS: BEEF, LAMB, PORK and others—Con.											
		PORK, Fresh Cooked—Con.											
		Pan fried:											
9	624	Lean and fat	3.1 oz	89	45	334	21	0	0	27	10	13	3
9	625	Lean only from #624	2.4 oz	67	54	178	19	0	0	11	3.7	4.8	1.3
		Leg, roasted:											
9	626	Lean and fat, piece 2½ × 2½ × ¾″	3 oz	85	53	250	21	0	0	18	6	8	2
9	627	Lean only from #626	3 oz	85	60	187	24	0	0	9	3.2	4.2	1.1
		Rib, roasted:											
9	628	Lean and fat, piece 2½ × 2½ × ¾″	3 oz	85	51	270	21	0	0	20	7	9	2
9	629	Lean only	3 oz	85	57	210	24	0	0	12	4.1	5.3	1.4
		Shoulder, braised:											
9	630	Lean and fat, 3 pieces 2½ × 2½ × ¼″	3 oz	85	47	293	23	0	0	22	8	10	2
9	631	Lean only	3 oz	85	54	208	27	0	0	10	4	5	1.3
9	1088	Spareribs, cooked, yield from 1 lb raw with bone	6.25 oz	177	40	703	51	0	0	54	20.8	25.1	6.2
9	1095	Rabbit, roasted (1 cup meat=140g)	3 oz	85	59	175	26	0	0	7	2.1	1.9	1.4
		VEAL, cooked:											
9	632	Veal cutlet, braised or broiled, 4⅛ × 2¼ × ½″	3 oz	85	60	166	27	0	0	6	1.6	2.0	.5
9	633	Veal rib roasted, lean, 2 pieces 4⅛ × 2¼ × ¼″	3 oz	85	65	151	22	0	0	6	1.8	2.3	.6
9	634	Veal liver, pan-fried	3 oz	85	53	208	25	3	0	10	3.6	1.6	1.5
9	1096	Venison (Deer meat) roasted	3.5 oz	100	65	158	30	0	0	3	1.3	.9	.6
		MEATS: POULTRY and POULTRY PRODUCTS											
		CHICKEN, cooked:											
		Fried, batter dipped:[78]											
10	635	Breast (5.6 oz with bones)	1 ea	140	52	364	35	13	<1	19	5	8	4
10	636	Drumstick (3.4 oz with bones)	1 ea	72	53	193	16	6	<1	11	3	5	3
10	637	Thigh	1 ea	86	52	238	19	8	<1	14	4	6	3
10	638	Wing	1 ea	49	46	159	10	5	<1	11	3	4	3
		Fried, flour coated:[78]											
10	639	Breast (4.2 oz with bones)	1 ea	98	57	218	31	2	<1	9	2.4	3.4	1.9
10	1212	Breast, without skin	1 ea	86	60	161	29	<1	0	4	1.1	1.5	.9
10	640	Drumstick (2.6 oz with bones)	1 ea	49	57	120	13	1	<1	7	1.8	2.7	1.6
10	641	Thigh	1 ea	62	54	162	17	2	<1	9	2.5	3.6	2.1
10	1099	Thigh, without skin	1 ea	52	59	113	15	1	<1	5	1.5	2.0	1.3
10	642	Wing	1 ea	32	49	103	8	1	<1	7	1.9	2.8	1.6
		Roasted:											
10	643	All types of meat	1 c	140	64	266	41	0	0	10	2.9	3.7	2.4
10	644	Dark meat	1 c	140	63	286	38	0	0	14	3.7	5.0	3.2
10	645	Light meat	1 c	140	65	242	43	0	0	6	1.8	2.2	1.4
10	646	Breast, without skin	½ ea	86	65	142	27	0	0	3	.9	1.1	.7
10	647	Drumstick	1 ea	44	67	76	13	0	0	2	.7	.8	.6
10	648	Thigh	1 ea	62	59	153	16	0	0	10	2.9	3.8	2.1
10	1100	Thigh, without skin	1 ea	52	63	109	14	0	0	6	1.6	2.2	1.3
10	649	Stewed, all types:	1 c	140	67	248	38	0	0	9	2.6	3.3	2.2
10	656	Canned, boneless chicken	5 oz	142	69	235	31	0	0	11	3.1	4.5	2.5
10	1102	Chicken gizzards, simmered	1 ea	22	67	34	6	<1	0	1	.2	.2	.2
10	1101	Chicken hearts, simmered	1 ea	3.3	65	6	1	<1	0	<1	.1	.1	.1
10	650	Chicken liver, simmered	1 ea	20	68	30	5	2	0	1	.4	.3	.2

[78] Fried in vegetable shortening.

(Computer code number is for West Diet Analysis program)

GRP KEY: 1 = BEV   2 = DAIRY   3 = EGGS   4 = FAT/OIL   5 = FRUIT   6 = BAKERY   7 = GRAIN   8 = FISH   9 = BEEF   10 = POULTRY
11 = SAUSAGE   12 = MIXED/FAST   13 = NUTS/SEEDS   14 = SWEETS   15 = VEG/LEG   16 = MISC   22 = SOUP/SAUCE

Chol (mg)	Calc (mg)	Iron (mg)	Magn (mg)	Phos (mg)	Pota (mg)	Sodi (mg)	Zinc (mg)	VT-A (RE)	Thia (mg)	Ribo (mg)	Niac (mg)	V-B6 (mg)	Fola (µg)	VT-C (mg)
92	4	.75	23	190	323	64	1.74	3	.91	.25	4.58	.35	4	<1
71	3	.67	21	178	305	57	1.61	2	.84	.22	4.03	.34	4	<1
79	5	.85	18	210	280	50	2.43	2	.54	.27	3.89	.33	9	<1
80	6	.95	21	239	317	54	2.77	2	.59	.3	4.2	.38	10	<1
69	9	.76	16	190	313	37	1.67	3	.5	.24	4.17	.3	7	<1
67	10	.85	18	218	360	40	1.9	3	.54	.26	4.6	.34	7	<1
93	6	1.4	16	162	286	74	3.43	3	.46	.26	4.43	.23	3	<1
95	6	1.64	19	189	339	85	4.16	3	.5	.3	5	.35	4	<1
214	83	3.27	43	462	566	165	8.14	5	.72	.68	9.69	.62	7	0
73	17	2.02	17	192	255	31	2.02	2	.05	.14	6.09	.29	8	0
100	20	.99	24	213	288	76	4.33	t	.05	.29	7.16	.28	13	0
97	10	.82	20	176	264	82	3.81	t	.05	.25	6.4	.23	12	0
280	10	4.45	22	373	372	112	6.69	4784[79]	.21	2.86	14.4	.73	272	18
112	7	4.47	24	226	335	54	2.75	0	.18	.60	6.71	.32[80]	4[80]	0
119	28	1.75	34	258	282	385	1.33	28	.16	.2	14.7	.6	8	0
62	12	.97	14	106	134	194	1.67	19	.08	.16	3.67	.2	6	0
80	16	1.24	18	134	165	248	1.75	25	.1	.2	4.92	.23	8	0
39	10	.63	8	59	68	157	.67	17	.05	.07	2.58	.15	3	0
88	16	1.17	29	228	253	74	1.07	15	.08	.13	13.5	.57	4	0
78	14	.98	27	212	237	68	.93	6	.07	.11	12.7	.55	4	0
44	6	.66	11	86	112	44	1.42	12	.04	.11	2.96	.17	4	0
60	8	.93	15	116	147	55	1.56	18	.06	.15	4.31	.21	5	0
53	7	.76	14	103	134	49	1.45	11	.05	.13	3.70	.20	4	0
26	5	.4	6	48	57	25	.56	12	.02	.04	2.14	.13	1	0
125	21	1.69	35	273	340	120	2.94	22	.1	.25	12.8	.65	8	0
130	21	1.86	33	250	336	130	3.92	30	.1	.32	9.17	.5	11	0
118	21	1.49	38	302	345	108	1.73	12	.09	.16	17.4	.84	5	0
73	13	.89	25	196	220	64	.86	5	.06	.1	11.8	.52	3	0
41	5	.57	11	81	108	42	1.4	8	.03	.1	2.67	.17	4	0
58	8	.83	14	108	137	52	1.46	30	.04	.13	3.95	.19	4	0
49	6	.68	12	95	124	46	1.34	10	.04	.12	3.39	.18	4	0
116	20	1.63	29	210	252	98	2.79	21	.07	.23	8.56	.37	8	0
88	20	2.2	17	158	196	714	2.13	48	.02	.18	8.99	.5	4	3
43	2	.91	4	34	39	15	.96	12	.01	.05	.87	.03	12	<1
8	1	.30	1	7	4	2	.24	<1	<.01	.02	.09	.01	3	<1
126	3	1.7	2	62	28	10	.87	983	.03	.35	.89	.12	154	3

[79] Value varies widely.
[80] Values estimated from other game meat.

(For purposes of calculations, use "0" for t, <1, <.1, <.01, etc.)

Table A–1   Food Composition

Grp	Computer Code No.	Food Description	Measure	Wt (g)	H₂O (%)	Ener (cal)	Prot (g)	Carb (g)	Dietary Fiber (g)	Fat (g)	Fat Breakdown (g) Sat	Mono	Poly
		MEATS: POULTRY and POULTRY PRODUCTS—Con.											
		DUCK, roasted:											
10	1293	Meat with skin, about 2.7 cups	½ duck	382	52	1287	73	0	0	108	37	49	14
10	651	Meat only, about 1.5 cups	½ duck	221	64	445	52	0	0	25	9.2	8.2	3.2
		GOOSE, domesticated, roasted:											
10	1294	Meat only, 4.2 cups	½ goose	591	57	1406	171	0	0	75	27	26	9
10	1295	Meat w/skin, about 5.5 cups	½ goose	774	52	2362	195	0	0	170	53	79	20
		TURKEY, roasted, meat only:											
10	652	Dark meat	3 oz	85	63	159	24	0	0	6	2.1	1.4	1.8
10	653	Light meat	3 oz	85	66	133	25	0	0	3	.9	.5	.7
10	654	All types, chopped or diced	1 c	140	65	238	41	0	0	7	2.3	1.5	2.0
10	655	All types, sliced	3 oz	85	65	145	25	0	0	4	1.4	.9	1.2
10	1103	Ground turkey, cooked	3.5 oz	100	60	229	24	0	0	14	3.8	5.0	3.3
		Turkey breast:											
10	1104	Barbecued	1 oz	28	70	40	6	0	0	1	.4	.5	.3
10	1105	Hickory smoked	1 oz	28	70	35	6	1	0	1	.3	.3	.3
10	1106	Gizzard, cooked	1 ea	67	65	109	20	<1	0	3	.7	.5	.7
10	1107	Heart, cooked	1 ea	16	64	28	4	<1	0	1	.3	.2	.3
10	1108	Liver, cooked	1 ea	75	66	127	18	3	0	4	1.4	1.1	1.1
		Poultry food products (see also items in sausages and lunchmeats section):											
10	658	Chicken roll, light meat	2 pce	57	69	90	11	1	0	4	1.2	1.7	.9
10	659	Gravy and turkey, frozen package	5 oz	142	85	95	8	7	<1	4	1.2	1.4	.7
10	660	Turkey loaf, breast meat	2 pce	42	72	46	10	0	0	1	.2	.2	.1
10	661	Turkey patties, breaded, fried	1 ea	64	50	181	9	10	<1	12	3	4.8	3
10	662	Turkey, frozen, roasted, seasoned	3 oz	85	68	130	18	3	0	5	1.6	1	1.4
		MEATS: SAUSAGES and LUNCHMEATS (see also Poultry food products)											
		Beerwurst/beer salami:											
11	1072	Beef	1 pce	23	54	75	3	<1	0	7	2.8	3.3	.2
11	1074	Pork	1 pce	23	62	55	3	<1	0	4	1.4	2.1	.5
11	1075	Berliner	1 pce	23	61	53	4	1	0	4	1.4	1.8	.4
		Bologna:											
11	1297	Beef	1 pce	23	55	72	3	<1	0	7	2.7	3.1	.2
11	663	Beef and pork	1 pce	28	54	89	3	1	0	8	3.0	3.8	.7
65	1298	Pork	1 pce	23	61	57	4	<1	0	5	1.6	2.3	.5
11	664	Turkey	1 pce	28	66	56	4	<1	0	4	1.5	1.9	1.2
11	665	Braunschweiger sausage	2 pce	57	48	205	8	2	0	18	6.2	8.5	2.1
11	1073	Brotwurst, link	1 ea	70	51	226	10	2	0	20	7.0	9.3	2.0
11	666	Brown-and-serve sausage links, cooked	1 ea	13	45	50	2	<1	0	5	1.7	2.2	.5
11	1089	Cheesefurter/cheese smokie	1 ea	43	53	141	6	1	0	13	4.5	5.9	1.3
11	1090	Corned beef loaf, jellied	1 pce	28	67	46	7	0	0	2	.8	.9	.1
		Frankfurters (see also #657):											
11	1077	Beef, large link, 8/pkg.	1 ea	57	54	184	6	1	0	17	6.8	8.2	.7
11	1078	Beef and pork, large link, 8/pkg.	1 ea	57	54	183	6	1	0	17	6.1	7.8	1.6
11	667	Beef and pork, smaller link, 10/pkg.	1 ea	45	54	145	5	1	0	13	4.8	6.2	1.2
10	657	Chicken frankfurter, 10/pkg.	1 ea	45	58	115	6	3	0	9	2.5	3.8	1.8
11	668	Turkey, smaller link, 10/pkg.	1 ea	45	63	102	6	1	0	8	2.7	3.3	2.1
		Ham:											
11	669	Ham lunchmeat, canned, 3 x 2 x ½"	1 pce	21	52	70	3	<1	0	6	2.3	3.0	.8
11	670	Chopped ham, packaged	2 pce	22	61	98	7	<1	0	8	2.6	3.9	.9

(Computer code number is for West Diet Analysis program)

GRP KEY: 1 = BEV 2 = DAIRY 3 = EGGS 4 = FAT/OIL 5 = FRUIT 6 = BAKERY 7 = GRAIN 8 = FISH 9 = BEEF 10 = POULTRY
11 = SAUSAGE 12 = MIXED/FAST 13 = NUTS/SEEDS 14 = SWEETS 15 = VEG/LEG 16 = MISC 22 = SOUP/SAUCE

Chol (mg)	Calc (mg)	Iron (mg)	Magn (mg)	Phos (mg)	Pota (mg)	Sodi (mg)	Zinc (mg)	VT-A (RE)	Thia (mg)	Ribo (mg)	Niac (mg)	V-B6 (mg)	Fola (µg)	VT-C (mg)
320	43	10.3	62	595	780	227	7.12	241	.67	1.03	18.4	.70	25	0
198	26	5.97	44	449	557	143	5.75	51	.57	1.04	11.3	.55	22	0
569	84	17.0	148	1828	2291	447	16.0	71	.54	2.31	24.1	2.75	13	0
708	104	21.9	169	2091	2546	543	16.0	162	.60	2.50	32.3	2.89	17	0
72	27	1.99	21	174	247	67	3.8	0	.05	.21	3.1	.3	8	0
59	16	1.14	24	186	259	54	1.73	0	.05	.12	5.81	.46	5	0
107	35	2.49	37	298	418	99	4.34	0	.09	.26	7.62	.64	10	0
64	21	1.51	23	181	254	60	2.64	0	.05	.16	4.63	.39	6	0
69	25	1.93	24	196	270	83	2.86	0	.05	.17	4.82	.39	7	0
16	2	.12	7	74	57	156	.35	0	.01	.03	2.73	.11	1	<1
13	1	.20	7	79	59	208	.30	0	.01	.03	2.75	.11	1	<1
155	10	3.64	13	86	141	37	2.79	37	.02	.22	2.06	.08	36	1
36	2	1.10	4	33	29	9	.84	1	.01	.14	.52	.05	13	<1
469	8	5.85	11	204	146	48	2.32	2806	.04	1.07	4.46	.39	499	1
28	24	.55	10	89	129	331	.41	14	.04	.07	3	.31	2	0
26	20	1.32	11	115	87	787	.99	18	.03	.18	2.55	.14	2	0
17	3	.17	9	97	118	608	.48	0	.02	.05	3.54	.15	2	0[81]
40	9	1.41	12	173	176	512	1.5	7	.06	.12	1.47	.13	3	0
45	4	1.4	20	207	253	578	2.37	0	.04	.14	5.3	.24	5	0
13	2	.31	3	24	42	214	.61	0	.03	.03	.66	.05	1	3
13	2	.17	3	24	58	285	.40	0	.13	.04	.75	.08	1	7
11	3	.27	3	30	65	298	.57	0	.09	.05	.72	.05	1	2
13	3	.32	2	19	36	230	.46	0	.01	.03	.61	.04	1	4
16	3	.43	3	26	51	289	.55	0	.05	.04	.73	.05	1	6[82]
14	3	.18	3	33	65	272	.47	0	.12	.04	.90	.06	1	8
28	23	.43	4	37	56	248	.49	0	.02	.05	1.04	.05	1	<1
89	6	5.32	6	96	113	652	1.62	2406	.14	.87	4.78	.19	57	5[82]
44	34	.72	11	94	197	778	1.47	0	.18	.16	2.31	.09	2	20
9	1	.1	2	14	25	105	.15	0	.05	.02	.40	.03	1	0
29	25	.46	5	76	89	465	.97	3	.11	.07	1.25	.05	1	8
12	3	.58	3	18	25	294	1.08	0	<.01	.03	.46	.04	1	2
27	7	.76	7	47	90	584	1.21	0	.03	.06	1.44	.06	2	14
29	6	.66	7	49	95	639	1.05	0	.11	.07	1.50	.08	2	15
23	5	.52	6	39	75	504	.83	0	.09	.05	1.18	.06	2	12[82]
45	43	.9	8	48	38	616	1	17	.03	.05	1.39	.09	2	0
39	58	.77	8	83	88	454	1	17	.04	.08	1.7	.10	2	<1
13	1	.15	2	17	45	271	.31	0	.08	.04	.66	.04	1	<1
21	3	.4	5	58	119	573	.77	0	.23	.07	1.4	.13	2	1[82]

[81]If sodium ascorbate is added, product contains 11 mg ascorbic acid.
[82]Values based on products containing added ascorbic acid or sodium ascorbate. If none added, ascorbic acid content would be negligible.

(For purposes of calculations, use "0" for t, <1, <.1, <.01, etc.)

Table A–1   Food Composition

Grp	Computer Code No.	Food Description	Measure	Wt (g)	H₂O (%)	Ener (cal)	Prot (g)	Carb (g)	Dietary Fiber (g)	Fat (g)	Fat Breakdown (g) Sat	Mono	Poly
		MEATS: SAUSAGES and LUNCHMEATS—Con.											
		Ham—Con.											
11	671	Ham lunchmeat, regular	2 pce	57	65	103	10	2	0	6	1.9	2.8	.7
11	672	Ham lunchmeat, extra lean	2 pce	57	70	75	11	1	0	3	.9	1.3	.3
11	673	Turkey ham	2 pce	57	72	73	11	1	0	3	1.0	.8	.8
11	1091	Keilbasa sausage	1 pce	26	54	81	3	1	0	7	2.6	3.4	.8
11	1092	Knockwurst sausage-link	1 ea	68	56	209	8	1	0	19	6.9	8.7	2.0
11	1093	Mortadella lunchmeat	1 pce	15	52	47	2	<1	0	4	1.4	1.7	.5
11	1097	Olive loaf lunchmeat	2 pce	57	58	133	7	5	<1	9	3.3	4.5	1.1
11	1080	Pastrami, turkey	2 pce	57	72	74	11	1	0	4	1.0	1.2	.9
11	1081	Pepperoni sausage, small slices	4 pce	22	27	109	5	1	0	10	3.6	4.6	1
11	1094	Pickle & pimento loaf	2 pce	57	57	149	7	3	<1	12	4.5	5.4	1.5
11	1082	Polish sausage	1 oz.	28	53	92	4	<1	0	8	2.9	3.8	.9
		Pork sausage, cooked:[83]											
11	674	Link, small	1 ea	13	45	48	3	<1	0	4	1.4	1.8	.5
11	1079	Patty	1 pce	27	45	100	5	<1	0	8	2.9	3.8	1.0
		Salami:											
11	675	Pork and beef	2 pce	57	60	143	8	1	0	11	4.6	5.2	1.1
11	676	Turkey	2 pce	57	66	111	9	<1	0	8	2.3	2.6	2.0
11	677	Dry, beef and pork	2 pce	20	35	85	5	1	0	7	2.4	3.4	.6
		Sandwich spreads:											
11	1300	Ham salad	1 c	240	63	518	21	26	<1	37	12.1	17.3	6.5
11	678	Pork and beef	1 tbsp	15	60	35	1	2	0	3	.9	1.1	.4
10	1296	Poultry sandwich spread	1 tbsp	13	60	25	2	1	0	2	.5	.4	.8
		Smoked link sausage:											
11	1083	Beef and pork	1 ea	68	39	265	15	1	0	22	7.7	10.0	2.6
11	1084	Pork	1 ea	68	52	229	9	1	0	21	7.2	9.7	2.2
11	1085	Summer sausage	1 pce	23	48	80	4	1	0	7	2.8	3.2	.4
11	1076	Turkey breakfast sausage	1 pce	28	60	65	6	0	0	4	1.6	1.8	1.2
11	679	Vienna sausage, canned	1 ea	16	60	45	2	<1	0	4	1.5	2.0	.3
		MIXED DISHES and FAST FOODS											
		MIXED DISHES:											
		Beef stew with vegetables:											
12	680	Homemade	1 c	245	82	220	16	15	3	11	4.4	4.5	.5
12	1109	Canned	1 c	245	83	194	14	18	1	8	3.1	3.1	.4
12	1116	Beef, macaroni & tomato sauce casserole	1 c	226	80	189	10	25	2	6	2.1	2.3	.4
12	681	Beef pot pie, homemade[84]	1 pce	210	55	515	21	39	1	30	8	13	7
12	682	Chicken à la king, home recipe	1 c	245	68	470	27	12	1	34	13	13	6
12	683	Chicken and noodles, home recipe	1 c	240	71	365	22	26	1	18	5	7	4
12	684	Chicken chow mein, canned	1 c	250	89	95	7	18	5	1	.1	.1	.8
12	685	Chicken chow mein, home recipe	1 c	250	78	255	23	10	4	11	4	4	3
12	686	Chicken pot pie, home recipe[84]	1 pce	232	57	545	23	42	2	31	10	16	7
12	1112	Chicken salad w/celery	.5 c	78	53	266	11	1	<1	25	4.1	7.2	12.0
12	687	Chili with beans, canned	1 c	255	76	286	15	30	8	14	6	6	1
12	688	Chop suey with beef and pork	1 c	250	75	300	26	13	2	17	4	7	4
12	689	Corn pudding[85]	1 c	250	76	271	11	32	9	13	6.3	4.3	1.7
12	690	Cole slaw[86]	1 c	120	82	84	2	15	2	3	.5	.9	1.6
12	1110	Corned beef hash-canned	1 c	220	67	382	18	22	1	10	4.2	4.9	.5
12	1113	Egg salad	1 c	183	66	438	19	3	<1	39	8.4	13.2	13.5

[83] Cooked weight is half the weight of raw sausage.

[84] Crust made with vegetable shortening and enriched flour.

[85] Recipe: 55% yellow corn, 23% whole milk, 14% egg, 4% sugar, 3% salt, and 1% pepper.

[86] Recipe: 41% cabbage; 12% celery; 12% table cream; 12% sugar; 7% green pepper; 6% lemon juice; 4% onion; 3% pimento; 3% vinegar; 2% each for salt, dry mustard, and white pepper.

(Computer code number is for West Diet Analysis program)

GRP KEY: 1=BEV   2=DAIRY   3=EGGS   4=FAT/OIL   5=FRUIT   6=BAKERY   7=GRAIN   8=FISH   9=BEEF   10=POULTRY
11=SAUSAGE   12=MIXED/FAST   13=NUTS/SEEDS   14=SWEETS   15=VEG/LEG   16=MISC   22=SOUP/SAUCE

A

Chol (mg)	Calc (mg)	Iron (mg)	Magn (mg)	Phos (mg)	Pota (mg)	Sodi (mg)	Zinc (mg)	VT-A (RE)	Thia (mg)	Ribo (mg)	Niac (mg)	V-B6 (mg)	Fola (μg)	VT-C (mg)
32	4	.56	11	140	188	746	1.21	0	.49	.14	2.98	.19	2	16[82]
27	4	.43	10	124	198	810	1.09	0	.53	.13	2.74	.26	2	15[82]
32	5	1.56	12	138	163	548	1.58	0	.04	.15	2.72	.16	4	0
17	11	.38	4	38	70	280	.52	0	.06	.06	.75	.05	1	6
39	7	.62	8	67	136	687	1.13	0	.23	.10	1.86	.11	2	18
8	3	.21	2	15	24	187	.32	0	.02	.02	.40	.02	<1	4
22	62	.31	11	72	169	842	.78	0	.17	.15	1.04	.13	1	5
30	5	.81	10	142	155	569	1.46	0	.05	.15	2.48	.16	4	<1
8	2	.31	4	26	76	449	.55	0	.07	.06	1.09	.06	—	<1
21	54	.58	10	79	193	787	.79	<1	.17	.14	1.16	.11	1	8
20	3	.41	4	39	67	248	.55	0	.14	.04	.98	.05	1	0
11	4	.16	2	24	47	168	.33	0	.1	.03	.59	.04	1	<1
22	9	.34	5	50	97	349	.68	0	.20	.07	1.22	.09	2	<1
37	7	1.51	9	65	112	604	1.21	0	.14	.21	2.02	.12	1	7[82]
46	11	.93	9	73	125	535	1.25	0	.06	.15	2.23	.14	5	<1
16	2	.3	4	28	76	372	.64	0	.12	.06	.97	.1	0	6[82]
88	19	1.42	23	286	359	2187	2.64	42	1.04	.29	5.02	.36	3	14
6	2	.12	1	9	16	152	.15	1	.03	.02	.26	.02	<1	0
4	1	.08	3	4	24	49	.25	6	<.01	.01	.22	.01	1	<1
46	20	.79	13	110	228	1020	1.92	0	.48	.18	3.08	.24	2	1
48	7	.99	8	73	129	642	1.44	0	.18	.12	2.19	.12	2	13
16	2	.47	3	23	53	334	.47	0	.04	.07	.94	.07	1	5
23	5	.52	6	52	76	191	.97	0	.03	.08	1.42	.08	1	—
8	2	.14	1	8	16	152	.26	0	.01	.02	.26	.02	<1	0
71	29	2.9	40	184	613	292	5.3	569	.15	.17	4.7	.28	37	17
15	23	3.18	39	56	417	992	4.23	262	.07	.12	2.43	.20	31	7
22	30	2.39	37	118	562	974	2.07	111	.19	.17	3.51	.30	23	16
42	29	3.8	6	149	334	596	3.17	517	.29	.29	4.8	.24	29	6
221	127	2.5	20	358	404	760	1.8	272	.1	.42	5.4	.23	11	12
103	26	2.4	37	247	211	600	2.14	130	.05	.17	4.3	.16	9	1
8	45	1.3	14	85	418	725	1.3	28	.05	.1	1	.09	12	13
75	58	2.50	28	293	473	718	2.12	50	.08	.23	4.3	.41	19	10
56	70	3.0	25	232	343	594	2.0	735	.32	.32	4.9	.46	29	5
48	16	.66	11	80	137	199	.80	31	.03	.08	3.25	.17	4	1
43	119	8.75	115	393	932	1330	5.10	86	.12	.27	.91	.34	41	4
68	60	4.80	32	248	425	1053	3.58	60	.28	.38	5.0	.32	22	33
230	100	1.40	38	143	402	138	1.26	89	1.03	.32	2.47	.30	63	7
10[87]	54	.70	12	38	218	28	.24	98	.08	.07	.33	.18	32	39
132	29	4.40	3	147	440	1354	4.38	0	.12	.40	4.60	.41	15	8
629	94	3.39	21	282	211	428	2.24	300	.12	.45	.16	.18	74	0

[82]Values based on products containing added ascorbic acid or sodium ascorbate. If none added, ascorbic acid content would be negligible.
[87]From dairy cream in recipe.

(For purposes of calculations, use "0" for t, <1, <.1, <.01, etc.)

Table A–1   Food Composition

Grp	Computer Code No.	Food Description	Measure	Wt (g)	H₂O (%)	Ener (cal)	Prot (g)	Carb (g)	Dietary Fiber (g)	Fat (g)	Fat Breakdown (g) Sat	Mono	Poly
		MIXED DISHES and FAST FOODS—Con.											
		MIXED DISHES—Con.											
12	691	French toast, home recipe[88]	1 pce	65	53	123	5	15	1	4	1.1	1.4	1.1
12	1355	Green pepper, stuffed	1 ea	172	76	217	10	16	1	13	5.3	5.2	.6
		Lasagna:											
12	1346	With meat	1 pce	245	64	398	26	30	2	20	9.2	7.2	1.5
12	1111	Without meat	1 pce	218	64	316	20	30	2	14	6.9	4.7	1.3
12	1117	Frozen entree	1 pce	205	73	275	17	19	1	12	6.3	4.2	1.2
		Macaroni and cheese:											
12	692	Canned[89]	1 c	240	80	230	9	26	1	10	5	3	1
12	693	Home recipe[90]	1 c	200	58	430	17	40	1	22	10	7	4
12	1115	Macaroni salad-no cheese	1 c	141	61	371	3	18	1	33	5.1	9.5	17.2
		Meat loaf:											
12	1120	Beef	1 pce	87	62	193	16	4	<1	12	4.8	5.2	.6
12	1119	Beef and pork (1/3)	1 pce	87	59	212	15	5	<1	15	5.5	6.3	1.2
12	1303	Moussaka (lamb and eggplant)	1 c	250	79	250	21	16	6	11	3.6	4.3	1.9
12	715	Potato salad with mayonnaise and egg[91]	1 c	250	76	358	7	28	4	21	4	6	9
12	694	Quiche lorraine, ⅛ of 8″ quiche[84]	1 pce	176	47	600	13	29	1	48	23	18	4
		Spaghetti (enriched) in tomato sauce:											
		With cheese:											
12	695	Canned	1 c	250	80	190	6	39	3	2	.4	.4	.5
12	696	Home recipe	1 c	250	77	260	9	37	3	9	3	3.6	1.2
		With meatballs:											
12	697	Canned	1 c	250	78	260	12	39	3	10	2	4	3
12	698	Home recipe	1 c	248	70	330	19	39	3	12	4	4	2
12	716	Spinach soufflé[92]	1 c	136	74	218	11	3	4	18	7	7	3
12	717	Tuna salad[93]	1 c	205	63	383	33	19	2	19	3	6	9
12	1121	Tuna noodle casserole, recipe	1 c	202	73	251	21	24	<1	7	2.0	1.5	3.2
12	1270	Waldorf salad	1 c	142	58	424	4	13	4	42	5.6	11.2	23.1
		FAST FOODS and SANDWICHES: see end of this appendix for additional Fast Foods.											
		Burrito:[94]											
12	699	Beef and bean	1 ea	175	54	390	21	40	5	18	7	7	2
12	700	Bean	1 ea	174	55	322	13	47	8	10	4	3	2
		Cheeseburger:											
12	701	Regular	1 ea	112	46	300	15	28	1	15	7	6	1
12	702	4-oz patty	1 ea	194	46	524	30	40	2	31	15	12	1
12	703	Chicken patty sandwich	1 ea	157	52	436	25	34	1	22	6	10	5
12	704	Corn dog	1 ea	111	45	330	10	27	<1	20	8	10	1
12	705	Enchilada, cheese	1 ea	163	63	320	10	29	3	19	11	6	.8
12	706	English muffin with egg, cheese, bacon	1 ea	138	49	360	18	31	2	18	8	8	.7
		Fish sandwich:											
12	707	Regular, with cheese	1 ea	140	43	420	16	39	1	23	6	7	8
12	708	Large, without cheese	1 ea	170	48	470	18	41	1	27	6	9	10

[84]Crust made with vegetable shortening and enriched flour.
[88]Recipe: 35% whole milk, 32% white bread, 29% egg, and cooked in 4% margarine.
[89]Made with corn oil.
[90]Made with margarine.
[91]Recipe: 62% potatoes; 12% egg; 8% mayonnaise; 7% celery; 6% sweet pickle relish; 2% onion; 1% each for green pepper, pimiento, salt, and dry mustard.
[92]Recipe: 29% whole milk, 26% spinach, 13% egg white, 13% cheddar cheese, 7% egg yolk, 7% butter, 4% flour, 1% salt and pepper.
[93]Made with drained chunk light tuna, celery, onion, pickle relish, and mayonnaise-type salad dressing.
[94]Made with a 10½″-diameter flour tortilla.

(Computer code number is for West Diet Analysis program)

GRP KEY: 1=BEV   2=DAIRY   3=EGGS   4=FAT/OIL   5=FRUIT   6=BAKERY   7=GRAIN   8=FISH   9=BEEF   10=POULTRY
11=SAUSAGE   12=MIXED/FAST   13=NUTS/SEEDS   14=SWEETS   15=VEG/LEG   16=MISC   22=SOUP/SAUCE

Chol (mg)	Calc (mg)	Iron (mg)	Magn (mg)	Phos (mg)	Pota (mg)	Sodi (mg)	Zinc (mg)	VT-A (RE)	Thia (mg)	Ribo (mg)	Niac (mg)	V-B6 (mg)	Fola (μg)	VT-C (mg)
73	79	1.08	12	82	96	189	.47	57	.15	.17	1.09	.04	18	<1
38	15	2.32	23	91	227	210	2.58	29	.11	.10	2.96	.22	14	83
56	460	3.08	41	393	507	783	3.23	168	.22	.33	3.64	.35	16	7
30	457	2.38	35	345	424	760	1.93	168	.21	.28	2.01	.22	14	7
90	246	2.48	52	253	437	967	1.25	97	.19	.33	2.70	.29	25	6
24	199	1.0	31	182	139	730	1.20	72	.12	.24	1.0	.02	8	<1
24	27	1.14	23	50	162	315	.34	40	.10	.07	.67	.07	7	3
98	29	1.90	19	123	227	340	3.50	26	.06	.18	3.19	.18	8	1
97	33	1.39	18	128	238	392	2.86	26	.19	.19	3.07	.19	8	1
143	129	2.75	44	245	695	485	3.29	125	.25	.32	4.78	.35	44	7
170	48	1.63	39	130	635	1323	.78	83	.19	.15	2.23	.35	17	25
44	362	1.8	37	322	240	1086	1.20	232	.20	.40	1.8	.05	10	1
285	211	1.4	23	276	283	653	1.95	454	.11	.32	1.2	.15	17	<1
3	40	2.8	21	88	303	955	1.12	120	.35	.28	4.5	.13	6	10
8	80	2.3	26	135	408	955	1.3	140	.25	.18	2.3	.20	8	13
23	53	3.3	20	113	245	1220	2.39	100	.15	.18	2.3	.12	5	5
89	124	3.7	40	236	665	1009	2.45	159	.25	.30	.4	.20	10	22
184	230	1.34	37	231	202	763	1.29	675	.09	.31	.48	.12	62	3
27	35	2.0	40	365	365	824	1.15	55	.06	.14	13.3	.17	15	5
52	37	1.94	31	182	224	869	.97	34	.14	.17	8.59	.24	13	1
22	44	.98	41	88	279	246	.69	41	.10	.06	.37	.16	19	6
52	165	2.7	61	274	388	516	3.30	58	.26	.29	4.36	.73	48	5
15	181	2.53	76	243	427	1030	2.37	58	.26	.23	2.40	1.01	55	5
44	135	2.30	22	174	219	672	2.53	65	.26	.24	3.70	.11	20	1
104	236	4.45	43	320	407	1224	5.27	128	.33	.49	7.37	.23	23	3
68	44	1.87	30	173	194	2732	1.00	16	.29	.26	9.21	.37	18	4
37	34	1.94	22	303	164	1252	1.44	<1	.28	.17	3.27	.11	2	3
44	324	1.31	50	133	240	784	2.51	186	.09	.42	1.91	.39	34	1
213	197	3.10	28	290	201	832	1.86	160	.46	.50	3.71	.15	35	1
56	132	1.85	29	223	274	667	.95	25	.32	.27	3.30	.10	24	3
90	61	2.23	34	246	375	621	.88	15	.35	.24	3.52	.12	43	1

(For purposes of calculations, use "0" for t, <1, <.1, <.01, etc.)

Table A–1   Food Composition

Grp	Computer Code No.	Food Description	Measure	Wt (g)	H₂O (%)	Ener (cal)	Prot (g)	Carb (g)	Dietary Fiber (g)	Fat (g)	Fat Breakdown (g) Sat	Mono	Poly
		MIXED DISHES and FAST FOODS—Con.											
		FAST FOODS and SANDWICHES—Con.											
		Hamburger with bun:											
12	709	Regular	1 ea	98	46	245	12	28	1	11	4	5	1
12	710	4-oz patty	1 ea	174	50	445	25	38	1	21	7	12	1
12	711	Hotdog/frankfurter and bun	1 ea	85	53	260	8	21	1	15	5	7	2
12	712	Cheese pizza, ⅛ of 15″ round[95]	1 pce	120	46	290	15	39	2	9	4	3	1
		SANDWICHES:											
		Avocado, cheese, tomato & lettuce:											
12	1276	On white bread, firm	1 ea	205	59	464	15	39	7	29	9.1	11.8	6.0
12	1278	On part whole wheat	1 ea	195	60	432	14	33	8	29	8.7	11.8	6.0
12	1277	On whole wheat	1 ea	209	58	459	16	39	13	29	9.1	11.9	6.2
		Bacon, lettuce & tomato sandwich:											
12	1137	On white bread, soft	1 ea	135	54	333	11	30	2	19	5.2	7.4	5.5
12	1139	On part whole wheat	1 ea	135	54	327	12	28	3	19	4.9	7.5	5.5
12	1138	On whole wheat	1 ea	149	53	355	13	34	8	20	5.4	7.7	5.7
		Cheese sandwich, grilled:											
12	1140	On white bread, soft	1 ea	117	37	399	17	28	1	24	12.7	7.6	2.3
12	1142	On part whole wheat	1 ea	117	37	393	18	27	3	24	12.5	7.7	2.3
12	1141	On whole wheat	1 ea	131	38	420	20	33	7	25	12.9	7.9	2.6
		Chicken salad sandwich:											
12	1143	On white bread, soft	1 ea	99.7	44	300	10	28	1	16	3.0	4.9	7.5
12	1145	On part whole wheat	1 ea	99.7	44	294	11	27	3	16	2.8	5.0	7.5
12	1144	On whole wheat	1 ea	114	44	321	12	33	8	17	3.2	5.2	7.8
12	1146	Corned beef & swiss cheese on rye	1 ea	147	45	429	27	25	5	24	9.4	8.2	5.0
		Egg salad sandwich:											
12	1147	On white bread, soft	1 ea	111	47	325	9	28	1	19	3.9	6.2	7.7
12	1149	On part whole wheat	1 ea	111	47	319	10	27	3	19	3.7	6.3	7.7
12	1148	On whole wheat	1 ea	125	47	346	12	33	7	20	4.1	6.4	8.0
		Ham sandwich:											
12	1279	On rye bread	1 ea	116	55	242	16	25	5	9	1.9	3.2	2.8
12	1151	On white bread, soft	1 ea	122	54	262	16	28	1	9	2.2	3.4	2.7
12	1153	On part whole wheat	1 ea	122	54	256	17	27	3	9	2.0	3.5	2.7
12	1152	On whole wheat	1 ea	136	53	283	18	33	7	10	2.4	3.7	3.0
		Ham & cheese sandwich:											
12	1280	On soft white bread	1 ea	151	51	369	22	29	1	18	7.8	6.0	3.0
12	1282	On part whole wheat bread	1 ea	151	51	363	23	28	3	18	7.6	6.1	3.0
12	1281	On whole wheat	1 ea	165	50	390	25	33	7	19	8.0	6.2	3.3
12	1150	Ham & swiss on rye	1 ea	145	51	350	24	26	5	17	7.0	5.3	3.1
		Ham salad sandwich:											
12	1154	On white bread, soft	1 ea	125	48	345	10	34	1	19	4.8	7.2	5.9
12	1156	On part whole wheat	1 ea	125	48	339	11	33	3	19	4.6	7.3	6.0
12	1155	On whole wheat	1 ea	139	47	366	12	38	7	20	5.0	7.5	6.2
12	1157	Patty melt sandwich: ground beef & cheese on rye:	1 ea	177	45	567	32	25	5	38	14.1	13.9	6.5
		Peanut butter & jam sandwich:											
12	1158	On soft white bread	1 ea	100	27	347	12	45	3	15	2.8	6.8	4.3
12	1160	On part whole wheat	1 ea	100	27	341	12	44	5	15	2.5	6.9	4.3
12	1159	On whole wheat	1 ea	114	29	368	14	50	9	16	3.0	7.1	4.6
12	1161	Reuben sandwich, grilled: corned beef, swiss cheese, sauerkraut on rye:	1 ea	233	61	480	28	29	7	28	10.2	10.0	6.2
		Roast beef sandwich:											
12	713	On a bun	1 ea	150	52	345	22	34	1	13	4	7	2
12	1162	On soft white bread	1 ea	122	51	286	17	28	1	11	2.5	3.7	4.4

[95] Crust made with vegetable shortening and enriched flour.

(Computer code number is for West Diet Analysis program)

GRP KEY: 1 = BEV   2 = DAIRY   3 = EGGS   4 = FAT/OIL   5 = FRUIT   6 = BAKERY   7 = GRAIN   8 = FISH   9 = BEEF   10 = POULTRY
11 = SAUSAGE   12 = MIXED/FAST   13 = NUTS/SEEDS   14 = SWEETS   15 = VEG/LEG   16 = MISC   22 = SOUP/SAUCE

A

Chol (mg)	Calc (mg)	Iron (mg)	Magn (mg)	Phos (mg)	Pota (mg)	Sodi (mg)	Zinc (mg)	VT-A (RE)	Thia (mg)	Ribo (mg)	Niac (mg)	V-B6 (mg)	Fola (µg)	VT-C (mg)
32	56	2.20	19	107	202	463	2.0	14	.23	.24	3.80	.12	16	1
71	75	4.84	38	225	404	763	5.01	28	.38	.38	7.85	.28	24	2
23	59	1.71	13	83	113	745	1.19	<1	.29	.19	2.48	.07	17	12
56	220	1.60	36	216	230	699	1.81	106	.34	.29	4.20	.04	40	2
32	312	3.02	54	242	557	556	1.69	160	.41	.43	3.98	.25	74	11
32	299	3.09	66	274	562	518	1.87	160	.36	.40	4.02	.29	76	11
32	279	3.52	105	353	608	660	2.46	160	.35	.37	4.18	.36	91	11
21	81	2.22	22	138	253	647	1.06	50	.42	.25	3.71	.10	35	13
21	80	2.57	36	181	269	661	1.30	50	.42	.26	4.13	.15	41	13
21	60	3.00	76	260	315	803	1.89	50	.41	.23	4.29	.21	55	13
55	424	1.82	25	489	158	1155	2.24	214	.28	.38	2.14	.06	25	<1
55	424	2.17	39	531	174	1169	2.49	214	.28	.38	2.56	.10	30	<1
55	404	2.61	78	610	219	1311	3.07	214	.26	.35	2.72	.17	45	<1
25	80	1.94	18	102	136	401	.76	18	.28	.21	3.73	.11	22	1
25	79	2.30	32	144	152	415	.00	18	.28	.22	4.15	.15	28	1
25	59	2.73	71	223	197	557	1.59	18	.27	.19	4.31	.22	43	1
85	331	3.98	32	310	174	1045	4.37	85	.23	.41	3.65	.14	25	0
164	96	2.49	17	133	119	447	.92	90	.29	.29	2.14	.07	38	<1
164	95	2.85	31	176	135	461	1.16	90	.29	.29	2.56	.11	44	<1
164	75	3.28	71	255	180	603	1.75	90	.28	.26	2.72	.18	59	<1
29	49	1.94	25	203	311	1261	1.91	4	.74	.30	4.50	.32	23	14
29	80	2.17	25	191	271	1199	1.50	4	.80	.31	4.94	.29	23	14
29	79	2.52	39	234	287	1213	1.74	4	.80	.32	5.36	.33	29	14
29	59	2.96	78	313	333	1355	2.33	4	.79	.29	5.52	.40	44	14
56	256	2.28	31	405	318	1610	2.44	88	.81	.42	4.96	.31	26	14
56	256	2.64	45	447	334	1624	2.69	88	.81	.42	5.38	.35	31	14
56	236	3.07	84	526	379	1766	3.27	88	.79	.39	5.54	.42	46	14
55	325	1.99	35	376	342	1336	3.03	77	.75	.40	4.52	.34	25	14
27	77	2.00	18	134	156	887	1.02	19	.52	.25	3.36	.11	21	4
27	77	2.36	32	177	172	901	1.26	19	.52	.25	3.78	.15	26	4
27	57	2.79	71	256	217	1043	1.85	19	.51	.22	3.94	.22	41	4
107	228	3.33	40	423	410	923	6.63	139	.25	.45	6.08	.31	26	<1
0	83	2.23	55	153	246	403	1.06	1	.30	.21	5.39	.12	42	<1
0	82	2.59	69	195	262	417	1.30	1	.30	.21	5.81	.16	47	<1
0	62	3.02	108	274	308	559	1.89	1	.28	.18	5.97	.23	62	<1
85	358	5.20	44	328	313	1642	4.55	133	.25	.43	3.80	.24	27	12
55	60	4.04	38	222	338	757	3.66	32	.39	.33	6.02	.28	42	2
30	80	2.86	23	157	298	757	2.63	8	.31	.29	5.10	.21	23	<1

(For purposes of calculations, use "0" for t, <1, <.1, <.01, etc.)

Table A–1   Food Composition

Grp	Computer Code No.	Food Description	Measure	Wt (g)	H₂O (%)	Ener (cal)	Prot (g)	Carb (g)	Dietary Fiber (g)	Fat (g)	Fat Breakdown (g)		
											Sat	Mono	Poly
		MIXED DISHES and FAST FOOD—Con.											
		SANDWICHES—Con.											
		Roast Beef—Con.											
12	1164	On part whole wheat bread	1 ea	122	51	280	18	27	3	11	2.3	3.8	4.4
12	1163	On whole wheat bread	1 ea	136	50	307	19	32	7	12	2.7	3.9	4.7
		Tuna salad sandwich:											
12	1165	On soft white	1 ea	116	47	309	13	32	2	14	2.6	4.1	6.6
12	1167	On part whole wheat bread	1 ea	116	47	303	14	31	3	14	2.4	4.2	6.7
12	1166	On whole wheat bread	1 ea	130	47	331	15	37	8	15	2.8	4.4	6.9
		Turkey sandwich:											
12	1168	On soft white bread	1 ea	122	52	277	18	28	1	10	2.1	3.2	4.5
12	1170	On part whole wheat	1 ea	122	52	271	18	26	3	11	1.9	3.3	4.5
12	1169	On whole wheat	1 ea	136	51	298	20	32	7	11	2.3	3.4	4.8
		Turkey ham sandwich:											
12	1272	On rye bread	1 ea	116	55	239	15	25	5	9	1.9	2.6	3.3
12	1273	On soft white bread	1 ea	122	55	259	16	29	1	9	2.2	2.8	3.2
12	1275	On part whole wheat	1 ea	122	54	253	16	28	3	9	2.0	2.9	3.2
12	1274	On whole wheat	1 ea	136	53	281	18	33	7	10	2.4	3.1	3.5
12	714	Taco, corn tortilla, beef filling	1 ea	78	52	207	14	10	1	13	5	5	2
		Tostada:											
12	1114	With refried beans	1 ea	157	69	212	10	26	7	9	3.6	2.5	2.3
12	1118	With beans & beef	1 ea	192	67	332	18	20	4	21	9.4	7.2	2.6
12	1354	With beans & chicken	1 ea	157	67	249	19	19	4	11	4.4	3.5	2.9
		Vegetarian Foods:											
12	1175	Nuteena	1 ea	34	52	89	7	3	1	6	—	—	—
12	1171	Proteena	1 pce	67	58	160	8	5	1	12	—	—	—
12	1172	Redi-burger	1 pce	71	56	140	17	5	2	6	—	—	—
12	1173	Vege-Burger	1 pce	68	57	130	14	5	1	6	—	—	—
12	1174	Breakfast links	.5 c	108	73	110	22	4	1	1	—	—	—
		NUTS, SEEDS and PRODUCTS											
		Almonds:											
13	1365	Dry roasted, salted	1 c	138	3	810	23	33	18	71	6.8	46.2	15.0
13	718	Slivered, packed, unsalted	1 c	135	4	795	27	28	15[96]	70	7	46	15
		Whole, dried, unsalted:											
13	719	Cup	1 c	142	4	837	28	29	17[96]	74	7	48	16
13	720	Ounce	1 oz	28	4	167	6	6	3[96]	15	1	10	3
13	721	Almond butter	1 tbsp	16	1	101	2	3	1	9	1	6	2
13	722	Brazil nuts, dry (about 7)	1 oz	28	3	186	4	4	3	19	5	7	7
		Cashew nuts:											
		Dry roasted, salted											
13	723	Cup	1 c	137	2	787	21	45	8	63	13	37	11
13	724	Ounce	1 oz	28	2	163	4	9	2	13	3	8	2
		Oil roasted, salted:											
13	725	Cup	1 c	130	4	748	21	37	8	63	12	37	11
13	726	Ounce	1 oz	28	4	163	5	8	2	14	3	8	2

[96]Values reported for dietary fiber in almonds vary from 7.0 to 14.3g/100g.

(Computer code number is for West Diet Analysis program)

GRP KEY: 1 = BEV 2 = DAIRY 3 = EGGS 4 = FAT/OIL 5 = FRUIT 6 = BAKERY 7 = GRAIN 8 = FISH 9 = BEEF 10 = POULTRY
11 = SAUSAGE 12 = MIXED/FAST 13 = NUTS/SEEDS 14 = SWEETS 15 = VEG/LEG 16 = MISC 22 = SOUP/SAUCE

Chol (mg)	Calc (mg)	Iron (mg)	Magn (mg)	Phos (mg)	Pota (mg)	Sodi (mg)	Zinc (mg)	VT-A (RE)	Thia (mg)	Ribo (mg)	Niac (mg)	V-B6 (mg)	Fola (µg)	VT-C (mg)
30	79	3.22	37	200	314	771	2.87	8	.31	.29	5.52	.25	29	<1
30	59	3.65	76	279	359	912	3.46	8	.29	.26	5.68	.32	44	<1
25	80	2.27	23	133	199	559	.65	22	.28	.21	5.43	.14	30	2
25	80	2.63	37	176	215	573	.89	22	.28	.22	5.85	.19	36	2
25	60	3.06	76	255	260	715	1.48	22	.26	.19	6.01	.25	51	2
29	76	1.87	23	192	223	1151	1.00	8	.29	.24	6.82	.23	23	<1
29	76	2.23	37	235	239	1165	1.24	8	.28	.24	7.24	.27	28	<1
29	56	2.66	77	314	285	1307	1.83	8	.27	.21	7.40	.34	43	<1
35	50	3.04	27	214	273	986	2.37	4	.25	.32	4.46	.21	24	0
35	81	3.28	26	203	233	924	1.96	5	.31	.34	4.90	.18	24	<1
35	80	3.63	40	245	249	938	2.20	5	.30	.34	5.32	.23	29	<1
35	60	4.06	80	324	295	1080	2.79	5	.29	.31	5.48	.29	44	<1
45	85	1.29	23	141	183	141	2.89	27	.03	.13	2.49	.16	13	1
15	177	1.93	62	195	422	618	1.55	74	.06	.14	.85	1.01	47	6
62	186	2.16	52	247	442	483	3.57	132	.08	.24	2.94	.67	37	6
53	162	1.69	48	242	358	474	1.94	81	.07	.19	4.53	.73	34	3
<1	11	1.96	—	—	43	203	—	<1	1.65	.17	3.77	.20	—	<1
0	21	1.20	40	111	200	120	.87	10	.47	.58	.14	.45	60	—
0	22	1.60	31	99	280	460	1.20	26	.64	.50	7.80	.50	23	—
0	19	1.40	13	56	120	370	1.20	10	.60	.40	6.70	.80	17	—
0	32	2.70	24	105	110	190	1.10	10	.53	.68	5.00	.56	27	—
0	389	5.25	419	756	1063	1076	6.76	0	.18	.83	3.89	.10	88	1
0	359	4.94	400	702	988	15	3.94	0	.28	1.05	4.54	.15	79	1
0	378	5.20	420	738	1034	15[97]	4.15	0	.30	1.11	4.77	.16	83	1
0	75	1.04	84	147	208	3[97]	.83	0	.06	.22	.96	.03	17	<1
0	43	.59	49	84	121	2[98]	.49	0	.02	.1	.46	.01	0	<1
0	50	.97	64	170	170	<1	1.30	t	.28	.04	.46	.07	1	<1
0	62	8.22	356	671	774	877[99]	7.67	0	.27	.27	1.92	.35	95	0
0	13	1.70	74	139	160	181[99]	1.59	0	.06	.06	.4	.07	20	0
0	53	5.33	332	554	689	814[100]	6.18	0	.55	.23	2.34	.33	88	0
0	12	1.16	72	121	151	177[100]	1.35	0	.12	.05	.51	.07	19	0

[97] Salted almonds contain 1108 mg sodium per cup, 221 mg per ounce.
[98] Salted almond butter contains 72 mg sodium per tablespoon.
[99] Dry-roasted cashews without salt contain 21 mg sodium per cup, or 4 mg per ounce.
[100] Oil-roasted cashews without salt contain 22 mg sodium per cup, or 5 mg per ounce.

A

(For purposes of calculations, use "0" for t, <1, <.1, <.01, etc.)

Table A–1   Food Composition

	Computer Code								Dietary		Fat Breakdown (g)		
Grp	No.	Food Description	Measure	Wt (g)	H₂O (%)	Ener (cal)	Prot (g)	Carb (g)	Fiber (g)	Fat (g)	Sat	Mono	Poly
NUTS, SEEDS and PRODUCTS—Con.													
		Cashew nuts, unsalted:											
13	1366	Dry roasted	1 c	137	2	787	21	45	8	64	12.6	37.4	10.7
13	1367	Oil roasted	1 c	130	4	748	21	37	8	63	12.4	36.9	10.6
13	727	Cashew butter	1 tbsp	16	3	94	3	4	1	8	2	5	1
13	728	European chestnuts, roasted, 1 c = approx 17 kernels	1 c	143	40	350	5	76	19	3	.6	1.1	1.2
		Coconut:											
		Raw:											
13	729	Piece 2 × 2 × ½″	1 pce	45	47	159	2	7	5	15	13	.6	.2
13	730	Shredded/grated, unpacked[101]	1 c	80	47	283	3	12	9	27	24	1	.3
		Dried, shredded/grated:											
13	731	Unsweetened	1 c	78	3	515	5	19	12	50	45	2	.6
13	732	Sweetened	1 c	93	16	466	3	44	9	33	29	1	.4
		Filberts (hazelnuts), chopped:											
13	733	Cup	1 c	115	5	727	15	18	7	72	5	57	7
13	734	Ounce	1 oz	28	5	179	4	4	2	18	1	14	2
		Macadamia nuts, oil roasted:											
		Salted:											
13	735	Cup	1 c	134	2	962	10	17	7	103	15	81	2
13	736	Ounce	1 oz	28	2	204	2	4	1	22	3	17	.4
13	1368	Unsalted	1 c	134	2	962	10	17	7	103	15.4	80.9	1.8
		Mixed nuts:											
13	737	Dry roasted, salted	1 c	137	2	814	24	35	12	70	10	43	15
13	738	Oil roasted, salted	1 c	142	2	876	24	30	13	80	12	45	19
13	1369	Oil roasted, unsalted	1 c	142	2	876	24	30	13	80	12.4	45.0	18.9
		Peanuts:											
		Oil roasted, salted:											
13	739	Cup	1 c	144	2	837	38	27	13	71	10	35.2	22.4
13	740	Ounce	1 oz	28	2	163	7	5	2	14	2	7	4
13	1370	Oil roasted, unsalted	1 c	144	2	837	38	27	13	71	9.9	35.2	22.4
		Dried, unsalted:											
13	741	Cup	1 c	146	7	827	38	24	13	72	10	36	23
13	742	Ounce	1 oz	28	7	161	7	5	3	14	2	7	4
13	743	Peanut butter	1 tbsp	16	2	94	4	3	1	8	1.5	4.0	2.3
		Pecans, halves:											
		Dried, unsalted:											
13	744	Cup	1 c	108	5	720	8	20	7[102]	73	6	46	18
13	745	Ounce	1 oz	28	5	190	2	5	2[102]	19	1.5	12	5
13	1372	Dry roasted, salted	¼ c	28	1	187	2	6	2	18	1.5	11.5	4.6
13	746	Pine nuts/piñons, dried	1 oz	28	6	161	3	5	2	17	3	7	7
		Pistachio nuts:											
13	747	Dried, shelled	1 oz	28	4	164	6	7	1	14	2	9	2
13	1373	Dry roasted, salted, shelled	1 c	128	2	776	19	35	14	68	8.6	45.7	10.3

[101]1 c packed = 130 g.
[102]Dietary fiber data calculated/derived from data on other nuts.

(Computer code number is for West Diet Analysis program)

GRP KEY: 1=BEV   2=DAIRY   3=EGGS   4=FAT/OIL   5=FRUIT   6=BAKERY   7=GRAIN   8=FISH   9=BEEF   10=POULTRY
11=SAUSAGE   12=MIXED/FAST   13=NUTS/SEEDS   14=SWEETS   15=VEG/LEG   16=MISC   22=SOUP/SAUCE

Chol (mg)	Calc (mg)	Iron (mg)	Magn (mg)	Phos (mg)	Pota (mg)	Sodi (mg)	Zinc (mg)	VT-A (RE)	Thia (mg)	Ribo (mg)	Niac (mg)	V-B6 (mg)	Fola (µg)	VT-C (mg)
0	62	8.22	356	671	774	21	7.67	0	.27	.27	1.92	.35	95	0
0	53	5.33	332	554	689	22	6.18	0	.55	.23	2.34	.33	88	0
0	7	.09	41	73	87	2[103]	.83	0	.05	.03	.26	.04	11	0
0	42	1.30	47	153	846	3	.82	4	.35	.25	1.92	.71	100	37
0	6	1.09	14	51	160	9	.50	0	.03	.01	.24	.02	12	2
0	12	1.94	26	90	285	16	.88	0	.05	.02	.43	.04	21	3
0	20	2.59	70	161	423	29	1.57	0	.05	.08	.47	2.34	7	1
0	14	1.79	47	100	313	244	1.69	0	.03	.02	.44	.29	9	1
0	216	3.76	328	359	512	3	2.76	8	.57	.13	1.31	.7	83	1
0	53	.93	81	89	126	1	.68	2	.14	.03	.32	.17	20	<1
0	60	2.41	157	268	441	348[104]	1.47	1	.28	.15	2.71	.33	79	0
0	13	.51	33	57	94	74[104]	.31	<1	.06	.03	.57	.07	17	0
0	60	2.41	157	268	441	9	1.47	1	.28	.15	2.71	.33	79	0
0	96	5.07	308	596	817	917[105]	5.21	2	.27	.27	6.44	.41	69	1
0	153	4.56	334	659	825	926[105]	7.22	3	.71	.32	7.19	.34	118	1
0	153	4.56	334	659	825	16	7.22	3	.71	.32	7.19	.34	118	1
0	126	2.63	266	744	982	624[106]	9.55	0	.364	.156	20.6	.367	181	0
0	24	.51	52	145	191	121[106]	1.86	0	.07	.03	4	.07	35	0
0	126	2.63	266	744	982	8.6	9.55	0	.364	.156	20.6	.367	181	0
0	85	4.72	263	559	1047	23	4.78	0	.97	.19	20.7	.43	153	0
0	17	.92	51	109	204	5	.93	0	.19	.04	4.02	.08	30	0
0	5.5	.27	25	52	115	77[107]	.4	0	.02	.02	2.1	.06	13	0
0	39	2.30	138	314	423	1[108]	5.91	14	.92	.14	.96	.20	42	1
0	10	.61	36	83	111	<1	1.55	4	.24	.04	.25	.05	11	1
0	10	.62	38	86	105	221	1.61	4	.09	.04	.26	.05	12	1
0	2	.87	67	10	178	20	1.22	1	.35	.06	1.24	.08	19	<1
0	38	1.93	45	143	310	2[109]	.38	7	.22	.05	.31	.06	17	<1
0	90	4.06	166	609	1242	998	1.74	30	.54	.32	1.80	.27	74	0

A

[103] Salted cashew butter contains 98 mg sodium per tablespoon.
[104] Macadamia nuts without salt contain 9 mg sodium per cup, or 2 mg per ounce.
[105] Mixed nuts without salt contain about 15 mg sodium per cup.
[106] Peanuts without salt contain 22 mg sodium per cup, or 4 mg per ounce.
[107] Peanut butter without added salt contains 3 mg sodium per tablespoon.
[108] Salted pecans contain 816 mg sodium per cup, or 214 mg per ounce.
[109] Salted pistachios contain approx 221 mg sodium per ounce.

(For purposes of calculations, use "0" for t, <1, <.1, <.01, etc.)

Table A–1   Food Composition

Grp	Computer Code No.	Food Description	Measure	Wt (g)	H₂O (%)	Ener (cal)	Prot (g)	Carb (g)	Dietary Fiber (g)	Fat (g)	Fat Breakdown (g) Sat	Mono	Poly
		NUTS, SEEDS and PRODUCTS—Con.											
		Pumpkin kernels:											
13	748	Dried, unsalted	1 oz	28	7	154	7	5	2	13	2.5	4	6
13	1374	Roasted, salted	1 c	227	7	1185	75	31	9	96	18.1	29.7	43.6
13	749	Sesame seeds, hulled, dried	¼ c	38	5	221	10	4	6	21	3	8	9
		Sunflower seed kernels:											
13	750	Dry	¼ c	36	5	205	8	7	2	18	2	3	12
13	751	Oil roasted	¼ c	34	3	208	7	5	2	19	2	4	13
13	752	Tahini (sesame butter)	1 tbsp	15	3	91	3	3	2	8	1	3	4
		Black walnuts, chopped:											
13	753	Cup	1 c	125	4	759	30	15	7	71	5	16	47
13	754	Ounce	1 oz	28	4	172	7	3	2	16	1	4	11
		English walnuts, chopped:											
13	755	Cup	1 c	120	4	770	17	22	7	74	7	17	47
13	756	Ounce	1 oz	28	4	182	4	5	2	18	2	4	11
		SWEETENERS and SWEETS: see also Dairy (milk desserts) and Baked Goods											
14	757	Apple butter	2 tbsp	35	52	66	<1	17	<1	<1	.1	<.1	.1
14	1124	Butterscotch topping	3 tbsp	50	33	156	1	41	0	<1	—	—	—
		Cake frosting:											
14	1127	Canned, average of all types	2.5 tbsp	39	15	160	0	24	0	7	1.7	2.9	1.7
14	1123	Prepared from mix	2.5 tbsp	39	15	167	0	28	0	6	—	—	—
		Candy:											
14	1128	Almond Joy® candy bar	1 oz	28	7	151	2	19	1.9	8	6.7	.6	.1
14	758	Caramel, plain or chocolate	1 oz	28	8	115	1	22	<1	3	2.2	.3	.1
		Chocolate (see also, #784, 785, 971):											
		Milk chocolate:											
14	759	Plain	1 oz	28	1	145	2	16	1	9	5.4	3	.3
14	760	With almonds	1 oz	28	2	150	3	15	1	10	4.4	4.7	1.0
14	761	With peanuts	1 oz	28	1	155	5	10	2	12	3.5	5.2	2.7
14	762	With rice cereal	1 oz	28	2	140	2	18	1	7	4.4	2.5	.2
14	763	Semisweet chocolate chips	1 c	170	1	860	7	97	5	61	36	20	2
14	764	Sweet dark chocolate	1 oz	28	1	150	1	16	1	10	5.9	3.3	.3
14	1133	English toffee candy bar	1 ea	32	2	220	1	11	<1	19	7	7	2
14	765	Fondant candy, uncoated (mints, candy corn, other)	1 oz	28	3	105	0	27	0	0	0	0	0
14	766	Fudge, chocolate	1 oz	28	8	115	1	21	2	3	2.1	1	.1
14	767	Gum drops	1 oz	28	12	98	0	25	0	<1	t	t	.1
14	768	Hard candy, all flavors	1 oz	28	1	109	0	28	0	0	0	0	0
14	769	Jelly beans	1 oz	28	6	104	t	26	0	<.1	t	t	.1
14	1134	M&M's Plain choc. candies®	48 grm	48	1	237	3	33	<1	10	5	3	3
14	1135	M&M's Peanut choc. candies®	47 grm	47.3	2	240	5	28	1	12	5	5	2
14	1130	MARS® bar	1 ea	50	7	240	4	30	1	11	4.8	4.4	.8
14	1129	MILKY WAY® candy bar	1 ea	60	7	260	3	43	<1	9	5.4	3.0	.3
14	1132	REESE's® peanut butter cup	2 ea	45	4	240	6	22	2	14	5.2	5.4	2.4
14	1131	SNICKERS® candy bar, 2.2oz size	1 ea	61.2	7	290	7	37	2	14	—	—	—
14	1125	Caramel topping	3 tbsp	50	31	155	1	39	<1	—	—	—	—
14	771	Gelatin salad/dessert	½ c	120	84	70	2	17	<1	0	0	0	0
		Honey:											
14	772	Cup	1 c	339	17	1030	1	279	0	0	0	0	0
14	773	Tablespoon	1 tbsp	21	17	65	<.1	17	0	0	0	0	0

(Computer code number is for West Diet Analysis program)

GRP KEY: 1 = BEV 2 = DAIRY 3 = EGGS 4 = FAT/OIL 5 = FRUIT 6 = BAKERY 7 = GRAIN 8 = FISH 9 = BEEF 10 = POULTRY
11 = SAUSAGE 12 = MIXED/FAST 13 = NUTS/SEEDS 14 = SWEETS 15 = VEG/LEG 16 = MISC 22 = SOUP/SAUCE

A

Chol (mg)	Calc (mg)	Iron (mg)	Magn (mg)	Phos (mg)	Pota (mg)	Sodi (mg)	Zinc (mg)	VT-A (RE)	Thia (mg)	Ribo (mg)	Niac (mg)	V-B6 (mg)	Fola (µg)	VT-C (mg)
0	12	4.25	152	333	229	5[110]	2.12	11	.06	.09	.50	.03	26	<1
0	98	33.9	1212	2600	1830	1305	16.9	88	.25	.66	3.60	.20	115	0
0	49	2.93	130	291	153	15	2.23	<1	.27	.03	1.76	.30	38	0
0	42	2.44	128	254	248	1	1.82	2	.83	.10	1.62	.46	85	<1
0	19	2.26	43	385	163	205[111]	1.76	2	.11	.10	1.40	.40	79	<1
0	21	.83	53	119	69	5	1.57	1	.24	.02	.85	.06	15	1
0	73	3.84	253	580	655	1	4.28	37	.27	.14	.86	.70	83	1
0	16	.87	57	132	149	0	.97	8	.06	.03	.20	.16	19	<1
0	113	2.93	203	380	602	12	3.28	15	.46	.18	1.25	.67	79	4
0	27	.69	48	90	142	3	.78	4	.11	.04	.30	.16	19	1
0	5	.25	2	13	89	1	.01	0	<.01	.01	.08	.01	<1	1
14	56	.10	3	23	34	66	.12	<1	0	.04	0	<.01	.06	0
0	—	—	—	—	—	91	—	0	—	—	—	—	—	—
0	—	—	—	—	—	84	—	0	—	—	—	—	—	—
0	20	.5	16	42	92	48	.43	3	.01	.05	.14	.05	2.1	.1
1	42	.4	6	35	54	64	.15	<1	.01	.05	.1	<.01	0	t
6	50	.4	16	61	96	23	.37	10	.02	.1	.1	.02	<1	t
5	61	.56	33	77	125	23	.48	8	.03	.13	.31	.02	4	t
3	32	.68	35	87	155	19	.68	8	.11	.07	2.2	.05	16	t
6	48	.2	13	57	100	46	.29	8	.01	.08	.1	.01	<1	t
0	51	5.8	230	178	593	24	2.39	3	.1	.14	.9	.04	22	t
0	7	.6	32	41	86	5	.42	1	.01	.04	.1	.01	5	t
0	0	.20	11,5	0	50	90	.24	5	.053	.05	.10	.04	1	0
0	2	.1	—	2	1	57	.1	0	<.01	<.01	.01	.01	0	0
1	22	.3	14	24	42	54	.16	16	.01	.03	.1	.01	2	t
0	2	.1	—	—	1	10	0	5	0	<.01	.01	0	0	0
0	6	.1	<1	2	1	7	0	0	0	0	0	0	0	0
0	1	.30	—	1	11	7	0	0	0	<.01	.01	—	0	0
0	79	.76	30	65	171	41	.57	13	.03	.12	.27	.01	5	—
0	59	.67	38	64	162	29	.66	<1	.03	.09	1.48	.03	5	—
0	85	.55	37	63	176	85	.59	<1	.02	.16	.48	.01	5	—
14	86	.49	22	80	167	140	.45	25	.03	.15	.20	.01	7	1
3	35	.68	47	87	168	92	.9	8	.03	.05	2.12	.06	17	—
0	70	.49	39	75	209	170	.69	5	.03	.11	1.84	.02	6	—
0	28	.10	3	23	33	152	—	<1	0	.05	0	—	—	0
0	2	.10	<1	23	91	55	.03	0	.01	.01	.20	<.01	0	0
0	17	1.70	7	20	173	17	.40	0	.02	.14	1.0	.06	32	3
0	1	.11	<1	1	11	1	.02	0	<.01	.01	.06	<.01	2	<1

[110]Salted pumpkin/squash kernels contain approximately 163 mg sodium per ounce.
[111]Unsalted sunflower seeds contain 1 mg sodium per ¼ cup.

(For purposes of calculations, use "0" for t, <1, <.1, <.01, etc.)

Table A–1   Food Composition

Grp	Computer Code No.	Food Description	Measure	Wt (g)	H₂O (%)	Ener (cal)	Prot (g)	Carb (g)	Dietary Fiber (g)	Fat (g)	Sat	Mono	Poly
		SWEETENERS and SWEETS—Con.											
		Jams or preserves:											
14	774	Tablespoon	1 tbsp	20	29	54	<1	14	<1	<.1	0	t	t
14	775	Packet	1 ea	14	29	38	<.1	10	<1	<.1	0	t	t
		Jellies:											
14	776	Tablespoon	1 tbsp	18	28	49	<.1	13	<1	<.1	t	t	t
14	777	Packet	1 ea	14	28	39	<.1	10	<1	<.1	t	t	t
14	1136	Marmalade	1 tbsp	20	29	52	<1	14	<1	0	0	0	0
14	770	Marshmallows	4 ea	28	17	90	t	23	0	0	0	0	0
14	1126	Marshmallow creme topping	3 tbsp	50	20	158	<1	40	0	0	0	0	0
14	778	Popsicles, 3 oz when fluid	1 ea	95	80	70	0	18	0	0	0	0	0
		Sugars:											
14	779	Brown sugar	1 c	220	2	820	0	212	0	0	0	0	0
		White sugar, granulated:											
14	780	Cup	1 c	200	1	770	0	199	0	0	0	0	0
14	781	Tablespoon	1 tbsp	12	1	45	0	12	0	0	0	0	0
14	782	Packet	1 ea	6	1	25	0	6	0	0	0	0	0
14	783	White sugar, powdered, sifted	1 c	100	<1	385	0	99	0	0	0	0	0
		Syrups:											
		Chocolate:											
14	784	Thin type	2 tbsp	38	37	85	1	22	1	<1	.2	.1	.1
14	785	Fudge type	2 tbsp	38	25	125	2	21	1	5	3	2	.2
14	786	Molasses, blackstrap[112]	2 tbsp	40	24	85	0	22	0	0	0	0	0
14	787	Pancake table syrup (corn and maple)	¼ c	84	25	244	0	64	0	0	0	0	0
		VEGETABLES AND LEGUMES											
15	788	Alfalfa seeds, sprouted	1 c	33	91	10	1	1	1	<1	t	t	.1
15	789	Artichokes, cooked globe (300 g with refuse)	1 ea	120	84	60	4	13	10	<1	<.1	t	.1
		Artichoke hearts:											
15	1177	Cooked from frozen	9 oz	240	87	108	7	22	18	1	.3	<.1	.5
15	1176	Marinated	6 oz	170	59	168	4	13	11	14	2.0	3.0	7.7
		Asparagus, green, cooked:											
		From raw:											
15	790	Cuts and tips	½ c	90	92	23	2	4	2	<1	.1	t	.1
15	791	Spears, ½″ diam at base	4 spears	60	92	15	2	3	1	<1	<.1	t	.1
		From frozen:											
15	792	Cuts and tips	1 c	180	91	50	5	9	3	1	.2	t	.3
15	793	Spears, ½″ diam at base	4 spears	60	91	17	2	3	1	<1	.1	t	.1
15	794	Canned, spears, ½″ diam at base	4 spears	80	95	11	2	2	1	1	.1	t	.2
15	795	Bamboo shoots, canned, drained slices	1 c	131	94	25	2	4	3	1	.1	t	.2
		Beans (see also Great northern, #855; Kidney beans, #860; Navy beans, #876; Pinto beans, #898; Refried beans, #921; Soybeans, #925):											
15	796	Black beans, cooked	1 c	172	66	227	15	41	15	1	.2	.1	.4
		Canned beans (white/navy):											
15	803	Beans w/pork and tomato sauce	1 c	253	73	247	13	49	14	3	1.0	1.1	.3
15	804	Beans w/pork and sweet sauce	1 c	253	71	282	13	53	14	4	1.4	1.6	.5
15	805	Beans with frankfurters	1 c	257	70	366	17	40	18	17	6	7	2
		Lima beans:											
15	797	Thick seeded (Fordhooks), cooked from frozen	½ c	85	74	85	5	16	5	<1	.1	t	.1

[112]Light molasses would contain about 66 mg calcium, 2.1 mg iron, 18 mg magnesium, and 366 mg potassium for 2 tbsp.

(Computer code number is for West Diet Analysis program)

GRP KEY: 1 = BEV   2 = DAIRY   3 = EGGS   4 = FAT/OIL   5 = FRUIT   6 = BAKERY   7 = GRAIN   8 = FISH   9 = BEEF   10 = POULTRY
11 = SAUSAGE   12 = MIXED/FAST   13 = NUTS/SEEDS   14 = SWEETS   15 = VEG/LEG   16 = MISC   22 = SOUP/SAUCE

Chol (mg)	Calc (mg)	Iron (mg)	Magn (mg)	Phos (mg)	Pota (mg)	Sodi (mg)	Zinc (mg)	VT-A (RE)	Thia (mg)	Ribo (mg)	Niac (mg)	V-B6 (mg)	Fola (μg)	VT-C (mg)
0	4	.20	1	2	18	2	.01	t	<.01	.01	.04	<.01	2	<1
0	3	.14	<1	1	13	1	<.01	t	<.01	.01	.03	<.01	1	<1
0	2	.12	<1	1	16	4	0	t	<.01	<.01	.04	<.01	2	1
0	1	.09	<1	1	12	3	0	t	<.01	<.01	.03	<.01	2	1
0	7	.12	1	3	12	4	—	1	<.01	<.01	.02	<.01	1	1.2
0	1	.45	1	2	2	25	<.01	0	0	<.01	.01	<.01	0	0
0	16	.8	2	6	16	29	<.01	0	0	<.01	.02	—	0	2
0	0	.01	—	0	4	11	0	0	0	0	0	0	0	0
0	187	4.80	135	56	757	97	.08	0	.02	.07	.20	0	0	0
0	3	.10	<1	.1	7	5	.04	0	0	0	0	0	0	0
0	<1	.01	<1	t	t	t	<.01	0	0	0	0	0	0	0
0	<1	<.01	<1	t	t	t	<.01	0	0	0	0	0	0	0
0	0	.08	<1	0	4	2	<.01	0	0	0	0	0	0	0
0	6	.75	26	49	85	36	.39	1	.02	.02	.11	<.01	3	0
0	38	.50	18	60	82	42	.39	13	.08	.08	.08	<.01	3	0
0	274[112]	10.1[112]	103[112]	34	1171[112]	38	0	0	.08	.08	.80	.11	6	0
0	2	.06	2	8	14	38	.08	0	0	0	0	t	<1	0
0	11	.32	9	23	26	2	.30	5	.03	.04	.16	.01	12	3
0	54	1.55	72	103	425	114	.59	22	.08	.08	1.20	.13	61	12
0	50	1.34	74	146	634	127	.86	39	.15	.38	2.20	.21	285	12
0	39	1.62	48	102	438	900	.54	28	.06	.17	1.38	.15	149	52
0	22	.59	17	55	279	4	.43	75	.09	.11	.95	.13	88	25
0	14	.4	11	37	186	2	.29	50	.06	.07	.63	.09	59	16
0	41	1.15	23	99	392	7	1.01	147	.12	.19	1.87	.16	176	44
0	14	.38	8	33	131	2	.34	49	.04	.06	.62	.06	59	15
0	11	.5	8	30	122	278[113]	.32	38	.05	.07	.7	.04	69	13
0	10	.42	6	33	105	9	.30	1	.03	.03	.18	—	40	1
0	47	3.60	121	241	611	1	1.92	1	.42	.10	.87	.12	256	0
17	141	8.30	88	297	759	45	2.60	31	.13	.12	1.26	.18	57	8
17	155	4.20	87	266	673	1113	3.80	29	.12	.15	.89	.22	95	8
15	123	4.45	71	267	604	849	4.79	40	.15	.14	2.32	.12	77	6
0	19	1.16	29	54	347	1105	.37	16	.06	.05	.91	.10	55	11

[112] Light molasses would contain about 66 mg calcium, 2.1 mg iron, 18 mg magnesium, and 366 mg potassium for 2 tbsp.
[113] Special dietary pack contains 3 mg sodium.

(For purposes of calculations, use "0" for t, <1, <.1, <.01, etc.)

Table A–1   Food Composition

Grp	Computer Code No.	Food Description	Measure	Wt (g)	H$_2$O (%)	Ener (cal)	Prot (g)	Carb (g)	Dietary Fiber (g)	Fat (g)	Fat Breakdown (g) Sat	Mono	Poly
VEGETABLES and LEGUMES—Con.													
		Lima Beans—Con.											
15	798	Thin seeded (baby), cooked from frozen	½ c	90	72	94	6	18	8	<1	.1	t	.1
15	799	Cooked from dry, drained	1 c	188	70	217	15	39	18	1	.2	.1	.3
		Snap beans/green beans, cuts and french style:											
15	800	Cooked from raw	1 c	125	89	44	2	10	3	<1	.1	t	.2
15	801	Cooked from frozen	1 c	135	92	36	2	8	4	<1	<.1	t	.1
15	802	Canned, drained	1 c	136	93	26	2	6	2	<1	<.1	t	.1
		Bean sprouts (mung):											
15	806	Raw	1 c	104	90	31	3	6	3	<1	<.1	t	.1
15	807	Cooked, stir fried	1 c	124	84	62	5	13	3	<1	<.1	.1	.1
15	808	Cooked, boiled, drained	1 c	124	93	26	3	5	3	<1	<.1	t	<.1
		Beets:											
		Cooked from fresh:											
15	809	Sliced or diced	½ c	85	91	26	1	6	2	<.1	t	t	t
15	810	Whole beets, 2″ diam	2 beets	100	91	31	1	7	2	<.1	t	t	t
		Canned:											
15	811	Sliced or diced	½ c	85	91	27	1	6	2	<1	t	t	<.1
15	812	Pickled slices	½ c	114	82	74	1	19	2	<1	t	t	<.1
15	813	Beet greens, cooked, drained	1 c	144	89	40	4	8	3	<1	<.1	.1	.1
		Black-eyed peas: see Peas											
		Broccoli:											
15	817	Raw, chopped	1 c	88	91	24	3	5	3	<1	.1	t	.1
15	818	Raw, spears	1 spear	151	91	42	5	8	6	1	.1	<.1	.3
		Cooked from raw:											
15	819	Spears	1 spear	180	91	50	5	9	7	<1	.1	<.1	.3
15	820	Chopped	1 c	156	91	44	5	8	6	<1	.1	<.1	.3
		Cooked from frozen:											
15	821	Spear, small piece	1 spear	30	91	8	1	2	1	<.1	t	t	t
15	822	Chopped	1 c	184	91	51	6	10	6	<1	<.1	t	<.1
		Brussels sprouts:											
15	823	Cooked from raw	1 c	156	87	60	6	14	6	1	.2	.1	.4
15	824	Cooked from frozen	1 c	155	87	65	6	13	5	1	.1	.1	.3
		Cabbage, common varieties:											
15	825	Raw, shredded or chopped	1 c	70	92	16	1	4	2	<1	t	t	.1
15	826	Cooked, drained	1 c	150	94	32	1	7	4	<1	.1	<.1	.2
		Chinese cabbage:											
15	1178	Bok-choy, raw, shredded	1 c	70	95	9	1	2	1	<1	t	t	.1
15	827	Bok choy, cooked, drained	1 c	170	96	20	3	3	3	<1	<.1	t	.1
15	828	Pe-Tsai, raw, chopped	1 c	76	94	11	1	2	2	<1	<.1	t	.1
		Cabbage, red, coarsely chopped:											
15	829	Raw	1 c	70	92	19	1	4	2	<1	t	t	.1
15	830	Cooked	½ c	75	94	16	1	3	4	<1	t	t	.1
15	831	Savoy cabbage, coarsely chopped, raw	1 c	70	91	20	1	4	2	<.1	t	t	<.1

(Computer code number is for West Diet Analysis program)

GRP KEY: 1=BEV 2=DAIRY 3=EGGS 4=FAT/OIL 5=FRUIT 6=BAKERY 7=GRAIN 8=FISH 9=BEEF 10=POULTRY
11=SAUSAGE 12=MIXED/FAST 13=NUTS/SEEDS 14=SWEETS 15=VEG/LEG 16=MISC 22=SOUP/SAUCE

A

Chol (mg)	Calc (mg)	Iron (mg)	Magn (mg)	Phos (mg)	Pota (mg)	Sodi (mg)	Zinc (mg)	VT-A (RE)	Thia (mg)	Ribo (mg)	Niac (mg)	V-B6 (mg)	Fola (µg)	VT-C (mg)
0	25	1.76	50	101	370	26	.50	15	.06	.05	.69	.11	58	5
0	32	4.50	82	208	955	4	1.79	0	.30	.10	.79	.30	156	0
0	58	1.60	32	48	373	4	.45	83[114]	.09	.12	.77	.07	42	12
0	61	1.11	29	33	151	17	.84	71[115]	.07	.10	.56	.08	42	11
0	36	1.22	18	26	147	339[116]	.39	47[117]	.02	.08	.27	.05	43	6
0	14	.95	22	56	154	6	.43	2	.09	.13	.78	.09	63	14
0	16	2.40	38	70	200	14	1.12	3	.17	.22	1.49	.10	72	20
0	15	.81	18	34	125	12	.58	2	.06	.13	1.01	.05	35	14
0	9	.53	31	26	266	42	.21	1	.03	.01	.23	.03	49	5
0	11	.62	37	31	312	49	.25	1	.03	.01	.27	.03	86	6
0	13	1.55	13	15	126	233[118]	.18	1	.01	.04	.15	.05	22	4
0	13	.47	17	19	169	301	.30	1	.03	.06	.29	.03	35	3
0	165	2.74	97	58	1308	346	.72	734	.17	.42	.72	.19	47	36
0	42	.78	22	58	286	24	.36	136[119]	.06	.10	.56	.14	62	82
0	72	1.33	38	99	490	41	.60	233[119]	.10	.18	.96	.24	107	141
0	83	1.51	43	106	525	47	.68	250[119]	.10	.2	1.03	.26	90	134
0	72	1.24	37	92	456	40	.59	217[119]	.09	.18	.90	.22	78	116
0	15	.18	6	16	54	7	.09	57[119]	.02	.02	.14	.04	9	12
0	94	1.12	37	101	331	44	.55	348[119]	.10	.15	.84	.19	55	74
0	56	1.88	32	87	491	17	.50	112	.17	.12	.95	.31	94	97
0	38	1.15	37	84	504	36	.55	91	.16	.18	.83	.27	157	71
0	32	.40	10	16	172	12	.12	9	.04	.02	.21	.07	40	33
0	50	.59	23	38	308	29	.24	13	.09	.08	.34	.10	31	36
0	74	.56	13	26	176	<1	.29	210	.03	.05	.35	.07	57	32
0	158	1.77	18	49	630	57	.43	437	.05	.11	.73	.30	32	44
0	59	.23	10	22	181	7	.17	91	.03	.04	.30	.18	60	21
0	36	.35	11	29	144	8	.15	3	.05	.02	.21	.15	19	40
0	28	.27	8	21	105	6	.11	2	.03	.01	.15	.11	9	26
0	25	.28	20	29	161	20	.26	70	.05	.02	.21	.13	32	22

[114] Data is for green varieties; yellow beans contain 10 RE per cup.
[115] Data is for green varieties; yellow beans contain 15 RE per cup.
[116] Dietary pack contains 3 mg sodium per cup.
[117] For green varieties; yellow beans contain 14 RE per cup.
[118] Dietary pack contains 39 mg sodium.
[119] Vitamin A for whole plant: leaves are 1600 RE/100 g raw; flower clusters are 300/100 g raw; stalks are 40 RE/100 g raw.

(For purposes of calculations, use "0" for t, <1, <.1, <.01, etc.)

Table A–1   Food Composition

Grp	Computer Code No.	Food Description	Measure	Wt (g)	H$_2$O (%)	Ener (cal)	Prot (g)	Carb (g)	Dietary Fiber (g)	Fat (g)	Fat Breakdown (g) Sat	Mono	Poly
		VEGETABLES and LEGUMES—Con.											
		Carrots:											
		Raw:											
15	832	Whole, 7½ × 1⅛″	1 carrot	72	88	31	1	7	2	<1	t	t	.1
15	833	Grated	½ c	55	88	24	1	6	2	<1	t	t	<.1
		Cooked, sliced, drained:											
15	834	Cooked from raw	½ c	78	87	35	1	8	3	<1	<.1	t	.1
15	835	Cooked from frozen	½ c	73	90	26	1	6	3	<.1	t	t	<.1
15	836	Canned, sliced, drained	½ c	73	93	17	<1	4	1	<1	<.1	t	.1
15	837	Carrot juice	½ c	123	89	49	1	11	2	<1	<.1	t	.1
		Cauliflower:											
15	838	Raw, flowerets	½ c	50	92	12	1	2	1	<.1	t	t	<.1
		Cooked, drained, flowerets:											
15	839	From raw	½ c	62	92	15	1	3	1	<1	t	t	.1
15	840	From frozen	1 c	180	94	34	3	7	3	<1	.1	<.1	.2
		Celery, pascal type, raw:											
15	841	Large outer stalk, 8 × 1½″ (at root end)	1 stalk	40	95	6	<1	1	1	<.1	t	t	t
15	842	Diced	½ c	60	95	11	<1	2	1	<.1	t	t	<.1
		Chard, swiss:											
15	1179	Raw, chopped	1 c	36	93	7	1	1	1	<1	t	t	<.1
15	1180	Cooked	1 c	175	93	35	3	7	4	<1	<.1	t	.1
		Chick-peas (see Garbanzo, #854)											
		Collards, cooked, drained:											
15	843	From raw	1 c	128	92	35	2	8	4	<1	.1	<.1	.1
15	844	From frozen	1 c	170	88	63	3	14	6	1	.1	.1	.3
		Corn:											
		Cooked, drained:											
15	845	From raw, on cob, 5″ long	1 ear	77	70	83	3	19	3	1	.2	.3	.5
15	846	From frozen, on cob, 3½″ long	1 ear	63	73	59	2	14	3	<1	.1	.1	.2
15	847	Kernels, cooked from frozen	½ c	82	76	67	2	17	3	<.1	t	t	<.1
		Canned:											
15	848	Cream style	½ c	128	79	93	2	23	2	<1	.1	.2	.3
15	849	Whole kernel, vacuum pack	1 c	210	77	166	5	41	3	1	.2	.3	.5
		Cowpeas; (see Black-eyed peas, #814–816)											
15	850	Cucumbers with peel, ⅛″ thick, 2⅛″ diam	6 slices	28	96	4	<1	1	<1	<.1	t	t	t
		Dandelion greens:											
15	851	Raw	1 c	55	86	25	1	5	1	<1	<.1	<.1	.2
15	852	Chopped, cooked, drained	1 c	105	90	35	2	7	1	1	.2	<.1	.4
15	853	Eggplant, cooked	1 c	160	92	45	1	11	6	<1	.1	<.1	.2
15	854	Garbanzo beans (chick-peas), cooked	1 c	164	60	269	15	45	11	4	.4	1.0	2.0
15	855	Great northern beans, cooked	1 c	177	69	210	15	37	11	1	.3	<.1	.3
15	856	Escarole/curly endive, chopped	1 c	50	94	9	1	2	1	<1	t	t	<.1
15	857	Jerusalem artichokes, raw slices	1 c	150	78	114	3	26	2	<.1	—	t	t
		Kale, cooked, drained:											
15	858	From raw	1 c	130	91	42	3	7	4	1	.1	<.1	.3
15	859	From frozen	1 c	130	90	39	4	7	3	1	.1	<.1	.3
15	860	Kidney beans, canned	1 c	256	77	216	13	39	19	<1	.1	.1	.4
		Kohlrabi:											
15	1181	Raw slices	1 c	140	91	38	2	9	2	<1	t	t	.1
15	861	Cooked	1 c	165	90	48	3	11	2	<1	t	t	.1

(Computer code number is for West Diet Analysis program)

GRP KEY: 1=BEV   2=DAIRY   3=EGGS   4=FAT/OIL   5=FRUIT   6=BAKERY   7=GRAIN   8=FISH   9=BEEF   10=POULTRY
11=SAUSAGE   12=MIXED/FAST   13=NUTS/SEEDS   14=SWEETS   15=VEG/LEG   16=MISC   22=SOUP/SAUCE

Chol (mg)	Calc (mg)	Iron (mg)	Magn (mg)	Phos (mg)	Pota (mg)	Sodi (mg)	Zinc (mg)	VT-A (RE)	Thia (mg)	Ribo (mg)	Niac (mg)	V-B6 (mg)	Fola (µg)	VT-C (mg)
0	19	.36	11	32	233	25	.14	2025	.07	.04	.67	.11	10	7
0	15	.28	8	24	178	19	.11	1547	.05	.03	.51	.08	8	5
0	24	.48	10	24	177	52	.23	1915	.03	.04	.40	.19	11	2
0	21	.35	7	19	115	43	.18	1292	.02	.03	.32	.09	8	2
0	19	.47	6	17	131	176[120]	.19	1006	.01	.02	.40	.08	7	2
0	29	.56	17	51	358	36	.22	3159	.11	.07	.47	.27	5	11
0	14	.29	7	23	178	7	.09	1	.04	.03	.32	.12	33	36
0	17	.26	7	22	200	4	.15	1	.04	.04	.34	.13	32	34
0	31	.74	16	43	250	33	.23	4	.07	.10	.56	.16	74	56
0	16	.16	5	10	115	35	.05	5	.02	.02	.13	.04	11	3
0	25	.25	7	15	170	55	.08	8	.03	.03	.19	.06	13	4
0	18	.65	29	17	136	77	.16	259	.01	.03	.14	.03	20	11
0	102	3.96	150	58	961	313	.59	1198	.06	.15	.63	.12	57	32
0	29	.21	9	10	168	21	.14	349	.03	.07	.37	.07	8	16
0	54	.38	16	19	307	37	.26	638	.05	.12	.68	.12	129	28
0	2	.47	25	79	192	13	.37	17[121]	.17	.06	1.24	.18	36	5
0	2	.38	18	47	158	3	.40	13[121]	.11	.04	.96	.14	19	3
0	2	.25	15	39	114	4	.29	20[121]	.06	.06	1.05	.18	19	2
0	4	.49	22	65	172	365[122]	.68	12[121]	.03	.07	1.23	.08	57	6
0	11	.88	48	134	390	572[123]	.97	51[121]	.09	.15	2.46	.12	104	17
0	4	.08	3	5	42	1	.07	1	.01	.01	.09	.02	4	1
0	103	1.71	20	36	218	42	.62	770	.11	.14	.39	.02	64	19
0	147	1.89	26	44	244	46	.80	1229	.14	.18	.50	.04	82	19
0	10	.56	21	35	397	5	.24	10	.12	.03	.96	.14	23	2
0	80	4.74	78	275	477	11	2.51	4	.19	.10	.86	.23	282	2
0	121	3.77	88	293	692	4	1.55	<1	.28	.10	1.21	.21	181	2
0	26	.42	8	14	157	11	.40	103	.04	.04	.20	.01	71	3
0	21	5.10	26	117	644	6	.11	3	.30	.09	1.95	.11	15	6
0	94	1.17	23	36	296	30	.31	962	.07	.09	.70	.18	30	53
0	179	1.22	23	36	417	20	.23	826	.06	.15	.87	.11	31	33
0	62	3.22	73	240	658	873	1.41	0	.27	.23	1.17	.06	129	3
0	34	.56	27	64	490	28	.32	5	.07	.03	.56	.21	14	87
0	41	.66	31	74	561	34	.32	6	.07	.03	.64	.18	13	89

[120]Dietary pack contains 31 mg sodium.
[121]For yellow varieties; white varieties contain only a trace of vitamin A.
[122]Dietary pack contains 4 mg sodium per ½ cup.
[123]Dietary pack contains 6 mg sodium per cup.

(For purposes of calculations, use "0" for t, <1, <.1, <.01, etc.)

A

Table A–1   Food Composition

Grp	Computer Code No.	Food Description	Measure	Wt (g)	H₂O (%)	Ener (cal)	Prot (g)	Carb (g)	Dietary Fiber (g)	Fat (g)	Fat Breakdown (g) Sat	Mono	Poly
		VEGETABLES and LEGUMES—Con.											
		Leeks:											
15	1183	Raw, chopped	1 c	104	83	63	2	15	2	<1	.1	<.1	.4
15	1182	Cooked, chopped	.5 c	52	91	16	<1	4	2	<1	t	t	.1
15	862	Lentils, cooked from dry	1 c	198	70	230	18	40	10	1	.1	.1	.4
		Lentils, sprouted:											
15	1288	Stir fried	3.5 oz	100	69	101	9	21	4	<1	.1	.1	.2
15	1289	Raw	1 c	77	67	81	7	17	3	<1	<.1	.1	.2
		Lettuce:											
		Butterhead/Boston types:											
15	863	Head, 5″ diam	1 head	163	96	21	2	4	3	<1	<.1	t	.2
15	864	Leaves, 2 inner or outer	2 leaves	15	96	2	<1	<1	<1	<.1	t	t	t
		Iceberg/crisphead:											
15	865	Head, 6″ diam	1 head	539	96	70	5	11	9	1	.1	<.1	.5
15	866	Wedge, ¼ of head	1 wedge	135	96	18	1	3	2	<1	<.1	t	.1
15	867	Chopped or shredded	1 c	56	96	7	1	1	1	<1	t	t	.1
15	868	Loose leaf, chopped	1 c	56	94	10	1	2	1	<1	t	t	.1
		Romaine:											
15	869	Chopped	1 c	56	95	9	1	1	1	<1	t	t	.1
15	870	Inner leaf	1 leaf	10	95	2	<1	<1	<1	<.1	t	t	t
		Mushrooms:											
15	871	Raw, sliced	½ c	35	92	9	1	2	1	<1	t	t	.1
15	872	Cooked from raw, pieces	½ c	78	91	21	2	4	2	<1	<.1	t	.1
15	873	Canned, drained	½ c	78	91	19	1	4	2	<1	<.1	t	.1
		Mustard greens:											
15	874	Cooked from raw	1 c	140	94	21	3	3	3	<1	t	.2	.1
15	875	Cooked from frozen	1 c	150	94	29	3	5	3	<1	t	.2	.1
15	876	Navy beans, cooked from dry	1 c	182	63	259	16	43	16	1	.3	.1	.4
		Okra, cooked:											
15	877	From fresh pods	8 pods	85	90	27	2	6	2	<1	<.1	t	<.1
15	878	From frozen slices	½ c	92	91	34	2	8	2	<1	.1	.1	.1
		Onions:											
15	879	Raw, chopped	1 c	160	90	61	2	14	3	<1	<.1	<.1	.1
15	880	Raw, sliced	1 c	115	90	44	1	10	2	<1	<.1	<.1	.1
15	881	Cooked, drained, chopped	½ c	105	88	46	1	11	2	<1	<.1	<.1	.1
15	882	Dehydrated flakes	¼ c	14	4	45	1	12	1	<.1	t	t	<.1
		Spring onions:											
15	883	Chopped, bulb and top	½ c	50	90	16	1	4	1	.1	t	t	<.1
15	1185	Green tops only, chopped	1 c	100	92	34	2	6	3	<1	.1	.1	.2
15	1184	White part only, chopped	1 c	100	92	50	1	10	3	<1	<.1	t	.1
15	884	Onion rings, breaded, prepared f/frozen	2 rings	20	29	81	1	8	<1	5	1.7	2.2	1
		Parsley:											
15	885	Raw, chopped	½ c	30	88	10	1	2	2	<.1	t	t	<.1
15	886	Raw, sprigs	10 sprigs	10	88	3	<1	1	1	<.1	t	t	t
15	887	Freeze dried	¼ c	1	2	4	<1	1	1	<.1	t	t	<.1
15	888	Parsnips, sliced, cooked	1 c	156	78	125	2	30	5	1	.1	.2	.1
		Peas:											
		Black-eyed peas, cooked:											
15	814	From dry, drained	1 c	171	70	198	13	36	21	1	.2	.1	.4
15	815	From fresh, drained	1 c	165	76	160	5	33	12	1	.2	<.1	.3
15	816	From frozen, drained	1 c	170	66	224	14	40	14	1	.3	.1	.5
15	889	Edible-pod, peas, cooked	1 c	160	89	67	5	11	4	<1	.1	<.1	.2

(Computer code number is for West Diet Analysis program)

A

GRP KEY: 1 = BEV   2 = DAIRY   3 = EGGS   4 = FAT/OIL   5 = FRUIT   6 = BAKERY   7 = GRAIN   8 = FISH   9 = BEEF   10 = POULTRY
11 = SAUSAGE   12 = MIXED/FAST   13 = NUTS/SEEDS   14 = SWEETS   15 = VEG/LEG   16 = MISC   22 = SOUP/SAUCE

Chol (mg)	Calc (mg)	Iron (mg)	Magn (mg)	Phos (mg)	Pota (mg)	Sodi (mg)	Zinc (mg)	VT-A (RE)	Thia (mg)	Ribo (mg)	Niac (mg)	V-B6 (mg)	Fola (µg)	VT-C (mg)
0	61	2.18	29	36	187	21	.17	10	.06	.03	.42	.24	67	13
0	16	.57	7	9	45	5	.12	2	.01	.01	.10	.08	16	2
0	37	6.59	71	356	731	4	2.50	2	.34	.14	2.10	.35	358	3
0	14	3.10	35	153	284	9	1.60	4	.22	.09	1.20	.16	84	13
0	19	2.47	28	133	248	8	1.16	4	.18	.10	.87	.15	77	13
0	52	.49	18	38	419	8	.42	158	.10	.10	.49	.11	119	13
0	5	.05	2	3	39	1	.04	15	.01	.01	.05	.01	11	1
0	102	2.70	49	108	852	48	1.19	178	.25	.16	1.01	.22	302	21
0	26	.68	12	27	213	12	.30	45	.06	.04	.25	.05	76	5
0	11	.28	5	11	89	5	.12	19	.03	.02	.11	.02	31	2
0	38	.78	6	14	148	5	.19	106	.03	.04	.22	.03	60	10
0	20	.62	3	25	162	4	.19	146	.06	.06	.28	.03	76	13
0	4	.11	1	5	29	1	.03	26	.01	.01	.05	.06	14	2
0	2	.43	4	36	130	1	.30	0	.04	.16	1.44	.03	7	1
0	5	1.36	9	68	278	2	.68	0	.06	.23	3.48	.07	14	3
0	9	.62	6	52	101	332	.56	0	.05	.17	1.25	.06	10	0
0	104	1.56	21	57	283	22	.30	424	.06	.09	.61	.18	20	35
0	152	1.68	20	36	209	38	.30	671	.06	.08	.39	.16	20	21
0	128	4.5	107	285	669	2	1.93	<1	.37	.11	.97	.30	255	1
0	54	.38	48	48	274	4	.47	49	.11	.05	.74	.16	39	14
0	88	.62	47	42	215	3	.57	47	.09	.11	.72	.04	134	11
0	32	.35	16	53	251	5	.30	0	.07	.03	.24	.19	30	10
0	23	.25	12	38	181	3	.22	0	.05	.02	.17	.13	22	7
0	23	.25	12	37	174	3	.22	0	.04	.02	.17	.14	16	5
0	36	.22	13	42	227	3	.26	0	.01	.01	.03	.22	23	11
0	36	.74	10	19	138	8	.20	20	.03	.04	.26	.03	32	9
0	56	2.20	21	39	260	7	.22	400	.07	.10	.60	0	80	51
0	40	.89	16	40	230	7	.25	<1	.07	.03	.33	.10	36	27
0	6	.34	4	16	26	75	.08	5	.06	.03	.72	.02	3	<1
0	39	1.86	13	12	161	12	.22	156	.02	.03	.21	.05	55	27
0	13	.62	4	4	54	4	.07	52	.01	.01	.07	.02	18	9
0	2	.75	5	8	88	5	.09	89	.02	.03	.15	.02	22	2
0	58	.90	46	108	573	16	.40	0	.13	.08	1.10	.15	91	20[124]
0	42	4.30	91	266	476	6	2.20	3	.35	.1	.85	.17	356	1
0	211	1.85	86	84	690	7	1.7	131	.17	.24	2.3	.11	210	4
0	40	3.60	85	208	638	9	2.42	13	.42	.11	1.24	.16	240	5
0	67	3.15	42	89	383	6	.60	30	.21	.12	.86	.23	48	77

[124] Value for Vitamin C is highest right after harvest and drops after that.

(For purposes of calculations, use "0" for t, <1, <.1, <.01, etc.)

Table A–1   Food Composition

Grp	Computer Code No.	Food Description	Measure	Wt (g)	H$_2$O (%)	Ener (cal)	Prot (g)	Carb (g)	Dietary Fiber (g)	Fat (g)	Sat	Mono	Poly
		VEGETABLES and LEGUMES—Con.											
		Peas—Con.											
		Green peas:											
15	890	Canned, drained	½ c	85	82	59	4	11	4	<1	.1	<.1	.1
15	891	Cooked from frozen	½ c	80	80	63	4	11	4	<1	<.1	t	.1
15	892	Split, green, cooked from dry	1 c	196	69	231	16	41	10	1	.1	.2	.3
		Peas and carrots:											
15	1187	Cooked from frozen	½ c	80	86	38	2	8	3	<1	.1	<.1	.2
15	1186	Canned, with liquid	½ c	128	88	48	3	11	4	<1	.1	<.1	.2
		Peppers, hot:											
15	893	Hot green chili, canned	½ c	68	92	17	1	4	1	<.1	t	t	<.1
15	894	Hot green chili, raw	1 pepper	45	88	18	1	4	1	<.1	t	t	<.1
15	895	Jalapenos, chopped, canned	½ c	68	90	17	1	3	2	<1	.4	t	.2
		Peppers, sweet, green:											
15	896	Whole pod (90 g with refuse), raw	1 pod	74	92	20	1	5	1	<1	.1	t	.1
15	897	Cooked, chopped (1 pod cooked = 73 g)	½ c	68	92	19	1	5	1	<1	<.1	t	.1
		Peppers, sweet, red:											
15	1286	Raw, chopped	½ c	50	92	14	<1	3	1	<1	<.1	t	.1
15	1287	Cooked, chopped	½ c	68	92	19	1	5	1	<1	<.1	t	.1
15	898	Pinto beans, cooked from dry	1 c	171	64	235	14	44	20	1	.2	.2	.3
15	1191	Poi - two finger	1 c	240	72	269	1	65	6	<1	.1	<.1	.1
		Potatoes:[125]											
		Baked in oven, 4¾ × 2⅓″ diam:											
15	899	With skin	1 potato	202	71	220	5	51	5	<1	.1	t	.1
15	900	Flesh only	1 potato	156	75	145	3	34	2	<1	<.1	t	.1
15	901	Skin only	1 ea	58	47	115	2	27	2	<.1	t	t	<.1
		Baked in microwave, 4¾ × 2⅓″ diam:											
15	902	With skin	1 potato	202	72	212	5	49	5	<1	.1	t	.1
15	903	Flesh only	1 potato	156	74	156	3	36	2	<1	<.1	t	.1
15	904	Skin only	1 ea	58	64	77	3	17	2	<.1	t	t	<.1
		Boiled, about 2½″ diam:											
15	905	Peeled after boiling	1 potato	136	77	119	3	27	2	<1	<.1	t	.1
15	906	Peeled before boiling	1 potato	135	78	116	2	27	2	<1	<.1	t	.1
		French fried, strips 2-3½″ long, frozen:											
15	907	Oven heated	10 strips	50	53	111	2	17	1	4	2.1	1.8	.3
15	908	Fried in veg oil	10 strips	50	38	158	2	20	1	8	2.5	1.6	3.8
15	1188	Fried in veg. and animal oil	10 strips	50	38	158	2	20	1	8	3.4	4.0	.5
15	909	Hashed brown, from frozen	1 c	156	56	340	5	44	3	18	7	8	2
		Mashed:											
15	910	Home recipe with milk[126]	1 c	210	78	162	4	37	3	1	.7	.3	.1
15	911	Home recipe with milk and margarine	1 c	210	76	222	4	35	3	9	2.2	3.7	2.5
15	912	Prepared from flakes; water, milk, margarine, salt added	1 c	215	76	239	4	28	2	13	3.0	5.4	3.7
		Potato products, prepared:											
		Au gratin:											
15	913	From dry mix	1 c	245	79	228	6	32	4	10	6.3	3	.3
15	914	From home recipe[127]	1 c	245	74	322	12	28	4	19	12	5	1

[125]Vitamin C varies with length of storage. After 3 months of storage approximately two-thirds of the ascorbic acid remains; after 6 to 7 months, about one-third remains.
[126]Recipe: 84% potatoes, 15% whole milk, 1% salt.
[127]Recipe: 55% potatoes, 30% whole milk, 9% cheddar cheese, 3% butter, 2% flour, 1% salt.

(Computer code number is for West Diet Analysis program)

GRP KEY: 1 = BEV   2 = DAIRY   3 = EGGS   4 = FAT/OIL   5 = FRUIT   6 = BAKERY   7 = GRAIN   8 = FISH   9 = BEEF   10 = POULTRY
11 = SAUSAGE   12 = MIXED/FAST   13 = NUTS/SEEDS   14 = SWEETS   15 = VEG/LEG   16 = MISC   22 = SOUP/SAUCE

A

Chol (mg)	Calc (mg)	Iron (mg)	Magn (mg)	Phos (mg)	Pota (mg)	Sodi (mg)	Zinc (mg)	VT-A (RE)	Thia (mg)	Ribo (mg)	Niac (mg)	V-B6 (mg)	Fola (µg)	VT-C (mg)
0	17	.81	15	57	147	186[128]	.60	65	.10	.07	.62	.05	38	8
0	19	1.25	23	72	134	70	.75	77	.23	.14	1.18	.09	47	8
0	26	2.52	71	195	710	4	1.96	1	.37	.11	1.74	.09	127	1
0	18	.75	13	39	127	55	.36	621	.18	.06	.92	.07	21	7
0	29	.97	18	58	128	332	.74	739	.10	.07	.74	.11	24	8
0	5	.34	8	12	143	10	.02	42[129]	.01	.03	.54	.08	35	46
0	8	.54	11	21	153	3	.14	35[129]	.04	.04	.43	.13	11	109
0	18	1.90	8	12	92	995	.13	116	.02	.03	.34	.14	35	9
0	7	.34	7	14	131	1	.09	47	.05	.02	.38	.18	16	66
0	6	.31	7	12	113	1	.08	40	.04	.02	.32	.16	10	51
0	5	.23	5	10	89	1	.06	285	.03	.02	.26	.12	11	95
0	6	.31	7	12	113	1	.08	256	.04	.02	.32	.16	11	116
0	82	4.47	95	273	800	3	1.85	<1	.32	.16	.68	.27	294	4
0	37	2.11	58	94	439	28	2.04	5	.31	.10	2.64	—	—	10
0	20	2.75	55	115	844	16	.65	0	.22	.07	3.32	.70	22	26
0	8	.55	39	78	610	8	.45	0	.16	.03	2.18	.47	14	20
0	20	2.20	25	59	332	12	.28	0	.07	.07	1.78	.35	13	8
0	22	2.50	54	212	903	16	.73	0	.24	.07	3.46	.70	24	31
0	8	.64	39	170	641	11	.51	0	.20	.04	2.54	.50	19	24
0	27	3.44	22	48	377	9	.30	0	.04	.04	1.29	.28	10	9
0	7	.42	30	60	515	6	.41	0	.14	.03	1.96	.41	14	18
0	10	.42	26	54	443	7	.37	0	.13	.03	1.77	.36	12	10
0	4	.67	11	43	229	15	.21	0	.06	.02	1.15	.12	8	6
0	10	.38	17	47	366	108	.19	0	.09	.01	1.63	.12	15	5
0	10	.38	17	47	366	108	.19	0	.09	.01	1.63	.12	15	5
0	24	2.36	27	112	680	53	.50	0	.17	.03	3.78	.20	26	10
4	55	.57	39	100	628	636	.60	12	.19	.08	2.35	.49	17	14
4[130]	54	.55	37	97	607	619	.58	41	.18	.11	2.27	.47	17	13
4[130]	92	.40	30	108	428	733	.51	176	.30	.14	1.91	.26	15	25
12	203	.78	37	233	537	1076	.59	76	.05	.20	2.30	.10	3	8
56[131]	292	1.56	48	277	970	1064	1.69	93	.16	.28	2.43	.43	25	24

[128] Dietary pack contains 1.7 mg sodium.
[129] Data is for green chili peppers; red varieties contain 809 RE vitamin A per ½ cup; 484 RE per whole pepper.
[130] Data is for margarine; if butter is used, cholesterol = 25 mg for 29 total mg.
[131] Data is for butter; if margarine is used, cholesterol = 37 mg.

(For purposes of calculations, use "0" for t, <1, <.1, <.01, etc.)

Table A–1   Food Composition

Grp	Computer Code No.	Food Description	Measure	Wt (g)	H₂O (%)	Ener (cal)	Prot (g)	Carb (g)	Dietary Fiber (g)	Fat (g)	Fat Breakdown (g) Sat	Mono	Poly
		VEGETABLES and LEGUMES—Con.											
		Potato Products—Con.											
		Potato salad (see Mixed Dishes #715)											
		Scalloped:											
15	915	From dry mix	1 c	245	79	228	5	31	3	11	6.5	3.0	.5
15	916	Home recipe[132]	1 c	245	81	210	7	26	3	9	5.5	2.6	.4
15	1192	Potato puffs, cooked from frozen	.5 c	62	53	138	2	19	1	7	3.2	2.7	.5
15	917	Potato chips (14 chips = about 1 oz)	14 chips	28	2	148	2	15	1	10	2.6	1.8	5.2
		Pumpkin:											
15	918	Cooked from raw, mashed	1 c	245	94	50	2	12	4	<1	.1	t	t
15	919	Canned	1 c	245	90	83	3	20	5	1	.4	.1	<.1
15	920	Red radishes	10 radishes	45	95	7	<1	2	1	<1	t	t	t
15	921	Refried beans, canned	1 c	253	72	270	16	47	22	3	1	1.2	.4
15	1375	Rutabaga, cooked cubes	.5 c	85	90	29	1	7	1	<1	<.1	<.1	.1
15	922	Sauerkraut, canned with liquid	1 c	236	92	44	2	10	4	<1	.1	<.1	.1
		Seaweed:											
15	923	Kelp, raw	1 oz	28	82	12	1	3	1	<1	.1	<.1	t
15	924	Spirulina, dried	1 oz	28	5	82	16	7	1	2	.8	.2	.6
15	925	Soybeans, cooked from dry	1 c	172	63	298	29	17	5	15	2.2	3.4	8.7
		Soybean products:											
15	926	Miso	½ c	138	46	283	16	39	7	8	1.2	1.9	4.7
15	927	Tofu	½ c	124	85	94	10	2	2	6	.9	1.3	3.4
		Spinach:											
15	928	Raw, chopped	1 c	56	92	12	2	2	2	<1	<.1	t	.1
		Cooked, drained:											
15	929	From raw	1 c	180	91	41	5	7	4	<1	.1	t	.2
15	930	From frozen (leaf)	1 c	190	90	53	6	10	5	<1	.1	t	.2
15	931	Canned, drained solids	1 c	214	92	50	6	7	6	1	.2	<.1	.5
		Spinach soufflé (Mixed Dishes)											
		Squash, summer varieties, cooked slices:											
15	932	Varieties averaged	1 c	180	94	36	2	8	3	1	.1	<.1	.2
15	933	Crookneck	1 c	180	94	36	2	8	3	1	.1	<.1	.2
15	934	Zucchini	1 c	180	95	29	1	7	4	<.1	t	t	<.1
		Squash, winter varieties, cooked:											
		Average of all varieties, baked:											
15	935	Mashed	1 c	245	89	96	2	21	7	2	.3	.1	.7
15	936	Baked cubes	1 c	205	89	79	2	18	6	1	.3	.1	.5
		Acorn squash:											
15	937	Baked, mashed	1 c	245	83	137	3	36	7	<1	<.1	t	.1
15	1218	Boiled, mashed	1 c	245	90	83	2	22	6	<1	<.1	t	.1
15	938	Butternut, baked cubes	1 c	205	88	83	2	22	6	<1	<.1	t	.1
		Butternut squash:											
15	1219	Baked, mashed	1 c	245	88	99	2	26	7	<1	<.1	t	.1
15	1193	Cooked from frozen	1 c	240	88	94	3	24	7	<1	<.1	t	.1
		Hubbard squash:											
15	1194	Baked, mashed	1 c	240	85	120	6	26	6	1	.3	.1	.6
15	1195	Boiled, mashed	1 c	236	91	70	4	15	7	1	.2	.1	.4
15	1196	Spaghetti squash, baked or boiled	1 c	155	92	45	1	10	4	<1	.1	<.1	.2
15	1189	Succotash, cooked from frozen	1 c	170	74	158	7	34	9	2	.3	.3	.7

[132]Recipe: 59% potatoes, 36% whole milk, 2% butter, 2% flour, 1% salt.

(Computer code number is for West Diet Analysis program)

GRP KEY: 1 = BEV   2 = DAIRY   3 = EGGS   4 = FAT/OIL   5 = FRUIT   6 = BAKERY   7 = GRAIN   8 = FISH   9 = BEEF   10 = POULTRY
11 = SAUSAGE   12 = MIXED/FAST   13 = NUTS/SEEDS   14 = SWEETS   15 = VEG/LEG   16 = MISC   22 = SOUP/SAUCE

Chol (mg)	Calc (mg)	Iron (mg)	Magn (mg)	Phos (mg)	Pota (mg)	Sodi (mg)	Zinc (mg)	VT-A (RE)	Thia (mg)	Ribo (mg)	Niac (mg)	V-B6 (mg)	Fola (μg)	VT-C (mg)
27	88	.93	34	137	497	835	.61	51	.05	.14	2.52	.10	3	8
29[133]	140	1.41	46	154	926	821	.98	46	.17	.23	2.58	.44	21	26
0	19	.97	12	30	236	462	.19	1	.12	.05	1.34	.14	.10	4
0	7	.34	17	43	369	133[134]	.30	0	.04	.01	1.19	.14	13	12
0	37	1.40	22	74	564	3	.45	265	.08	.19	1.01	.16	33	12
0	64	3.41	56	85	504	12	.42	5404	.06	.13	.9	.14	30	10
0	9	.13	4	8	104	11	.13	t	<.01	.02	.14	.03	12	10
0	118	4.5	99	214	994	1071	3.45	0	.12	.14	1.23	.28	150	15
0	36	.40	18	42	244	15	.26	0	.06	.03	.54	.08	13	19
0	72	3.47	31	46	401	1561	.44	4	.05	.05	.34	.31	4	35
0	48	.81	34	12	25	66	.35	3	.01	.04	.13	—	51	—
0	34	8.08	55	33	386	297	—	16	.68	1.04	3.63	.10	—	3
0	175	8.84	148	421	886	1	1.98	2	.27	.49	.69	.40	93	3
0	92	3.78	58	211	226	5032	4.58	12	.13	.35	1.19	.3	46	0
0	130	6.65	127	120	150	9	1.00	11	.10	.06	.24	.06	19	<1
0	55	1.52	44	27	312	44	.30	448	.04	.11	.41	.11	109	16
0	244	6.42	157	100	838	126	1.37	1750	.17	.43	.88	.44	262	40
0	277	2.89	131	91	566	163	1.33	1756	.11	.32	.80	.28	204	23
0	271	4.92	162	94	740	683[135]	.99	1878	.03	.30	.83	.21	209	31
0	48	.64	44	69	346	2	.71	52[136]	.08	.07	.92	.12	36	9
0	48	.64	44	69	346	2	.71	52[136]	.09	.09	.92	.17	36	10
0	23	.63	40	72	455	5	.32	43[136]	.07	.07	.77	.14	30	8
0	34	.81	20	49	1071	2	.64	872	.21	.06	1.72	.18	69	24
0	28	.67	16	41	895	3	.54	730	.17	.05	1.43	.15	57	20
0	108	2.28	104	111	1071	11	.42	105	.41	.03	2.16	.48	46	26
0	65	1.37	63	67	645	6	.27	63	.25	.02	1.30	.29	28	16
0	84	1.23	59	55	582	7	.27	1435	.15	.04	1.99	.25	39	31
0	100	1.47	71	66	697	8	.32	1715	.18	.04	2.38	.30	47	37
0	46	1.40	22	34	319	4	.29	801	.12	.09	1.11	.17	29	8
0	41	1.13	53	55	859	19	.36	1450	.18	.11	1.34	.41	39	23
0	23	.67	32	33	504	12	.22	945	.10	.07	.79	.24	23	15
0	33	.52	17	21	182	28	.31	17	.06	.03	1.26	.15	12	6
0	25	1.51	39	119	451	77	.76	39	.13	.12	2.22	.16	57	10

[133]Data is for butter; if margarine is used cholesterol = 15 mg.
[134]If no salt added, sodium = 2 mg.
[135]Dietary pack contains 58 mg sodium.
[136]Applies to squash including skin; flesh has no appreciable vitamin A value.

(For purposes of calculations, use "0" for t, <1, <.1, <.01, etc.)

Table A–1   Food Composition

Grp	Computer Code No.	Food Description	Measure	Wt (g)	H₂O (%)	Ener (cal)	Prot (g)	Carb (g)	Dietary Fiber (g)	Fat (g)	Fat Breakdown (g) Sat	Mono	Poly
		VEGETABLES and LEGUMES—Con.											
		Sweet potatoes:											
		Cooked, 5 × 2" diam:											
15	939	Baked in skin, peeled	1 potato	114	73	118	2	28	3	<1	<.1	t	.1
15	940	Boiled without skin	1 potato	151	73	160	2	37	5	<1	.1	t	.2
15	941	Candied, 2½ × 2"	1 pce	105	67	144	1	29	2	3	1.4	.7	.2
		Canned:											
15	942	Solid pack, mashed	1 c	265	74	258	5	59	6	<1	.1	t	.2
15	943	Vacuum pack, mashed	1 c	255	76	233	4	54	5	1	.1	t	.2
15	944	Vacuum pack, 2¾ × 1"	1 pce	40	76	36	1	8	1	<1	t	t	<.1
		Tomatoes:											
15	945	Raw, whole, 2⅗" diam	1 tomato	123	94	26	1	6	2	<1	<.1	<.1	.2
15	946	Raw, chopped	1 c	180	94	38	2	8	3	<1	.1	.1	.2
15	947	Cooked from raw	1 c	240	92	65	3	14	4	1	.1	.2	.4
15	948	Canned, solids and liquid	1 c	240	94	47	2	10	3	1	.1	.1	.2
15	949	Tomato juice, canned	1 c	244	94	42	2	10	2	<1	t	t	.1
		Tomato products, canned:											
15	950	Paste	1 c	262	74	220	10	49	11	2	.3	.4	.9
15	951	Puree	1 c	250	87	102	4	25	6	<1	<.1	<.1	.1
15	952	Sauce	1 c	245	89	74	3	18	4	<1	.1	.1	.2
15	953	Turnips, cubes, cooked from raw	½ c	78	94	14	1	4	2	<1	t	t	<.1
		Turnip greens, cooked:											
15	954	From raw (leaves and stems)	1 c	144	94	29	2	6	4	<1	.1	t	.1
15	955	From frozen (chopped)	½ c	82	90	24	3	4	4	<1	.1	t	.1
15	956	Vegetable juice cocktail, canned	1 c	242	94	46	2	11	2	<1	<.1	<.1	.1
		Vegetables, mixed:											
15	957	Canned, drained	1 c	163	87	77	4	15	6	<1	.1	<.1	.2
15	958	Frozen, cooked, drained	1 c	182	83	107	5	24	7	<1	.1	t	.1
		Water chestnuts, canned:											
15	959	Slices	½ c	70	86	35	1	9	2	<.1	t	t	t
15	960	Whole	4 ea	28	86	14	<1	4	1	<1	t	t	t
15	1190	Watercress, fresh, chopped	.5 c	17	95	2	<1	<1	<1	<1	t	t	t
		MISCELLANEOUS											
		Baking powders for home use:											
		Sodium aluminum sulfate:											
16	962	With monocalcium phosphate monohydrate	1 tsp	3	2	5	t	1	0	0	0	0	0
16	963	With monocalcium phosphate monohydrate, calcium sulfate	1 tsp	3	1	5	t	1	0	0	0	0	0
16	964	Straight phosphate	1 tsp	4	2	5	t	1	0	0	0	0	0
16	965	Low sodium	1 tsp	4	1	5	t	1	0	0	0	0	0
16	1204	Baking soda	1 tsp	3	1	0	0	0	0	0	0	0	0
16	966	Basil, ground	1 tbsp	5	6	11	1	3	1	<1	—	—	—
16	961	Carob flour	1 c	103	3	185	5	92	34	1	.1	.2	.2

(Computer code number is for West Diet Analysis program)

GRP KEY: 1 = BEV   2 = DAIRY   3 = EGGS   4 = FAT/OIL   5 = FRUIT   6 = BAKERY   7 = GRAIN   8 = FISH   9 = BEEF   10 = POULTRY
11 = SAUSAGE   12 = MIXED/FAST   13 = NUTS/SEEDS   14 = SWEETS   15 = VEG/LEG   16 = MISC   22 = SOUP/SAUCE

A

Chol (mg)	Calc (mg)	Iron (mg)	Magn (mg)	Phos (mg)	Pota (mg)	Sodi (mg)	Zinc (mg)	VT-A (RE)	Thia (mg)	Ribo (mg)	Niac (mg)	V-B6 (mg)	Fola (µg)	VT-C (mg)
0	32	.52	23	63	397	12	.33	2488	.08	.14	.7	.28	26	28
0	32	.8	15	41	278	20	.4	2575	.08	.21	1	.36	22	26
0[137]	27	1.2	12	27	198	73	.16	440	.02	.04	.41	.17	12	7
0	77	3.4	61	133	536	191	.54	3857	.07	.23	2.4	.48	42	13
0	56	2.27	57	125	796	136	.46	2036	.09	.14	1.89	.49	42	67
0	9	.36	9	20	125	21	.07	319	.02	.02	.3	.08	7	11
0	6	.55	14	30	273	11	.11	77	.07	.06	.77	.10	18	22[138]
0	9	.81	20	43	400	16	.16	112	.11	.09	1.13	.14	27	34[138]
0	14	1.34	34	74	670	26	.26	178	.17	.14	1.80	.23	31	55
0	63[139]	1.45	29	46	529	390[140]	.38	145	.11	.07	1.76	.22	35	36
0	22	1.41	27	46	537	881[141]	.34	136	.12	.08	1.64	.27	49	45
0	92	7.84	134	207	2442	170[142]	2.1	647	.41	.5	8.44	1	40	111
0	37	2.32	60	99	1051	49[143]	.54	340	.18	.14	4.29	.38	39	88
0	34	1.88	46	78	908	1481[144]	.6	240	.16	.14	2.82	.33	39	32
0	18	.17	6	15	106	39	.16	0	.02	.02	.23	.05	7	9
0	198	1.15	32	41	293	41	.29	792	.07	.1	.59	.26	171	40
0	125	1.59	21	27	184	12	.34	654	.04	.06	.38	.06	32	18
0	27	1.02	27	41	467	883	.48	283	.1	.07	1.76	.34	38	67
0	44	1.71	26	68	474	243	.67	1899	.07	.08	.94	.13	39	8
0	46	1.49	40	93	308	64	.89	779	.13	.22	1.55	.14	35	6
0	3	.61	3	14	82	6	.27	t	.01	.02	.25	—	8	1
0	1	.25	1	5	33	2	.11	t	<.01	.01	.1	—	3	<1
0	20	.03	4	10	56	7	.03	80	.02	.02	.03	.02	34	7
0	58	0	t	87	5	329	0	0	0	0	0	0	0	0
0	183	0	—	45	4	290	0	0	0	0	0	0	0	0
0	239	0	—	359	6	312	0	0	0	0	0	0	0	0
0	207	0	—	314	891	t	0	0	0	0	0	0	0	0
0	0	—	—	—	—	821	—	0	0	0	0	0	0	0
0	95	1.89	18	22	154	2	.26	42	.01	.01	.31	—	—	3
0	359	3.03	56	81	852	36	.94	2	.06	.48	1.95	.38	30	<1

[137] For recipe using margarine; if butter is used, cholesterol = 8 mg.

[138] Year-round average. From June through October, ascorbic acid is approximately 32 mg and 47 mg, respectively, for one tomato and 1 c chopped tomato. From November through May, market samples average around 12 and 18 mg, respectively.

[139] Calcium is added as a firming agent.

[140] Dietary pack contains 31 mg sodium.

[141] If no salt is added, sodium content is 24 mg.

[142] If salt is added, sodium content is 2070 mg.

[143] If salt is added, sodium content is 998 mg.

[144] With salt added.

(For purposes of calculations, use "0" for t, <1, <.1, <.01, etc.)

Table A–1 Food Composition

Grp	Computer Code No.	Food Description	Measure	Wt (g)	H$_2$O (%)	Ener (cal)	Prot (g)	Carb (g)	Dietary Fiber (g)	Fat (g)	Fat Breakdown (g) Sat	Mono	Poly
		MISCELLANEOUS—Con.											
		Catsup:											
16	967	Cup	1 c	245	67	255	4	67	4	1	.2	.2	.4
16	968	Tablespoon	1 tbsp	15	67	16	<1	4	<1	<.1	t	t	t
16	1200	Cayenne (red pepper)	1 tbsp	5.3	8	17	1	3	2	1	.2	.2	.4
16	969	Celery seed	1 tsp	2	6	9	<1	1	<1	1	<.1	.3	.1
16	970	Chili powder	1 tsp	3	8	8	<1	1	1	<1	.1	.1	.2
		Chocolate:											
16	971	Baking, unsweetened	1 oz	28	2	145	4	7	4	15	9	5	.5
		For other chocolate items, see Sweeteners and Sweets											
16	972	Coriander, fresh	¼ c	4	93	<1	<1	<1	<1	<.1	<.01	<.01	.01
16	1197	Cornstarch	1 tbsp	8	8	20	<.1	5	<.1	<.1	t	t	t
16	973	Cinnamon	1 tsp	2	10	6	<1	2	1	<.1	t	t	t
16	974	Curry powder	1 tsp	2	10	6	<1	1	<1	<1	t	.2	<.1
16	1202	Dill weed, dried	1 tbsp	3.1	7	8	1	2	<1	<1	—	—	—
		Garlic:											
16	975	Cloves	4 cloves	12	59	18	1	4	<1	<.1	t	t	<.1
16	976	Powder	1 tsp	3	6	9	<1	2	<1	<.1	t	t	t
16	977	Gelatin, dry, plain	1 envelope	7	13	25	6	0	1	0	0	0	0
16	978	Ginger root, raw, sliced	5 slices	11	87	8	<1	2	<1	<.1	t	t	t
16	1198	Horseradish, prepared	1 tbsp	15	87	6	<1	1	<1	<1	t	t	t
16	1199	Hummous/Humous	1 c	246	65	420	33	50	4	21	3.1	8.8	7.8
16	979	Mustard, prepared, (1 packet =1 tsp)	1 tsp	5	80	4	<1	<1	<1	<1	t	.2	t
		Miso (see #926 under Vegetables and Legumes, Soybean products)											
		Olives:											
16	980	Green	10 olives	39	78	45	<1	<1	1	6	.6	3.6	.3
16	981	Ripe, pitted	10 olives	45	80	52	<1	3	1.5	5	.6	3.6	.4
16	982	Onion powder	1 tsp	2.1	5	5	<1	2	<1	<.1	t	t	t
16	983	Oregano, ground	1 tsp	2	7	5	<1	1	<1	<1	t	t	.1
16	984	Paprika	1 tsp	2	10	6	<1	1	<1	<1	t	t	.2
16	985	Pepper, black	1 tsp	2	11	5	<1	1	<1	<.1	<.1	<.1	<.1
		Pickles:											
16	986	Dill, medium, 3¾ × 1¼" diam	1 pickle	65	92	12	<1	3	1	<1	<.1	t	<.1
16	987	Fresh pack, slices, 1½" diam × ¼"	4 slices	30	79	20	<1	5	<1	<.1	t	t	t
16	988	Sweet, medium	1 pickle	35	65	41	<1	11	<1	.1	t	t	<.1
16	989	Pickle relish, sweet	1 tbsp	15	63	20	<.1	5	<1	<.1	t	t	<.1
16	1201	Sage, ground	1 tbsp	2	8	6	<1	1	<1	<1	.1	<.1	<.1
		Popcorn (see Grain Products, #539-541)											
22	1347	Salsa, from recipe	.85 c	184	91	79	2	9	3	5	.7	3.4	.5
16	990	Salt	1 tsp	6	0	0	0	0	0	0	0	0	0
		Salt substitute:											
16	1205	Morton Salt Substitute	1 tbsp	6	0	0	0	<1	0	0	0	0	0
16	1206	No Salt, packet, Norcliff Thayer	1 packet	.75	0	0	0	0	0	0	0	0	0
16	1207	Light Salt, Morton	1 tsp	6	0	0	0	0	0	0	0	0	0
16	991	Vinegar, cider	1 tbsp	15	94	2	0	1	0	0	0	0	0
		Yeast:											
16	992	Baker's, dry, active, package	1 package	7	5	20	3	3	2	<1	t	.1	t
16	993	Brewer's, dry	1 tbsp	8	5	25	3	3	3	<.1	t	t	0

GRP KEY: 1=BEV 2=DAIRY 3=EGGS 4=FAT/OIL 5=FRUIT 6=BAKERY 7=GRAIN 8=FISH 9=BEEF 10=POULTRY
11=SAUSAGE 12=MIXED/FAST 13=NUTS/SEEDS 14=SWEETS 15=VEG/LEG 16=MISC 22=SOUP/SAUCE

Chol (mg)	Calc (mg)	Iron (mg)	Magn (mg)	Phos (mg)	Pota (mg)	Sodi (mg)	Zinc (mg)	VT-A (RE)	Thia (mg)	Ribo (mg)	Niac (mg)	V-B6 (mg)	Fola (µg)	VT-C (mg)
0	47	1.72	54	96	1178	2906	.56	250	.22	.18	3.3	.44	37	37
0	3	.11	3	6	72	178	.04	15	.01	.01	.21	.03	2	2
0	8	.41	8	16	107	7	.13	221	.02	.05	.46	—	—	4
0	38	.90	10	11	30	4	.14	<1	.01	.01	.1	—	—	<1
0	7	.37	4	8	50	26	.07	91	.01	.02	.21	—	1	2
0	22	1.9	82	109	235	1	1.01	1	.02	.1	.38	.01	18	0
0	4	.08	1	1	22	1	—	11	<.01	<.01	.03	<.01	.4	<1
0	.12	.08	.16	.7	.16	.5	<.01	0	0	0	0	0	0	0
0	28	.86	1	1	11	1	.05	1	<.01	<.01	.03	.02	—	1
0	10	.59	5	7	31	1	.08	2	<.01	<.01	.07	—	—	<1
0	50	1.50	13	16	110	6	.10	—	.01	.01	.09	.05	—	—
0	22	.2	3	18	48	2	1.06	0	.02	.01	.08	.40	<1	4
0	2	.08	2	12	31	1	.07	0	.01	<.01	.02	.57	2	<1
0	1	0	2	0	2	6	0	0	0	0	0	<.01	0	0
0	2	.05	5	3	46	1	.22	0	<.01	<.01	.08	.02	2	1
0	9	.10	4	5	44	14	.18	0	.01	<.01	.06	.01	2	1
0	124	3.87	71	275	427	599	2.70	6	.23	.13	1.01	.98	146	19
0	4	.1	3	4	7	63	.03	0	<.01	.01	.07	<.01	0	<1
0	24	.6	9	6	21	936	.03	12	<.01	<.01	.01	.01	<1	<1
0	40	1.49	2	1	4	392	.10	18	<.01	<.01	.02	<.01	.3	.4
0	8	.06	3	7	20	1	.05	0	01	<.01	.01	.03	3	<1
0	24	.66	4	3	25	<1	.07	10	<.01	t	.09	—	—	1
0	4	.50	4	7	49	1	.09	127	.01	.04	.32	—	—	2
0	9	.61	4	4	26	1	.03	<1	<.01	<.01	.02	0	—	0
0	6	.34	7	14	199	833	.09	21	.01	.02	.04	<.01	1	1
0	3	.20	2	6	20	201	.02	4	t	.01	.02	<.01	0	1
0	1	.21	1	4	11	329	.03	4	<.01	.01	.06	.01	<1	<1
0	3	.13	1	2	30	107	.01	2	t	t	<.01	0	0	1
0	33	.56	9	2	21	0	.09	12	.02	.01	.11	—	—	1
0	18	.86	19	41	347	191	.20	150	.09	.07	.93	.16	28	39
0	14	<.01	2	3	.3	2132	t	0	0	0	0	0	0	0
0	30	0	t	28	2800	t	0	0	0	0	0	0	0	0
0	—	—	—	—	385	0	—	0	0	0	0	0	0	0
0	<1	0	4	0	1500	1100	0	0	0	0	0	0	0	0
0	1	.09	<1	1	15	t	02	0	0	0	0	0	0	0
0	4	1.1	16	90	140	4	.43	t	.17	.38	2.7	.14	266	t
0	17[145]	1.39	18	140	152	10	.63	t	1.25	.34	3.16	.4	313	t

[145] Value varies from 6 to 60 mg.

(For purposes of calculations, use "0" for t, <1, <.1, <.01, etc.)

Table A–1   Food Composition

Grp	Computer Code No.	Food Description	Measure	Wt (g)	H₂O (%)	Ener (cal)	Prot (g)	Carb (g)	Dietary Fiber (g)	Fat (g)	Fat Breakdown (g)		
											Sat	Mono	Poly
SOUPS, SAUCES, AND GRAVIES													
		SOUPS, canned, condensed:											
		Unprepared, condensed:											
22	1210	Cream of celery	1 c	251	85	180	3	18	1	11	2.8	2.6	5.0
22	1215	Cream of chicken	1 c	251	82	233	7	19	<1	15	4.2	.8	3.0
22	1216	Cream of mushroom	1 c	251	81	257	4	19	<1	19	5.2	3.6	8.9
22	1220	Onion	1 c	246	86	114	8	16	1	3	.5	1.5	1.3
		Prepared with equal volume of whole milk:											
22	994	Clam chowder, New England	1 c	248	85	163	9	17	1	7	3.0	2.3	1.1
22	1209	Cream of celery	1 c	248	87	165	6	15	<1	10	4.0	2.5	2.7
22	995	Cream of chicken	1 c	248	85	191	7	15	<1	12	5	4	2
22	996	Cream of mushroom	1 c	248	85	205	6	15	<1	14	5	3	5
22	1214	Cream of potato	1 c	248	87	148	6	17	<1	6	3.8	1.7	.6
22	1213	Oyster stew	1 c	245	89	134	6	10	0	8	5.1	2.1	.3
22	997	Tomato	1 c	248	85	160	6	22	<1	6	2.9	1.6	1.1
		Prepared with equal volume of water:											
22	998	Bean with bacon	1 c	253	84	173	8	23	3	6	1.5	2.2	1.8
22	999	Beef broth, bouillon, consommé	1 c	240	98	16	3	<1	0	1	.3	.2	t
22	1000	Beef noodle	1 c	244	92	84	5	9	<1	3	1.2	1.2	.5
22	1001	Chicken noodle	1 c	241	92	75	4	9	1	2	.7	1.1	.6
22	1002	Chicken rice	1 c	241	94	60	4	7	1	2	.5	.9	.4
22	1208	Chili beef soup	1 c	250	85	169	7	22	1	7	3.3	2.8	.3
22	1003	Clam chowder, Manhatten	1 c	244	92	78	2	12	1	2	.4	.4	1.3
22	1004	Cream of chicken	1 c	244	91	115	3	9	<1	7	2.1	3.3	1.5
22	1005	Cream of mushroom	1 c	244	90	130	2	9	1	9	2.4	1.7	4.2
22	1006	Minestrone	1 c	241	91	80	4	11	1	3	.5	.7	1.1
22	1211	Onion soup	1 c	241	93	57	4	8	<1	2	.3	.8	.7
22	1007	Split pea with ham	1 c	253	82	189	10	28	1	4	1.8	1.8	.6
22	1008	Tomato	1 c	244	90	86	2	17	<1	2	.4	.4	1.0
22	1009	Vegetable beef	1 c	244	92	79	6	10	1	2	.9	.8	.1
22	1010	Vegetarian vegetable	1 c	241	92	70	2	12	2	2	.3	.8	.7
		SOUPS, dehydrated:											
		Unprepared, dry products:											
22	1011	Bouillon	1 packet	6	3	14	1	1	<1	1	.3	.2	t
22	1012	Onion	1 packet	7	4	20	1	4	<1	<1	.1	.2	.1
		Prepared with water:											
22	1299	Beef broth/bouillon	1 c	244	97	20	1	2	<1	1	.3	.3	<.1
22	1376	Chicken broth/bouillon	1 c	244	97	21	1	1	<1	1	.3	.4	.4
22	1013	Chicken noodle	¾ c	188	94	40	2	6	<1	1	.2	.4	.3
22	1122	Cream of chicken	1 c	261	91	107	2	13	1	5	3.4	1.2	.4
22	1014	Onion	¾ c	184	96	20	1	4	<1	<1	.1	.3	.1
22	1217	Split pea	1 c	255	87	133	8	23	1	2	.4	.7	.3
22	1015	Tomato vegetable	¾ c	189	94	41	1	8	<1	1	.3	.3	.1
		SAUCES											
		From dry mixes, prepared with milk:											
22	1016	Cheese sauce	1 c	279	77	305	16	23	<1	17	9	5	2
22	1017	Hollandaise	1 c	259	84	240	5	14	—	20	12	6	1
22	1019	White sauce	1 c	264	81	240	10	21	<1	13	6	5	2
		From home recipe:											
22	1019	White sauce, medium[146]	1 c	250	73	395	10	24	<1	30	9	12	7
		Ready to serve:											
22	1020	Barbeque sauce	1 tbsp	16	81	10	<1	2	<1	<1	<.1	.1	.1
22	1021	Soy sauce	1 tbsp	18	71	9	1	2	0	t	0	0	0

[146]Made with enriched flour, margarine, and whole milk.

(Computer code number is for West Diet Analysis program)

GRP KEY: 1 = BEV 2 = DAIRY 3 = EGGS 4 = FAT/OIL 5 = FRUIT 6 = BAKERY 7 = GRAIN 8 = FISH 9 = BEEF 10 = POULTRY
11 = SAUSAGE 12 = MIXED/FAST 13 = NUTS/SEEDS 14 = SWEETS 15 = VEG/LEG 16 = MISC 22 = SOUP/SAUCE

A

Chol (mg)	Calc (mg)	Iron (mg)	Magn (mg)	Phos (mg)	Pota (mg)	Sodi (mg)	Zinc (mg)	VT-A (RE)	Thia (mg)	Ribo (mg)	Niac (mg)	V-B6 (mg)	Fola (µg)	VT-C (mg)
28	80	1.25	13	75	246	1899	.30	61	.06	.10	.67	.03	5	<1
20	68	1.21	5	75	174	1973	1.26	112	.06	.12	1.64	.03	3	<1
3	64	1.05	9	84	167	2032	1.19	0	.06	.17	1.62	.03	7	2
0	53	1.35	5	22	138	2116	1.23	0	.07	.05	1.21	.10	31	3
22	187	1.48	23	157	300	992	1.3	40	.07	.24	1.03	.13	12	4
32	186	.69	22	151	309	1010	.20	68	.07	.25	.44	.06	9	1
27	180	.67	18	152	273	1046	.68	94	.07	.26	.92	.07	8	1
20	178	.59	20	156	270	1076	.64	38	.08	.28	.81	.06	15	2
22	166	.54	17	160	323	1060	.68	67	.08	.24	.64	.09	9	1
32	167	1.04	21	162	235	1040	10.3	45	.07	.23	.34	.06	7	4
17	159	1.82	23	148	450	932	.29	109	.13	.25	1.52	.16	21	68
3	81	2.05	44	132	403	952	1.03	89	.09	.03	.57	.04	32	2
1	15	.41	9	31	130	782	.6	0	<.01	.05	1.87	.07	2	0
5	15	1.1	6	46	100	952	1.54	63	.07	.06	1.07	.04	4	<1
7	17	.78	7	36	55	900	.55	71	.05	.06	1.39	.01	2	<1
7	17	.75	1	22	101	815	.26	66	.02	.02	1.13	.02	1	<1
12	43	2.40	30	148	525	1035	1.40	503	.06	.08	1.07	.16	10	4
2	27	1.64	10	41	188	578	.98	98	.03	.04	.82	.10	10	4
10	34	.61	3	37	88	986	.63	56	.03	.06	.82	.02	2	<1
2	46	.5	5	49	100	1032	.59	0	.05	.09	.7	.02	3	1
2	34	.92	7	56	312	911	.74	234	.05	.04	.94	.10	16	1
0	26	.67	2	11	69	1053	.61	0	.03	.02	.60	.05	15	1
8	22	2.28	48	213	399	1008	1.32	44	.15	.08	1.48	.07	3	1
0	13	1.76	8	34	263	872	.24	69	.09	.05	1.42	.11	15	67
5	17	1.11	6	41	173	956	2	189	.04	.05	1.03	.08	11	2
0	21	1.08	7	35	209	823	.46	301	.05	.05	.92	.06	11	1
1	4	.06	3	19	27	1019	0	<1	<.01	.02	.27	.01	2	0
<1	10	.14	3	23	47	627	.06	<1	.02	.04	.4	.01	2	<1
0	10	.02	7	24	37	1362	.07	.5	<.01	.02	.36	0	0	.01
1	15	.08	4	13	25	1484	.01	4	.01	.03	.20	.02	—	<1
2	24	.37	5	24	23	957	.15	5	.05	.04	.66	.01	1	<1
3	76	—	—	96	215	1184	—	—	—	.20	—	.05	—	—
0	9	.14	6	22	48	635	.06	<1	.02	.04	.36	<.01	2	<1
3	22	1.01	46	134	238	1220	.59	5	.22	.15	1.34	.05	15	—
0	6	.47	15	23	78	856	.13	15	.04	.03	.59	.04	2	5
53	569	.3	32	438	552	1565	.95	117	.15	.56	.3	.1	12	2
52	124	.9	—	127	124	1564	—	220	.05	.18	.1	.5	—	t
34	425	.3	30	256	444	797	1.15	92	.08	.45	.5	.06	16	3
32	292	.9	35	238	381	888	1.05	340	.15	.43	.8	.1	12	2
0	3	.13	1	3	27	128	.03	14	<.01	<.01	.06	.02	1	1
0	3	.36	6	20	32	1029	.07	0	.01	.02	.61	.03	3	0

(For purposes of calculations, use "0" for t, <1, <.1, <.01, etc.)

Table A–1   Food Composition

Grp	Computer Code No.	Food Description	Measure	Wt (g)	H$_2$O (%)	Ener (cal)	Prot (g)	Carb (g)	Dietary Fiber (g)	Fat (g)	Fat Breakdown (g) Sat	Mono	Poly
SOUPS, SAUCES and GRAVIES—Con.													
		SAUCES—Con.											
		Spaghetti sauce: canned:											
22	1377	Plain	1 c	249	75	272	5	40	3	12	1.7	6.1	3.3
22	1378	With meat	.8 c	206	75	220	8	27	1	10	2.5	4.5	1.5
22	1379	With mushrooms	.75 c	185	75	162	2	9	2	5	.6	2.3	1.2
22	1380	Teriyaki sauce	1 tbsp	18	84	15	1	3	0	<1	t	t	<.1
		GRAVIES:											
		Canned:											
22	1022	Beef	1 c	233	87	123	9	11	<1	5	2.7	2.2	.2
22	1023	Chicken	1 c	238	85	189	5	13	<1	14	3.4	6.1	3.6
22	1024	Mushroom	1 c	238	89	120	3	13	<1	6	1	3	2.4
		From dry mix:											
22	1025	Brown	1 c	258	92	75	2	13	<1	2	.8	.7	.1
22	1026	Chicken	1 c	260	91	85	3	14	<1	2	.5	.9	.4

(Computer code number is for West Diet Analysis program)

GRP KEY: 1 = BEV 2 = DAIRY 3 = EGGS 4 = FAT/OIL 5 = FRUIT 6 = BAKERY 7 = GRAIN 8 = FISH 9 = BEEF 10 = POULTRY
11 = SAUSAGE 12 = MIXED/FAST 13 = NUTS/SEEDS 14 = SWEETS 15 = VEG/LEG 16 = MISC 22 = SOUP/SAUCE

Chol (mg)	Calc (mg)	Iron (mg)	Magn (mg)	Phos (mg)	Pota (mg)	Sodi (mg)	Zinc (mg)	VT-A (RE)	Thia (mg)	Ribo (mg)	Niac (mg)	V-B6 (mg)	Fola (μg)	VT-C (mg)
0	70	1.62	60	90	957	1236	.53	306	.14	.15	3.75	.40	39	28
17	36	2.80	15	106	444	1045	1.05	189	.20	.16	3.40	.27	13	2
0	22	1.50	22	45	500	744	.51	362	.12	.12	1.40	.24	19	14
0	4	.31	11	28	41	690	.02	0	<.01	.01	.23	.02	4	0
7	14	1.63	5	70	189	1305	2.33	0	.07	.08	1.54	.02	5	0
5	48	1.1	5	69	260	1375	1.91	264	.04	.1	1.06	.02	3	0
0	17	1.6	—	36	252	1357	1.66	0	.08	.15	1.6	.05	0	0
3	67	.2	10	44	57	1076	.31	0	.04	.09	.8	0	0	0
3	39	.3	—	47	62	1134	.32	0	.05	.15	.8	.03	—	3

A

(For purposes of calculations, use "0" for t, <1, <.1, <.01, etc.)

Table A–1 Food Composition

Grp	Computer Code No.	Food Description	Measure	Wt (g)	H₂O (%)	Ener (cal)	Prot (g)	Carb (g)	Dietary Fiber (g)	Fat (g)	Sat	Mono	Poly
ARBY'S													
12	1402	Bac'n Cheddar, deluxe	1 ea	229	56	532	29	35	<1	33	8	14	11
		Roast beef sandwiches:												
12	1403	Regular	1 ea	147	51	353	22	32	<1	15	7	5	2
12	1404	Junior	1 ea	85	48	218	13	21	<1	11	4	5	2
12	1405	Super	1 ea	246	58	529	33	46	<1	28	3	11	9
12	1406	Deluxe	1 ea	247	62	486	26	43	<1	23	9	8	5
12	1407	Beef 'n Cheddar	1 ea	198	57	451	25	42	<1	20	7	8	4
		Chicken sandwiches:												
12	1408	Chicken breast sandwich	1 ea	184	52	489	23	48	<1	26	4	8	14
12	1409	Chicken salad sandwich	1 ea	156	53	386	18	33	<1	20	—	—	—
12	1410	Chicken salad & croissant	1 ea	150	50	472	22	16	<1	36	—	—	—
12	1411	Roast Chicken club sandwich	1 ea	234	44	513	31	40	<1	29	5	8	14
12	1412	Hot ham and cheese sandwich	1 ea	162	62	330	23	33	<1	15	4	7	3
12	1413	Turkey deluxe sandwich	1 ea	221	61	399	27	36	<1	20	4	4	12
		Baked potatoes:												
12	1414	Plain	1 ea	241	75	240	6	50	6	2	0	.5	1
12	1415	Deluxe, w/butter & sour cream	1 ea	312	74	463	8	53	6	25	12	8	3
12	1416	W/broccoli & cheese	1 ea	340	70	417	11	55	6	18	7	7	8
12	1417	W/mushrooms & cheese	1 ea	347	70	515	15	58	6	27	6	11	9
12	1418	Taco	1 ea	425	70	619	23	73	6	27	11	9	3
		Milkshakes:												
12	1419	Chocolate	1 ea	340	74	451	10	77	<1	12	3	7	2
12	1420	Jamocha	1 ea	326	75	368	9	59	0	11	3	6	2
12	1421	Vanilla	1 ea	312	75	330	11	46	0	12	4	5	2

Source: Arby's Inc., Atlanta Georgia for the basic nutrients. Values for dietary fiber, magnesium, phosphorus, potassium, zinc, vitamin A (in RE's), B6, folacin, some of the fatty acids, and percent water are estimates calculated from known values for major ingredients.

Grp	Code No.	Food Description	Measure	Wt	H₂O	Ener	Prot	Carb	Fiber	Fat	Sat	Mono	Poly
BURGER KING													
		Croissant sandwiches:												
12	1422	With egg, bacon & cheese	1 ea	119	49	335	15	20	<1	24	13	8	2
12	1423	With egg, sausage & cheese	1 ea	163	49	538	19	20	<1	41	20	12	3
12	1424	With egg, ham & cheese	1 ea	145	58	335	18	20	<1	20	12	7	1
		Whopper sandwiches:												
12	1425	Whopper	1 ea	265	57	640	27	42	<1	41	16	19	4
12	1426	Whopper w/cheese	1 ea	289	57	723	31	43	<1	48	20	20	3
12	1427	Double beef	1 ea	351	56	850	46	52	<1	52	20	24	5
12	1428	Double w/cheese	1 ea	374	55	950	51	54	<1	60	24	28	4
12	1429	Whopper, Junior	1 ea	136	52	370	15	31	<1	17	6	8	1
12	1430	Whopper, Junior w/cheese	1 ea	158	55	420	17	32	<1	20	9	8	1
12	1431	Hamburger	1 ea	109	46	275	15	29	<1	12	5	6	<1
12	1432	Cheeseburger	1 ea	120	45	317	17	30	<1	15	7	6	1
12	1433	Bacon double cheeseburger	1 ea	159	41	510	33	27	<1	31	14	15	2
12	1434	Chicken sandwich	1 ea	230	46	688	26	56	<1	40	11	17	10
12	1435	Chicken tenders	1 ea	95	50	204	20	10	0	10	3	4	2
12	1436	Ham & cheese sandwich	1 ea	230	59	471	24	44	<1	23	10	8	4
12	1437	Whaler fish sandwich	1 ea	189	45	488	19	45	<1	27	6	9	10
12	1438	Whaler sandwich w/cheese	1 ea	201	45	530	21	46	<1	30	7	9	10
12	1439	French fries, regular	1 svg	74	37	227	3	24	<1	13	5	4	1
12	1440	Onion rings, regular	1 svg	79	37	274	4	28	<1	16	5	7	4
		Milkshakes:												
12	1441	Chocolate, medium	1 ea	273	76	320	8	46	<1	12	—	—	—
12	1442	Vanilla, medium	1 ea	273	74	321	9	49	<1	10	—	—	—

GRP KEY: 1 = BEV   2 = DAIRY   3 = EGGS   4 = FAT/OIL   5 = FRUIT   6 = BAKERY   7 = GRAIN   8 = FISH   9 = BEEF   10 = POULTRY
11 = SAUSAGE   12 = MIXED/FAST   13 = NUTS/SEEDS   14 = SWEETS   15 = VEG/LEG   16 = MISC   22 = SOUP/SAUCE

Chol (mg)	Calc (mg)	Iron (mg)	Magn (mg)	Phos (mg)	Pota (mg)	Sodi (mg)	Zinc (mg)	VT-A (RE)	Thia (mg)	Ribo (mg)	Niac (mg)	V-B6 (mg)	Fola (μg)	VT-C (mg)
83	120	2.5	—	—	422	1672	3	85	.4	.48	7	—	—	1
39	32	2	16	120	368	588	3	t	.27	.43	6.23	.20	14	0
23	16	1	8	60	197	345	1.5	t	.13	.24	4	.10	7	0
47	48	2.5	25	190	503	798	3.8	60	.34	.4	7	.30	21	1.2
59	100	6.30	25	190	500	1288	3.8	10	.30	.34	5	.30	22	t
52	76	2	24	260	335	955	3	60	.27	.4	6	.22	19	0
45	64	2	30	180	330	1099	1.5	0	.20	.5	7	.38	18	5
30	—	—	—	—	—	630	—	—	—	—	—	—	—	—
12	—	—	—	—	—	725	—	—	—	—	—	—	—	—
75	120	2	—	—	430	1423	2.3	—	.47	.57	8	—	—	0
45	80	1.5	31	405	312	1350	.9	60	.4	.32	4	.31	26	24
39	64	1.5	30	250	346	1047	1.5	91	.27	.4	7	.52	20	5
0	0	1.80	80	175	1333	58	0	0	.08	.13	2.7	1.08	30	33
40	520	1.5	83	200	1420	203	0	60	.08	.13	2.7	1.10	33	33
22	80	1.5	97	400	1455	361	0	60	.08	.16	2.7	1.15	60	45
47	200	1.5	91	440	1445	923	.9	227	.13	.24	2.7	1.25	36	33
145	450	3.60	105	530	1425	1065	4.7	860	.38	.26	8	1.40	38	63
36	200	.4	48	350	410	341	1.5	91	.11	.65	.7	.14	14	0
35	200	0	36	350	525	262	1.5	91	.11	.65	.7	.14	14	0
32	240	0	36	350	686	281	1.5	91	.11	.65	0	.14	37	0
249	136	2.00	20	249	182	762	1.5	150	.32	.30	2	.06	24	t
293	145	2.90	19	292	284	1042	2.4	150	.36	.32	4	.06	24	t
262	136	2.20	24	317	256	987	1.9	150	.49	.32	3	.06	24	t
94	80	4.90	43	237	547	842	4.5	60	.33	.41	7	.40	35	14
117	210	4.90	47	360	570	1126	5.1	85	.34	.48	7	.40	35	14
188	91	7.30	60	387	760	1080	8.5	60	.34	.56	10	.50	45	14
211	222	7.30	65	510	730	1535	9.1	85	.35	.63	10	.50	45	14
41	40	2.80	24	127	275	486	2.3	30	.23	.25	4	.20	17	6
52	105	2.80	27	189	287	628	2.6	85	.23	.29	4	.20	17	6
37	37	2.70	23	124	235	509	2.4	15	.23	.25	4	.12	18	3
48	102	3.80	26	186	247	651	2.6	70	.23	.29	4	.13	24	3
104	168	3.80	37	328	363	728	5.1	85	.31	.42	6	.30	30	t
82	79	3.30	54	274	375	1423	1.2	13	.45	.31	10	.40	18	t
47	18	.70	24	236	200	636	.6	5	.08	.08	7	.34	10	t
70	195	3.20	42	384	419	1534	2.4	85	.87	.42	6	.31	25	7
84	t	2.20	40	249	366	592	.1	20	.28	.21	4	.13	3	t
95	112	2.20	43	311	378	734	1.1	40	.27	.24	4	.13	3	t
14	t	.50	21	114	360	160	.3	0	.10	.30	7.5	.23	20	t
0	124	.80	18	195	173	665	.4	—	t	t	t	.07	8	t
—	260	1.60	46	262	567	202	1.0	—	.13	.55	t	—	—	t
—	295	t	32	284	505	205	1.0	—	.11	.57	t	—	—	t

Table A–1   Food Composition

Grp	Computer Code No.	Food Description	Measure	Wt (g)	H₂O (%)	Ener (cal)	Prot (g)	Carb (g)	Dietary Fiber (g)	Fat (g)	Fat Breakdown (g)		
											Sat	Mono	Poly
BURGER KING—Con.													
		Pies:											
12	1443	Apple pie	1 ea	125	51	305	3	44	<1	12	—	—	—
12	1444	Cherry pie	1 ea	128	42	357	4	55	<1	13	—	—	—
12	1445	Pecan pie	1 ea	113	20	459	5	64	1	20	3	11	5

Source: Burger King Corporation for basic nutrients. Values for dietary fiber and percent water, calculated from known values for major ingredients.

Grp	Computer Code No.	Food Description	Measure	Wt (g)	H₂O (%)	Ener (cal)	Prot (g)	Carb (g)	Dietary Fiber (g)	Fat (g)	Sat	Mono	Poly
DAIRY QUEEN													
		Ice cream cones:											
12	1446	Small	1 ea	85	65	140	3	22	0	4	2	1	<1
12	1447	Regular	1 ea	142	65	240	6	38	0	7	—	—	—
12	1448	Large	1 ea	213	65	340	9	57	0	10	—	—	—
		Dipped ice cream cones:											
12	1449	Small	1 ea	92	58	190	3	25	<1	9	—	—	—
12	1450	Regular	1 ea	156	58	340	6	42	<1	16	—	—	—
12	1451	Large	1 ea	234	58	510	9	64	<1	24	—	—	—
		Sundaes:											
12	1452	Small	1 ea	106	60	190	3	33	<1	4	—	—	—
12	1453	Regular	1 ea	177	60	310	5	56	<1	8	—	—	—
12	1454	Large	1 ea	248	60	440	8	78	<1	10	—	—	—
12	1455	Banana split	1 ea	383	67	540	9	103	<1	11	—	—	—
12	1456	Peanut buster parfait	1 ea	305	52	740	16	94	<1	34	—	—	—
12	1457	Hot fudge brownie delight	1 ea	266	55	600	9	85	<1	25	—	—	—
12	1458	Strawberry shortcake	1 ea	312	61	540	10	100	<1	11	—	—	—
12	1459	Buster bar	1 ea	149	45	460	10	41	<1	29	—	—	—
12	1460	Dilly bar	1 ea	85	55	210	3	21	<1	13	—	—	—
12	1461	DQ ice cream sandwich	1 ea	60	47	140	3	24	<1	4	—	—	—
		Milkshakes:											
12	1462	Small	1 ea	291	63	490	10	82	<1	13	—	—	—
12	1463	Regular	1 ea	418	63	710	14	120	<1	19	—	—	—
12	1464	Large	1 ea	489	63	831	16	140	<1	22	—	—	—
		Malted milkshakes:											
12	1465	Small	1 ea	291	60	520	10	91	<1	13	—	—	—
12	1466	Regular	1 ea	418	60	760	14	134	<1	18	—	—	—
12	1467	Large	1 ea	489	60	889	16	157	<1	21	—	—	—
12	1468	Float	1 ea	397	76	410	5	82	0	7	—	—	—
12	1469	Freeze	1 ea	397	72	500	9	89	0	12	—	—	—
		Mr. Misty:											
12	1470	Regular	1 ea	330	81	250	0	63	0	0	0	0	0
12	1471	Kiss	1 ea	89	81	70	0	17	0	0	0	0	0
12	1472	Freeze	1 ea	411	72	500	9	91	0	12	—	—	—
12	1473	Float	1 ea	411	78	390	5	74	0	7	—	—	—
12	1474	Chicken sandwich	1 ea	202	46	608	27	46	<1	34	8	15	17
12	1475	Fish fillet sandwich	1 ea	177	52	430	20	45	<1	18	4	6	6
12	1476	Fish fillet sandwich w/cheese	1 ea	191	51	483	23	46	<1	22	7	7	6
		Hamburgers:											
12	1477	Single	1 ea	148	51	360	21	33	<1	16	6	7	1
12	1478	Double	1 ea	210	52	530	36	33	<1	28	10	13	2
12	1479	Triple	1 ea	272	52	710	51	33	<1	45	17	21	4
		Cheeseburgers:											
12	1480	Single	1 ea	162	51	410	24	33	<1	20	8	8	1
12	1481	Double	1 ea	239	51	650	43	34	<1	37	15	14	2
12	1482	Triple	1 ea	301	52	820	58	34	<1	50	20	20	3

GRP KEY: 1 = BEV   2 = DAIRY   3 = EGGS   4 = FAT/OIL   5 = FRUIT   6 = BAKERY   7 = GRAIN   8 = FISH   9 = BEEF   10 = POULTRY
11 = SAUSAGE   12 = MIXED/FAST   13 = NUTS/SEEDS   14 = SWEETS   15 = VEG/LEG   16 = MISC   22 = SOUP/SAUCE

Chol (mg)	Calc (mg)	Iron (mg)	Magn (mg)	Phos (mg)	Pota (mg)	Sodi (mg)	Zinc (mg)	VT-A (RE)	Thia (mg)	Ribo (mg)	Niac (mg)	V-B6 (mg)	Fola (μg)	VT-C (mg)
4	t	1.20	t	31	122	412	.2	4	.27	.16	.6	.03	7	5
6	t	1.10	12	37	166	204	.2	15	.24	.16	.5	.03	4	8
4	24	1.10	16	84	204	374	<1	16	.28	.18	.6	.06	15	t
10	100	.40	13	100	134	45	.47	25	.03	.17	t	.04	2	t
15	150	.70	20	200	220	80	.49	49	.06	.34	t	.06	3	t
25	250	1.40	30	300	330	115	1.0	98	.12	.51	t	.09	4	t
10	100	.40	13	100	134	55	.47	25	.03	.17	t	.04	2	t
20	150	.70	20	200	220	100	.70	49	.06	.34	t	.06	3	t
30	250	1.40	30	300	330	145	1.0	98	.12	.51	t	.09	4	t
10	100	.40	13	150	145	75	.45	25	.03	.17	.17	.03	2	t
20	200	1.10	26	200	290	120	.90	49	.06	.34	.3	.06	4	t
30	250	1.40	40	300	435	165	1.35	98	.12	.43	.4	.09	6	t
30	250	1.80	60	350	670	150	2.1	160	.15	.51	.4	.80	9	15
30	250	1.80	50	450	500	250	1.5	74	.15	.43	2	.10	7	t
20	200	1.80	30	300	300	225	.90	74	.12	.34	.3	.06	4	t
25	250	1.80	—	300	—	215	—	98	.23	.51	t	—	—	12
10	100	1.10	—	250	—	175	—	25	.12	.17	2	—	—	t
10	100	.40	—	100	—	50	—	25	.03	.17	t	—	—	t
5	60	.04	—	60	—	40	—	15	.03	.07	.4	—	—	t
35	350	1.80	30	400	480	180	.10	123	.15	.60	.3	.14	3	t
50	450	2.70	43	500	690	260	.14	184	.23	.77	.4	.20	4	t
60	550	3.60	60	600	960	304	.20	200	.30	.94	.4	.28	6	t
35	350	2.70	30	400	480	180	.10	123	.15	.60	.4	.14	3	t
50	450	4.50	43	600	690	260	.14	184	.30	.85	.8	.20	4	t
60	550	5.40	60	700	960	304	.20	200	.37	.90	.8	.28	6	t
20	200	1.10	—	200	—	85	—	40	.06	.26	t	—	—	t
30	300	1.80	—	350	—	180	—	98	.15	.51	t	—	—	t
0	t	t	—	t	—	10	—	0	t	t	t	—	—	t
0	t	t	—	t	—	10	—	—	t	t	t	—	—	t
30	300	1.40	—	200	—	140	—	98	.12	.51	t	—	—	t
20	200	.70	—	200	—	95	—	49	.06	.26	t	—	—	t
78	150	5.4	15	250	200	725	.5	20	.6	.59	.8	.16	9	2.4
40	150	3.6	20	150	370	674	.3	<1	.6	.42	8	.16	40	<1
49	250	3.6	22	200	370	870	.3	100	.67	.51	8	.16	20	<1
45	100	3.60	33	150	290	630	4.5	10	.30	.17	5	.18	16	t
85	100	6.30	45	300	410	660	6.4	20	.45	.34	9	.28	23	t
135	100	9.00	60	450	532	690	8.2	28	.60	.51	14	.33	29	t
50	200	3.60	35	250	300	790	5.0	110	.30	.17	5	.20	20	t
95	350	6.30	50	500	443	980	7.3	160	.45	.43	9	.30	30	t
145	350	9.00	65	700	550	1010	9.2	200	.60	.60	14	.55	37	t

A

Table A–1   Food Composition

Grp	Computer Code No.	Food Description	Measure	Wt (g)	H₂O (%)	Ener (cal)	Prot (g)	Carb (g)	Dietary Fiber (g)	Fat (g)	Fat Breakdown (g) Sat	Mono	Poly
		DAIRY QUEEN—Con.											
		Hotdogs:											
12	1483	Regular	1 ea	100	50	280	11	21	<1	16	6	7	2
12	1484	With cheese	1 ea	114	49	330	15	21	<1	21	8	8	2
12	1485	With chili	1 ea	128	55	320	13	23	2	20	8	8	2
		Super hotdogs:											
12	1486	Regular	1 ea	175	48	520	17	44	<1	27	9	12	3
12	1487	With cheese	1 ea	196	48	580	22	45	<1	34	11	13	3
12	1488	With chili	1 ea	218	53	570	21	47	2	32	11	13	3
12	1489	French fries, small	1 svg	71	47	200	2	25	<1	10	4	3	<1
12	1490	French fries, large	1 svg	113	47	320	3	40	<1	16	7	5	1
12	1491	Onion Rings	1 svg	85	28	280	4	31	<1	16	5	7	4

Source: International Dairy Queen Inc., Minneapolis, MN for basic nutrients. Values for dietary fiber, magnesium, potassium, zinc, fatty acids, vitamin A (RE's), B6, folacin and percent water, calculated from known values for the major ingredients.

Grp	Computer Code No.	Food Description	Measure	Wt (g)	H₂O (%)	Ener (cal)	Prot (g)	Carb (g)	Dietary Fiber (g)	Fat (g)	Fat Breakdown (g) Sat	Mono	Poly
		JACK IN THE BOX											
12	1492	Breakfast Jack sandwich	1 ea	126	49	307	18	30	<1	13	—	—	—
12	1493	Canadian crescent	1 ea	134	42	472	19	25	<1	31	—	—	—
12	1494	Sausage crescent	1 ea	156	38	584	22	28	<1	43	—	—	—
12	1495	Supreme crescent	1 ea	146	38	547	20	27	<1	40	—	—	—
12	1496	Pancakes breakfast platter	1 ea	231	45	612	15	87	<1	22	8.6	7.6	3.5
12	1497	Scrambled egg breakfast platter	1 ea	249	51	662	24	52	<1	40	17.1	16	4.7
12	1498	Hamburger	1 ea	98	44	276	13	30	<1	12	—	—	—
12	1499	Cheeseburger	1 ea	113	44	323	16	32	<1	15	—	—	—
12	1500	Jumbo Jack	1 ea	205	57	485	26	38	<1	26	—	—	—
12	1501	Jumbo Jack w/cheese	1 ea	246	56	630	32	45	<1	35	—	—	—
12	1502	Bacon cheeseburger supreme	1 ea	231	45	724	34	44	<1	46	—	—	—
12	1503	Swiss & baconburger	1 ea	231	52	643	33	31	<1	43	—	—	—
12	1504	Ham & swiss burger	1 ea	203	44	638	36	37	<1	39	—	—	—
12	1505	Chicken supreme	1 ea	228	52	601	31	39	<1	36	—	—	—
12	1506	Moby Jack sandwich	1 ea	137	40	444	16	39	<1	25	—	—	—
12	1583	Double cheeseburger	1 ea	149	64	467	21	33	—	27	12.3	11.6	3.1
		Tacos:											
12	1508	Regular	1 ea	81	57	191	8	16	<1	11	—	—	—
12	1509	Super	1 ea	135	63	288	12	21	<1	17	—	—	—
12	1513	Taco salad	1 ea	358	81	377	31	10	1	24	—	—	—
12	1516	French fries	1 svg	68	40	221	2	27	<1	12	—	—	—
12	1517	Hash brown potatoes	1 svg	62	60	116	2	11	<1	7	3.6	3.2	.4
12	1518	Onion rings	1 svg	108	28	382	5	39	<1	23	—	—	—
		Milkshakes:											
12	1519	Chocolate	1 ea	322	77	330	11	55	0	7	—	—	—
12	1520	Strawberry	1 ea	328	77	320	10	55	0	7	—	—	—
12	1521	Vanilla	1 ea	317	76	320	10	57	0	6	—	—	—
12	1522	Apple turnover	1 ea	119	38	410	4	45	<1	24	—	—	—

Source: Jack in the Box Restaurants, Foodmaker, Inc., San Diego, CA for basic nutrients. Some values for dietary fiber, magnesium, phosphorus, potassium, zinc, vitamin A (RE's), B6, folacin, and fatty acids calculated from known values for major ingredients.

GRP KEY:　1=BEV　2=DAIRY　3=EGGS　4=FAT/OIL　5=FRUIT　6=BAKERY　7=GRAIN　8=FISH　9=BEEF　10=POULTRY
　　　　　　　11=SAUSAGE　12=MIXED/FAST　13=NUTS/SEEDS　14=SWEETS　15=VEG/LEG　16=MISC　22=SOUP/SAUCE

Chol (mg)	Calc (mg)	Iron (mg)	Magn (mg)	Phos (mg)	Pota (mg)	Sodi (mg)	Zinc (mg)	VT-A (RE)	Thia (mg)	Ribo (mg)	Niac (mg)	V-B6 (mg)	Fola (µg)	VT-C (mg)
45	80	1.40	21	100	130	830	1.4	t	.12	.14	3	.08	20	<1
55	150	1.40	24	200	140	990	1.9	85	.12	.17	3	.08	24	<1
55	80	1.80	38	150	170	985	1.8	60	.15	.26	4	.17	30	<1
80	150	2.70	24	150	210	1365	2.8	t	.23	.26	5	.14	35	<1
100	250	1.40	38	300	220	1605	2.5	100	.23	.26	5	.16	39	<1
100	150	2.70	48	250	250	1595	2.5	60	.23	.43	6	.25	45	<1
10	t	.34	16	60	450	115	t	0	.06	t	.8	.16	15	9
15	t	1.08	24	100	700	185	.3	0	.09	.03	1.2	.30	25	15
15	20	.72	16	60	110	140	.3	15	.09	t	.4	.08	10	2
203	170	3.10	24	310	190	871	1.8	120	.47	.41	3	.11	—	<1
226	125	3.40	—	—	—	851	—	135	.50	.40	3.6	—	—	3
187	170	2.90	—	—	—	1012	—	—	.60	.51	4.6	—	—	t
178	150	2.70	—	—	—	1053	—	—	.64	.54	4.2	—	—	t
99	100	1.8	36	633	237	888	1.9	69	.03	.75	7	.19	3	6
354	200	5.4	55	483	635	1188	3.0	252	.3	.77	5	.34	30	4.8
29	70	2.70	20	115	165	521	1.8	9	.36	.24	3.2	.10	—	1
42	160	2.70	22	194	177	749	2.3	57	.36	.27	3.3	.10	—	1
64	97	6.90	35	208	390	905	3.7	—	.51	.21	7	.25	—	5
110	250	4.50	49	411	499	1665	4.8	—	.53	.34	12	.31	—	5
70	310	4.90	—	—	—	1307	—	—	.56	.51	8.8	—	—	3
99	230	4.70	—	—	—	1354	—	—	.45	.41	6.8	—	—	3
117	268	6.10	—	—	—	1330	—	—	.76	.48	7.6	—	—	10
60	240	3.00	—	—	—	1582	—	—	.52	.37	10.6	—	—	4
47	160	2.20	30	263	246	820	1.1	—	.40	.25	2.8	.08	—	<1
72	400	2.7	—	—	—	842	—	—	.15	.34	6	—	—	—
21	100	1.10	35	146	257	460	1.2	—	.07	.17	1.0	.13	—	<1
37	150	1.60	45	198	347	765	1.8	—	.12	.08	1.4	.18	—	2
102	280	4.30	—	—	—	1436	—	141	.18	.53	6	—	—	7
8	10	.50	23	75	360	164	.26	<1	.07	.03	1.20	.18	—	3
3	40	.36	—	—	—	211	—	0	.06	.03	1.2	—	—	4
27	30	1.40	16	69	109	407	.40	<1	.21	.12	1.80	.06	—	3
25	350	.70	55	330	650	270	1.20	—	.15	.59	.60	.18	—	3
25	350	.40	40	328	613	240	1.10	—	.15	.43	.40	.16	—	3
25	350	.30	38	312	599	230	1.00	<1	.15	.34	.40	.20	—	<1
15	11	1.40	10	33	69	350	.20	—	.23	.12	2.50	.03	—	<1

A

Table A–1　Food Composition

Grp	Computer Code No.	Food Description	Measure	Wt (g)	H$_2$O (%)	Ener (cal)	Prot (g)	Carb (g)	Dietary Fiber (g)	Fat (g)	Fat Breakdown (g) Sat	Mono	Poly
KENTUCKY FRIED CHICKEN													
		Original Recipe:											
12	1253	Center breast	1 ea	95	52	236	24	7	<1	14	4	7	2
12	1251	Side breast	1 ea	69	39	199	16	7	<1	12	3	5	3
12	1250	Drumstick	1 ea	47	53	117	12	3	<1	7	2	3	2
12	1252	Thigh	1 ea	88	49	257	18	7	<1	18	4	7	4
12	1249	Wing	1 ea	42	44	136	10	4	<1	9	2	4	2
		Dinners:											
12	1254	2 pce dinner, white	1 ea	322	64	604	30	48	1	32	7	12	10
12	1255	2 pce dinner, dark	1 ea	346	65	643	35	46	1	35	8	13	11
12	1256	2 pce dinner, combination	1 ea	341	63	661	33	48	1	38	8	14	11
		Extra crispy recipe:											
12	1261	Center breast	1 ea	104	39	297	24	14	<1	16	4	7	4
12	1259	Side breast	1 ea	84	39	286	17	14	<1	18	5	7	4
12	1258	Drumstick	1 ea	58	51	155	13	5	<1	9	2	4	2
12	1260	Thigh	1 ea	107	45	343	20	13	<1	23	6	10	6
12	1257	Wing	1 ea	53	36	201	11	9	<1	14	4	6	3
		Dinners:											
12	1262	2 pce dinner, white	1 ea	348	60	755	33	60	1	43	10	16	12
12	1263	2 pce dinner, dark	1 ea	375	62	765	38	55	1	54	11	16	13
12	1264	2 pce dinner, combination	1 ea	371	60	902	36	58	1	48	12	18	14
12	1265	Mashed potatoes	⅓ c	80	81	60	2	12	<1	1	<1	<1	<1
12	1266	Chicken gravy	⅓ c	78	76	59	2	4	<1	4	1	2	<1
12	1267	Dinner roll	1 ea	21	31	61	2	11	<1	1	<1	<1	<1
12	1268	Corn on the cob	1 ea	143	70	176	5	32	2	3	<1	1	1
12	1269	Coleslaw	⅓ c	79	76	103	1	12	<1	6	1	2	3
12	1381	Kentucky nuggets	1 ea	16	44	46	3	2	<1	3	1	2	<1
		Kentucky nugget sauces:											
12	1382	Barbeque	2 tbsp	30	51	35	<1	7	—	1	<1	<1	<1
12	1383	Sweet & sour	2 tbsp	30	50	58	<1	13	—	1	<1	<1	<1
12	1384	Honey	1 tbsp	15	50	49	0	12	—	<1	—	—	—
12	1385	Mustard	2 tbsp	30	52	36	1	6	—	1	—	—	—
12	1386	Kentucky fries	1 svg	119	45	268	5	33	<1	13	3	8	1
12	1387	Mashed potatoes & gravy	⅓ c	86	80	62	2	10	<1	1	<1	<1	<1
12	1388	Buttermilk biscuit	1 ea	75	27	269	5	32	<1	14	4	8	1
12	1389	Potato salad	⅓ c	90	76	141	2	13	1	9	1	3	5
12	1390	Baked beans	⅓ c	89	71	105	5	18	6	1	<1	<1	<1
12	1391	Chicken Little sandwich	1 ea	57	52	177	6	17	1	9	2	3	3

Source: Kentucky Fried Chicken Corporation

Grp	No.	Food Description	Measure	Wt (g)	H$_2$O (%)	Ener (cal)	Prot (g)	Carb (g)	Dietary Fiber (g)	Fat (g)	Sat	Mono	Poly
LONG JOHN SILVER'S													
		Fish, batter fried:											
12	1523	Fish & fryes, 3 pce	1 ea	350	55	853	43	64	<1	48	—	—	—
12	1524	Fish & fryes, 2 pce	1 ea	260	53	651	30	53	<1	36	—	—	—
12	1525	Fish dinner, 3 pce	1 ea	540	60	1180	47	93	<1	70	—	—	—
		Fish, breaded & fried:											
12	1526	Fish dinner, 3 pce	1 ea	450	60	940	35	84	<1	52	—	—	—
12	1527	Fish dinner, 2 pce	1 ea	400	60	818	26	76	<1	46	—	—	—
		Chicken:											
12	1528	Chicken plank dinner, 3 pce	1 ea	370	60	885	32	72	<1	51	—	—	—
12	1529	Chicken plank dinner, 4 pce	1 ea	440	60	1037	41	82	<1	59	—	—	—
12	1530	Chicken nugget dinner, 6 pce	1 ea	300	60	699	23	54	<1	45	—	—	—
12	1531	Clam chowder	1 svg	185	85	128	7	15	<1	5	—	—	—
12	1532	Clam dinner	1 ea	460	60	955	22	100	<1	58	—	—	—
12	1533	Fish & chicken dinner	1 ea	460	60	935	36	73	<1	55	—	—	—

GRP KEY: 1 = BEV 2 = DAIRY 3 = EGGS 4 = FAT/OIL 5 = FRUIT 6 = BAKERY 7 = GRAIN 8 = FISH 9 = BEEF 10 = POULTRY
11 = SAUSAGE 12 = MIXED/FAST 13 = NUTS/SEEDS 14 = SWEETS 15 = VEG/LEG 16 = MISC 22 = SOUP/SAUCE

A

Chol (mg)	Calc (mg)	Iron (mg)	Magn (mg)	Phos (mg)	Pota (mg)	Sodi (mg)	Zinc (mg)	VT-A (RE)	Thia (mg)	Ribo (mg)	Niac (mg)	V-B6 (mg)	Fola (µg)	VT-C (mg)
87	30	1.17	28	205	267	631	.72	6	.08	.11	7.57	.31	8	2
70	50	.98	19	151	176	558	.77	4	.06	.08	5.66	.20	6	1
63	12	.80	13	95	122	207	1.29	3	.04	.09	2.38	.09	4	1
109	34	1.45	22	169	217	566	1.65	5	.08	.16	4.03	.17	9	2
55	22	.68	10	76	86	302	.58	3	.03	.04	2.28	.10	4	1
133	142	3.31	61	326	643	1528	1.88	77	.22	.19	10.0	.50	39	37
180	116	3.90	66	363	720	1441	3.47	77	.25	.32	8.46	.46	42	37
172	126	3.78	64	344	684	1536	2.76	77	.24	.27	8.36	.47	41	37
79	62	1.29	29	218	244	584	.77	6	.11	.11	7.89	.30	11	2
65	57	1.12	21	157	188	564	.88	5	.12	.13	5.37	.24	9	2
66	11	.95	14	100	147	263	1.32	4	.07	.11	3.07	.16	6	1
109	49	1.49	24	185	228	549	1.73	7	.12	.19	5.35	.17	11	2
59	16	.65	12	77	100	312	.67	3	.06	.09	2.94	.11	5	1
132	143	6.03	65	333	689	1544	2.08	77	.31	.29	10.4	.56	43	37
183	130	4.09	70	383	776	1480	3.58	77	.32	.38	10.4	.54	46	37
176	135	6.40	68	361	729	1529	2.93	77	.31	.35	10.3	.49	45	37
<1	21	.28	14	41	218	228	.16	5	.01	.04	.96	.11	7	5
2	9	.48	2	10	21	398	.04	1	.01	.03	.47	<.01	2	<1
1	21	.53	6	28	29	118	.20	1	.10	.04	.98	.01	7	<1
<1	7	.79	53	134	323	12	.99	27	.14	.11	1.80	.22	71	2
4	29	.19	9	20	115	171	.13	28	.03	.03	.20	.07	10	19
12	2	.13	4	29	33	140	.22	30	.02	.03	1.00	.04	1	2
1	6	.24	5	10	75	450	.05	37	.01	.01	.19	.02	3	<1
1	5	.16	2	5	39	148	.02	6	.01	.02	.04	.01	1	<1
t	1	.11	<1	<1	6	10	<.01	0	.01	<.01	.04	t	1	3
1	10	.26	6	15	23	346	.09	1	.02	.01	.16	.02	3	1
1	24	.94	28	78	606	81	.31	0	.17	.06	2.70	.18	20	3
1	19	.35	9	28	137	297	.11	5	.01	.04	1.00	.08	8	1
1	77	1.22	9	264	95	521	.29	30	.28	.13	1.80	.03	8	<1
11	10	.32	15	32	256	396	.29	27	.07	.02	.60	.19	7	3
1	54	1.43	29	90	229	387	1.29	10	.06	.04	.50	.07	32	2
20	39	1.40	10	105	114	398	.93	6	.15	.14	1.65	.07	11	<1
106	—	—	—	—	—	2025	—	—	—	—	—	—	—	—
75	—	—	—	—	—	1352	—	—	—	—	—	—	—	—
119	—	—	—	—	—	2797	—	—	—	—	—	—	—	—
101	—	—	—	—	—	1900	—	—	—	—	—	—	—	—
76	—	—	—	—	—	1526	—	—	—	—	—	—	—	—
25	—	—	—	—	—	1918	—	—	—	—	—	—	—	—
25	—	—	—	—	—	2433	—	—	—	—	—	—	—	—
25	—	—	—	—	—	853	—	—	—	—	—	—	—	—
17	—	—	—	—	—	611	—	—	—	—	—	—	—	—
27	—	—	—	—	—	1543	—	—	—	—	—	—	—	—
56	—	—	—	—	—	2076	—	—	—	—	—	—	—	—

Table A–1 Food Composition

Grp	Code No.	Food Description	Measure	Wt (g)	H₂O (%)	Ener (cal)	Prot (g)	Carb (g)	Dietary Fiber (g)	Fat (g)	Fat Breakdown (g) Sat	Mono	Poly
LONG JOHN SILVER'S—Con.												
12	1534	Oyster dinner	1 ea	360	60	789	17	78	<1	45	—	—	—
12	1535	Scallop dinner	1 ea	320	60	747	17	66	<1	45	—	—	—
12	1536	Seafood platter	1 ea	410	60	976	29	85	<1	58	—	—	—
12	1537	Batter fried shrimp dinner	1 ea	300	60	711	17	60	<1	45	—	—	—
12	1538	Fish sandwich platter	1 ea	400	60	835	30	84	<1	42	—	—	—
		Salads:											
12	1539	Ocean chef	1 ea	320	85	229	27	13	2	8	—	—	—
12	1540	Seafood	1 ea	480	85	426	19	22	2	30	—	—	—
12	1541	Cole slaw	1 svg	98	70	182	1	11	<1	15	—	—	—
12	1542	Fries	1 svg	85	42	247	4	31	<1	12	—	—	—
12	1543	Hush puppies	1 ea	47	37	145	3	18	<1	7	—	—	—

Source: Long John Silver's Inc., Lexington, KY.

Grp	Code No.	Food Description	Measure	Wt (g)	H₂O (%)	Ener (cal)	Prot (g)	Carb (g)	Dietary Fiber (g)	Fat (g)	Sat	Mono	Poly
McDONALD'S												
		Sandwiches:											
12	1221	Big Mac	1 ea	215	48	560	25	43	1	32	10	21	2
12	1591	McDLT Sandwich	1 ea	234	59	580	26	36	1.4	37	12	17	9
12	1222	Quarter Pounder	1 ea	166	49	410	23	34	1	21	8	11	1
12	1223	Quarter Pounder w/cheese	1 ea	194	48	520	29	35	1	29	11	16	1
12	1224	Filet-O-Fish sandwich	1 ea	142	44	440	14	38	<1	26	5	10	11
12	1225	Hamburger	1 ea	102	46	260	12	31	<1	10	4	5	1
12	1226	Cheeseburger	1 ea	116	45	310	15	31	<1	14	5	8	1
12	1227	French fries	1 svg	68	37	220	4	26	1	12	3	8	.5
12	1228	Chicken McNuggets	6 ea	112	49	270	20	17	<1	15	4	10	2
		Sauces:											
12	1229	Hot Mustard	1 ea	30	53	70	.5	8	<1	4	<1	1	1
12	1230	Barbecue	1 ea	30	51	50	.3	12	<1	<1	<1	<1	<1
12	1231	Sweet & sour	1 ea	32	50	60	<1	14	<1	<1	<1	<1	<1
		Lowfat Milkshakes:											
12	1232	Chocolate	10 fl oz	293	70	320	12	66	<1	2	.8	.9	<1
12	1233	Strawberry	10 fl oz	293	72	320	11	67	<1	1	.6	.6	<1
12	1234	Vanilla	10 fl oz	293	73	290	11	60	<1	1	.63	.67	<1
		Sundaes:											
12	1235	Hot fudge	1 ea	169	60	240	7	51	<1	3	2	1	<1
12	1236	Strawberry	1 ea	171	62	210	6	49	<1	1	1	4	<1
12	1237	Hot Caramel	1 ea	174	57	270	7	59	<1	3	2	1	<1
12	1238	Vanilla cone	1 ea	80	65	100	4	22	<1	1	<1	<1	<1
		Pies:											
12	1239	Apple pie	1 ea	83	45	260	2	30	<1	15	5	9	1
12	1240	Apple Bran Muffin	1 ea	85	44	190	5	46	3	0	0	0	0
		Cookies, package:											
12	1241	McDonaldland cookies	1 pkg	56	3	290	4	47	<1	9	2	7	<1
12	1242	Chocolate chip cookies	1 pkg	56	3	330	4	42	2	16	5	10	<1
		Breakfast items:											
12	1243	English muffin, w/butter	1 ea	59	42	170	5	27	<1	5	2	2	1
12	1244	Egg McMuffin	1 ea	138	51	290	8.2	28	<1	11	4	6	1
12	1245	Hot cakes w/butter & syrup	1 ea	176	46	410	8	74	<1	9	4	3	3
12	1246	Scrambled eggs	1 ea	100	70	140	12	1	<1	10	3	5	1
12	1247	Pork Sausage	1 svg.	48	43	180	8	0	<1	16	6	9	2
12	1248	Hash brown potato patty	1 ea	53	56	130	1	15	1	7	3	4	<1
12	1392	Sausage McMuffin	1 ea	117	38	370	17	27	<1	22	8	12	2
12	1393	Sausage McMuffin w/egg	1 ea	167	47	440	23	28	<1	27	9	15	3
12	1394	Biscuit with spread	1 ea	75	27	260	5	32	<1	13	3	9	1

GRP KEY: 1 = BEV 2 = DAIRY 3 = EGGS 4 = FAT/OIL 5 = FRUIT 6 = BAKERY 7 = GRAIN 8 = FISH 9 = BEEF 10 = POULTRY
11 = SAUSAGE 12 = MIXED/FAST 13 = NUTS/SEEDS 14 = SWEETS 15 = VEG/LEG 16 = MISC 22 = SOUP/SAUCE

A

Chol (mg)	Calc (mg)	Iron (mg)	Magn (mg)	Phos (mg)	Pota (mg)	Sodi (mg)	Zinc (mg)	VT-A (RE)	Thia (mg)	Ribo (mg)	Niac (mg)	V-B6 (mg)	Fola (µg)	VT-C (mg)
55	—	—	—	—	—	763	—	—	—	—	—	—	—	—
37	—	—	—	—	—	1579	—	—	—	—	—	—	—	—
95	—	—	—	—	—	2161	—	—	—	—	—	—	—	—
127	—	—	—	—	—	1297	—	—	—	—	—	—	—	—
75	—	—	—	—	—	1402	—	—	—	—	—	—	—	—
64	—	—	—	—	—	986	—	—	—	—	—	—	—	—
113	—	—	—	—	—	1086	—	—	—	—	—	—	—	—
12	—	—	—	—	—	367	—	—	—	—	—	—	—	—
13	—	—	—	—	—	.6	—	—	—	—	—	—	—	—
—	—	—	—	—	—	405	—	—	—	—	—	—	—	—
103	256	4	41	338	268	950	5.04	88	.48	.41	6.81	.285	23	2
109	225	4	45	321	414	990	6	188	.39	.36	7	.26	30	7
86	142	4	38	258	334	660	5.3	45	.36	.29	6.7	.28	24	3
118	296	3.7	42	315	356	1150	6	190	.37	.39	6.7	.24	24	3
50	165	1.8	27	227	149	1030	.88	36	.30	.15	3.00	.10	20	.1
37	122	2.29	20	129	145	500	2.13	15	.28	.16	3.84	.12	17	2
53	197	2.3	23	205	157	750	2.60	112	.30	.21	3.86	.12	21	2
0	9	.61	27	101	564	70	.32	0	.13	0	1.8	.22	19	2
56	14	1	27	293	313	580	.923	0	.12	.12	8.3	.394	11	0
5	15	.22	6	15	23	250	.09	1.6	.01	.01	.15	.01	3	.45
0	13	.31	5	10	75	340	.05	15	.01	.01	.17	.02	3	2.34
0	11	.17	2	5	39	190	.02	32	0	.01	.08	.01	.6	.64
10	322	.84	47	319	555	240	1.21	92	.13	.52	.41	.148	15	0
10	327	.1	36	302	509	170	1.07	92	.13	.48	.31	.148	11	0
10	327	.10	35	339	521	170	1.09	92	.13	.48	.31	.148	36	0
6	235	.48	36	243	422	170	1.01	65	.08	.35	.30	.138	11	0
5	191	.16	29	188	302	95	.838	65	.07	.29	.25	.056	21	1
13	222	.1	31	243	356	180	.916	88	.08	.35	.26	.054	14	0
3	112	.23	13	120	136	70	.482	87	.04	.18	.37	.046	2	0
0	11	.71	6	26	38	240	.16	0	.06	.02	.32	.02	5	11
0	31	.6	—	—	—	230	—	.7	.02	.08	.4	—	—	.7
0	9	2.1	11	72	50	300	.325	0	.25	.18	2.54	.03	6	0
4	24	2.2	27	102	160	280	.50	0	.18	.21	2.47	.03	6	0
9	151	1.61	13	69	66	270	.50	31	.33	.14	2.47	.04	16	0
226	256	2.77	26	322	168	740	1.92	151	.47	.33	3.71	.21	30	0
21	114	2.08	23	412	154	640	.56	52	.32	.33	2.82	.099	7	0
399	57	2.08	13	269	138	290	1.69	157	.07	.26	.05	.20	66	0
48	8	.67	8	86	115	350	1.33	0	.27	.10	2.31	.165	1	0
9	6	.27	13	65	238	330	.164	0	.06	.02	.85	.124	6	2
64	235	2.3	24	189	219	830	1.71	72	.60	.29	4.8	.15	23	0
263	263	3.34	30	291	298	980	2.39	150	.64	.42	4.8	.20	33	0
1	75	1.31	9	264	95	730	.292	0	.23	.11	1.65	.03	8	0

Table A–1   Food Composition

Grp	Computer Code No.	Food Description	Measure	Wt (g)	H₂O (%)	Ener (cal)	Prot (g)	Carb (g)	Dietary Fiber (g)	Fat (g)	Fat Breakdown (g) Sat	Mono	Poly
McDONALD'S—Con.													
		Breakfast Items—Con.											
12	1395	Biscuit w/sausage	1 ea	123	32	440	13	32	<1	29	9	17	3
12	1396	Biscuit w/sausage & egg	1 ea	180	43	529	20	33	<1	35	11	20	3
12	1397	Biscuit w/bacon, egg & cheese	1 ea	156	41	440	18	33	<1	26	8	16	2
		Salads:											
12	1398	Chef salad	1 ea	283	84	230	21	8	2	13	6	7	1
12	1399	Shrimp salad	1 ea	262	88	104	14	6	2	3	1	2	<1
12	1400	Garden salad	1 ea	213	91	110	7	6	2	7	3	3	<1
12	1401	Chunky Chicken salad	1 ea	250	88	140	23	5	2	3	1	2	1

Source: McDonald's Corporation, Oak Brook, Illinois. Some values for Salads estimated from known values for major ingredients.

Grp	Computer Code No.	Food Description	Measure	Wt (g)	H₂O (%)	Ener (cal)	Prot (g)	Carb (g)	Dietary Fiber (g)	Fat (g)	Sat	Mono	Poly
TACO BELL													
		Burritos:											
12	1544	Bean	1 ea	191	58	357	13	54	8	10	3	5	2
12	1545	Beef	1 ea	191	58	403	22	39	2	17	7	7	2
12	1546	Bean & beef	1 ea	191	58	381	17	46	5	14	7	6	1
12	1547	Burrito supreme	1 ea	241	66	413	18	46	5	18	8	8	2
12	1548	Double beef supreme	1 ea	255	66	457	24	42	2	22	10	10	2
12	1549	Enchirito	1 ea	213	61	382	20	31	5	20	9	8	1
12	1550	Fajita (steak taco)	1 ea	135	65	234	15	20	2	11	5	4	1
		Tacos:											
12	1551	Regular	1 ea	78	55	183	10	11	1	11	5	3	1
12	1552	Taco bellgrande	1 ea	163	63	355	18	18	2	23	11	6	1
12	1553	Taco light	1 ea	170	59	410	19	18	2	29	12	8	5
12	1554	Soft taco	1 ea	92	52	228	12	18	2	12	5	4	1
		Tostadas:											
12	1555	Regular	1 ea	156	67	243	10	27	7	11	4	4	1
12	1556	Beefy tostada	1 ea	198	69	322	15	22	4	20	10	8	1
12	1557	Bellbeefer	1 ea	177	63	312	17	32	<1	13	6	4	2
12	1558	Mexican pizza	1 ea	223	55	575	21	40	5	48	31	14	2
12	1559	Taco salad with salsa	1 ea	595	73	941	36	63	5	61	19	18	12
		Nachos:											
12	1560	Regular	1 ea	106	40	356	7	38	<1	19	12	5	1
12	1561	Bellgrande	1 ea	287	58	649	22	61	6	35	12	20	3
12	1562	Pintos & cheese	1 ea	128	69	190	9	19	7	9	4	4	1
12	1563	Taco sauce	1 ea	3.7	96	2	<1	<1	<1	<1	<1	<1	<1
12	1564	Salsa	1 ea	9.7	95	18	1	4	1	<1	<1	<1	<1
12	1565	Cinnamon Crispas	1 ea	47.3	1	259	3	27	<1	15	4	2	1

Source: Taco Bell Corporation, California for most nutrient values. Values for Dietary fiber, mono-unsaturated fat, magnesium, phosphorus, zinc, folacin, Vitamin B6, Vitamin A in REs, and percentage water are estimates calculated from known values of major ingredients.

Grp	Computer Code No.	Food Description	Measure	Wt (g)	H₂O (%)	Ener (cal)	Prot (g)	Carb (g)	Dietary Fiber (g)	Fat (g)	Sat	Mono	Poly
WENDY's													
		Hamburgers:											
12	1566	Single, on white bun, no toppings	1 ea	119	41	350	21	29	<1	16	7	9	1
12	1568	Double, on white bun, no toppings	1 ea	197	44	560	41	32	<1	34	7	13	8
12	1569	Big classic	1 ea	241	63	470	26	36	2	25	7	10	5
		Cheeseburgers:											
12	1570	Bacon cheeseburger	1 ea	147	46	460	29	23	<1	28	13	13	2
12	1571	Single, w/all toppings	1 ea	215	50	548	30	32	2	33	13	12	5
12	1572	Double, w/all toppings	1 ea	291	50	735	48	27	2	48	18	18	6

GRP KEY: 1 = BEV   2 = DAIRY   3 = EGGS   4 = FAT/OIL   5 = FRUIT   6 = BAKERY   7 = GRAIN   8 = FISH   9 = BEEF   10 = POULTRY
11 = SAUSAGE   12 = MIXED/FAST   13 = NUTS/SEEDS   14 = SWEETS   15 = VEG/LEG   16 = MISC   22 = SOUP/SAUCE

A

Chol (mg)	Calc (mg)	Iron (mg)	Magn (mg)	Phos (mg)	Pota (mg)	Sodi (mg)	Zinc (mg)	VT-A (RE)	Thia (mg)	Ribo (mg)	Niac (mg)	V-B6 (mg)	Fola (µg)	VT-C (mg)
49	83	1.98	18	359	235	1080	1.33	0	.49	.21	3.96	.12	12	0
275	116	3.16	25	490	321	1250	3.16	88	.53	.35	3.99	.199	36	0
253	185	2.56	21	496	250	1230	1.67	162	.36	.33	2.47	.11	47	0
128	256	1.51	35	200	400	490	1.40	514	.31	.29	3.6	.04	60	14
193	65	1.33	60	180	420	480	1.90	372	.13	.10	1.08	.06	60	13
83	149	1.26	18	80	280	160	.40	391	.10	.16	.59	.06	60	14
78	24	1	20	140	350	230	.66	458	.22	.17	8.5	.34	61	20
9	147	3.47	65	210	428	888	2.05	65	.037	2.02	1.98	1.00	55	53
57	114	3.73	35	225	313	1051	4.00	100	.398	2.14	3.44	.23	27	2
36	111	2.15	50	220	370	958	2.67	80	.49	.42	3.09	.59	38	2
33	153	3.6	50	227	432	921	3.00	185	.41	2.12	2.89	.52	40	27
57	145	4	52	230	431	1053	4.00	200	.43	2.2	3.68	.30	30	9
54	269	2.84	61	263	423	1243	3.51	157	.256	.418	2.3	.61	29	28
14	117	3.03	24	150	207	485	3.18	133	.403	.341	3.71	.17	15	3
32	84	1.10	16	100	159	276	2.12	42	.05	.142	1.07	.12	10	1
56	182	1.91	18	100	334	472	2.12	132	.11	.29	2.02	.12	13	5
56	155	2.4	18	100	316	594	2.12	128	.2	.33	2.5	.12	13	5
32	116	2.27	18	100	178	516	2.12	42	.39	.22	2.74	.12	10	1
16	179	1.53	62	195	401	596	1.55	84	.061	.169	.626	1.01	47	45
40	185	1.96	43	206	408	764	2.97	152	.24	.29	1.61	.56	31	6
39	174	2.36	22	125	299	855	2.10	121	.16	.30	1.73	.12	<1	5
81	453	3.08	80	400	449	1364	5.40	355	.36	.39	2.00	1.11	60	7
80	398	7.1	130	460	1212	1662	5.59	450	.51	.75	4.8	1.30	140	77
9	178	.99	40	200	158	423	.80	27	.03	.16	.09	.14	4	2
36	297	3.48	100	400	674	997	4.30	280	.104	.34	2.17	.98	33	58
16	156	1.42	110	156	385	642	2.17	87	.05	.146	.396	.21	68	52
0	2	.07	—	—	13	126	—	19	<.01	<.01	.06	—	—	<1
0	36	.60	—	—	376	376	—	112	.02	.14	—	—	—	2
1	37	1.26	—	—	36	127	—	<1	.138	.084	.966	—	—	<1
65	100	4.50	20	118	265	420	2.10	—	.38	.34	6	.12	<1	<1
125	48	6.30	42	339	431	575	8.35	—	.22	.43	9.00	.47	29	<1
80	40	4.55	34	200	470	900	5.11	60	.26	.25	4.80	.25	30	12
65	136	3.60	33	296	332	860	5.14	82	.27	.28	5.70	.24	25	1
84	177	4.00	33	339	430	864	4.41	111	.34	.35	5.29	.25	28	6
165	180	5.40	50	470	620	883	8.80	112	.36	.53	10.0	.46	31	6

Table A–1   Food Composition

Grp	Computer Code No.	Food Description	Measure	Wt (g)	H₂O (%)	Ener (cal)	Prot (g)	Carb (g)	Dietary Fiber (g)	Fat (g)	Fat Breakdown (g) Sat	Mono	Poly
		WENDY'S—Con.											
		Baked potatoes:											
12	1573	Plain	1 ea	250	75	250	6	52	5	<1	<1	<1	<1
12	1574	W/bacon & cheese	1 ea	350	71	570	19	57	5	30	12	11	6
12	1575	W/broccoli & cheese	1 ea	365	74	500	13	54	5	25	9	8	5
12	1576	W/cheese	1 ea	350	71	590	17	55	5	34	13	13	7
12	1577	W/chili & cheese	1 ea	400	72	510	22	63	8	20	13	7	<1
12	1578	W/sour cream & chives	1 ea	310	71	460	7	53	5	24	10	8	3
12	1579	Chili	1 c	256	77	230	21	16	5	9	3	4	<1
12	1580	French fries	1 svg	106	43	306	4	38	<1	15	7	5	2
12	1581	Frosty dairy dessert	1 c	216	35	354	7	53	0	13	5	3	2
12	1582	Chocolate chip cookie	1 ea	64	5	320	3	40	1	17	6	6	5

Source: Wendy's International, for most nutrient values. Some of the values for Dietary fiber, the types of fatty acids, magnesium, phosphorus, zinc, Vitamin B6, Vitamin A in REs, and percentage water for estimates calculated from known values of major ingredients.

A

GRP KEY: 1 = BEV   2 = DAIRY   3 = EGGS   4 = FAT/OIL   5 = FRUIT   6 = BAKERY   7 = GRAIN   8 = FISH   9 = BEEF   10 = POULTRY
11 = SAUSAGE   12 = MIXED/FAST   13 = NUTS/SEEDS   14 = SWEETS   15 = VEG/LEG   16 = MISC   22 = SOUP/SAUCE

Chol (mg)	Calc (mg)	Iron (mg)	Magn (mg)	Phos (mg)	Pota (mg)	Sodi (mg)	Zinc (mg)	VT-A (RE)	Thia (mg)	Ribo (mg)	Niac (mg)	V-B6 (mg)	Fola (μg)	VT-C (mg)
0	40	2.7	67	169	1360	60	.65	0	.28	.10	3.82	.70	68	36
22	200	3.7	80	406	1380	180	2.53	150	.225	.17	4.64	.866	33	36
22	250	3.6	83	373	1550	2.19	.865	350	.31	.255	4	.861	66	90
22	350	3.6	78	49.7	1380	2.22	.609	200	.225	.255	3.3	.80	33	36
22	250	6.1	111	498	1590	810	3.78	172	.32	.26	4.1	.9	50	36
15	40	2.7	70	185	1420	230	.9	100	.225	.13	3	.79	32	36
30	60	4.50	60	320	565	960	3.78	200	.12	.17	3.00	.26	40	9
15	13	1.02	45	197	689	105	.51	0	.15	.04	2.96	.27	33	12
45	257	.86	43	238	518	194	.92	143	.11	.45	.31	.12	17	<1
5	10	1.09	15	62	100	235	.46	0	.06	.07	.4	.03	6	0

A

Recommended Nutrient Intakes for Canadians (RNI)

The U.S. recommendations for nutrient intakes appear in the RDA tables on the inside front cover. The U.S. RDA used on food labels are on the inside front cover, page c. The Canadian recommendations are here, in Tables B–1 and B–2. Some lines have been shaded to ease reading across them.

■ **TABLE B–1**
Recommended Nutrient Intakes for Canadians, 1990

				Fat-Soluble Vitamins		
Age	Sex	Weight (kg)	Protein (g/day)[a]	Vitamin A (RE/day)[b]	Vitamin D (μg/day)[c]	Vitamin E (mg/day)[d]
Months						
0–4	Both	6.0	12[f]	400	10	3
5–12	Both	9.0	12	400	10	3
Years						
1	Both	11	13	400	10	3
2–3	Both	14	16	400	5	4
4–6	Both	18	19	500	5	5
7–9	M	25	26	700	2.5	7
	F	25	26	700	2.5	6
10–12	M	34	34	800	2.5	8
	F	36	36	800	2.5	7
13–15	M	50	49	900	2.5	9
	F	48	46	800	2.5	7
16–18	M	62	58	1000	2.5	10
	F	53	47	800	2.5	7
19–24	M	71	61	1000	2.5	10
	F	58	50	800	2.5	7
25–49	M	74	64	1000	2.5	9
	F	59	51	800	2.5	6
50–74	M	73	63	1000	5	7
	F	63	54	800	5	6
75+	M	69	59	1000	5	6
	F	64	55	800	5	5
Pregnancy (additional amount needed)						
1st trimester			5	0	2.5	2
2nd trimester			15	0	2.5	2
3rd trimester			24	0	2.5	2
Lactation (additional amount needed)			20	400	2.5	3

Recommended intakes of energy and of certain nutrients are not listed in this table because of the nature of the variables upon which they are based. The figures for energy are estimates of average requirements for expected patterns of activity (see Table B–2). For nutrients not shown, the following amounts are recommended based on at least 2000 kcal/day and body weights as given: thiamin, 0.4 mg/1000 cal (0.48/5000 kJ); riboflavin, 0.5 mg/1000 cal (0.6 mg/5000 kJ); niacin, 7.2 NE/1000 cal (8.6 NE/5000 kJ); vitamin B_6, 15 μg, as pyridoxine, per gram of protein. Recommended intakes during periods of growth are taken as appropriate for individuals representative of the midpoint in each age group. All recommended intakes are designed to cover individual variations in essentially all of a healthy population subsisting upon a variety of common foods available in Canada.

Source: Health and Welfare Canada, *Nutrition Recommendations: The Report of the Scientific Review Committee* (Ottawa: Canadian Government Publishing Centre, 1990), Table 20, p. 204. Reproduced with permission of the Minister of Supply and Services Canada 1991.

| Water-Soluble Vitamins | | | Minerals | | | | | |
Vitamin C (mg/day)[e]	Folate (μg/day)	Vitamin B$_{12}$ (μg/day)	Calcium (mg/day)	Phosphorus (mg/day)	Magnesium (mg/day)	Iron (mg/day)	Iodine (μg/day)	Zinc (mg/day)
20	25	0.3	250	150	20	0.3[g]	30	2[h]
20	40	0.4	400	200	32	7	40	3
20	40	0.5	500	300	40	6	55	4
20	50	0.6	550	350	50	6	65	4
25	70	0.8	600	400	65	8	85	5
25	90	1.0	700	500	100	8	110	7
25	90	1.0	700	500	100	8	95	7
25	120	1.0	900	700	130	8	125	9
25	130	1.0	1100	800	135	8	110	9
30	175	1.0	1100	900	185	10	160	12
30	170	1.0	1000	850	180	13	160	9
40	220	1.0	900	1000	230	10	160	12
30	140	1.0	700	850	200	12	160	9
40	220	1.0	800	1000	240	9	160	12
30	180	1.0	700	850	200	13	160	9
40	230	1.0	800	1000	250	9	160	12
30	185	1.0	700	850	200	13[i]	160	9
40	230	1.0	800	1000	250	9	160	12
30	195	1.0	800	850	210	8	160	9
40	215	1.0	800	1000	230	9	160	12
30	200	1.0	800	850	210	8	160	9
0	200	0.2	500	200	15	0	25	6
10	200	0.2	500	200	45	5	25	6
10	200	0.2	500	200	45	10	25	6
25	100	0.2	500	200	65	0	50	6

[a]The primary units are expressed per kilogram of body weight. The figures shown here are examples.
[b]One retinol equivalent (RE) corresponds to the biological activity of 1 μg of retinol, 6 μg of beta-carotene, or 12 μg of other carotenes.
[c]Expressed as cholecalciferol or ergocalciferol.
[d]Expressed as δ-α-tocopherol equivalents, relative to which β- and γ-tocopherol and α-tocotrienol have activities of 0.5, 0.1, and 0.3, respectively.
[e]Cigarette smokers should increase intake by 50 percent.
[f]The assumption is made that the protein is from breast milk or is of the same biological value as that of breast milk, and that between 3 and 9 months, adjustment for the quality of the protein is made.
[g]Based on the assumption that breast milk is the source of iron.
[h]Based on the assumption that breast milk is the source of zinc.
[i]After menopause, the recommended intake is 8 mg/day.

■ TABLE B–2
Average Energy Requirements for Canadians

Age	Sex	Average Height (cm)	Average Weight (kg)	Requirements[a] (cal/kg)[b]	(MJ/kg)[b]	(cal/day)	(MJ/day)	(cal/cm)	(MJ/cm)
Months									
0–2	Both	55	4.5	120–100	0.50–0.42	500	2.0	9	0.04
3–5	Both	63	7.0	100–95	0.42–0.40	700	2.8	11	0.05
6–8	Both	69	8.5	95–97	0.40–0.41	800	3.4	11.5	0.05
9–11	Both	73	9.5	97–99	0.41	950	3.8	12.5	0.05
Years									
1	Both	82	11	101	0.42	1100	4.8	13.5	0.06
2–3	Both	95	14	94	0.39	1300	5.6	13.5	0.06
4–6	Both	107	18	100	0.42	1800	7.6	17	0.07
7–9	M	126	25	88	0.37	2200	9.2	17.5	0.07
	F	125	25	76	0.32	1900	8.0	15	0.06
10–12	M	141	34	73	0.30	2500	10.4	17.5	0.07
	F	143	36	61	0.25	2200	9.2	15.5	0.06
13–15	M	159	50	57	0.24	2800	12.0	17.5	0.07
	F	157	48	46	0.19	2200	9.2	14	0.06
16–18	M	172	62	51	0.21	3200	13.2	18.5	0.08
	F	160	53	40	0.17	2100	8.8	13	0.05
19–24	M	175	71	42	0.18	3000	12.6		
	F	160	58	36	0.15	2100	8.8		
25–49	M	172	74	36	0.15	2700	11.3		
	F	160	59	32	0.13	1900	8.0		
50–74	M	170	73	31	0.13	2300	9.7		
	F	158	63	29	0.12	1800	7.6		
75 +	M	168	69	29	0.12	2000	8.4		
	F	155	64	23	0.10	1500	6.3		

[a]Requirements can be expected to vary within a range of ±30%.
[b]First and last figures are averages at the beginning and at the end of the 3-month period.

Source: Health and Welfare Canada, *Nutrition Recommendations: The Report of the Scientific Review Committee* (Ottawa: Canadian Government Publishing Centre, 1990), Tables 5 and 6, pp. 25, 27.
Reproduced with permission of the Minister of Supply and Services Canada 1991.

Aids to Calculation

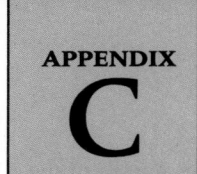

Contents

Conversion Factors

Percentages

Ratios

Weights and Measures

Many mathematical problems have been worked out for you as examples at appropriate places in the text. This appendix aims to help with the use of the metric system and with those problems not fully explained elsewhere.

■ Conversion Factors

Conversion factors are useful mathematical tools in everyday calculations, like the ones encountered in the study of nutrition. Skill in the use of conversion factors is especially desirable as the United States and Canada "go metric."

A conversion factor is a fraction in which the numerator (top) and the denominator (bottom) express the same quantity in different units. For example, 2.2 pounds (lb) and 1 kilogram (kg) are equivalent; they express the same weight. The conversion factor used to change pounds to kilograms or vice versa is:

$$\frac{2.2 \text{ lb}}{1 \text{ kg}} \text{ or } \frac{1 \text{ kg}}{2.2 \text{ lb}}.$$

Because both factors equal 1, measurements can be multiplied by the factor without changing the value of the measurement. Thus the units can be changed.

The correct factor to use in a problem is the one with the unit you are seeking in the numerator (top) of the fraction. Following are two examples of problems commonly encountered in nutrition study; they illustrate the usefulness of conversion factors.

Example 1 Convert the weight of 130 pounds to kilograms.

1. Choose the conversion factor in which the unit you are seeking is on top:

$$\frac{1 \text{ kg}}{2.2 \text{ lb}}.$$

2. Multiply 130 pounds by the factor:

$$130 \text{ lb} \times \frac{1 \text{ kg}}{2.2 \text{ lb}} = \frac{130 \text{ kg}}{2.2} = \begin{array}{l} 59 \text{ kg (rounded off to the} \\ \text{nearest whole number).} \end{array}$$

Example 2 How many grams (g) of saturated fat are contained in a 3-ounce (oz) hamburger?

1. Appendix A shows that a 4-ounce hamburger contains 7 grams of saturated fat. You are seeking grams of saturated fat; therefore, the conversion factor is:

$$\frac{7 \text{ g saturated fat}}{4 \text{ oz hamburger}}.$$

2. Multiply 3 ounces of hamburger by the conversion factor:

$$3 \text{ oz hamburger} \times \frac{7 \text{ g saturated fat}}{4 \text{ oz hamburger}} = \frac{3 \times 7}{4} = \frac{21}{4}$$

$$= 5 \text{ g saturated fat (rounded off to the nearest whole number).}$$

Energy Units
1 cal[a] = 4.2 kJ
1 MJ = 240 cal
1 kJ = 0.24 cal
1 g carbohydrate = 4 cal = 17 kJ
1 g fat = 9 cal = 37 kJ
1 g protein = 4 cal = 17 kJ
1 g alcohol = 7 cal = 29 kJ

■ Percentages

A percentage is a comparison between a number of items (perhaps your intake of energy) and a standard number (perhaps the number of calories recommended for your age and sex—your energy RDA). The standard number is the number you divide by. The answer you get after the division must be multiplied by 100 to be stated as a percentage (*percent* means "per 100").

[a]Note: Throughout this book and in the Appendixes, the term *calorie* is used to mean kilocalorie. Thus, when converting the calories of foods listed in Appendixes A or D to kilojoules, do not enlarge the calorie values—they are kilocalorie values.

Example 3   What percentage of the RDA for energy is your energy intake?

1. Find your energy RDA (inside front cover). We'll use 2100 calories to demonstrate.
2. Total your energy intake for a day—for example, 1200 calories.
3. Divide your calorie intake by the RDA calories:

1200 cal (your intake) ÷ 2100 cal (RDA) = 0.573.

4. Multiply your answer by 100 to state it as a percentage:

$0.573 \times 100 = 57.3 =$ 57% (rounded off to the nearest whole number).

In some problems in nutrition, the percentage may be more than 100. For example, suppose your daily intake of vitamin A is 3200 RE and your RDA (male) is 1000 RE. Your intake as a percentage of the RDA is more than 100 percent (that is, you consume more than 100 percent of your vitamin A RDA). The following calculations show your vitamin A intake as a percentage of the RDA:

$3200 \div 1000 = 3.2$.
$3.2 \times 100 = 320\%$ of RDA.

Sometimes the comparison is between a part of a whole (for example, your calories from protein) and the total amount (your total calories). In this case, the total number is the one you divide by.

Example 4   What percentages of your total calories for the day come from protein, fat, and carbohydrate?

1. Using Appendix A and your diet record, find the total grams of protein, fat, and carbohydrate you consumed—for example, 60 grams protein, 80 grams fat, and 285 grams carbohydrate.
2. Multiply the number of grams by the number of calories from 1 gram of each energy nutrient (conversion factors):

$60 \text{ g protein} \times \dfrac{4 \text{ cal}}{1 \text{ g protein}} = 240 \text{ cal}.$

$80 \text{ g fat} \times \dfrac{9 \text{ cal}}{1 \text{ g fat}} = 720 \text{ cal}.$

$285 \text{ g carbohydrate} \times \dfrac{4 \text{ cal}}{1 \text{ g carbohydrate}} = 1140 \text{ cal}.$

$240 + 720 + 1140 = 2100 \text{ cal}.$

3. Find the percentage of total calories from each energy nutrient (see example 3):

- Protein: $240 \div 2100 = 0.114 \times 100 = 11.4 = 11\%$ of cal.
- Fat: $720 \div 2100 = 0.342 \times 100 = 34.2 = 34\%$ of cal.
- Carbohydrate: $1140 \div 2100 = 0.542 \times 100 = 54.2 = 54\%$ of cal.
- $11\% + 34\% + 54\% = 99\%$ of cal (total).

The percentages total 99 percent rather than 100 percent because a little was lost from each number in rounding off. This is a reasonable error.

■ Ratios

A ratio is a comparison of two or three values in which one of the values is reduced to 1. A ratio compares identical units and so is expressed without units. For example, the P:S ratio is a comparison of the grams of polyunsaturated fat to the grams of saturated fat in the diet.

Example 5   Find the P:S ratio of your diet.

1. Using Appendix A and your diet record, find the grams of polyunsaturated fat and the grams of saturated fat that you consumed. Say they are 32 grams polyunsaturated fat and 25 grams saturated fat.
2. Divide the polyunsaturated fat grams by the saturated fat grams:

Polyunsaturated fat (g) ÷ saturated fat (g).

$32 \text{ g} \div 25 \text{ g} = 1.28$.

3. The P:S ratio is usually expressed as correct to one decimal place: $1.28 = 1.3$.

The P:S ratio of your diet is 1.3:1 (read as "one point three to one" or simply "one point three"). A ratio greater than 1 means that the first value (in this case, grams of polyunsaturated fat) is greater than the second (saturated fat). If it were less than 1, you would know that the second value was the greater.

Research is beginning to find that diets low in saturated fats and high in monounsaturated fatty acids may protect against heart disease. Consequently, the polyunsaturated to monounsaturated to saturated (P:M:S) ratio may be more meaningful than the P:S ratio.[1]

■ Weights and Measures

Length
1 inch (in) = 2.54 centimeters (cm).
1 foot (ft) = 30.48 centimeters.
1 meter (m) = 39.37 inches.

Temperature

Steam	⊥	100° C	212° F	⊥ Steam
Body temperature		37° C	98.6° F	Body temperature
Ice		0° C	32° F	Ice
	Celsius[a]		Fahrenheit	

To convert Fahrenheit temperature (t_F) to Celsius:

$$t_F = 9/5\ t_C + 32.$$

To convert Celcius temperature (t_C) to Fahrenheit:

$$t_C = 5/9\ (t_F - 32).$$

Volume

1 liter (l) = 1.06 quarts (qt) or 0.85 imperial quart.
1 liter = 1000 milliliters (ml).
1 milliliter = 0.034 fluid ounces.
1 gallon = 3.79 liters.
1 quart = 0.95 liter or 32 fluid ounces.
1 cup (c) = 8 fluid ounces, or about 250 ml.
1 tablespoon (tbsp) = 15 milliliters.
3 teaspoons (tsp) = 1 tablespoon.
1 teaspoon (tsp) = about 5 g or 5 ml.
16 tablespoons = 1 cup.
4 cups = 1 quart.

Weight

1 ounce (oz) = approximately 28 grams (g).
16 ounces = 1 pound (lb).
1 pound = 454 grams.
1 kilogram (kg) = 1000 grams or 2.2 pounds.
1 gram = 1000 milligrams (mg).
1 milligram = 1000 micrograms (μg).

■ Nutrient Units

To convert IU (International Units) found on supplement labels to the units used in the RDA tables:

Vitamin A
From animal sources:
.3 μg = 1 IU
1 RE[a] = 3.33 IU
From vegetables and fruits:
.6 μg = 1 IU
1 RE = 10 IU

Vitamin D₃
1 μg = 40 IU

Vitamin E
1 mg = 1 IU
1 α TE[b] = 1 IU

Sodium
To convert milligrams of sodium to grams of salt:
mg sodium ÷ 400 = g of salt
The reverse is also true:
g salt × 400 = mg sodium

■ Notes

1. F. H. Mattson, A changing role for dietary monounsaturated fatty acids, *Journal of the American Dietetic Association* 89 (1989): 387–391.

[a]Retinol equivalents.
[b]Alpha-tocopherol equivalents.

[a]Also known as *centigrade*.

Food Exchange Systems

Contents

The U.S. Exchange System

The Canadian Food Group System

For an introduction to the use of food group plans and exchange systems, see Chapter 2. The details of the U.S. and Canadian exchange systems, are presented here.

■ The U.S. Exchange System

The U.S. Exchange System divides the foods suitable for use in planning a healthy diet into six lists—the starch/bread, meat/meat alternate, vegetable, fruit, milk, and fat lists.[1] These lists are shown in Tables D–1 through D–6. Following these lists are three other sets of foods: free foods, combination foods, and foods for occasional use (Tables D–7, D–8, and D–9).

■ TABLE D–1
Starch/Bread List

(15 g carbohydrate, 3 g protein, trace fat, 80 cal)

Amount	Food
Cereals/Grains/Pasta	
⅓ c	Bran cereals, concentrated✔
½ c	Bran cereals, flaked✔
½ c	Bulgur, cooked
½ c	Cooked cereals
2½ tbsp	CornMeal, dry
3 tbsp	Grape-Nuts
½ c	Grits, cooked
¾ c	Other ready-to-eat unsweetened cereals
½ c	Pasta, cooked
1½ c	Puffed cereals
⅓ c	Rice, white or brown, cooked
½ c	Shredded Wheat
3 tbsp	Wheat germ✔
Dried Beans/Peas/Lentils	
¼ c	Baked beans✔
⅓ c	Beans and peas, cooked, such as kidney, white, split, black-eyed✔
⅓ c	Lentils, cooked✔
Starchy Vegetables	
½ c	Corn✔
1 cob	Corn, on the cob, 6" long✔
½ c	Lima beans✔

■ TABLE D–1
Starch/Bread List   (continued)

Amount	Food
½ c	Peas, green, canned or frozen✔
½ c	Plantains✔
1 small (3 oz)	Potatoes, baked
½ c	Potatoes, mashed
¾ c	Squash, winter (acorn, butternut)
⅓ c	Yams, sweet potatoes, plain
Bread	
½ (1 oz)	Bagels
2 (⅔ oz)	Bread sticks, crisp, 4" × ½"
1 c	Croutons, low-fat
½	English muffins
½ (1 oz)	Frankfurter or hamburger buns
½ loaf	Pita, 6" across
1 (1 oz)	Plain rolls, small
1 slice (1 oz)	Raisin, unfrosted
1 slice (1 oz)	Rye, pumpernickel✔
1	Tortillas, 6" across
1 slice (1 oz)	White (including French, Italian)
1 slice (1 oz)	Whole-wheat
Crackers/Snacks	
8	Animal crackers
3	Graham crackers, 2½" square
¾ oz	Matzoth
5 slices	Melba toast
24	Oyster crackers
3 c	Popcorn, popped, no fat added
¾ oz	Pretzels
4	Rye crisp, 2" × 3½"
6	Saltine-type crackers
2 to 4 (¾ oz)	Whole-wheat crackers, no fat added (crisp breads)
Starch Foods Prepared with Fat	
(Count as 1 starch/bread serving, plus 1 fat serving.)	
1	Biscuits, 2½" across
½ c	Chow mein noodles
1 (2 oz)	Corn bread, 2" cube
6	Crackers, round butter type
10 (1½ oz)	French fries, 2" to 3½" long

✔3 g or more dietary fiber per serving. Average fiber contents of whole-grain products is 2 g/serving. For starch foods not on this list, the general rule is that ½ c cereal, grain, or pasta is 1 serving; 1 oz of a bread product is 1 serving.

■ TABLE D–1
Starch/Bread List (continued)

Amount	Food
1	Muffins, plain, small
2	Pancakes, 4″ across
¼ c	Stuffing, bread, prepared
2	Taco shells, 6″ across
1	Waffles, 4½″ square
4 to 6 (1 oz)	Whole-wheat crackers, fat added

■ TABLE D–2
Meat/Meat Alternate Lists

(Lean meat = 7 g protein, 3 g fat, 55 cal. Medium-fat meat = 7 g protein, 5 g fat, 75 cal. High-fat meat = 7 g protein, 8 g fat, 100 cal.)

Lean Meat and Alternates

Category	Amount	Food
Beef:	1 oz	USDA Good or Choice grades of lean beef, such as round, sirloin, and flank steak; tenderloin; chipped beef⬏
Pork:	1 oz	Lean pork, such as fresh ham; canned, cured, or boiled ham⬏ Canadian bacon⬏ tenderloin
Veal:	1 oz	All cuts are lean except for veal cutlets (ground or cubed); examples of lean veal: chops and roasts
Poultry:	1 oz	Chicken, turkey, Cornish hen (without skin)
Fish:	1 oz	All fresh and frozen fish
	2 oz	Crab, lobster, scallops, shrimp, clams (fresh or canned in water)⬏
	6 medium	Oysters
	¼ c	Tuna⬏, canned in water
	1 oz	Herring, uncreamed or smoked
	2 medium	Sardines, canned
Wild Game:	1 oz	Venison, rabbit, squirrel
	1 oz	Pheasant, duck, goose (without skin)
Cheese:	¼ c	Any cottage cheese
	2 tbsp	Grated Parmesan
	1 oz	Diet cheeses⬏ (fewer than 55 cal/oz)
Other:	1 oz	95% fat-free lunch meats
	3 whites	Egg whites
	¼ c	Egg substitutes, fewer than 55 cal per ¼ c

Medium-Fat Meat and Alternates

Beef:	1 oz	Most beef products fall into this category; examples: all ground beef, roasts (rib, chuck, rump), steak (cubed, porterhouse, T-bone), meatloaf
Pork:	1 oz	Most pork products fall into this category; examples: chops, loin roast, Boston butt, cutlets

■ TABLE D–2
**Meat/Meat Alternate
Lists** (continued)

(Lean meat = 7 g protein, 3 g fat, 55 cal. Medium-fat meat = 7 g protein, 5 g fat, 75 cal. High-fat meat = 7 g protein, 8 g fat, 100 cal.)

Category	Amount	Food
Lamb:	1 oz	Most lamb products fall into this category; examples: chops, leg, roast
Veal:	1 oz	Cutlet, ground or cubed, unbreaded
Poultry:	1 oz	Chicken (with skin), domestic duck or goose (well-drained of fat), ground turkey
Fish:	¼ c	Tuna,⬏ canned in oil and drained
	¼ c	Salmon,⬏ canned
Cheese:		Skim or part-skim milk cheeses, such as:
	¼ c	Ricotta
	1 oz	Mozzarella
	1 oz	Diet cheeses⬏ (56 to 80 cal/oz)
Other:	1 oz	86% fat-free lunch meat⬏
	1	Eggs (high in cholesterol, limit to 3 per week)
	¼ c	Egg substitutes (56 to 80 cal per ¼ c)
	4 oz	Tofu, 2 ½″ × 2¾″ × 1″
	1 oz	Liver, hearts, kidneys, sweetbreads (high in cholesterol)

High-Fat Meat and Alternates[a]

Beef:	1 oz	Most USDA Prime cuts of beef, such as ribs, corned beef⬏
Pork:	1 oz	Spareribs, ground pork, pork sausages⬏ (patties or links)
Lamb:	1 oz	Patties, ground lamb
Fish:	1 oz	Any fried fish product
Cheese:	1 oz	All regular cheeses,⬏ such as American, blue, Cheddar, Monterey, Swiss
Other:	1 oz	Lunch meats,⬏ such as bologna, salami, pimento loaf
	1 oz	Sausage,⬏ such as Polish, Italian
	1 oz	Knockwurst, smoked
	1 oz	Bratwurst⬏
	1 (10/lb)	Frankfurters⬏ (turkey or chicken)
	1 tbsp	Peanut butter (contains unsaturated fat)

Count as 1 high-fat meat plus 1 fat exchange:

1 frank	(10/lb)	Frankfurters⬏ (beef, pork, or combination)

⬏400 mg or more sodium per exchange. Meats contribute no fiber to the diet.
[a]These items are high in saturated fat, cholesterol, and calories, and should be used no more than three times per week.

If beans are used as a meat substitute:

Dried beans,⬗ peas,⬗ lentils⬗	1 c (cooked)	2 starch/bread, 1 lean meat

⬗3 g or more dietary fiber per serving.

■ TABLE D–3
Vegetable List

(5 g carbohydrate, 2 g protein, 25 cal)
All portion sizes, except as otherwise noted, are ½ c of any cooked vegetable or vegetable juice, 1 c of any raw vegetable

Artichokes, ½ medium	Mushrooms, cooked
Asparagus	Okra
Bean sprouts	Onions
Beans (green, wax, Italian)	Pea pods
Beets	Rutabagas
Broccoli	Sauerkraut
Brussels sprouts	Spinach, cooked
Cabbage, cooked	Summer squash (crookneck)
Carrots	Tomatoes, 1 large
Cauliflower	Tomato/vegetable juice
Eggplant	Turnips
Green peppers	Water chestnuts
Greens (collard, mustard, turnip)	Zucchini, cooked
Kohlrabi	
Leeks	

Starchy vegetables such as corn, peas, and potatoes are found on the Starch/Bread List.
For free vegetables, see the Free Food List (Table D–7).

400 mg or more sodium per serving. Most vegetable servings contain 2 to 3 g dietary fiber.

■ TABLE D–4
Fruit List

(15 g carbohydrate, 60 cal)
All portion sizes, unless otherwise noted, are ½ c fresh fruit or fruit juice, ¼ c dried fruit.

Amount	Food
Fresh, Frozen, and Unsweetened Canned Fruit	
1	Apples, raw, 2" across
½ c	Applesauce, unsweetened
4	Apricots, medium, raw
½ c (4 halves)	Apricots, canned
½	Bananas, 9" long
¾ c	Blackberries, raw
¾ c	Blueberries, raw
⅓	Cantaloupe, 5" across
1 c	Cantaloupe, cubes
12	Cherries, large, raw
½ c	Cherries, canned
2	Figs, raw, 2" across
½ c	Fruit cocktail, canned
½	Grapefruit, medium
¾ c	Grapefruit, segments
15	Grapes, small
⅛	Honeydew melon, medium
1	Honeydew melon, cubes
1	Kiwis, large
¾ c	Mandarin oranges
½	Mangoes, small
1	Nectarines, 1½" across
1	Oranges, 2½" across
1 c	Papayas
1 peach (¾ c)	Peaches, 2¾" across
½ c (2 halves)	Peaches, canned

■ TABLE D–4
Fruit List (continued)

(15 g carbohydrate, 60 cal)
All portion sizes, unless otherwise noted, are ½ c fresh fruit or fruit juice, ¼ c dried fruit.

Amount	Food
½ large or 1 small	Pears
½ c (2 halves)	Pears, canned
2	Persimmons, medium, native
¾ c	Pineapple, raw
⅓ c	Pineapple, canned
2	Plums, raw, 2" across
½	Pomegranates
1 c	Raspberries, raw
1¼ c	Strawberries, raw, whole
2	Tangerines, 2½" across
1¼ c	Watermelon, cubes
Dried Fruit	
4 rings	Apples
7 halves	Apricots
2½ medium	Dates
1½	Figs
3 medium	Prunes
2 tbsp	Raisins
Fruit Juice	
½ c	Apple juice/cider
⅓ c	Cranberry juice cocktail
⅓ c	Grape juice
½ c	Grapefruit juice
½ c	Orange juice
½ c	Pineapple juice
⅓ c	Prune juice

3 g or more dietary fiber per serving. Average fiber contents of fresh, frozen, and dry fruits: 2 g/serving.

■ TABLE D–5
Milk List

(Nonfat and very low-fat milk = 12 g carbohydrate, 8 g protein, trace fat, 90 cal. Low-fat milk = 12 g carbohydrate, 8 g protein, 5 g fat, 120 cal. Whole milk = 12 g carbohydrate, 8 g protein, 8 g fat, 150 cal.)

Amount	Food
Nonfat and Very Low-Fat Milk	
1 c	Nonfat milk
1 c	½% milk
1 c	1% milk
⅓ c	Dry nonfat milk
½ c	Evaporated nonfat milk
1 c	Low-fat buttermilk
8 oz	Plain nonfat yogurt
Lowfat Milk	
1 c fluid	2% milk
8 oz	Plain low-fat yogurt, with added nonfat milk solids

D

■ TABLE D–5
Milk List   (continued)

(Nonfat and very low-fat milk = 12 g carbohydrate, 8 g protein, trace fat, 90 cal. Low-fat milk = 12 g carbohydrate, 8 g protein, 5 g fat, 120 cal. Whole milk = 12 g carbohydrate, 8 g protein, 8 g fat, 150 cal.)

Amount	Food
Whole Milk	
1 c	Whole milk
½ c	Evaporated whole milk
8 oz	Whole plain yogurt

■ TABLE D–6
Fat List

(5 g fat, 45 cal)

Amount	Food
Unsaturated Fats	
⅛ medium	Avocados
1 tsp	Margarine
1 tbsp	Margarine, diet[a]
1 tsp	Mayonnaise
1 tbsp	Mayonnaise, reduced calorie[a]
	Nuts and seeds:
6 whole	Almonds, dry roasted
1 tbsp	Cashews, dry roasted
20 small or 10 large	Peanuts
2 whole	Pecans, walnuts
2 tsp	Pumpkin seeds
1 tbsp	Other nuts and seeds (without shells)
1 tsp	Oil (corn, cottonseed, safflower, soybean, sunflower, olive, peanut)
10 small or 5 large	Olives[a]
1 tbsp	Salad dressing, all varieties[a]
2 tsp	Salad dressing, mayonnaise type
1 tbsp	Salad dressing, mayonnaise type, reduced calorie
2 tbsp	Salad dressing, reduced calorie[b]
Saturated Fats	
1 slice	Bacon[a]
1 tsp	Butter
½ oz	Chitterlings
2 tbsp	Coconut, shredded
2 tbsp	Coffee whitener, liquid
4 tsp	Coffee whitener, powder
1 tbsp	Cream (heavy, whipping)
2 tbsp	Cream (light, coffee, table)

■ TABLE D–6
Fat List (continued)

(5 g fat, 45 cal)

Amount	Food
2 tbsp	Cream (sour)
1 tbsp	Cream cheese
¼ oz	Salt pork[a]

[a]If more than one or two servings are eaten, these foods provide 400 mg or more sodium.
[b]Two tablespoons of low-calorie salad dressing is a free food.
✔400 mg or more sodium per serving.

■ TABLE D–7
Free Foods

A free food is any food or drink that contains fewer than 20 cal/serving. No serving size is specified for foods that can be used freely. For items that have a specific serving size, use moderation (2–3 servings per day).

Amount	Food
Drinks	Bouillon, low-sodium
	Bouillon✔ or broth without fat
	Carbonated drinks, sugar-free
	Carbonated water
	Club soda
1 tbsp	Cocoa powder, unsweetened
	Coffee/tea
	Drink mixes, sugar-free
	Tonic water, sugar-free
Nonstick Pan Spray	
Fruit:	
½ c	Cranberries, unsweetened
½ c	Rhubarb, unsweetened
Vegetables (raw, 1 c)	Cabbage
	Celery
	Chinese cabbage✔
	Cucumbers
	Green onions
	Hot peppers
	Mushrooms
	Radishes
	Zucchini✔
Salad Greens	Endive
	Escarole
	Lettuce
	Romaine
	Spinach
Salad Dressing	
2 tbsp	Any low-calorie type

■ TABLE D−7
Free Foods   (continued)

Amount	Food
Sweet Substitutes	Candy, hard, sugar-free
	Gelatin, sugar-free
	Gum, sugar-free
2 tsp	Jam/jelly, sugar-free
1 to 2 tbsp	Pancake syrup, sugar-free
	Sugar substitutes (saccharin, aspartame)
2 tbsp	Whipped topping
Condiments	
1 tbsp	Catsup
	Horseradish
	Mustard
	Pickles,⌇ dill, unsweetened
2 tbsp	Salad dressing, low-calorie
1 tbsp	Taco sauce
	Vinegar
Seasonings	Basil, fresh
	Celery seeds
	Chili powder
	Chives
	Cinnamon
	Curry
	Dill
	Flavoring extracts (almond, butter, lemon, peppermint, vanilla, walnut, etc.)
	Garlic
	Garlic powder
	Herbs
	Hot pepper sauce
	Lemon
	Lemon juice
	Lemon pepper
	Lime
	Lime juice
	Mint
	Onion powder
	Oregano
	Paprika
	Pepper
	Pimento
	Soy sauce⌇
	Soy sauce, low-sodium ("lite")
	Spices
¼ c	Wine, used in cooking
	Worcestershire sauce

⌖ 3 g or more dietary fiber per serving.
⌇ 400 mg or more sodium per serving.

■ TABLE D−8
Combination Foods

This is a list of average values for some typical combination foods that can help you fit these foods into your meal plan. Ask your dietitian for information about any other foods you'd like to eat. The *American Diabetes Association/American Dietetic Association Family Cookbooks* and the *American Diabetes Association Holiday Cookbook* have many recipes and further information about many foods, including combination foods. Check your library or local bookstore.

Food	Amount	Exchanges
Casseroles, homemade	1 c (8 oz)	2 starch, 2 medium-fat meat, 1 fat
Cheese pizza,⌇ thin crust	¼ of 15 oz, or ¼ of 10"	2 starch, 1 medium-fat meat, 1 fat
Chili with beans,⌖ ⌇ commercial	1 c (8 oz)	2 starch, 2 medium-fat meat, 2 fat
Chow mein,⌖ ⌇ without noodles or rice	2 c (16 oz)	1 starch, 2 vegetable, 2 lean meat
Macaroni and cheese⌇	1 c (8 oz)	2 starch, 1 medium-fat meat, 2 fat
Soups:		
Bean⌖ ⌇	1 c (8 oz)	1 starch, 1 vegetable, 1 lean meat
Chunky, all varieties⌇	10¾-oz can	1 starch, 1 vegetable, 1 medium-fat meat
Cream,⌇ made with water	1 c (8 oz)	1 starch, 1 fat
Vegetable⌇ or broth⌇	1 c (8 oz)	1 starch
Spaghetti and meatballs,⌇ canned	1 c (8 oz)	2 starch, 1 medium-fat meat, 1 fat
Sugar-free pudding, made with nonfat milk	½ c	1 starch

⌇ 400 mg or more sodium per serving.
⌖ 3 g or more dietary fiber per serving

■ TABLE D−9
Foods for Occasional Use

The following list includes average exchange values for some foods high in sugar and fat. People are advised to use them only occasionally and in moderate amounts.

Food	Amount	Exchanges
Angel food cake	1/12 cake	2 starch
Cake, no icing	1/12 cake, or a 3" square	2 starch, 2 fat
Cookies	2 small, 1¾" across	1 starch, 1 fat
Frozen fruit yogurt	⅓ c	1 starch

■ TABLE D–9
Foods for Occasional Use   (continued)

Food	Amount	Exchanges
Gingersnaps	3	1 starch
Granola	¼ c	1 starch, 1 fat
Granola bars	1 small	1 starch, 1 fat
Ice cream, any flavor	½ c	1 starch, 2 fat
Ice milk, any flavor	½ c	1 starch, 1 fat
Sherbet, any flavor	¼ c	1 starch
Snack chips,✔ all varieties	1 oz	1 starch, 2 fat
Vanilla wafers	6 small	1 starch, 1 fat

✔ If more than one serving is eaten, these foods have 400 mg or more sodium.

■ The Canadian Food Group System

The Canadian Food Group System is similar to the U.S. Exchange System, but the serving sizes and some of the foods listed are different. This food group system, as explained in the handbook *Good Health Eating Guide,* is a revision of the Canadian exchange system of meal planning.[2] Features of the new system similar to those of the exchange system include the following:

■ Foods are divided into six groups according to carbohydrate, protein, and fat content.
■ Foods are interchangeable within a group.
■ Most foods are eaten in measured amounts.
■ An energy value is given for each food group.

Additional features of the food group system include the following:

■ Protein foods low in fat are emphasized in the protein foods group. Protein foods containing extra fat are identified.
■ The user is able to distinguish between complex and simple carbohydrates (starches and sugars).

Tables D–10 through D–16 present the Canadian Food Group System.

■ **TABLE D–11**
Protein Foods Group

(7 g protein, 3 g fat, 55 cal)

Food	Measure	Mass (weight)
Cheese		
All types, made from partly skim milk (e.g., mozzarella, part-skim)	1 piece, 5 cm × 2 cm × 2 cm (2″ × ¾″ × ¾″)	25 g
Cottage cheese, all types	50 ml (¼ c)	55 g
Fish		
Anchovies (see ''Extras,'' Table G–17)		
Canned, drained (e.g., chicken haddie, mackerel, salmon, tuna)	50 ml (¼ c)	30 g
Cod tongues/cheeks	75 ml (⅓ c)	50 g
Fillet or steak (e.g., Boston blue, cod, flounder, haddock, halibut, perch, pickerel, pike, salmon, shad, sole, trout, whitefish)	1 piece, 6 cm × 2 cm × 2 cm (2½″ × ¾″ × ¾″)	30 g
Herring	⅓ fish	30 g
Octopus	50 ml (¼ c)	40 g
Sardines	2 medium or 3 small	30 g
Seal, walrus	1 slice, 6 cm × 4 cm × 1 cm (2½″ × 1½″ × ½″)	25 g
Smelts	2 medium	30 g
Squid	50 ml (¼ c)	40 g
Shellfish		
Clams, mussels, oysters, scallops, snails	3 medium	30 g
Crab, lobster, flaked	50 ml (¼ c)	30 g
Shrimp, fresh	5 large	30 g
Frozen	10 medium	30 g
Canned	18 small	30 g
Dry pack	50 ml (¼ c)	30 g
Meat and Poultry (e.g., beef, chicken, ham, lamb, pork, turkey, veal, wild game)		
Back bacon	3 slices, thin	25 g
Chop	½ chop, with bone	35 g
Minced or ground, lean	30 ml (2 tbsp)	25 g
Sliced, lean	1 slice, 10 cm × 5 cm × 5 mm (4″ × 2″ × ¼″)	25 g
Steak, lean	1 piece, 4 cm × 3 cm × 2 cm (1½″ × 1¼″ × ¾″)	25 g
Organ Meats		
Hearts, liver	1 slice, 5 cm × 5 cm × 1 cm (2″ × 2″ × ½″)	25 g
Kidneys, sweetbreads, chopped	50 ml (¼ c)	25 g
Tongue	1 slice, 80 cm × 6 cm × 5 mm (3¼″ × 2½″ × ¼″)	25 g
Tripe, 1 piece = 4 cm × 4 cm × 8 mm (1½″ × 1½″ × ⅜″)	5 pieces	50 g
Soyabean		
Bean curd or tofu, 1 block = 6 cm × 6 cm × 4 cm (2½″ × 2 ½″ × 1½″)	½ block	70 g
The following choices contain extra fat, so use them less often.		
Cheese		
Cheeses, all types made from whole milk (e.g., brick, Brie, Camembert, Cheddar, Edam, Tilsit)	1 piece, 5 cm × 2 cm × 2 cm (2″ × ¾″ × ¾″)	25 g
Cheese, coarsely grated (e.g., Cheddar)	75 ml (⅓ c)	25 g
Cheese, dry, finely grated (e.g., Parmesan)	45 ml (3 tbsp)	15 g
Cheese, ricotta	50 ml (¼ c)	55 g

D

■ TABLE D–11
Protein Foods Group   (continued)

Food	Measure	Mass (weight)
Eggs		
Eggs, in shell, raw or cooked	1 medium	50 g
Eggs, without shell, cooked or poached in water	1 medium	45 g
Eggs, scrambled	50 ml (¼ c)	55 g
Fish		
Eel	5 cm, 4-cm diameter (2", 1½" diameter)	50 g
Meat		
Bologna	1 slice, 5 mm, 10-cm diameter (¼", 4" diameter)	40 g
Canned lunch meats	1 slice, 85 mm × 45 mm × 10 mm (3½" × 1¾" × ½")	40 g
Corned beef, canned	1 slice, 75 mm × 55 mm × 5 mm (3" × 2¼" × ¼")	25 g
Corned beef, fresh	1 slice, 10 cm × 5 cm × 5 mm (4" × 2" × ¼")	25 g
Ground beef, medium-fat	30 ml (2 tbsp)	25 g
Meat spreads, canned	45 ml (3 tbsp)	35 g
Pâté (see ''Fats and oils group,'' Table G–16)		
Sausages, garlic, Polish or knockwurst	1 slice, 1 cm, 5-cm diameter (½", 2" diameter)	50 g
Sausages, pork, links	1 link	25 g
Spareribs or shortribs, with bone	10 cm × 6 cm (4" × 2½")	65 g
Stewing beef	1 cube, 25 mm (1")	25 g
Summer sausage or salami	1 slice, 5 mm, 10-cm diameter (¼", 4" diameter)	40 g
Wieners	½ medium	25 g
Miscellaneous		
Blood pudding	1 slice, 5 cm × 1 cm (2" × ½")	25 g
Peanut butter, all kinds	15 ml (1 tbsp)	15 g

■ TABLE D–12
Starchy Foods Group

(15 g carbohydrate (starch), 2 g protein, 68 cal)

Food	Measure	Mass (weight)
Breads		
Bagels	½	25 g
Bread crumbs	50 ml (¼ c)	25 g
Bread cubes	250 ml (1 c)	25 g
Bread sticks, 11 cm × 1 cm (4½" × ½")	2	20 g
Brewis, cooked	50 ml (¼ c)	45 g
English muffins, crumpets	½	25 g
Flour	40 ml (2½ tbsp)	20 g
Hamburger buns	½	30 g
Hot dog buns	½	30 g
Kaiser rolls	½	25 g
Matzoth, 15 cm (6") square	1	20 g
Melba toast, rectangular	4	15 g
Pita, 20-cm (8") diameter	¼	25 g
Plain rolls	1 small	25 g
Raisin	1 slice	25 g
Rusks	2	20 g
Rye, coarse or pumpernickel, 10 cm × 10 cm × 8 mm (4" × 4" × ⅜")	½ slice	25 g

■ **TABLE D–12**
Starchy Foods Group   (continued)

Food	Measure	Mass (weight)
Tortillas, 15 cm (6″)	1	20 g
White (French and Italian)	1 slice	25 g
Whole-wheat, cracked wheat, rye, white enriched	1 slice	25 g
Cereals		
Bran flakes, 40% bran	125 ml (½ c)	20 g
Cooked cereals, cooked	125 ml (½ c)	125 g
Dry	30 ml (2 tbsp)	20 g
Cornmeal, cooked	125 ml (½ c)	125 g
Dry	30 ml (2 tbsp)	20 g
Ready-to-eat unsweetened cereal	250 ml (1 c)	20 g
Shredded Wheat, biscuits, bite size	125 ml (½ c)	20 g
Shredded Wheat biscuits, rectangular or round	1	20 g
Wheat germ	75 ml (⅓ c)	30 g
Cookies and Biscuits		
See "Prepared Foods" (below).		
Grains		
Barley, cooked	125 ml (½ c)	120 g
Dry	30 ml (2 tbsp)	20 g
Bulgur, kasha, cooked, moist	125 ml (½ c)	70 g
Cooked, crumbly	75 ml (⅓ c)	40 g
Dry	30 ml (2 tbsp)	20 g
Rice, cooked, loosely packed	125 ml (½ c)	105 g
cooked, tightly packed	75 ml (⅓ c)	70 g
Tapioca, pearl and granulated, quick cooking, dry	30 ml (2 tbsp)	15 g
Pastas		
Macaroni, cooked	125 ml (½ c)	70 g
Noodles, cooked	125 ml (½ c)	80 g
Spaghetti, cooked	125 ml (½ c)	70 g
Starchy Vegetables		
Beans and peas, dried, cooked	125 ml (½ c)	80 g
Breadfruit	1 slice	75 g
Corn, canned, whole kernel	125 ml (½ c)	85 g
Canned, creamed	75 ml (⅓ c)	60 g
Corn, on the cob, 13 cm, 4-cm diameter (5″, 1½″ diameter)	1 small cob	140 g
Cornstarch	30 ml (2 tbsp)	15 g
Plantains	⅓ small	50 g
Popcorn, unbuttered, large kernel	750 ml (3 c)	20 g
Potatoes, whipped	125 ml (½ c)	105 g
Potatoes, whole, 13 cm, 5-cm diameter (5″, 2″ diameter)	½	95 g
Yams, sweet potatoes, 13 cm, 5-cm diameter (5″, 2″ diameter)	½	75 g
Prepared Foods		
Baking powder biscuits, 5-cm diameter (2″ diameter)	1	30 g
Cookies, plain (e.g., digestive, oatmeal)	2	20 g
Cupcake, un-iced, 5-cm diameter (2″ diameter)	1 small	35 g
Doughnuts, cake type, plain, 7-cm diameter (2¾″ diameter)	1	30 g
Muffins, plain, 6-cm diameter (2½″ diameter)	1 small	40 g
Pancakes, homemade using 50 ml (¼ c) batter	1 small	50 g
Potatoes, french fries, 5 cm × 9 cm (2″ × 3½″)	10	65 g
Soup, canned, prepared with equal volume of water	250 ml (1 c)	260 g
Waffles, homemade, using 50 ml (¼ c) batter	1 small	35 g

D

■ TABLE D–13
Milk Group

Type of Milk	Carbohydrate	Protein	Fat	Energy
Nonfat	6 g	4 g	0 g	40 cal
2%	6 g	4 g	2 g	58 cal
Whole	6 g	4 g	4 g	76 cal

Food	Measure	Mass (weight)
Buttermilk	125 ml (½ c)	125 g
Evaporated milk	50 ml (¼ c)	50 g
Milk	125 ml (½ c)	125 g
Powdered milk, regular	30 ml (2 tbsp)	15 g
Instant	50 ml (¼ c)	15 g
Unflavoured yogurt	125 ml (½ c)	125 g

■ TABLE D–14
Fruits and Vegetables Group

(10 g carbohydrate (simple sugar), 1 g protein, 44 cal)

Food	Measure	Mass (weight)
Fruits (fresh, frozen without sugar, canned in water)		
Apples, raw	½ medium	75 g
Raw, without skin and core	½ medium	65 g
Sauce	125 ml (½ c)	120 g
Apricots, raw	2 medium	115 g
Canned, in water	4 halves, plus 30 ml (2 tbsp) liquid	110 g
Bake-apples (cloudberries), raw	125 ml (½ c)	120 g
Bananas, 15 cm (6″), with peel	½ small	75 g
Peeled	½ small	50 g
Blackberries, raw	125 ml (½ c)	70 g
Canned, in water	125 ml (½ c), includes 30 ml (2 tbsp) liquid	100 g
Blueberries, raw	125 ml (½ c)	120 g
Boysenberries, raw	125 ml (½ c)	70 g
Canned, in water	125 ml (½ c), includes 30 ml (2 tbsp) liquid	100 g
Cantaloupe, wedge with rind, 13-cm (5″) diameter	¼	240 g
Cubed or diced	250 ml (1 c)	160 g
Cherries, raw, with pits	10	75 g
Raw, without pits	10	70 g
Canned, in water, with pits	75 ml (⅓ c), includes 30 ml (2 tbsp) liquid	90 g
Canned, in water, without pits	75 ml (⅓ c), includes 30 ml (2 tbsp) liquid	85 g
Crabapples, raw	1 small	55 g
Cranberries, raw	250 ml (1 c)	100 g
Figs, raw	1 medium	50 g
Canned, in water	3 medium, plus 30 ml (2 tbsp) liquid	100 g
Foxberries, raw	250 ml (1 c)	100 g
Fruit, mixed, cut up	125 ml (½ c)	120 g
Fruit cocktail, canned, in water	125 ml (½ c), includes 30 ml (2 tbsp) liquid	120 g
Gooseberries, raw	250 ml (1 c)	150 g
Canned, in water	250 ml (1 c), includes 30 ml (2 tbsp) liquid	230 g
Grapefruit, raw, with rind	½ small	185 g
Raw, sectioned	125 ml (½ c)	100 g
Canned, in water	125 ml (½ c), includes 30 ml (2 tbsp) liquid	120 g
Grapes, raw, slip skin	125 ml (½ c)	75 g
Raw, seedless	125 ml (½ c)	75 g
Canned, in water	75 ml (⅓ c), includes 30 ml (2 tbsp) liquid	115 g
Guavas, raw	½	50 g
Honeydew melon, raw, with rind	⅒	225 g
Cubed or diced	250 ml (1 c)	170 g
Huckleberries, raw	125 ml (½ c)	70 g
Kiwis, raw, with skin	2	155 g

■ TABLE D–14
Fruits and Vegetables Group   (continued)

Food	Measure	Mass (weight)
Kumquats, raw	3	60 g
Loganberries, raw	125 ml (½ c)	70 g
Loquats, raw	8	130 g
Lychee fruit, raw	8	120 g
Mandarin oranges, raw, with rind	1	135 g
Raw, sectioned	125 ml (½ c)	100 g
Canned, in water	125 ml (½ c), includes 30 ml (2 tbsp) liquid	100 g
Mangoes, raw, without skin and seed	⅓	65 g
Diced	75 ml (⅓ c)	65 g
Nectarines	½ medium	75 g
Oranges, raw, with rind	1 small	90 g
Raw, sectioned	125 ml (½ c)	90 g
Papayas, raw, with skin and seeds	¼ medium	150 g
Raw, without skin and seeds	¼ medium	100 g
Cubed or diced	125 ml (½ c)	100 g
Peaches, raw, with seed and skin, 6-cm (2½) diameter	1 large	130 g
Raw, sliced, diced	125 ml (½ c)	100 g
Canned, in water, halves or slices	125 ml (½ c), includes 30 ml (2 tbsp) liquid	120 g
Pears, raw, with skin and core	½	90 g
Raw, without skin and core	½	85 g
Canned, in water, halves	2 halves, plus 30 ml (2 tbsp) liquid	90 g
Persimmons, raw, native	1	30 g
Raw, Japanese	¼	50 g
Pineapple, raw, sliced	1 slice, 8-cm diameter, 2 cm thick (3⅓" diameter, ¾" thick)	75 g
Raw, diced	125 ml (½ c)	75 g
Canned, in juice, diced	75 ml (⅓ c), includes 15 ml (1 tbsp) liquid	55 g
Canned, in juice, sliced	1 slice, plus 15 ml (1 tbsp) liquid	55 g
Canned, in water, diced	125 ml (½ c), includes 30 ml (2 tbsp) liquid	100 g
Canned, in water, sliced	2 slices, plus 15 ml (1 tbsp) liquid	100 g
Plums, raw, prune type	2	60 g
Damson	6	65 g
Japanese	1	70 g
Canned, in apple juice	2, plus 30 ml (2 tbsp) liquid	70 g
Canned, in water	3, plus 30 ml (2 tbsp) liquid	100 g
Pomegranates, raw	½	140 g
Raspberries, raw, black or red	125 ml (½ c)	65 g
Canned, in water	125 ml (½ c), includes 30 ml (2 tbsp) liquid	100 g
Saskatoons (see Blueberries)	250 ml (1 c)	150 g
Strawberries, raw	250 ml (1 c)	150 g
Canned, in water	250 ml (1 c), includes 30 ml (2 tbsp) liquid	240 g
Tangelos, raw	1	205 g
Tangerines, raw	1	115 g
Raw, sectioned	125 ml (½ c)	100 g
Watermelon, raw, with rind	1 wedge, 125-mm triangle, 22 mm thick (5" triangle, 1" thick)	310 g
Cubed or diced	250 ml (1 c)	160 g
Dried Fruit		
Apples	5 pieces	15 g
Apricots	4 halves	15 g
Banana flakes	30 ml (2 tbsp)	15 g
Currants	30 ml (2 tbsp)	15 g
Dates, without pits	2	15 g
Peaches	½	15 g
Pears	½	15 g
Prunes, raw, with pits	2	15 g
Raw, without pits	2	10 g
Stewed, no liquid	2	20 g
Stewed, with liquid	2, plus 15 ml (1 tbsp) liquid	35 g
Raisins	30 ml (2 tbsp)	15 g

D

■ **TABLE D–14**
Fruits and Vegetables Group   (continued)

Food	Measure	Mass (weight)
Juices (no sugar added or unsweetened)		
Apricot, grape, guava, mango, prune	50 ml (¼ c)	55 g
Apple, carrot, papaya, pear, pineapple, pomegranate	75 ml (⅓ c)	80 g
Grapefruit, loganberry, orange, raspberry, tangelo, tangerine	125 ml (½ c)	130 g
Tomato, tomato-based mixed vegetables	250 ml (1 c)	255 g
Vegetables (fresh, frozen, or canned)		
Artichokes, Jerusalem, mature or late season[a]	2 small	50 g
Beets, diced or sliced	125 ml (½ c)	85 g
Carrots, diced	125 ml (½ c)	75 g
Parsnips, mashed	125 ml (½ c)	80 g
Peas, fresh or frozen	125 ml (½ c)	80 g
Canned	75 ml (⅓ c)	55 g
Pumpkin, mashed	125 ml (½ c)	45 g
Rutabagas, mashed	125 ml (½ c)	85 g
Sauerkraut	250 ml (1 c)	235 g
Snow peas	10 pods	100 g
Squash, yellow or winter, mashed	125 ml (½ c)	115 g
Succotash	75 ml (⅓ c)	55 g
Tomatoes, canned	250 ml (1 c)	240 g
Turnips, mashed	125 ml (½ c)	115 g
Vegetables, mixed	125 ml (½ c)	90 g
Water chestnuts	8 medium	50 g

[a]Jerusalem artichokes contain inulin, which converts to carbohydrate during storage, in or out of the ground. Jerusalem artichokes in early season (autumn) are low in carbohydrate, but in late season (winter/spring) they become a fruits and vegetables choice.

D

■ TABLE D–15
Extra Vegetables Group

(½ c = 3.5 g carbohydrate, 14 cal.)

Artichokes, globe or French
Artichokes, Jerusalem, early season[a]
Asparagus
Bamboo shoots
Bean sprouts, mung or soyabean
Beans, string, green, or yellow
Bitter melon (balsam pear)
Bok choy
Broccoli
Brussels sprouts
Cabbage
Cauliflower
Celery
Chard
Cucumbers
Eggplant
Endive
Fiddleheads
Greens: beet, collard, dandelion, mustard, turnip, etc.
Kale
Kohlrabi
Leeks
Lettuce
Mushrooms
Okra
Onions, green or mature
Parsley
Peppers, green or red
Radishes
Rhubarb
Shallots
Spinach
Sprouts: alfalfa radish, etc.
Tomatoes, raw
Vegetable marrow
Watercress
Zucchini

If eaten in large amounts, the following foods must be counted as 1 fruits and vegetables choice:

Brussels sprouts, cooked, 250 ml (1 c)	155 g
Eggplant, cooked, diced, 250 ml (1 c)	200 g
Kohlrabi, cooked, diced, 250 ml (1 c)	140 g
Leeks, cooked, edible parts of 4 leeks	100 g
Okra, cooked, sliced, 250 ml (1 c)	160 g
Onion, mature, cooked, 250 ml (1 c)	210 g
Rhubarb, cooked, no sugar added, 250 ml (1 c)	244 g
Tomatoes, raw, 2 medium (6-cm, or 2½", diameter) *or* 1 large (13-cm, or 5", diameter)	270 g

[a]Jerusalem artichokes contain inulin, which converts to carbohydrate during storage, in or out of the ground. Jerusalem artichokes in early season (autumn) are low in carbohydrate, but in late season (winter/spring) they become a fruits and vegetables choice.

■ TABLE D–16
Fats and Oils Group

(5 g fat, 45 cal)

Food	Measure	Mass (Weight)
Avocado pears	⅛	30 g
Bacon, side, crisp	1 slice	5 g
Butter	5 ml (1 tsp)	5 g
Cheese spread	15 ml (1 tbsp)	15 g
Coconut, fresh	45 ml (3 tbsp)	15 g
Dried	15 ml (1 tbsp)	10 g
Cream, half and half (cereal), 10%	30 ml (2 tbsp)	30 g
Light (coffee), 20%	15 ml (1 tbsp)	15 g
Sour, 12 to 14%	45 ml (3 tbsp)	35 g
Whipping, 32 to 37%	15 ml (1 tbsp)	15 g
Cream cheese	15 ml (1 tbsp)	15 g
Gravy	30 ml (2 tbsp)	30 g
Lard	5 ml (1 tsp)	5 g
Margarine	5 ml (1 tsp)	5 g
Nuts, shelled:		
Almonds	8	20 g
Brazil nuts	2	5 g
Cashews	5	10 g
Filberts, hazelnuts	5	10 g
Macadamia	3	5 g
Peanuts	10	10 g
Pecans	5 halves	5 g
Pignolias, pine nuts	25 ml (5 tsp)	10 g
Pistachios, shelled	20	10 g
In shell	20	20 g
Pumpkin and squash seeds	20 ml (4 tsp)	10 g
Sesame seeds	15 ml (1 tbsp)	10 g
Sunflower seeds, shelled	15 ml (1 tbsp)	10 g
In shell	45 ml (3 tbsp)	15 g
Walnuts	4 halves	10 g
Oil, cooking and salad	5 ml	5 g
Olives, green	10	45 g
Ripe	7	40 g
Pâté, liverwurst, meat spreads	15 ml (1 tbsp)	15 g
Salad dressing: blue, French, Italian, mayonnaise, Thousand Island	5 ml (1 tsp)	5 g
Salt pork, raw or cooked	5 ml	5 g
Sesame oil	5 ml	5 g

D

■ **TABLE D–17**
Extras

(May be used without measuring)

Beverages
Bouillon from cube, powder or liquid
Bouillon or clear broth
Coffee, clear
Consommé
Herbal teas, unsweetened
Mineral water
Soda water, club soda
Sugar-free soft drinks
Tea, clear
Water

Condiments
Chowchow, unsweetened tomato pickles
Garlic
Gelatin, unsweetened
Ginger root
Horseradish, uncreamed
Lemon juice or lemon wedges
Lime juice or lime wedges
Mustard
Parsley
Pickles, unsweetened dill pickles or sour cucumber pickles
Pimentos
Soya sauce
Vinegar
Worcestershire sauce

Herbs and spices
Cinnamon, marjoram, pepper, salt, thyme, etc.

Miscellaneous
Artificial sweetener, such as cyclamate or saccharin
Baking powder, baking soda
Dulse
Flavorings and extracts (e.g., vanilla)
Rennet

■ **TABLE D–17**
Extras   (continued)

(2.5 g carbohydrate, 15 cal, limited to amount indicated)

Food	Measure
Anchovies	2 fillets
Barbecue sauce	15 ml (1 tbsp)
Bran, natural	30 ml (2 tbsp)
Brewer's yeast	5 ml (1 tsp)
Carob powder	5 ml (1 tsp)
Catsup	5 ml (1 tsp)
Chili sauce	5 ml (1 tsp)
Cocoa powder	5 ml (1 tsp)
Cranberry sauce, unsweetened	15 ml (1 tbsp)
Dietetic fruit spreads	5 ml (1 tsp)
Marschino cherries	1
Nondairy coffee whitener	5 ml (1 tsp)
Nuts, chopped pieces	5 ml (1 tsp)
Relishes	5 ml (1 tsp)
Sugar substitutes, granular	5 ml (1 tsp) (3 to 4 packages)
Whipped toppings	15 ml (1 tbsp)
Yogurt, plain	30 ml (2 tbsp)

■ *Notes*

1. The U.S. Exchange System presented here is based on material in *Exchange Lists for Meal Planning*, 1986, prepared by committees of the American Diabetes Association and the American Dietetic Association, with permission of both organizations.
2. The tables for the Canadian Food Group System are taken from *Good Health Eating Guide* (Toronto: Canadian Diabetes Association, 1981), and are used with the association's permission.

Nutrition Resources

Contents

Books

Journals

Addresses

People interested in nutrition often want to know where, in their own town or county, they can find reliable nutrition information. Wherever you live, there are several sources you can turn to:

- The Department of Health may have a nutrition expert.
- The local extension agent is often an expert.
- The food editor of your local paper may be well informed.
- The dietitian at the local hospital had to fulfill a set of qualifications before he or she became an R.D. (see Controversy 1).
- There may be knowledgeable professors of nutrition or biochemistry at a nearby college or university.

The syndicated column on nutrition by J. Mayer and J. Dwyer, which appears in many newspapers, presents well-researched, reliable answers to current questions. The column by R. Alfin-Slater and D. B. Jelliffe is also accurate and trustworthy. In addition, you may be interested in building a nutrition library of your own. Books you can buy, journals you can subscribe to, and addresses you can write to for general information are given below.

■ *Books*

A 54-page list of references with critiques of each, *Nutrition References and Book Reviews*, is available for purchase from the Chicago Nutrition Association. (See "Addresses," below).

This 532-page paperback has a chapter on each of 59 topics, including energy, obesity, all the nutrients, several diseases, malnutrition, growth and its assessment, immunity, alcohol, fiber, exercise, drugs, and toxins. The only major omissions seem to be nutrition and food intake and national nutrition status surveys. Watch for an update; these come out every several years. The most recent update is:

- *Nutrition Reviews' Present Knowledge in Nutrition*, 6th ed. (Washington, D.C.: Nutrition Foundation, 1990).

This 1694-page volume is a major technical reference book on nutrition topics. It contains encyclopedic articles on the nutrients, foods, the diet, metabolism, malnutrition, age-related needs, and nutrition in disease.

- R. S. Goodhart, M. E. Shils, and V. R. Young, eds., *Modern Nutrition in Health and Disease*, 7th ed. (Philadelphia: Lea and Febiger, 1988).

Another book that readers may wish to add to their libraries is the latest edition of *Recommended Dietary Allowances*, available from the National Academy of Sciences (see "Addresses," below). The Canadian equivalent is *Recommended Nutrient Intakes for Canadians*, available by mail from the Canadian Government Publishing Centre, Supply and Services Canada, Ottawa, Ontario K1A 0S9, Canada.

We also recommend two of our own books that explore current nutrition and fitness topics:

- Whitney, E. N., Hamilton, E. M. N., and Rolfes, S. R., *Understanding Nutrition*, 5th ed. (St. Paul: West, 1990).
- L. K. DeBruyne, F. S. Sizer, and E. N. Whitney, *The Fitness Triad: Motivation, Nutrition, and Training* (St. Paul: West, 1991).

Another of our books provides information pertinent to each stage of life:

- L. K. DeBruyne, S. R. Rolfes, and E. N. Whitney, *Life Span Nutrition: Conception through Life* (St. Paul, Minn.: West, 1990).

■ *Journals*

Nutrition Today, the publication of the Nutrition Today Society, is an excellent magazine for the interested layperson. It makes a point of raising controversial issues and providing a forum for conflicting opinions. References are seldom printed in the magazine but are available on request. Six issues per year are published. Order from the Director of Membership Services, Nutrition Today Society. (See "Addresses," below.)

The *Journal of the American Dietetic Association,* the official publication of the ADA, contains articles of interest to dietitians and nutritionists, news of legislative action on food and nutrition, and a very useful section of abstracts of articles from many other journals of nutrition and related areas. There are twelve issues per year, available from the American Dietetic Association. (See "Addresses," below.)

Nutrition Reviews, a publication of the Nutrition Foundation, Inc., does much of the work for the library researcher, compiling recent evidence on current topics and presenting extensive bibliographies. Twelve issues per year are available from the Nutrition Foundation. (See "Addresses," below.)

Nutrition and the M.D. is a monthly newsletter that provides up-to-date, easy-to-read, and practical information on nutrition for health care providers. It is available from PM, Inc. (See "Addresses," below.)

Other journals that deserve mention here are *Food Technology, Journal of Nutrition, American Journal of Clinical Nutrition,* and *Journal of Nutrition Education. FDA Consumer,* a government publication with many articles of interest to the consumer, is available from the Food and Drug Administration. (See "Addresses," below.) Many other journals of value are referred to throughout this book.

Some of this book's Controversies, as well as other articles of interest to consumers, are available as individual booklets called *Nutrition Clinics.* You can write for a free publication list from the J. B. Lippincott Company. (See "Addresses," below.) Many of the other organizations listed below will also provide publication lists free on request.

■ *Addresses*

U.S. Government

The U.S. Department of Agriculture (USDA) has several divisions. The USDA's Food Safety and Inspection Service (FSIS) inspects and analyzes domestic and imported meat, poultry, and meat and poultry food products; establishes standards for, and approves recipes and labels of, processed meat and poultry products; and monitors the meat and poultry industries for violations of inspection laws. To obtain publications or ask questions, write or call:

- FSIS Consumer Inquiries
  USDA
  Washington, DC 20250
  (202) 472-4485
  USDA also maintains a Meat and Poultry Hotline:
  1-800-535-4555

The USDA's Agricultural Research Service (ARS) conducts research to fulfill the diverse needs of agricultural users—from farmers to consumers—in the areas of crop and animal production, protection, processing, and distribution; food safety and quality; and natural resources conservation. Write to the Information Division, ARS, USDA (same address).

The USDA's Human Nutrition Information Service (HNIS) maintains the USDA's Nutrient Data Bank; conducts the Nationwide Food Consumption Survey; monitors the nutrient content of the U.S. food supply; provides nutrition guidelines for education and action programs; collects and disseminates food and nutrition materials; and conducts nutrition education research. Write to:

- HNIS, USDA
  6505 Belcrest Road
  Federal Building No. 1, Room 325-A
  Hyattsville, MD 20782

The USDA's Food and Nutrition Service (FNS) administers the Food Stamp Program; the national School Lunch and School Breakfast programs; the Special Supplemental Food Program for Women, Infants, and Children (WIC); and the food distribution, Child Care Food, summer food service, and special milk programs. Write to:

- FNS, USDA
  500 12th Street SW
  Washington, DC 20250

The USDA's Agricultural Marketing Service (AMS) operates a variety of marketing programs and services—several of interest to consumers—that include developing grades and standards for the trading of food and other farm products and carrying out grading services on request from packers and processors; inspecting egg products for wholesomeness; administering marketing orders that aid in the marketing of milk, fruits, vegetables, and related specialty crops like nuts; and administering truth-in-seed labeling and other regulatory programs. Write to:

- Information Division
  AMS, USDA
  Washington, DC 20250

The USDA's *Food News for Consumers*, a quarterly newsletter, is available from the U.S. Government Printing Office (address below).

Other U.S. Government addresses are:

- Food and Drug Administration (FDA)
  5600 Fishers Lane
  Rockville, MD 20852
- The Food and Nutrition Information Education Resources Center (FNIERC)
  National Agriculture Library
  10301 Baltimore Boulevard, Room 304
  Beltsville, MD 20705
  (301) 344–3719
- National Academy of Sciences/National Research Council (NAS/NRC)
  2101 Constitution Avenue NW
  Washington, DC 20418
- National Center for Health Statistics (NCHS)
  U.S. Department of Health and Human Services (USDHHS)
  Public Health Service
  3700 East-West Highway
  Hyattsville, MD 20782
- U.S. Government Printing Office
  The Superintendent of Documents
  Washington, DC 20402

Canadian Government

- Department of Community Health
  1075 Ste-Foy Road, 7th Floor
  Quebec, Quebec G1S 2M1, Canada
- Home Economics Directorate
  880 Portage Avenue, 2nd Floor
  Winnipeg, Manitoba R3G 0P1, Canada
- Nutrition Programs
  446 Jeanne Mance Building
  Tunney's Pasture
  Ottawa, Ontario K1A 1B4, Canada
- Nutrition Services
  P.O. Box 488
  Halifax, Nova Scotia B3J 3R8, Canada
- Nutrition Services
  P.O. Box 6000
  Fredericton, New Brunswick E3B 5H1, Canada
- Public Health Resource Service
  15 Overlea Boulevard, 5th Floor
  Toronto, Ontario M4H 1A9, Canada

Consumer and Advocacy Groups

- Action for Children's Television (ACT)
  46 Austin Street
  Newtonville, MA 02160

- Center for Science in the Public Interest (CSPI)
  1755 S Street NW
  Washington, DC 20009
- Children's Foundation
  1420 New York Avenue NW, Suite 800
  Washington, DC 20005
- Community Nutrition Institute
  1146 19th Street NW
  Washington, DC 20036
- The Consumer Information Center
  Department 609K
  Pueblo, CO 81009
- Food Research and Action Center (FRAC)
  2011 I Street NW
  Washington, DC 20006
- National Council against Health Fraud, Inc.
  P.O. Box 1276
  Loma Linda, CA 92354
- National Self-Help Clearinghouse
  33 West 42nd Street, Room 1227
  New York, NY 10036
- Nutrition Information Service
  234 Webb Building
  Birmingham, AL 35294

Professional and Service Organizations, Publishers

- Al-Anon Family Group Headquarters
  P.O. Box 182
  Madison Square Station
  New York, NY 10010
- Alcoholics Anonymous World Services
  P.O. Box 459
  Grand Central Station
  New York, NY 10017
- American Academy of Pediatrics
  P.O. Box 1034
  Evanston, IL 60204
- American Anorexia/Bulimia Association, Inc.
  418 East 76 Street
  New York, NY 10021
  (212) 734–1114
- American College of Nutrition
  100 Manhattan Avenue #1606
  Union City, NJ 07087
- American College of Sports Medicine
  P.O. Box 1440
  Indianapolis, IN 46204
- American Council on Science and Health
  1995 Broadway
  New York, NY 10023
- American Dental Association
  211 East Chicago Avenue
  Chicago, IL 60611

E

- American Diabetes Association
  1660 Duke Street
  Alexandria, VA 22314
  (800) 232–3472
- American Dietetic Association
  216 West Jackson Boulevard, Suite 800
  Chicago, IL 60606
  (312) 899–0040
- American Heart Association
  7320 Greenville Avenue
  Dallas, TX 75231
- American Home Economics Association
  2010 Massachusetts Avenue NW
  Washington, DC 20036
- American Institute for Cancer Research
  803 West Broad Street
  Falls Church, VA 22046
- American Institute of Nutrition
  9650 Rockville Pike
  Bethesda, MD 20014
- American Medical Association
  Nutrition Information Section
  535 North Dearborn Street
  Chicago, IL 60610
- American National Red Cross
  Food and Nutrition Consultant
  National Headquarters
  Washington, DC 20006
- American Public Health Association
  1015 Fifteenth Street NW
  Washington, DC 20005
- American Society for Clinical Nutrition
  9650 Rockville Pike
  Bethesda, MD 20014
- Anorexia Nervosa and Related
  Eating Disorders, Inc.
  P.O. Box 5102
  Eugene, OR 97405
- Canadian Diabetes Association
  78 Bond Street
  Toronto, Ontario M5B 2J8, Canada
  (416) 362–4440
- Canadian Dietetic Association
  480 University Avenue, Suite 601
  Toronto, Ontario M5G 1V2 Canada
  (416) 596–0857
- Chicago Nutrition Association
  8158 Kedzie Avenue
  Chicago, IL 60652
- High Blood Pressure Information Center
  120/80, National Institutes of Health (NIH)
  Bethesda, MD 20205
  (703) 558–4880
- Institute of Food Technologists
  221 North LaSalle Street
  Chicago, IL 60601

- La Leche League International, Inc.
  9616 Minneapolis Avenue
  Franklin Park, IL 60131
- J. B. Lippincott Company
  East Washington Square
  Philadelphia, PA 19105
- March of Dimes Birth Defects Foundation (National Headquarters)
  1275 Mamaroneck Avenue
  White Plains, NY 10605
- National Anorexic Aid Society
  5796 Karl Road
  Columbus, OH 43229
  (614) 436–1112
- National Clearinghouse for Alcohol Information
  Box 2345
  Rockville, MD 20850
- National Council on Alcoholism
  733 Third Avenue
  New York, NY 10017
- National Nutrition Consortium
  1635 P Street NW, Suite 1
  Washington, DC 20036
- National Osteoporosis Foundation
  2100 M Street NW, Suite 602
  Washington, DC 20037
  (202) 223–2226
- Nutrition Foundation, Inc.
  1126 Sixteenth Street NW, Suite 111
  Washington, DC 20036
- Nutrition Today Society
  428 East Preston Street
  Baltimore, MD 21202
- Overeaters Anonymous (OA)
  2190 190th Street
  Torrance, CA 90504
  (213) 320–7941
- PM, Inc. (Publisher of *Nutrition and the M.D.*)
  14545 Friar, #106
  Van Nuys, CA 91411
- Society for Nutrition Education
  1700 Broadway, Suite 300
  Oakland, CA 94612
- Technical Information Center
  Office on Smoking and Health
  5600 Fishers Lane, Room 1–16
  Rockville, MD 20857

Trade Organizations

Trade organizations produce many excellent free materials on nutrition. Naturally, they also promote their own products. The student must learn to differentiate between slanted and valid information. We find the brief reviews in *Contemporary Nutrition*

(General Mills), *Dairy Council Digest*, Ross Laboratories' *Dietetic Currents*, and R. A. Seelig's reviews from the United Fresh Fruit and Vegetable Association to be generally reliable and very useful.

- ABC Corporation
1330 Avenue of the Americas
New York, NY 10019
- American Egg Board
1460 Renaissance Street
Park Ridge, IL 60068
- American Meat Institute
P.O. Box 3556
Washington, DC 20007
- Beech-Nut Nutrition Hotline
(800) 523-6633
- Best Foods
Division of CPC International
Consumer Service Department
Internation Plaza
Englewood Cliffs, NJ 07623
- Borden Farm Products
Borden Company, Consumer Affairs
180 East Broad Street
Columbus, OH 43215
- Campbell Soup Company
Food **Service Products** Division
375 Memorial Avenue
Camden, NJ 08101
- Del Monte Teaching Aids
P.O. Box 9075
Clinton, IA 52736
- Egg Nutrition Center
2501 M Street NW, Suite 410
Washington, DC 20037
- Fleischmann's Margarines
Standard Brands, Inc.
625 Madison Avenue
New York, NY 10022
- General Foods Consumer Center
250 North Street
White Plains, NY 10625
- General Mills
P.O. Box 113
Minneapolis, MN 55440
- Gerber Products Company
445 State Street
Fremont, MI 49412
- H. J. Heinz
Consumer Relations
P.O. Box 57
Pittsburgh, PA 15230
- Hunt-Wesson Foods
Educational Services
1645 West Valencia Drive
Fullerton, CA 92634

- Kellogg Company
Department of Home Economics Services
Battle Creek, MI 49016
- McGraw-Hill Films
Association Films, Inc.
600 Grand Avenue
Ridgefield, NJ 07657
- Mead Johnson Nutritionals
2404 Pennsylvania Avenue
Evansville, IN 47721
- Meat and Poultry Hotline
(800) 535-4555
- National Dairy Council
6300 North River Road
Rosemont, IL 60018
- Nestlé Company
Home Economics Division
100 Bloomingdale Road
White Plains, NY 10605
- NutraSweet/Simplesse Company
P.O. Box 830
Deerfield, IL 60015
(800) 321−7254
- Oscar Mayer Company
Consumer Service
P.O. Box 1409
Madison, WI 53701
- Pillsbury Company
1177 Pillsbury Building
608 Second Avenue South
Minneapolis, MN 55402
- The Potato Board
1385 South Colorado Boulevard, Suite 512
Denver, CO 80222
- Procter and Gamble Company
One Procter and Gamble Plaza
Cincinnati, OH 45202
- Rice Council
P.O. Box 22802
Houston, TX 77027
- Ross Laboratories
Director of Professional Services
625 Cleveland Avenue
Columbus, OH 43216
- Sister Kenny Institute
Chicago Avenue at 27th Street
Minneapolis, MN 55407
- Soy Protein Council
1800 M Street NW
Washington, DC 20036
- Sunkist Growers
Consumer Service, Division BB
P.O. Box 7888, Valley Annex
Van Nuys, CA 91409

E

- United Fresh Fruit and Vegetable Association
727 North Washington Street
Alexandria, VA 22314
- Vitamin Information Bureau
383 Madison Avenue
New York, NY 10017
- Vitamin Nutrition Information Service (VNIS)
Hoffmann-LaRoche
340 Kingsland Avenue
Nutley, NJ 07110
- Wheat Flour Institute
600 Maryland Avenue
Washington, DC 20024

- Interreligious Taskforce on U.S. Food Policy
110 Maryland Avenue NE
Washington, DC 20002
- Meals for Millions/Freedom from Hunger Foundation
1800 Olympic Boulevard
P.O. Drawer 680
Santa Monica, CA 90406
- Oxfam America
115 Broadway
Boston, MA 02116
- Worldwatch Institute
1776 Massachusetts Avenue NW
Washington, DC 20036

Organizations Concerned with World Hunger

- Bread for the World
802 Rhode Island Avenue NE
Washington, DC 20018
- The Hunger Project
2015 Steiner Street
San Francisco, CA 94115
- Institute for Food and Development Policy
1885 Mission Street
San Francisco, CA 94103

United Nations

- Food and Agriculture Organization (FAO)
North American Regional Office
1325 C Street SW
Washington, DC 20025
- World Health Organization (WHO)
1211 Geneva 27
Switzerland

E

Self-Study Forms

This appendix contains the forms needed to complete the self-study exercises presented throughout the book. Form 1 starts on the next page. You may want to copy form 1 on a copy machine that can enlarge it to ease your task in recording foods.

F

■ FORM 1
Nutrient Intakes (Use One Form for Each Day)

Food	Approximate Measure or Weight	Energy[a] (cal)	Prot[b] (g)	Carb[b] (g)	Fiber[b] (g)	Fat[b] (g)	Fat Breakdown Sat (g)	Fat Breakdown Mono (g)	Fat Breakdown Poly (g)	Chol[a] (mg)	Calcium[a] (mg)	Iron[c] (mg)	Magn[a] (mg)	Phos[a] (mg)	Potas[a] (mg)	Sodium[a] (mg)	Zinc[b] (mg)	Vit A[a] (RE)	Thia[c] (mg)	Ribo[c] (mg)	Niac[b] (mg)	V-B$_6$[b] (mg)	Fol[a] (µg)	Vit C[b] (mg)
Totals																								

[a]Compute these values to the nearest whole number.
[b]Compute these values to one decimal place.
[c]Compute these values to two decimal places.

■ FORM 2
Average Daily Energy and Nutrient Intakes

Day	Energy (cal)	Protein (g)	Carb (g)	Fiber (g)	Fat (g)	Sat (g)	Mono (g)	Poly (g)	Chol (mg)	Calcium (mg)	Iron (mg)	Magn (mg)	Phos (mg)	Potas (mg)	Sodium (mg)	Zinc (mg)	Vit A (RE)	Thia (mg)	Ribo (mg)	Niac (mg)	V B₆ (mg)	Fol (µg)	Vit C (mg)
							Fat Breakdown																
1																							
2																							
3																							
Total																							
Average daily intake (divide total by 3)																							

■ FORM 3
Comparison with Standard Intakes

Day	Energy (cal)	Prot (g)	Fat (g)	Carb (g)	Fiber (g)	Chol (mg)	Calcium (mg)	Iron (mg)	Magn (mg)	Phos (mg)	Potas (mg)	Sodium (mg)	Zinc (mg)	Vit A (RE)	Thia (mg)	Ribo (mg)	Niac (mg)	V B₆ (mg)	Fol (µg)	Vit C (mg)
Average daily intake (from Form 2)																				
Standard[a]			X	X	25	<300														
Intake as percentage of standard[b]																				

[a]Taken from RDA (inside front cover) or *Recommended Nutrient Intakes for Canadians* (Appendix B).
[b]For example, if your intake of protein was 50 g and the standard for a person your age and sex was 46 g, then you consumed (50 ÷ 46) × 100, or 109 percent of the standard.

■ FORM 4
Percentage of Calories from Protein, Fat, and Carbohydrate

From Form 3:

Protein: _____g/day × 4 cal/g = (P)_____ cal/day.

Fat: _____g/day × 9 cal/g = (F)_____ cal/day.

Carbohydrate: _____g/day × 4 cal/g = (C)_____ cal/day.

If you consumed an alcoholic beverage you must include its calories, (see note [a]):

Alcohol: (A)_____ cal/day.

                      Total cal/day = (T)_____ cal/day.

Percentage of calories from protein:

$\dfrac{(P)}{(T)}$ × 100 = _____% of total calories.

Percentage of calories from fat:

$\dfrac{(F)}{(T)}$ × 100 = _____% of total calories.

Percentage of calories from carbohydrate:

$\dfrac{(C)}{(T)}$ × 100 = _____% of total calories.

Percentage of calories from alcohol, if any:

$\dfrac{(A)}{(T)}$ × 100 = _____% of total calories.

Note: The four percentages can total 99, 100, or 101, depending on the way in which figures were rounded off earlier.

[a]To find out how many calories in a beverage are from alcohol, look up the beverage in Appendix H. Figure out how many calories are from carbohydrate (multiply carbohydrate grams times 4), fat (fat grams times 9), and protein (protein grams times 4). The remaining calories are from alcohol.

F

■ **FORM 5**
Food Selection Scorecard

Food Group and Recommended Intake	Your Intake from Group (Specify Food and Amount)	Your Score
Fruits and vegetables—4 or more portions (½ c cooked edible portion or 3 to 4 oz raw); at least 1 raw daily.		
1 portion vitamin A–rich dark green or deep orange fruit or vegetable (any food with more than your RDA) = 10 points (no more than 10 points allowed).		
1 portion vitamin C–rich fruit or vegetable (any food with more than your RDA) = 10 points (no more than 10 points allowed).		
Other fruits and vegetables, including potatoes = 2.5 points each.		
Subtotal (no more than 25 points allowed)		
Breads and cereals—4 or more portions of whole-grain or enriched (1 oz dry-weight cereal or 1-oz slice bread or equivalent grain product).		
1 portion cereal or 2 bread equivalents = 10 points (no more than 10 points allowed).		
Other bread equivalents = 5 points each.		
Subtotal (no more than 25 points allowed)		
Milk and milk products—2 or more portions (8 oz fluid milk; calcium equivalents are 1⅓ oz hard cheese, 1⅓ c cottage cheese, 1 pint ice milk or ice cream).		
1 portion = 12.5 points.		
Subtotal (no more than 25 points allowed)		
Meat and meat substitutes—2 or more portions of meat (2 to 3 oz cooked lean meat, fish, poultry; protein equivalents are 2 eggs, 2 oz hard cheese, or ½ c cottage cheese) and 2 portions legumes or nuts (¾ c cooked legumes, 4 tbsp peanut butter, 1 oz nuts or sunflower seeds); count cheese either in milk group or in meat group, not both.		
2 portions meat = 12.5 points.		
2 portions legumes = 12.5 points.		
Subtotal (no more than 25 points allowed)		
Grand total (no more than 100 points)		

The above are foundation foods. Additional foods are those that do not fit into the above groupings but add flavor, interest, variety, and (often) calories. List those eaten:

_____

_____

_____

_____

F

■ FORM 6
Calculation of Iron Absorbed from Meals

Three factors go into the calculation of the amount of iron absorbed from a meal: first, how much of the iron in the meal was heme and how much was nonheme iron; second, how much vitamin C was in the meal; and third, how much total meat, fish, and poultry (MFP) was consumed. (It is assumed your iron stores are moderate; otherwise, you'd have to take this into consideration, too.) Write down the foods you eat at a typical meal, look up their iron content in Appendix A, and then answer these six questions:

1. How much iron was from animal tissues (MFP)? _____ mg.
2. 40% of (1), on the average, is heme iron: (1) _____ mg × 0.40 = _____ mg heme iron.
3. How much iron was from other sources? _____ mg.
4. This (3), plus 60% of (1), is nonheme iron: (3) _____ mg + 0.60 × (1) _____ mg = _____ mg nonheme iron.
5. How much vitamin C was in the meal? Less than 25 mg is low; 25 to 75 mg is medium; more than 75 mg is high. _____ mg.
6. How much MFP was in the meal? Less than 1 oz lean MFP is low; 1 to 3 oz is medium; more than 3 oz is high.* _____ oz.

Now calculate:
You absorbed 23% of the heme iron, or (2) _____ mg × 0.23 = _____ mg heme iron absorbed.

Now, take your best score from (5) and (6). If either vitamin C or MFP was high or if both were medium, the availability of your nonheme iron was high. If neither was high, but one was medium, the availability of your nonheme iron was medium. If both were low, your nonheme iron had poor availability. You absorbed:

- High availability: 8% of the nonheme iron.
- Medium availability: 5% of the nonheme iron.
- Poor availability: 3% of the nonheme iron.

Now calculate:
You absorbed _____ % of the nonheme iron, or (4) _____ mg × _____ = _____ mg nonheme iron absorbed.
Your total: _____ mg nonheme iron absorbed.
Add the two together:

- _____ mg heme iron absorbed.
- _____ mg nonheme iron absorbed.

Total = _____ mg iron absorbed.
The RDA assumes you will absorb 10% of the iron you ingest. Thus, if you are a man of any age or a woman over 50 years old (RDA 10 mg), you need to absorb 1 mg per day; if you are a woman 11 to 50 years old (RDA 15 mg), you need to absorb 1.5 mg per day. If you have higher menstrual losses than the average woman, you may need still more.

---

*Note on #6: We have adapted the calculation of Monsen and coauthors, stating it in ounces. Her actual numbers are less than 23 g cooked meat, low; 23 to 46 g, medium; and 69 g or more, high.

Source: E. R. Monsen and coauthors, Estimation of available dietary iron, *American Journal of Clinical Nutrition* 31 (1978): 134–141.

■ FORM 7
Diet Planning by Exchange Groups

Exchange List	Number of Exchanges[b]	Amounts to Be Delivered[a]			
		Carbohydrate ____g	Protein ____g	Fat ____g	Energy ____cal
Starch/bread					
Meat					
Vegetable					
Fruit					
Milk					
Fat					
	Total actually delivered[c]				

[a]From step 2 and 3, page 315.
[b]From steps 4, 5, and 6.
[c]From step 7.

■ FORM 8
Meal patterns

Exchange List	Total Exchanges to Be Consumed Daily[a]	Exchanges Consumed at Each Meal				
		Breakfast	Lunch	Snack	Dinner	Snack
Starch/bread						
Meat						
Vegetable						
Fruit						
Milk						
Fat						

[a]From Form 7, column 2.

F

■ FORM 9
Nutrient Density of Foods

Food Item	Size of Serving I Would Eat	A Amount of Nutrient #1 (⎯⎯) That One Serving Would Supply (% of my RDA)	B Amount of Nutrient #2 (⎯⎯) That One Serving Would Supply (% of my RDA)	C Amount of Nutrient #3 (⎯⎯) That One Serving Would Supply (% of my RDA)	D Amount of Food Energy That One Serving Would Supply (% of my RDA)	E F G A/D B/D C/C	Nutrient Score E + F + G

▌▌▌ I N D E X

The standalone page numbers A, B, and C are for the tables beginning on the inside front cover. The standalone page numbers X, Y, and Z are for the tables ending on the inside back cover. The page numbers preceded by A through F are appendix page numbers. The page numbers followed by *n* indicate entries and footnotes. The boldfaced page numbers are the pages on which the boxed definitions appear.

West's NutriPro™

You can purchase your West's NutriPro™ Software Package using the order form below. It is available through West Publishing Company. The package was developed by ESHA Research and and consists of one disk (see below for options) and *The Student Manual to Accompany West's NutriPro™.*

NutriPro™ runs on either the IBM PC, PS/2 and compatible machines or the Macintosh (either require a minimum of 512K). It is a menu driven program that allows you to analyze your nutritional and health status. Using the computer, you can plan a diet and exercise program to achieve or maintain your desired weight and nutient intake. NutriPro™ is a fast, flexible program filled with diet analysis and planning options.

To order by phone, call: 1-800-328-9352
Specify IBM PC and compatible either
5-1/4" disk: 0-314-85178-X
3-1/2" disk: 0-314-85161-5
Macintosh disk: 0-314-00157-3

ORDER FORM

Complete form and return with payment to:
West Publishing Company
C.O.P Department
P.O. Box 64833
St. Paul, MN 55164-1803

❏ Send one West's NutriPro™ manual and Macintosh disk (ISBN:0-314-00157-3)
❏ Send one West's NutriPro™ manual and DOS based 3-1/2" disk (ISBN: 0-314-85161-5)
❏ Send one West's NutriPro™ manual and DOS Based 5-1/4" disk (ISBN: 0-314-85178-X)
I have enclosed a check payable to West Publishing Company for **$29.95 plus** the local tax of $_____. Total amount $_____.

Or, charge to: ❏ Master Card ❏ Visa. Credit Card #:_____
Expiration Date: _____

Name:_____

Street Address:_____

City:_____State:_____Zip:_____

Order subject to approval of vendor. Applicable local tax to be added.
Price subject to change without notice.

Please allow 6 to 8 weeks for delivery.

1983 Metropolitan Height and Weight Tables

Weights at ages 25 to 29 based on lowest mortality. Weights in pounds according to frame (in indoor clothing weighing 5 pounds for men or 3 pounds for women), shoes with 1-inch heels. For frame size standards, see Chapter 9, Table 9–1.

Men					Women				
Height		Small Frame	Medium Frame	Large Frame	Height		Small Frame	Medium Frame	Large Frame
(ft)	(inches)				(ft)	(inches)			
5	2	128–134	131–141	138–150	4	10	102–111	109–121	118–131
5	3	130–136	133–143	140–153	4	11	103–113	111–123	120–134
5	4	132–138	135–145	142–156	5	0	104–115	113–126	122–137
5	5	134–140	137–148	144–160	5	1	106–118	115–129	125–140
5	6	136–142	139–151	146–164	5	2	108–121	118–132	128–143
5	7	138–145	142–154	149–168	5	3	111–124	121–135	131–147
5	8	140–148	145–157	152–172	5	4	114–127	124–138	134–151
5	9	142–151	148–160	155–176	5	5	117–130	127–141	137–155
5	10	144–154	151–163	158–180	5	6	120–133	130–144	140–159
5	11	146–157	154–166	161–184	5	7	123–136	133–147	143–163
6	0	149–160	157–170	164–188	5	8	126–139	136–150	146–167
6	1	152–164	160–174	168–192	5	9	129–142	139–153	149–170
6	2	155–168	164–178	172–197	5	10	132–145	142–156	152–173
6	3	158–162	167–182	176–202	5	11	135–148	145–159	155–176
6	4	162–176	171–187	181–207	6	0	138–151	148–162	158–179

Source: Reproduced with permission of Metropolitan Life Insurance Company. Source of basic data: *1979 Build Study,* Society of Actuaries and Association of Life Insurance Medical Directors of America, 1980.

Body Weights: Rules of Thumb for People 18 to 25 Years of Age

Men

For 5 ft, consider 110 lb a reasonable weight.
For each inch over 5 ft, add 5 lb.
Example: A man 5 ft 8 inches tall would start at 110 lb, add 40, and arrive at a reasonable weight of 150 lb.

Women

For 5 ft, consider 100 lb a reasonable weight.
For each inch over 5 ft, add 5 lb.
For each year under 25 (down to 18), subtract 1 lb.
Example: A woman 21 years old, 5 ft 4 inches tall, would start at 100 lb, add 20, and subtract 4, arriving at a reasonable weight of 116 lb.

Acceptable Weight for Height Based on Body Mass Index (BMI)

To determine your acceptable weight range, find your height in the top line. Look down the column below it and find the range represented by the color blue. Look to the left column to see what weights are accepta‑ble for you.

Men
Height, m (in)

Weight kg (lb)	1.47 (58)	1.50 (59)	1.52 (60)	1.55 (61)	1.57 (62)	1.60 (63)	1.63 (64)	1.65 (65)	1.68 (66)	1.70 (67)	1.73 (68)	1.75 (69)	1.78 (70)	1.80 (71)	1.83 (72)	1.85 (73)	1.88 (74)	1.90 (75)	1.93 (76)
39 (85)																			
41 (90)																			
43 (95)																			
45 (100)																			
48 (105)																			
50 (110)																			
52 (115)																			
54 (120)																			
57 (125)																			
59 (130)																			
61 (135)																			
64 (140)																			
66 (145)																			
68 (150)																			
70 (155)																			
73 (160)																			
75 (165)																			
77 (170)																			
79 (175)																			
82 (180)																			
84 (185)																			
86 (190)																			
88 (195)																			
91 (200)																			
93 (205)																			
95 (210)																			
98 (215)																			
100 (220)																			
102 (225)																			
104 (230)																			
107 (235)																			
109 (240)																			
111 (245)																			
113 (250)																			
116 (255)																			
118 (260)																			
120 (265)																			
122 (270)																			
125 (275)																			
136 (300)																			
159 (350)																			
181 (400)																			

Key:

- ☐ Underweight
- ■ Acceptable weight
- ■ Marginal overweight
- ☐ Overweight
- ■ Severe overweight
- ☐ Morbid obesity

Note: For more information on the body mass index, see Chapter 9.

Source: Adapted from M. I. Rowland, A nomogram for computing body mass index, Dietetic Currents 16 (1989): 9, used and reprinted with permission of Ross Laboratories, Columbus, OH 43216. Copyright 1989 Ross Laboratories.

Y